Ocular Disease

Diagnosis and Treatment

Ocular Disease
Diagnosis and Treatment

SECOND EDITION

Editor-in-Chief

DANIEL K. ROBERTS, O.D.

*Associate Professor of Optometry, Department of Clinical Education,
Illinois College of Optometry, Illinois Eye Institute, Chicago*

Founding Editor

JACK E. TERRY, M.S., O.D., Ph.D.

*Associate Professor of Pharmacology, Marshall University School
of Medicine, Huntington; Chief, Optometry Service, Department
of Veterans Affairs Medical Center, Huntington, West Virginia;
Clinical Assistant Professor of Optometry, The Ohio State
University College of Optometry, Columbus*

BUTTERWORTH-HEINEMANN
Boston • Oxford • Johannesburg • Melbourne • New Delhi • Singapore

Copyright © 1996 by Butterworth–Heinemann

ℛ A member of the Reed Elsevier group

All rights reserved.

Every effort has been made to ensure that the drug dosage schedules within this text are accurate and conform to standards accepted at the time of publication. However, as treatment recommendations vary in the light of continuing research and clinical experience, the reader is advised to verify drug dosage schedules herein with information found on product information sheets. This is especially true in cases of new or infrequently used drugs.

∞ Recognizing the importance of preserving what has been written, Butterworth–Heinemann prints its books on acid-free paper whenever possible.

Library of Congress Cataloging-in-Publication Data
Ocular disease : diagnosis and treatment / editor in chief, Daniel K.
  Roberts ; founding editor, Jack E. Terry. -- 2nd ed.
      p.   cm.
    Includes bibliographical references and index.
    ISBN 0-7506-9062-3 (hard cover : alk. paper)
    1. Eye--Diseases. 2. Optometrists. I. Roberts, Daniel K., 1962–.
  II. Terry, Jack E.
    [DNLM: 1. Eye Diseases--diagnosis. 2. Eye Diseases--therapy.
  3. Optometry--methods.   WW 141 0202 1996]
  RE46.383 1996
  617.7—dc20
  DNLM/DLC
  for Library of Congress   95-51004
                                                                          CIP

British Library Cataloguing-in-Publication Data
A catalogue record for this book is available from the British Library.

The publisher offers discounts on bulk orders of this book.
For information, please write:
Manager of Special Sales
Butterworth–Heinemann
313 Washington Street
Newton, MA 02158–1626
Tel: 617-928-2500
Fax: 617-928-2620

For information on all our medical publications available, contact our
World Wide Web home page at: http://www.bh.com/bh/

10 9 8 7 6 5 4 3 2 1

Printed in the United States of America

*To the students and practitioners who use
this textbook, as well as their patients,
whom it is ultimately intended to benefit*

Contents

Contributing Authors

Gregory S. Abel, O.D.
Clinical Assistant Professor of Optometry, Indiana University School of Optometry, Bloomington; formerly at the Southern California College of Optometry, Ocular Disease and Special Testing Service, Fullerton
23. Uveitis

Kevin L. Alexander, O.D., Ph.D.
Clinical Associate Professor of Optometry, The Ohio State University College of Optometry, Columbus; Retina Vitreous Associates, St. Vincent Medical Center, Toledo, Ohio
5. Fluorescein Angiography

Rex Ballinger, O.D.
Eye Clinic, Veterans Affairs Medical Center, Baltimore
24. Diseases of the Retina and Vitreous

Sherry J. Bass, O.D.
Professor of Clinical Sciences, Ocular Disease and Specialty Testing Services, State University of New York, State College of Optometry, New York
13. Electrodiagnosis

Debra J. Bezan, M.Ed., O.D.
Professor of Optometry, Northeastern State University College of Optometry; Staff Optometrist, W.W. Hastings Hospital, Tahlequah, Oklahoma
21. Diseases of the Lids and Lashes

Chris J. Cakanac, O.D.
Clinical Instructor in Ophthalmology, University of Pittsburgh School of Medicine, Pittsburgh; Associate Medical Staff, Jeannette District Memorial Hospital, Jeannette, Pennsylvania
18. Ophthalmic Radiology

Leland W. Carr, O.D.
Clinical Professor of Optometry, The Pacific University College of Optometry, Forest Grove; Clinical Director of Optometry, Southeast Health Center, Multnomah County Health Department, Portland, Oregon
10. Evaluation of Disorders of Ocular Alignment and Motility

Michael A. Chaglasian, O.D.
Associate Professor of Optometry, Illinois College of Optometry, Chicago; Attending Staff, Glaucoma Service, Illinois Eye Institute, Chicago
25. Glaucoma

John E. Conto, O.D., F.A.A.O.
Associate Professor of Optometry, Department of Clinical Education, Illinois College of Optometry, Chicago; Attending Module Chief, Primary Care Service, Illinois Eye Institute, Chicago
9. Evaluation of Pupillary Disorders; 15. Evaluation and Postoperative Management of the Cataract Patient

T. Michael Goen, O.D.
Adjunct Associate Professor of Optometry, Indiana University School of Optometry, Bloomington; Department of Surgery, Biloxi Veterans Administration Medical Center, Biloxi, Mississippi
20. Sphygmomanometry

Gregory W. Good, O.D., Ph.D.
Professor of Clinical Optometry, The Ohio State University College of Optometry, Columbus
1. Visual Acuities; 7. Color Vision

William L. Jones, O.D.
Professor of Optometry, University of Houston College of Optometry, Houston; Optometry Section, Veterans

Affairs Medical Center, Albuquerque, New Mexico
  4. Ophthalmoscopy

Michelle M. Marciniak, O.D.
Assistant Professor of Optometry, Department of Clinical Education, Illinois College of Optometry, Chicago; Attending Optometrist, Surgical Service, Veterans Affairs Medical Center-West Side, Chicago
  16. Clinical Laboratory Testing

Dennis E. Mathews, O.D.
Vitreo Retinal Foundation, Memphis, Tennessee
  19. Neurologic Testing

Richard E. Meetz, O.D., M.S.
Clinical Assistant Professor of Optometry, Indiana University School of Optometry, Bloomington
  2. Slit Lamp Biomicroscopy

Gerald G. Melore, O.D., M.P.H.
Clinical Professor of Optometry, The Pacific University College of Optometry, Forest Grove; Chief, Optometry Service, Veterans Affairs Medical Center, Portland, Oregon
  11. Evaluation of the Lacrimal System

Kenneth J. Myers, Ph.D., O.D.
Professor of Clinical Optometry, Ferris State University College of Optometry, Big Rapids; Chief of Optometry, VA Outpatient Clinic, Department of Veterans Affairs Medical Center, Grand Rapids, Michigan
  3. Tonometry

Gary E. Oliver, O.D.
Associate Clinical Professor of Optometry, Department of Clinical Sciences, and Chief, Ocular Disease and Special Testing Service, State University of New York State College of Optometry, New York
  22. Diseases of the Conjunctiva, Cornea, and Sclera

Neil A. Pence, O.D.
Assistant Professor of Optometry and Director, Continuing Education, Indiana University School of Optometry, Bloomington
  12. Carotid Artery Disease and Ophthalmodynamometry

Sara L. Penner, O.D.
Associate Professor of Optometry, Illinois College of Optometry, Chicago; Adjunct Assistant Professor of Optometry, Indiana University School of Optometry, Bloomington; Clinical Associate Professor of Optometry, Ferris State University College of Optometry, Big Rapids, Michigan; Chief of Optometry, Veterans Affairs

Medical Center, Fort Wayne, Indiana
  16. Clinical Laboratory Testing

Hurbert D. Riley, O.D.
Assistant Professor of Optometry, Indiana University School of Optometry, Bloomington
  2. Slit Lamp Biomicroscopy

Daniel K. Roberts, O.D.
Associate Professor of Optometry, Department of Clinical Education, Illinois College of Optometry, Illinois Eye Institute, Chicago
  6. Gonioscopy and Fundus Contact Lens; 19. Neurologic Testing

John P. Schoessler, O.D., Ph.D.
Acting Dean, The Ohio State University College of Optometry, Columbus
  8. Visual Fields

Donald A. Seibert, O.D.
Adjunct Clinical Assistant Professor of Optometry, Illinois College of Optometry, Chicago; Attending Optometrist, Optometry Service, Department of Veterans Affairs Medical Center, Huntington, West Virginia
  8. Visual Fields

Jerome Sherman, O.D.
Distinguished Teaching Professor, Department of Clinical Sciences, State University of New York State College of Optometry, New York
  13. Electrodiagnosis; 14. Ophthalmic Ultrasonography

Jack E. Terry, M.S., O.D., Ph.D.
Associate Professor of Pharmacology, Marshall University School of Medicine, Huntington; Chief, Optometry Service, Department of Veterans Affairs Medical Center, Huntington, West Virginia; Clinical Assistant Professor of Optometry, The Ohio State University College of Optometry, Columbus
  1. Visual Acuities; 3. Tonometry; 6. Gonioscopy and Fundus Contact Lens; 7. Color Vision; 18. Ophthalmic Radiology; 20. Sphygmomanometry

Ruth A. Trachimowicz, Ph.D., O.D.
Assistant Professor of Anatomy, Illinois College of Optometry, Chicago
  9. Evaluation of Pupillary Disorders

Diane P. Yolton, Ph.D., O.D.
Professor of Optometry, The Pacific University College of Optometry, Forest Grove, Oregon
  17. Ocular Microbiology and Cytology

I

Ophthalmic Diagnostic Procedures

1

Visual Acuities

GREGORY W. GOOD AND JACK E. TERRY

The measurement of visual acuity is a fundamental component of any eye examination. Traditionally, the patient reads from a printed or projected chart consisting of dark letters on a bright background to determine the smallest letter size that is discernible. Although acuity testing can become routine, its results are extremely significant, and it must be performed with care.

In cases of uncorrected refractive error, measuring visual acuities provides the clinician with an initial appraisal of the magnitude of the optical correction that will be required. Visual acuity measurement is also of considerable importance in detecting certain eye diseases and monitoring their course. Additionally, acuity measurements can be a factor in legal accountability. Recording entrance visual acuities provides a safeguard against later claims that a particular course of treatment caused a reduction in vision.

In analyzing a patient with reduced acuity, the examiner must consider the various elements of the visual system and determine whether the poor vision is caused by uncorrected refractive error, opacities in the ocular media, disturbances in the integrity of the retina, lesions in the visual pathway or cortex, or a combination of factors. An example is greatly reduced acuity in the presence of a mature cataract. The question arises whether the cataract is the sole cause of the decreased acuity or whether other factors are contributing to the reduction in acuity (e.g., macular degeneration).

PRINCIPLES OF VISUAL ACUITY TESTING

In common use, the term *visual acuity* implies acuteness or sharpness of vision.[1] Traditionally, visual acuity testing consists of presenting the subject with high-contrast optotypes of gradually decreasing size to the point where they can no longer be resolved. The measure of visual acuity is then defined by the reciprocal of the visual angle of the elements of the smallest optotype discernible.

There is wide variability in the type of target and the testing paradigm used to measure visual acuity. However, the fundamental task required of the patient has classically been assigned to one of four categories[2]: (1) detection, (2) resolution, (3) recognition, and (4) localization. Clinical visual acuity testing methods concentrate on resolution and recognition. Visual resolution refers to the ability to discern two adjacent targets as separate entities. Figure 1-1 illustrates examples of resolution acuity targets.

Of targets used for measuring resolution acuity, the grating pattern has received the most clinical use. A high-contrast grating of dark and light bars of equal width is presented. The spatial frequency then is increased until the grating can no longer be differentiated from a homogeneous, gray background. The grating can be presented at various orientations in a forced choice format to overcome a changing patient criterion. The critical detail is given by the angular width of a single bar.

Visual acuity testing with gratings is clinically useful because it does not require the subject to be knowledgeable of certain symbols. Through a technique called preferential viewing, which is discussed in a later section, grating targets are often used when testing infants and other patients incapable of a verbal or written response.

Visual resolution is, in principle, the basis for clinical acuity testing when letters or numerals are used. However, because clinical testing typically uses a chart from which patients must properly name letters or numbers, the psychological recognition of that letter or number is required. Therefore, this type of visual acuity testing is more appropriately termed recognition acuity testing. The ease and quickness of testing with letter charts have made recognition acuity testing the typical method for clinical use.

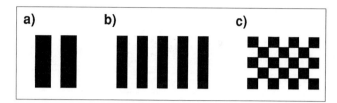

FIGURE 1-1
Examples of resolution acuity targets are (a) Konig bars, (b) square wave grating, and (c) checkerboard pattern.

There is wide variation in significant design features of the many visual acuity charts in use today. Diversity in the letters used, the design of the letters, the progression of letter sizes, and the amount of letter separation have led to misinterpretation and confusion over the meaning of specific visual acuity measures. Since 1979, however, much progress has been made in the standardization of visual acuity testing.[3]

THEORETICAL LIMIT TO VISUAL ACUITY

The measured visual acuity is a function of both the optical and neural components of the eye. In the absence of refractive error and ocular disease, foveal visual acuity could be limited by other optical factors (e.g., diffraction through the pupil and the optical aberrations of the eye) or neural factors (e.g., photoreceptor spacing or neural grain). Even in the most ideal conditions, the resolution limit imposed by the eye's optical system is 50–60 cycles/degree.[4] Diffraction through the pupil and the optical aberrations of the eye create a limit to the fineness of detail that can be focused on the retina. This theoretical limit closely matches the psychophysically measured visual acuity at high luminance using normal viewing.[5]

The resolution of the neural system alone can be obtained using techniques that bypass the optics of the eye. By focusing twin beams of coherent radiation at the pupillary plane of the eye, interference fringes are produced on the retina (Figure 1-2). The frequency of the fringes depends on the lateral separation of the twin beams within the pupil. As the separation of the beams is increased, a finer grating of high modulation is produced. Using this method, investigators have found that the maximum resolving capability of the retina for vertical gratings is similar to that found with normal viewing.[6,7] This is to be expected, because there would be little advantage in having a photoreceptor configuration that is capable of discerning detail finer than that which can be imaged onto the retina. The general agreement between the opti-

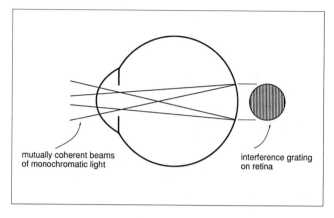

FIGURE 1-2
Laser-generated interference fringes are created by focusing twin beams of mutually coherent laser light into the pupil. Finer patterns are created by increasing the separation of the beams within the pupil.

cal and neural limits to visual acuity, at approximately 60 cycles/degree, has led to the notion that the retina has evolved based on the spatial frequency cutoff imposed by the optical elements of the eye.[8]

BASIC CLINICAL TESTING

Visual acuity should be evaluated at the beginning of each examination session. This will normally follow the case history but must precede any investigative or diagnostic procedure. This testing provides useful information concerning the functional integrity of the entire visual system. Additionally, it provides legal documentation of the patient's visual status before any testing or treatment.

When measurement of unaided visual acuity is necessary, it should always be done before aided visual acuity is tested. This will minimize any learning effects and provide a more accurate measurement. Using this same logic requires that the worse of the two eyes be tested first. However, which eye has the worse visual acuity is often not known at the beginning of the examination sequence. To help eliminate recording errors made by switching the two monocular results, it is prudent for the examiner to habitually test one eye first (conventionally the *right* eye).

One of the most common methods of recording visual acuity is with the Snellen fraction. Visual acuity is represented as a fraction, *a/b*, where *a* equals the viewing distance and *b* equals the distance at which the smallest discernible letter subtends 5 minutes of arc. Using a test distance of 20 feet, visual acuity is then recorded as 20/20, 20/40, 20/200, etc., depending on the size of the smallest test letter read. When metric units are used, it is common practice to use 6 meters as the standard test distance (6/6, 6/12, 6/60, etc.). Even if the size of the examination room does not allow a testing distance of 20 feet, the acuity is frequently recorded in 20/X notation. This is easily handled with projected charts by optically adjusting the letter sizes until they subtend the appropriate angle. With a test distance of 12 feet, for example, the chart projector is adjusted to minify the letters to 12/20ths of their size for the 20-foot test distance; then, although the letters are smaller than they would be for a 20-foot testing distance, their angular subtense is the same. Although testing distances are frequently shortened in the clinical setting, a fractional equivalent using "20" as the numerator is typically used, e.g., 20/20 instead of the technically correct 12/12 designation.

When using printed acuity charts (instead of projected charts), it is better to record the acuity using the actual test distance used. As an example, if a patient read letters that subtend the 5-minute angle at 80 feet at a test distance of 10 feet, the acuity would be recorded as 10/80 (an 80-foot letter read at 10 feet). This eliminates any ambiguity in the interpretation of the acuity measurement during future review of the record but can easily be converted to the more conventional 20/160 equivalent Snellen recording, if needed.

Using the 20/X notation to designate visual acuity whatever the test distance may create confusion and recording errors. Bailey[3] explained the problem by pointing out that visual acuity is actually a single dimension (the minimum angle of resolution), and therefore argued that only a single number is required. For this purpose, he proposed a logarithmic scaling system (Visual Acuity Rating Scale).

When testing with a line of letters, exact visual acuity is often expressed by indicating the fraction of letters correctly identified for a given line. If over half the letters in a line are read correctly, credit is given for that line. Letters missed in that row or read correctly in the next row are indicated by a "–" or "+" designation. For example, a result of "20/60 +2 of 5" indicates that the entire line of letters subtending 3 minutes of critical detail was read correctly as well as two of the five letters on the next smaller row. This designation increases the sensitivity of the recording and provides a better indication of visual abilities. This method is especially meaningful when using charts designed with a geometric size progression and an equal number of test letters within each row.

Decimal notation is also used to designate visual acuity. Decimal acuity is determined by "dividing out" the Snellen fraction. For example, 20/20 acuity is designated as 1.0, 20/40 as 0.5, and 20/200 acuity as 0.1. The disadvantage in using decimal notation is that it erroneously implies a percentage of vision.

The most common cause of reduced visual acuity is simple refractive error. Peters[9] compiled a table presenting expected uncorrected visual acuities for various sphero/cylindrical errors for patients within three different age groups (Table 1-1). An understanding of the relationship between refractive error and uncorrected visual acuity can aid the clinician in the refractive evaluation of the patient.

A pinhole aperture is frequently used to neutralize refractive error to determine if a visual acuity deficit is optically based.[10] Viewing through a 1-mm pinhole will decrease the size of the blur circle on the retina and partially offset even large amounts of ametropia. Best corrected potential acuity is often not demonstrated with the pinhole because of diffraction and reduced retinal illumination; however, any substantial improvement indicates that at least some of the visual acuity deficit is optical in nature. Because many patients have difficulty with alignment of a single, small aperture, multiple pinhole devices are available to overcome this inconvenience.

Standardization

Numerous charts exist for evaluating visual acuities. Significant differences in the design features among charts in common use provide some limit to the meaningfulness of most visual acuity measures. One problem is the varying discriminability of different letters. Ginsburg[11] explained these differences by showing the spatial frequency components of letters necessary for their identification. He reported the letter "L" to require resolution of only 1.5 cycles/letter for its identification, whereas the letter "E" requires 2.5 cycles/letter (Figure 1-3). For a letter subtending 5 minutes of arc, these values correspond to 18 cycles/degree (20/33 grating acuity) and 30 cycles/degree (20/20 grating acuity), respectively.

Differences in the style of the letters from one chart to another also add to this problem. For example, the use of serifs by some manufacturers, as well as variable height and width dimensions, can lead to inconsistencies. Sloan letters use a framework of 5 units high × 5 units wide, while British letters use a framework of 5 units high × 4 units wide.[3]

In an early attempt at the standardization of visual acuity methods, the International Ophthalmological Congress in 1909 adopted the Landolt ring (also known as the Landolt C, Figure 1-4) as the standard optotype.[12] The ring may be presented with the gap placed to the left, right, up, down, or obliquely. By its design, it induces a forced choice response by the patient, reduces artifacts and secondary cues, and is unaffected by meridional blurring. In a presentation using four possible orientations, the patient

TABLE 1-1

Visual Acuity and Refractive Error. (The number in the table represents the denominator of the Snellen fraction (20/X) for the indicated uncorrected refractive error and patient age.)

Diopter Sphere	Diopter Minus Cylinder						
	0.0	0.50	1.00	1.50	2.00	3.00	4.00
−2.00	200	200	200	200 or poorer			
−1.50	80–100	100	100	200			
−1.00	60	70	80	100	100	200	
−0.50	30–40	50	60	70	80	100	200
0.00	20	25–30	40–50	60	70	100	200
+0.50	20	20	30	50	60	80	100
+1.00	20	20	25	40	50–60	80	100
+1.50 a	20	20	25	40	50	70	100
b	20	25	25–30	40	50	70–80	100
c	30	25–30	30–40	50	60	80	100
+2.00 a	20	25	25	30–40	50	70	100
b	25	25	30	40	50	70	100
c	50–60	40	40–50	50–60	60–70	80	100
+3.00 a	25	25	30	30–40	50	70	100
b	40	30	40	50	60	70–80	100
c	200	80	70–80	80	80	100	200
+4.00 a	40–50	30	30	40–50	60	80	100–200
b	70	50–60	50–60	60	70	100	200
+5.00 a	70	50	40–50	60	70–80	100	200
b	200	80	80	80–100	100	200	200

Patient age: a = 5–15 years; b = 25–35 years, c = 45–55 years.
Source: Adapted with permission from IM Borish. Visual Acuity. In Clinical Refraction (3rd ed). Chicago: Professional Press, 1970:371.

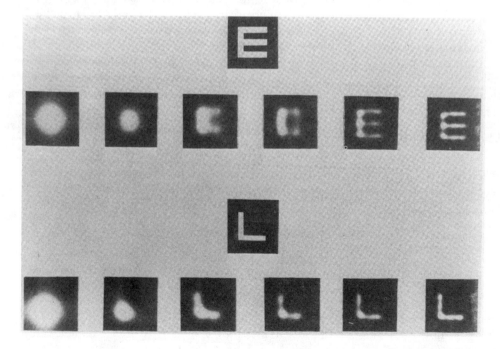

FIGURE 1-3

Fourier synthesis of Snellen letters E and L in increments of 0.5 cycles per letter width. The E requires a minimum of 2.5 cycles per letter for indentification, whereas the L requires a minimum of only 1.5 cycles/letter. (Reprinted with permission from AP Ginsburg. Spatial filtering and vision: implications for normal and abnormal vision. In LM Proenza, JM Enoch, A Jampolsky [eds], Clinical Applications of Visual Psychophysics. Cambridge: Cambridge University Press, 1981.)

Ocular Disease

Diagnosis and Treatment

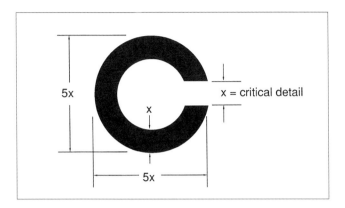

FIGURE 1-4

Specifications for the Landolt ring. The ring is constructed in a 5 unit high × 5 unit wide matrix with the stroke width and gap equal to 1 unit.

should correctly guess the gap position 25% of the time. The acuity is then defined by the row at which 62.5% (halfway between chance and 100% correct) of the letters are read correctly.

Although the Landolt ring is the optotype of choice for accurate visual acuity testing, it may be impractical for routine clinical use. The patient or the examiner may lose his or her place because of the similarity of the targets. Also, left and right may be ambiguous to some patients. Letter charts are useful because testing is easy and patients are generally familiar with them.

Since 1979 there has been much activity internationally to standardize visual acuity testing in both chart layout and general methodology.[3] Three authoritative groups have developed standards that address most of the short-comings (Table 1-2). Although small differences in the standards exist among the three bodies, there is general agreement on many of the important concepts.

The Landolt ring is the standard optotype. Letter charts are permissible if the specific optotypes are shown to be of comparable difficulty to the Landolt ring. There are differences in the recommended number of optotypes for a given size row; however, all three organizations recognize that multiple presentations (at least five) are necessary. Additionally, a 0.1 log unit size progression was unanimously chosen. With this stipulation each row should be approximately 0.8 times the size of the next larger row. Specifications concerning spacing of letters and rows are also standardized.

Standardizing these design features for test charts provides for a more meaningful measure of visual acuity, especially for visual acuities of 20/100 or worse. Typical projected charts have only one or two letters at these larger sizes, as well as inappropriately large steps in letter size (e.g., 20/400 to 20/200 to 20/100).

The three organizations agree that the chart luminance be at least 80 cd/m². Providing this minimum level of luminance is particularly important for older patients, whose relatively small pupil size and clouded media can significantly reduce retinal illumination. Standard test distance has also been consistently specified as 4 meters. A distance shorter than 20 feet, or 6 meters, is preferred because examination lanes are routinely shorter than these dimensions.[13] The 4-meter distance is particularly useful in that a vergence of exactly –0.25 diopters is manifest at the spectacle plane of the patient. The examiner can easily compensate for this by adding –0.25 diopters to a refractive result determined at this distance.

TABLE 1-2

Testing Visual Acuity Standards

	Working Group 39[a] *NAS-NRC*	*C.O.U.*[b]	*I.S.O.*[c]
Standard optotype	Landolt ring, 4-choice	Landolt ring, 4-choice	Landolt ring, 8-choice
Alternative optotypes	Encouraged	Encouraged	Accepted
Test distance	4 meters	4 meters	4 meters
Size progression	0.1 log unit (ratio 1.2589)	0.1 log unit (ratio 1.2589)	0.1 log unit (ratio 1.2589)
Criterion for specifying V.A.	7 of 10 optotypes (or 6 of 8)	3 of 5 optotypes or over 50% of total presented	3 of 5 optotypes or 60% of total presented
Chart luminance	85 ±5 cd/m²	≥ 80 cd/m²	80–320 cd/m²

[a]National Academy of Sciences–National Research Council Committee on Vision Working Group 39.
[b]Consilium Ophthalmologicum Universale.
[c]International Organization for Standardization.
Source: Adapted from IL Bailey. Measurement of Visual Acuity—Towards Standardization. In Vision Science Symposium: A Tribute to Gordon G. Heath. Bloomington, IN: Indiana University, 1988;215–30.

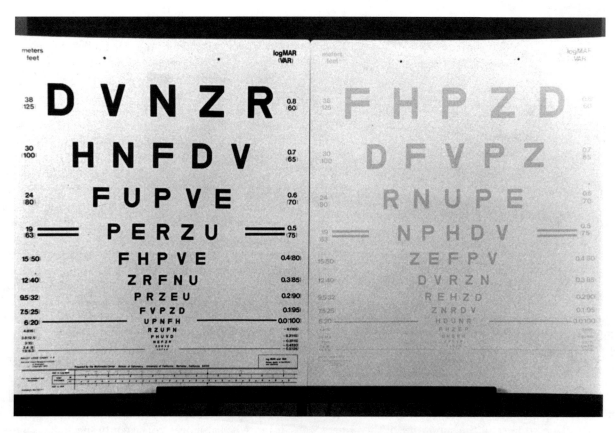

FIGURE 1-5
High- and low-contrast Bailey-Lovie logMAR visual acuity charts.

An example of a chart following the recommendations just outlined is the Bailey-Lovie logMAR visual acuity chart (Figure 1-5). When situations arise requiring accurate acuity measurement, standardized charts such as this one should be used. Examples of when standardized methods are most important include examinations involving determination of acuity levels for admittance into military or police programs or for driver's and pilot's license examinations.

Nearpoint Testing

The measurement of visual acuity at the nearpoint can be used to assess the angular size of detail discernible at the nearpoint as well as providing a functional measure of the size of print the patient is capable of reading. As with distance acuity testing, the two factors important in specifying the nearpoint visual acuity are test distance and size of the target.

Many different types of nearpoint acuity charts have been developed; these include single letter, individual word, or continuous text charts in upper case and lower-case styles. Various designations are used to specify the sizes of the letters on different charts.

Equivalent Snellen

Equivalent Snellen charts are the equivalent of a photographic reduction of a distance acuity chart. The different sized rows are designated by the equivalent Snellen notation for the row when used at the proper viewing distance (usually 40 cm). Figures in a row marked "20/20" would then subtend an angle of 5 minutes to the eye at this test distance.

Other charts use a Snellen fraction notation but specify acuity using distances marked in inches, typically 14 inches. When used at this working distance, the row subtending 5 minutes of arc is designated as "14/14."

Jaeger Acuity

Letters on a Jaeger chart are presented in different sizes ranging from J1 (0.5 mm high) to J20 (19.5 mm high) in ascending order. J1 subtends 5 minutes of arc for a test distance of 45 cm. Although Jaeger charts are widely

TABLE 1-3
Comparison of Nearpoint Visual Acuity Charts

Sample Text	Mail Order Small Bible		Want Ads Phone Book		Newspapers Magazines	Books Adult	Children	
Equivalent Snellen	20/20	20/25	20/30	20/40	20/50	20/70	20/100	20/200
Jaeger	1+	1	2	3	5	7	10	16
Point	3	4	5	6	8	10	14	26
M notation	.4M	.5M	.6M	.8M	1M	1.4M	2M	4M

used, they have disadvantages compared with most other nearpoint charts.[12] For example, Jaeger notation is not standardized. Therefore, different manufacturers have produced charts that vary in the exact letter size for a specific Jaeger designation. Additionally, Jaeger designations are not linear. There is a nongeometric progression in letter size for the different designations. This limits the usefulness of the chart in predicting visual performance or comparing the nearpoint visual acuity finding to that found at distance.

M Notation

Sizes of figures on a chart using "M" notation are marked by the distance in meters at which the figures subtend 5 minutes of arc. Acuity is then recorded by specifying the test distance in centimeters over the appropriate "M" designation. For example, a nearpoint acuity of 40/1M denotes a working distance of 40 cm. The smallest letter read subtends an angle of 5 minutes at 1 meter. The acuity measurement using M notation can be easily converted to the Snellen equivalent: (1) Express both the numerator and denominator in centimeters; (2) multiply both by the ratio 20/numerator. The resultant ratio expresses the acuity measurement in the more typical Snellen notation. Using the previous example: (1) 40/1M = 40/100; (2) $40 \times 20/40 = 20$; $100 \times 20/40 = 50$; (3) 40/1M = 20/50.

Point System

The point system is used in the printing industry to express letter size. Each "point" is equal to 1/72nd of an inch, or 0.35 mm. Acuity measurements using this system are functionally based, since the point size read tells the examiner what size of print and therefore what type of document (e.g., newspaper, Bible, or large print books) can be read by the patient. The testing distance must again be recorded when using this system of measurement. If the test distance were 20 cm and 8-point print were read, the visual acuity would be recorded as 8-point print @ 20 cm. A comparison of these different systems and some common examples are given in Table 1-3.

TESTING ACUITY IN PEDIATRIC PATIENTS

Visual acuity testing in young children can be challenging for the clinician. Testing may require special methods and testing materials to accurately determine visual function. Lippman[14] reported that testing time can be reduced and testing efficiency improved by decreasing the test distance from 20 feet to 10 feet. Clinicians often must provide special encouragement and reward cooperative behavior with small prizes.

Conventional visual acuity charts are not appropriate for young children who are not able to read letters or numbers. Additionally, children who have not yet developed directionality concepts may have difficulty with orientation-specific optotypes (e.g., tumbling E, Landolt ring).

Marsh-Tootle described a strategy for visual acuity testing based upon a child's level of development.[15] She categorized acuity tests into basic, medium, and advanced levels and recommended testing at the highest level the child can complete. A partial listing of these tests is given in Table 1-4.

Basic Level: Preferential Looking Cards

Very young children, even infants, may be tested using the technique of preferential looking. When two objects are presented to an infant in a setting free of distractions, the infant is most likely to look at the more visually interesting object.[16] This observation provides the basis for preferential looking techniques.[17-19] Two targets of equal average brightness are presented to the infant. One target consists of a black-and-white line grating, while the other is a uniform gray target. If the infant can resolve the grating pattern, he or she will look at it in lieu of the gray field. If the grating cannot be resolved, no preference will be exhibited. Grating targets with different spatial frequencies are presented to the infant while the examiner watches the infant's eye movement response. If the infant looks at the grating pattern preferentially to the uniform gray target, a positive response is recorded. Finer and finer grating targets are presented until threshold resolution is

TABLE 1-4
Pediatric Visual Acuity Tests for Different Levels of Ability

Test	Availability
Basic level	
Preferential Looking	
Teller Acuity Cards	Vistech (513) 454-1399
Medium level	
LH Symbol Test	Lighthouse (800) 453-4923
Broken Wheel Test	Bernell (800) 348-2225
H-O-T-V Chart	Lighthouse (800) 453-4923
Advanced level	
Psychometric Acuity	
S Chart	Merton Flom, O.D., Ph.D
	College of Optometry
	University of Houston
	Houston, TX 77204
	(713) 743-1957
Bailey-Lovie Chart	School of Optometry
	University of California
	Berkeley, CA 94720
	(510) 642-0229

Source: Adapted with permission from W Marsh-Tootle. Clinical Methods of Testing Visual Acuity in Amblyopia. In RP Rutstein (ed), Problems in Optometry: Amblyopia. Philadelphia: Lippincott, 1991:208–36.

reached, i.e., the point at which the infant fixates the two targets randomly. By knowing the angular subtense of the grating, an approximation of the visual acuity may be determined.

The preferential looking test works well for infants aged 6–12 months. Older infants may become less attentive and respond more poorly to the patterns.

Although the preferential looking test is desirable for preverbal children and infants, it may overestimate visual acuity (relative to recognition acuity) in some cases.[15,20] Strabismic amblyopia and ocular conditions with foveal hypoplasia may yield better visual acuity with grating targets than with conventional optotypes. Since grating targets cover a relatively large retinal area, imprecise retinal localization does not necessarily reduce visual acuity in the same manner as with small, individual optotypes.

Teller Acuity Cards (Vistech Consultants, Dayton, OH) are commercially available (see Table 1-4 and Figure 1-6). These are hand-held preferential looking acuity cards that can be used without elaborate testing facilities.

Medium Level

LH Symbol Test

The LH symbol test presents four easy to name symbols: house, apple, ring/ball, and square/block/brick. The symbols were chosen because when blurred, each will be seen as a ball or ring. The newer versions of the chart conform to visual acuity measurement standards by presenting the symbols with the appropriate separations and by incorporating a geometric progression of row sizes.

H-O-T-V Test

The H-O-T-V test is a four-letter modification of the STYCAR test in which letters have been chosen for their lateral symmetry.[21] The child can name the letters or point to a match on a hand-held key card. It is therefore very useful for a child of any age who is nonverbal or other-

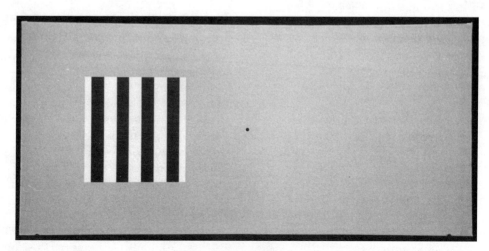

FIGURE 1-6
Preferential looking card. (Teller Acuity Cards, Vistech Consultants, Dayton, OH.)

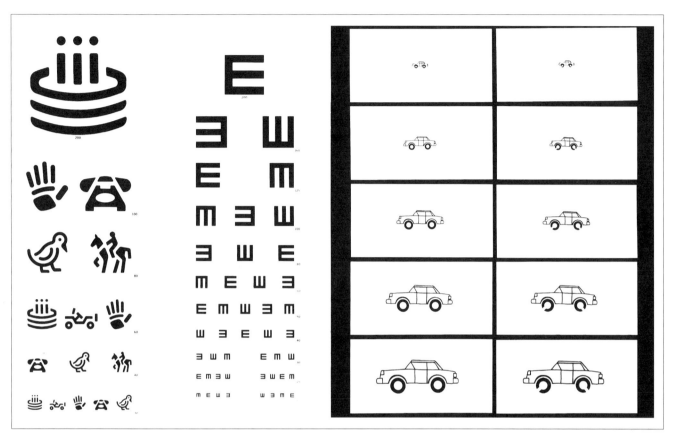

FIGURE 1-7

Examples of preliterate visual acuity charts are (left to right) Allen figures, tumbling E, and broken wheel. (Reprinted with permission from PP Schmidt. Comparisons of preliterate visual acuity tests in preschool children. Binocular Vision Q 1991;6:37–42.)

wise reluctant to give verbal answers. It has been shown to have a very low rate of untestability.[14] Fern and Manny[22] recommended this test as the test of choice for preschoolers. The optotypes are presented in high contrast using Snellen designs without directional components.

Broken Wheel

The broken wheel test is designed for children aged 3 years and older and is a modification of the Landolt ring test.[23] The test uses a forced choice design where the child must determine which of two cars has "broken wheels" (Figure 1-7). The test is understood by preschoolers and has a high testability rate.[24] Additionally, the use of the Landolt ring as the distinguishing feature eliminates varying difficulty among chart optotypes and allows for accurate calibration. Six pairs of charts ranging from visual acuities of 20/100 to 20/20 are included for the recommended test distance of 10 feet.

The H-O-T-V and broken wheel tests are the preferred visual acuity charts for young children who are unable or unwilling to be tested using advanced ability charts. The tumbling E and Allen figure charts have been used by many clinicians for testing preschool age children; however, recent studies have shown that visual acuity testing using these charts is less reliable than testing using the H-O-T-V or broken wheel tests.[24–26]

Tumbling E

The tumbling E acuity test is one that can be given to any cooperative patient (child or adult) who may be unfamiliar with letters. The E's are presented in one of four orientations (right, left, up, or down) (see Figure 1-7). Patients must respond by identifying the proper orientation. They may do so by verbalizing this to the examiner or by simply pointing toward the direction in which the "legs" of the E's are displayed. Although the tumbling E was once considered the unofficial standard test[27] for preschool and younger school age children who do not respond to letters, Schmidt[25] found responses using the test on 3-, 4-, and 5-year-old children inconsistent enough to make it "unusable." One difficulty with the test is the right-left confusion many children show before approximately age 7 years. Simons[28] therefore recommended that when the tumbling E test is used, responses should be restricted to three responses (up, down, or sideways) to avoid left-right reversals.

Allen Figures

The Allen figures test was designed to be used with a child who cannot respond to Snellen letters or the tumbling E.[29] It consists of black-and-white drawings of familiar figures (e.g., telephone, chicken, hand). The figures for this test were selected because they were thought to be recognizable to the average 3-year-old.

In a study of preschool children, Schmidt[25] found fewer untestable individuals using the Allen figure cards than when using the broken wheel or tumbling E. DeYoung-Smith and Baker[26] reported that the Allen figures tended to show better acuity than other acuity tests for children and that they failed to confirm a diagnosis of amblyopia in 51% of their cases (17 of 33). The test does not conform to Snellen design principles and may be subject to cultural influence in the recognition of the figures.[22] Additionally, the smallest line on the chart is designated 20/30. For these reasons Allen figures should be used only when children are untestable using more standardized methods.

Advanced Level

Most children above 6 or 7 years of age can be tested using the same recognition-type charts used for adults. For standardized testing, the charts should be of high contrast, have consistent spacing between letters and rows where appropriate, and have a logarithmic progression of row size.[3] Fern and Manny[22] made similar recommendations for visual acuity charts for preschool children.

AMBLYOPIA

Amblyopia is the condition in which visual acuity is decreased in an otherwise normal appearing eye even after refractive correction because one or more of the following was present in the patient before the age of 6 years[30]:

1. Amblyogenic anisometropia
2. Constant unilateral strabismus
3. Amblyogenic bilateral isometropia
4. Amblyogenic astigmatism
5. Image degradation

Careful examination to check for amblyopia in children is especially important, since it may be present with no obvious signs or symptoms.

The assessment of visual acuities is often challenging in patients with amblyopia. Frequently the amblyopic patient will have a large region of confusion in which some letters will be correctly identified but others will be missed. The patient may find the first and last letters of a row to be easily identifiable while the middle letters may be missed or read out of order.[31] This is an example of the crowding effect (phenomenon). The crowding effect is experienced to some degree by all observers but is more pronounced in individuals with amblyopia.[32,33] Better visual acuity is often measured in amblyopia when isolated rows and letters are used rather than a full Snellen chart.

Flom[31] described the crowding effect as having three components: (1) contour interaction, (2) divided attention within a complex display, and (3) unsteady and inaccurate fixational eye movements. Contour interaction is demonstrated by presenting a line or border close to an object of regard. Recognition of an acuity letter begins to degrade when the separation between the acuity letter and the competing contour is approximately five times the critical detail of the letter (i.e., one letter width).[34] More degradation in recognition occurs as the competing contour approaches the letter, until there is a separation of approximately one to two times the letter's critical detail. This is the distance at which the maximum effect of contour interaction occurs.

Even if adjacent optotypes are presented outside the area where contour interaction has an effect, performance may be reduced because of the unconscious division of the patient's attention among the optotypes. Additionally, poor fixational control in amblyopia[35] prevents consistent, accurate positioning of an acuity target onto the fovea. These effects may be related to the abnormally high spatial uncertainty found in strabismic and anisometropic amblyopia and the spatial distortion found in strabismic amblyopia.[31]

Visual acuity measurement with amblyopia requires patience and consistency of testing procedures. Accuracy is extremely important, especially when a patient is undergoing vision therapy, during which periodic measurements are necessary to evaluate progress. Test conditions during any therapy period should remain constant throughout and should be recorded for later reference. Weymouth[36] recommended making many measurements and plotting a frequency-of-seeing curve. Flom[37] developed a visual acuity chart ideally suited for this purpose. Eight Landolt rings are presented for a given size letter

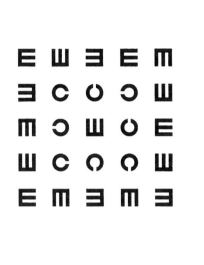

FIGURE 1-8

Flom's "S" chart. Eight Landolt rings are presented in four possible orientations. The "E's" give uniform crowding to the pattern. A constant letter separation of five times the critical detail size is used at all acuity levels. (Courtesy of Merton Flom, O.D., Ph.D.)

with uniform spacing and constant contour interaction (Figure 1-8). The patient must identify the orientation (right, left, up, or down) for each of the eight rings. Testing should begin with letters that are large enough such that all eight rings can be identified correctly for two successive letter sizes. Smaller and smaller charts are then presented until only two or less of the rings are properly specified, again for two successive letter sizes. The number of correct responses for each slide is plotted on the recording sheet as shown in Figure 1-9. A best-fit S-shaped curve is then drawn through the data points. The visual acuity is considered that point at which this line crosses the 5 correct response level (the 50% correct response level after considering that on average, two of the eight letters should be correctly identified simply by guessing).

This chart meets many of the recommendations for standardized visual acuity testing and is ideally suited for testing visual acuity in amblyopia. The chart has an equal number of optotypes (eight) at each acuity level, all with the same level of difficulty. A geometric progression of letter sizes is used, which allows accurate measurement even at very reduced visual acuity levels. The relative spacing is consistent at all letter sizes, thereby ensuring constant contour interaction. Additionally, the test can

be administered over many patient visits without the worry of the patient memorizing the chart.

The testing of visual acuity with low light levels may be appropriate for amblyopic patients to help determine the cause of reduced acuity. Von Noorden and Burian[38,39] demonstrated that patients with functional amblyopia demonstrated little or no reduction in visual acuity under low luminance conditions. Normal subjects showed a small but consistent reduction, whereas patients with organic disorders showed a large reduction. These investigators suggested measuring visual acuity while the subject is viewing the test chart through a 3.0 neutral-density filter and comparing this finding with that measured without the filter. Caloroso and Flom,[40] however, reported that visual acuity did decrease with low luminance for amblyopes, but agreed that the reduction was less than that for normal subjects. Additionally, they found that normal subjects fixating parafoveally responded in a manner similar to that of the amblyopes under low luminance. This suggests that eccentric fixation may be the cause of this phenomenon. Callahan[41] suggested that the interpretation of this test was ambiguous and should be used with caution because a reduction in acuity may not be seen under low illumination for some organic disorders.

Laser interferometric acuity has also been shown to be useful in the evaluation of amblyopes. Gstalder and Green[42] reported that laser-generated gratings yielded better visual acuity measurements than did Snellen testing in their amblyopic subjects. The spatial redundancy in the grating pattern is thought to partially negate the effects of unsteady or eccentric fixation. Additionally, the retinal contrast of the grating will be relatively high regardless of fluctuations in accommodation. Because of this, the visual acuity measurement using laser gratings may have prognostic value in determining the benefit of therapy in amblyopia. Selenow et al.[43] measured pretherapy grating acuity on 39 amblyopes. They found the posttherapy Snellen acuity to be within two lines of the initial laser visual acuity measurement in 90% of their subjects. They suggested using interference fringes to measure visual acuity in the initial evaluation of amblyopic subjects to help determine the potential posttherapy visual acuity.

OBJECTIVE TECHNIQUES

Various objective methods for assessing visual acuity have been used through the years. Only two, optokinetic nystagmus and visual evoked potentials, continue to receive frequent clinical use. Additionally, although by definition these tests require no subjective response, patient cooperation is required to obtain meaningful results.

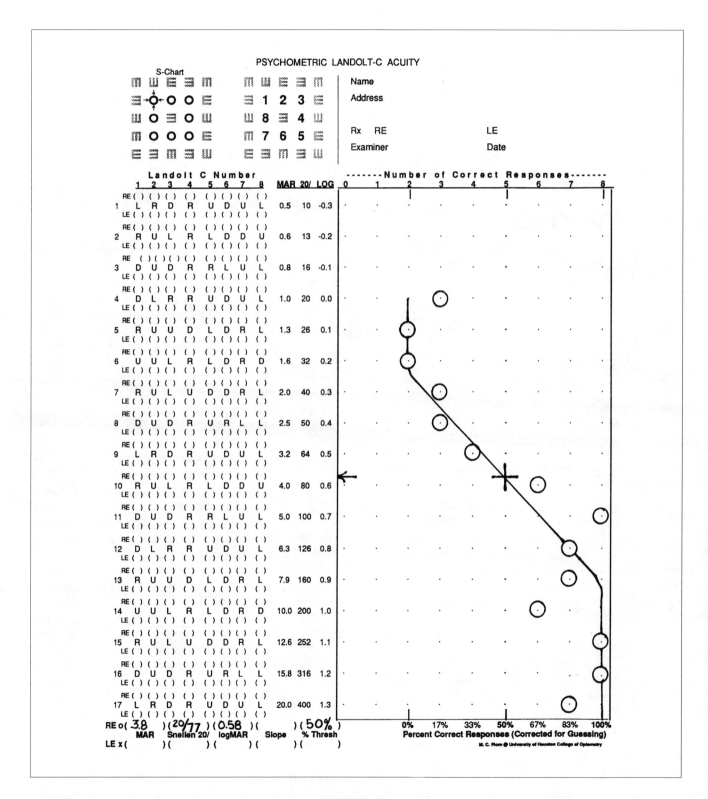

FIGURE 1-9

Landolt ring visual acuity series recording sheet. A series of targets is presented with a gradual decrease in size. The orientations of the rings are given on the left to aid the examiner in scoring. The number of correct responses for each size target are graphed on the right. The level of visual acuity is specified by where the best-fit S-shaped line crosses the 5 correct level. (Courtesy of Merton Flom, O.D., Ph.D.)

Optokinetic Nystagmus

By rotating a drum that has an evenly spaced series of black and white stripes before an observer, an alternating smooth and jerky eye movement response known as optokinetic nystagmus may be induced.[44] The speed of the moving target should not exceed 4 degrees per second.[12] The level of acuity is defined by the angular subtense of the finest grating target at which the nystagmoid movement can be elicited. Modifications of this basic technique include monitoring eye movements by electro-oculography.[45]

Visual Evoked Potentials

Visual evoked potentials (VEPs) are measures of the electrical activity of the visual cortex in response to visual stimulation. Recordings are obtained through an electrode placed on the scalp directly overlying the occipital cortex. Electrical responses to a repeating visual stimulus are recorded and averaged to retrieve the small visual response from the larger, unsynchronized background activity of the brain.

Much research has been conducted to investigate the relationship between the amplitude of the VEP and visual acuity.[46] Original testing was done with a full-field flashing target. Using this type of stimulus, the correlation between response amplitude and visual acuity was low. A much higher correlation is found when testing is done using patterned stimuli. Here, the patient typically views reversing checkerboard patterns of different sizes. The amplitude of the evoked response is then plotted versus the size of the checks, and a regression line is fit to the data. The visual acuity is defined by the check size corresponding to the zero amplitude of response along this regression line. Current instrumentation allows for the use of a more advanced technique ("sweep VEP") to quickly and efficiently determine visual acuity. This method is used most frequently with uncommunicative patients, such as infants, when other methods for determining visual acuity are unsuccessful and a loss of acuity is suspected. Additionally, assessment of visual acuity using VEPs is done to evaluate suspected malingerers. The visual evoked potential is discussed in more detail in Chapter 13.

SPECIALIZED TESTS

Contrast Sensitivity Function

In conventional visual acuity testing, patients are shown optotypes of high contrast in decreasing dimensions until the visual detail is no longer resolvable. Contrast is defined as the absolute value of the difference in luminance of the target background (L_B) and target detail (L_D) divided by the luminance of the target background (L_B):

$$\text{Contrast} = (L_B - L_D)/L_B$$

For a typical visual acuity chart, contrast is greater than 85%. Here, acuity levels give one measure of vision—the smallest image of high contrast that can be resolved by the visual system. Targets of this type are ideally suited for use during subjective refractive evaluation because optical blur mainly affects the high frequency spatial components of the retinal image. These measurements may be poor predictors of functional visual performance, however, because most visual objects in daily life are larger in size and possibly of low contrast.[11]

Contrast sensitivity testing measures the amount of contrast necessary for resolution of images of various sizes. Typically, grating targets (patterns of light and dark bars) with a sine wave luminance profile are presented to the patient at various spatial frequencies. At each spatial frequency the contrast of the grating is modified to the "threshold" of visibility. By plotting the threshold contrast values at different spatial frequencies, a contrast sensitivity function (CSF) (visual modulation transfer function) is determined.[47] The importance of this type of testing is that the visual system appears to be composed of independent channels for the detection of spatial detail of varying size.[48,49] These independent channels may be affected differently by various disease conditions. The complete CSF measures the sensitivity for these different channels and is not as limited as customary visual acuity testing.

The contrast sensitivity of the normal visual system is highest with medium spatial frequencies (between 3 and 8 cycles/degree). The sensitivity to contrast then drops off for higher and lower spatial frequencies. The high-frequency drop appears to be a result of diffraction and the optical aberrations of the eye.[4] There is a gradual reduction in retinal contrast at the higher spatial frequencies until approximately 50 cycles/degree, where the retinal image becomes a uniform gray. Sensitivity also drops at spatial frequencies below 4 cycles/degree. This is thought to be a function of the lateral inhibition mechanism of the visual system.[47] The gradual change in retinal illumination across the wide bars at the lower frequencies decreases the inhibitory and excitatory effects for adjacent retinal elements. This creates a reduction in the magnitude of the visual response.

The CSF can be affected by optical degradation or by diseases of the retina, the visual pathways, or the visual cortex. An opacity within the ocular media may affect vision more adversely than indicated by traditional visual acuity testing.[50] For example, reduction in retinal contrast caused by a nuclear cataract may significantly

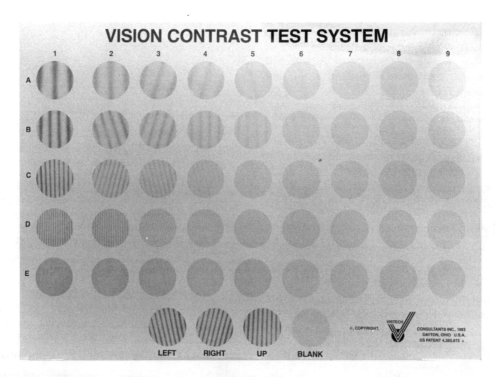

FIGURE 1-10

Vistech sine wave grating chart. The subject views the chart from 10 feet and reports the orientation of the grating targets (tilted left or right, vertical, or blank). The contrast of the sine wave gratings decreases from left to right, and the spatial frequency increases from top to bottom. (Courtesy of Vistech Consultants, Dayton, OH.)

decrease visual performance in a low contrast environment, although Snellen acuity may remain near normal in this case because high contrast optotypes are used. Contrast sensitivity testing thus may give the practitioner additional information that is helpful in determining more realistic levels of disability.

Reductions in contrast sensitivity that are independent of conventional visual acuity changes have also been reported for glaucoma,[51,52] other forms of optic nerve disease,[53,54] diabetes,[55,56] and Parkinson's disease.[57,58] Often, however, responses overlap in normal and abnormal patients, making diagnosis difficult using CSF testing alone. Nevertheless, contrast sensitivity testing has become more commonplace in clinical practice and is useful clinically in determining the visual effect of an abnormal ocular condition across all spatial frequencies, monitoring disease progression, or further investigating patients' visual complaints that are not explained by standard visual acuity testing or other means.

There are several methods for measuring contrast sensitivity clinically. Arden plates[52] were the first clinically convenient method developed. These plates consist of sinusoidal gratings of gradually increasing contrast using six different spatial frequencies. The gratings are uncovered slowly from low to high contrast until the patient can just detect the grating. Scores for each test plate are summed to give an overall numerical rating of contrast sensitivity.

Vistech Consultants developed a single, large test chart upon which gratings of decreasing contrast are presented for several spatial frequencies (Figure 1-10).[59] Testing is performed with a viewing distance of 10 feet using a "four alternative" testing procedure. This technology has also been incorporated into a table-top instrument that is capable of testing contrast sensitivity at distance and near, using high or low light levels, with or without a peripheral glare source.

Although the Vistech wall chart is a moderately simple and inexpensive way to measure contrast sensitivity on untrained patients, its test-retest reliability is reportedly less than desirable.[60,61] This is apparently because of the limited steps of contrast at each spatial frequency and the lack of a true criterion-free testing procedure.

Several manufacturers have available computer-controlled systems that present gratings on the face of a cathode ray tube (CRT). Although the CRT systems are generally more expensive than the others mentioned, they can provide a larger test field and have the capability of testing contrast sensitivity to temporally modulated targets.

Visual acuity charts printed at low contrast provide contrast sensitivity information using a more conventional testing mode. Less information can be extracted from this test versus measuring a complete CSF across numerous spatial frequencies. As with conventional acuity testing, the endpoint represents the smallest detail that can be resolved at a given level of contrast. However, the test is easily administered, well understood by patients, requires less testing time, and appears to have an excellent test-retest reliability.[61]

The Bailey-Lovie[62] and the Regan[63] charts are examples of conventional visual acuity charts produced in both high and low contrast. Both charts follow a logarithmic size progression and present the same number of letters on each row. Brown and Lovie-Kitchin[61] reported a 2.5-line difference in results for the high-contrast (90%) and low-contrast (8%) Bailey-Lovie charts for normal subjects with different degrees of refractive error. Although the Regan charts are available in high (96%), medium (7%), and low (4%) contrasts, Regan reported that only the two higher contrast levels are needed for routine clinical use.[64]

The Pelli-Robson Letter Sensitivity Chart[65] presents letters of constant size but with decreasing contrast from 90% to less than 1% at a 1-meter test distance. The letter size and test distance were chosen to indicate the patient's overall sensitivity to contrast. Although this test will not provide a detailed assessment of contrast sensitivity to all target sizes, Pelli et al.[65] argued that coupled with the high contrast visual acuity measure, sufficient additional information is provided by this test to determine if a patient's vision falls within the normal range.

Glare Testing

Difficulty with night driving or problems seeing under glare conditions are complaints frequently expressed by patients. Normal visual acuity testing using ideal examination room lighting may reveal only a small, if any, decrement, which may not be consistent with the severity of the subjective complaint. Clinical measurements of the susceptibility to disability glare may be useful especially in assessing the need for cataract surgery in patients maintaining relatively good visual acuity (20/20 to 20/50).

Comparing Snellen visual acuity measurements as tested with and without simultaneously shining a peripheral light source (situated 15–30 degrees off the line of sight) into the eye is a method for measuring the effects of glare. Using a penlight[66] for the peripheral glare source is an inexpensive method recommended for this purpose. A significant drop

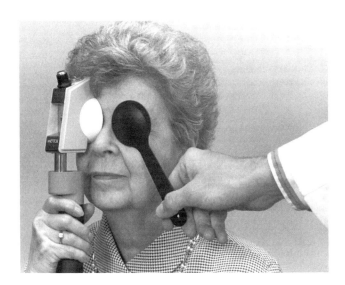

FIGURE 1-11
The subject views an ordinary visual acuity chart through the Brightness Acuity Tester (Mentor Ophthalmics, Norwell, MA). A reduction in visual acuity greater than 3 lines indicates abnormal glare sensitivity.

in measured visual acuity to 20/100 or worse with this technique may indicate an abnormal glare sensitivity.

Several instruments providing a consistent glare source have been developed to help standardize glare testing. Nadler and Miller[67,68] designed a glare tester using a tabletop projector with a built-in viewing screen. A 20/400 Landolt ring is presented in steps of gradually decreasing contrast from 80% to 2.5% in the center of the screen. The brightly illuminated periphery serves to create glare. The contrast sensitivities for the Landolt rings with and without the peripheral glare source serve to indicate the degree of visual disability present.

The Brightness Acuity Tester (BAT) (Mentor Ophthalmics, Norwell, MA) is a relatively inexpensive, hand-held instrument designed to test the effects of glare (Figure 1-11). A standard visual acuity chart is viewed through a small hole located at the apex of the reflecting hemisphere. The equiluminous glare source presents light to the eye from all directions except for the central 10 degrees. The instrument is adjustable to three different brightness levels. Outdoor visual acuity has been predicted best with the instrument on level two.[69] At this level, a decrease of three lines or more of measured visual acuity is considered abnormal.

The Vistech MCT 8000 (Vistech Consultants, Dayton, OH) is a table-top instrument designed to measure contrast sensitivity and is also capable of measuring the effects of a peripheral glare source. Because the unit is self-contained, testing can be accomplished in a small area and does not require an examination lane.

Neumann et al.[69] compared the three instruments just discussed and others for their usefulness. They found the BAT to most accurately predict (within one line of measurement 73% of the time) Snellen acuity under glare conditions outdoors. This instrument was used easily by patients and was relatively inexpensive. However, it lacked versatility in that clinical use was limited to glare and photostress testing. The Vistech (56%) and Miller-Nadler (47%) instruments predicted outdoor visual acuity less accurately but were more versatile overall.

Elliott and Bullimore[70] compared these instruments along with the Berkeley Glare Test[71] using both high- and low-contrast visual acuity charts as well as with the Pelli-Robson contrast sensitivity chart. The results were compared to those obtained with the van den Berg Straylightmeter.[72] The van den Berg Straylightmeter measures the forward light scatter within the eye using three rings of flickering light-emitting diode sources positioned at angular distances of 3.5 degrees, 10 degrees, and 28 degrees. The patient adjusts a central 1-degree circular target flickering in counterphase fashion to the peripheral rings. The setting at which the patient observes no flicker of the central circular target indicates the degree of forward scatter present in the eye.

Elliott and Bullimore[70] found that measuring glare using a low-contrast visual acuity chart (Regan or Bailey-Lovie Charts) or the Pelli-Robson contrast sensitivity chart yields results more highly correlated with the van den Berg Straylightmeter measurements. The results with the Vistech MCT 8000 and Miller-Nadler instruments yielded lower correlations presumably due to non-uniform target size progression and/or shortfalls in the recommended psychophysical testing methods.

Photostress Test

The time required to recover visual acuity after the macula is exposed to a bright light source has been used as an indicator of macular integrity. Magder[73] reported active cases of central serous retinopathy in which visual acuity was very slow to recover after the macular area was bleached during ophthalmoscopy. A macular condition that affects the outer retinal layers as well as regeneration of the photopigment within the photoreceptors' outer segments will prolong photostress recovery, whereas an optic nerve lesion will not.

Although variations of the photostress test are described, most are similar to that presented by Glaser et al.[74] After best corrected visual acuity is measured, the patient is asked to monocularly view for 10 seconds a bright light source held close to the eye. The patient is then asked to begin reading down the acuity chart until he or she is able to resolve the line immediately above the level of best acuity. The photostress recovery time is the time in seconds that it takes the patient to read three letters in this row. A recovery time under 50 seconds is considered normal. Glaser et al.[74] reported an average recovery time of 27 seconds in 179 normal eyes with 99% recovering in under 50 seconds. The average recovery time for 63 eyes with various maculopathies was 150 seconds, while for 20 eyes with optic nerve disease the average recovery time was 36 seconds. This testing may be useful clinically to differentiate between macular (prolonged recovery) and optic nerve (normal recovery) disease when ophthalmoscopic clues are not evident.

POTENTIAL ACUITY MEASUREMENT

The prediction of postsurgical visual acuity is an important component of the presurgical evaluation of a patient with cataract.[75] It is helpful in assessing the risk-to-benefit ratio and relating expected outcomes to patients. Present methods routinely used to measure retinal function in the presence of a cataract fall into two categories. Several instruments attempt to "bypass" the optics of the eye. Other techniques use unpatterned, full-field light stimuli and require only that light reaches the retina. The degree of focus is irrelevant.

The laser interferometer produces an interference grating upon the retina by focusing mutually coherent light sources in the plane of the pupil. A mild to moderate cataract is thus "bypassed" allowing high-contrast gratings to be focused onto the retina.[76,77] The Rodenstock Retinometer (Rodenstock, München-Hamburg, Germany) a laser interferometer that attaches easily to a Zeiss slit lamp. The instrument is adjustable for intensity, grating frequency, and grating orientation. The focused laser light sources are moved back and forth across the pupil to find an area of relative clarity within the lens. The patient must indicate whether the grating can be appreciated instead of a uniform background. Having the patient indicate the grating orientation adds objectivity to the test. The grating frequency may be increased in steps to measure a grating acuity from 20/660 to 20/20.

The Randwal White Light Interferometer (Randwal Instruments, Southbridge, MA) is similar to the laser interferometer in that the patient is shown gratings of various frequencies. With the white light interferometer, however, a grating pattern is produced by the interaction of the mutually coherent first-order components of the diffraction spectrum of a moiré fringe pattern.[78] The cloudy media is "bypassed" by focusing these slit images into the plane of the pupil. Since the grating is produced by a white light source, the white light interferometer is less expensive than the laser model. Also, the Randwal White Light Interferometer is portable and requires no supporting base (Figure 1-12).

The Potential Acuity Meter (Mentor Ophthalmics, Norwell, MA) is another instrument that "bypasses" cloudy ocular media.[79] However, this instrument does not use interference. With the Potential Acuity Meter (PAM) the patient views a normal acuity letter target projected onto the retina through an extremely small exit pupil (0.15 mm diameter).

Techniques that use an unpatterned light stimulus to predict retinal function include visualization of entopic phenomena, the full-field flash visual evoked potential (VEP), and electroretinogram (ERG). Because a focused retinal image is not required for these tests, testing can be accomplished even in the presence of dense opacification of the ocular media.

The visualization of Purkinje's tree is a gross indicator of retinal function. Gently moving a penlight or other bright source over the sclera produces a visual perception of the retinal vasculature. The diffuse, moving light directed through the sclera creates an unstabilized shadow of the vessels onto the photoreceptors so that the shadow image does not fade from view. If the patient can describe a branching pattern such as a tree, cobweb, or dried river bed, and reports no darkened central area in the image, some reassurance of gross retinal function is provided. However, using this method Sinclair et al.[80] reported that 13 of 17 patients with visual acuity of 20/50 or worse after cataract surgery were able to visualize Purkinje's tree preoperatively, whereas 10 of the 116 patients with better than 20/50 resultant visual acuity could not. Therefore this test is relatively unreliable in predicting poor macular function (visual acuity of 20/50 or worse).

Blue field entoptoscopy will provide an estimate of the integrity of the macular area by allowing the patient to visualize shadows of leukocytes flowing in the perifoveal capillary circulation.[81] The patient views an intense blue field that diffusely illuminates the retina. A dense cataract is not a great obstacle with this method and may even facilitate testing by providing more uniform illumination. Good macular function is predicted if the patient reports seeing at least 15 corpuscles. A negative result is when only a few or no corpuscles are seen. Sinclair et al.[80] reported excellent results with blue field entoptoscopy: 48 of 50 patients with postoperative visual acuity better than 20/40 responded positively with the instrument before surgery. Only 1 of 10 subjects with resultant visual acuity of 20/50 or worse gave a positive response preoperatively. Other investiga-

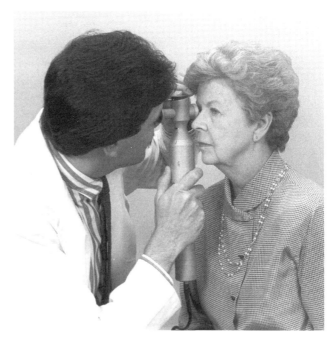

FIGURE 1-12
The examiner (left) aligns the IRAS Interferometer (Randwal Instruments, Southbridge, MA) into the subject's pupil.

tors have also reported clinically useful results using the blue field entoptoscope; however, the level of success is generally lower than that reported by Sinclair et al.[80]

Electrodiagnostic testing using the electroretinogram and visual evoked potentials has also been found useful for assessing retinal function in the presence of media opacities (see Chapter 13). The electroretinogram (ERG) reflects the electrical activity within the layers of the retina as measured at the surface of the cornea. An abnormal ERG finding is indicative of abnormal visual functioning. However, since the full-field flash ERG represents the summation of the response for the entire retina, a normal ERG can be found in many conditions where an abnormality is confined to the macular area. Age-related macular degeneration and macular scarring from a chorioretinal infection are two examples of conditions in which full-field flash ERG responses are normal yet central visual acuity may be extremely low. The ERG is therefore most predictive in cases where a widespread retinal abnormality affects central and peripheral visual function.

The VEP test is much more useful than the ERG in assessing macular integrity. The visual response is monitored by placing an electrode on the scalp over the occipital cortex. Because the macula projects to the brain surface and is disproportionately represented within the cortex, the

TABLE 1-5

Comparison of Methods for Postoperative Visual Acuity Estimation in Patients with Cataracts

	Prevalence*	Accuracy	Mean Sensitivity	Specificity	Predictive Value	
					Positive	Negative
Laser interferometry	0.21	0.78	0.55	0.84	0.47	0.89
Visual evoked potential	0.43	0.81	0.59	0.91	0.84	0.77
Blue field entoptoscopy	0.13	0.76	0.77	0.76	0.36	0.94
Potential acuity meter (PAM)	0.20	0.74	0.74	0.72	0.40	0.98

*The criterion for poor visual acuity varied among the different studies, but was generally worse than 20/40 or 20/50.
Source: Adapted from JV Odom, G Chao, GW Weinstein. Preoperative prediction of postoperative visual acuity in patients with cataracts: a quantitative review. Doc Ophthalmol 1988;70:5–17. With permission of Kluwer Academic Publishers.

VEP is dominated by macular function. Visual acuity can be determined by measuring the electrical response evoked during the viewing of an alternating checkerboard pattern. Checkerboards with finer and finer check sizes are successively presented until no further response is recorded. The response amplitude is plotted versus check size, and the check size corresponding to zero amplitude of response along a regression line connecting data points represents the visual acuity of the subject. To determine the macular integrity, or potential acuity, of a patient with a dense media opacity, a different testing method for the VEP is needed because very cloudy media will reduce the contrast of the fine checkerboard pattern to subthreshold levels. Therefore, a steady-state visual evoked potential is recorded using a bright, unpatterned stimulus flashing at 10 Hz. The patient response is evaluated based on the primary and secondary components of the recorded waveform. This method has been shown to be comparable in sensitivity and specificity to methods that "bypass" the optics of the eye.[82] Additionally, the predictive accuracy for this test does not decrease with denser lenticular opacities as do the predictive accuracies of those methods requiring a focused retinal image.

Odom et al.[83] presented a quantitative review of the literature for several methods used to assess retinal integrity in patients with cataracts. Data were compiled from 52 reports that attempted to predict postoperative visual acuity using the methods previously described. The compiled statistics are presented in Table 1-5. As shown, none of the listed tests can perfectly predict postsurgical visual performance. This is to be expected, not only because of difficulties in administering these tests, but also because of complications of surgery, including cystoid macular edema, posterior capsular opacification, or optical irregularities involving the intraocular lens or cornea.

All these tests have a moderately high negative predictive value (NPV), meaning the majority of patients demonstrating potential for good acuity before surgery

end up with good acuity postoperatively. That the PAM method shows the highest NPV is to be expected. The PAM test is a letter recognition acuity test. If the patient can read letters from an acuity chart before surgery using the PAM apparatus, and no significant surgical complications are encountered, good resultant letter acuity is expected.

Several authors have reported a tendency for measurements with an interferometer to overestimate resultant visual acuity in patients with macular irregularities.[77,84,85] With a grating target only a small portion of the grating need be visible for proper resolution. Because the grating generally covers a relatively large retinal area (2 or 3 degrees), an individual with a small remaining island of vision within the macular or paramacular region will more likely "see" a fine grating than a small acuity letter.[85] With a small island of vision, the stable fixation necessary to recognize letters in a conventional visual acuity chart may be difficult to maintain.

The main shortcoming of potential acuity measurements is the underprediction of postsurgical visual acuity. Odom et al.[83] reported all methods except the VEP to show positive predictive values (PPVs) less than 50%, which indicates that less than 50% of the individuals failing the presurgical visual acuity test have poor acuity postsurgically. When the resultant acuity is better than predicted, both the patient and surgeon are pleasantly surprised. A problem surfaces, however, when a poor potential acuity measurement results in a decision not to have surgery; thus, the potential increase in visual function afforded by surgery may be needlessly lost. It is therefore important to thoroughly investigate those cases where poor acuity is predicted by initial testing.

The VEP appears to be vastly superior to the other tests in terms of PPV. An abnormal visual signal recorded during VEP testing appears to be the best indicator of abnormal macular processing and poor visual acuity. This is especially true when a dense media opacity is present. Ideally, those individuals who perform poorly on a device that "bypasses" the optics of the eye should be retested using the VEP. Unfortunately, this is usually not feasible for a private practitioner because of the cost and availability of the equipment, as well as the need for an experienced individual to interpret the testing results. However, the blue field entoptoscope uses a bright, unpatterned light stimulus similar to the VEP. This type of stimulus is especially useful with a dense media opacity. Therefore, using the blue field entoptoscope in conjunction with an interferometer or the PAM creates a useful testing protocol to determine potential visual function.

REFERENCES

1. Cline D, Hofstetter HW, Griffin JR. Dictionary of Visual Science (3rd ed). Radnor, PA: Chilton, 1980.
2. Riggs LA. Visual Acuity. In CH Graham (ed), Vision and Visual Perception. New York: Wiley, 1965;321–49.
3. Bailey IL. Measurement of Visual Acuity—Towards Standardization. In Vision Science Symposium: A Tribute to Gordon G. Heath. Bloomington, IN: Indiana University, 1988;215–30.
4. Campbell FW, Gubisch RW. Optical quality of the human eye. J Physiol (Lond) 1966;186:558–78.
5. Van Nes FL, Bouman MA. Spatial modulation transfer in the human eye. J Opt Soc Am 1967;57:401–6.
6. Westheimer G. Modulation thresholds for sinusoidal light distributions on the retina. J Physiol (Lond) 1960;152:67–74.
7. Campbell FW, Green DG. Optical and retinal factors affecting visual resolution. J Physiol (Lond) 1965;181:576–93.
8. Yellot JI, Wandell BA, Cornsweet TN. The Beginnings of Visual Perception: The Retinal Image and Its Initial Encoding. In JM Brookhart, VB Mountcastle (eds), Handbook of Physiology: Section I: The Nervous System: Vol III: Sensory Processes, Part 1. Bethesda, MD: American Physiological Society, 1984;7:257–316.
9. Peters HB. The relationship between refractive error and visual acuity at three age levels. Am J Optom 1961;38:194–8.
10. Amos JF, Noorden LC. The Eye Not Correctable to 20/20. In JF Amos (ed), Diagnosis and Management in Vision Care. Boston: Butterworth-Heinemann, 1987;11:267–8.
11. Ginsburg AP. Spatial Filtering and Vision: Implications for Normal and Abnormal Vision. In LM Proenza, JM Enoch, A Jampolsky (eds), Clinical Applications of Visual Psychophysics. Cambridge: Cambridge University Press, 1981;70–106.
12. Borish IM. Clinical Refraction (3rd ed). Chicago: Professional Press, 1970.
13. Hofstetter HW. From 20/20 to 6/6 or 4/4? Am J Optom 1973;50:212–21.
14. Lippman O. Vision screening of young children. Am J Public Health 1971;61:1586–601.
15. Marsh-Tootle W. Clinical Methods of Testing Visual Acuity in Amblyopia. In RP Rutstein (ed), Problems in Optometry: Amblyopia. Philadelphia: Lippincott, 1991:208–36.
16. Fantz RL. Pattern vision in young infants. Psychol Res 1958;8:43–7.
17. Teller DY, Morse R, Borton R, Regal D. Visual acuity for vertical and diagonal gratings in human infants. Vision Res 1975;14:1433–9.
18. Dobson V, Teller DY, Lee CP, Wade B. A behavioral method for efficient screening of visual acuity in young infants. I: Preliminary laboratory development. Invest Ophthalmol Vis Sci 1978;17:1142–50.
19. Fulton AB, Manning KA, Dobson V. A behavioral method for efficient screening of visual acuity in young infants. II: Clinical application. Invest Ophthalmol Vis Sci 1978;17:1151–7.
20. Harris SJ, Hansen RM, Fulton AB. Assessment of acuity of amblyopic subjects using face, grating, and recognition stimuli. Invest Ophthalmol Vis Sci 1986;27:1184–7.
21. Sheridan MD. Vision screening of very young or retarded children. Br Med J 1960;2:453–6.
22. Fern KD, Manny RE. Visual acuity of the preschool child: A review. Am J Optom Physiol Opt 1986;63:319–45.
23. Richman JE, Petito GT, Cron MT. Broken wheel acuity test: A new and valid test for preschool and exceptional children. J Am Optom Assoc 1984;55:561–5.
24. Schmidt PP. Allen figure and broken wheel visual acuity measurement in preschool children. J Am Optom Assoc 1992;63:124–30.
25. Schmidt PP. Comparisons of testability of preliterate visual acuity tests in preschool children. Binocular Vision Q 1991;6:37–42.
26. DeYoung-Smith MA, Baker JD. A comparative study of visual acuity tests. Am Orthop J 1986;36:160–4.
27. Hatfield EM. Methods and standards for screening preschool children. Sight-saving Rev 1979;49(Summer):71–83.
28. Simons K. Visual acuity norms in young children. Surv Ophthalmol 1983;28:84–92.
29. Allen HF. A new picture series for preschool vision testing. Am J Ophthalmol 1957;44:38–41.
30. Ciuffreda KJ, Levi DM, Selenow A. Amblyopia: Basic and Clinical Aspects. Boston: Butterworth-Heinemann, 1991;13–7.
31. Flom M. Contour Interaction and the Crowding Effect. In RP Rutstein (ed), Problems in Optometry: Amblyopia. Philadelphia: Lippincott, 1991:237–57.
32. Stuart JA, Burian HM. A study of separation difficulty: Its relationship to visual acuity in normal and amblyopic eyes. Am J Ophthalmol 1962;53:471–7.
33. Maraini G, Pasino L, Peralta S. Separation difficulty in amblyopia. Am J Ophthalmol 1963;56:922–5.
34. Flom MC, Weymouth FW, Kahneman D. Visual resolution and contour interaction. J Opt Soc Am 1963;53:1026–32.
35. Cuiffreda K. Eye Movements. In KJ Cuiffreda, DM Levi, A Selenow (eds), Amblyopia: Basic and Clinical Aspects. Boston: Butterworth-Heinemann, 1991:165–241.
36. Weymouth FW. Visual Acuity in Children. In MJ Hirsch, RE Wick (eds), Vision of Children. Philadelphia: Chilton, 1963;119–43.

37. Flom MC. New concepts in visual acuity. Opt Weekly 1966;57 (July 14):63–8.
38. von Noorden GK, Burian HM. Visual acuity in normal and amblyopic patients under reduced illumination: I. Behavior of visual acuity with and without neutral density filter. Arch Ophthalmol 1959;61:533–5.
39. von Noorden GK, Burian HM. Visual acuity in normal and amblyopic patients under reduced illumination: II. The visual acuity at various levels of illumination. Arch Ophthalmol 1959;62:396–9.
40. Caloroso E, Flom MC. Influence of luminance on visual acuity in amblyopia. Am J Optom 1969;46:189–95.
41. Callahan WP. Investigations of amblyopia. Trans Canad Ophthalmol Soc 1961;25:186–95.
42. Gstalder RJ, Green DG. Laser interferometric acuity in amblyopia. J Pediatr Ophthalmol 1971;8:251–6.
43. Selenow A, Ciuffreda KJ, Mozlin R, Rumpf D. Prognostic value of laser interferometric visual acuity in amblyopia therapy. Invest Ophthalmol Vis Sci 1986;27:273–7.
44. Barany R. The clinical aspects and theory of train nystagmus. Arch Augenheilk 1921;88:139–42.
45. Dayton GO, Jones MH, Aiu P, Rawson RA, et al. Developmental study of coordinated eye movements in the human infant, I. Visual acuity in the newborn human: A study based on induced optokinetic nystagmus recorded by electro-oculography. Arch Ophthalmol 1964;71:865–70.
46. Tyler CW, Apkarian P, Levi DM, Nakayama K. Rapid assessment of visual function: An electronic sweep technique for the pattern visual evoked potential. Invest Ophthalmol Vis Sci 1979;18:703–13.
47. Cornsweet TN. Visual Perception. New York: Academic, 1970:311–64.
48. Campbell FW, Robson JG. Application of Fourier analysis to the visibility of gratings. J Physiol (Lond) 1968;197:551–66.
49. Blakemore C, Campbell FW. Adaptation to spatial stimuli. J Physiol (Lond) 1969;200:11–3.
50. Hess R, Woo G. Vision through cataracts. Invest Ophthalmol Vis Sci 1978;17:428–35.
51. Atkin A, Bodis-Wollner I, Wolkstein M, et al. Abnormalities of central contrast sensitivity in glaucoma. Am J Opthalmol 1979;88:205–11.
52. Arden GB, Jacobson JJ. A simple grating test for contrast sensitivity: Preliminary results indicate value in screening for glaucoma. Invest Ophthalmol Vis Sci 1978;17:23–32.
53. Regan D, Silver R, Murray TJ. Visual acuity and contrast sensitivity in multiple sclerosis—hidden visual loss: An auxiliary diagnostic test. Brain 1977;100:563–79.
54. Hess RF, Plant G. The Psychophysical Loss in Optic Neuritis: Spatial and Temporal Aspects. In RF Hess, G Plant (eds), Optic Neuritis. Cambridge: Cambridge University Press, 1986:109–51.
55. Hyvärinen L, Laurinen P, Rovamo J. Contrast sensitivity in evaluation of visual impairment due to diabetes. Acta Ophthalmol 1983;61:94–101.
56. Sokol S, Moskowitz A, Skarf B, et al. Contrast sensitivity in diabetics with and without background retinopathy. Arch Ophthalmol 1985;103:51–4.
57. Regan D, Neima D. Low-contrast letter charts in early diabetic retinopathy, ocular hypertension, glaucoma and Parkinson's disease. Br J Ophthalmol 1984;68:885–9.
58. Bodis-Wollner I, Mitra S, Bobak P, et al. Low frequency distortion in temporal surface in Parkinson's disease. Invest Ophthalmol Vis Sci 1984;25(Suppl):313.
59. Ginsburg AP. A new contrast sensitivity vision test chart. Am J Optom Physiol Opt 1984;61:403–7.
60. Rubin GS. Reliability and sensitivity of clinical contrast sensitivity tests. Clin Vision Sci 1988;2:169–77.
61. Brown B, Lovie-Kitchin JE. High and low contrast acuity and clinical contrast sensitivity tested in a normal population. Optom Vision Sci 1989;66:467–73.
62. Bailey IL, Lovie JE. New design principles for visual acuity letter charts. Am J Optom Physiol Opt 1976;53:740–5.
63. Regan D, Neima D. Low-contrast letter charts as a test of visual function. Ophthalmology 1983;90:1192–1200.
64. Regan D. Low-contrast letter charts and sinewave grating tests in ophthalmological and neurological disorders. Clin Vision Sci 1988;2:235–50.
65. Pelli DG, Robson JG, Wilkins AJ. The design of a new letter chart for measuring contrast sensitivity. Clin Vision Sci 1988;2:187–99.
66. Maltzmann BA, Horan C, Rengel A. Penlight test for glare disability of cataracts. Ophthalmic Surg 1988;19:356–8.
67. LeClaire J, Nadler MP, Weiss S, Miller D. A new glare tester for clinical testing: Results comparing normal subjects and variously corrected aphakic patients. Arch Ophthalmol 1982;100:153–8.
68. Hirsch RP, Nadler MP, Miller D. Glare measurement as a predictor of outdoor vision among cataract patients. Ann Ophthalmol 1984;16:965–8.
69. Neumann AC, McCarty GR, Locke J, Cobb B. Glare disability devices for cataractous eyes: A consumer's guide. J Cataract Refract Surg 1988;14:212–6.
70. Elliott DB, Bullimore MA. Assessing the reliability, discriminative ability, and validity of disability glare tests. Invest Ophthalmol Vis Sci 1993;34:108–19.
71. Bailey IL, Bullimore MA. A new test for the evaluation of disability glare. Optom Vis Sci 1991;68:911–7.
72. van den Berg TJTP. On the relation between glare and straylight. Doc Ophthalmol 1991;78:177–81.
73. Magder H. Test for central serous retinopathy based on clinical observations and trial. Am J Ophthalmol 1960;49:147–50.
74. Glaser JS, Savino PJ, Sumers KD, et al. The photostress recovery test in the clinical assessment of visual function. Am J Ophthalmol 1977;83:255–60.
75. Sherman J, Davis E, Schnider C, et al. Presurgical prediction of postsurgical visual acuity in patients with media opacities. J Am Optom Assoc 1988;59:481–8.
76. Green DG. Testing the vision of cataract patients by means of laser generated interference fringes. Science 1970;168:1240–2.
77. Faulkner W. Laser interferometric prediction of postoperative visual acuity in patients with cataracts. Am J Ophthalmol 1983;95:626–36.

78. Lotmar W. Apparatus for the measurement of retinal visual acuity by moiré fringes. Invest Ophthalmol Vis Sci 1980;19:393–400.

79. Minkowski JS, Palese M, Guyton DL. Potential acuity meter using a minute aerial pinhole aperture. Ophthalmol 1983; 90:1360–8.

80. Sinclair SH, Loebl M, Riva CE. Blue field entoptic phenomenon in cataract patients. Arch Ophthalmol 1979;97: 1092–5.

81. Riva CE, Loebl M. Autoregulation of blood flow in the capillaries of the human macula. Invest Ophthalmol Vis Sci 1977;16:568–71.

82. Odom JV, Chao G, Hobson R, Weinstein GW. Prediction of post cataract extraction visual acuity: 10 Hz visually evoked potentials. Ophthalmic Surg 1988;19:212–8.

83. Odom JV, Chao G, Weinstein GW. Preoperative prediction of postoperative visual acuity in patients with cataracts: A quantitative review. Doc Ophthalmol 1988;70:5–17.

84. Green DG, Cohen MM. Laser interferometry in the evaluation of potential macular function in the presence of opacities in the ocular media. Trans Am Acad Ophthalmol Otolaryngol 1971;75:629–35.

85. Loshin DS, White J. Contrast sensitivity: The visual rehabilitation of the patient with macular degeneration. Arch Ophthalmol 1984;102:1303–6.

Preface

Since the publication of the first edition of *Ocular Disease*, optometry has remained a rapidly changing profession with ever-expanding roles for the optometrist in the diagnosis and management of ophthalmic pathology. As students, residents, and existing practitioners prepare themselves for these extended roles in health care, educational resources dedicated to the subject of ocular disease are essential. While a variety of textbooks have been produced that are concerned with various aspects of ophthalmic pathology, the second edition of *Ocular Disease* is intended to remain an introductory text emphasizing fundamental clinical techniques as well as the more common clinical conditions to which they pertain.

Although basic components of the first edition were used, the second edition has been altered significantly to update and improve the text. Most chapters have been completely rewritten. In some instances, chapters have been renamed and reorganized to provide a new emphasis consistent with contemporary optometry. Completely new chapters have also been added to the text.

The second edition is divided into two parts. The first part, Ophthalmic Diagnostic Procedures, includes 20 chapters dedicated to clinical procedures that are useful to the primary care practitioner. Some of the clinical techniques discussed are basic to every eye examination; others are more advanced procedures used only when specific clinical conditions are suspected or identified. Chapters on the more basic techniques include Visual Acuities; Slit Lamp Biomicroscopy; Tonometry; Ophthalmoscopy; Gonioscopy and Fundus Contact Lens; and Visual Fields. Chapters discussing more advanced techniques include Fluorescein Angiography; Electrodiagnostic Testing; and Ocular Microbiology and Cytology.

The techniques covered in the first part are presented at an introductory level so that the student may learn fundamental concepts. A significant amount of material in this section is devoted to the presentation of specific clinical entities to assist the reader in learning the application of the clinical techniques as well as building knowledge in the area of ocular disease. This helps make the book a very practical and useful resource. Since many diseases are covered in significant detail, this book is also a useful reference for the practitioner simply wanting to refresh his or her memory on a particular topic.

Part II, Treatment and Management of Common Ocular Disorders, consists of five chapters that are of fundamental importance to the student, resident, or practicing optometrist. This section is a major change from the first edition and discusses clinical presentation and management in five particular areas. The individual chapters include Diseases of the Lids and Lashes; Diseases of the Conjunctiva, Cornea, and Sclera; Uveitis; Diseases of the Retina and Vitreous; and Glaucoma. This section builds the reader's knowledge of ocular disease and increases the usefulness of the text as a basic reference source. The more pertinent and common clinical entities encountered by the practicing primary care optometrist have been included in this section.

As with any book of its kind, the second edition of *Ocular Disease: Diagnosis and Treatment* would not have been possible without the participation of and assistance from dozens of individuals. Twenty-eight authors contributed to the book, all of them experts in the field of optometry. We are most indebted to these individuals, who sacrificed their valuable time for this project.

We also thank those people who reviewed portions of the book or offered their advice, including Drs. Paul Abplanalp, Mike Chaglasian, Lynn Conrad, Susan Cotter, John E. Conto, Mary Flynn, Helen Gabriel, David Lee, Iris Matsukado, Leonard Messner, Stephanie Messner, Mike Patella, Sara L. Penner, Pete Russo, and Bruce Teitelbaum.

We are grateful to the Media Production staff of the Illinois College of Optometry, who helped prepare many of the new illustrations for the second edition, including Tom Brady, Al Pouch, and Becky Reyes. We are extremely appreciative of Tom Brady, who diligently prepared many of the new line drawings. We also thank David Maish for preparation of a few of the line drawings as well. Many thanks also go to the Learning Resources staff at the Illinois College of Optometry, who helped during various phases of the project. Included are Gerald Dujsik, Director of Learning Resources, and his staff: Johnetta Coleman, Laurie Curtis, Sandra Engram, and Peter Weil. We also thank Dr. Angela Berry, Kerri Shoener, and Dr. Ashley Tracy, who provided clerical assistance within the work study program at the College. We are indebted to Bernie Roberts for clerical assistance as well. Sandra Brown, Gladys Christmas, Lillian Skinner, and Ella Wilson, the staff in the Academic Support Center at the College, helped type chapters for the second edition. Their efforts are also appreciated.

Our genuine thanks go to Dr. David Greenberg, Vice President for Academic Affairs and Dean, and Dr. Dennis Siemsen, Associate Dean for Patient Care and Chairman, Department of Clinical Education, at the Illinois College of Optometry, who provided their support of the project from beginning to end. Without their support this book would not have been possible.

We also thank Elizabeth Willingham and the staff at Silverchair Science + Communications for their hard work and assistance during production of the book. Last, but certainly not least, we thank the editors and staff at Butterworth-Heinemann, who provided their support and assistance throughout the project. Special thanks go to Barbara Murphy, Kathleen Higgins, and Karen Oberheim. We appreciate their professional manner, guidance, and dedication to the project affectionately known as "OD2."

D.K.R.
J.E.T.

2

Slit Lamp Biomicroscopy

Hurbert D. Riley and Richard E. Meetz

Slit lamp biomicroscopy has dynamically enhanced the diagnostic capabilities of all who master its use and should be a part of every patient's comprehensive eye examination. It affords the optometrist the means to perform a swift, yet careful examination of the anterior parts of the eye. In addition, with the aid of a tonometer, gonioscopy lens, Hruby lens, and other fundus lenses, many other procedures can easily be incorporated into the general examination.

The concept of using only a binocular microscope would be limited if it were not for its adjustable slit illumination system. The ability to focus a fine slit of light on a transparent tissue and see that tissue stereoscopically and in great detail under differing degrees of magnification is what makes slit lamp biomicroscopy truly unique. Although there have been some later modifications, for the most part, the slit lamp illumination system has remained unchanged from Gullstrand's 1911 design.

Diffuse illumination, perhaps better described as broad or wide beam illumination, deserves a discussion separate from other types of direct illumination. The terminology *diffuse illumination* has been carried over from earlier writings when slit lamps consisted of an illumination source and a biomicroscope that could be focused or unfocused independently.[1] Use of an unfocused, widely dispersed beam of light would diffusely illuminate the entire anterior part of the eye and its adnexa. The biomicroscope could then be focused anywhere from the eyelids to the iris or front of the lens. Modern slit lamp biomicroscopes are designed to have their light source and microscope coincident with one another and in focus in the same plane. Some current models do have interchangeable diffusing filters and are mainly used to photograph the anterior segment of the eye.

ILLUMINATION TYPES

Diffuse or Broad-Beam Direct Illumination

With diffuse or broad-beam direct illumination, a broad, unnarrowed beam of light is directed at the eye from an angle of approximately 45 degrees. The biomicroscope is positioned directly in front of the patient's eye and focused on the anterior lid or cornea under low to medium magnification (7–10×), permitting general inspection of anterior segment structures (Figure 2-1). Routine slit lamp examination generally includes an initial scanning of the lid margins, palpebral and bulbar conjunctiva, cornea, and iris with diffuse illumination. Abnormalities detected in this manner may then be evaluated further with additional illumination types and magnification.

Diffuse or broad-beam illumination is excellent for the measurement of tear breakup time (BUT) using a blue filter and fluorescein dye. In this technique, fluorescein dye is instilled into the conjunctival cul-de-sac and the patient then is asked to initially blink several times followed by cessation of blinking. Observation is then made for the first appearance of a dark spot or streak within the uniform, yellow-green tear film, indicating dry spot formation. The BUT is the time interval between the last blink and the development of a dry spot.[2] If the dark area always appears in the same location, this most likely is not a true tear breakup but rather "negative staining."[3] This occurs when there is an epithelial defect that does not allow the tear film to spread uniformly and consequently permits premature separation of the tear film layer. Examples of conditions that may cause epithelial irregularities include epithelial basement membrane dystrophy, microcystic edema, and wound healing sites containing rough edges.[4]

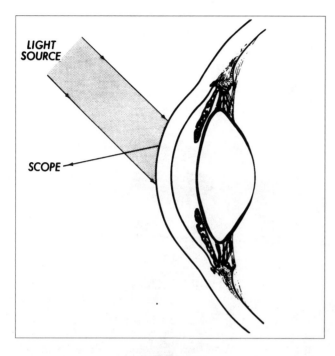

FIGURE 2-1
Broad-beam direct illumination. (Reprinted with permission from JB Eskridge, JP Schoessler, GE Lowther. A specific biomicroscopy procedure. J Am Optom Assoc 1973;44:400–9.)

Use of diffuse, broad-beam illumination with fluorescein dye is also helpful in assessing the extent of giant papillary conjunctivitis (GPC). The fluorescein dye collects around the papillae of the everted upper tarsal conjunctiva, making it somewhat easier to appreciate their elevations.[5]

Diffuse illumination is commonly used in contact lens fitting. With the aid of the blue filter and sodium fluorescein dye, the bearing, movement, and positioning of a contact lens as well as related corneal staining can be evaluated.

Diffuse illumination (using white light) may be used to demonstrate rose bengal staining of devitalized tissue in conditions such as keratoconjunctivitis sicca and herpes simplex.[6] A system for scoring rose bengal staining of the bulbar conjunctiva and cornea has been suggested by van Bijsterveld.[7] Here, the ocular surface is divided into three regions: the cornea, the nasal bulbar conjunctiva, and the temporal bulbar conjunctiva. Each of the three sectors is then graded separately (according to the level of staining) with a value ranging from 0 to 3. A maximum total score for the anterior ocular surface is therefore 9. Applying this grading system to the diagnosis of keratoconjunctivitis sicca, van Bijsterveld has found scores of 3.5 to be fairly sensitive.

Diffuse, broad-beam illumination is helpful when viewing the bulbar conjunctival and episcleral blood vessels. When differentiating between conjunctival and scleral (episcleral) injection, it can be appreciated that conjunctival vessels are more superficial and move with friction from the eyelid, whereas superficial and deep episcleral vessels show minimal to no movement with the overlying conjunctiva. Deeper episcleral injection may also give an overall purplish hue when viewed grossly. Abelson et al.[8] proposed a standardized grading system for judging different types of injection (Figure 2-2; Table 2-1).

Direct Focal Illumination

For direct focal illumination, the light beam may be a slit of variable length and width or a circular section. The bulbar and palpebral conjunctiva, cornea, limbus, aqueous, depth of the angles, iris, lens, and anterior vitreous

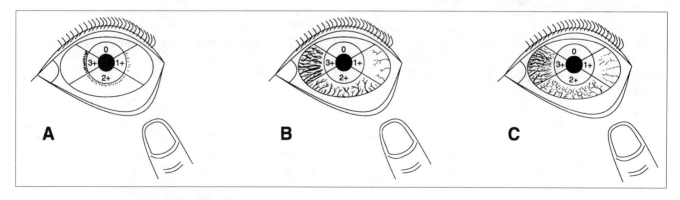

FIGURE 2-2
Grades of ocular surface injection. A. Ciliary injection. B. Episcleral injection. C. Conjunctival injection. (Adapted with permission from MB Abelson, IJ Udell, JH Weston. Standardization of ocular surface injection intensity. Ann Ophthalmol 1981;13:1225.)

TABLE 2-1
Grades of Ocular Surface Injection

Grade	Severity
0	White and quiet
½	Slight, usually normal
1 to 1+	Mild
2 to 2+	Moderate
3 to 3+	Severe

Source: Based in part on MB Abelson, IJ Udell, JH Weston. Standardization of ocular surface injection intensity. Ann Ophthalmol 1981;13:1225.

may be examined with this type of illumination. For observation of the anterior structures, the angle between the light source and biomicroscope can vary from 25 to 60 degrees. For deeper structures, such as the crystalline lens (especially if the pupil is not dilated), it is better if they are separated only 10–20 degrees.

Optic Section
With the optic section, it is possible to detect changes in corneal and conjunctival thickness, to assess the depth of foreign bodies, scars, and opacities, to estimate the anterior chamber depth, and to localize the depth of opacification within the crystalline lens (Figure 2-3). The biomicroscope should be directly in front of the patient's eye, the illumination source at about 45 degrees. The slit should be barely open (0.5–1.0 mm wide × 7–10 mm high) and focused on the cornea. Magnification should be low to medium (7–10×). With the patient fixating to stabilize any eye movement, the cornea may be scanned in a horizontal direction. To maintain a clear, distortion-free view, the illumination source must always be swung to a position on the same side of the cornea being examined.

With a clearly focused optic section slightly temporal to the center of the cornea, magnification increased to about 16×, and brightness increased, the following layers may be delineated (anterior to posterior): (1) Tear film—thin, bright line; (2) epithelium—thin, darker line; (3) Bowman's membrane—thin, brighter line; (4) stroma—wide, gray, granular zone; (5) endothelium—thin, bright line.

To attain an optic section of the crystalline lens, the angular separation between the illumination source and biomicroscope is reduced to approximately 10–20 degrees and the vertical slit height is reduced to approximate the diameter of the pupil. Initially the iris can be focused on and then the beam moved just inside the pupil margin. When the beam enters the pupil, the crystalline lens will appear sectioned. By focusing the biomicroscope's joystick with one hand and controlling the direction or angle of the light source with the other hand, the differ-

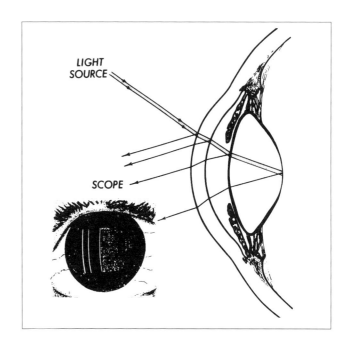

FIGURE 2-3
Optic section direct illumination. (Reprinted with permission from JB Eskridge, JP Schoessler, GE Lowther. A specific biomicroscopy procedure. J Am Optom Assoc 1973;44:400–9.)

ent layers of the lens can be brought into focus and the anatomic location of any opacities can be determined. Furthermore, the degree of nuclear opalescence and color can be evaluated and graded via the Lens Opacities Classification System II (LOCS II).[9] Different magnifications may be used, but medium to high magnifications give the best detail.

van Herick Technique of Angle Estimation
The van Herick method of angle estimation uses an optic section. This technique is used to judge the relationship between the peripheral iris and cornea and can be helpful in determining the likelihood of angle closure glaucoma. Magnification is set at 16–20× with the biomicroscope placed directly in front of the eye. The viewing angle between the biomicroscope and illumination source is 60 degrees. A long, thin, vertical optic section is formed perpendicular to the horizontal corneal limbal junction. The sharply focused beam is then positioned in the cornea as close to the limbus as possible while a clear full-thickness section of the cornea is maintained. Placing the optic section any farther inward into the cornea will result in a false angle estimation. With this arrangement, a darker zone can be seen between the posterior aspect of the corneal optic section and the location where the light beam hits the iris. The van Herick angular grade is derived from

FIGURE 2-4

van Herick method of angle estimation. A vertical optic section of the cornea is placed just inside the limbus. The distance between the posterior aspect of the optic section and the location where the light beam hits the iris (A) is then compared with the thickness of the corneal optic section (B). The smaller the distance "A," the more narrow the angle. (Courtesy of Daniel K. Roberts, O.D.)

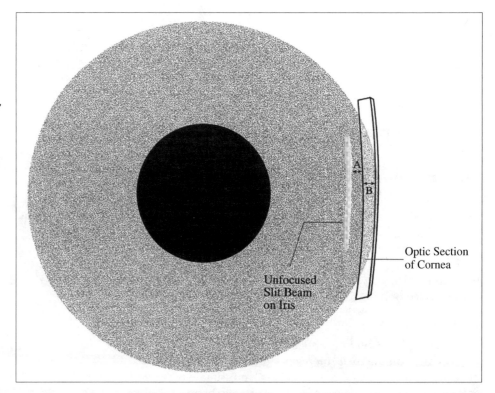

Optic Section of Cornea

Unfocused Slit Beam on Iris

the ratio or fractional component of the dark zone relative to the corneal thickness (Figure 2-4). When the dark zone is the same width as the cornea (ratio = 1:1), the angle is wide open and graded as 4. The angle is incapable of closure in this situation[10] (Table 2-2). Narrow angles of less than grade 2 should be examined gonioscopically. The superior and inferior angles may vary as much as two grades from the laterals.

Parallelepiped Beam

For a parallelepiped beam, the biomicroscope should be directly in front of the patient's eye and the illumination source at about 45 degrees. The angle may be varied, however. A parallelepiped beam is essentially an optic section, except the slit width is greater (2–4 mm versus 0.5–1.0 mm), providing a more three-dimensional view of the cornea (Figure 2-5) or crystalline lens. As with the optic section, when scanning the cornea, the illumination source should be directed from the side of the cornea that is being examined so that a clear, undistorted view is maintained.

During examination of the cornea, the parallelepiped beam is helpful in identifying a number of normal and abnormal entities; these included are tear debris, stromal and epithelial edema, corneal nerves, neovascularization, scarring and opacification, and pigmentation.

Evaluating hydrophilic soft contact lens wearers for corneal striae is useful for the detection of early corneal edema. Corneal striae appear in the posterior stroma or Descemet's membrane.[11] The best observation technique is the use of a parallelepiped beam, with a slit width of 2–3 mm and a height of 6–7 mm. The illumination source angle is 40–60 degrees and the biomicroscope is placed directly in front of the patient's eye. High magnification (16–20×) and high illumination are used. One should concentrate mainly against the backdrop of the pupil area. Striae may occasionally be mistaken for corneal nerves, which do appear in the posterior stroma. However, nerves will bifurcate or even trifurcate and may pass in a horizontal or oblique direction, whereas striae are almost always vertical without bifurcation.

The width of corneal striae varies from very thin and threadlike to a more thickened appearance. They increase in number with the degree of edema and are grayish white. Striae are completely reversible within a few hours after contact lens removal.[12] It should be pointed out that application of digital pressure on the globe through the lid will cause the striae lines to momentarily disappear.[11] Corneal striae first appear at 4–6% corneal thickening and increase in quantity to 9% thickening.[12] Severe corneal edema (>15%)[13] will cause larger foldlike lines to develop in

TABLE 2-2
van Herick Angle Estimation and Grading Method

Angle Grade	Risk of Closure	Cornea-to-Angle Ratio
4	Wide open angle; incapable of closure. Iris-to-cornea angular separation equals 35–45 degrees	Anterior chamber depth (shadow) is equal to or greater than the corneal thickness.
3	Moderately open angle; incapable of closure. Iris-to-cornea angular separation equals 20–35 degrees	Anterior chamber depth (shadow) is between ¼ and ½ the corneal thickness
2	Moderately narrow angle; closure possible. Iris-to-cornea angular separation equals 20 degrees	Anterior chamber depth (shadow) is equal to ¼ the corneal thickness
1	Extremely narrow angle; closure probable. Iris-to-cornea angular separation equals 10 degrees	Anterior chamber depth (shadow) is equal to less than ¼ the corneal thickness
0	Basically closed angle; closure is imminent. Iris-to-cornea angular separation equals 0 degrees	Anterior chamber depth (shadow) is only a very narrow slit or the peripheral iris is in contact with the posterior cornea

Source: Adapted with permission from HD Hoskins Jr, MA Kass. Becker-Shaffer's Diagnosis and Therapy of the Glaucomas (6th ed). St. Louis: Mosby, 1989.

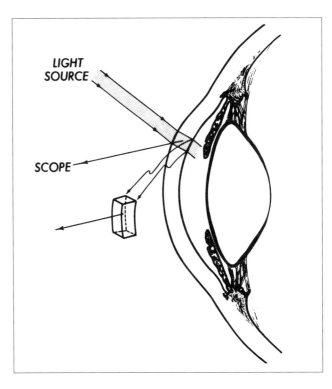

FIGURE 2-5
Parallelepiped direct illumination. (Reprinted with permission from JB Eskridge, JP Schoessler, GE Lowther. A specific biomicroscopy procedure. J Am Optom Assoc 1973;44:400–9.)

Descemet's membrane and the endothelial cell layer. These folds represent a more severe "buckling" of the posterior cornea. They are usually oriented vertically, although they may be seen to cross one another obliquely.[14] Few offices have a pachometer to gauge corneal thickness changes; hence, a grading system of corneal striae is helpful[15] (Table 2-3).

The use of a parallelepiped beam to investigate the anterior vitreous is helpful in the evaluation of possible existing retinal detachments or tears. With the pupil dilated, a parallelepiped beam is focused on the back surface of the crystalline lens. Using the joystick to control fine focusing, the slit lamp is advanced into the anterior vitreous. This area is carefully scanned for brown pigment granules, which when present with a retinal break constitute "Shafer's sign." Pigment in the anterior vitreous in the absence of previous intraocular surgery is almost pathognomonic of a retinal break.[16,17] It is believed that the pigment granules come from the retinal pigment epithelium when a tear or detachment occurs. To differ-

entiate between pigment granules and red blood cells, the red-free (green) filter is used. Red blood cells will absorb the red-free light and appear black, making them invisible. The pigment granules do not absorb the red-free light and remain visible.[3]

Conical Beam

Conical beam illumination is used to detect floating aqueous cells and flare via the Tyndall effect.[18] Examination of the anterior chamber for cells and flare must be per-

TABLE 2-3
Grades of Corneal Striae

Grade	Observed Number
0	None
1	<5
2	5–10
3	10–20
4	Too many to count

Source: Adapted with permission from DD Koch, MC de Sanabria, FB Scanning, JW Soper. Adverse Effects to Contact Lens Wear. Thorofare, NJ: Slack, 1984.

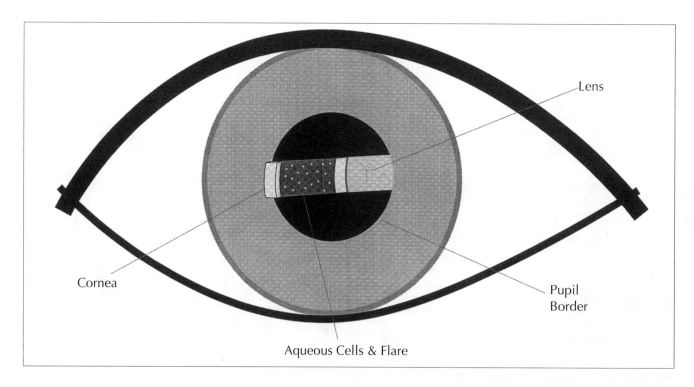

FIGURE 2-6

Evaluation of the anterior chamber for cells and flare. A small beam of light is directed (45–60 degrees temporally) into the pupil and focused between the cornea and anterior lens surface. Cells and flare are illuminated within the aqueous beam against the backdrop of the dark pupillary zone. (Courtesy of Daniel K. Roberts, O.D.)

formed before pupillary dilation or applanation tonometry. Dilation often results in an increase in the number of cells, and fluorescein dye used in applanation tonometry causes an increased appearance of flare.[19]

The traditional method of locating and grading cells and flare is to reduce the beam to a small circular pattern with the light source 45–60 degrees temporally and directed into the pupil.[20] The brightest illumination possible is ideal. The biomicroscope is positioned directly in front of the patient's eye, and high magnification should be used. The examiner must be allowed a period of time to dark adapt. The conical beam is focused between the cornea and the anterior lens surface, and observation is concentrated on the dark zone between the out-of-focus cornea and lens. This zone is normally optically empty and appears black. Flare (protein escaping from leaking capillaries) makes the normally optically empty zone appear gray or milky. Cells (white blood cells) will reflect the light and appear as white dots. Because the area of illumination is small, it is helpful to either oscillate the light source with the joystick from left to right while focused in the anterior chamber or to quickly focus from

the posterior cornea to the anterior lens surface while oscillating the light source.[20]

The following is a less traditional technique, but one that works well clinically and is superior when grading the severity of inflammation. A parallelepiped beam approximately 2 mm wide and 4 mm high is used[21] to focus on the iris. The focus is then pulled back into the anterior chamber. The examiner then views the zone between the out-of-focus cornea and the light passing through the pupil. The convection currents of the aqueous will move any protein or cells into this zone (Figure 2-6). A system for grading cells and flare is presented in Table 2-4.

Cells and flare in the anterior chamber are usually diagnostic of inflammation. However, if no cells or flare are seen but inflammation is suspected, using the "consensual pupillary reflex" test,[22] "Henkind" test,[21] or "consensual pain reflex" test, all one and the same, can be beneficial in confirming a diagnosis. The patient completely covers the eye in question so no light can enter. The patient then reports any discomfort when a bright slit lamp beam is shown into the "good eye." If pain is reported, there likely is a smol-

TABLE 2-4
Grades of Anterior Chamber Cells and Flare

Grade	Aqueous Cells	Grade	Flare
0	None	0	Optically empty when compared bilaterally
1	2–5 seen in 45 seconds to 1 minute	1	Faint: Hazy when compared bilaterally
2	5–10 at once	2	Moderate: Iris detail still clear
3	Scattered through-out beam, 20 or more	3	Marked: Iris detail becoming hazy
4	Dense cells in beam, more than can be counted	4	Dense haze: Obvious fibrin collecting on iris

Source: Adapted with permission from LJ Catania. Primary Care of the Anterior Segment (2nd ed). E. Norwalk, CT: Appleton & Lange, 1995.

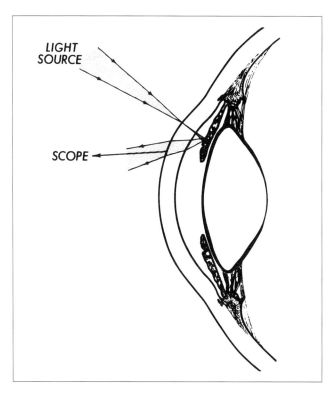

FIGURE 2-7
Retro-illumination of the cornea. (Reprinted with permission from JB Eskridge, JP Schoessler, GE Lowther. A specific biomicroscopy procedure. J Am Optom Assoc 1973;44:400-9.)

dering inflammation that has not completely resolved or one that is about to develop.[22]

Retro-Illumination or Transillumination

For retro-illumination and transillumination, the alignment and angular separation of the biomicroscope and the illumination source will vary. The light beam is reflected off a structure such as the iris, crystalline lens, or retina, and the biomicroscope is focused on a more anterior structure (Figure 2-7). To retro-illuminate or transilluminate the iris or crystalline lens, low to medium magnification (7–10×) and a slit beam 1–2 mm wide and 4–5 mm high is used. The biomicroscope and light source are placed in direct alignment with each other and positioned in front of the eye. The slit is focused just inside the edge of the pupil border and on the anterior surface of the lens. In the presence of iris atrophy or loss of pigment along the posterior layers, tissue defects may be visualized via the passage of light reflected from the retina through the compromised areas. The iris should be transilluminated in patients who have numerous pigment deposits on the endothelium.[3] Furthermore, retro-illumination of the crystalline lens is required for classification and grading of both cortical and posterior subcapsular cataracts via the LOCS II.[9]

The cornea is probably the most common structure viewed in retro-illumination. Keratic precipitates that appear white by direct illumination are dark under retro-illumination (Figure 2-8). This technique is valuable for observing deposits on the corneal endothelium and invading blood vessels. According to some authors,[23] this is the only way by which tiny rodlike fibrin flecks may be seen on the back of the cornea, which warn that a resolving anterior uveitis is still active.

Indirect Lateral or Proximal Illumination

For indirect lateral or proximal illumination, the biomicroscope is placed directly in front of the patient's eye with the illumination source at about 45 degrees. A parallelepiped beam is used and is sharply focused on a given structure such as the cornea. The dark area just lateral or proximal to the parallelepiped is the indirect or proximal zone of illumination and it is this area of the cornea that is surveyed through the biomicroscope. This type of illumination is commonly used for observation and detection of pathologic changes such as keratic precipitates on the endothelium (Figures 2-8 and 2-9), or microcystic edema and faint corneal infiltrates of the epithelium.

FIGURE 2-8
Keratic precipitates as seen with direct parallelepiped, indirect or proximal, and retro-illumination. (Modified with permission from JE Terry. Slit Lamp Biomicroscopy. In JE Terry [ed], Ocular Disease: Detection, Diagnosis and Treatment. Springfield, IL: Thomas, 1984;175.)

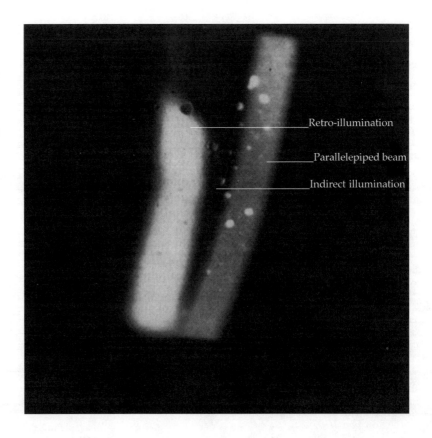

Retro-illumination

Parallelepiped beam

Indirect illumination

Sclerotic Scatter

For sclerotic scatter, the illumination source is positioned at 45 degrees, and a 2- to 3-mm wide beam is placed vertically at the corneal limbus. The biomicroscope is positioned directly in front of the patient's eye with magnification set at low to medium (7–10×) to allow the entire cornea to be observed. Because of the internal reflection of light throughout the cornea, visualization of a variety of corneal lesions is possible (Figure 2-10). For example, anterior or posterior corneal pigmentation may be highlighted, as well as scarring or other types of opacification.

The most common use of sclerotic scatter is for the detection of corneal edema secondary to wearing rigid contact lenses. Central corneal clouding (CCC)[24] is the term most often used to describe this condition. Although this is still occasionally observed, it does not occur as frequently with rigid gas permeable (RGP) lenses as with older polymethyl methacrylate (PMMA) lenses. Although CCC may be observed through the biomicroscope, it is best visualized with the naked eye. As with other types of illuminations, magnification that is too great often inhibits overall perspective. The central clouding is best seen against the dark background of the pupil with the examiner viewing from the opposite side. Central corneal clouding will appear as a gray haze against the dark pupil. The more significant the edema, the more well delineated this zone will be.

It is not uncommon to see CCC during the adaptation period in patients who are beginning to wear contact lenses.[25] If CCC continues beyond this period it must be regarded as a sign of a poor physical fit and changes in lens design are needed. Observation for CCC must be done immediately after contact lens removal, since epithelial edema resolves rapidly, usually within 15 minutes.[26,27] However, its effects may last longer (i.e., 26 hours may be needed before the corneal tissue is completely oxygenated).[28]

Edema secondary to hydrophilic soft contact lenses is different because the entire cornea is covered by the lens. The epithelium may take on a misty, nonlustrous appearance. As previously noted, striate lines develop as the corneal thickness increases; these are best detected using a parallelepiped beam and direct illumination.

Specular Reflection

Endothelial cells of the cornea are only visible using specular reflection, which is the most difficult illumination to

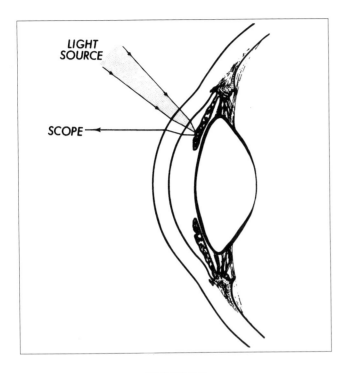

FIGURE 2-9
Indirect or proximal illumination of the iris. The examiner's gaze is directed just lateral to the focused light beam. (Reprinted with permission from JB Eskridge, JP Schoessler, GE Lowther. A specific biomicroscopy procedure. J Am Optom Assoc 1973;44: 400–9.)

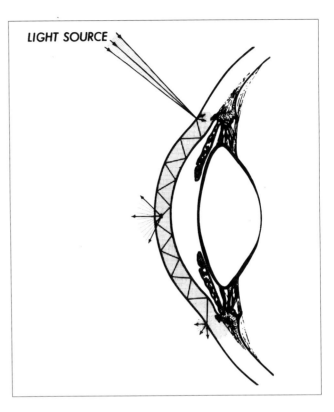

FIGURE 2-10
Sclerotic scatter illumination. (Reprinted with permission from JB Eskridge, JP Schoessler, GE Lowther. A specific biomicroscopy procedure. J Am Optom Assoc 1973;44:400–9.)

master. Prealigned illumination and microscopic systems, which focus in the same plane, are important for all types of illumination, but are most critical in accomplishing specular reflection (Figure 2-11).

Whenever the illumination system and the biomicroscope are at equal angles of incidence and reflection, both the front and back surfaces of the cornea will be seen. The basic requirements for specular reflection include a 60-degree angular separation between the illumination source and biomicroscope, high magnification, high illumination, and a parallelepiped beam of light. To set up for this illumination the biomicroscope is placed directly in front of the patient's eye and the illumination source at 60 degrees. With a parallelepiped beam focused at the corneal limbus, the beam of light is slowly advanced centrally across the cornea until a dazzling reflection of the filament is visualized. This reflection is only seen through one ocular of the slit lamp. Keeping the reflected light within the biomicroscope's field of view, the focus is then moved back toward the endothelial cells. There will be a point where two images of the filament are seen, one bright and the other ghostlike or

copper-yellow in color. If the biomicroscope is critically focused on the latter, a mosaic of hexagonal endothelial cells will be seen. It should be noted that even with 40× magnification the endothelial cells do not appear as large as most texts show. Both the front and back surfaces of the crystalline lens can also be viewed using specular reflection.

GENERAL EXAMINATION PROCEDURE

The table and slit lamp are adjusted for the patient. The patient is seated with the head positioned against the chin and forehead rests. Patient fixation should be directed at the fixation light, some part of the slit lamp, or just past the top of the examiner's shoulder or ear. To begin general examination of the eye, the illumination source is set at 35–45 degrees with the diaphragm wide open. The biomicroscope is positioned directly in front of the patient's eye, and a low magnification (10×) is initially used. The sequence followed is variable depending on individual

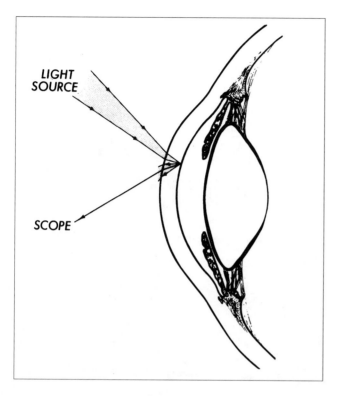

FIGURE 2-11
Specular reflection illumination of the cornea. (Reprinted with permission from JB Eskridge, JP Schoessler, GE Lowther. A specific biomicroscopy procedure. J Am Optom Assoc 1973;44: 400–9.)

preferences; however, routine examination should generally include the following:

1. The upper lid and lashes are scanned from the temporal to the nasal edge, then the lower lid is scanned from the nasal aspect back temporally.
2. The patient is instructed to look up. The lower lid is retracted and then the lower bulbar conjunctiva, palpebral conjunctiva, and cornea are scanned.
3. The patient is instructed to look down. The upper lid is retracted, and the upper bulbar conjunctiva and cornea are examined.
4. The patient is instructed to look to the extreme right while the nasal bulbar conjunctiva and sclera are scanned. Then the temporal bulbar conjunctiva and sclera are observed while the patient looks to the extreme left.
5. The biomicroscope is positioned directly in front of the eye, the illumination source is set at 60 degrees, the magnification and brightness are adjusted moderate to high, and the slit width is reduced to an optic

section. The temporal and nasal angles are then estimated using the van Herick technique.
6. The slit width is adjusted to a 2- to 3-mm wide parallelepiped beam, and the entire cornea and iris are scanned.
7. Using both a parallelepiped and optic section, the crystalline lens and anterior vitreous are examined.

The sequence is then repeated in a similar fashion on the opposite eye.

Fundus Examination

Without the use of additional lenses, examination with the slit lamp biomicroscope is limited to the anterior portions of the globe. With the aid of the Hruby lens and a variety of plus-powered condensing lenses, funduscopic and posterior vitreal examination is also routinely performed.

Hruby Lens

The Hruby lens is available in both a contact and noncontact version. The noncontact Hruby lens is a high powered, plano-concave, –55 D lens that is available for some slit lamp biomicroscopes as an attachment that can be rotated into the line of sight (Figure 2-12). The lens is aligned and focused by following a grooved track or rail, which is positioned directly in front of the eye. Use of the Hruby lens generally requires that the illumination source and biomicroscope be in direct alignment in the straight-ahead position. A dilated pupil is necessary.[29] The beam height and width should be set similar to a parallelepiped beam to minimize reflections.

With the Hruby lens examination, a posterior segment image is achieved by effectively neutralizing the optical power of the eye and extending the focus of the biomicroscope back to the retina. The view is erect but is subject to reflections and a restricted field of 5–8 degrees (just larger than one disk diameter). This, plus the need for precise patient fixation and cooperation, may make Hruby lens evaluation a difficult procedure for screening the posterior pole. Therefore, it is used primarily for evaluation of the macula and optic nerve head.[30] With the development of the double aspheric hand-held indirect lenses, routine use of the Hruby lens has been considerably reduced.

For a contact Hruby lens the biomicroscopy set-up is the same as for the noncontact Hruby lens except that a high-minus lens is placed in direct apposition to the cornea. Further discussion on examination with the contact Hruby lens is given in Chapter 6.

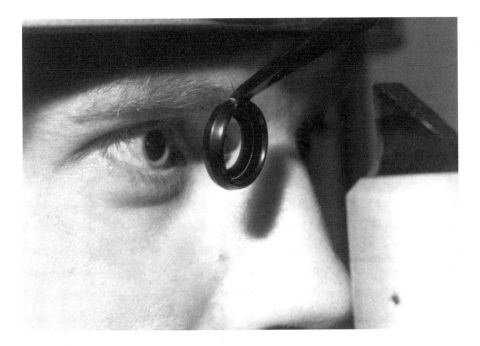

FIGURE 2-12
Example of a noncontact Hruby lens attached to a Zeiss slit lamp. (Courtesy of Daniel K. Roberts, O.D.)

Aspheric Biomicroscopy Indirect Fundus Lenses

Fundus examination with the aid of the biomicroscope and a strong convex lens was first described by El Bayadi[31] and later by Rotter.[32] Both techniques used a strong plano-convex lens in a preset mount affixed to the slit lamp.

In 1959, Rosen[33] discussed a technique using a spherical +55 D hand-held lens in combination with a slit lamp biomicroscope to examine the fundus. However, it never gained popularity. In 1982 Volk Optical developed and began to manufacture a double aspheric +60 D hand-held lens for binocular indirect ophthalmoscopy of newborn infants.[34] In 1985 Lundberg[35] described the use of a biconvex aspheric (conoid) +60 D hand-held lens used in conjunction with a slit lamp to examine the fundus. The acceptance of this lens influenced the development of other slit lamp biomicroscope indirect lenses, i.e., the +90 D and +78 D lenses. The indirect funduscopic lenses form an inverted and perverted virtual image in front of the condensing lens.

With these indirect fundus lenses magnification increases as the power of the lens decreases, similar to that found with condensing lenses used for binocular indirect ophthalmoscopy (see Chapter 4). The +60 D lens gives greater magnification and is preferred by some for examination of the optic nerve and macula. The +90 D lens produces less magnification and a larger field of view (30–40 degrees).[30] However, the slit lamp biomicroscope permits variable magnification, which helps neutralize this magnification problem. An increased field of view permits easier examination of the peripheral fundus. The +78 D lens obviously falls between the +60 D and +90 D lenses in terms of magnification and field of view. It is about the same as the +60 D lens and slightly larger than the +90 D lens (Figure 2-13). The +78 D lens is usually preferred by the novice, who finds it is easier to hold and manipulate. One report has given preference to the +78 D lens over the others in the study of the nerve fiber layer.[36]

One potential disadvantage of the +60 D lens is its longer focal length and the extent that the slit lamp must be pulled away from the patient to focus on the virtual image in front of the condensing lens. Some older model slit lamps may not have enough of a range to bring this image into clear focus. Even the +90 D lens when used on some patients can be challenging because of their forwardly positioned orbits.

All three lenses are available either clear or with a yellow tint. The yellow tint filters the wavelengths below 480 nm, enhancing patient comfort and acceptance. The yellow tint causes a slight color shift in the appearance of the retina, which could result in misinterpretation of optic nerve pallor and makes detection of macular edema more difficult.[30] In lieu of an actual tint to the condensing lens itself, other products are also available to provide yellow illumination. One example is a filter that attaches directly to the slit lamp; another is a removable yellow filter that can be attached to the condensing lens itself.

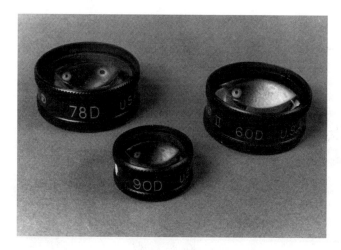

FIGURE 2-13
The Volk 60 D, 78 D, and 90 D aspheric biomicroscopy indirect fundus lenses.

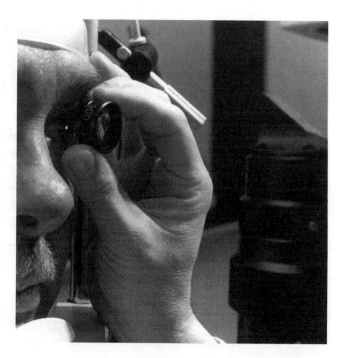

FIGURE 2-14
Examination with the 90 D hand-held indirect fundus lens.

A good working knowledge of binocular indirect ophthalmoscopy (BIO) is highly useful. The alignment and movement of the lens is much the same. With the pupil maximally dilated, the patient is seated at the slit lamp and instructed to look straight forward or past the top of the examiner's ear. With the magnification set on low, the slit lamp illumination source and the biomicroscope are adjusted so they are in direct alignment ("click" position). The slit is opened 3–4 mm wide and 6–7 mm high and focused within the center of the patient's pupil. The entire slit lamp is pulled back about an inch while keeping the slit beam aligned within the pupil. The lens is held between the thumb and index finger as the examiner observes from outside the biomicroscope (Figure 2-14). The lens is inserted into the path of light so the light comes to a focus in the center of the pupil. With the +78 D or +90 D lenses, this is 1.0–1.5 cm from the patient's eye. The index finger is placed against the patient's brow and the other three fingers are braced on the cheek or forehead rest. While viewing through the biomicroscope, the examiner adjusts the slit lamp forward or backward, focusing on the aerial image of the retina. Adjusting the lens toward or away from the eye will help to refine the focus and fill the entire lens with the image of the posterior segment. Slightly tilting or rotating the lens may help to move any reflections out of the line of sight. Once a retinal image is obtained, the optic nerve head is usually examined first. Then, the remainder of the posterior pole is scanned for any abnormalities (Figure 2-15).

Examination of the peripheral retina requires maximum dilation and is not done on a routine basis with biomicroscopic fundus lenses. It may be performed after exam-

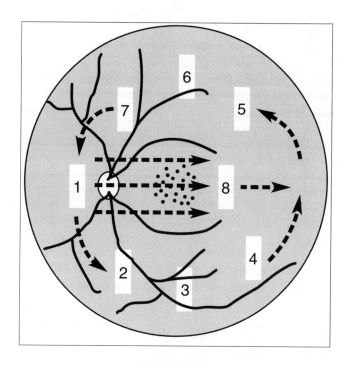

FIGURE 2-15
Suggested procedure for examining the posterior pole with a hand-held funduscopic lens.

ination with the binocular indirect ophthalmoscope, however, when a more magnified stereoscopic view is needed. As an example, to examine the superior peripheral retina the patient looks up as far as possible and the bottom of the lens is tilted slightly in toward the cheek. Because of inversion of the image, the most peripheral retina will be seen in the inferior part of the lens. When the superior-nasal or superior-temporal quadrants are to be examined, the patient's gaze is shifted in the appropriate direction, and the slit lamp may be slightly rotated to the right or left in the opposite direction. As the slit lamp is rotated, the condensing lens is likewise rotated around the same axis to maintain its perpendicular alignment. To examine the three o'clock or nine o'clock fundus regions, a greater lateral rotation of the slit lamp may be required. During inferior gazes, the examiner must retract the upper lid with the middle or ring finger while the lens is being held between the thumb and index fingers. Similar to binocular indirect ophthalmoscopy, to examine any particular region of the peripheral fundus the patient's gaze is shifted in the direction of the fundus area, the condensing lens is held perpendicular, and the slit lamp observation system is positioned opposite to the quadrant of interest.

REFERENCES

1. Schmidt TAF. History of the Development of the Slit-Lamp Microscope. In AG Haag Streit (ed), On Slit Lamp Microscopy: Theory and Practice. Liebefeld, Switzerland: Haag-Streit, 1975.
2. Lemp MA. Factors affecting tear film breakup in normal eyes. Arch Ophthalmol 1973;89:103–5.
3. Fingeret M, Casser L, Woodcome HT. Atlas of Primary Eyecare Procedures. Norwalk, CT: Appleton & Lange, 1990.
4. Lemp MA. Tear Deficiencies. In TD Duane (ed), Clinical Ophthalmology (Vol 4). Hagerstown: Harper & Row, 1980.
5. Allansmith MR, Korb DR, Greiner JV, et al. Giant papillary conjunctivitis in contact lens wearers. Am J Ophthalmol 1977;83:697–708.
6. Kanski JJ. Clinical Ophthalmology (2nd ed). Oxford: Butterworth-Heinemann, 1989.
7. van Bijsterveld OP. Diagnostic tests in the sicca syndrome. Arch Ophthalmol 1969;82:10–4.
8. Abelson MB, Udell IJ, Weston JH. Standardization of ocular surface injection intensity. Ann Ophthalmol 1981;13:1225.
9. Chylack LT Jr, Leske MC, McCarthy D, et al. Lens opacities classification system II (LOCS II). Arch Ophthalmol 1989;107:991–7.
10. van Herick W, Shaffer RN, Schwartz A. Estimation of width of angle of anterior chamber. Am J Ophthalmol 1969;68:626–9.
11. Sarver MD. Striate corneal lines among patients wearing hydrophilic contact lenses. Am J Optom Arch Am Acad Optom 1971;48:762–3.
12. Polse KA, Sarver MD, Harris MG. Corneal edema and vertical striae accompanying the wearing of hydrogel lenses. Am J Optom Arch Am Acad Optom 1975;52:185–91.
13. Klyce SD, Farris RL, Dabezies OHJ. Corneal Oxygenation in Contact Lens Wearers. In OHJ Dabezies (ed), Contact Lenses: The CLOA Guide to Basic Science and Clinical Practice (Vol 1). Orlando: Grune & Statton, 1986.
14. Holden BA. High Magnification Examination and Photography with the Slit Lamp. In RH Brandreth (ed), Clinical Slit Lamp Biomicroscopy. San Leandro: Balco, 1978.
15. Koch DD, de Sanabria MC, Scanning FB, Soper JW. Adverse Effects of Contact Lens Wear. Thorofare, NJ: Slack, 1984.
16. Hamilton AM, Taylor W. Significance of pigment granules in the vitreous. Br J Ophthalmol 1972;56:700–2.
17. Shafer DM. Controversial Aspects of the Management of Retinal Detachment. In CL Schepens, CDJ Regan (eds), Retina Foundation. Institute of Biological and Medical Sciences Monographs and Conferences (Vol. 3). Boston: Little, Brown, 1965.
18. Leitman M W, Gartner S, Henkind P. Manual for Eye Examination and Diagnosis. Oradell, NJ: Medical Economics, 1975.
19. Schlaegel TF Jr. Symptoms and Signs of Uveitis. In T Duane (ed), Clinical Ophthalmology (Vol 4). Philadelphia: Harper & Row, 1982.
20. Fingeret M, Potter JW. Uveitis. In JD Bartlett, SD Jaanus (eds), Clinical Ocular Pharmacology (2nd ed). Stoneham: Butterworth, 1989.
21. Catania LJ. Primary Care of the Anterior Segment (2nd ed). East Norwalk, CT: Appleton & Lange, 1995.
22. Au Y-K, Henkind P. Pain elicited by consensual pupillary reflex: A diagnostic test for acute iritis. Lancet 1981;2:1254–5.
23. Goar EL, Krieger AA, Kronfeld PC, et al. Slit Lamp Biomicroscopy: A Manual (2nd ed). Omaha: Douglas Printing, 1954.
24. Mandell RB, Polse KA. Corneal thickness changes accompanying central corneal clouding. Am J Optom Arch Am Acad Optom 1971;48:129–32.
25. Mandell RB, Polse KA. Corneal thickness changes as a contact lens fitting index—experimental results and a proposed model. Am J Optom Arch Am Acad Optom 1969;46:479–91.
26. Schoessler JP, Lowther GE. Slit lamp observations of corneal edema. Am J Optom Arch Am Acad Optom 1971;48:666–71.
27. Hill RM, Uniacke CA, Schoessler JP. Resolution of epithelial edema: Compared physiologically and histologically. Am J Optom Arch Am Acad Optom 1970;47:217–21.
28. Hill RM, Shoessler J. Epithelial edema: Respiratory characteristics of the lesion. Am J Optom Arch Am Acad Optom 1968;45:241–5.
29. Bock WC. Fundus contact lens and Hruby lens. J Am Ophthalmol Assoc 1977;48:1425–9.
30. Barker FM. Vitreoretinal biomicroscopy: A comparison of techniques. J Am Optom Assoc 1987;58:985–92.

31. El Bayadi G. New method of slit-lamp micro-ophthal-moscopy. Br J Ophthalmol 1953;37:625–8.

32. Rotter H. Technique of biomicroscopy of the posterior eye. Am J Ophthalmol 1956;42:409–15.

33. Rosen E. Biomicroscopic examination of the fundus with a +55D lens. Am J Ophthalmol 1959;48:782–7.

34. Jackson J, Fisher M. Evaluation of the posterior pole with a 90D lens and the slit-lamp biomicroscope. South J Optom 1987;5:80–3.

35. Lundberg C. Biomicroscopic examination of the ocular fundus with +60 diopter lens. Am J Ophthalmol 1985;99:490–1.

36. Litwak AB. Nerve fiber layer in glaucoma. Presented at the Section on Disease Symposium: Glaucoma 1990s Strategies for Diagnosis and Management. Annual American Academy of Optometry Meeting, Nashville, TN, 1990.

3

Tonometry

KENNETH J. MYERS AND JACK E. TERRY

SIGNIFICANCE OF INTRAOCULAR PRESSURE

Tonometers assess intraocular pressure (IOP) indirectly by measuring the force needed to alter corneal contour to a predetermined configuration. For the same force, higher IOPs allow less corneal deformation and lower IOPs allow more. Early tonometry used finger palpation, but highly accurate measurements can now be made using a variety of tonometers.[1]

Because elevated IOP is a major glaucoma risk factor, IOP measurement is essential.[2] However, except for very elevated IOPs from angle closure, an elevated IOP is only one risk factor (albeit a major one), not a diagnosis of glaucoma.[3-5] Eyes vary in their ability to withstand elevated IOP without the development of damage to the optic nerve head and visual field defects.[6] Most eyes with IOP over 21 mm Hg do not develop glaucoma.[7-9] A difference between eyes of 4–5 mm Hg indicates increased risk of glaucoma, as does a daily variation of over 10 mm Hg.[10] Whereas eyes with high IOP have a greater chance of an initial field defect, the correlation with further field changes is poor.[11] Patients with IOPs of over 30 mm Hg do have an increased risk factor of about 15× for developing field loss, and most practitioners today will begin treatment at this IOP level.[3] Thus, additional information is needed beyond an IOP measurement, and these include a careful history, age, race, visual fields status, disc and cup evaluation, gonioscopy findings, and nerve fiber layer evaluation.

Tonometry usually cannot be used to differentiate ocular hypertension from glaucoma or eyes that will stay stable from those that will develop visual field loss except when the IOP is very elevated. Repeat IOP measurements are often needed because some eyes have IOP spikes long enough to produce optic nerve damage. In spite of the uncertainty with which IOP readings must often be interpreted, IOP measurement remains a vital part of ocular assessment for all patients for which IOP can be determined.

Intraocular pressure is measured as the height, in millimeters of mercury (mm Hg), to which the mercury in a column would be raised were it connected to the eye's anterior chamber. The IOP level results from a balance between aqueous inflow and outflow rates. Aqueous is formed by the ciliary body processes and released into the posterior chamber. It then circulates between the iris and lens into the anterior chamber, where it next flows through the angle's trabecular meshwork and into Schlemm's canal. It then drains into the general venous circulation via the aqueous veins.

The distribution of IOPs in the nondiseased population of all ages is not gaussian (symmetrical) but skewed toward higher pressures with more instances of IOPs over 21 mm Hg than under 9 mm Hg. There is a further shift toward higher IOPs with age along with an increased incidence of glaucoma.[12] The average IOP of normal eyes is about 15.5 mm Hg, with the upper limit of normal somewhat arbitrarily set at 21 mm Hg (two standard deviations above average IOP) for the gaussian IOP distribution and at 24 mm Hg for the skewed (actual) IOP distribution[13,14] (Table 3-1). Daily IOP variations of 3–4 mm Hg are common among normal persons. The IOP is higher in many eyes in the morning. The IOP declines throughout the day, but there are wide variations, with some eyes showing a reverse cycle. Some open angle glaucoma patients have IOP spikes of 10 mm Hg or more and IOP may need to be measured at different times to detect these spikes. Some investigators attribute many cases of presumed "low tension glaucoma" to these spikes. The IOP difference between eyes is

TABLE 3-1
Intraocular Pressure (Normal Population Statistical Values)

	Two SD (97.5%)	Three SD (99.9%)
Gaussian	21 mm Hg	22 mm Hg
Skewed	24 mm Hg	30 mm Hg

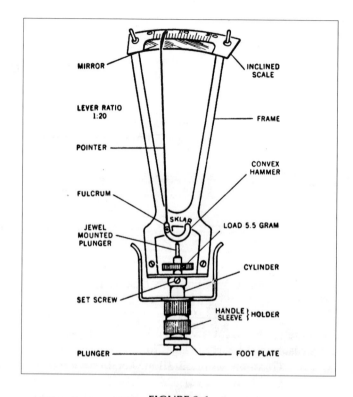

FIGURE 3-1
Diagram of the Sklar Jewel model Schiotz tonometer.
(Courtesy of Sklar Instruments, West Chester, PA.)

usually less than 5 mm Hg, and in most patients it is typically less than 3 mm Hg. Thus, IOP differences between eyes of 4–5 mm Hg or greater should be fully investigated, even if both are in the normal range.[15]

As with blood pressure, IOP can vary depending on an individual's posture. In addition, exercise provides a temporary reduction in IOP, as does ingestion of alcohol or marijuana.[16-18] Medications can alter IOP. For example, systemic beta-blockers can lower IOP, and topical steroids can elevate IOP in predisposed individuals ("steroid responders").[19,20] Hypertensive patients treated with beta-blockers can therefore show normal IOPs and enlarged cups because of previously high IOP, whereas patients recently treated with steroids can show elevated IOPs but normal cups.

Keeping the preceding information about intraocular pressure in mind, a single IOP reading can be misleading, and it is impossible to establish a clear cutoff point for normal IOPs such as 21 mm Hg. It should be remembered that the frequency of demonstrable visual field loss in eyes with IOPs over 21 mm Hg varies from only 0.4% to 8.0% after 4–14 years of follow-up.[21]

MEASUREMENT OF IOP

Indentation Tonometry

Indentation, or impression, tonometers rest a small plunger of known weight on the cornea and measure the plunger's depth of impression as an indication of IOP. Although there are several varieties of these tonometers, only the Schiotz and pneumatic types will be discussed.

Schiotz Tonometry

The Schiotz tonometer is designed with a calibrated weight on an indenting plunger, which is placed on the cornea. Depth of impression is shown by a needle pointer (Figure 3-1). Different weights can be used (5.5, 7.5, 10.5, and 15.0 g) to cover large IOP ranges. Scale readings are then converted to IOP (Figure 3-2, Table 3-2) using furnished tables.

The Schiotz tonometer must be kept clean between uses to prevent its plunger from sticking. For sterilization, the footplate or entire tonometer can be soaked in alcohol for 5–10 minutes before use, but care must be taken to fully flush and remove this or any other sterilizing fluids, because solutions may adhere to tonometer parts and later drain onto the cornea during measurement. As recommended by the Centers for Disease Control (CDC), acceptable sterilizing solutions are 70% ethanol or isopropanol, 3% hydrogen peroxide, or a 1:10 dilution of common household bleach.[22,23] The instrument should be rinsed thoroughly with tap water and dried before use.

To obtain a measurement with the Schiotz tonometer, the cornea is anesthetized and the patient is placed in a supine position with the eyes fixed on a ceiling target or the patient's thumb held overhead. It is best to start with the lightest weight (5.5 g) to minimize aqueous displacement from within the eye. Because intraocular pressures are typically under 20 mm Hg, a midrange scale reading will usually result with this weight. Heavier weights can be used if the initial scale

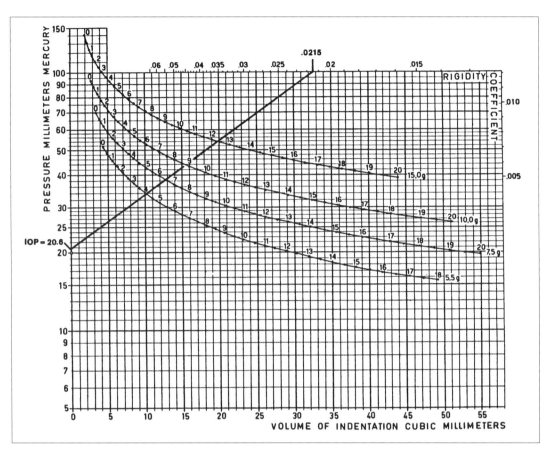

FIGURE 3-2

Nomograms are available to convert Schiotz tonometer scale readings into millimeters of mercury. For example, using the 5.5-g weight, a scale reading of 4.0, and the standard ocular rigidity of 0.0215, the resulting intraocular pressure is 20.6 mm Hg. (Courtesy of Ostertag Optical Service, St. Louis, MO.)

reading is very low (indicative of a high IOP). The Schiotz tonometer is gently lowered onto the central cornea and, once the footplate makes contact, the instrument handle is allowed to "float" (Figure 3-3) without pressure being applied either upward or downward. After stabilization, the reading is taken while the needle pointer is aligned with its mirror reflection (to eliminate parallax). The measurement is recorded as a fraction with the scale reading as the numerator and the accessory weight as the denominator. This is then converted to millimeters of mercury with the aid of the conversion chart (e.g., 4/5.5 = 20.6 mm Hg).

Although not the standard for general office IOP measurement today, the Schiotz tonometer is useful when a Goldmann or other applanation tonometer is unavailable or when the presence of an irregular corneal surface precludes the use of other devices.

Common sources of error when using the Schiotz tonometer include poor calibration, improper footplate application, and lid squeezing. Like all indentation tonometers, Schiotz readings are influenced by "ocular rigidity," since as indentation proceeds, corneal forces related to tissue tension develop that oppose further surface distortion. This "ocular rigidity" varies from eye to eye and also increases with age. As another potential source of error, a large volume of aqueous may be displaced during Schiotz indentation tonometry, thereby producing falsely lower IOPs upon remeasurement. This is in contrast to the minimal aqueous displacement that occurs with applanation tonometry.

Pneumatic Tonometry

A pneumatic indentation tonometer or pneumatonograph (PTG) measures IOP by creating an equilibrium

TABLE 3-2
Calibration Scale for Schiotz Tonometers

Scale Reading	Pressure (mm Hg) for Various Loads			
	5.5 g	7.5 g	10.0 g	15.0 g
2.0	29.0	42.1	59.1	94.3
2.5	26.6	38.8	54.7	88.0
3.0	24.4	35.8	50.6	81.8
3.5	22.4	33.0	46.9	76.2
4.0	20.6	30.4	43.4	71.0
4.5	18.9	28.0	40.2	66.2
5.0	17.3	25.8	37.2	61.8
5.5	15.9	23.8	34.4	57.6
6.0	14.6	21.9	31.8	53.6
6.5	13.4	20.1	29.4	49.9
7.0	12.2	18.5	27.2	46.5
7.5	11.2	17.0	25.1	43.2
8.0	10.2	15.6	23.1	40.2
8.5	9.4	14.3	21.3	38.1
9.0	8.5	13.1	19.6	34.6
9.5	7.8	12.0	18.0	32.0
10.0	7.1	10.9	16.5	29.6
10.5	6.5	10.0	15.1	27.4
11.0	5.9	9.0	13.8	25.3
11.5	5.3	8.3	12.6	23.3
12.0	4.9	7.5	11.5	21.4
12.5	4.4	6.8	10.5	19.7
13.0	4.0	6.2	9.5	18.1

Source: Reprinted with permission of the American Academy of Ophthalmology, "Tonometer Calibration. An Attempt to Remove Discrepancies Found in the 1954 Calibration Scale for Schiotz Tonometer," Transactions of the American Academy of Ophthalmology and Otolaryngology, San Francisco, 1957;61:108–23.

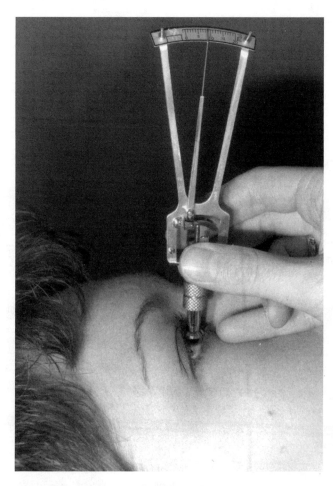

FIGURE 3-3
Shiotz tonometry. As the footplate of the tonometer is allowed to contact the cornea, the handle is lowered to a midway position. The examiner then notes the position of the needle on the scale. (Courtesy of Daniel K. Roberts, O.D.)

between the forces acting on a probe's thin membrane (i.e., instrument gas pressure on one side and IOP on the other side). The PTG's probe consists of a hollow plunger that slides on a porous sleeve through whose walls Freon 12 gas flows. The gas cushions and propels the plunger until its flat tip, covered with a silicone rubber (Silastic) membrane, contacts the cornea. On contact, gas flow is impeded, causing the tip to be propelled with greater force, thus commencing applanation. At first, the tip's membrane "seals" onto the cornea, and increasing gas pressure causes further applanation. With further pressure, this "seal" is reduced and some gas escapes until equilibrium is reached. At this point IOP is recorded.[21]

The PTG can operate in most positions, although readings do vary.[24] It has been found sufficiently accurate for eyes with deformed or edematous central corneas when the plunger is applied to the juxtalimbal area. For this

purpose, Breitfeller and Krohn[25] have calculated the following correction factors: For sitting patients, subtract 1 mm Hg when measurement is taken at the corneal apex and subtract 2 mm Hg for limbal measurement; for supine patients, subtract 3 mm Hg (apex or limbal reading).

Applanation Tonometry

Applanation tonometers press a small, flat probe onto the corneal apex and measure the area flattened by a known, fixed force (Maklalov Tonomat) or the force required to flatten a fixed area (Goldmann and noncontact tonometers). The errors that occur with indentation tonometry because of "ocular rigidity" are not as significant, since far less aqueous is displaced because of the small area applanated. Applanation tonometers are accurate and have gained widespread acceptance.

Goldmann Tonometer

The Goldmann tonometer is widely used and measures the force required to applanate a corneal area 3.06 mm in diameter. The device is usually mounted on a slit lamp, but hand-held versions are available for nursing home, hospital, and field use, and for litter or wheelchair patients. Its flat, plastic applanating probe (about 7 mm in diameter) contains a split prism mounted on a spring-loaded arm, the tension of which is adjusted by a drum wheel calibrated to read IOP values in millimeters of mercury (scale reading multiplied by 10). The applanation diameter of 3.06 mm was chosen to balance tear film tension and corneal bending forces and to produce a convenient 10-to-1 ratio between IOP in millimeters of mercury and applanating force in grams. The tear meniscus around the flattened corneal apex defines the area of applanation and is visualized using fluorescein dye and a blue light.[26]

The probe must be sterilized between patients (or eyes when ocular infection is suspected). The only methods approved by the CDC are to immerse the probe in 70% ethanol or isopropanol, 3% hydrogen peroxide, or a 1:10 bleach solution, the same solutions approved for use on the Schiotz tonometer.[22,23] The probe must be soaked for at least 5–10 minutes. It should be noted that alcohol dissolves the cement holding the biprism in place and also degrades the optics by crazing the biprism's surface. Of the three CDC methods, 3% hydrogen peroxide produces the least tip damage.[27] Many practitioners either immerse the probe in the sterilizer solution or suspend the probe tip in a solution held in a small cup. Tips are stored in these cups between use and then flushed with sterile saline and blotted dry before use. A good practice is to have two tips so that one tip may be soaking while the other is in use.

To perform Goldmann tonometry the cornea is anesthetized and fluorescein dye instilled into the conjunctival cul-de-sac. It is common practice to use a combination solution for this purpose.[28] With the Goldmann tonometer rotated into position, the blue slit lamp filter is clicked into place and the instrument's illumination aperture is fully opened. The illumination arm is rotated outward to about 60 degrees so that the probe tip is fully illuminated. Eyepiece magnification should be low and the tonometer's drum wheel scale set at 1 g of force (10 mm Hg) so the probe arm is flexed forward. The patient should keep his or her forehead against the headrest with both eyes fully open. Because of the blink response, some examiners routinely hold the lids using care not to press on the globe and falsely elevate the IOP. To reduce patient apprehension, the probe can be

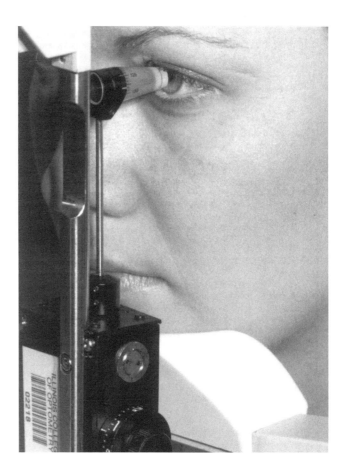

FIGURE 3-4
Measurement of IOP with the Goldmann applanation tonometer. The drum scale indicates 13 mm Hg. (Courtesy of Daniel K. Roberts, O.D.)

kept well inferior and temporal to the line of sight and only shifted in front of the corneal apex once it is very close. This also helps avoid touching the upper lashes on approach and inducing a blink. Once close to the corneal apex, the probe tip is moved into contact with the ocular surface (Figure 3-4). The examiner should look for a faint limbal glow as well as flexure of the probe arm as this occurs. Further inward joystick movement should not be made at this point or the slack in the probe's area will be exceeded, causing a distorted mire pattern. The mires are then viewed through the slit lamp oculars as the joystick is adjusted to center the blue-green semicircles. The drum wheel is adjusted until the inner edges of the semicircles just touch (Figure 3-5). The cardiac pulse of some patients will produce pulsating semicircles, and the average IOP can be taken by adjusting the drum wheel for equal amounts of overlap and underlap during these cardiac pulsations.

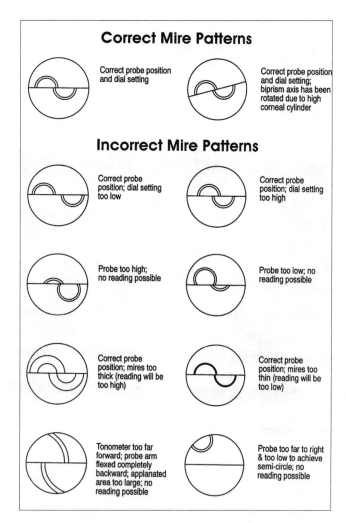

FIGURE 3-5

Normal and abnormal configurations of the fluorescein mires with Goldmann applanation tonometry.

Normally, the semicircles should be perfectly shaped. If not, inaccurate readings may result. Fluorescein mires that are too thick can cause overestimation of IOP and mires that are too thin can result in underestimation. For this reason, it is important to instill an appropriate amount of fluorescein dye into the eye before measurement.

It should be noted that the probe arm sleeve, which holds the tonometer tip, has one white and one red line along its outer surface. In addition, the probe has degree markings from 0 to 180. With the probe inserted into the sleeve, the white line should be aligned with the 180-degree sleeve marking so that the semicircles are vertically oriented. For fairly spherical corneas, measurements may be taken with the semicircles in any

alignment, but if corneal astigmatism exceeds 3 diopters, measurements should be taken at a meridian 43 degrees from that of lowest power. The white and red lines are exactly 43 degrees apart (see Figure 3-4), so for a highly astigmatic cornea, the red line should be aligned with the scale marking corresponding to the lowest power meridian. An example is "K" readings: 42.00 @ 121 and 45.75 @ 031. Align the 121-degree marking on the probe with the red line on the sleeve.

Goldmann tonometers are considered highly accurate and are used as a standard to evaluate new tonometers. As Grolman has shown, however, there is variability in readings obtained with a Goldmann tonometer even when the examiner repeats readings on the same eye with the same Goldmann tonometer.[29] The standard deviation (error) of the difference of these paired, same-eye measurements can range from about 1 mm Hg for a single examiner and Goldmann instrument to 3 or 4 mm Hg when different skilled examiners use different, certified Goldmann tonometers on the same eye. This intra- and inter-instrument Goldmann variability is sometimes overlooked when a new tonometer is compared with a Goldmann, where all "errors" in paired readings are attributed to the tested tonometer and not the Goldmann. This may therefore under estimate the accuracy of the tested tonometer.

Hand-Held Goldmann Tonometry

Several hand-held, battery-powered Goldmann tonometers are available for use on wheelchair or litter patients or at non-office locations. These operate on the same principles; however, their measurement techniques depend on each instrument's design. The examiner views a magnified mire pattern through a window opposite the probe, which is illuminated from below (Figure 3-6). Applanation force is adjusted by a circular dial from which IOP is read. This instrument's probe is counterbalanced, allowing it to be used on supine or reclining patients.

Noncontact Tonometry

The noncontact tonometer (NCT) was introduced in 1972 by the American Optical Co.[30] A second-generation version (NCT II) with essentially the same features has been followed by a new version (XPERT NCT) that uses a video monitor to align the instrument with the cornea and has a less forceful and quieter air puff (Figure 3-7). All three versions have been widely accepted and used throughout the world. Topcon has also developed a noncontact tonometer (CT-20), which is essentially identical in function to the XPERT NCT. Studies have found these tonometers to be accurate,

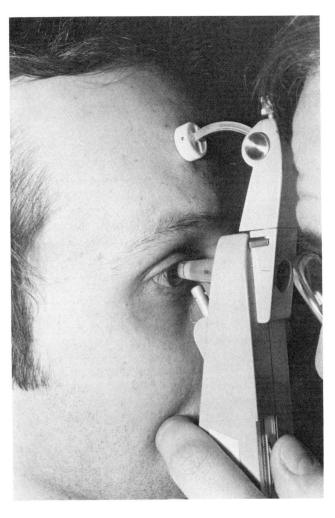

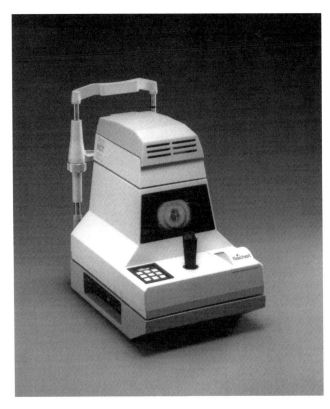

FIGURE 3-7

The XPERT NCT uses a video monitor to align the instrument with the cornea. (Photo courtesy of Reichert Ophthalmic Instruments, Buffalo, NY.)

FIGURE 3-6

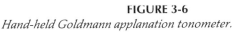

Hand-held Goldmann applanation tonometer.

safe, convenient, and easily operated by support personnel because subjective judgment is not required.[31–37] All noncontact tonometers use a stream of air whose pressure increases with time to progressively applanate a small circular area of the corneal apex. The degree of applanation is monitored by an infrared beam reflected from the corneal apex into a photocell whose output reaches a peak at applanation. At this peak signal the air puff pressure is measured and correlated with IOP in millimeters of mercury via internal logic and then displayed. Successive measurements can be made and then printed along with an average reading.

Noncontact tonometry is ideal for rapid and accurate IOP measurement of large numbers of patients as well as for regular office use. Many studies have validated the accuracy of the NCT, NCT II, and XPERT NCT, but, because these instruments take only milliseconds

to measure IOP, there may be slight variation from reading to reading on the same eye as a result of actual IOP changes produced by the ocular pulse. The average of three noncontact IOP readings has been found to compare closely with mid-pulse (average) measurements with a Goldmann device.

Highly irregular or edematous corneas may not be measurable with noncontact tonometers under usual circumstances; however, fairly accurate IOP readings may be obtained by placing a thin (<0.15 mm), soft contact lens on the cornea before measurement. Such a thin, soft contact lens usually only elevates the IOP reading by 1–2 mm Hg, so that when IOP measurement is critical to treatment decisions, such a technique can be useful.

Patient apprehension can occasionally cause elevated readings during noncontact tonometry because the patient squeezes the lids tightly together just before measurement. This effect can often be reduced by demonstrating the air puff on the patient's closed eyelid to show its mild pressure. Because the eye is not mechanically contacted by a probe during noncontact tonometry, there are no concerns regarding sterilization and risk of infection.

The Pulsair noncontact tonometer (Keeler Instruments, Broomall, PA) has an air-emitting probe that is attached by a cord so it may be transported to a patient, leaving the main unit at some distance. Brencher et al.[38] compared the Pulsair, XPERT NCT, and Topcon CT-10 and found the results with the Pulsair differed more from Goldmann readings than the results with the other two tonometers. Armstrong[39] found some high variability among Pulsair readings on the same eye and a slight tendency to overestimate low IOPs. In addition, there was a greater tendency to underestimate higher IOPs compared with Goldmann readings. Pearce et al.[40] reported that measurements with a second-generation instrument (Pulsair 2000) deviate less from Goldmann measurements than those of the first version.

Mackay-Marg Tonometer

The Mackay-Marg tonometer is used less frequently today although some corneal specialists still find it of use for IOP measurement of very scarred, edematous, or irregular corneas not well measured by other tonometer types.[41] It uses a small, central spring-loaded sensor set within a metal guard that is displaced when the cornea is contacted by the instrument's probe. This displacement is then correlated with IOP. Whereas earlier versions of this instrument required interpretation of a graph for determination of IOP, newer models calculate readings internally and display them digitally.

Tono-Pen Tonometer

The Tono-Pen (Mentor Ophthalmics, Norwell, MA) is a small, battery-powered, hand-held portable tonometer using the Mackay-Marg principle. On contact with the cornea the device emits a beep when an acceptable reading is obtained and displays the IOP in digital form. Additional readings can be taken, stored, and then displayed as an average and percentage of variability. A disposable latex cover on the tip can be changed after each patient (Figure 3-8).

The Tono-Pen's chief advantage is portability, objective measurement, and patient acceptance. However, some studies have shown it must be carefully used, since inaccurate readings result from poor technique. Farrar et al.[42] concluded the Tono-Pen was not accurate enough to obtain diurnal IOP curves reliably, and others have found statistically significant differences from Goldmann readings. Holec-Iwasko et al.[43] found the

device can give falsely elevated readings after argon laser trabeculoplasty because of residual ocular methylcellulose and concluded that the substance must be irrigated from the eye before IOP measurement. Armstrong compared the Tono-Pen with the Goldmann tonometer and found it tended to overestimate low and normal IOPs. Whereas mean differences were less than 1 mm Hg, the variability was higher, with a standard deviation of paired differences of 3 mm Hg. Of the 188 eyes he studied, Armstrong[40] found 30% had Tono-Pen readings differing by more than 3 mm Hg from Goldmann results, and 7% differed by more than 5 mm Hg. Kooner et al.[44] reported that the Tono-Pen systematically underestimated IOPs in the 16–30 mm Hg range compared with Goldmann readings.

TONOMETER STANDARDIZATION AND COMPARISON

Variations in IOP readings frequently result from artifactual influences such as aqueous massage (displacement), abnormal ocular rigidity, and corneal irregularity. In addition, calibration error can affect IOP measurements. Different tonometers can yield different readings on the same eye, but if properly calibrated and applied, these differences should be small.

Several studies have found that mean IOPs determined with the Goldmann and Schiotz tonometers are essentially the same. However, individual variations between them can be significant, leading Bengtsson[45] to conclude the Schiotz tonometer often fails to detect moderately increased IOPs detected with Goldmann tonometry. Other studies have shown the NCT, NCT II, and XPERT NCT devices to be highly accurate and essentially equal to the Goldmann instrument. Most tonometer studies use the Goldmann as the standard and attribute differences in readings to be an error of the test tonometer, not the Goldmann. But a calibrated Goldmann tonometer, used by a trained and skilled operator will, itself, produce a variety of readings on the same eye as summarized by Grolman, who reviewed various Goldmann repeatability studies.[29-46]

Whereas a Goldmann reading is rarely doubted, that reading is still an indirect assessment of IOP and subject to many influences. And unlike noncontact tonometry, Goldmann results are critically dependent on operator skills. As Grolman pointed out, the most intimately related index of a tonometer's accuracy when compared with the Goldmann is its standard

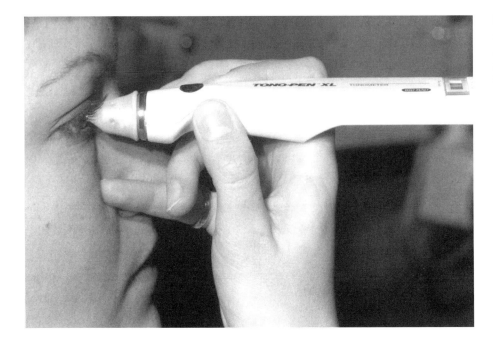

FIGURE 3-8
Measurement of IOP with the Tono-Pen XL Tonometer. (Courtesy of Daniel K. Roberts, O.D.)

deviation of matched pair differences (S_d) between its readings and those of the Goldmann. S_d measures the variability resulting from patient physiology, the two instruments, their operators, IOP changes between matched pairs of readings, and the effect of the first measurement upon the second.

Grolman's analysis disclosed that the S_d of the Goldmann tonometer is largely influenced by the protocol of the repeatability study used.[29] The literature shows a range extending from S_d = 0.9 mm Hg for a skilled operator immediately remeasuring the same eye with the same Goldmann, to S_d = 3.0 mm Hg for two skilled operators using two different but certified Goldmanns, with brief intervals between measurements on the same eyes. Thus a tonometer that, when tested against a Goldmann tonometer, gives an S_d equal to that for a Goldmann-versus-Goldmann test using the same protocol is essentially identical in performance to the Goldmann. And since a Goldmann itself has an S_d = 0.9 mm Hg for immediate remeasures, no new tonometer will have a lower S_d even if identical to the Goldmann and may, depending upon the test protocol, have an S_d of 3.0 mm Hg even if identical to the Goldmann. Therefore, the fact that new tonometers do not exactly agree with Goldmann results must be viewed relative to the Grolman analysis of Goldmann-versus-Goldmann repeatability studies.

TONOMETER STERILIZATION

Because the human immunodeficiency virus (HIV) has been isolated from the tears and conjunctival cells of AIDS patients, special care must be taken to sterilize tonometers that contact the eye. Although the spread of the AIDS virus by tonometry has not been documented, the CDC has recommended specific guidelines for sterilization.[22,23] The once-common practice of swabbing the Goldmann probe with alcohol is not CDC approved. Lingel and Coffey[27] have reviewed the effects of the three CDC-approved tonometer sterilization methods on the optics and clarity of the Goldmann biprism. With these three methods, the probe is initially wiped clean and then soaked in 70% ethanol or isopropanol, a 1:10 dilution of common household bleach, or 3% hydrogen peroxide for a minimum of 5–10 minutes. It was found that the alcohol solutions can dissolve the biprism cement and therefore are not ideal. Hydrogen peroxide produced the least damage to the biprism optics and image clarity. Some practitioners now use a small plastic cup to hold the sterilization fluid; the cover of the cup has holes into which the probes are placed to suspend just their tips in the fluid. This allows the tips to be kept in sterilizing solution at all times and reduces the slight swelling found when probes are totally immersed in the various fluids. All of the CDC-approved sterilization solutions must be flushed away with sterile saline and the probe patted dry with sterile cotton before use.

TONOGRAPHY

Tonography is a method whereby the eye's resistance to outflow is estimated by tracking IOP as it returns to normal levels after being mechanically elevated by a weighted tonometer. After a set time (usually 4 minutes) the IOP is remeasured and an estimate of outflow facility is made. A number of studies have assessed the value of tonography.[47,48] Unfortunately, it measures an ophthalmic variable related only indirectly to glaucoma (i.e., facility of outflow) and it evaluates only one of the physical signs of glaucoma, elevated IOP. Furthermore, nonglaucomatous normal subjects reveal wide variations in outflow facility. Podos and Becker[49] estimated that at least 85% of patients with abnormalities of aqueous outflow as shown by tonography will not demonstrate glaucoma damage within 5 or more years. They indicated that tonography is only an adjunct to other examination techniques. It has become accepted that tonography alone cannot differentiate glaucoma from ocular hypertension and it is not currently used on a routine clinical basis.[50]

REFERENCES

1. Carter JH. Tonometry in optometric practice—the current status. J Am Optom Assoc 1977;48:1391–400.
2. Armaly MF, Krueger DE, Maunder LR, et al. Biostatistical analysis of the collaborative glaucoma study. I. Summary report of the risk factors for glaucomatous visual-field defects. Arch Ophthalmol 1980;98:2163–71.
3. Sommer A. Intraocular pressure and glaucoma. Am J Ophthalmol 1989;107:186–8.
4. Armaly MF. Lessons to be learned from the collaborative glaucoma study. Surv Ophthalmol 1980;25:139–44.
5. Sponsel WE. Tonometry in question: Can visual screening tests play a more decisive role in glaucoma diagnosis and management? Surv Ophthalmol 1989;33(Supp):291–300.
6. Leske MC, Rosenthal J. Epidemiologic aspects of open-angle glaucoma. Am J Epidemiol 1979;109:250–72.
7. Perkins ES. The Bedford glaucoma survey. I. Long-term follow-up of borderline cases. Br J Ophthalmol 1973;57:179–85.
8. Bengtsson B. The prevalence of glaucoma. Br J Ophthalmol 1981;65:46–9.
9. Hollows FC, Graham PA. Intra-ocular pressure, glaucoma, and glaucoma suspects in a defined population. Br J Ophthalmol 1966;50:570–86.
10. Davanger M. The difference in ocular pressure in the two eyes of the same person. In individuals with healthy eyes and in patients with glaucoma simplex. Acta Ophthalmol 1965;43:299–313.
11. Vogel R, Crick RP, Newson RB, et al. Association between intraocular pressure and loss of visual field in chronic simple glaucoma. Br J Ophthalmol 1990;74:3–6.
12. National Society to Prevent Blindness. Glaucoma Detection and Treatment. Proceedings of the First National Glaucoma Conference, Tarpon Springs, Florida, January 1980.
13. Kolker AE, Hetherington J. Becker-Shaffer's Diagnosis and Therapy of the Glaucomas. St. Louis: Mosby, 1976.
14. Moses RA. Adler's Physiology of the Eye (6th ed). St. Louis: Mosby, 1975.
15. Hollows FC, Graham PA. A Critical Review of Methods of Detecting Glaucoma. In LB Hurt (ed), Glaucoma. London: Williams & Wilkins, 1966:24–44.
16. Anderson DR, Grant WM. The influences of position of intraocular pressure. Invest Ophthalmol 1973;12:204–12.
17. Armaly MF. Glaucoma. Arch Ophthalmol 1975; 93:146–62.
18. Marcus DF, Krupin T, Podos SM, Becker B. The effect of exercise on intraocular pressure. I. Human beings. Invest Ophthalmol 1970;9:749–52.
19. Bulpitt CJ, Hodes C, Everitt MG. Intraocular pressure and systemic blood pressure in the elderly. Br J Ophthalmol 1975;59:717–20.
20. Kahn HA, Leibowitz HM, Ganley JP, et al. The Framingham Eye Study: 2. Association of ophthalmic pathology with single variables previously measured in the Framingham Heart Study. Am J Epidemiol 1977;106:33–41.
21. Kitazawa Y, Horie T, Aaki S, et al. Untreated ocular hypertension: A long-term prospective study. Arch Ophthalmol 1977;95:1180–4.
22. Centers for Disease Control. Recommendations for preventing possible transmission of human T-lymphotropic virus type III/lymphadenopathy-associated virus from tears. MMWR 1985;34:533–4.
23. Centers for Disease Control. Recommendations for prevention of HIV transmission in health-care settings. MMWR 1987;36(25):35–185.
24. Moses RA, Grodzki WJ. The pneumatonograph. Arch Ophthalmol 1979;97:547–52.
25. Breitfeller JM, Krohn DL. Limbal pneumatonometry. Am J Ophthalmol 1980;89:344–52.
26. Roper DL. Applanation tonometry with and without fluorescein. Am J Ophthalmol 1980;90:668–71.
27. Lingel NJ, Coffey B. Effects of disinfecting solutions recommended by the Centers for Disease Control on Goldmann tonometer biprisms. J Am Optom Assoc 1992;63:43–8.
28. Hales RH. Combined solution of fluorescein and anesthetic for applanation tonometry. Am J Ophthalmol 1967;64:158–60.

29. Grolman B. Tonometer Performance. Proceedings of the 13th Hellenic Ophthalmological Congress, Kavala, Greece, June 5, 1980.
30. Grolman B. A new tonometer system. Am J Optom Arch Am Acad Optom 1972;49:646–60.
31. Wittenberg S. Repeated applanation tonometry with the NCT. J Am Optom Assoc 1973;44:50–6.
32. Myers KJ. Repeatability of IOP measurement with the non-contact tonometer. Am J Optom Physiol Opt 1974;51:39–48.
33. Wittenberg S. Effect of working distance on intraocular pressure as measured with the NCT. Am J Optom Physiol Opt 1974;51:325–30.
34. Shields MB. The non-contact tonometer. Its value and limitations. Surv Ophthalmol 1980;24:211–9.
35. Myers KJ, Scott CA. The non-contact ("air puff") tonometer: variability and corneal staining. Am J Optom Physiol Opt 1975;52:36–46.
36. Sagan W, Schwaderer K. Non-contact tonometry by assistants. Am J Optom Physiol Opt 1975;52:228–90.
37. Myers KJ, Lalle P, Litwak A, et al. XPERT® NCT®—A clinical evaluation. J Am Optom Assoc 1990;61:863–9.
38. Brencher HL, Kohl P, Reinke AR, Yolton RL. Clinical comparison of air-puff and Goldmann tonometers. J Am Optom Assoc 1991;62:395–402.
39. Armstrong TA. Evaluation of the Tono-Pen and the Pulsair tonometers. Am J Ophthalmol 1990;109:716–20.
40. Pearce CD, Kohl P, Yolton RL. Clinical evaluation of the Keeler PULSAIR 2000 tonometer. J Am Optom Assoc 1992;63:106–10.
41. Kaufman HE, Wind CA, Waltman SR. Validity of MacKay-Marg electronic applanation tonometer in patients with scarred irregular corneas. Am J Ophthalmol 1970;69:1003–7.
42. Farrar SM, Miller KN, Shields MB, Stoup CM. An evaluation of the Tono-Pen for the measurement of diurnal intraocular pressure. Am J Ophthalmol 1989;107:411–6.
43. Holec-Iwasko S, Shin DH, Parrow KA, et al. The influence of residual methylcellulose solution on Tono-Pen® readings. Am J Ophthalmol 1990;109:602–3.
44. Kooner KS, Cooksey JC, Barron JB, et al. Tonometer comparison: Goldmann vs Tono-Pen. Ann Ophthalmol 1992;24:29–36.
45. Bengtsson B. Comparison of Schiotz and Goldmann tonometry in a population. Acta Ophthalmol 1972;50:445–57.
46. Grolman B, Myers KJ, Lalle P. How reliable is the Goldmann tonometer as a standard? J Am Optom Assoc 1990;61:857–62.
47. Fisher RP. Value of tonometry and tonography in the diagnosis of glaucoma. Br J Ophthalmol 1972;56:200–4.
48. Takeda Y, Azuma I. Diurnal variations in outflow facility. Ann Ophthalmol 1978;10:1575–80.
49. Podos SM, Becker B. Tonography—current thoughts. Am J Ophthalmol 1973;75:733–5.
50. Pohjanpelto PEJ. The value of tonography [letter]. Arch Opthalmol 1978;96:729.

4

Ophthalmoscopy

William L. Jones

Ophthalmoscopy is the examination of the eye by means of an optical instrument known as an ophthalmoscope. Jan Purkinje described the technique of ophthalmoscopy in 1823,[1] but it was not until 1850 that Herman von Helmholtz[2] introduced the ophthalmoscope. Helmholtz's monograph on ophthalmoscopy was published in 1851 and soon became widely accepted.[1] His ophthalmoscope was improved shortly after its introduction by the addition of two movable discs with lenses for easier focusing. Later Epkins and Donders developed a perforated mirror that allowed a greater degree of illumination with the direct ophthalmoscope.[3] The technical advances from candlelight, to gaslight, to external electric light, to built-in electric light gradually improved the capabilities and convenience of the ophthalmoscope. In 1852, Ruete[4] devised the indirect method of ophthalmoscopy, and the first binocular ophthalmoscope was made by Giraud-Teulon in 1861.[5] Zeiss and Bausch and Lomb later constructed large table-mounted binocular ophthalmoscopes that were popular for many years. However, it was not until Schepens in 1947[6] introduced his binocular head-mounted ophthalmoscope with a built-in light source that binocular indirect ophthalmoscopy became widespread in popularity.

DIRECT OPHTHALMOSCOPY

Basic Principles

The basic principle of direct ophthalmoscopy involves the focusing of light rays from the patient's fundus onto the observer's fundus. This is easily accomplished if both the patient's and the observer's eyes are emmetropic (Figure 4-1). The problem is obtaining adequate illumination of the patient's fundus. Because of the optics of the eye, the light source only illuminates that part of the fundus which is struck directly by light; the rest of the fundus remains dark (Figure 4-2). Therefore, the fundus can be adequately viewed only if the observed areas and the illuminated areas coincide. This can take place only if the light source and the observer's pupil are closely aligned optically (Figure 4-3). Since this normally does not take place, the pupil appears black to the naked eye. An elevated structure such as a tumor or retinal detachment allows the illuminating and observation beams to overlap, and therefore may sometimes be seen without the aid of an ophthalmoscope.

Field of View

The field of view during direct ophthalmoscopy is approximately 10 degrees for an emmetropic eye and is limited by the most oblique light rays that can pass from the patient's pupil into the observer's pupil. With the ophthalmoscope, maximum field of view is related to the diameter of its viewing aperture. Field of view can be increased maximally by dilating the patient's pupil or by bringing the observer's eye closer to the patient's eye. Smaller sections of pupil are used by the peripheral light rays, and thus the fundus image gradually decreases in luminosity toward the periphery of the illuminated fundus. Practically speaking, the field of vision is determined by the illuminating system and not by the viewing system.

Magnification

The magnification of the direct ophthalmoscope for an emmetropic patient viewed by an emmetropic observer is 15×. If the patient and observer have refractive errors, then the axial length and refractive power of both eyes, plus the compensating lenses of the ophthalmoscope, must all be used to calculate the resultant magnification. If the patient is myopic, then the eye has plus power and the ophthalmoscope requires a minus lens for viewing a clear

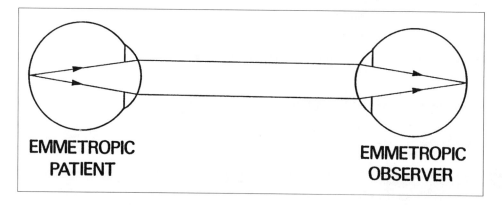

FIGURE 4-1
Conjugate retinal points can be accomplished with an emmetropic observer and an emmetropic patient, but without adequate illumination, fundus detail cannot be seen.

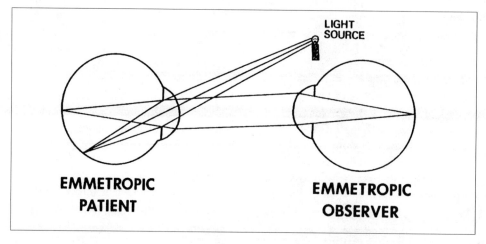

FIGURE 4-2
Nonalignment of the illumination source and the viewing axis results in the observer seeing a nonilluminated area of the fundus.

image. The combination results in a Galilean telescope, which enlarges fundus detail. The opposite effect is seen in a hyperopic eye (reverse telescope).

Refractive Error
If neither the patient nor the observer is emmetropic, then a single lens in the ophthalmoscope must equal the mathematical sum of the patient's and the observer's refractive errors. This problem can be eliminated by having the patient and the observer wear their optical corrections. A particular advantage to this is when one or both of the participants have a large refractive error or a high degree of astigmatism. However, for small to moderate refrac-

tive errors, it is more advantageous to remove the glasses to decrease the viewing distance, thus increasing the field of view.

Reflections
A serious problem with viewing the fundus is unwanted reflections. The brightest and most troublesome reflection is from the cornea; less bothersome is the reflection off the crystalline lens. Gullstrand,[7] in 1910, pointed out that to avoid both scattering and reflection of light rays into the viewing beam, both the illuminating and viewing beams must be totally separated across areas where interference might occur. Therefore, separation of the two

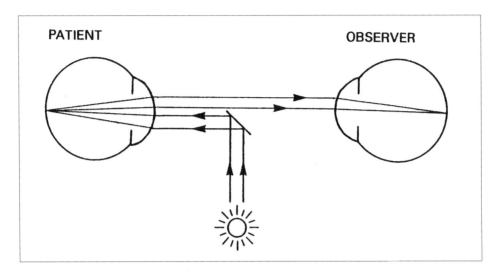

FIGURE 4-3

Alignment of the illumination and viewing beams is accomplished by use of a mirror or prism during direct ophthalmoscopy. Thus, the illuminated area of the fundus can be viewed by the observer.

beams must be maintained through the cornea and lens, yet overlap onto the retina. Bringing the illuminating and viewing beams close together will allow observation through a small pupil, but this increases reflections and scatter. With a dilated pupil, reflex-free viewing is more easily obtained because the beams can have greater separation. Most direct ophthalmoscopes have the illuminating beam situated below the viewing aperture. Modern ophthalmoscopes have a condensing lens to intensify the light beam and a diaphragm and projecting lens to limit the size of the light beam.

Accessory Functions

Accessory functions can be built into the ophthalmoscope to widen the diagnostic capabilities. A slit diaphragm can produce a narrow slit beam, which can be used to detect elevation or depression of retinal lesions. Here, a distortion of the beam occurs when it travels across an elevation or depression. The beam bows toward the observer on an elevated area and away from the observer in a depressed area. A pinhole diaphragm produces a narrow beam of light that can be used to reduce reflections, which is especially helpful when viewing through a small pupil. A small circle of light allows observation of fine retinal detail seen in the zone adjacent to the directly illuminated retina. This zone consists of areas of indirect and retroillumination that enhance observation. A fixation reticle can be used to discover eccentric fixation or eccentric viewing by the patient. This may be helpful in the evaluation of strabismic patients or those with macular lesions. In the latter case, it can be determined if the size of the functional deficit is larger than the size of the observed lesion. The stability of the eccentric viewing can also be determined.

Different types of filters can be very helpful in performing ophthalmoscopy. A blue filter can be used to enhance fluorescence during fluorescein angiography or to observe autofluorescence of optic nerve head drusen. It may also be used to observe fluorescein staining of the cornea. A red-free filter absorbs red light; therefore, red objects appear very dark. This is helpful when studying blood vessels and hemorrhages. Defects in the nerve fiber layer and retinal edema are more easily seen with red-free light because of the high fraction of shorter wavelengths that are readily scattered by superficial retinal layers. Crossed polarizing filters reduce reflection because light reflected back from the cornea is depolarized and blocked by the viewing filter, but light reflected from the retina (except for the internal limiting membranes) is polarized and remains visible. The chief drawback of polarizing filters is the substantial reduction in illumination that results from their use.

Technique

A number of general principles should be considered before ophthalmoscopy is initiated. The patient, whose eyes have been dilated, should be seated at a height at which the

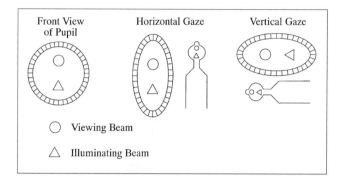

FIGURE 4-4

Rotating the direct ophthalmoscope when the patient looks in the far fields of gaze will enhance the entry of the illumination and viewing beams through the elliptically shaped pupil.

examiner can comfortably approach him or her. Room lights should be dimmed to reduce reflections from overhead lights and to improve viewing contrast. The patient should be instructed to remove his or her glasses, as previously discussed, and to look straight ahead or slightly up. The patient and examiner should attempt to keep both eyes open during the examination.

The ophthalmoscopic examination normally begins on the right eye of the patient. Hence, the examiner holds the scope with the right hand and uses the right eye to view through the instrument. The opposite should occur for the examination of the left eye (i.e., left eye, left hand, left eye).

The examiner should select the desired aperture for the particular examination conditions and then place the forefinger on the round lens dial. The scope is now brought to rest on and braced by the nose and cheek of the examiner.

The examination with the direct ophthalmoscope can now proceed with a +2 or +3 D lens placed within the scope. The examiner should hold the ophthalmoscope about 12–14 inches from the patient while focusing on the pupillary zone and observing the red reflex. This is an extremely important initial step. Should the reflex be absent or partially obstructed, the examiner should anticipate the presence of some type of media opacification within the eye. Examples are any form of corneal opacity, cataracts, or vitreal debris. Retinal changes, such as retinal detachment, may also interfere with the red reflex.

After the red reflex has been assessed, the examiner should move closer to the patient and rotate additional plus power into the ophthalmoscope aperture so that the anterior segment of the eye remains focused. The transparency of the cornea, anterior chamber, and lens can be studied and any opacity of these structures will appear dark against the red fundus reflex. In the case of a large,

dense corneal scar, enough light may be reflected back from the surface of the scar so that it appears white. Initially the examiner should step back from the patient to look at the front of the eye, then slowly move forward while changing focus to observe deeper structures within the globe. This makes it easy to examine the cornea, anterior chamber, lens, vitreous, and retina.

Description of Important Landmarks

Generally, an ophthalmoscopic examination of the fundus starts at the optic nerve head because localization of this structure provides immediate orientation. The optic disc should be examined for the cup-to-disc ratio, color, clarity of margins, spontaneous venous pulsations, and any abnormalities. The tissue around the disc is studied, with emphasis placed on the blood vessels, especially the superior and inferior temporal arcades. The vessels should be evaluated for their arteriovenous ratio, color, diameter, and course. The background retinal tissue is also examined. The macula is usually examined last because of the dazzling and discomfort that is experienced by the patient. The macula should be examined for the presence of a foveal reflex, color, pigmentation, and any abnormalities.

Peripheral Viewing

Peripheral viewing with a direct ophthalmoscope is limited because the pupil becomes too narrow for the viewing and illumination beams. Therefore, the wider the pupil, the farther out into the periphery the field of view. The equatorial region is usually the limit in peripheral viewing with the direct ophthalmoscope. A technique to aid in peripheral viewing has to do with the change in the pupil configuration on extreme eye gazes. When the patient looks to the right or left, the pupil is elongated vertically. In this situation the ophthalmoscope should be held vertically to facilitate the entrance of both beams into the eye. Likewise, a horizontal elongation of the pupil results during up or down gaze, and a horizontal orientation of the scope may be helpful (Figure 4-4).

Description of Fundus Abnormalities

Of major importance is the description of fundus lesions, which includes color, shape, size, elevation, and location. Size estimation of a lesion is usually accomplished by comparing it with a structure of known dimensions, such as the optic disc. Most fundus lesions are described relative to disc diameters (DDs) in size (e.g., a choroid nevus is "2 DDs by 3 DDs"). This is often done by viewing the optic disc first and then quickly relocating the lesion and comparing the two. Since the horizontal diameter of a normal optic disc is 1.5 mm, it is possible to translate DDs into millimeters. For future comparison, the size of a lesion

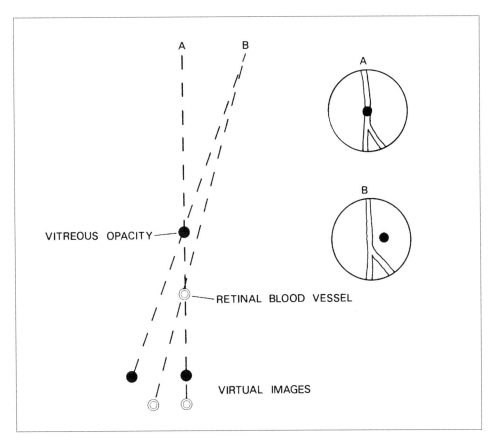

FIGURE 4-5

Viewing a vitreous opacity against a retinal blood vessel from the two different vantage points of A and B will give the opacity apparent motion and an apparent displacement. As the examiner initially views the vitreous opacity in A, it appears to move to the right of the blood vessel when he or she moves to the left (against motion).

can also be compared with the reticle dimensions projected on the fundus.

Elevation or depression of a fundus lesion may sometimes be determined by noting whether the entire lesion is in focus or whether parts seem to be out of focus. If an out-of-focus area can be brought into focus, then the two parts of the lesion are in two different focal planes. If the hazy area cannot be brought into focus, however, then the reason is optical disruption (e.g., flare and cells secondary to inflammation, vitreous changes, or a cataract). A change in focal planes is more easily detected by a presbyopic observer, since variable accommodation is not present. A 3 D difference in focal planes in an emmetropic eye converts into a linear depth equivalent of approximately 1 mm in a phakic eye and into approximately 2 mm in an aphakic eye.

Relative positions of lesions within the eye can be determined by using parallax to localize lesions. To use parallax, the observer moves his or her head and ophthalmoscope from side to side while fixating on an ocular structure to be used as the plane of regard. An object located in front of the plane of regard will seem to move in the opposite direction to the head movement, but an object located behind the plane of regard will seem to move in the same direction. The farther the object is located away from the plane of regard, the faster will be its relative speed of movement. For example, if the plane of regard is the iris, then a lesion in the anterior chamber or cornea will display "against motion," whereas "with motion" will be displayed by lesions in the lens and vitreous. Parallax can also be used to appreciate elevation of retinal lesions into the vitreous (Figure 4-5).

The location of fundus lesions during direct ophthalmoscopy is usually made in reference to the optic disc or fovea. For example, "a chorioretinal scar is located approximately 5 DDs superior and nasal to the optic nerve head." Sometimes there may be two lesions located close to each other, and it might be recorded that a pigmented lesion is just inferior to a hypopigmented area.

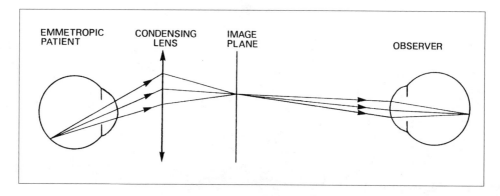

FIGURE 4-6
Schematic of binocular indirect ophthalmoscopy. Note that the image, which is real and invert-ed, is formed on the observer's side of the condensing lens.

INDIRECT OPHTHALMOSCOPY

Binocular Indirect Ophthalmoscopy

Basic Principles

Indirect ophthalmoscopy differs from direct ophthal-moscopy by the insertion of a lens between the patient and observer, which images the light from the patient's fundus to a plane on the observer's side of the lens (Fig-ure 4-6). Table 4-1 and Figure 4-7 are provided for a comparison between direct and binocular indirect oph-thalmoscopy. The real, aerial fundus image created by the condensing lens is inverted and is what the observ-er sees. To focus the diverging light from the real image on his or her own retina, the observer must use accom-modation, which limits how closely the observer can approach the image. Therefore, it requires a much greater distance between the patient and the observer. If the patient's eye is emmetropic, then the real image is brought to focus at the focal plane of the condensing lens; however, a myopic eye yields an image slightly in front of the focal plane, and a hyperopic eye yields an image slightly behind the focal plane.

Field of View

The field of view of a direct ophthalmoscope is about 10 degrees compared with 37 degrees for a binocular indi-rect ophthalmoscope. This translates into an area differ-ence that is twelve times greater while using the binocular indirect ophthalmoscope and a 20 D lens. Indirect oph-thalmoscopy has a greater field of view because the con-densing lens is able to capture more light rays escaping from the eye (Figure 4-8). The field of view is calculated from the ratio of the lens diameter to the focal length. Thus, both a larger diameter lens and a stronger-powered

TABLE 4-1
Comparison Between Direct and Indirect Ophthalmoscopy

Parameter	Direct	Indirect
Image	Virtual and erect	Real and inverted
Field of view	10 degrees	37 degrees (20 D)
Magnification	15×	Depends on the con-densing lens only: 5× (12 D) 3× (20 D) 2× (30 D)
Viewable area of fundus	60–70%	To the ora serrata without scleral depression and to mid pars plana with scleral depression.
Image brightness	0.5–4.0 watts	Up to 18 watts
Working distance	1–2 cm	Arm's length from lens to observer. Lens to patient distance depends on the focal length of the lens: 12 D > 20 D > 30 D
Stereopsis	None	Excellent: 12 D > 20 D > 30 D

lens will increase the field of view. However, since stronger lenses generally are manufactured with smaller diame-ters, a stronger lens may not always increase the field of view. In direct ophthalmoscopy, the field of view is deter-mined by the patient's and observer's pupils, but in indi-rect ophthalmoscopy, the limitation is determined solely by the patient's pupil. An interesting situation occurs in the examination of a 20 D myope, for an image of the fun-

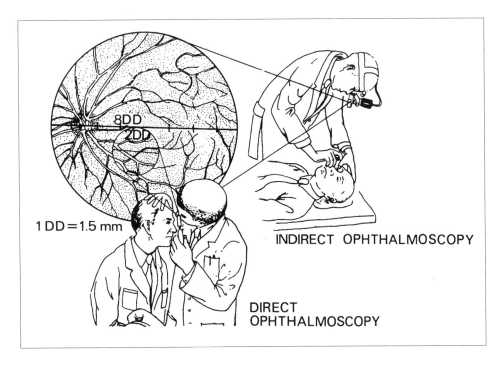

FIGURE 4-7

Comparison of the fundus area visible during direct and binocular indirect ophthalmoscopy. (Reprinted with permission from WC Blount. Direct and indirect ophthalmoscopy, for a more accurate baseline evaluation in air crew members. Aviat Space Environ Med 1977;48:269.)

dus would be produced 5 cm in front of the eye without the help of an ophthalmoscopy lens. The image could be viewed with the naked eye, but the field of view would be limited by the patient's pupil, and it would be quite small. With the lens in place before the patient's eye, the view becomes much larger and, hence, emphasizes the importance of lens diameter in increasing the field of view.[8]

Refractive Error

Refractive error compensation in indirect ophthalmoscopy is accomplished without additional corrective lenses. Only small changes in the observer's accommodation are needed to overcome significant patient refractive errors. The presbyopic observer can make small changes in the distance between the lens and himself or herself to compensate for refractive error variation.[8]

Magnification

Magnification in indirect ophthalmoscopy is determined by the power of the condensing lens and the viewing distance between the aerial image and the observer. Magnification with regard to lens power can be expressed as the ratio of the focal power of the eye over the focal power

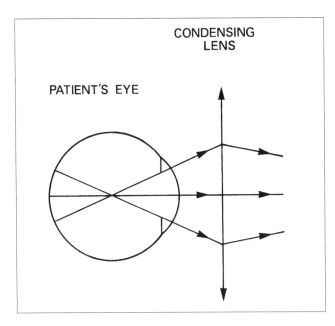

FIGURE 4-8

A condensing lens used with indirect ophthalmoscopy is able to capture more light rays escaping from the eye than is possible with direct ophthalmoscopy.

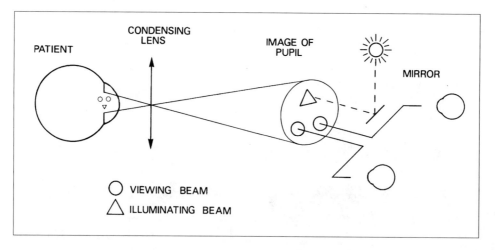

FIGURE 4-9

Schematic demonstrating the imaging of the pupil and the placement of the illumination and viewing beams within the image during binocular indirect ophthalmoscopy.

of the lens. If the assumption is made that the power of the eye is 60 D, then dividing this by the power of the condensing lens will give the magnification. A 20 D lens will produce 3× magnification, and 2× is produced by a 30 D lens. The aerial image viewed at 25 cm produces no further magnification, since this is the reference distance of magnification. A more typical viewing distance is 40 cm, and the ratio of the reference distance over the actual observer's distance would produce approximately 0.6× magnification. Thus, a 20 D lens used at a 40-cm viewing distance would result in an overall magnification of approximately 1.9× (60/20 × 25/40 = 1.9).

As the magnification is reduced, the field of view increases by a factor of four. This accounts for the difference between indirect ophthalmoscopy using a 20 D lens and direct ophthalmoscopy. The obvious price to pay for increasing the field of view is a loss of magnification. Extra magnification can be obtained by decreasing the viewing distance, but this requires accommodation by the examiner. Therefore, to help decrease viewing distance (from the examiner to the real aerial image), a +2 D trial lens can be placed in front of an ophthalmoscope's oculars, or reading glasses can be worn.

Latitude of Beam Placement and Interpupillary Distance

In indirect ophthalmoscopy, the illuminating beam is directed by a mirror into the condensing lens, which focuses it in the patient's pupil for maximum fundus illumination (Figure 4-9). Greater flexibility for positioning of the illumination and observation beams is available with indirect ophthalmoscopy, which allows for the inclusion of two observation beams and, thus, stereoscopic viewing. The flexibility of beam placement increases with the use of higher-powered lenses by increasing the magnification of the patient's pupil (see Figure 4-9). Most indirect ophthalmoscopes are designed to have the observing beams (one from each eye) separated by 15–20 mm, and the magnified pupil diameter must be equal to or greater than the beam separation for binocular viewing. An observer using a 20 D condensing lens would have a difficult time imaging through a 2-mm pupil, but switching to a 30 D lens would allow an easier view. To achieve binocular vision of the fundus, the observer's interpupillary distance (PD) must "fit" into the aerial image produced by the condensing lens. This is made possible by optically reducing the observer's PD with the use of mirrors or prisms on the ophthalmoscope. The greater the PD used, the greater will be the effects of stereopsis.

The luminosity of the fundus image is equal from edge to edge, and this is the reason most fundus cameras are based on the indirect optical system. The luminosity of the indirect image decreases with an increase in the power of the condensing lens. The light intensity can be increased to compensate for the reduction in image brightness when using stronger lenses.

Illumination

Many technical advances in light sources have been made in modern ophthalmoscopes. These light sources can deliver high-intensity light to the subject's eye. There has been some concern about the possibility of retinal damage from the high-intensity light used in indirect ophthalmoscopy, but a study by Robertson and Erickson[9] of prolonged indirect ophthalmoscopy on human eyes failed to reveal any long-term retinal damage. However, there were some short-term changes consisting of irregular bending and twisting of photoreceptor outer segments and transient corneal edema. Attempts have been made to reduce the infrared radiation through the use of fiberoptics, dichroic mirrors, and tinted condensing lenses such as the Volk yellow-tinted lenses that absorb light in both blue and infrared wavelengths.

Reflections

Reflections and light scatter are problems in indirect ophthalmoscopy, and binocular viewing requires a larger pupil than monocular viewing to meet Gullstrand's original ophthalmoscope design. Moving the beams closer together will facilitate viewing through a small pupil but will increase reflections and reduce stereopsis. The advantage of the indirect ophthalmoscope is the ability to change the distance between the illuminating beam and viewing beams by tilting the mirror on the scope. During indirect ophthalmoscopy, the illumination is focused in the plane of the pupil to better satisfy Gullstrand's requirements, for this will be the smallest diameter of the beam. Because a 14 D condensing lens has a longer focal length, it is held a greater distance from the eye than a 30 D lens to place the smallest diameter of the beam in the pupil.

Indirect Ophthalmoscopy Condensing Lens

The indirect ophthalmoscopy lens is designed to decrease peripheral aberrations that increase with stronger and larger lenses. To overcome this problem, most condensing lenses are made of an aspheric design. This results in a lens with two different curves, the steeper curve on the examiner's side of the lens. The illumination beam produces reflections and scatter on the condensing lens surface that can be minimized by antireflective coatings. If the lens is held perpendicular to the line of viewing, it produces reflections on the front and rear surfaces in the center of the lens. These reflections can be directed out of the line of light by a slight tilt of the lens. Observation of the reflections can be helpful for determining the proper orientation of the condensing lens (i.e., the steeper curvature on the examiner's side). When facing the proper direction, the two reflections will be approximately equal in size. When opposite to this, one reflection will be significantly larger than the other. To help assist with proper orientation, modern condensing lenses have a silver or white ring painted on the edge of the lens holder's flange that faces the patient.

Technique

Adjustments

The ophthalmoscopic oculars, which are generally $+2\,D$ lenses, are positioned perpendicular to the pupillary axis and as close to the observer's eyes as possible. Adjustments can be made in the interpupillary distance while viewing an object at about 2 feet or by viewing one's thumb held in the midline at arm's length. The oculars are then positioned so that the object or thumb is seen in the middle of each viewing window. The eyes are alternately opened and closed to check this. Horizontal diplopia may be seen if the interpupillary distance is incorrect. An observation of vertical diplopia indicates that the instrument is tilted. Some binocular indirect ophthalmoscopes have linkage screws that allow for vertical alignment of the oculars in front of the eyes.

The light beam is directed into the upper half of the field of view so that the illumination and optical axis are separated. The lower half of the lens is used for viewing, thus reducing unwanted reflections (see Figure 4-9). These gross adjustments should not be made while shining the light into the patient's eye because of the discomfort to the patient. Fine adjustments may be required once the examination has begun.

Condensing Lens and Hand Placement

The condensing lens is held in either hand between the thumb and forefinger, and one or more of the remaining fingers are placed on the patient's head for stability. It is best to be ambidextrous; however, the lens is usually held in the dominant hand, and the opposite hand can be used to hold the patient's lids apart. The third finger of the hand holding the condensing lens can be used to hold one lid of the eye being examined, and many examiners use the thumb of the opposite hand to hold the opposing lid. By flexing or extending either the digits holding the lens or the fingers placed on the patient's head, it is possible to adjust the distance between the condensing lens and the patient's eye for the best possible view.

Since a lower power condensing lens has a longer focal length, the lens must be held farther away from the eye for optimal viewing. The most convex surface of the condensing lens faces the observer, and the advantage of this steep curvature is to direct reflections away from the viewing axis with slight tilting of the lens. Two reflections of the light source can be seen originating from the front and back surfaces of the lens, which can be separated by tilting the lens. Other annoying reflections can also be directed out of the line of sight by tilting the lens.

Excessive lens tilt will induce astigmatic distortion of the fundus image and should be avoided. However, induced astigmatism can be advantageous when viewing the peripheral fundus. By inducing astigmatism with the condensing lens at 90 degrees to the astigmatism produced during observation of the fundus periphery, it is possible to reduce peripheral optical distortions. The degree of induced astigmatism increases with greater lens tilt, and the observer can vary the tilt to obtain the clearest focus. Although ideal positioning of the condensing lens becomes second nature for an experienced ophthalmoscopist, students are encouraged to experiment with different lens positions and tilts while learning the procedure of binocular indirect ophthalmoscopy. Considerable practice is usually required before one becomes comfortable with the technique.

The selection of a particular condensing lens is dependent on many circumstances and the structures the examiner desires to see. If the observer wants to increase stereopsis or magnification, then a lower power lens is needed, such as a 14 D lens. A peripheral view of the fundus is more easily obtained with a higher power lens (30 D). Since a higher power lens uses less pupillary area, it produces a more stable image and, thus, is advantageous for examining uncooperative patients and children. In performing ophthalmodynamometry, it is advantageous to have a magnified view of the optic disc vessels, and the use of a low-power lens is indicated.

Patient Preparation

Pupillary dilation is usually accomplished with instillation of an anticholinergic agent such as tropicamide 0.5% or 1% and a sympathomimetic agent such as phenylephrine hydrochloride 2.5%. It generally takes about 20 minutes to obtain full dilation. Shorter or longer pupillary dilation times may be required depending on amount of iris pigmentation. If the clinician attempts ophthalmoscopy before there is adequate paralysis of the pupillary sphincter muscle, the pupil will constrict under the intense illumination, and viewing of the fundus will be difficult.

The patient can be either supine or seated, but many clinicians prefer to have the patient in the supine position. It is easier to hold the condensing lens steady while standing over the patient, and it is easier to rotate around the eye.

Patient Examination

The center of the condensing lens is held over the pupil near the eye, and the light is directed into the lens. The lens is raised until the image fills the lens. The entire optical system must be kept on a rigid axis, which uses the pupil as its center of rotation. To change the fundus view, the observer's head and the condensing lens must rotate

in the same direction, with the lens moving less distance than the head. It is necessary for the examiner to move the entire torso to maintain the proper distance and optical axis. An effective procedure is to have the patient move his or her eyes to the 12-o'clock position, at which point the observer starts the examination and continues as the patient is instructed to move his or her eyes in a clockwise direction. The same procedure is performed on the contralateral eye. By repeating the same procedure on every patient, it becomes easier to remember the location of fundus detail.

During the examination, the patient's eye may become dry from the prolonged exposure to the bright light and the lack of blinking. Therefore, the patient must be permitted to blink periodically. The fundus must be viewed as quickly as possible because the light is very bright and uncomfortable for the patient. It is best to use the lowest light intensity that still allows a good view of the fundus. The highest light intensity settings are generally reserved for viewing through media opacities (e.g., cataracts, corneal opacification, and vitreous hemorrhage).

Fundus Orientation

One must remember that during indirect ophthalmoscopy, the fundus image is inverted within the condensing lens. Therefore, when viewing the posterior pole, a lesion seen above and nasal to the optic disc in relation to the patient's head is actually located below and temporal to the optic disc. The temporal and nasal locations are generally not difficult to remember because of the fovea localizing the temporal region, but the superior and inferior regions may be more easily confused. When viewing the fundus periphery, the image within the condensing lens is likewise reversed.

Three landmarks are generally used to localize lesions in indirect ophthalmoscopy: the optic disc, the equator, and the ora serrata. The optic disc and ora serrata are easy to recognize, but the equator is not as easily delineated. Its approximate location, however, is delineated by the retinal zone containing the vortex veins. As in direct ophthalmoscopy, measurement of retinal distance is usually made in disc diameters (DDs) (e.g., a retinal hole is "2 DDs from the ora serrata at 3 o'clock.")

Correct orientation is a must in order to localize a lesion in the periphery. A straight line must be imagined from the observer's eye through the condensing lens to the lesion. If the examiner believes that a lesion is located at 2 o'clock in the fundus, then he or she should stand at the 8-o'clock position. If the lesion is then seen at 2 o'clock in the lens relative to the patient's head, then

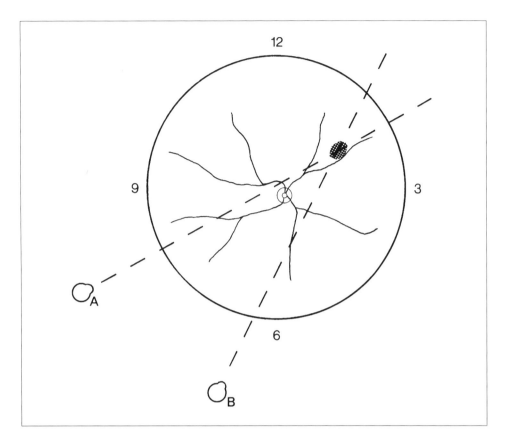

FIGURE 4-10

Fundus orientation is important for localizing fundus detail. At viewpoint A, the patient looks at the 2-o'clock position, and the observer sees the lesion at 2 o'clock, thus indicating proper localization. At viewpoint B, the patient looks at the 2-o'clock position, but the observer sees the lesion more towards 1 o'clock, thus indicating improper localization.

there is a straight optical line, and the lesion is truly at that position (Figure 4-10).

Peripheral Viewing

When viewing the periphery, the pupil becomes elliptical and much smaller in diameter along the short axis. This may make it impossible to direct both viewing beams and the illumination beam into the patient's pupil. This can be remedied by tilting the observer's head 45 degrees, which may allow the illumination beam and one viewing beam to enter the pupil (Figure 4-11). This will eliminate stereopsis, but will allow a more peripheral view of the fundus. Also, it is helpful to increase the viewing distance when examining through a small pupil by moving farther away from the condensing lens; the closer one is to the pupil, the less the chances of intercepting the angle of exiting rays.

Elevation Determination by Parallax

Parallax can be helpful when performing indirect ophthalmoscopy to determine the elevation of intraocular structures. Even though stereopsis is possible with binocular indirect ophthalmoscopy, sometimes the elevation of a lesion is so slight that the examiner is not sure whether any elevation is truly present. By moving the condensing lens from side to side, a relative parallax movement can be elicited. A vitreous opacity may be seen over a retinal vessel, and slight movements of the lens may make the opacity change its position relative to the vessel. The farther away from the vessel, the faster the relative movement of the opacity.

Proximal Illumination

Proximal illumination can be of great value in studying retinal lesions by positioning so that the object is visual-

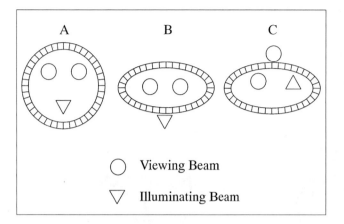

FIGURE 4-11

The examiner can more easily view the fundus periphery by tilting his or her head 45 degrees to allow the illumination beam and one viewing beam to enter an elliptical pupil. A. Both beams easily pass through the large pupillary aperture present in primary gaze. B. Without tilting of the examiner's head, the illumination beam and at least one of the viewing beams do not readily pass through the patient's elliptical pupil. C. The illumination beam and one of the viewing beams easily pass through the pupil with tilting of the examiner's head.

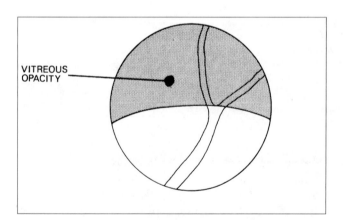

FIGURE 4-12

Proximal illumination is accomplished by placing the object of interest just within the shadow on the fundus.

ized just adjacent to the illuminated area. The examiner can accomplish this by rotating his or her head slightly downward and moving the condensing lens down slightly. This will place a part of the image seen in the lens in shadow. Ideally, the lesion is positioned just within the shadow (Figure 4-12). This technique is especially useful

in differentiating between a retinal hole and hemorrhage, both of which appear red on direct illumination. Any opacity such as blood will block the light reflected back from the choroid and sclera and appear darker, but a retinal hole will appear even more luminous than before (Figure 4-13).

Viewing Around Media Opacities

The need to see around a media opacity, such as a corneal scar, cataract, or vitreous opacity, that does not totally obscure the view of the fundus can be partially fulfilled by moving the lens in a circular pattern around the opacity to see structures that are directly behind it. Some of the views obtained in this manner may be very poor in quality, and the examiner may need to search for a while to find the best view possible. Of course, even a poor quality view is better than no view at all.

Fundus Drawings

Fundus drawing is an art that requires some skill. The examiner must be able to view the fundus and rearrange what is seen so that it is drawn true to form. With practice, this becomes easier to do, although it may take many separate views of the fundus to confirm one orientation. It must be remembered during fundus drawing that the image in the condensing lens is inverted and perverted. One method of performing a fundus drawing is to place a drawing chart on the patient's chest with the 12-o'clock position pointing at the patient's feet. Now the observer can draw exactly what is seen, and all relationships will be correctly maintained. When standing at the 12-o'clock position relative to the patient's head (during examination of the inferior fundus) the examiner draws exactly what is seen at the 6-o'clock portion of the chart (closest to the patient's chin). At the end of the examination, rotating the chart to its 12-o'clock position will obtain the proper relationships. Color coding and symbols make it much easier to identify structures in a fundus drawing (Table 4-2).

Scleral Depression

Scleral depression is the technique of indenting the globe to bring into view peripheral structures that were not visible during routine ophthalmoscopy and to highlight details of a fundus lesion. The depression device is usually a scleral depressor probe that has either a handle or thimble attachment (Figure 4-14). A cotton-tipped applicator can be used if no specialized device is available. This depression technique allows the examiner to view as far anterior as the middle pars plana region of the ciliary body. Scleral depression is useful in detecting retinal holes by moving the depressor under the hole (rolling the hole) to

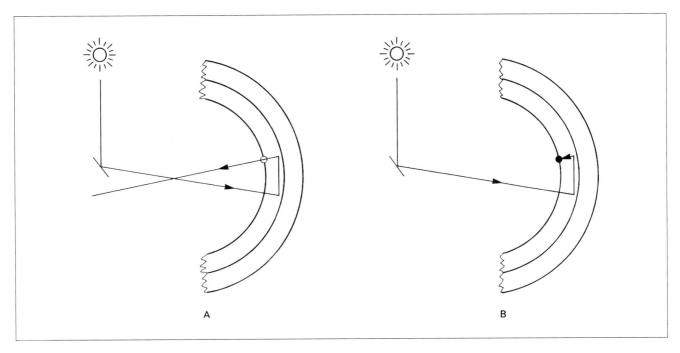

FIGURE 4-13

A. An example of a retinal hole seen during proximal illumination of the fundus. The hole will appear more luminous because it allows more of the light that is reflected from the choroid and sclera to pass toward the observer. B. A retinal hemorrhage will appear darker than its surroundings because it blocks more of the reflected light than the surrounding retina.

TABLE 4-2
Example Color Coding for Fundus Drawings

Color	Pathologic Entity
Red	Attached retina, retinal arteries, retinal hemorrhage
Blue	Detached retina, retinal veins
Blue outlining red	Retinal holes
Black	Retinal pigmentation, old chorio- retinitis, choroidal pigmentation seen through attached retina, demarcation lines, melanoma
Brown	Choroidal pigmentation seen through detached retina
Yellow	Chorioretinal exudation, active inflammatory infiltration or debris, macular edema
Green	Opacities in media, including vitreous hemorrhage
/ / /	Nonpigmented lattice
X X X	Pigmented lattice
(((	Scleral buckle

observe the edge of the hole as it is being lifted upward. Additionally, the topographic detail of numerous other fundus lesions and anomalies can be evaluated with scleral depression.

Generally, indentation of the globe can be performed through the eyelid, but if this does not allow adequate positioning, then the probe can be placed directly into the conjunctival fornix. A properly sterilized probe should be used if the tip is placed directly onto the conjunctival surface, and topical anesthesia should be obtained with an agent such as 0.5% proparacaine hydrochloride.

Scleral depression is an advanced technique that requires proficient use of the binocular indirect ophthalmoscope. During the procedure the probe is held in either hand (and the condensing lens in the opposite hand) dependent on the particular fundus location of interest. Although some patients may report mild discomfort during scleral depression, it should not be painful. Typically, only a minimal amount of pressure is needed to actually indent the globe. Care should be taken to allow adequate blinking and to avoid "pinching" of the lid tissue during the technique. Any perforation of the globe, secondary to either trauma or a recent surgical technique, is an absolute contraindication to scleral depression. Precaution should also be maintained with patients who have intraocular lenses, as

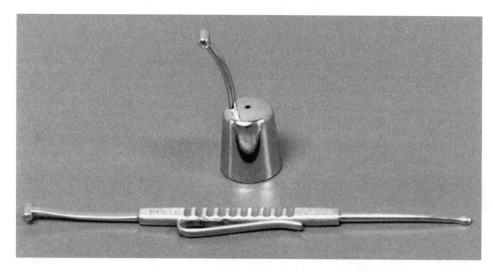

FIGURE 4-14
Thimble and stick scleral depressors. (Courtesy of Daniel K. Roberts, O.D.)

distortion of the globe potentially could cause dislocation of the lens.

Monocular Indirect Ophthalmoscopy

Monocular indirect ophthalmoscopy was more commonly performed before the advent of more routine pupillary dilation. Whereas the monocular indirect ophthalmoscope (MIO) uses optical principles similar to those of the binocular indirect ophthalmoscope, it produces only a monocular view of the fundus. A separate condensing lens is not used with the MIO. Rather, the instrument itself is placed close to the eye and necessary lenses are incorporated into the instrument's housing. The primary advantage of the MIO is that it can provide a fairly wide field of view of the fundus through a relatively small pupil. Consequently, greater overall perspective when viewing the fundus can be acquired than with direct ophthalmoscopy, and a more peripheral view of the fundus can also be obtained. This is accomplished in part by placement of the instrument's illumination source very close to the examiner's line of sight.

With the incorporation of "small pupil" features on many modern binocular indirect ophthalmoscopes, the MIO has become less useful. Nevertheless, the MIO may be preferred in some situations where pupillary dilation is not possible. Principle disadvantages of the MIO are less light intensity, no stereopsis, and a smaller field of view compared with the binocular indirect ophthalmo-

scope. The magnification of the MIO is approximately 5×, compared with 15× for the direct ophthalmoscope, and 3× for the binocular indirect ophthalmoscope (using a 20-D condensing lens). The image obtained with the MIO is inverted, similar to that of the BIO.

INTERPRETATION

Pupillary Reflex

As mentioned, an important initial step in the direct ophthalmoscopic examination is evaluation of the pupil reflex (red reflex). Here, the pupil is retroilluminated with light reflected from the fundus. Many types of media opacification, as well as some retinal pathologic states (e.g., retinal detachment, retinal tumors) can interfere with the evenness or color of the pupillary reflex. To observe the pupillary reflex, the direct ophthalmoscope is held approximately 10–15 cm from the eye and an appropriate amount of plus is dialed into the instrument, which brings the pupillary plane into focus. Cataracts are the most common media opacification that interfere with the pupillary reflex (Figure 4-15). By moving the ophthalmoscope to the right or to the left, parallax can be used to localize opacification that is in front of or behind the iris plane. Lenticular opacities will appear to move in the same direction (with motion) as that of the ophthalmoscope, whereas corneal opacification will appear to move in the opposite direction (against motion).

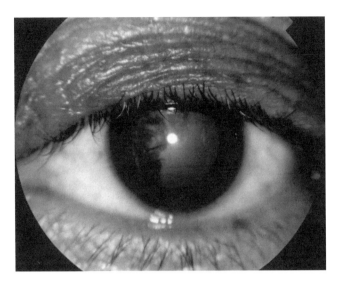

FIGURE 4-15
Lens opacities commonly interrupt the red pupillary reflex during ophthalmoscopy. In this example, a cortical cataract interrupts the reflex nasally. (Courtesy of Sara Penner, O.D.)

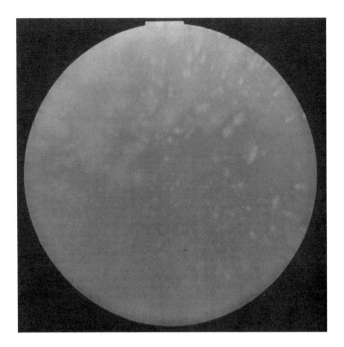

FIGURE 4-16
Ophthalmoscopic appearance of asteroid hyalosis.

Vitreous Opacities

Examination of the vitreous is a fundamental component of the ophthalmoscopic examination. With direct ophthalmoscopy, vitreal opacities may be evident during evaluation of the pupillary reflex. Individual, small opacities may appear dark or semitransparent against the red reflex, whereas their true color will become evident as they are focused on directly. Because of their location behind the pupillary plane, vitreal opacities will demonstrate "with motion" during movement of the ophthalmoscope from side to side. The farther posterior in the vitreous an opacity is located with regard to the iris, the greater the relative movement. More diffuse opacification such as a vitreal hemorrhage may result in an overall dimming of the pupillary reflex instead of an uneven or spotty degradation. With direct examination, however, individual corpuscles may be evident with careful observation. Vitreal opacities of all types may be more or less evident with the indirect ophthalmoscope. Because of relative magnification differences, small opacities may not be easily visualized with the indirect ophthalmoscope. Greater peripheral views may allow better visualization of some opacities with the indirect ophthalmoscope, however.

Vitreal floaters secondary to vitreal syneresis and posterior vitreal detachment (PVD) are the most common vitreous opacities. A PVD is a separation of the vitreous cortex from the retinal surface in an anterior direction all the way up to the posterior margin of the vitreous base (an area of tenacious attachment of the vitreous cortex straddling the ora serrata). When the posterior vitreal (hyaloid) face detaches, it often pulls free a glial ring from around the optic disc, which may then be perceived by the patient as a circular or broken circle floater. Whereas the posterior hyaloid face is usually difficult to see ophthalmoscopically, the annular opacity adherent to the membrane may be quite evident to the examiner. Typically, the ring floater is present within the middle of the vitreal cavity because of the anterior displacement of the posterior vitreal face following detachment. The collapse of the vitreous body following a PVD allows for contraction of vitreal fibrils, leading to additional floaters (aside from the annular ring). These vitreal floaters may also cast retinal shadows and subsequently produce patient symptoms. Ophthalmoscopically, they may appear as isolated, irregularly shaped lines, or they may intertwine in a cobweb-shaped fashion.

Asteroid hyalosis, a condition consisting of calcium soap spheres within the vitreous cavity, is also frequently found (Figure 4-16). These harmless vitreal opacities may be strikingly evident to the examiner, while causing few, if any, patient symptoms. Occasionally, they are so evident ophthalmoscopically that they prevent adequate visualization of fundus details.

Examination of the optic nerve during ophthalmoscopy should include delineation of cup-to-disc ratio, color, mar-

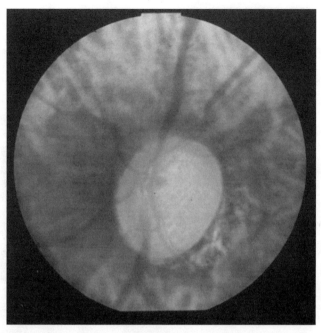

FIGURE 4-17

A glaucomatous optic disc showing marked pallor, laminar dots, and a 0.9 cup-to-disc ratio with extension of the cup to the inferior disc margin. The atrophy to the inferior disc margin should result in a superiorly located nerve fiber bundle visual field defect. Also note the presence of a choroidal crescent temporal to the optic disc.

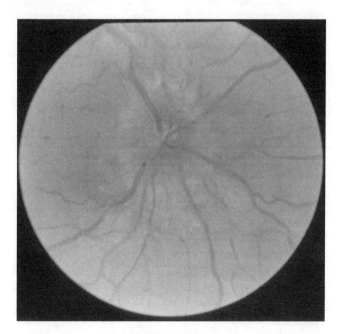

FIGURE 4-18

Papilledema. Note that the disc is swollen and exhibits very indistinct margins. The disc was very hyperemic and no spontaneous venous pulsations were present.

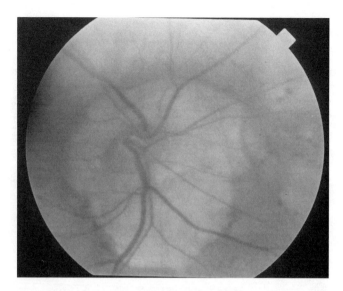

FIGURE 4-19

Inferior nasal tilting of the optic nerve head. Extensive peripapillary atrophy is also present in this example.

gin clarity, shape, and presence of spontaneous venous pulsations. Pallor to the optic disc may be a sign of optic atrophy which may result from a number of conditions including ischemic optic neuropathy, optic nerve tumor, demyelinating disease, or trauma. An increase in the cup of the optic disc classically results from glaucoma (Figure 4-17). A swollen optic nerve typically is elevated with indistinct margins and congested venules. Peripapillary hemorrhages may also be present, and spontaneous venous pulsations may be absent. The term *papilledema* refers to optic disc edema occurring secondary to increased intracranial pressure. Papilledema (Figure 4-18) is typically bilateral and may result from such entities as intracranial tumor, infections, hydrocephalus, and pseudotumor cerebri (benign intracranial hypertension). Optic disc edema unrelated to intracranial pressure may have a number of causes, such as angle closure glaucoma, optic neuritis (inflammation from any cause), and optic nerve ischemia. Pseudo-edema (pseudopapilledema) of the optic disc is commonly caused by optic disc drusen. Tilting of the optic nerve head is a common congenital anomaly frequently found in high myopia or in otherwise normal eyes. Discs in highly myopic eyes are usually tilted temporally. They appear vertically elongated and their nasal margin is elevated relative to the temporal. Inferior or inferonasal tilting (Figure 4-19) commonly occurs as a congenital defect and may be associated with an inferior or inferonasal scleral crescent, which is often referred to as a Fuchs' coloboma.

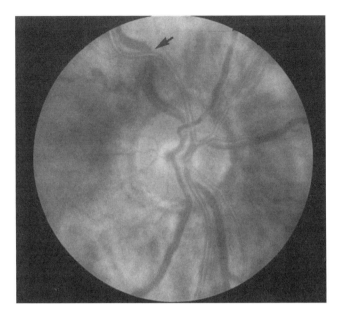

FIGURE 4-20
Arteriovenous compression (arrow) secondary to arteriolosclerosis.

Retinal Vessels

The retinal vessels are composed of arterioles, venules, and capillaries. These retinal vessels (except for the capillaries) travel in a branching pattern away from the optic disc. Ophthalmoscopic examination of the fundus should always include a careful evaluation of the retinal vessels, noting their course, width, and color. Commonly, a general comparison is made between the widths of arterioles and venules (arteriovenous, or A/V ratio). Normally the arterioles are approximately two-thirds (0.6 or 0.7) the diameter of the venules. A common cause for changes in this ratio is arteriolosclerosis (see Chapter 20), which typically results in arteriolar narrowing (e.g., A/V ratio = 0.5). The width of the arteriolar light reflex (ALR) is noted during ophthalmoscopy as a ratio relative to the overall arteriolar diameter. Normally, the ALR is about one-third the width of the arteriole. Arteriolosclerosis may cause a widening of the ALR and therefore an increase in its width relative to arteriole diameter (e.g., ALR ratio = 0.6 or 2/3).

A change in the color of the vessel walls may result from a number of conditions. Sheathing refers to an opacification or whitening of the vessel walls and can result from conditions such as embolic occlusion, Eale's disease, multiple sclerosis, sarcoidosis, pars planitis, or any retinal inflammatory condition. Sheathing may appear as a thin whitish outline to the retinal vessels, or the entire vessel may be white with no blood column visible (pipestem sheathing). Arteriolosclerosis can lead to a gradual opacification of the arteriolar walls, which is described as either a copper wire, or even more advanced, a silver wire appearance.

Intersections of the arterioles and venules are known as arteriovenous (A/V) crossings. The arteriole usually crosses over the venule, but occasionally the venule will be found above the arteriole. The arterioles and venules share a common adventitial sheath at these crossings and this keeps them firmly attached to each other. "Hardening" of the arteriole wall, which occurs in arteriolosclerosis, can cause an arteriole to impinge on the wall and lumen of an adjacent vein, which may result in some characteristic physical A/V crossing changes (see Figures 20-9 and 20-10), which include such findings as banking (mild ballooning of a venule's distal aspect at a crossing site), tapering (narrowing of a venule's proximal aspect at a crossing), compression (a lowering of an underlying venule into the retina (Figure 4-20), humping (an elevation of an overlying venule), and deviation (a right-angle deviation of a venule at a crossing).

Arterioles and venules may become abnormally straightened or tortuous in a number of retinal conditions and such abnormalities should be noted at ophthalmoscopic examination. Hypertension and arteriolosclerosis can cause arterioles to become attenuated and straight. Venous tortuosity commonly occurs with central or branch retinal vein occlusion. Tortuosity is most often found as a congenital anomaly but can also occur secondary to such disorders as diabetic retinopathy, hyperviscosity syndromes, and hypoperfusion retinopathy.

The Macula

Careful examination of the macula is always an integral component of the general ophthalmoscopic evaluation. The integrity of this fundus region is of obvious importance because of its unique anatomic structure and its role in the discrimination of fine visual detail. The macula can be involved in a number of different diseases and may exhibit a wide variety of pathologic clinical appearances.

The center of the macula, or fovea, is usually located by first focusing on the optic disc, then shifting gaze temporally approximately 1.5–2.0 DDs. The fovea is recognized by its lack of vasculature and by its pinpoint light reflex (foveal reflex). The foveal light reflex is caused by the curvature of the foveal region, which essentially behaves like a concave mirror. Although loss of the foveal light reflex can occur secondary to pathologic conditions affecting macular anatomic detail, it should be remembered that a significant percentage of patients normally

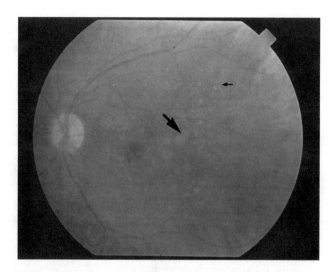

FIGURE 4-21
Drusenoid changes associated with age-related macular degeneration. Small hard drusen (small arrow) and larger, soft, confluent drusen (large arrow) are present.

do not exhibit a foveal light reflex. Hence, its absence should not automatically be construed as abnormal.

Commonly found within the macular region of healthy eyes are drusen. Macular drusen may exhibit a wide variety of clinical appearances but are typically small, round, yellow-white deposits located at the level of the retinal pigment epithelium (RPE) and Bruch's membrane. They may be found in patients in almost all age groups but are more common in the elderly. Vision is typically unaffected. Whereas drusenoid changes are typically mild and of no significance, they may be one component of the degenerative process known as age-related macular degeneration. Here they may be larger (soft drusen), greater in number, confluent, and associated with pigment epithelial degeneration (Figure 4-21). Drusenoid changes may be dominantly inherited (familial or dominant drusen) and appear quite prominently in relatively young patients between 20 and 30 years of age. Metamorphopsia and decreased vision may occur as drusen become larger and more confluent.

Examination of the macula should include observation not only for drusen, but for the presence of thinning, thickening, pigmentary hyperplasia or atrophy, hemorrhage, exudate, edema, and epiretinal membrane formation. Macular conditions commonly found in adult patients include age-related macular degeneration, macular hole formation, central serous retinopathy, and posttraumatic changes. Hereditary macular diseases are seen infrequently, but include Stargardt's disease (fundus flavimaculatus), vitel-

liform dystrophy (Best's disease), rod or cone dystrophies, patterned dystrophy, and X-linked juvenile retinoschisis.

Retinal Hemorrhage

Retinal hemorrhages are red unless they are viewed with a red-free light; then they will appear black. Hemorrhages may be shaped like dots, blots, flames, splinters, domes, or boats. Dot- and blot-shaped hemorrhages are usually found in the middle layers of the retina. Flame- and splinter-shaped hemorrhages are located in the nerve fiber layer, which is responsible for producing their striated appearance. Dome-shaped hemorrhages result from bleeding in the subsensory retinal space or beneath the pigment epithelium. These relatively thick hemorrhages cause the sensory retina to elevate over them. Hemorrhage above the RPE appears red, but the thicker the layer of blood, the darker red it will become. Hemorrhage beneath the RPE loses its red color and appears dark gray or green because of the translucent nature of the RPE. Boat-shaped hemorrhages have been called subhyaloid, preretinal, or subinternal limiting membrane hemorrhages and have this characteristic appearance because of the effects of gravity on the pool of blood. The hemorrhage appears as a red pool of blood with a flat or slightly concave upper margin and sometimes it may break through into the vitreous, producing a red smokestack appearance. Small retinal hemorrhages may sometimes exhibit a white center and are then referred to as Roth's spots. Retinal hemorrhages result from a wide variety of pathologic processes affecting the eye. Common causes include diabetes, hypertension, and vein occlusion.

Retinal Exudates

Retinal exudates occur secondary to the leakage of components of the blood plasma from the retinal vasculature. Visible exudates do not consist of this serous leakage in its entirety, but rather of materials (proteins, fats, and other constituents) that precipitate out of this fluid. Exudates are generally yellow, shiny, and can be almost any shape. When leakage from a particular site is significant enough, a ring of exudate (circinate exudative ring) may form around that location. Exudates occurring in the macular region may accumulate in Henle's fiber layer and form what is referred to as a macular star (Figure 4-22). Exudates may occur anywhere in the fundus secondary to many fundus conditions. They are most frequently encountered in diabetic retinopathy, but other disease conditions include hypertensive retinopathy, anemia, age-related macular degeneration, Coat's disease, and macroarterial aneurysm. Retinal exudates that are temporary may

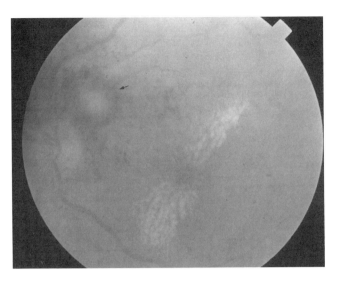

FIGURE 4-22
Retinal exudates in the macular area are forming a partial macular star. Note the juxtapapillary hemorrhage surrounding an infarcted area of retina (arrow).

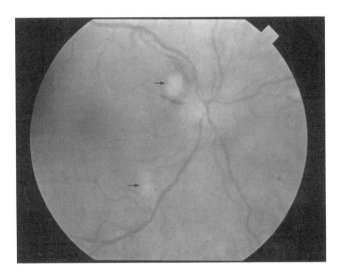

FIGURE 4-23
Cotton wool spots occurring in hypertensive retinopathy (arrows). Flame-shaped (splinter) hemorrhages are also present.

resolve without sequelae, but longstanding exudation (especially involving the macula) can result in permanent visual dysfunction.

Cotton Wool Spots

Cotton wool spots are the result of small infarctions of the nerve fiber and ganglion cell layers of the retina. The infarction causes swelling of these tissue layers, which produces a white, hazy spot in the superficial retina (Figure 4-23). The involved nerve fibers become nonfunctional and a small scotoma may be demonstrated. The whitish discoloration eventually disappears, but the involved nerve fibers may remain nonfunctional. Cotton wool spots may occur anywhere throughout the fundus, but are commonly found in the posterior pole with conditions such as diabetes, hypertension, collagen vascular disease, AIDS, and leukemia.

Neovascularization

Neovascularization of the fundus generally occurs secondary to two basic mechanisms. The first occurs along the superficial retina or optic nerve in response to retinal hypoxia (Figure 4-24). Here, the oxygen-starved tissue probably releases an angiogenic (vessel forming) stimulus, which causes new fragile blood vessels to form adjacent to areas of tissue hypoxia in an attempt to supply oxygen. Whereas new vessels result from a reparative

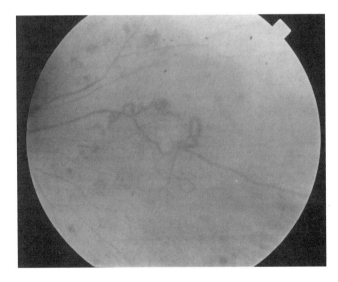

FIGURE 4-24
Retinal neovascularization in proliferative diabetic retinopathy.

attempt, their fragile walls can lead to retinal or vitreal hemorrhage. In addition, tractional retinal detachment can occur. Retinal neovascularization of this type may result from many causes, but most commonly from diabetes, retinal vein occlusion, and sickle cell disease. The second type of neovascularization occurs beneath the RPE secondary to almost any condition that alters the integrity of Bruch's membrane. Here, the so-called subretinal

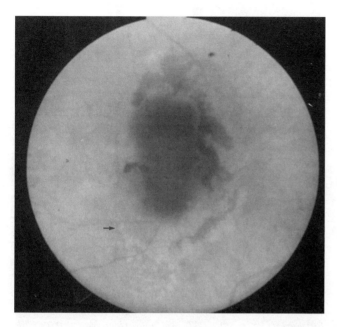

FIGURE 4-25
Macular hemorrhaging from a subretinal neovascular membrane occurring in age-related macular degeneration. The neovascular membrane is hidden beneath the hemorrhages. Note the drusenoid changes characteristic of this disorder (arrow).

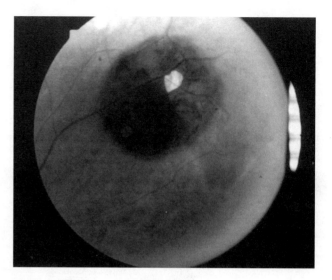

FIGURE 4-26
A congenital hypertrophy of the pigment epithelium, which is flat, black in color, and has sharp margins. Also note that there is a window-like defect in the lesion, referred to as a lacuna. Lacunae represent zones of chorioretinal atrophy and are characteristic of these congenital lesions. (Courtesy of Scott Robison, O.D.)

neovascular membrane (SRNVM) originates from the choriocapillaris and penetrates Bruch's membrane to grow within the subpigment epithelial space. Hemorrhagic leakage from the SRNVM causes degeneration and scarring of the overlying RPE and photoreceptor layers (Figure 4-25). Subretinal neovascularization most commonly results from age-related macular degeneration. Other causes include histoplasmosis, angioid streaks, high myopia, and trauma.

Congenital Hypertrophy of the Retinal Pigment Epithelium

Congenital hypertrophy of the pigment epithelium is a common, benign fundus anomaly consisting of a hypertrophied pigment epithelial cell layer containing large, densely packed pigment granules. The resultant hyperpigmented lesions are typically round, well-circumscribed, black, and flat; have distinct margins; and are sometimes surrounded by a lighter halo (Figure 4-26). The halo is caused by a loss of pigment granules in the epithelial cells adjacent to the lesion and is pathognomonic for this entity. Areas of depigmentation, known as lacunae, are often present with these lesions. These areas of prominent chori-

oretinal atrophy may increase in number or size over time. Congenital hypertrophy of the RPE may occur anywhere throughout the fundus and is variable in size. Multiple lesions may occur in a single eye and when clustered together they are commonly referred to as grouped pigmentation of the RPE or bear tracks. These lesions are benign in nature and can be found anywhere in the retina, even adjacent to the optic disc as a pigmented crescent.

Acquired Hyperplasia of the Retinal Pigment Epithelium

Retinal pigment epithelial hyperplasia is a common fundus finding that may occur secondary to almost any type of retinal disease. The retinal pigment epithelial cells and their pigment granules increase in number, yielding increased pigmentation in the involved area. Areas of hyperplasia may be almost any shape or size. The margins of these lesions are irregular. This helps differentiate them from congenital hypertrophy of the RPE, which is usually round and well circumscribed. Disorders that commonly produce significant RPE hyperplasia include toxoplasmosis retinochoroiditis, lattice degeneration, trauma, retinitis pigmentosa, and age-related macular degeneration.

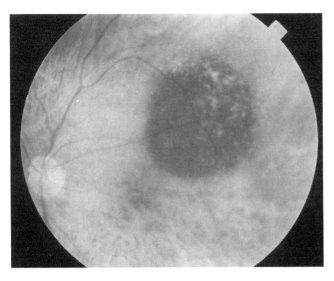

FIGURE 4-27

A large choroidal nevus is seen superotemporal to the macula. It has distinctive mottling which is caused by drusen formation and pigment epithelial degeneration. The lesion is essentially flat and has indistinct margins.

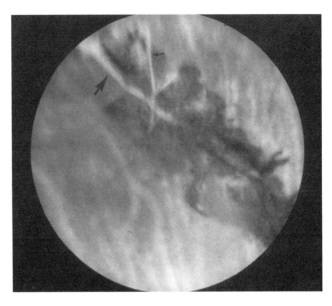

FIGURE 4-28

Perivascular lattice degeneration within the midperipheral retina. The lesion is hyperpigmented and radial in orientation. The central radial vessel is white and sclerosed (large arrow). Vessels crossing through the lesion perpendicularly are also sclerosed (small arrow).

Choroidal Nevus

A choroidal nevus is a benign accumulation of melanocytes within the choroid. This process begins in the suprachoroid but can extend through the entirety of the choroidal layer. The thicker the nevus, the darker it will appear in the fundus. Choroidal nevi can be found in any location of the ocular fundus. They are typically slate gray and elevated. Mottling on the surface of nevi is common and is caused by drusen formation and RPE degeneration (Figure 4-27). These lesions are usually 1–3 DDs in size. They may grow slowly, but usually they remain stable for years. Choroidal nevi that are over 10 mm in diameter or over 3 mm in elevation should be suspected of being malignant until proven otherwise.

Chorioretinal Atrophy

Chorioretinal atrophy describes the nonspecific degeneration of choroid and retina. As a result of the loss of the choriocapillaris and the RPE layers, areas of chorioretinal atrophy appear white because the underlying sclera is visible. Commonly, regions of chorioretinal atrophy exhibit RPE hyperplasia at the borders of the lesion. Larger choroidal vessels may still be visible within the base

of these lesions. A common example of chorioretinal atrophy is the lesion known as pavingstone degeneration. The punched-out, white lesions (lacunae) that occur within areas of congenital hypertrophy of the RPE are also exemplary of chorioretinal atrophy (see Figure 4-26). Chorioretinal atrophy is also common in various forms of macular degeneration and high myopia.

Lattice Degeneration

Lattice degeneration is a very common vitreoretinal degeneration of the peripheral retina. It is characterized by a circumferentially oriented, elongated band of retinal thinning usually located between the equator and ora serrata. The lesions are usually 1–4 DDs in length and about 0.25–0.75 DD in width; however, they can be as long as an entire quadrant and as wide as a disc diameter. Whereas a circumferential pattern is usually present, a radial orientation is also possible. Lattice lesions are often hyperpigmented, and blood vessels crossing these areas may be sclerosed and white (Figure 4-28). Progressive thinning within the base of lattice lesions often leads to atrophic hole formation, which may cause retinal detachment. The borders of lattice degeneration are often fairly well demarcated and may be highlighted during scleral depression.

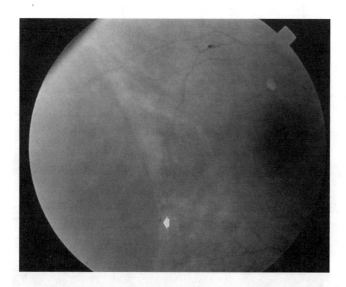

FIGURE 4-29
A retinoschisis is seen in the temporal region of the fundus denoted by a subtle curved demarcation line (arrow). The dark area to the right is the macula. The retinoschisis is very bullous and has a taut, smooth appearance. Note the loss of choroidal detail beneath the retinoschisis.

The vitreous immediately overlying lattice lesions is degenerated and liquefied.

Acquired Retinoschisis

Acquired retinoschisis is a specific disorder commonly affecting the peripheral retina. It is characterized by a splitting of the sensory retina (usually at the outer plexiform layer) into two layers. The inner layer then billows forward into the vitreous cavity, appearing as a smooth, taught, possibly bullous, membrane that does not undulate with eye movements (as seen in retinal detachments) (Figure 4-29). The inner layer may have a variable elevation and can be highly transparent except for the retinal blood vessels that it supports. Occasionally, blood vessels coursing through the inner layer of a retinoschisis are sclerotic and white. Small, whitish flecks (snowflakes) are sometimes attached to the inner layer, which make it more visible. Retinoschises extend from the ora serrata, with their posterior borders semicircular in configuration and pointing toward the posterior pole. The cavity created by the separated retinal tissue is filled with a viscous fluid that does not tend to dissect the sensory retina easily. Therefore, progression of a retinoschisis is usually slow, if it occurs at all. Holes can develop in both the inner and outer layers of a retinoschisis. Inner layer breaks by themselves do not lead to retinal detachment; however,

outer layer breaks, especially when coexistent with inner layer breaks, may do so.

Atrophic Retinal Hole

An atrophic retinal hole is characterized by atrophy and loss of sensory retinal tissue above the RPE. Usually, these lesions are round and appear red. They may be quite variable in size but are typically less than 1 DD. Atrophic holes often are surrounded by a variable sized, whitish cuff because of the accumulation of fluid around the margin of the free retinal edge or due to degenerative fibrosis of the retinal tissue. Atrophic holes may be isolated but also frequently develop within areas of lattice degeneration.

Retinal Tears

Retinal tears are characterized by a tractional separation of the sensory retina from the underlying RPE. Commonly, this is caused by a posterior vitreal detachment. Tears usually develop in areas of greater than normal vitreoretinal adhesion, such as occurs at the edges of lattice degeneration and at retinal tufts. Retinal tears may have various shapes including horseshoe, linear, and round. Because of their configuration, horseshoe-shaped and linear tears are very prone to further tearing and subsequent retinal detachment (Figure 4-30). On the other hand, round retinal breaks (operculated retinal breaks) result in a completely dislocated plug of tissue, which floats in the overlying vitreous and no longer causes tension on the margins of the retinal break (Figure 4-31). Subsensory retinal fluid is often present adjacent to the edges of retinal breaks and may give a whitish discoloration to the retina. Localized retinal detachment may occur in the region of the break, which can lead to total retinal detachment.

Retinal Detachment

Retinal detachment occurs when the sensory retina separates from the underlying pigment epithelium. Clinically, a retinal detachment may be characterized by a relatively shallow or bullous elevation of the sensory retina into the vitreous cavity. The elevated membrane often has a whitish appearance and may contain a number of folds (Figure 4-32). The fluid beneath a retinal detachment is not as viscous as that within a retinoschisis cavity, and therefore the sensory retinal membrane will undulate on eye movement. If the posterior leading margin of a retinal detachment is stationary for a few months, hyperplasia of the underlying RPE may occur at the border, leading to a pigmented demarcation

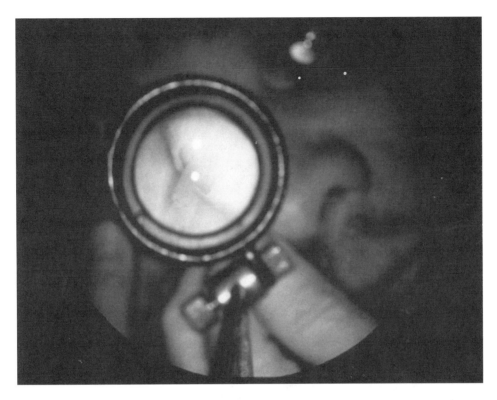

FIGURE 4-30

A horseshoe-shaped tear can be seen in the condensing lens of the binocular indirect ophthalmoscope during scleral depression. The flap is about one fourth the size of the underlying break, which is outlined by slightly elevated white edges. Note that the tip of the flap has pigment clumps and whitish retinal degeneration, which denotes previous longstanding vitreous traction. There is a surrounding localized detachment, which can be seen by noting the shadow being cast by the uplifted retina along the posterior border of the break.

line. This is an apparent attempt to prevent further progression. If a detached retina periodically advances beyond an existing demarcation line, then multiple, parallel pigmented lines may be found. Demarcation lines at the posterior border of a retinal detachment may occasionally be white due to retinal fibrosis.

Longstanding retinal detachments have a different physical appearance than ones of recent onset. The retina becomes more translucent secondary to atrophy and resultant thinning. The detachment also may become less elevated and have an appearance similar to a retinoschisis. This is because of fibrotic changes, which contract the sensory retinal membrane. Pigmented or white demarcation lines are common with longstanding retinal detachments. Retinal detachments produced by a retinal break are referred to as rhegmatogenous detachments and those not associated with a break are known as nonrhegmatogenous retinal detachments. Discovery of a retinal detachment should always be followed by thorough investigation for its cause, as this will influence the treatment modality. Nonrhegmatogenous retinal detachments may be caused by many different entities, among which are proliferative neovascular retinopathy, choroidal tumors, scleritis, and choroiditis.

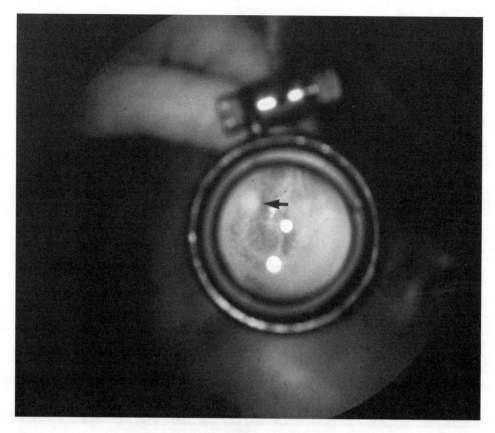

FIGURE 4-31

An operculated retinal tear in the far periphery. The operculum (arrow), the underlying round break with white margins, and a surrounding pigmented demarcation line are seen. The view is through the condensing lens during binocular indirect ophthalmoscopy.

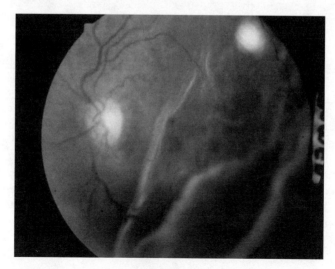

FIGURE 4-32

An extensive retinal detachment of the temporal fundus that has extended into the macula. Note the undulating folds of the detachment. (Courtesy of Sun Ma, O.D.)

REFERENCES

1. Albert DM, Miller WH. Jan Purkinje and the ophthalmoscope. Am J Ophthalmol 1973;76:494–9.
2. von Helmholtz H. Description of an ophthalmoscope for examining the retina in the living eye. [Translation.] Arch Ophthalmol 1951;46:565–83.
3. Rucker WF. A History of the Ophthalmoscope. Rochester, NY: Whiting Printers and Stationers, 1971.
4. Ruete CGT. Der Augenspiegel und das Optometer für practische Aerzte. Göttingen, Prussia: Dieterich, 1852.
5. Giraud-Teulon, MALF. Ophthalmoscopie binocularie ou s'exercant par le concours des yeux associés. N N Ocul 1961;45:233–50.
6. Schepens CL. A new ophthalmoscope: demonstration. Trans Am Acad Ophthalmol Otolaryngol 1947;51:298–301.
7. Gullstrand A. Neue Methoden der reflexosen Ophthalmoskopie. Ber Dtsch Ophthalmol Gesellsch 1910;36:75–80.
8. Colenbrander A. Principles of Ophthalmoscopy. In TD Duane (ed), Clinical Ophthalmology (vol 1). Hagerstown, MD: Harper & Row, 1979;1–21.
9. Robertson DM, Erickson GJ. The effect of prolonged indirect ophthalmoscopy on the human eye. Am J Ophthalmol 1979;87:652–61.

5

Fluorescein Angiography

KEVIN L. ALEXANDER

Since its introduction as a clinical diagnostic technique in the 1960s,[1] fluorescein angiography has become a mainstay in the diagnosis and management of retinal disease. Fluorescein angiography has progressed from a crude laboratory technique used to investigate normal retinal vasculature to a highly refined clinical diagnostic procedure. In recent years angiographic techniques have evolved to include digital enhancement of a video picture to provide instant results for analysis.

Normal retinal structures and numerous retinal conditions have been studied with fluorescein angiography, and the angiographic appearance of disease states has been well documented. While fluorescein interpretation of the more common disorders is presented in this chapter, more comprehensive sources are available for additional study.[2-4]

Fluorescein angiography is indicated in the evaluation of a variety of retinal vascular, inflammatory, and degenerative conditions. The technique provides another method of retinal analysis, demonstrating structural changes or characteristics not always visible with ophthalmoscopy. Table 5-1 lists common conditions in which fluorescein angiography may aid in diagnosis and management.

ANATOMIC CONCEPTS

The angiographic appearance of the retina results from two separate vascular systems: the uveal system and the retinal system. These two vascular systems are separated by the retinal pigment epithelium (RPE).

Uvea

The uvea consists of the choroid and iris. The choroid lies beneath Bruch's membrane, whose inner and outer layers form the basement membrane of the retinal pigment epithelium and of the choriocapillaris, respectively. The choriocapillaris is supplied by the posterior ciliary arteries. The endothelial cells of the choriocapillaris are fenestrated, allowing blood (and fluorescein) to enter the extracellular space. This differs anatomically from retinal vessels, which are not fenestrated and do not normally leak.

Iris

Although the iris stroma is highly vascularized, the capillaries are not fenestrated and do not generally leak fluorescein except in diseased states. The study of the iris with fluorescein angiography may therefore be indicated in conditions such as diabetes, uveitis, iris tumors, ischemic ocular syndrome, and retinal vascular occlusive disease in which rubeosis may occur.

Retinal Pigment Epithelium

The RPE is a single layer of cells separating the outer retina from the choroid. Its dense pigmentation serves as an optical filter with the greatest density at the fovea, decreasing toward the periphery. The RPE serves as a part of the blood–retinal barrier because of the tight junctions (zonula occludens) between cells. Any breakdown in these tight junctions will lead to leakage of fluid or blood into the subsensory retinal space. Figure 5-1 shows the relationship of the RPE and the choriocapillaris.

Retina

The vasculature of the retina is composed of the central retinal artery and the central retinal vein and their respective branches. Unlike the choriocapillaris, retinal capil-

TABLE 5-1

Examples of Conditions in Which Fluorescein Angiography Aids in Diagnosis or Management

1. Age-related macular degeneration
2. Angioid streaks
3. Anterior ischemic optic neuropathy
4. Branch retinal vein occlusion
5. Central retinal vein occlusion
6. Central serous chorioretinopathy
7. Choroidal melanoma
8. Cystoid macular edema
9. Degenerative myopia
10. Diabetic retinopathy
11. Ischemic ocular syndrome
12. Macroarterial aneurysm
13. Macular hemorrhage of unknown etiology
14. Pigment epithelial detachment
15. Presumed ocular histoplasmosis syndrome
16. Retinal telangiectasia
17. Rubeosis iridis
18. Sickle cell retinopathy
19. Tumors of the ciliary body and iris
20. Tumors of the retina

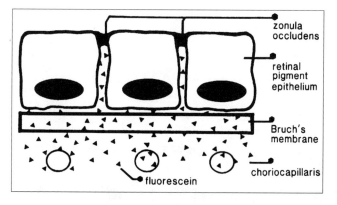

FIGURE 5-1

Relationship between the retinal pigment epithelium and the choriocapillaris.

laries are not fenestrated and therefore do not normally leak fluorescein into the extravascular space. Additionally, there is a 500-μ capillary-free zone in the macula that is supplied almost entirely by the choriocapillaris. Occasionally the macula will also be supplied by a cilioretinal artery.

PROCEDURE FOR FLUORESCEIN ANGIOGRAPHY

Equipment and Materials

The underlying principle making fluorescein angiography possible is the property of fluorescence. When sodium fluorescein is exposed to blue light between 465 and 490 nm, fluorescein molecules fluoresce, emitting a yellow-green light between 520 and 530 nm.

Ophthalmic fluorescein angiography is accomplished with any one of a number of excellent 35-mm fundus cameras on the market. These cameras are capable of making at least one exposure per second. Importantly, the fluorescein camera is equipped with matched filters. A blue exciter filter allows the camera to emit blue light into the patient's eye, causing the sodium fluorescein to fluoresce.

A yellow barrier filter blocks extraneous reflected blue light while allowing the yellow-green light emitted by sodium fluorescein molecules to pass to the camera. Figure 5-2 illustrates the photographic principles of fluorescein angiography.

The film should be a high-speed (ASA 400) and fine-grained film such as Kodak T Max or Tri-X Pan. Color photography is technically possible to perform but of somewhat limited value.

Sodium fluorescein is a pharmacologically inert dye that fluoresces when exposed to visible light, emitting light of a longer wavelength. Sodium fluorescein for intravenous administration is available in 5%, 10%, and 25% concentrations. Five milliliters of 10% fluorescein gives satisfactory fluorescence. Three milliliters of 25% sodium fluorescein may be preferable because a small bolus of dye lessens the likelihood of nausea during the procedure.[5]

Angiography with oral fluorescein is possible but only of value in a limited number of cases, primarily where leakage is expected to be found late in the study.[6] Because oral fluorescein is absorbed slowly into the bloodstream through the gastrointestinal system, it is impossible to obtain the bolus of dye that is needed early in the study to delineate initial filling phases.

Technique

The patient should be maximally dilated, and written informed consent must always be obtained. The patient is seated comfortably at the fundus camera with the camera at a height comfortable for both the photographer and the patient. Name tag and baseline photographs should be taken before injection of the drug. Baseline photographs consist of a red-free photograph and a photograph with

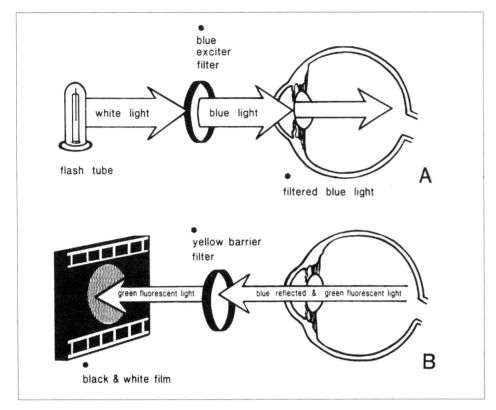

FIGURE 5-2
Fluorescein photography principles. A. The blue exciter filter passes blue light, which stimulates fluorescence of sodium fluorescein. B. The yellow barrier filter blocks extraneous blue light and passes yellow-green fluorescent light, which is recorded on film. (Adapted with permission from A Patz. Interpretation of the fundus fluorescein angiogram. Int Ophthalmol Clin 1977;17:17.)

both the exciter and barrier filters in place. The latter combination, which simply yields a black image, ensures that the filters are properly matched.

An antecubital vein is identified and sodium fluorescein is injected into the vein via a 21-gauge butterfly needle (Figure 5-3). Injection should be done rapidly over 5–7 seconds and the camera timer started immediately. The butterfly needle/syringe should be left in place during the initial few minutes in case an intravenous line is necessary for emergency purposes.

Exposures are taken approximately every second for the first 20 seconds, then at 3-, 5-, and 10-minute intervals. Late views, longer than 10 minutes, are rarely required but may be useful in detecting subtle leakage. The film is processed and the negative read directly or printed as a contact sheet or transparency (Figure 5-4) from which results may be read.

Adverse Reactions

Practitioners should be alert to the occasional adverse reaction to sodium fluorescein. These include (1) mild nausea and vomiting, (2) urticaria (hives), (3) vasovagal (systemic hypotension) response, and (4) extravasation (injection to subcutaneous tissues).[7]

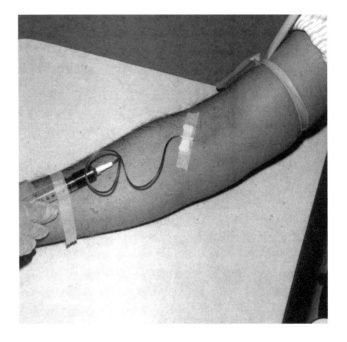

FIGURE 5-3
Injection of sodium fluorescein. A 21-gauge butterfly needle is used.

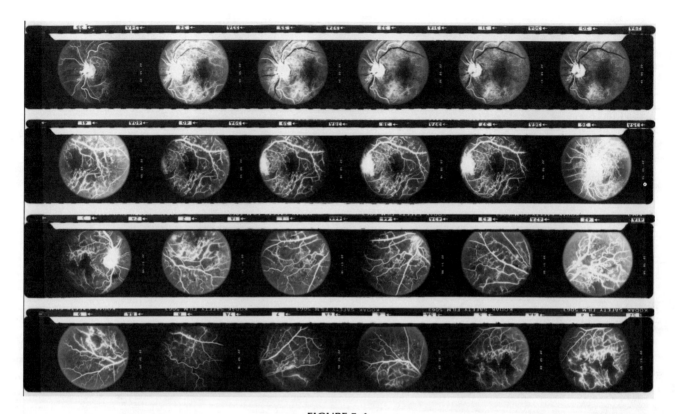

FIGURE 5-4

Positive contact print of a fluorescein angiogram. The frames progress sequentially from the upper right and then leftward. The latest frame in this series is in the lower-left corner. (Courtesy of Indre Rudaitis, O.D.)

Nausea and vomiting are managed with the emesis basin. Patients exhibiting urticaria may benefit by oral or parenteral diphenhydramine HCl (Benadryl). Vasovagal reactions need to be recognized immediately, and the patient should be allowed to lie recumbent with the feet elevated. Blood pressure should be monitored and will usually stabilize within a few minutes. Extravasation is avoided by good technique; however, if fluorescein is injected subcutaneously, the resultant burning and local irritation is treated with ice packs and direct pressure for a few minutes.

An emergency tray including 1:1000 epinephrine, diphenhydramine HCl, aminophylline, and hydrocortisone should be readily available.[8] Additionally, oxygen should be accessible and all personnel should be trained in cardiopulmonary resuscitation. Emergency phone numbers should be posted. All patients may expect a slight yellow discoloration of the skin for 12–24 hours and bright yellow urine for 24–36 hours.

Reading the Angiogram

During the evaluation of an angiogram, color fundus photographs should be available. This will allow the clinician to rapidly compare angiographic findings with the ophthalmoscopic appearance.

The first step in reading an angiogram is to orient the photographs properly and identify the eye to be studied. It is helpful then to inspect the overall quality of the angiogram, noting whether the frames are evenly exposed and of good contrast.

Next, it is important to determine the time taken for dye to travel from arm to eye, as well as filling times for all major retinal vascular branches. It should be determined whether the times are normal or delayed. Areas of hypofluorescence or hyperfluorescence should then be identified and evaluated for change over the course of the study. The angiographic results should be studied to arrive at an overall clinical impression and to determine whether they are consistent with the working diagnosis.

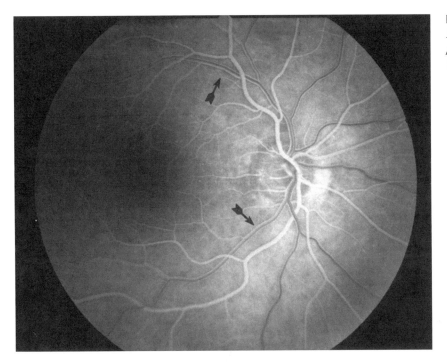

FIGURE 5-5
Normal angiogram—laminar phase. Note laminar flow in veins (arrows).

NORMAL ANGIOGRAPHIC FINDINGS

Early Views

Choroidal filling begins 10–20 seconds after injection. Because the choroidal vascular system is fenestrated, fluorescein enters the extravascular space quickly and appears as a generalized "flush" or hyperfluorescence. The choroidal hyperfluorescence is relatively blocked at the macula due to the denser pigmentation and xanthophyll.[9]

The arteriolar phase begins 1–2 seconds after choroidal filling, and all branches should fill simultaneously. Any delay in filling of the arteriolar tree should be considered abnormal. Because the retinal capillaries are not fenestrated, fluorescein does not normally leak into the extravascular space.

The capillary phase is theoretically present, but in actuality is not well delineated because of the small architecture of this vascular network. It occurs between the arteriolar and venous phases.

Venous filling is divided into two phases: laminar and complete. The laminar venous phase is represented by the characteristic flow pattern in which the blood closest to the vessel wall fluoresces initially. This can be observed within the larger venules as a bright outline of fluorescence along the walls of the vessel, bounding a darker line centrally (Figure 5-5). As more blood converges on the

larger venules from smaller tributaries, complete venous filling occurs, laminar flow is less discernible, and the entire vessel fluoresces. The entire process of filling usually takes place within the first 45–60 seconds.

Late Views

After the initial 30–60 seconds, photographs are typically taken at 3 minutes and again 7–10 minutes into the study (Figure 5-6). By this time, the dye has made multiple transits of the vascular system (recirculation phase). Early leakage will be evident by this phase. Subtle leakage such as that resulting from mild macular edema secondary to diabetes may not show up until 10 or 20 minutes or longer.

ABNORMAL FLUORESCEIN FINDINGS

Abnormalities of the fluorescein angiogram are the result of alteration or disruption of the normal anatomy of the choroid and retina. The terms hypofluorescence and hyperfluorescence have evolved to describe fluorescein patterns. The extent to which an area hypofluoresces or hyperfluoresces is gauged relative to the normal background fluorescein pattern.

In general, hypofluorescence is a result of either (1) blocked fluorescence (i.e., the obstruction of visibility

FIGURE 5-6
Normal angiogram—late phase.

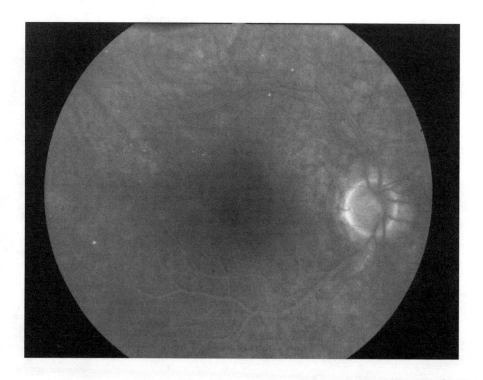

of the dye by blood or other opaque substances), or (2) a filling defect, which prevents fluorescein from reaching an area (nonperfusion). The best way to identify the type or cause of hypofluorescence is by comparing the angiogram with the ophthalmoscopic appearance of the eye. If the darkened area on the angiogram on a positive print corresponds to an ophthalmoscopically visible structure, then the hypofluorescence is possibly a result of blockage. If nothing is visible ophthalmoscopically, then the hypofluorescence is likely a result of nonperfusion of the area (filling defect).

Hyperfluorescence results from (1) fluorescein reaching an abnormal location because of alterations in retinal architecture, (2) abnormal blood vessels, or (3) transmitted fluorescence, which is caused by a defect in a tissue overlying a normally fluorescent structure. Artifactual fluorescence results from mismatched exciter and barrier filters. The term *autofluorescence* applies to structures possessing the innate property of fluorescence, an example of which is optic disc drusen. Pseudofluorescence results from reflected light from fluorescein found in the vitreous late in a study.

Hypofluorescence

Blocked Fluorescence

Hypofluorescence may be caused by choroidal or retinal fluorescence being blocked by blood, exudate, edema, scar tissue, pigment, or other substances, which lie in front of portions of the choroid or retina. Choroidal fluorescence is normally blocked in the macular area by the yellowish xanthophyll and lipofusion pigments. These pigments absorb the blue exciting light, resulting in the characteristic dark area of the avascular zone normally found on angiograms (see Figure 5-6).

Hemorrhage effectively blocks fluorescence and may occur in a subretinal (sub-RPE), intraretinal, or preretinal location. Subretinal hemorrhage may occur in degenerative or inflammatory conditions and is frequently the result of a subretinal neovascular membrane (Figure 5-7). Subretinal hemorrhage blocks choroidal fluorescence and may obscure the presence of an underlying subretinal neovascular membrane. Intraretinal hemorrhages arising from the vessels located in the inner nuclear layer will block choroidal fluorescence while not interrupting retinal fluorescence. Such intraretinal hemorrhages are common in diabetes or venous occlusion (Figure 5-8). Tiny dot hemorrhages may be difficult to distinguish from microaneurysms without the aid of fluorescein angiography.

Preretinal hemorrhage, commonly observed in proliferative diabetic retinopathy, totally obscures fluorescence from both the choroid and retina. The flame-shaped hemorrhages (located within the retinal nerve fiber layer) seen in hypertensive retinopathy and vein occlusion will likewise block choroidal and retinal fluorescence in early views but may be difficult to see in late views due to

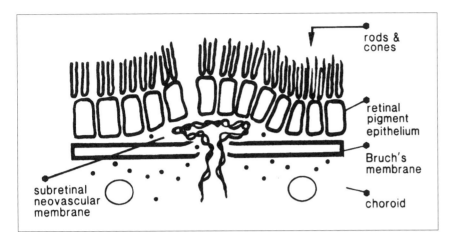

A

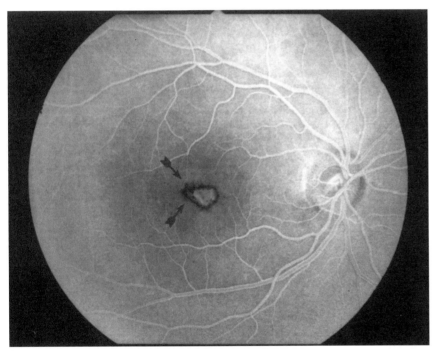

B

FIGURE 5-7
A. Subretinal neovascularization is characterized by the growth of neovascular vessels from the choroid into the subretinal pigment epithelial space. B. Well-delineated subretinal neovascular membrane visible in the early venous phase. Subretinal hemorrhage surrounding the membrane blocks choroidal fluorescence and part of the subretinal membrane (arrows).

the abundant retinal edema sometimes observed with these conditions.

Hard exudates associated with diabetes, Coat's disease, or exudative maculopathy result in a degree of blockage that depends on the density of the accumulated material. Diffuse or cystoid edema associated with diabetic retinopathy, vascular occlusive disease, or after cataract surgery may block fluorescence early in the angiographic study, especially when the fluid is turbid. Edema will hyperfluoresce late in the study, however.

Pigment hyperplasia from inflammatory disease, such as presumed ocular histoplasmosis syndrome, occurring

primarily at the level of the pigment epithelium, will result in blockage of choroidal fluorescence. Such hyperpigmentation may be associated with adjacent areas of pigment loss that hyperfluoresce (Figure 5-9). Pigment and scar tissue resulting from thermal injury such as cryotherapy or photocoagulation will block fluorescence. However, scar tissue tends to hyperfluoresce in late views because of eventual fluorescein staining.

Choroidal Filling Defects
Choroidal vascular filling defects occur as a result of either nonperfusion or absence of choroidal tissue. The clinical

FIGURE 5-8
Intraretinal blot hemorrhages block choroidal fluorescence (arrows) during the venous phase in a patient with background diabetic retinopathy. The tiny points of hyperfluorescence are microaneurysms, which ophthalmoscopically appear similar to dot hemorrhages.

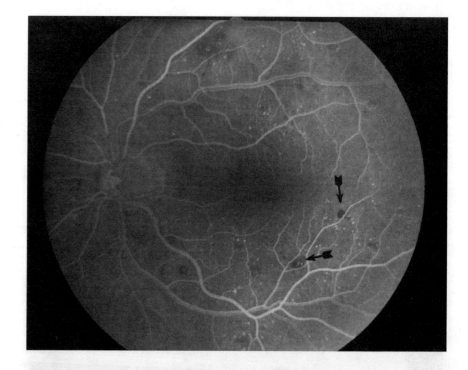

FIGURE 5-9
Presumed ocular histoplasmosis (inactive). Note area of blocked fluorescence resulting from hyperpigmentation surrounded by a ring of hyperfluorescence resulting from hypopigmentation (large arrowhead). Several small hyperfluorescent spots are also present caused by focal loss of pigment (small arrows). Hyperfluorescent areas caused by loss of the pigment epithelial layer are often referred to as "window defects."

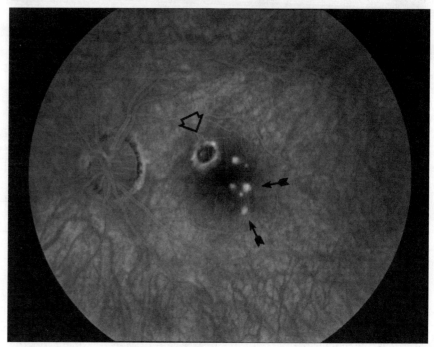

hallmark differentiating nonperfusion from loss of choroid is scleral visibility. When the choroid is absent, the sclera is visible ophthalmoscopically.

Nonperfusion of choroidal tissue may be a result of embolic occlusion, which results in a dark triangular area on angiograms. Isolated areas of nonperfusion may be easily overlooked because the pigment epithelium normally attenuates choroidal fluorescence.

Loss of choroidal tissue may be seen in congenital, hereditary, or degenerative conditions. For example, the choroid is absent when a congenital coloboma is present, thus allowing the sclera to be easily observed through the retina.

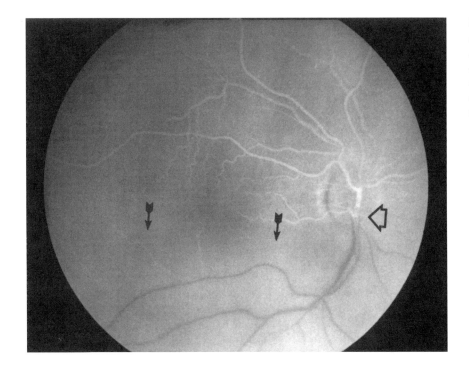

FIGURE 5-10
Branch retinal artery occlusion. Note the absence of filling in the inferior retina (small arrows) because of an arterial plaque in the nerve head region (large arrowhead).

Colobomas appear dark in the early views of an angiogram, but tend to hyperfluoresce during late views because of fluorescein binding to the sclera ("staining"). Choroidal rupture secondary to trauma will result in a similar angiographic appearance.

Dystrophies or degenerations of the pigment epithelium, choriocapillaris, and choroid will affect choroidal fluorescence depending on the extent of atrophy or loss of choroidal tissue. Central areolar atrophy often causes changes of the choriocapillaris, as well as the pigment epithelium, resulting in poor choroidal fluorescence. Similarly, choroideremia, Stargardt's disease, and retinitis pigmentosa may adversely affect the choriocapillaris, resulting in hypofluorescence.

Retinal Filling Defects

Both central retinal artery and central retinal vein occlusion produce hypofluorescence early in an angiographic study. Most often, some degree of patency has returned to the occluded vessels by the time the angiogram is performed.

In central retinal (or branch) artery occlusion, early views show nonperfusion of large areas of the retina (Figure 5-10). These areas are often edematous, and a plaque may be observed at an arteriolar bifurcation. The ophthalmoscopic picture usually corresponds to the angiographic view. Although blood flow may be reestablished, the infarcted area may continue to appear hypofluores-

cent in subsequent angiograms due to necrosis and atrophy of the retinal tissue.

Blockage of the central retinal vein or one of its branches results in a classic retinal appearance of feathered hemorrhage, exudate, and edema. Most often the diagnosis of central retinal (or branch) vein occlusion can be made with the ophthalmoscope. However, fluorescein angiography can be useful in helping to identify areas of retinal capillary nonperfusion as well as edema, neovascularization, and collateral vessels (Figure 5-11). It is important to remember that the extensive hemorrhage seen early in venous occlusive disease frequently obscures underlying details. In this case, fluorescein angiography may be deferred until the hemorrhage has cleared somewhat.

Capillary nonperfusion appears as a dark area of hypofluorescence and is most frequently observed in diabetic retinopathy (Figure 5-12).

Optic Nerve Filling Defects

Filling defects occur in the optic nerve as a result of capillary nonperfusion or an absence of tissue. An example is seen in optic atrophy in which the atrophic, chalky-white disc will appear dark angiographically because of an absence of capillaries.

Because it produces occluded sclerotic arterioles, anterior ischemic optic neuropathy causes a filling defect. Such a disc is edematous and frequently surrounded by flame-

FIGURE 5-11
*Branch retinal vein occlusion—
venous phase. Note blocked fluorescence caused by hemorrhage
(arrows pointing up) and capillary nonperfusion (arrow pointing down). (Courtesy of Leonard
V. Messner, O.D.)*

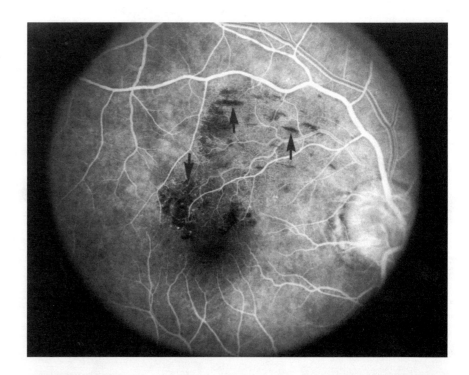

FIGURE 5-12
*Extensive capillary nonperfusion
in a patient with proliferative diabetic retinopathy. Arrows denote
a few locations where it is most
marked. Pronounced alteration of
the capillary plexus is present,
including widespread formation
of microaneurysms. (Courtesy of
Indre Rudaitis, O.D.)*

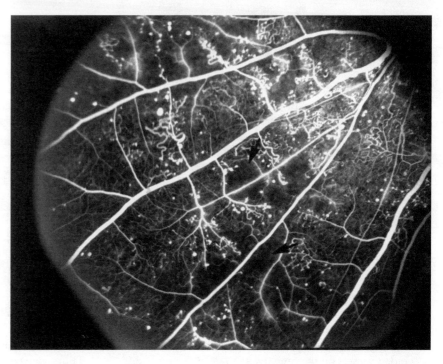

shaped hemorrhages. The disc appears hypofluorescent
in the early views, but often hyperfluoresces late in the
study because of edema.

An optic pit appears dark during early angiographic phases because of an absence of tissue. Optic pits are frequently associated with serous elevation of the sensory retina.

Hyperfluorescence

Hyperfluorescence appears as a light area on a positive
print and is caused by (1) leakage of dye from abnormal
blood vessels, (2) accumulation of dye in an abnormal space
or staining of existing tissues, or (3) greater visibility of dye
due to an attenuation or loss of overlying structures.

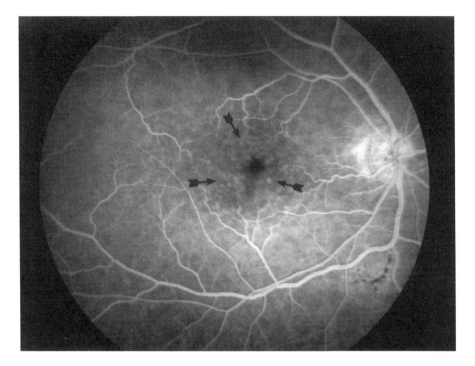

FIGURE 5-13
Relatively early angiographic view of cystoid macular edema. Note the generalized blurring of structures within the macula caused by leakage of dye into the extracellular spaces. Arrows denote relatively focal areas of leakage.

Leakage

Fluorescein leakage occurs when there is a breakdown of the blood–retinal barrier. Leakage is therefore extravascular and is most frequently observed late in the angiogram after blood vessels have emptied available dye. Leakage should not be confused with staining, which also is observed late in the study. Staining occurs when fluorescein binds with tissue during its normal transit through the retina and choroid. Structures that commonly stain are the sclera, normal optic nerve, drusen, and glial scarring.

Retinal edema appears angiographically as late hyperfluorescence because of the gradual accumulation of dye in the extracellular space. Due to its unique architectural structure, retinal edema is commonly pronounced within the macular area but occurs elsewhere as well (Figure 5-13). Edema within the macular region may appear as a diffuse hyperfluorescence or it may be cystic (cystoid macular edema). Edema of the background fundus or macula commonly occurs secondary to diabetic retinopathy and venous occlusion. Macular edema (diffuse or cystic) may also occur after cataract extraction.

Fluorescein pooling occurs in potential spaces, such as those formed by the detachment of the sensory retina from the pigment epithelium, or by the detachment of the pigment epithelium from Bruch's membrane. Sensory retinal detachments tend to result in a hyperfluorescent zone with diffuse borders, whereas RPE detachments cause a hyperfluorescent area with distinct borders. With central serous chorioretinopathy, a focal disruption in the RPE allows fluid to elevate the sensory retina and collect in the subsensory retinal space. Angiographically, this is demonstrated by an early spot of focal fluorescence that then may acquire a "smokestack" appearance as dye permeates the subsensory retinal space (Figure 5-14). RPE detachments are characterized angiographically by a well-delineated zone of hyperfluorescence occurring diffusely throughout the area of detachment that gradually intensifies (Figure 5-15). The hyperfluorescence observed with both subsensory and sub-RPE detachments persists very late in the angiographic study.

Abnormal Vessels

Abnormal vessels within the fundus include aneurysms, neovascularization, arteriolar-venous shunts, and telangiectatic vessels.

Subretinal neovascularization associated with age-related macular degeneration or inflammatory disease is typically well delineated 1–2 seconds before the retinal arterioles fill and then leaks diffusely as the study progresses (see Figure 5-7). The clinician must always be aware that associated hemorrhage often obscures subretinal neovascularization and makes identification difficult.

FIGURE 5-14

A. Central serous chorioretinopathy is characterized by a focal disruption in the retinal pigment epithelium (RPE), which allows fluorescein dye to leak into the subsensory retinal space. B. A small hyperfluorescent spot is present at the site of RPE disruption (arrow) in a patient with central serous chorioretinopathy. C. During late stages of the angiogram, leakage of dye into the subsensory retinal space creates a "smokestack" appearance (large arrowhead). The entire zone of serous sensory retinal elevation is faintly delineated by hyperfluorescence (small arrows). Visual acuity is 20/25.

A
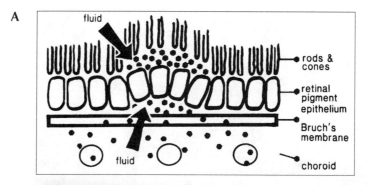

B
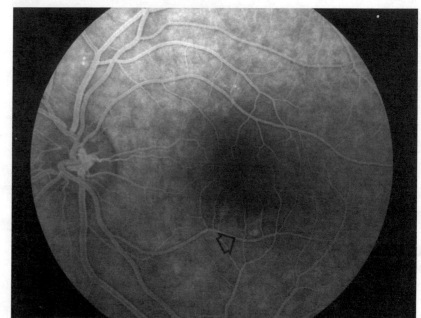

C
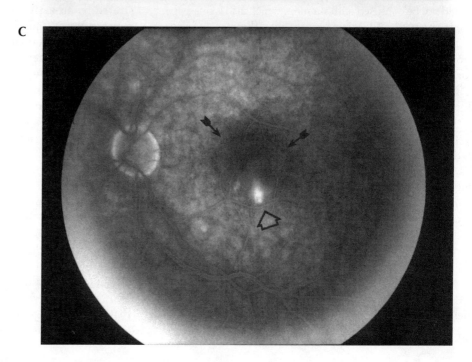

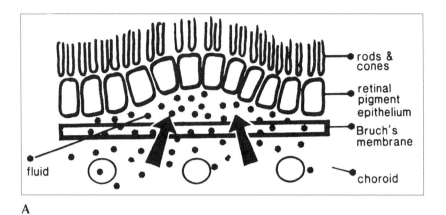

A

FIGURE 5-15
A. Detachment of the retinal pigment epithelium (RPE) allows accumulation of serous fluid within the sub-RPE space.
B. Early focal hyperfluorescence within a well-delineated RPE detachment. Fluorescence occurs diffusely throughout the region of the detachment and gradually increases in intensity. Fluorescence may persist for hours after the completion of the angiogram. (Figure 5-15B courtesy of Leonard V. Messner, O.D.)

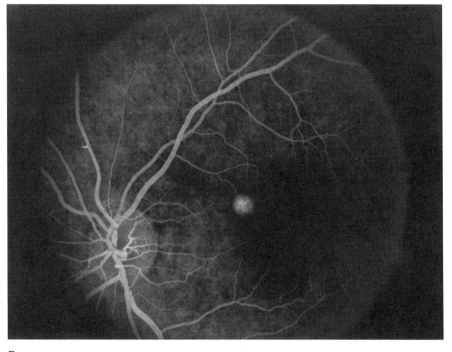

B

Microaneurysmal dilatation occurs most often with diabetic retinopathy (see Figures 5-8 and 5-12). Such microaneurysms represent localized abnormal dilation of vessels within the capillary bed and may appear ophthalmoscopically similar to a dot hemorrhage. Fluorescein angiography aids identification, since microaneurysms are hyperfluorescent. Microaneurysms may also be associated with central retinal vein occlusions and are often observed near areas of neovascularization. Aneurysms tend to leak late during angiography.

Retinal neovascularization is associated with proliferative diabetic retinopathy, as well as other retinal vascular conditions such as venous occlusion and sickle cell retinopathy. Neovascularization is identified in early angiographic views by a lacy network of surface retinal vessels that fill rapidly (Figure 5-16). These vessels leak diffusely in late views.

Collateral or shunt vessels may develop after vascular occlusion. They may also be found with diabetic retinopathy. Collateral (vein to vein) and shunt (artery to vein) vessels are differentiated from neovascularization by an absence of leakage.

Retinal telangiectasis is seen in congenital malformations, Coat's disease, Leber's miliary aneurysms, and degenerative processes, and with epiretinal membrane formation. These vessels are easily identified by early

FIGURE 5-16
A. Disc neovascularization in proliferative diabetic retinopathy appears as a lacy hyperfluorescent network (arrows) during early venous phase. B. Later in the angiogram pronounced hyperfluorescence results from leakage of dye.

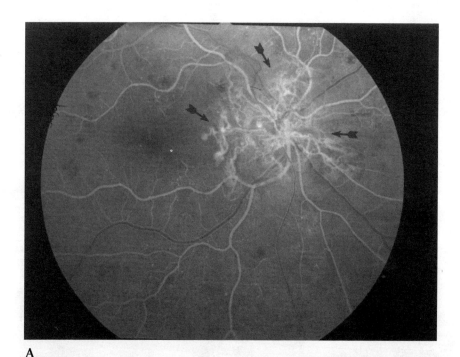

A

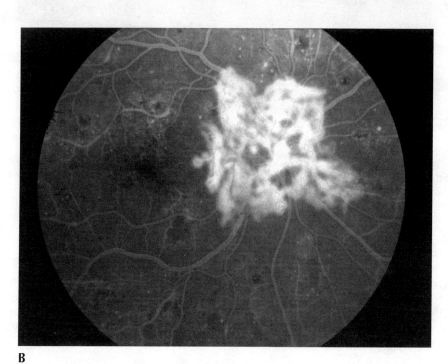

B

hyperfluorescence during angiographic study. They may also leak during later views.

Hyperfluorescence from a solid tumor is likely a result of increased vascularity in the area. Such hyperfluorescence generally is caused by leakage into the extravascular space, which is not observed until late during angiography.

Transmission (Window) Defects
Transmission, or window, defects occur when there is a loss or thinning of overlying tissue, allowing choroidal fluorescence to be easily observed. The loss of pigment epithelium, either because of atrophy or inflammation, gives rise to the classic "window defect" (Figure 5-17).

FIGURE 5-17
A. Retinal pigment epithelial (RPE) "window defects." Loss or thinning of RPE cells allows visualization of choroidal fluorescence. B. Multiple pigment epithelial window defects caused by atrophy of pigment epithelium in age-related macular degeneration.

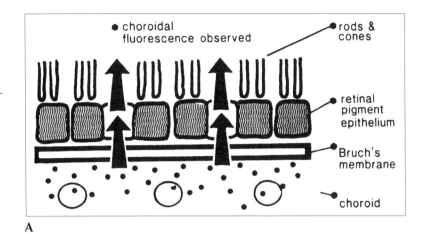

A

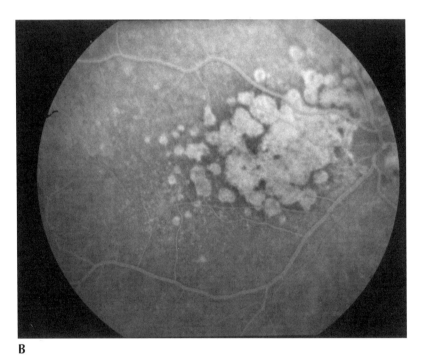

B

Transmission defects also occur with drusen, angioid streaks, and pigment epithelial loss from all causes.

REFERENCES

1. Novotny HR, Alvis DL. A method of photographing fluorescence in circulating blood in the human retina. Circulation 1961;24:82–6.
2. Schatz H, Burton TC, Yannuzi LA, Robb MF. Interpretation of Fundus Fluorescein Angiography. St. Louis: Mosby, 1978.
3. Wessing A. Fluorescein Angiography of the Retina. St. Louis: Mosby, 1969.
4. Berkow JW, Kelley JS, Orth DH. Fluorescein Angiography: A Guide to the Interpretation of Fluorescein Angiograms. Manuals Program, American Academy of Ophthalmology, 1984.
5. Aaberg TM. Fluorescein Angiography. In GA Peyman, DR Sanders, MF Goldberg (eds), Principles and Practice of Ophthalmology (Vol 2). Philadelphia: Saunders, 1980.
6. Alexander LJ. Primary Care of the Posterior Segment. East Norwalk, CT: Appleton & Lange, 1989;78.
7. George TW. Method of Fluorescein Angiography. In A Patz, SL Fine (eds), Interpretation of the Fundus Fluorescein Angiogram. Int Ophthalmol Clin 1977;17:21–33.
8. Anand R. Fluorescein angiography. Part 1. Technique and normal study. J Ophthal Nurs Tech 1989;8:48–52.
9. Federman JL, McGuire JI. Intravenous Fluorescein Angiography. In T Duane (ed), Clinical Ophthalmology (Vol 3). Philadelphia: Lippincott, 1989;5–7.

6

Gonioscopy and Fundus Contact Lens

Daniel K. Roberts and Jack E. Terry

Gonioscopy is the ophthalmic technique by which the angle of the anterior chamber is visualized under dynamic, in vivo conditions. This examination procedure is performed with various goniolenses, which are essentially contact lenses with or without reflecting mirrors and are used in conjunction with the slit lamp or a hand-held illuminator and magnifier. Use of the goniolens is necessary because the angle structures cannot be viewed by direct inspection, since the overlying sclera and the corneoscleral limbus are opaque. In addition, the light rays originating from the drainage angle undergo total internal reflection because of the limitation of the critical angle (46 degrees) associated with the cornea-to-air refractive index interface.[1] Hence, the rays are reflected back into the eye as seen in Figure 6-1.

While gonioscopy is not routinely performed on patients, it is commonly used on patients suspected of having glaucoma so that the proper classification can be made rationally (e.g., open, narrow, closed, pigmentary, secondary, and so forth).[2] It is of particular importance inasmuch as findings of the angle tissue (primarily the functioning portion of the trabeculum overlying Schlemm's canal) and an evaluation of the distance of the root of the iris from the trabeculum are the fundamental bases for a distinction between angle-closure glaucoma and open-angle glaucoma (e.g., actual or potential angle block). However, it must be realized that gonioscopy does not assist in differentiating primary open-angle glaucoma from ocular hypertension because of the relatively normal angles of the anterior chambers in both conditions (i.e., the widths may range from wide open to narrow in both populations). Another valuable function of gonioscopy is an evaluation of the angle before dilation is initiated. The oblique illumination (flashlight test)[3] and van Herick[4] slit lamp procedures have been summarized[5] and shown to afford highly specific and sensitive results when compared

with gonioscopy.[6] However, it must be realized that the chamber angle structural elements are being indirectly assessed in these secondary evaluation methods. Hence, gonioscopy offers the practitioner the only means with which to study the angle width firsthand so that a more justifiable decision can be made regarding the appropriateness of pupil dilation in patients having very narrow angles as found on the flashlight and van Herick tests.

Gonioscopy has also been shown to be useful in localizing and estimating the extent of involvement of iris or ciliary body masses, since the area behind the iris (posterior chamber), ciliary processes, zonules, and the equator of the lens can often be seen through the widely dilated pupil. Additionally, this technique affords an opportunity to evaluate suspected foreign bodies in the recesses of the anterior chamber angle[7,8] as well as the extent of peripheral anterior synechiae.[9]

GONIOSCOPIC ANATOMY

To become proficient at the gonioscopic examination, the practitioner must first have a thorough understanding of iridocorneal angle anatomy (Figure 6-2). Aside from having knowledge of the basic structures, it must be realized that even the normal chamber angle has immense variability and only with sufficient experience will one be able to accurately assess the angle appearance. To prevent confusion it is helpful for the examiner to follow a systematic approach in order to localize and identify the normal and abnormal structural appearance of the angle. A typical manner in which to proceed is to first start at the iris and then progress toward the corneal side of the angle. Specific structures to be identified along the way are the pupil border, peripheral iris, ciliary body, scleral spur, trabecular meshwork, and Schwalbe's line. These

93</>

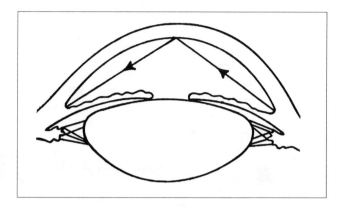

FIGURE 6-1
Since light rays from the anterior chamber angle strike the cornea-to-air interface at an angle greater than the critical angle, they are reflected internally. (Adapted with permission from LG Gray. Fundamentals of gonioscopy. Rev Optom 1977;(Oct.):52.)

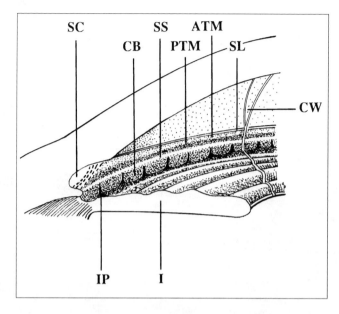

FIGURE 6-2
Schematic representation of gonioscopic anatomy. (I = iris; IP = iris process; CB = ciliary body; SS = scleral spur; SC = Schlemm's canal; PTM = posterior trabecular meshwork; ATM = anterior trabecular meshwork; SL = Schwalbe's line; CW = corneal wedge.)

have been described as the six cardinal features of the iridocorneal angle and should be understood and evaluated in detail.[10,11]

Pupil Border

Aside from allowing for rapid orientation, the practitioner should routinely evaluate the pupil border for certain pathologic features. Some of these include posterior synechiae, neovascularization, sphincter atrophy, iris cysts, and the white dandruff-like flecks that may accumulate along the pupil border in pseudoexfoliation syndrome.

Peripheral Iris

Several aspects of the peripheral iris should be evaluated. First of all, the anterior stromal surface is examined for neovascularization, atrophy, hypoplasia, tumors, and so forth. With regard to the anatomic relationship between the far peripheral iris and the inner wall of the eye, three aspects should be studied.[10–13] These include (1) the angular approach, (2) the curvature or configuration of the last iris roll, and (3) the location of the insertion of the iris root (Figure 6-3).

The angular approach is the estimated angular subtense between the anterior iris surface and the inner wall of the trabecular meshwork. According to Spaeth,[12] the tangent to the anterior iris surface is estimated at a location about one-third the distance from the most peripheral portion of the iris. Determination of this relationship is impor-

tant for assessing the probability of pupil block and subsequent angle closure. Angle closure is more likely the smaller the angular subtense.

The last roll of the peripheral iris greatly contributes to the depth and extent of the angle recess and is related to certain pathologic states of the angle. The peripheral iris can be posteriorly bowed, or concave, as in pigment dispersion syndrome, or convex, as found in the plateau iris configuration. The importance of noting this variable is highlighted with the example of plateau iris syndrome, where the angular approach may be normal yet angle closure is quite possible because of the tendency for the peripheral iris roll to occlude the angle (Figure 6-4). Here the primary mechanism for angle closure is quite different from pupillary block, which more commonly occurs in patients with a very narrow angular approach.

The final aspect of the peripheral iris to be studied is the iris insertion into the inner wall of the eye. Typically the iris root inserts into the ciliary body but may occasionally join the scleral spur or trabecular meshwork. When a very wide ciliary body band is present, differentiation must be made between a posteriorly located insertion of the iris on the ciliary body or the presence of an angle recession. Angle recession is secondary to blunt trauma and results when a tear occurs between the lon-

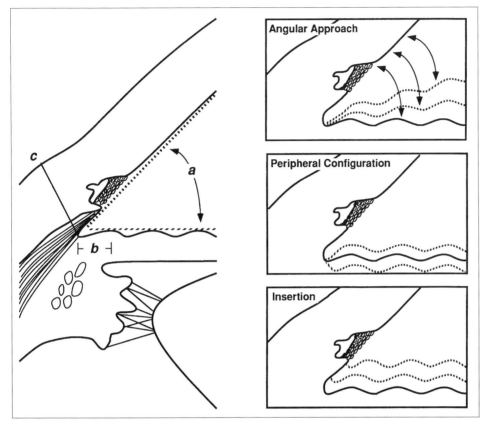

FIGURE 6-3

Three fundamental variables that determine the relationship between the iris and the inner wall of the eye: (a) angular approach; (b) configuration of the peripheral iris; (c) iris insertion. Diagrams on the right demonstrate how each of these may vary. (Adapted with permission from CL Spaeth. The normal development of the human anterior chamber angle: a new system of descriptive grading. Trans Ophthalmol Soc UK 1971;91:709–39.)

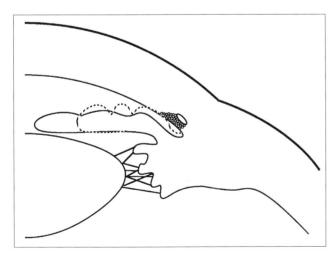

FIGURE 6-4

The plateau iris configuration illustrates the effect that a convex peripheral iris can have on the dynamics of pupil dilation (dotted line). The iris is not bowed along its entire extent and the anterior chamber is of normal depth centrally. Pupil block is absent in this example, but occlusion of the trabecular meshwork occurs nevertheless.

gitudinal and circular muscles of the ciliary body.[14] Gonioscopically, it may simply appear as a widening of the ciliary body band. The trauma associated with such lesions can lead to a secondary glaucoma in many instances. A high or anterior origin of the peripheral iris must be differentiated from peripheral anterior synechia (PAS), which occurs when the peripheral iris becomes attached abnormally to the inner wall of the angle, often blocking the outflow of aqueous humor. Synechiae form where the peripheral iris is pushed or pulled into the inner wall such as with angle closure glaucoma or the contraction of a fibrovascular membrane in the angle (Figure 6-5).

Ciliary Body Band

The gonioscopically visible ciliary body band represents the anterior end of the ciliary muscle which is bounded by the iris root posteriorly and the scleral spur anteriorly. In a normal eye its width varies considerably depending on a high or low iris insertion. A very wide band may indicate the presence of an angle recession as described in the previous section. A broad band is also commonly

FIGURE 6-5

Gonioscopic image of a relatively large, broad-based peripheral anterior synechia inserting anterior to Schwalbe's line. (PAS = peripheral anterior synechia; SL = Schwalbe's line; TM = trabecular meshwork; SS = scleral spur; CB = ciliary body.)

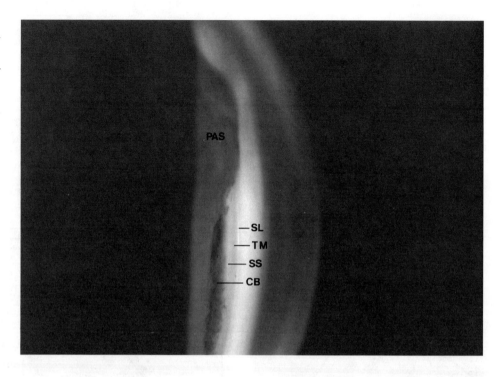

found in the very wide angle associated with the pigment dispersion syndrome. The color of the band has extreme variability as well. Contributing to the color is pigmentation within the ciliary muscle itself and the variability in the density and pigmentation of the overlying uveal meshwork.[15] The uveal meshwork is a thin layer of ropelike trabeculae that lines the anterior chamber angle from the iris root to the peripheral cornea. It may not be visible in some eyes; however, it can appear as a darkly pigmented, dense syncytium leading to greater or lesser visibility of other angle structures. In addition to the uveal meshwork, separate slender fibers arise from the peripheral iris and bridge the angle recess to attach near the scleral spur or anterior trabecular meshwork. These fine strands are referred to as iris processes and can also vary considerably in their density, color, and location of insertion (Figure 6-6).[16] In certain pathologic situations such as the Axenfeld-Rieger syndrome, exaggerated processes extend up to attach to Schwalbe's line. Unlike peripheral anterior synechiae, in which the iris becomes pathologically attached to the trabecular wall, iris processes do not impede aqueous outflow.

Another variability of the ciliary body band is the presence or absence of prominent blood vessels.[17] Normal blood vessels are more commonly observed in blue-eyed individuals, and they can be radially or circumferentially arranged. It is important to differentiate normal vessels from those of pathologic angle neovascularization.

Scleral Spur

The scleral spur, an extremely helpful localizing landmark, forms the anterior boundary of the ciliary body band and the posterior boundary of the trabecular meshwork. It acts as the insertion point for longitudinal ciliary muscle fibers and also serves as the posterior wall of the scleral sulcus, which forms a portion of Schlemm's canal. Clinically it appears as a whitish band of varying width. Whether it is visible in a wide open angle is somewhat dependent on the pigmentation and density of the overlying uveal meshwork.

Trabecular Meshwork

The trabecular meshwork consists of a porous network of trabecular sheets through which aqueous humor passes from the anterior chamber to Schlemm's canal. Gonioscopically, it extends from the scleral spur to Schwalbe's line. Its visibility and coloration vary markedly depending on pigmentation within the trabeculum and the density of the overlying uveal meshwork. When free of pigment, the region usually is light gray and has a fine granular texture. If significant pigmentation is present, the trabeculum may be clinically divided into anterior and posterior zones. Pigment accumulates predominantly in the posterior half of the meshwork, which approximates the more actively fil-

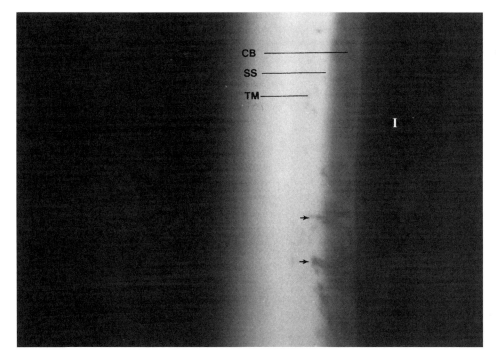

FIGURE 6-6
Gonioscopic image of iris processes (arrows). (I = iris; CB = ciliary body; SS = scleral spur; TM = trabecular meshwork.)

tering portion of the trabeculum. The anterior half may also contain some pigment but usually substantially less than the posterior trabeculum.

Schlemm's canal lies within the scleral sulcus and serves as a collection channel for aqueous humor that drains through the trabecular meshwork. Gonioscopically, it may sometimes be visualized as a faint gray line within the posterior trabeculum, but it is generally undetectable. Occasionally, blood may accumulate in Schlemm's canal, especially when intraocular pressure is very low, or episcleral venous pressure is high. This is visualized as a bright red band within the filtration portion of the posterior trabecular meshwork. Clinically, this may be a useful phenomenon for localizing the trabeculum, when accidental or intentional pressure is applied to the episcleral vessels with the rim of the gonioscopic lens.

Once the trabecular meshwork has been localized, evaluation is imperative for differentiation of the various glaucomas. When excessive pigmentation is present with associated elevated intraocular pressures, one must consider pigment dispersion glaucoma and pseudoexfoliative glaucoma (Figure 6-7). Abnormal vascularization of the trabeculum and adjacent structures would lead one to consider neovascular glaucoma. Similarly, a perfectly normal appearing, wide open angle with associated elevated pressures would indicate primary open-angle glaucoma.

Schwalbe's Line

Schwalbe's line marks the termination of Descemet's membrane and the most anterior extension of the trabecular meshwork. It normally appears as a thin, white, glistening line projecting slightly into the anterior chamber (see Figures 6-5 and 6-8). It is often difficult to detect clinically. However, localization may be aided by projecting a thin slit beam into the iridocorneal angle.[18] The optic section of the cornea will be seen to taper into a two-dimensional light beam at Schwalbe's line, because this is the junction between the transparent cornea and translucent trabeculum. The portion of the cornea between the interior and exterior edges of the optic section is referred to as the corneal wedge (see Figure 6-2). The slight protuberance of Schwalbe's line often provides a small shelf for accumulation of pigment along its anterior border, especially in the inferior quadrant. This is referred to as a Sampaolesi's line (see Figure 6-7). It is occasionally seen in normal eyes but is more common in patients with pigment dispersion syndrome or pseudoexfoliation syndrome.

In about 15% of patients, Schwalbe's line is prominent and anteriorly displaced.[19] In this instance the line is referred to by the term *posterior embryotoxon*, or simply, prominent anterior border ring of Schwalbe. It is conspicuous both externally (Figure 6-9) and during gonioscopic examination. It is a benign finding when it occurs alone, but in the congenital syndrome of Axenfeld-Rieger,

FIGURE 6-7
Dense pigment within the posterior trabecular meshwork in a patient with pigment dispersion syndrome (long arrow). Pigment has also collected along Schwalbe's line, which is referred to as a Sampaolesi's line (short arrow).

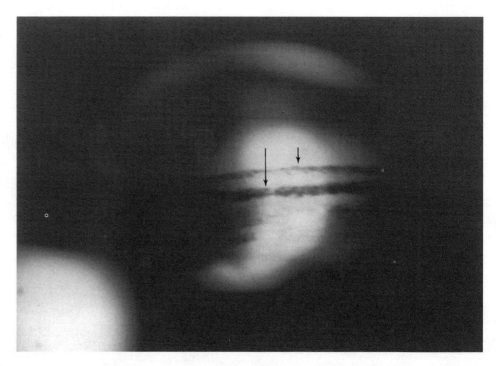

prominent iris processes adhere to the line with an associated increase in intraocular pressure caused by malformation of the angle.

TECHNIQUE

Gonioscopy lenses are used to examine the angle structures of the eye and are divided into two categories according to design—i.e., whether the angle is visualized directly or indirectly with the use of mirrors (Figure 6-10). The various goniolenses, however, are all some form of contact lens design. A brief description of the different lenses is given because the technique by which gonioscopy is performed is determined by the design of the lens.

The Goldmann three-mirror, or universal, lens has each mirror inclined at a slightly different angle so that, in addition to the angle structures of the anterior chamber, an evaluation of the ciliary body and retinal periphery can be obtained. The Zeiss, Sussman, and Thorpe four-mirror lenses have each mirror inclined at the same angle so that the examiner can view four quadrant sections of the angle without rotating the goniolens. These four indirect lenses all have in common a smooth, nonflanged base and hence are retained on the eye by finger pressure and the surface tension provided by the tear film or a solution of methylcellulose (depending on the instrument). The

patient is examined while seated at the slit lamp, and its light source and magnification are used.

A second gonioscopic lens design is that with a flanged or scleral haptic, which allows the lens to be retained between the lids. The most noted example of this variety is the Koeppe direct goniolens, which is applied over the cornea utilizing a layer of methylcellulose between the lens and cornea.

In addition, the patient is placed in a reclining posture, since the patient's head must be kept in a nearly horizontal position. The angle structures are then viewed through a hand-held gonioscopy microscope. Bright focal illumination is provided by a Barkan illuminator, which is held in the other hand. The Koeppe lens gives greater magnification of angle details than other designs.[20] However, in addition to the goniolens, a gonioscopy microscope (gonioscope) and illuminator must be purchased since the direct Koeppe method does not make use of the slit lamp.

Indirect Procedure

A number of advantages and disadvantages exist for the direct and indirect goniolenses and are summarized in Table 6-1. The following discussion will include the detailed angle evaluation procedures for the aforementioned lenses, with preferential analysis being given to the Goldmann indirect goniolens.

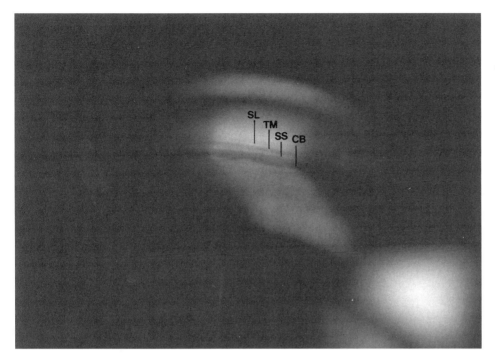

FIGURE 6-8
Gonioscopic image of a normal chamber angle illustrating a fairly prominent Schwalbe's line. (SL = Schwalbe's line; TM = trabecular meshwork; SS = scleral spur; CB = ciliary body.)

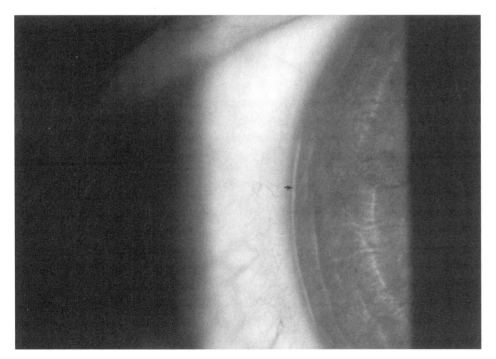

FIGURE 6-9
External photograph of a prominent, anteriorly displaced Schwalbe's line, also referred to as posterior embryotoxon (arrow).

Goldmann Goniolenses

The three Goldmann goniolenses (Figure 6-11) all have radius of curvatures of 7.4 mm but differing overall diameters of 15.5 and 18.5 mm (one- and two-mirror lenses versus the larger three-mirror lens). The three-mirror lens has one mirror to view the chamber angle, and the other two are used to observe the peripheral retina.

Initially, an adult patient should have one or two drops of 0.5% proparacaine instilled into the cul-de-sac. A small amount of a cushioning agent such as 1% methylcellulose or 1% carboxymethylcellulose (Celluvisc) solution is placed on the concave back surface of the Goldmann goniolens (Figure 6-12A). This permits some mechanical cushioning of the corneal epithelium and also completes

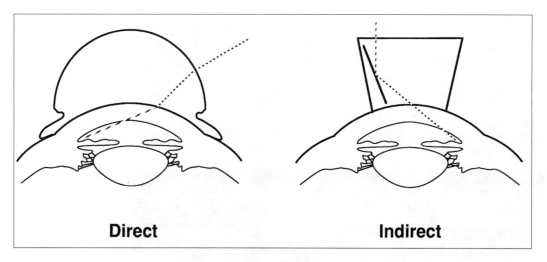

FIGURE 6-10
Schematic representation of the direct and indirect methods of gonioscopy.

the critical lens-cornea contact. If a commercially available agent such as Goniosol is used, the solution should be stored upside down to prevent air bubbles from coming out of the bottle into the concave surface of the goniolens. The patient is then positioned on the chin rest of the biomicroscope with the light turned on. The lens, being held between the thumb and forefinger of one hand, is brought close to the patient's eye while the index finger of the other hand, or the middle finger of the same hand, is used to draw down the lower lid as the patient looks upward. The lower edge of the lens is then inserted against the center of the lower lid border between the limbus and cul-de-sac fornix. The lens should be rotated so that the semicircular mirror (versus the two flat-edged mirrors) is placed in the 12-o'clock position. The upper lid is then drawn away from the globe. The goniolens is now angled inward, bringing its concave surface gently against the patient's cornea. The upper lid is slowly released to drop against the upper surface of the goniolens. The patient is encouraged to relax, to maintain the primary position of gaze, and to not squeeze his or her eyelids (Figure 6-12B and 6-12C).

An additional technique with which the examiner may feel comfortable is to position the patient at the illuminated slit lamp. The patient is then asked to look down, and the right upper lid is held securely against the orbital rim by the examiner's left index finger while the thumb on the same hand applies traction to the lower lid. The goniolens is held in the right hand with the semicircular mirror in the vertical position (for viewing the inferior angle). The patient is then instructed to look straight

TABLE 6-1
Some Contrasting Features of Direct and Indirect Gonioscopy

Feature	Direct	Indirect
Image	Virtual Erect	Virtual Inverted
Goniolens magnification	Magnified (1.5×)	Nonmagnified
Gonioscope magnification	Goniomicroscope-dependent	Biomicroscope-dependent
Illumination source	Focal illuminator	Biomicroscope
Stereopsis	Excellent	Good
Field of view	Larger	Smaller; limited by size of goniomirror
Angle detail	Fair	Excellent
Narrow angle observation	Excellent	Good
Lateral angle observation	Less difficult	More difficult
Patient position	Supine	Erect
Examiner position	Above patient	Slit lamp observation

Source: Modified with permission from LG Gray. Fundamentals of gonioscopy. Rev Optom 1977;10(Oct.):56.

ahead or slightly down. The lower edge of the goniolens is pivoted onto the cornea. The patient is then asked to look straight ahead while relaxing and not blinking. The examiner finally switches the grip of the lens to the other hand so that he or she can get into position behind the slit lamp.

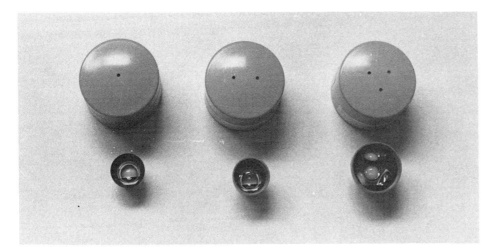

FIGURE 6-11
The one-, two-, and three-mirror Goldmann goniolenses and their identifying caps.

When slit lamp gonioscopy is being performed (Figure 6-12D) the microscope lamp and line of observation first are brought to coincidence on the reflecting surface positioned at the upper pole so that the lower angle can be studied. It may be necessary to tilt the lens at various points of examination to visualize better the more narrowed angles. Initial contact should be relatively light to avoid unknowingly manipulating open an angle that has been physiologically closed or to avoid artificially giving a narrow appearance to an open angle; hence, the lens should rest so lightly against the cornea that any less pressure would allow air bubbles to form. The slit lamp magnification can be varied depending on the structure being visualized, but moderate to high magnification (16–35×) is generally preferable. Diffuse or broad-beam illumination should first be used to identify the landmarks of the angle and major pathologic conditions. The beam can be narrowed to a thin slit to demonstrate the precise curvature of the iris surface into the angle. The entire circumference of the angle is inspected by rotating the goniolens and moving the light and line of observation to appropriate mirror positions.

Indirect slit lamp gonioscopy of the upper angle is at times more difficult than that of the lower. In addition, focusing into the medial and lateral areas is the most difficult for the novice gonioscopist because it affords the least latitude in aligning the light and observational axes. Indirect illumination may be useful in the horizontal recesses if it seems impossible to obtain direct illumination and visualization in good coordination. To avoid distortion of trabecular details by oblique inspection, the observer's line of sight should be nearly parallel to the surface of the iris. In narrow-angled eyes, however, the oblique view precludes critical evaluation of structures beneath the trabeculum (scleral spur, and so forth) and gives a foreshortened illusion of the extent of the meshwork.

The procedure to disengage the goniolens from the patient's eye is first to break the vacuum that has been created between the cornea and posterior lens surface (Figure 6-12E). This is accomplished by gently raising or rocking the lower lens edge to allow the entry of air. The lens can then be gently removed from the eye by a slight separation of the lids. The lens should not be pulled forcibly from the eye. Once the goniolens is removed, it is important to carefully and thoroughly rinse the viscous methylcellulose solution from the goniolens; it should not be allowed to dry on the lens. In addition, the eye should be lavaged with an irrigating solution to remove the excess methylcellulose (Figure 6-12F).

Zeiss Goniolens
The Zeiss four-mirror goniolens has an optic zone of 9.0 mm, which is significantly smaller than that of the Goldmann goniolenses. It also has a flatter (7.85 mm) posterior radius of curvature. All of its mirror surfaces are inclined at an angle of 64 degrees to view the chamber angle.

The Zeiss lens is held by the Unger handle, which acts in a tweezer-like fashion to cradle the lens. The handle is held between the thumb and index finger. The lens is placed on the anesthetized cornea with the tear film of the patient acting as the contact medium; no methylcellulose is necessary (Figure 6-13).

The examiner gently rests his or her remaining fingers against the cheek of the patient to provide stability. Careful attention is given to the interface between

FIGURE 6-12

Stepwise procedure for use of the Goldmann three-mirror lens. A. Cushioning agent is placed onto the concave surface of the lens. B, C. While the patient looks up, the lower lid is pulled down and the inferior lens edge is placed in contact with the globe. The lens is then angled forward until in complete contact with the cornea. D. Once the lens is in position, the slit beam is reflected into the angle via the semicircular mirror. The angle visualized is directly opposite the mirror position. E. For lens removal, the patient looks upward and the inferior lens edge is tilted upward. The examiner may apply slight pressure against the globe with his or her index finger to help break any vacuum that exists. F. The eye may be irrigated for removal of any remaining cushioning agent.

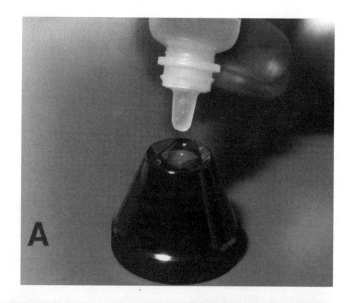

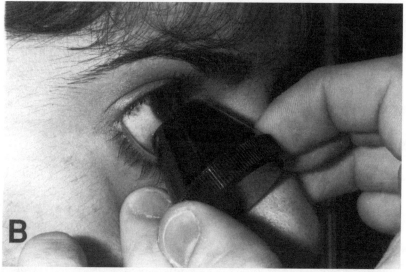

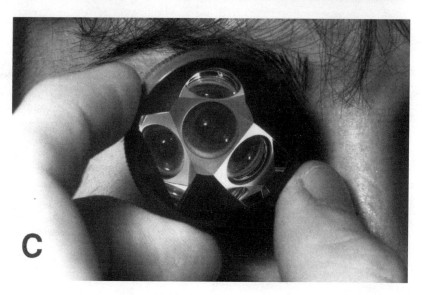

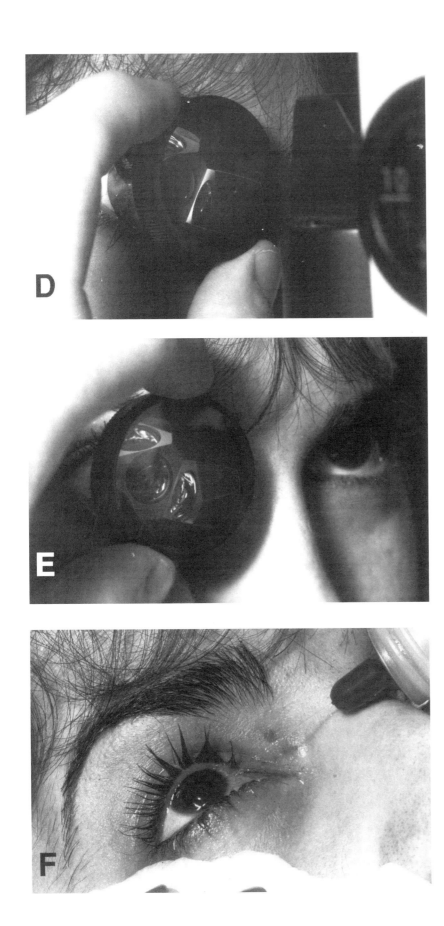

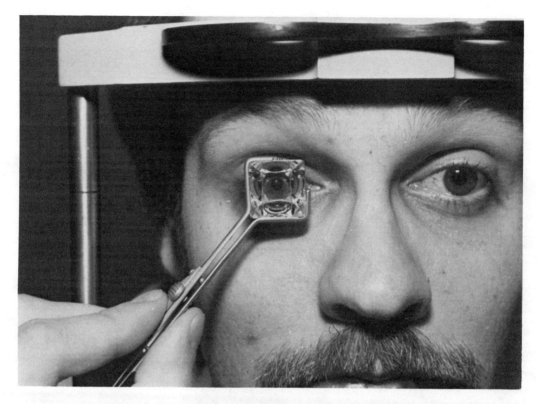

FIGURE 6-13
The Zeiss four-mirror goniolens is being held on the eye with the Unger holder.

the cornea and lens. When this is broken, or the lens is moved off-center, distortion of the angle anatomy can occur and error in judging the iridocorneal relationships can be made. A gentle, uniform pressure is required. When excessive or uneven pressure is applied, the examiner may observe folds in the posterior corneal surface (Figure 6-14). This phenomenon may provide very useful feedback for optimum positioning and pressure from the lens.

Although mastering use of the Zeiss lens is more difficult than mastering use of the Goldmann lens, it is preferred by many clinicians for routine gonioscopy because it allows for very rapid evaluation of the chamber angle. Because no methylcellulose is required, the steps of filling the lens with the cushioning agent and rinsing the eye are eliminated.

The technique for the Sussman four-mirror gonioscope (Figure 6-15), which is a variation of the Zeiss lens, is very similar except it is designed for direct hand-held use. The lens has a small diameter base like the Zeiss, but the viewing side has a rounded grip for ease of rotation and tilt.

Because of their small diameter bases, the Zeiss and Sussman goniolenses are especially well suited for compres-

sion gonioscopy to differentiate between appositional and synechial angle closure (discussed in a later section).

Direct Procedure

The procedures by which direct gonioscopy is performed are actually quite dissimilar from those of the indirect method, even though both render an evaluation of the anterior chamber angle. Initially, one or two drops of proparacaine 0.5% are instilled into each eye. The patient is then positioned supine in the examination chair, with the patient's head turned approximately 45 degrees toward the examiner and the eye under investigation straight ahead. Therefore, the doctor is standing next to the head of the patient, who is looking at the examiner's nose. The Koeppe lens (Figure 6-16) is held between the thumb and forefinger of the right hand (right eye examination) so that it can readily be rotated. The patient is again reminded to retain critical fixation of the examiner's nose. This allows the examiner to slowly move his or her head and correctly position the eye for lens insertion. Hence, the examiner moves up slightly, so that the patient's eyes are turned upward while the examiner uses the opposite

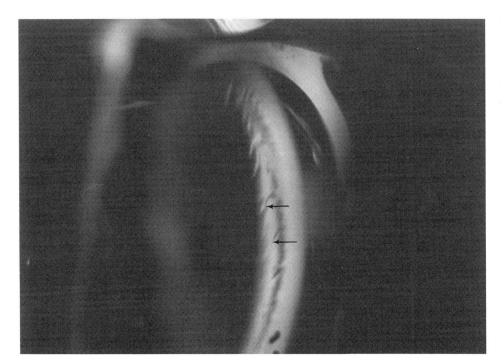

FIGURE 6-14
Folds (arrows) on the posterior corneal surface are observed when excessive or uneven pressure is applied with the Zeiss four-mirror goniolens. The angle is out of focus underlying the corneal folds in this photograph.

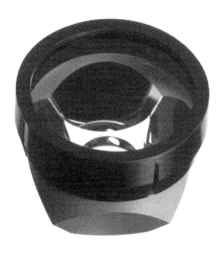

FIGURE 6-15
The Sussman four-mirror goniolens. (Manufactured by Ocular Instruments, Inc., Bellevue, WA.)

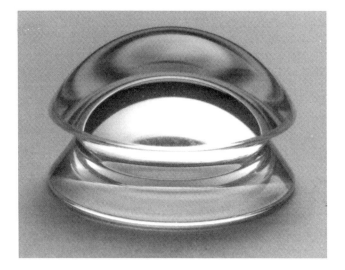

FIGURE 6-16
The Koeppe direct gonioscopic lens. (Manufactured by Ocular Instruments, Inc., Bellevue, WA.)

hand to pull down the lower lid. The lower edge of the lens is placed into the cul-de-sac while the top remains angled away from the superior limbus. The pressure exerted by the fingers holding down the lower lid is gently released. The same fingers are then used to lift the upper lid so that the lens can be pivoted back against the eye.

The space between the cornea and the posterior surface of the goniolens must be filled with either a solution of isotonic sodium chloride or 1% methylcellulose. This is accomplished when the examiner slightly lifts the nasal edge of the lens and allows the fluid to flow into the cavity. The index finger of the hand that was holding the

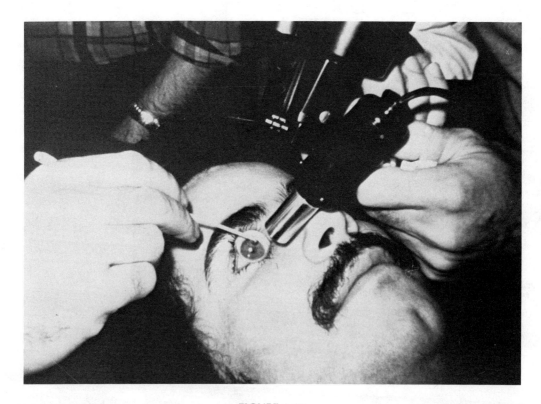

FIGURE 6-17
The direct Koeppe lens is positioned on the supine patient's right eye. The angle is illuminated through the goniolens with a direct focal illuminator while it is viewed simultaneously with a magnifier. An assistant may help position the lens. (Courtesy of L.G. Gray, O.D.)

upper lid is now placed on the dimple of the contact lens, which is pushed directly back toward the pupil. This creates a small relative vacuum due to the displaced excess fluid and aids in holding the lens on the eye and in preventing bubbles.

The patient is now repositioned so that his or her head is turned upright. This, again, is accomplished by the examiner leaning over the patient so that forward fixation is maintained. The lens can also be steadied by an assistant with an applicator, but this is not always mandatory. The magnification is provided by a supported overhead microscope, while the Barkan illuminator serves as the light source (Figure 6-17).

When an extremely narrow angle is being examined with the Koeppe lens, the gonioscopist needs simply to adjust the viewing angle of the hand-held microscope and illuminator. This repositioning normally does not require repositioning of the lens.

Indirect gonioscopy is better suited for general optometric practice because it only requires the use of equipment already available (i.e., a biomicroscope) once the goniolens is obtained. In addition, the patient can remain in a sitting position, and an assistant is not normally required. Campbell has determined that the Goldmann goniolens is almost as effective as the Koeppe goniolens in determining whether the angle is open or closed.[21]

CLASSIFYING ANGLE WIDTH

Aside from the detection and examination of angle abnormalities such as neovascularization, excessive pigmentation, tumors, inflammatory debris, and so forth, the clinician must become adept at grading the angle width. The importance of this skill is to not only determine whether the angle is closed at the time of examination, but also to determine the potential for closure. Several systems have been devised that attempt to correlate gonioscopic appearance with the potential for angle closure. None of them is perfect, and each emphasizes certain aspects of the iridocorneal anatomy (Table 6-2). The examiner must be aware of their limitations and realize that multiple variables must actually be considered when grading the angle.

TABLE 6-2
Comparison of Anterior Chamber Angle Grading Systems

Scheie (1957)[22]	Most Posterior Structure Visible	Interpretation
Grade of angle width is based on extent of visible structures. The fewer structures visible, the more likely is angle closure. Incidence of angle closure relatively high in grade III and IV narrow angles.	All structures with ease Ciliary body with difficulty Scleral spur Anterior trabecular meshwork Only Schwalbe's line	Wide open Grade I narrow Grade II narrow Grade III narrow Grade IV narrow

Shaffer (1960)[23]	Angular Approach	Interpretation
Emphasizes angular approach between iris and inner wall of the eye. Increased risk of angle closure when angle becomes smaller than 20 degrees. Angle closure probably inevitable with grade 1.	Wide open (20–45 degrees) Moderately narrow (20 degrees) Extremely narrow (10 degrees) Closed (0 degrees)	Grades 3–4 Grade 2 Grade 1 Grade 0

Spaeth (1971)[12]	Angular Approach	Configuration	Iris Insertion
Considers other variables important in addition to angular approach (peripheral iris configuration and iris insertion). Examples: The designation D40s indicates a fairly open angle with an anterior ciliary body insertion, a steep peripheral configuration, and 40-degree approach. Angle closure is more likely in a D20s angle than a D20r or D20q angle.	40 degrees 30 degrees 20 degrees 10 degrees 0 degrees	Concave or queer (q) Regular (r) Convex or steep (s)	E = posterior ciliary body D = anterior ciliary body C = scleral spur B = trabecular meshwork A = Schwalbe's line

Becker (1972)[27]	TM Width	Insertion on CB
Considers apparent width of trabeculum and site of iris insertion. Probability of angle closure increases the more anterior the insertion and the thinner the apparent width of the trabecular band. Examples: The designation 3-C indicates a wide trabeculum and a posterior iris insertion; angle closure is not possible. Angle closure is more likely in a 1-A angle than a 1-C angle.	3 = wide 2 = average 1 = narrow 0 = not visible	C = posterior B = middle A = anterior 0 = not visible

The Scheie[22] system is based exclusively on the extent of gonioscopically visible structures. Here, easy visibility of the entire ciliary body band implies a wide open angle. A grade-I narrow angle is characterized by slight narrowing, but part of the ciliary body band can be visualized. The narrowest angle is a grade IV, which implies possible closure of the angle.

One of the most popular grading systems is that devised by Shaffer.[23] It has been adopted jointly by the United States Public Health Service Committee on Glaucoma and the Symposium on Primary Glaucoma.[24] It is based exclusively on the estimated angular extent between the iris and the inner wall of the eye at the trabecular meshwork.

The angle is described as wide open (grade 3 to 4) when the angular width is between 20 and 45 degrees. The details of the trabeculum and recess can be visualized with either no or minimal tilting of the goniolens. The iris generally appears flat with little convexity. Physiologic pupillary

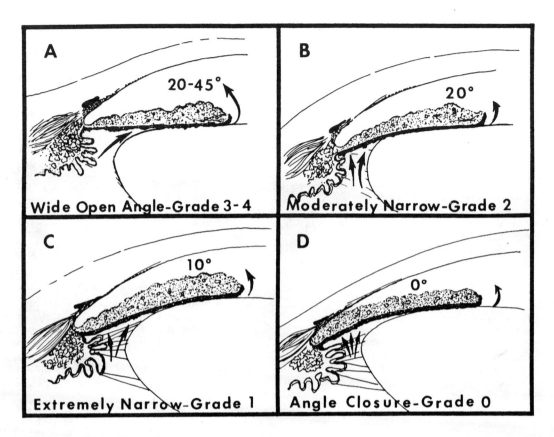

FIGURE 6-18

The various Shaffer grades (4 to 0) are shown diagrammatically in cross section from wide open to closed. (Modified with permission from HD Hoskins, MA Kass. Becker-Shaffer's Diagnosis and Therapy of the Glaucomas [6th ed]. St. Louis: Mosby, 1989;108–9.)

block and angle closure are impossible. Figure 6-18A schematically depicts such a wide open angle. A photographic example is shown in Figure 6-19.

The angle is classified as being moderately narrow (grade 2) when the iridocorneal angle is approximately 20 degrees. A moderately convex iris surface is often apparent, but trabecular details can usually be visualized without excessive tilting and manipulation of the goniolens. It must be remembered, however, that the goniolens may have to be slightly rotated toward the angle being examined so that the line of sight passes over the last roll of the iris (Figure 6-20).[25] The crystalline lens is slightly anterior to the ciliary body ring, and there is moderately broad contact between the posterior iris surface centrally and the anterior lens capsule. Closure of the angle is possible; the earlier in life such an angle is seen, the greater the likelihood of closure in later years.[26] Figure 6-18B shows such a moderately narrow angle in cross section. A photographic example is shown in Figure 6-21.

An anterior chamber angle is classified as extremely narrow (grade 1) when the iridocorneal angle is reduced to approximately 10 degrees and appears slitlike. The angle could close with iris edema or physiologic pupillary block. In any case, closure is usually considered inevitable in time.[26] The crystalline lens is anterior to the ciliary body ring, and a large area of the posterior iris surface is in contact with the anterior lens capsule. Figure 6-18C schematically depicts such an extremely narrow angle. An in vivo example is given in Figure 6-22.

An angle is considered to be closed (Shaffer grade 0) when the anterior iris surface is in contact with the trabeculum. Hence, no anatomic details of the trabecular area can be visualized. The lens is considerably anterior to the ciliary body ring, and the central posterior iris surface is snug against the majority of the anterior lens capsule. Figure 6-18D shows such a closed angle in cross section.

The Spaeth[12,13] system emphasizes three variables of the chamber angle to predict the probability of angle

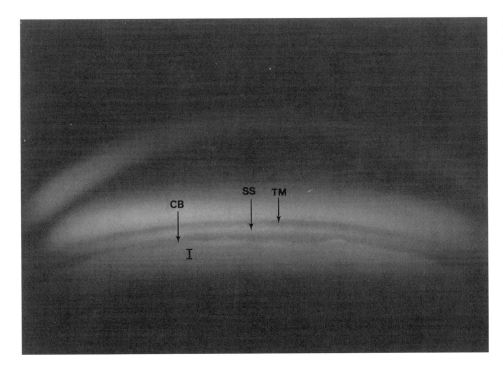

FIGURE 6-19
Gonioscopy of a wide-open anterior chamber angle. Angle closure is not possible. (I = iris; CB = ciliary body; SS = scleral spur; TM = trabecular meshwork.)

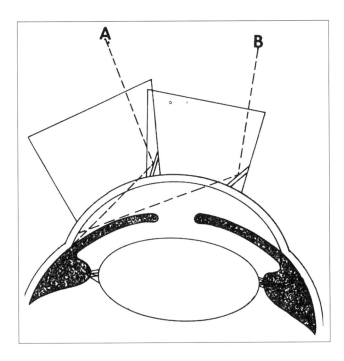

FIGURE 6-20

The goniolens may need to be rotated toward the angle being viewed, in the narrower grades, so that their depths can be more readily observed. This is represented on the illustration as a change from position B to A. (Modified with permission from HD Hoskins Jr. Interpretive gonioscopy in glaucoma. Invest Ophthalmol 1972;11:97–102.)

closure. These include (1) the angular approach, (2) the configuration of the peripheral iris, and (3) the insertion of the iris root. As shown earlier in Figure 6-3, the angular approach is estimated by tangents from the peripheral iris surface and the inner wall of the trabecular meshwork. The peripheral iris configuration may be convex, relatively flat, or concave. The apparent iris insertion may vary from the ciliary body up to Schwalbe's line.

It is felt that although their relative importance may vary, each of these variables may contribute significantly to the probability of angle closure and should be taken into consideration. An excellent example is the plateau iris configuration in which the angular approach may be quite large, but a steep, or convex, peripheral iris brings the iris into close proximity to the trabecular meshwork. Hence, on dilation it is possible that occlusion of the angle will occur (see Figure 6-4).

Becker[27] proposed a system that takes into consideration the width of the visible trabecular band and the point of insertion of the iris on the ciliary body. Numbers are used to designate trabecular width and letters are used to designate iris insertion. The designation 3-C indicates a wide open angle.

Recording the Angle

The anatomic characteristics of any given angle may vary in different regions around the circumference of the eye.

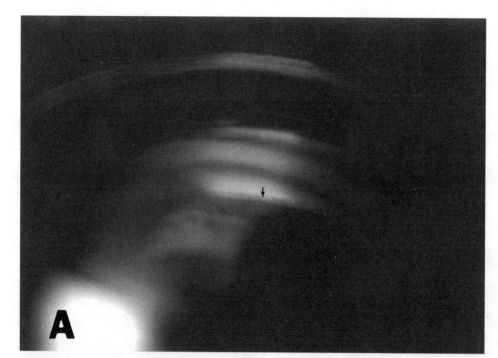

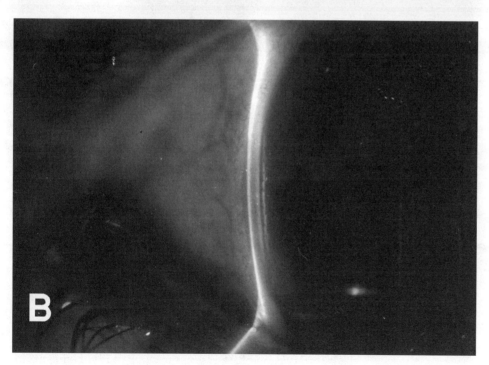

FIGURE 6-21
A. Gonioscopy of a moderately narrow angle. The trabecular meshwork (arrow) is seen without excessive tilting and manipulation of the goniolens. B. The van Herick method of angle estimation shows a relatively narrow separation between the cornea and iris.

The entire 360-degree circumference may be found to be fully open or, as is usual, the angle is narrower above (i.e., 12-o'clock position) than below. It is standard to rate the angle configuration by quadrants. This can be easily displayed by the use of a schematic set of three concentric circles in which the outermost circle represents Schwalbe's line and the middle represents the angle recess.[24] The position and height of synechiae are recorded by drawing radial lines to the anterior limit (Figure 6-23). In addition, the width and intensity of the pigment band of the trabeculum can be graded from 1 through 4, with the most advanced grade 4 filling in about one-half or more of the trabecular width.

General Comments

Campbell[21] evaluated the Koeppe, Goldmann three-mirror, and Zeiss four-mirror lenses on ten eyes with angle-closure glaucoma. He found that the most accurate way to determine whether the angle was open or closed with no artificial opening or distortion was with the Koeppe direct gonioscopy lens because of its wide base (12 mm) and high dome. This lens also provided the examiner with the best view into the extremely narrow angles over a convex iris.

Indirect gonioscopy can artificially narrow an open angle or open a closed angle with pressure from the examining lens. Force from the lens edge at or slightly anterior to the limbus can indent the cornea, change the angle curvature, and give the appearance of a narrower angle than actually exists. In addition, Bell's phenomenon can cause a change in ocular position and contribute to corneal compression and mechanical distortion of the angle.[28] Movement of the lens away from this position allows the angle to open to its original width. Conversely, goniolens pressure over the center of the cornea of the opposite angle can displace aqueous humor into the observed angle. This may give a false impression of a wider angle than is normally found.[28]

Conventional gonioscopy provides a static image of the angle configuration at the particular moment of examination. The extent of occlusion can be determined, but the type of closure cannot be accurately distinguished. The method of gonioscopy for distinguishing between appositional closure and synechial closure basically involves corneal indentation, which widens the anterior chamber angle (Figures 6-22 and 6-24).[9] The Zeiss four-mirror contact goniolens has been found to be best suited for this purpose. After viewing the unaltered angle, the lens is pressed directly against the corneal apex, which displaces aqueous humor to the periphery of the anterior chamber and consequently displaces the peripheral iris posteriorly and widens the angle. The area of appositional closure will be readily opened by this procedure; the peripheral iris will remain adherent to the inner wall of the eye in locations where there are peripheral anterior synechiae. This indentation technique allows the examiner an opportunity to widen a closed angle and see its structures. After forward pressure has been applied, it can then be gradually reduced, and the peripheral iris will be seen to bow forward to reproduce appositional closure. The Koeppe and Goldmann lenses, because of their large fluid-filled chambers, are not suited for indentation gonioscopy because external pressure applied to these lenses is transmitted to the limbal zone and may produce a narrowed angle.[28]

Bedside gonioscopy has been described and shown to provide an interpretable image.[29] This technique may be useful for an examination performed in a nursing home or hospital. The Goldmann goniolens (the larger one-mirror style) is filled with methylcellulose, quickly inverted, and placed on the patient's cornea while the patient is either relaxing in a supine position or in a wheelchair with his or her head tilted back. A bright ophthalmoscope in conjunction with a +25 D lens is used to focus accurately on the angle at about one-fourth inch from the contact lens.

FUNDUS CONTACT AND HRUBY LENSES

Examination of the fundus with the slit lamp biomicroscope offers the advantage of a binocular view as well as greater magnification than that afforded with the indirect ophthalmoscope. To accomplish this task, the refractive power of the eye must be neutralized with a high minus lens placed close to the eye in air or directly on the eye as a contact lens. The central area of the Goldmann goniolenses, as well as the Zeiss lens, serves as a fundus contact lens so that the variable illumination and magnification of the biomicroscope can be used to provide detailed examination of the posterior pole through a dilated pupil. Various fundus contact lenses have been designed solely for this examination purpose without being engineered for gonioscopy as well (Figure 6-25).

The fundus contact lens, sometimes referred to as a contact Hruby lens, has the advantages of superior optical view, magnification, and field of view. A slight disadvantage is that contact of this instrument with the eye necessitates use of a topical anesthetic and a cushioning agent.

The noncontact Hruby lens, which is also a high minus lens (50–55 D), can also be used to examine the posterior fundus in conjunction with the slit lamp biomicroscope. Because it is not placed directly on the eye, it can generally be used more quickly because no anesthetic and cushioning agent are required. Freedom of eye movement is also retained so that points farther removed from the posterior pole may be examined without the use of indirect viewing methods.

When desirable, the three mirrors of the Goldmann lens can be used in conjunction with the central contact lens to indirectly view the more anterior portions of the retina. Once again, this offers the advantage of high magnification and binocularity.

Technique

Fundus Contact Lens

The patient's eyes are initially widely dilated so that maximum field and stereopsis can be achieved. The cornea is then anesthetized with one drop of 0.5%

FIGURE 6-22
A. Gonioscopy of an extremely narrow angle. Essentially no details of the angle structures are seen without excessive tilting of the goniolens. B. Indentation gonioscopy with the Zeiss four-mirror goniolens causes deepening of the angle, thus revealing structures normally hidden by the anteriorly bowed iris. C. The anterior chamber depth is shallow centrally.

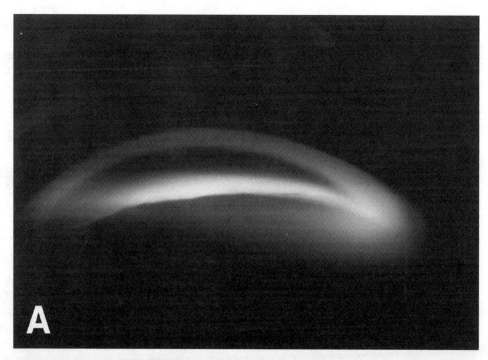

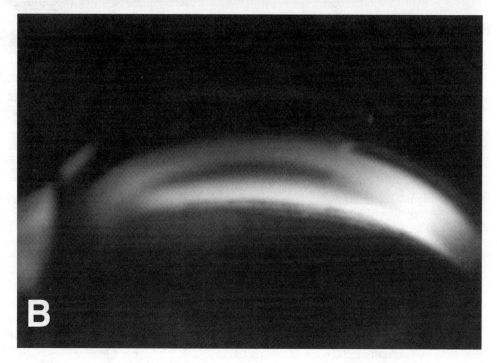

proparacaine. A methylcellulose solution is then dropped into the concave surface of the lens while care is taken that it is not accompanied by air bubbles. The lens can then be inserted into the lower cul-de-sac and rotated onto the cornea as previously described for indirect gonioscopy.

Assuming that the examiner desires to inspect the posterior pole, the slit lamp beam is narrowed both vertically and horizontally and directed through the central area of the lens. Initially using a low level of magnification and having the patient fixate straight ahead, the examiner focuses the microscope on the optic nerve head

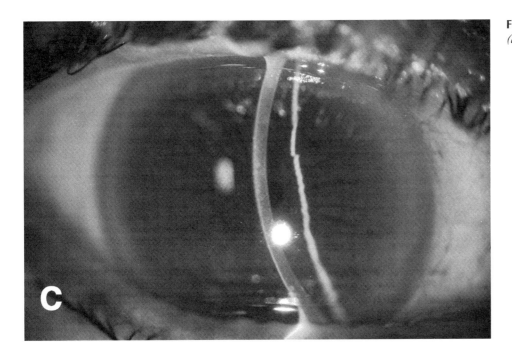

FIGURE 6-22
(continued)

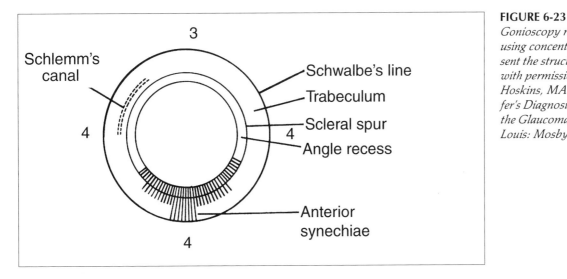

FIGURE 6-23
Gonioscopy recording system using concentric circles to represent the structures. (Modified with permission from HD Hoskins, MA Kass. Becker-Shaffer's Diagnosis and Therapy of the Glaucomas [6th ed]. St. Louis: Mosby, 1989;110–1.)

to gain an anatomic orientation. The examiner can then have the patient change his or her fixation slightly so that the area to be investigated can be brought into view. Once the correct localization has been achieved, the examiner may increase the magnification as needed. Slit width can be varied to enhance the perception of an area of depression or elevation as the beam is oscillated back and forth across the involved site.

The mirrors of the three-mirror lens can be used in the same basic fashion as indirect gonioscopy to examine a lesion that is not located in the posterior pole. Each mirror has a specific tilt that allows certain portions of the fundus to be visualized through a dilated pupil (Figure 6-26). The parabolic mirror, which is used to view the iridocorneal angle, will also allow inspection of the anterior fundus. The mirror labeled *b* in Figure 6-26 is angled so that anterior and equatorial fundus regions can be seen (Figure 6-27), and the mirror labeled *c* will help visualize an area of the retina from approximately 30 degrees to the equator.

FIGURE 6-24

The Forbes technique of indentation gonioscopy. A. The Zeiss four-mirror goniolens is positioned gently on the eye. B. Forward pressure is applied, which displaces aqueous and widens the angle, demonstrating whether synechial or appositional closure is present. (Adapted with permission from M Forbes. Gonioscopy with corneal indentation. A method for distinguishing between appositional closure and synechial closure. Arch Ophthalmol 1966;76:488–92.)

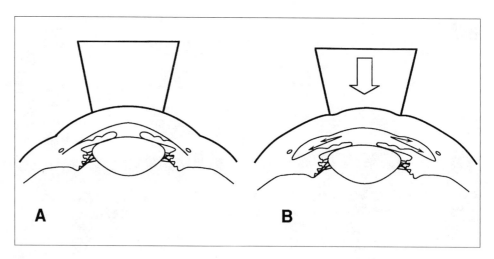

A   B

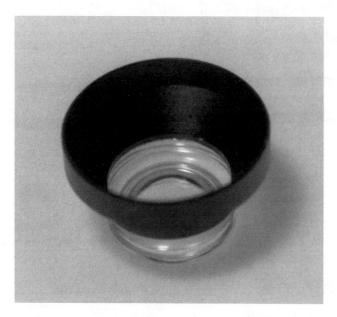

FIGURE 6-25

Example of a fundus contact lens, also referred to as a contact Hruby lens.

The relative area of the fundus that can be seen with each mirror can be increased substantially by tilting the lens to one side or by having the patient change his or her position of gaze. Taking this into consideration, there is actually some overlap of retinal area viewed with each mirror.

Similar to indirect gonioscopy, when a lesion of interest is located in the 6-o'clock meridian the proper mirror to allow inspection is placed in the 12-o'clock position. To aid in the appreciation of depth and contour already

afforded by this binocular system, the slit lamp beam can be placed 5–10 degrees off axis. The lens is removed from the eye in the manner previously described for gonioscopy.

Noncontact Hruby Lens

The patient's eyes are initially widely dilated, and the Hruby lens is then positioned such that the concave surface is directed toward the eye. The lens itself should be placed approximately 1.5 mm in front of the cornea. This positioning of the lens is achieved differently depending on the type of biomicroscope used. Some slit lamps provide an attachment to the headrest, which positions the lens properly by spring tension against the attachment (Figure 6-28). Other biomicroscopes use rails or tracks to position the lens at the proper location. The former method has the advantage of automatic positioning, while the latter method requires the examiner to move the lens forward or backward to the correct position. Once the lens is in the correct position, the examiner focuses the biomicroscope on the optic nerve head. As with fundus contact lenses, the biomicroscope should be on a low level of magnification to aid in focusing and anatomic orientation. At this point, the noncontact Hruby lens may be rocked slightly forward and backward to maximize the image clarity and field of view. Slit width and magnification may then be varied to evaluate the involved area.

As mentioned, the noncontact Hruby lens can generally be used more quickly than the fundus contact lens to evaluate features of the posterior pole such as optic nerve head elevation, cupping, pallor, and rim tissue integrity (Figure 6-29). Unfortunately, the slit lamp beam must be aimed fairly straight ahead through the lens so that the prismatic displacement of the beam is minimized.

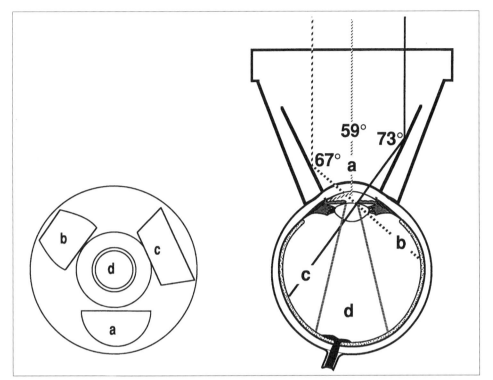

FIGURE 6-26
Left: Schematic representation of the mirrors and central lens of the universal (Goldmann) three-mirror lens. Right: Schematic demonstrating the fundus regions examined with each portion of the Goldmann three-mirror lens. (Adapted with permission from Ocular Instruments Inc., Bellevue, WA.)

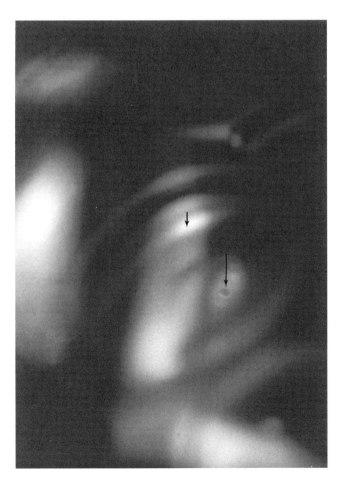

FIGURE 6-27
The fundus mirrors of the Goldmann three-mirror goniolens are excellent for detailed examination of peripheral retinal lesions. The example shows an equatorial retinal hole viewed with the Goldmann three-mirror lens (long arrow). The anterior chamber angle is also seen here but is out of focus (short arrow).

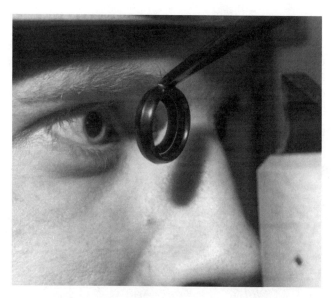

FIGURE 6-28
A noncontact Hruby lens attached to a Zeiss slit lamp.

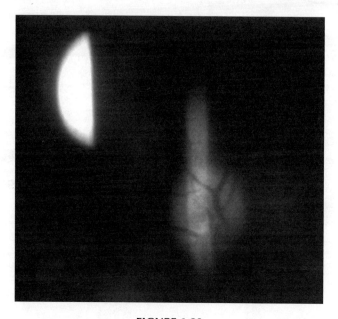

FIGURE 6-29
The Hruby lens is excellent for evaluating details of the optic nerve head, such as in this example of mild elevation from buried drusen.

Interpretation

A number of ocular disorders lend themselves to close scrutiny with the fundus contact lens, the Hruby lens, or both. The combination of high magnification and stereopsis is imperative in the evaluation of subtle changes of the posterior pole of the eye that cannot be examined ade-

quately with direct and indirect ophthalmoscopy. The fundus contact and Hruby lenses allow the practitioner to carefully examine the posterior vitreous for hemorrhage, cells, media haze, and membranes, which may not be visible by other means.

It is particularly helpful to use the high magnification and stereopsis provided by the fundus contact and Hruby lenses to detect the early patterns of cupping that occur in glaucomatous eyes. One should look for signs such as a focal loss of neural rim tissue most commonly at the inferior and superior poles of the nerve head. Stereopsis is especially important because this localized defect, referred to as notching, may not have corresponding pallor. Failure to detect focal or diffuse cupping that is greater than pallor is a common mistake when evaluating the glaucomatous nerve head without binocularity.

The fundus background and macula can be thoroughly examined for signs of inflammation, atrophy, holes, degeneration, or detachment. It is here that the value of the Hruby or fundus contact lens is evident. Changes in the macula, such as edema or early degenerative changes too subtle to be seen by other means, may be visualized. These lenses can be particularly important in the detection of diabetic macular retinal thickening, which is an important indicator of clinically treatable significant macular edema.

The Hruby and fundus contact lenses are valuable in differentiating two different clinical entities that manifest a similar appearance with direct and indirect ophthalmoscopy. Drusen and hard exudates, retinal holes and blot hemorrhages, and drusen of the nerve head and papilledema are just a few examples of entities that may be differentiated by the use of these lenses.

REFERENCES

1. Rubin ML. Optics for Clinicians (2nd ed). Gainesville: Triad Scientific Publishing, 1974;56.
2. Richardson KT. Diagnostic evaluation and therapeutic decision in the glaucomas. Br J Ophthalmol 1972;56:216–22.
3. Hoskins HD Jr, Kass MA. Becker-Shaffer's Diagnosis and Therapy of the Glaucomas (6th ed). St Louis: Mosby, 1989.
4. van Herick W, Shaffer RV, Schwartz A. Estimation of width of angle of anterior chamber. Incidence and significance of the narrow angle. Am J Ophthalmol 1969;68:626–9.
5. Terry JE. Mydriatic angle-closure glaucoma—mechanism, evaluation and reversal. J Am Optom Assoc 1977;48:159–68.
6. Vargas E, Drance SM. Anterior chamber depth in angle-closure glaucoma. Arch Ophthalmol 1973;90:438–9.
7. Cullen AP. Encapsulated foreign body of the angle. J Am Optom Assoc 1973;44:66–7.

8. Thorpe HE. Foreign bodies in the anterior chamber angle. Am J Ophthalmol 1966;61:1339–43.

9. Forbes M. Gonioscopy with corneal indentation. A method for distinguishing between appositional closure and synechial closure. Arch Ophthalmol 1966;76:488–92.

10. Fellman RL, Spaeth GL, Starita RJ. Gonioscopy: key to successful management of glaucoma. American Academy of Ophthalmology. Focal points 1984: Clinical Modules for Ophthalmologists No. 7. San Francisco: American Academy of Ophthalmology, 1984;1–8.

11. Fellman RL, Starita RJ, Lynn JR. Glaucoma series. In Henkind P (ed), Clinical Signs in Ophthalmology. St Louis: Mosby, 1987;9(1):1–12.

12. Spaeth GL. The normal development of the human anterior chamber angle: a new system of descriptive grading. Trans Ophthalmol Soc UK 1971;91:709–39.

13. Spaeth GL. Distinguishing between the normally narrow, the suspiciously shallow, and the particularly pathological, anterior chamber angle. Pers Ophthalmol 1977;1:205–14.

14. Shields MB. Textbook of Glaucoma (2nd ed). Baltimore: Williams & Wilkins, 1987.

15. Epstein DL. Chandler and Grant's Glaucoma (3rd ed). Philadelphia: Lea and Febiger, 1986.

16. Lichter PR, Shaffer RN. Iris processes and glaucoma. Am J Ophthalmol 1970;70:905–11.

17. Henkind P. Angle vessels in normal eyes. A gonioscopic evaluation in anatomic correlation. Br J Ophthalmol 1964;48:551–7.

18. Palmberg P. Gonioscopy. In R Ritch, MB Shields, T Krupin (eds), The Glaucomas (Vol 1). St. Louis: Mosby, 1989; 345–59.

19. Burian HM, Braley AE, Allen L. External and gonioscopic visibility of the ring of Schwalbe and the trabecular zone: an interpretation of the posterior corneal embryotoxon and the so-called congenital hyaline membranes on the posterior corneal surface. Trans Am Ophthalmol Soc 1954;52: 389–426.

20. Scheie HG, Albert DM. Adler's Textbook of Ophthalmology. Philadelphia: Saunders, 1969;436.

21. Campbell DG. A comparison of diagnostic techniques in angle-closure glaucoma. Am J Ophthalmol 1979;88:197–204.

22. Scheie H. Width and pigmentation of the angle of the anterior chamber. A system of grading by gonioscopy. Arch Ophthalmol 1957;58:510–2.

23. Shaffer RN. Gonioscopy, ophthalmoscopy, and perimetry. Trans Am Acad Ophthalmol Otolaryngol 1960;64:112–27.

24. Kolker AE, Hetherington J. Becker-Shaffer's Diagnosis and Therapy of the Glaucomas (4th ed). St. Louis: Mosby, 1976.

25. Hoskins HD Jr. Interpretive gonioscopy in glaucoma. Invest Ophthalmol 1972;11:97–102.

26. Kenney AH. Ocular Examination. St. Louis: Mosby, 1970:135.

27. Becker S. Clinical Gonioscopy: A Text and Stereoscopic Atlas. St. Louis: Mosby, 1972.

28. Schirmer KE. Gonioscopy and artifacts. Br J Ophthalmol 1967;51:50–3.

29. Sussman W. Ophthalmoscopic gonioscopy. Am J Ophthalmol 1968;66:549.

7

Color Vision

Gregory W. Good and Jack E. Terry

Although color discrimination is one of our most important visual abilities, clinicians rarely investigate this aspect of vision in other than a cursory manner. Adams and Haegerstrom-Portnoy[1] speculated that the reason for this is that should a congenital, and therefore stable, deficiency be found, the clinician is unable to remedy the condition and is generally helpless except for counseling the patient.

The detection and classification of acquired color vision deficiencies, however, can be used to diagnose a visual or systemic condition, serve as a measure of disease progression, or aid in determining when toxic levels of various medications are reached. Color vision status has frequently been shown to be a sensitive indicator of the intactness of the visual pathway.

This chapter will initially discuss present theories of color vision and will then address the classification of color deficiencies. The effects of ocular and systemic disease and drug toxicity on color perception will then be reviewed. Finally, clinical tests of color vision will be covered along with an evaluation protocol that allows a systematic approach to color vision analysis.

BASIC THEORIES OF COLOR VISION

Vision begins with the absorption of electromagnetic radiation by the photoreceptors within the retina. If only a single type of photoreceptor with a constant wavelength sensitivity were present, our visual world would be colorless because the visual system would not be able to differentiate stimuli of varying wavelengths. Only differences in stimulus intensity could be signaled to the higher cortical centers for interpretation.

Current color vision theory recognizes that photoreceptors within the human retina are differentially sensitive to the various components of the visible spectrum. The relative responses of the different photoreceptor types are compared, ultimately signaling a perception of color.

During the nineteenth century, two apparently incompatible theories arose to explain color vision processing. The trichromatic theory was developed from a stimulus perspective and received support from the results of color mixing and color matching experimentation. All colors of the spectrum could be matched exactly by mixing three (hence, trichromatic) appropriately chosen colors. The opponent color theory was developed to explain color perceptions and that subjects routinely name four unique, or primary, colors: red, yellow, green, and blue. Present-day "zone" theories incorporate components of both the trichromatic and opponent theories to explain color processing at different levels of the visual pathway.

Trichromatic Theory

Although in 1777, Palmer[2] hypothesized the presence of a three-receptor system in the retina, Thomas Young[3] is generally given credit for the trichromatic theory of color vision because of his lecture in 1801 to the Royal Society of London formally describing the theory using physiologic and physical terms.[4]

The trichromatic color vision theory was not widely accepted, however, until Helmholtz revived it approximately 60 years later.[5] Helmholtz succinctly stated that the retina is composed of three distinct types of nerve fibers, and that each type of fiber is sensitive across the entire visible spectrum but to different degrees. In addition, the three fiber types have maximum sensitivities within the visible spectrum in the red, green, and violet portions, respectively, and it is the interaction of these three fiber systems that gives rise to color perception. Helmholtz's fervent support of the trichromatic theory has led it to its well-known synonym, the Young-

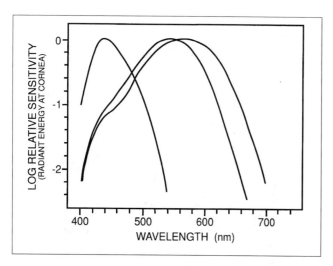

FIGURE 7-1

The calculated relative sensitivities (as measured at the cornea) for the short-wavelength–sensitive (SWS), middle-wavelength–sensitive (MWS), and long-wavelength–sensitive (LWS) cones are shown for the visible spectrum. The curves for each type of cone have been normalized to their own maxima. (Modified with permission from J Pokorny, VC Smith, G Verriest, AJLG Pinckers [eds], Congenital and Acquired Color Vision Defects. New York: Grune & Stratton, 1979;65.)

Helmholtz theory. Weale[6] has provided a summary of the early history of trichromatic theory.

Early experimental evidence for the theory was provided by Helmholtz,[5] Grassman,[7] and Maxwell.[8] More recent supporting evidence for the trichromatic theory has arisen as investigators have isolated and measured the absorption spectra of different cone types within primate and human retinas.[9,10] Figure 7-1 illustrates calculated spectral sensitivities of the three photoreceptors found within the retina of a human with normal color vision.[11] It is the presence of these three cone systems with different spectral sensitivities that provides the basis for human trichromatic color vision.

Opponent Theory

Although the trichromatic theory explains color phenomena from a color mixing and matching perspective, it inadequately explains the perception of colors under all viewing conditions. Simultaneous color contrast is one such phenomenon. The perception that colors are most intense when presented next to a contrasting color and that black appears its blackest when placed against a white background are examples that demonstrate

simultaneous contrast. Color afterimages also demonstrate that colors have a contrasting counterpart. To explain these phenomena that deal with the psychological aspects of color perception, Hering developed his opponent color theory.[12]

Hering proposed that opponent processing channels are present within the visual system. Red and green, yellow and blue, and white and black are signaled by antagonistic processing within three opponent mechanisms. Within a single processing channel, one color—for example, red—would be signaled by a higher frequency of response. Green, red's opponent color, would be signaled within the same channel, but by a lower frequency of response. Hering described this as dissimilative (breakdown) processing for red and assimilative (buildup) processing for green.

Hering's opponent theory explains how certain colors cannot be seen in combination. Reddish and greenish are never used together to describe the appearance of a color. A color may have the appearance of red or green, but not both simultaneously. When red and green are mixed equally, neither is seen. A new primary color, yellow, is perceived. Likewise, when blue and yellow are mixed equally, white is the resultant.

Zone Theory

Present-day theories of color vision incorporate aspects of both the trichromatic and opponent philosophies (Figure 7-2). Color processing begins with the absorption of light within the three types of retinal cones. Trichromatic processing occurs only at this very early portion of the visual process. Signals from the cones are then processed within three separate opponent channels.

The signals from the long-wavelength–sensitive (LWS) and middle-wavelength–sensitive (MWS) cones are added to form a luminance, or achromatic, channel. The short-wavelength–sensitive (SWS) cones have very little input into this channel. This agrees with color mixing experiments that show that blue light will add little additional brightness to a mixture although it will change the color drastically.

Signals from the LWS and MWS cones also combine in opponent fashion within the red-versus-green chromatic channel. Within a single nerve fiber in this channel, red light might cause inhibitory effects while green light causes excitation, or the opposite may be true. In either case, inputs from the LWS and MWS cones oppose one another. Similar opponent processing occurs within the blue-yellow chromatic channel. Signals from the LWS and MWS cones add and are processed as a single signal, which is opposed to that of the SWS cone.

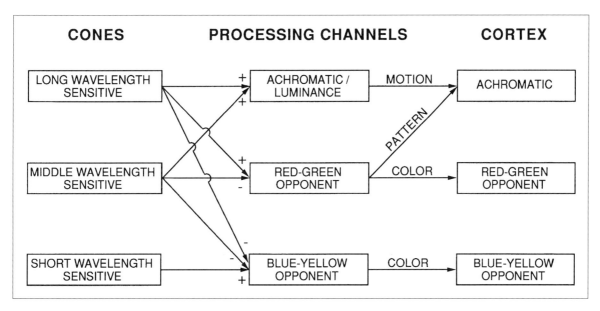

FIGURE 7-2
Diagram illustrating color processing from the photoreceptor level through the optic nerve to the cortex. The plus and minus signs are given only to show relative excitatory or inhibitory effects through the processing channels. Some processing fibers may receive opposite inputs from those illustrated. (Modified from E King-Smith. Psychological Methods for the Investigation of Acquired Colour Vision Deficiencies. In D Foster [ed], Vision and Visual Dysfunction. Vol 7, Inherited and Acquired Colour Vision Deficiencies. Boca Raton, FL: CRC Press, 1991;39.)

CLASSIFICATION OF COLOR VISION DEFICIENCIES

Most research investigating deficiencies in color vision discrimination has concentrated on hereditary defects. Hereditary color deficiencies can generally be attributed to an abnormality of one of the three types of photopigments within the retinal cones. Affected patients typically have normal visual acuity. The color defects are stable, bilateral, and relatively easy to classify.

Acquired color vision deficiencies are the result of physiologic insult within the visual system. They can result from damage at any level along the visual pathway. Because damage is rarely isolated to a single type of photoreceptor or color processing channel, the resulting color defect is often difficult to classify. However, because of physiologic differences among the three processing channels, acquired color vision losses are typically more prominent in one of the processing channels and can be classified using terminology similar to that for the hereditary defects. A decrease in visual acuity is more likely to accompany an acquired color deficiency, and an asymmetric loss of color vision between the two eyes is more frequently encountered.

HEREDITARY COLOR DEFICIENCIES

Normal human color vision is trichromatic in nature. The basis for trichromatic vision is the three retinal cone types, which exhibit differential wavelength sensitivities (see Figure 7-1). If there is either a reduction in the number of the cone types present (only two cone types present, dichromacy; only one cone type present, monochromacy) or an alteration in the specific wavelength sensitivity of one of the cone types (anomalous trichromacy), altered color vision discrimination results.

Classification of a color deficiency depends on the specific cone type affected. Protan defects are those in which the light-sensitive pigment within the LWS cones is absent (protanopic dichromacy) or is present but exhibits an abnormal spectral sensitivity (protanomalous trichromacy). *Deutan* and *tritan* are the terms used to specify similar defects in the MWS or SWS cone types, respectively. Although protan and deutan type defects can be differentiated with proper testing, the similarity of color confusions and inheritance patterns for these two classes has led us to generally refer to these defects as red-green defects. Similarly, a tritan type defect is commonly referred to as a blue-yellow defect.

Of the hereditary color defects, protan and deutan defects are by far the most prevalent (Table 7-1). They are inherited as X-linked recessive traits and therefore affect a greater proportion of men than women. For white men of European descent, approximately 8% exhibit a hereditary red-green color deficiency. Tritan defects are inherited in an autosomal dominant manner and are much more rare. Men and women are thought to be affected equally.

Color testing reveals that there is a wide range of color discrimination ability among individuals with defective color vision. Mild anomalous trichromats (all three cone types present, but one type with altered sensitivity) can perform many color vision tasks almost as well as persons with normal color vision. However, when comparing stimuli of differing wavelength composition, even these mild anomalous trichromats are distinctly different. Some anomalous trichromats demonstrate very poor color discrimination and function more like dichromats. It is therefore useful to classify anomalous trichromats according to their abilities to discriminate colors. Protanomalous and deuteranomalous trichromacy can be separated into mild and extreme classifications based on the color mixing performance on the Nagel anomaloscope.[13]

A characteristic that differentiates a dichromat from a trichromat (either normal or anomalous) is that dichromats demonstrate a "neutral point" within the visible spectrum. According to trichromatic color theory, a stimulus will be perceived as white when all three cone systems respond with near equal intensity. For a trichromat, a minimum of two widely separated wavelengths must be used to stimulate the three cones equally. For a dichromat, however, a single wavelength to which the two cone systems are equally sensitive can be chosen. When stimulated with light of this wavelength, the dichromat will perceive a white (or gray). The neutral points for a protanope, deuteranope,[14] and tritanope[15] are 498 nm, 492 nm, and 570 nm, respectively.

Protan Defects

Protan defects are characterized by an insensitivity in both color discrimination and luminous efficiency at the long wavelength end of the visible spectrum. Protanopes lack the normal LWS cones and therefore have only the MWS cones to detect the longer wavelengths (see Figure 7-1). Color discrimination for a given portion of the spectrum is not possible unless at least two types of receptors with different sensitivities are present. Because the SWS cones lack sensitivity to longer wavelengths, no color discrimination is possible at this portion of the visible spectrum for a protanope.

TABLE 7-1
Prevalence of Hereditary Color Vision Defects[a]

Defect	Males (%)	Females (%)
Red-green (X-linked recessive)		
Deuteranopic dichromacy	1	0.05[b]
Deuteranomalous trichromacy	5	0.25[b]
Protanopic dichromacy	1	0.05[b]
Protanomalous trichromacy	1	0.05[b]
Total	8	0.40
Blue-yellow (autosomal dominant)		
Tritan defect (tritanopic or tritanomaly)	0.005 (males = females)	
Achromatopsia		
Rod monochromacy (autosomal recessive)	0.003 (males = females)	
Incomplete (blue cone) monochromacy (X-linked recessive)	?	

[a]Approximate figures. Prevalence figures for red-green defects are for white population of European descent.
[b]Calculated figures based on overall female prevalence and percentages of red-green color vision defects for males.
For literature review and global incidence, see R Fletcher, J Voke. Defective Colour Vision. Bristol, England: Hilger, 1985;191–5.

If the intensities are modified to equalize brightness, protanopes cannot differentiate the colors of monochromatic lights from approximately 540 nm to 760 nm at the end of the visible spectrum.[13] However, because they are especially insensitive to red light, protan defectives may have a good color naming ability compared with deutan defectives. Protans are able to use brightness cues to help with color discrimination. Red colors are especially dark for patients with a protan defect. Therefore, when comparing a yellow with a red in our natural environment, although no color discrimination may be possible, the protan will name the colors correctly, calling the bright stimulus yellow and the dark stimulus red. In situations where brightness cues are minimized, however, green-yellow-red color confusions remain.

Protanomalous trichromats have an abnormal pigment within the LWS cones.[16,17] This abnormal pigment has a peak absorption shifted to shorter wavelengths relative to the normal LWS pigment. This, in turn, shifts the sensitivity of the LWS cones, reducing the luminous efficiency for longer wavelengths (similar to a protanope). The protanomalous trichromat does have color discrimination for the longer wavelengths, but it is reduced relative to a color vision normal.

Deutan Defects

Deutan defects are the most prevalent of hereditary color vision deficiencies. Deuteranopes totally lack the MWS cones. Similar to the protanope, deuteranopes also lack all color discrimination at the long wavelength end of the visible spectrum. Again, color discrimination is not possible unless at least two types of receptors with different sensitivities for a given portion of the spectrum are present. Since the deuteranope only has the LWS cones to detect the longer wavelengths, color discrimination is not possible past the point where the SWS cones lose sensitivity.

Deuteranomalous trichromats have an abnormal MWS pigment with the peak sensitivity shifted to longer wavelengths.[16,17] This reduces the difference in sensitivities between the MWS and LWS cones. Because of this, a deuteranomalous trichromat has color discrimination for the long wavelengths but it is reduced relative to a normal trichromat.

Although a deutan defective has a slightly reduced luminous efficiency to wavelengths in the middle of the visible spectrum, the overall shape of a deutan's relative luminous efficiency curve is approximately normal. A deuteranope therefore does not have a brightness cue to aid color naming as does a protanope. Because protan and deutan defectives have similar color confusions, differentiating between the two clinically can be difficult. Tests of color vision (e.g., the anomaloscope) can use the difference in luminous sensitivity as one method to discriminate between the two.

Tritan Defects

Hereditary defects involving the SWS cone are relatively rare and show an autosomal dominant inheritance pattern. Because of the rarity of the condition, relatively few investigators have thoroughly tested the color vision of large numbers of individuals with congenital tritan-type defects. Additionally, clinical tests to differentiate between the degrees and or types of tritan losses are not readily available. Although it seems clear that some tritan defectives exhibit dichromatic-type losses whereas others do not, confusion still exists whether true tritanomalous individuals exist.[18] Therefore, hereditary blue-yellow losses are simply called tritan defects, without specifying whether they are a dichromatic or an anomalous type. Tritan defectives show near normal luminous efficiency.[19]

Monochromacy

True monochromacy is an extremely rare condition. It is true color blindness. The term implies that no color discrimination is present. Visual perception is based solely on differences in brightness. The condition is present when only a single type of photoreceptor in the retina is functional.

Two types of monochromats have generally been reported. Rod monochromacy (also called complete achro-

matopsia) is a condition in which vision is dependent solely on rod function. Rod monochromats exhibit photophobia, visual acuity of around 20/200, and nystagmus.[20] The condition shows autosomal recessive inheritance.

Blue-cone monochromacy (incomplete achromatopsia) has also been identified. Subjects show a best visual acuity of 20/60 and a photopic spectral sensitivity similar to that of the SWS cones. It is thought that, through interaction with the rods, blue cone monochromats exhibit some color discrimination ability at intermediate brightness levels.[4] This condition shows X-linked recessive inheritance.

ACQUIRED COLOR DEFICIENCIES

Acquired color vision deficiencies may result from pathologic dysfunction anywhere along the visual pathway, extending from the retina to visual cortex. Although most disease processes are not so specific that they exclusively affect a single chromatic or achromatic visual processing channel, the physiologic differences in the size, number, and position of the nerve fibers and cell bodies making up the different channels can influence the amount of damage within one channel versus another.

Color vision performance can be a sensitive measure, indicating the relative integrity or function of the visual pathway. One reason for this is that the SWS cones are relatively few in number within the retina and may be especially vulnerable to certain disease processes.[21] In addition, they appear to have little input into luminance and visual acuity processing; therefore, a decrease in blue-yellow discrimination may appear before changes in visual acuity or visual field are noted.

Acquired color deficiencies differ from hereditary defects in that acquired losses (1) are more likely to be associated with visual acuity or field loss, (2) are more likely to be progressive, (3) differ in severity from one eye to the other, (4) cannot be classified as easily, and (5) are more likely to show a blue-yellow type defect. Because of these differences, a separate classification system and modified testing methods are required to properly investigate and describe acquired color deficiencies.

Classification

Verriest[22] developed a classification system for acquired color vision deficiencies based primarily on the chromatic discrimination loss exhibited by the patient (Table 7-2). A type I defect produces predominantly a red-green discrimination loss. It is caused by retinal disease affecting the photoreceptors, an example being a cone dys-

TABLE 7-2
Verriest Classification of Acquired Color Vision Defects

Type	Primary Confusion Axis	Progression of Vision Loss	Visual Acuity Loss	Probable Site of Action
I	Red-green	Progresses to complete achromatopsia (progression to scotopic luminous efficiency)	Moderate to severe	Photoreceptor (e.g., Stargardt's disease, cone dystrophy)
II	Red-green	Accompanying blue-yellow loss—retains photopic luminous efficiency loss of apparent saturation	Moderate to severe	Optic nerve (e.g., optic neuritis)
III	Blue-yellow	Progresses from mild confusions in blue region of color diagram to more complete blue-yellow defect	Mild to moderate	Various sites (e.g., cataract, glaucoma, ARMD)

ARMD = age-related macular degeneration.
Source: Adapted from G Verriest. Further studies on acquired deficiency of color discrimination. J Opt Soc Am 1963;53:185–95.

trophy. A reduction in visual acuity is expected as well as a change in luminous efficiency from photopic to primarily scotopic.

Verriest type II defects show primarily a red-green loss, but a milder blue-yellow loss may also be present. The luminous efficiency curve remains normal. A loss of apparent saturation of colors may be present. Optic neuritis is an example of a disease causing a type II defect.

Verriest type III defects are the most commonly encountered. They are characterized by a loss of discrimination along the blue-yellow axis. Visual acuity may be mildly or substantially affected. Luminous efficiency remains normal except for some sensitivity loss in the blue region. Nuclear cataract, glaucoma, and age-related macular degeneration are examples of conditions giving rise to a type III defect.

Kollner[23] also studied acquired color defects and developed a general guide to help identify the primary location of the causative lesion. Kollner's rule states that damage within the outer retinal layers is characterized by a blue-yellow defect, whereas damage of the inner retina and optic nerve gives rise to a red-green defect. Although this general rule is a useful memorization tool, it should be noted that numerous pathologic conditions give rise to color deficiencies contrary to these guidelines.

Ophthalmic disease conditions causing changes in color vision perception and discrimination are listed in Table 7-3. The main color confusion axis is listed as well as the Verriest classification. A similar presentation is given for various drugs and toxins in Table 7-4.

von Kries first classified color vision deficiencies in 1897.[24] He introduced the classification system for congenital defects using words from the Greek: protan = first, deutan = second, and tritan = third. In addition, von Kries developed a system of classification that could be applied to either congenital or acquired defects

TABLE 7-3
Acquired Color Vision Defects from Ophthalmic Disease*

Ophthalmic Condition	Main Confusion Axis	Verriest Type
Absorption		
Cataract	Blue-yellow	III
Outer retinal layers		
Retinitis pigmentosa	Blue-yellow	III
Macular degeneration		
ARMD	Blue-yellow	
Best's disease	Blue-yellow?	III?
Stargardt's disease	Red-green	I
Central serous retinopathy	Blue-yellow	III
Cone dystrophy	Red-green	I
Inner retinal layers		
Diabetes	Blue-yellow	III
Hypertensive retinopathy	Blue-yellow	III
Ganglion cell layer and optic nerve		
Glaucoma	Blue-yellow	III
Juvenile optic atrophy	Blue-yellow	III
Ischemic optic neuropathy	Blue-yellow	III
Optic neuritis	Red-green	II
Leber's hereditary optic atrophy	Red-green	II

ARMD = age-related macular degeneration.
*The main type of color deficiency is indicated. It should be noted, however, that acquired conditions are not as easily classified as congenital conditions.
Source: Adapted from R Fletcher, J Voke. Defective Colour Vision. Bristol, England: Hilger, 1985;217.

based on the presumed mechanism of the defect. Three classes of defects were described: absorption, alteration, and reduction.

An absorption defect is caused by a prereceptoral filtering of the incident light. Age-related pigmentary changes within the crystalline lens are an example of a condition

TABLE 7-4
Acquired Color Vision Defects Associated with Drugs and Toxins

| | Main Confusion Axis Verriest Type | | |
| | Red-Green | Red-Green | Blue-Yellow |
Drug	*I*	*II*	*III*
Antidiabetics (oral)		+	
Chlorpropamide		+	
Tolbutamide		+	
Antipyretics		+	
Ibuprofen		+	
Phenylbutazone		+	
Nitrofurane derivatives	+	+	
Furaltodone	+	+?	
Phenothiazine derivatives	+?		+
Quinoline derivatives	+	+	+
Chloroquine derivatives		+	+ +
Clioquinol		+ +	+
Quinidine		+	
Quinine	+	+	
Sulfonamides		+	
Salazosulfapyridine	+		
Tuberculostatics		+	
Dihydrostreptomycin	+		
Ethambutol		+	
Isoniazid		+	
Para-aminosalicylate (PAS)		+	
Rifampin		+	
Streptomycin		+	
Amoproxan		+	
Arsenicals		+	
Chloramphenicol		+	
Contraceptive agents (oral)	+		+ +
Cyanide		+	
Digitalis	+ +	+	+
Disulfiram		+	
Ergotamine		+	
Erythromycin			+
Ethanol		+	
Hexamethonium		+	
Indomethacin			+
Lead		+	
MAO inhibitors		+	
Mercaptopurine		+	
Penicillamine		+	
Thallium		+	
Tobacco amblyopia		+	+ +
Trimethadione			+
Vincristine		+	

Source: Modified with permission from J Birch, I Chisholm, P Kinnear et al. Acquired Color Vision Defects. In J Pokorny, V Smith, G Verriest et al. (eds), Congenital and Acquired Color Vision Defects. New York: Grune & Stratton, 1979;329–30.

that causes this type of defect. Yellow pigment within the lens reduces the patient's relative sensitivity to blue light and associated blue-yellow discrimination.

Alteration defects are those in which the patient will not agree with a color match made by a person with normal color vision. Anomalous trichromacy is an example of a condition that causes this type of defect. The patient has an abnormal visual pigment and will not accept a match made by a normal trichromat if the two test patches have different color compositions (metameric matching).

A patient with a reduction defect will agree with a metameric match made by a person with normal color vision. However, the match is not unique, as the patient will accept a wide range of combinations of the color mixture. An example of a condition causing a reduction defect is congenital dichromacy. A dichromat's photopigments are normal but reduced in number compared with a normal trichromat.

METHODS OF ANALYSIS

Based on their design and intent, color vision tests fall into various categories. Certain tests are designed to identify all individuals who have abnormal red-green color processing, and as such, may be appropriate only for screening for congenital defects. Some tests are designed to grade hue discrimination even in persons with normal color vision, whereas others identify only those individuals with a severe color defect. To properly interpret results, it is important to understand the theory behind the different color vision tests. Also, since no single test reveals all aspects of color vision performance, clinicians must use a battery of tests to properly diagnose and categorize color vision status. Testing should be done monocularly to identify any discrimination differences between the eyes. This is especially important when assessing acquired deficiencies.

COLOR VISION TESTING

Standard Illumination

The precision in chromaticity required for the various colors used in color vision tests mandates that a standard illuminant be used for all testing. Most color tests have been designed for use with standard illuminant C (correlated color temperature = 6774 K). This source approximates northern sky light and is most often obtained by using an incandescent source (100-W tungsten lamp) with a blue colored filter (Macbeth easel lamp, Figure 7-3). An

length distributions of light for color testing, Birch et al.[27] list several that are adequate. The fluorescent sources they describe produce full-spectrum light comparable with that from incandescent sources.

One disadvantage of the Macbeth easel lamp is that it provides an illumination of only approximately 100 lux. This is considered the minimum illumination for color testing. The recommended illumination level for the FM 100-hue and Panel D-15 tests is 270 lux. This level of illumination is provided with the True Daylight Illuminator. This commercially available testing unit (Richmond Products, Boca Raton, FL, 800-448-4538) provides 270 lux by using a daylight fluorescent bulb.

Color Naming

Requesting a patient to name the color of readily available objects is an unreliable test of chromatic discrimination. Different colored objects typically are also different in brightness. Therefore, a cue is added that allows many color vision–deficient individuals to name colors effectively. As an example, yellow objects are typically bright whereas red objects are typically dark. When comparing these objects in a naturally lit environment, many individuals with color vision deficiencies will be able to properly color name based on the brightness difference. Any test designed to evaluate chromatic discrimination must eliminate brightness cues.

In addition to the standard testing plates, the Dvorine pseudoisochromatic plates[28] include two desaturated color spots for color naming. Although the results of the naming of these colored spots are not useful in diagnosing a defect, the spots can be useful to demonstrate a child's color confusion to a parent or teacher.

Although it is not specifically a test of color naming, the "red cap test" is a related test that has been shown to be useful in the clinical setting. During this test the patient compares the amount of color perceived from a red pharmaceutical cap as it is presented within different areas of one eye's visual field, or when compared centrally in one eye relative to the other. If the red cap appears grayish or desaturated in color for one eye, or within one portion of the visual field, an optic nerve disorder may be present.

Pseudoisochromatic Plates

The ease of use and general familiarity by patients make the pseudoisochromatic plate test (see Figure 7-3) one of the most widely used types of clinical color vision tests. Individual plates have symbols composed of numerous small disks of varying colors and brightnesses. The backgrounds for the symbols are similarly configured but have

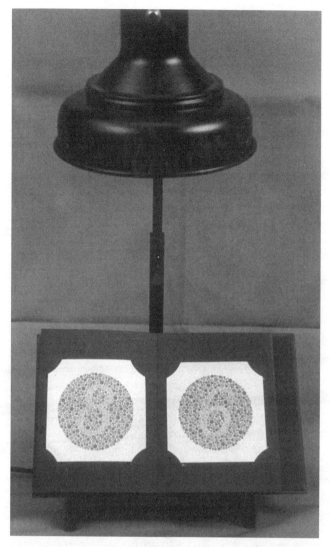

FIGURE 7-3
Ishihara pseudoisochromatic plates under a Macbeth lamp. The colors within the background of the plate are chosen to be subtly different from those of the numeral figure in order to discriminate between color vision normals (CVN) and color vision defectives (CVD). The design of the plate can be such that the figure is (1) seen by a CVN but not by a CVD (vanishing figure), (2) seen as a different number altogether by a CVN versus a CVD (confusion figure), or (3) seen by a CVD but not by a CVN (hidden digit).

alternative is to filter the light after reflection. "Color test glasses" consist of filters worn during testing to provide the proper quality of illumination[25] when used in conjunction with a 200-W incandescent source. Viewing through Kodak Wratten filters (No. 78AA) while using a 100-W incandescent lamp is also appropriate.[26] Although typical fluorescent sources do not exhibit proper wave-

colors that can be differentially discriminated by persons with normal versus defective color vision. Only small differences must be present between the symbol and background to make the plates sensitive enough to identify mild color defects, but these differences must be great enough to allow most subjects with normal color vision to pass.

To maximize the diagnostic effectiveness of pseudoisochromatic plates, the directions for use must be followed. A standard illuminant must be used, and only 3–5 seconds of exposure typically should be allowed for an individual plate. If patients are allowed to study the plate for an unlimited amount of time, even a patient with a severe color vision defect may be able to identify subtle chromatic or brightness differences and correctly identify the symbol.

Pseudoisochromatic plate tests are moderately effective in screening for congenital red-green color vision defects. Most are ineffective for evaluating acquired defects, grading the severity of a congenital defect, or discriminating between a protan or a deutan defect. None can be used to discriminate between severe anomalous trichromats and dichromats. Also, most of these tests do not have plates with blue-yellow screening capability. Accurate blue-yellow pseudoisochromatic plates are difficult to manufacture because of differences in luminous efficiency at the short wavelength end of the spectrum that are exhibited by persons with normal color vision.[27]

The Ishihara, Standard (Part 1), American Optical-H.R.R. (Hardy, Rand, Rittler), and Dvorine pseudoisochromatic plates are tests commonly found in the clinical setting. All show relatively good predictive efficiency in screening for congenital red-green defects. Of these, only the American Optical-H.R.R. plates have significant testing capability along the blue-yellow axis.

The Farnsworth F_2 plate (Plate 7-I) is a single plate with two overlapping squares, one yellow-green and one blue. A person with normal color vision will see both squares with the yellow-green square being predominant. Congenital red-green defectives see only the yellow-green square, whereas tritanopes see only the blue square. Incomplete tritanopes may see both squares, but, contrary to persons with normal color vision, the blue square will be dominant.[27] The F_2 plate is not commercially available but can be constructed using Munsell papers.[29] Adams et al.[30] reported the F_2 to be comparable to the American Optical-H.R.R. plates as a screening device and that it is appropriate for school-aged children past grade 1.

Using colors identical to those of the F_2 plate, Pease and Allen[31] developed a preferential viewing test. A small square is presented on one of two ends of a rectangular background. The test is an appropriate screening test for preschool-aged children who may have difficulty with the identification of test symbols. The Standard Pseudoisochromatic Plates (Part 2) are relatively new test plates designed specifically for acquired color deficiencies.[32]

In summary, pseudoisochromatic plates are excellent screening devices for congenital red-green color defects. However, they have limited effectiveness for use with acquired defects. Only the American Optical-H.R.R. and Standard Pseudoisochromatic Plates (Part 2) have significant blue-yellow testing capability. Additionally, even for red-green defects, pseudoisochromatic plates do not reliably grade the depth of the deficiency.

Nagel Anomaloscope

The Nagel Anomaloscope is the single instrument that can accurately differentiate protan versus deutan congenital-type defects and severe red-green anomalous trichromats from dichromats. The instrument presents a 1- to 2-degree bipartite field to the subject (Figure 7-4). The upper field consists of a mixture of monochromatic red and green lights. The lower is a monochromatic yellow light. The subject varies (1) the ratio of red versus green light in the upper field, and (2) the brightness of the lower yellow field until a perfect color and brightness match is obtained for the two fields.

Simple anomalous trichromats will have a small matching range similar to that of subjects with normal color vision. However, the center of the matching range will be shifted (Figure 7-5). Relative to a normal trichromat, a deuteranomalous trichromat will require extra green in the upper field to match the yellow lower field, whereas a protanomalous trichromat will require extra red in the upper field. Extreme anomalous trichromats are characterized by a relatively large matching range on the color scale. Deutan and protan dichromats will match over the entire range of red-green combinations. Deuteranopes can be discriminated from protanopes by the brightness setting for the yellow light.

The Nagel Anomaloscope is most useful in characterizing congenital red-green color defects. It is a moderately expensive instrument and therefore not often found in smaller clinics or in private offices.

Arrangement Tests

In arrangement color vision tests a patient is asked to arrange colored chips or caps according to color. The results can indicate specific color confusions of a patient and overall chromatic discrimination ability. These tests have colors from the entire color spectrum plus purples (red and violet mixtures) and thus are capable of identifying both red-green or blue-yellow color confusions.

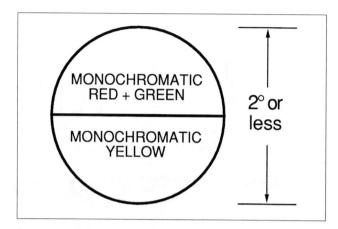

FIGURE 7-4

The viewing field for the modern version of the Nagel Anomaloscope is shown. Monochromatic red (approximately 670 nm) and green (approximately 540 nm) lights are mixed to exactly match a monochromatic yellow light (approximately 590 nm) in brightness and color. The red-to-green mixture and brightness settings will indicate the patient's specific red/green color vision status.

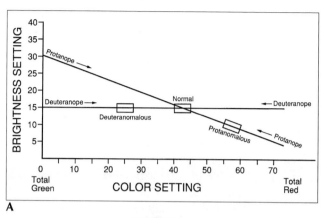

FIGURE 7-5

Possible anomaloscope test results for protan, deutan, and normal subjects. A. Persons with normal color vision will accept a relatively narrow red/green mixture ratio to exactly match a monochromatic yellow. Mild anomalous trichromats also have a relatively narrow red/green mixture but the matching range is shifted relative to the normal (more red required for protanomalous, more green required for the deuteranomalous). Extreme anomalous trichromats will have a larger matching range which may include one of the endpoints (monochromatic red, 670 nm, or monochromatic green, 540 nm), the normal mixture range, or both. Red/green dichromats will accept matches over the entire range, regardless of the red/green mixture. The abnormal luminous efficiency for protan defectives is demonstrated by the need to change the brightness setting as the red/green mixture is modified. B. Ranges of accepted color mixtures for various types of red/green color vision defects.

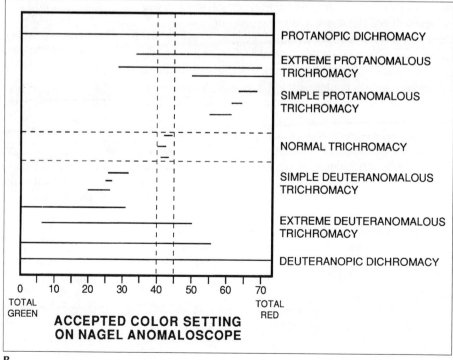

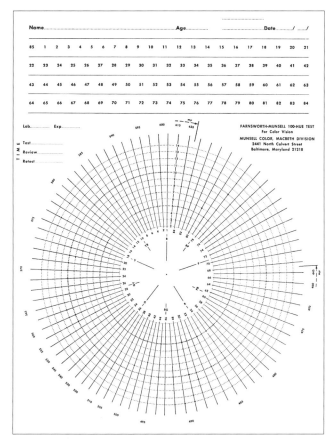

FIGURE 7-6
Farnsworth-Munsell 100-hue test recording sheet.

Farnsworth-Munsell 100-Hue Test

In the Farnsworth-Munsell (FM) 100-hue test, a total of 85 colored caps, which are numbered on their back surfaces, are presented from four individual boxes. The boxes are presented to the patient one at a time. The patient replaces the caps according to color using two fixed end colors within each box as references. A time limit is not typically used for this test.[27] A cap score is calculated for each cap by summing the absolute values of the differences of adjacent caps. For example, suppose the caps are replaced within the first box in the following order: . . . 3 – 6 – 7 – 8 – 4 – 5 – 9 – 10 – 11. . . . The cap score for cap 6 = (6 – 3) + (7 – 6) = 4. Similarly, the cap score for cap 8 = (8 – 7) + (8 – 4) = 5. A cap score of 2 indicates that the cap was arranged in perfect sequence relative to its neighbors (cap 10 in the example). The cap score is then plotted on the appropriate radial line of the circular scoring grid (Figure 7-6). Cap 1 is plotted at the 12-o'clock position of the diagram, with cap number positions increas-

ing in counterclockwise fashion. The innermost circle of the diagram represents a cap score of 2. With each successive circle the cap score increases by one. Cap scores are always positive numbers greater than or equal to 2. The change in color from one cap to the next is so small that some errors are expected even for normal trichomats with good color discrimination.

The axis representing the highest cap scores—hence, the main areas of confusion—is indicative of the classification of the defect. The results for deutan, protan, and tritan defects are shown in Figure 7-7. The overall indicator of color discrimination ability is given by the total error score. The error score for an individual cap is determined by subtracting 2, the perfect cap score, from the actual cap score. The total error score is then calculated by summing the error scores for all 85 caps.

The FM 100-hue test can be used in color vision normals as an indicator of fine color discrimination ability. In occupations requiring fine color discrimination, the FM 100-hue test can be used to screen the sensitivity of potential employees. Young adults with good color discrimination can have total error scores less than 25. All normal trichromats cannot be expected to score this well, however. Verriest[22] presented error scores for subjects of various ages with normal color vision (Table 7-5). His data indicate that color discrimination ability is widely variable and appears to worsen with age. When determining the significance of FM 100-hue testing results for an individual patient, this chart should be consulted to compare the data for persons of the same approximate age with normal color vision.

The FM 100-hue test is well suited to testing for and monitoring acquired color vision deficits. Because the colors represented are from the entire color spectrum including purples, the FM-100 has excellent blue-yellow testing capability. Also, a changing total error score can give an indication of the progression of the disease.

Farnsworth Panel D-15 Test

The Farnsworth Panel D-15 test is an arrangement test that uses only 16 colors. The test is similar in format to the FM 100-hue test but was designed to identify those individuals with a moderate to severe color vision deficit. There is a relatively large step in color from one cap to the next across the color spectrum. The first cap in the box is anchored and serves as the reference cap. Again, the subject must place the caps, which are numbered on their back surfaces, in the box according to color progression. Persons with normal color vision or those with only a mild color deficiency will pass this test. Approximately 50% of persons with congenital red-green color vision defects pass.

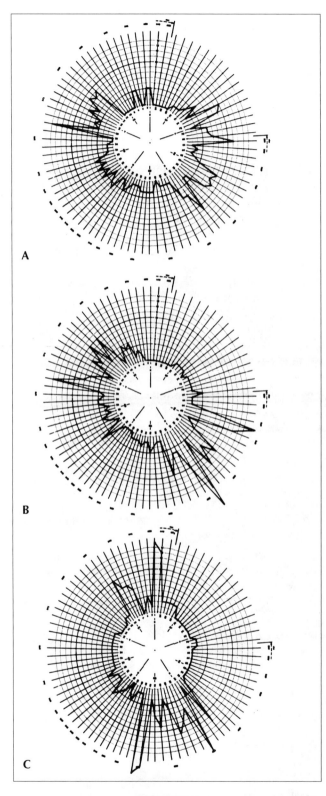

FIGURE 7-7

Sample Farnsworth-Munsell 100-hue test results for observers with congenital color vision deficiencies. A. Protan defects. B. Deutan defects. C. Tritan defects.

TABLE 7-5

Farnsworth-Munsell 100-Hue Test Error Scores for Normal Trichromats of Different Ages

Age (years)	Ninety-Fifth Percentile Error Score
10–14	160
15–19	100
20–24	74
25–29	92
30–34	106
35–39	120
40–44	134
45–49	144
50–54	154
55–59	164
60–64	174

Source: Data from G Verriest. Further studies on acquired deficiency of color discrimination. J Opt Soc Am 1963;53:185–95.

The Panel D-15 test is typically scored by connecting the dots on an answer sheet (Figure 7-8) in the order the caps were replaced in the box. If a patient makes two or more major errors it is considered a test failure. A major error is where more than one cap is skipped when replacing the caps "2" to "5," for example. A simple neighbor reversal (e.g., . . . 1 – 2 – 4 – 3 – 5 . . .) is considered a minor error. The type of defect is shown by the axis at which most of the lines cross the scoring circle. Although most young adults with normal color vision will make no errors on the test, the most typical major error made by a subject with normal color vision is skipping from cap 7 to cap 15 and then reversing the series.[27]

Bowman[33] and Vingrys and King-Smith[34] have developed quantitative scoring methods for the Panel D-15 test. These methods are based on the differences in chromaticity between the colored caps and yield a score representing the degree of color loss relative to perfect replacement.

Bowman's total color difference score[33] is a measure of the total color differences of adjacent caps for the Panel D-15 test results as measured in International Committee on Illumination (CIE)-LAB color space.[35] This method yields a quantitative assessment of the results and provides a number that can be used to specify the depth of a congenital defect[36] or to monitor the progression of an acquired defect.[37,38]

The method of Vingrys and King-Smith[34] calculates a total error score indicative of the degree of difference in arrangement relative to a perfect replacement. This method calculates its results by representing errors in cap replacement by vectors in the CIE-LUV color space.[35] The ends of the vectors terminate at the positions of the respective caps for each error in replacement. This method is advan-

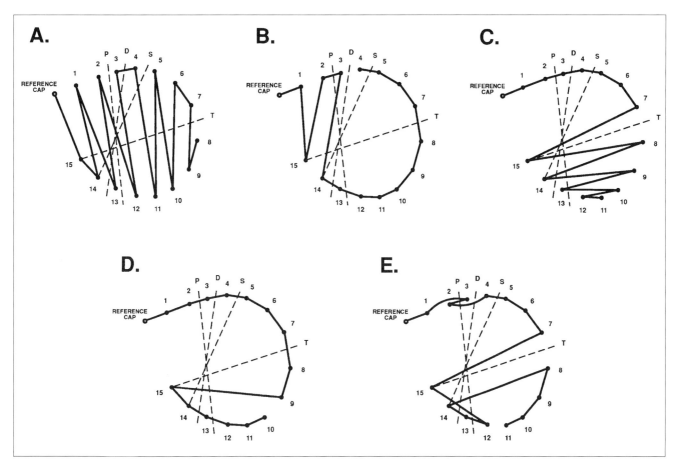

FIGURE 7-8

Sample Panel D-15 test results for various color vision defects. Theoretical axes of confusion are included (P = protan, D = deutan, S = scotopic, T = tritan). A. Protanope. B. Deuteranomalous. C. Tritan. D. Mild tritan. E. Same mild tritan as D, but results shown are for the desaturated version of the test.

tageous because it provides an angle of the primary confusion axis, as well as indices representing the significance of the replacement errors (C′-index) and the pureness of the axis of confusion (S′-index).

This method can be used to analyze results not only for the Panel D-15, but for the Desaturated Panel D-15 and FM 100-hue tests as well. It has been shown to accurately discriminate between congenital deutan and protan defects[34] and can be used to analyze results for acquired defects.[39]

A desaturated version of the Panel D-15 test is also available. The desaturated colors of this test make it much more difficult than the normal Panel D-15. The Desaturated Panel D-15 can be used in conjunction with the more saturated version to grade the severity of a congenital defect and chart the progression of acquired losses.[27]

The City University test is a plate test that uses the colors of the Panel D-15 test along with a gray and a yellow-green.[40] Four colors are presented surrounding a fifth. The subject chooses the peripheral sample that most nearly matches the central sample. Because the colors used in the test are from the Panel D-15 test, the two tests have similar difficulty.

TEST BATTERY

No single color vision test will provide the clinician with all the information necessary to describe a patient's color vision in terms of both diagnostic status and functional performance. Pseudoisochromatic plate tests may confirm that the patient has normal trichromatic vision, but they can-

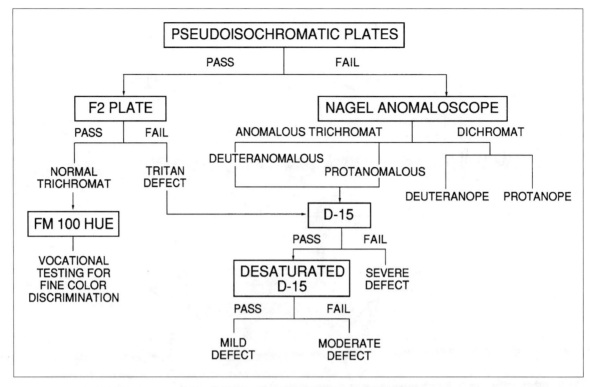

FIGURE 7-9

Color vision testing sequence to determine diagnosis of color vision status and overall color discrimination ability. (Adapted from Michael Kalloniatis, Department of Optometry, University of Melbourne, Carlton, Victoria, Australia, personal communication.)

not be used to grade overall color discrimination ability. The anomaloscope may identify a red-green anomalous trichromat, but it may not indicate if color confusions will be significant. A battery of tests is required to properly classify color vision status and grade the severity of a defect.

Adams and Haegerstrom-Portnoy[1] recommended to the practitioner a minimum testing battery of the pseudoisochromatic plates and the Panel D-15 test. The pseudoisochromatic plates will identify those individuals with a congenital red-green deficiency. The Panel D-15 can then be used to grade the deficiencies into mild and severe categories. The Panel D-15 will also provide the blue-yellow testing capability to identify relatively rare congenital tritan defects and most acquired defects.

Figure 7-9 illustrates a testing scheme for assessing congenital color vision status in a clinical environment where multiple color vision tests are available. As mentioned previously, the Nagel Anomaloscope is the only method that can reliably classify deutans and protans and discriminate extreme anomalous trichromats from red-green dichromats. The FM 100-hue test is useful in evaluating overall color discrimination ability, even in those subjects with normal trichromatic vision.

The classification and grading of acquired defects requires arrangement type tests. Lesions or trauma affecting the visual pathway will typically not be isolated within one color opponent channel. Testing using pseudoisochromatic plates may give ambiguous results or may even indicate normal processing. Pseudoisochromatic plates do best with congenital defects where the causes of the defects are based on abnormal visual pigments and color confusions are predictable. Pseudoisochromatic plates are unreliable when used alone to test for acquired color vision defects.

The Panel D-15, Desaturated Panel D-15, and the FM 100-hue tests all measure discrimination ability around the entire color circle and can be used to screen and grade acquired color vision deficiencies. The Panel D-15 test can be used initially to acquaint the patient with the testing sequence and to discriminate between mild and relatively severe defects. If no errors or only relatively few errors are made with the Panel D-15 test, the desaturated version may be used. If the Panel D-15 test shows extremely poor color discrimination, the desaturated version will provide no additional information. Although tedious and time consuming, the FM 100-hue test provides the most information concerning fine color discrimination and is recommended for grading severity and measuring the progression of acquired color vision deficiencies.

MANAGEMENT OF HEREDITARY COLOR VISION DEFECTS

Counseling a patient concerning his or her color vision defect is an important component to color vision testing. Affected patients know they are not color "blind" and should not be addressed as such. These patients can see colors and make discriminations based on color. However, when compared with persons with normal color vision, they will show discrimination deficits. Certain colors may be confused, especially pale or dark colors. Color discrimination is usually enhanced by illuminating colored objects with a bright, full spectrum light. A description of the genetic nature of the defect is usually appreciated. The patient should be told that the condition is stable and will not progress.

Protan defectives should be informed that they have an insensitivity to red light. This reduced sensitivity may lead to increased reaction times when driving. Automobile taillights and brake lights may be difficult to see, especially when there is poor visibility because of bad weather.

Because of the use of color coding in the classroom, early detection of any color discrimination loss in children is important. A child may be classified as having a learning disorder or may be ridiculed by classmates if colors are misnamed or inappropriately identified. Teachers and parents should be made aware of the expected deficits. Reds may be confused with greens or with browns and blacks. Additionally, blues may be confused with purples, and bluish-greens may appear gray.

With few exceptions, a congenital color vision deficiency rarely leads to major complications in lifestyle. It can, however, limit vocational opportunities (Table 7-6). An individual with a moderate or severe color deficit may not pass the visual standards for a job requiring the identification of color coding or signal lights (e.g., police officer, firefighter, civilian or military pilot, commercial driver). Therefore, it is useful to perform a complete analysis on any patient with a color vision deficiency so that proper information concerning the defect can be provided.

Partial improvement of the color discrimination loss of congenital red-green color defectives can be provided through the use of colored filters. A colored filter may alter the color and brightness of a visual scene, adding extra cues for the observer. A red filter with extremely low green transmission is typically used over the non-

TABLE 7-6
Vocations Requiring Good Color Discrimination*

Automobile body repair
Cartography
Ceramics (inspector, painter)
Color restoration
Cosmetology
Dentistry
Electrician
Electronics
Firefighting
Gemologist
Horticulturist
Interior design
Laboratory analysis (chemist, medical technologist, pathologist)
Law enforcement
Medicine
Military (certain specialties)
Quality control/inspection/color grading (e.g., fruit, vegetables, meat)
Metallurgist
Paint industry (production)
Pharmacy
Photography
Printing
Television repair
Textile industry (buying, dye matching, manufacturing)
Transportation (aviation, maritime, railroad)

*Normal color vision may be required for some occupations due to safety concerns or to the degree and nature of the color discriminations that are necessary. However, for many occupations, mild color vision defectives with good color discrimination may perform as well as normals.

dominant eye.[41] "Color" discrimination is enhanced by the lustre appearance of certain colors created by a substantial brightness difference between the retinal images of the two eyes. In her summary of the history of the use of colored filters to help persons with color vision defects, Schmidt[42] stated that these filters are most useful in occupations in which color discriminations are made from a limited and fixed range of colors.

Colored filters are made available to patients via the tinting of both rigid and soft contact lenses. Zeltzer[41] introduced the most well-known of these lenses, the X-chrom lens, in 1971 and presented a fitting strategy for the lens.[43] He stated that the lens is most useful with anomalous red-green defectives. However, Adams and Haegerstrom-Portnoy[1] believe that dichromats receive the most benefit. They recommended demonstrating the visual effects of these filtering lenses by using a Kodak Wratten No. 30 filter. Also, they recommended loaning this filter to the patient with a color vision defect for a trial period before deciding whether to fit the patient with the contact lens.

REFERENCES

1. Adams A, Haegerstrom-Portnoy G. Color deficiency. In J Amos (ed), Diagnosis and Management in Vision Care. Boston: Butterworth, 1987;671–711.
2. Palmer G. Theory of Colors and Vision. London: Leacroft, 1777. In DL MacAdam (ed), Sources of Color Science. Cambridge MA: MIT Press, 1970.
3. Young T. On the theory of light and colors. Philosophical Transactions of the Royal Society of London 1802;92:20–71.
4. Boynton R. Human Color Vision. New York: Holt, Rinehart & Winston, 1979;14–8.
5. Southall JPC (ed). Helmholtz's treatise on Physiological Optics (translated from 3rd German ed.), Vol. II. Rochester NY: Optical Society of America, 1924;141–6.
6. Weale R. Trichromatic ideas in the seventeenth and eighteenth centuries. Nature 1957;179:648–51.
7. Grassman H. On the theory of compound colours. Philosophic Magazine 1854;7:254–64.
8. Maxwell JC. On the theory of three primary colours. Lecture at the Royal Institution of Great Britain, May 17, 1861. In WD Niven (ed), Scientific Papers (Vol 1). London: Cambridge University Press, 1890;445–50.
9. Bowmaker JK, Dartnall HJA, Lythgoe JN, Mollon JD. The visual pigments of rods and cones in the rhesus monkey, Macaca mulatta. J Physiol (Lond) 1978;274:329–48.
10. Dartnall HJA, Bowmaker JK, Mollon JD. Human visual pigments: Microspectrophotometric results from the eyes of seven persons. Proc R Soc Lond [Biol] 1983;220:115–30.
11. Smith VC, Pokorny J, Starr SJ. Variability of color mixture data—I. Interobserver variability in the unit coordinates. Vision Res 1976;16:1087–94.
12. Hering E. Outlines of a theory of the light sense. Cambridge MA: Harvard University Press, 1964.
13. Pokorny J, Smith V, Verriest G. Congenital Color Defects. In J Pokorny, V Smith, G Verriest, A Pickners (eds), Congenital and Acquired Color Vision Defects. New York: Grune & Stratton, 1979;183–241.
14. Walls GL, Heath GG. Neutral points in 138 protanopes and deuteranopes. J Opt Soc Am 1956;46:640–9.
15. Cole BL, Henry GH, Nathan J. Phenotypical variations in tritanopia. Vision Res 1966;6:301–13.
16. von Kries J. Normal and Anomalous Color Systems. In JPC Southall (ed), Helmholtz's Treatise on Physiological Optics, (translated from 3rd German ed.), Vol II. Rochester NY: Optical Society of America, 1924;395–425.
17. Wald G. Defective color vision and its inheritance. Proc Natl Acad Sci USA 1966;55:1347–63.
18. Piantanida T. Genetics of Inherited Colour Vision Deficiencies. In D Foster (ed), Inherited and Acquired Colour Vision Deficiencies. Vol. 7. Boca Raton, FL: CRC Press, 1991;88–114.
19. Wright WD. The characteristics of tritanopia. J Opt Soc Am 1952;42:509–21.
20. Ruddock K. Psychophysics of Inherited Colour Vision Deficiencies. In D Foster (ed), Inherited and Acquired Colour Vision Deficiencies. Vol. 7. Boca Raton, FL: CRC Press, 1991;4–37.
21. Sperling HG. Vulnerability of the Blue-Sensitive Mechanism. In D Foster (ed), Inherited and Acquired Colour Vision Deficiencies, Vol. 7. Boca Raton, FL: CRC Press, 1991;72–87.
22. Verriest G. Further studies on acquired deficiency of color discrimination. J Opt Soc Am 1963;53:185–95.
23. Kollner H. Die storungen des Farbensinnes, ihre klinische Bedeutung und ihre Diagnose. Berlin: Karger, 1912.
24. von Kries J. Uber farbensysteme. Z Psychol Physiol Sinnesorg 1897;13:241–324.
25. Pokorny J, Smith VC, Trimble J. A new technique for proper illumination for color vision tests. Am J Ophthalmol 1977;84:429.
26. Higgins K, Moskowitz-Cook A, Knoblauch K. Color vision testing—an alternative source of illuminant C. Mod Probl Opthalmol 1978;19:113–21.
27. Birch J, Chisholm I, Kinnear P, et al. Clinical Testing Methods. In J Pokorny, V Smith, G Verriest, A Pickners (eds), Congenital and Acquired Color Vision Defects. New York: Grune & Stratton, 1979;83–135.
28. Dvorine I. Improvements in color vision in twenty cases. Am J Optom Physiol Opt 1946;23:302–21.
29. Taylor WOG. Constructing your own PIC test. Br J Physiol Opt 1975;30:22–4.
30. Adams AJ, Bailey JE, Harwood LW. Color vision screening: a comparison of the AO H-R-R and Farnsworth F-2 tests. Am J Optom Physiol Opt 1983;61:1–9.
31. Pease PL, Allen J. A new test for screening color vision: concurrent validity and utility. Am J Optom Physiol Opt 1988;65:729–38.
32. Ichikawa K, Ichikawa H, Tanabe S. Detection of acquired color vision defects by standard pseudoisochromatic plates II. Doc Opthalmol Proc Ser 1984;46:133–40.
33. Bowman KJ. A method of quantitative scoring of the Farnsworth Panel D-15. Acta Opthalmol 1982;60:907–16.
34. Vingrys AJ, King-Smith PE. A quantitative scoring technique for panel tests of color vision. Invest Ophthalmol Visual Sci 1988;29:50–63.
35. Commission Internationale De L'Eclairage (CIE). Recommendations on uniform color spaces, color-difference equations, psychometric color terms. Supplement 2 of CIE Publication 15 (E-1.3.1), 1971. Paris: Bureau Central de la CIE, 1978.
36. Steward JM, Cole BL. The Effect of Object Size on the Performance of Colour Ordering and Discrimination Tasks. In B Drum, G Verriest (eds), Colour Vision Deficiencies IX. Doc Ophthalmol Proc Ser 1989;52:79–88.
37. Bowman KJ, Cameron KD. A Quantitative Assessment of Colour Discrimination in Normal Vision and Senile Macular Degeneration Using Some Colour Confusion Tests. In G Verriest (ed), Colour Vision Deficiencies VII. Doc Ophthalmol Proc Ser 1984;39:363–70.
38. Collins MJ. Pre-age related maculopathy and the desaturated D-15 colour vision test. Clin Exp Optom 1986;69:223–7.
39. Bassi CJ, Galanis JC, Hoffman J. Comparison of the Farnsworth-Munsell 100-Hue, the Farnsworth D-15, and the L'Anthony D-15 desaturated color tests. Arch Ophthalmol 1993;111:639–41.

40. Fletcher R. A modified D-15 test. Mod Probl Opthalmol 1972;11:22–4.

41. Zeltzer H. The x-chrom lens. J Am Optom Assoc 1971;42:933–9.

42. Schmidt I. Visual aids for correction for red-green colour deficiencies. Can J Optom 1976;38:38–46.

43. Zeltzer HI. Recommended procedure for fitting the X-chrom lens. J Am Optom Assoc 1974;45:72–5.

8

Visual Fields

DONALD A. SEIBERT AND JOHN P. SCHOESSLER

Examination of the visual field has been performed for centuries. There are references to Hippocrates examining the visual fields of patients in ancient Greece.[1] Today the term *visual field* is used to describe the extent and sensitivity of the patient's visual world with both eyes. Each eye has its own field of vision, and the projection of one eye's field overlaps with the alternate eye's visual field in a synergistic manner, creating the entire binocular visual field (Figure 8-1).

Visual field testing is a comprehensive concept encompassing the many techniques for measuring the extent and sensitivity of the visual field. It can be performed using stimuli of different sizes, colors, luminance, and character. It has proved to be the most clinically useful test for detecting, diagnosing, and evaluating disturbances of the entire visual pathway.

Testing the visual field is a detection task. Clinicians are accustomed to measuring central visual acuity by asking the patient to interpret a letter or figure, but this is not a feasible method for testing the peripheral vision because visual acuity drops off too quickly. Instead, the detection of a stimulus in the periphery by the patient has proved to be the best method for clinical evaluation of the visual field.

Visual field testing has been classified into campimetric testing and perimetric testing. In the clinical setting, perimetric testing has become synonymous with visual field testing, although perimetry actually means measurement of the periphery.[1] Perimetric testing is designed in such a manner that the distance from the stimulus to the eye and therefore the angular size of the stimulus is held constant. In campimetric testing the angular size of the stimulus varies because the test plane is flat and therefore the peripheral stimuli have a different angular size than the central stimuli. In practical terms this means that a 30-degree stimulus on a perimetric machine is not the same as a 30-degree stimulus on a campimetric screen,

and results from the two machines should never be compared. Clinically, perimetric machines are bowl-shaped while campimetric testing is performed on a flat surface.

The patient may be tested kinetically with a moving stimulus or statically with a blinking stimulus. Kinetic testing involves moving the stimulus from peripheral to central vision at a slow rate of speed until it is observed by the patient. Static testing involves turning the stimulus on and off at a predetermined point and determining whether the patient perceives the light. Both methods have benefits and difficulties (see Central Visual Field Testing).

The apparatuses most commonly used today for testing the visual field are the tangent screen, the manual hemispheric projection perimeter of Goldmann (shortened clinically to a "Goldmann"), and, more recently, automated or computerized visual field testing machines (Figures 8-2, 8-3, and 8-4).

Visual field testing should be part of every vision analysis even if it only involves screening the patient with a confrontation test (see section on Confrontation Field Testing). The ease of administration coupled with the wealth of knowledge it provides makes visual field testing ideal for evaluating the visual pathway. The type of visual field testing that the practitioner chooses to perform may vary depending on the case history, visual acuity testing, ophthalmoscopy, patient ambulation, or previous examination.

RETINAL FUNCTION

Retinal Architecture and its Functional Significance to Visual Field Testing

The human retina (Table 8-1) is a ten-layer structure that can be thought of as three compartments or sections. The

FIGURE 8-1

A graphical representation of the limits of the normal visual field and the area of binocular vision.

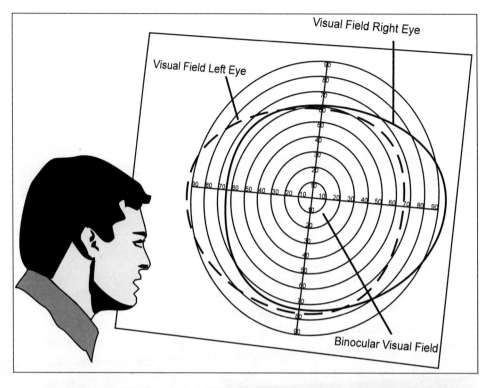

FIGURE 8-2

The tangent screen with an optional large X to aid patients with poor central vision.

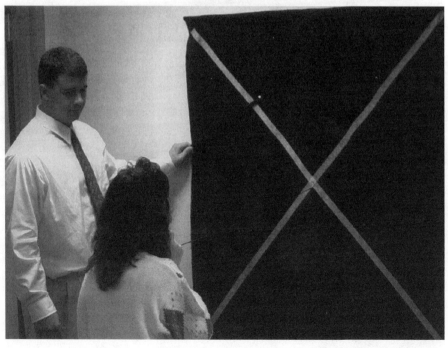

three sections consist of a receiving segment, an interconnecting section, and a transmitting section. The receiving (outer) section is made up of the retinal pigment epithelium (RPE), photoreceptors, and external limiting membrane. The interconnecting section continues forward from the outer plexiform layer to the inner nuclear layer. The transmitting section extends from the individual ganglion cells to the optic nerve.

As light passes through the inner retina to the outer receiving section, it stimulates the photoreceptors to transform light into an electrical signal, which rapidly moves up the retinal tree to the interconnecting layer and final-

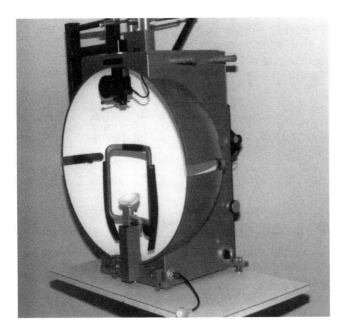

FIGURE 8-3
A typical Goldmann bowl.

ly to the transmitting layer, where it exits the eye through the optic nerve.

Sensitivity to light varies in different areas of the retina and generally decreases from central to peripheral regions. This variation in sensitivity is a function of three properties of the retina:

1. The concentration of photoreceptors varies at different locations within the retina. The central retina has the greatest concentration of photoreceptors and has the most sensitive visual acuity.

2. The type of photoreceptor found in each area of the retina affects its sensitivity. The rods are more sensitive to dim light but do not regenerate their pho-

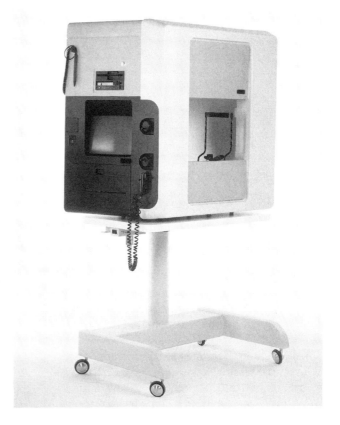

FIGURE 8-4
The automated Humphrey Visual Field Analyzer Model 640. (Courtesy of Humphrey Instruments, Inc., San Leandro, CA.)

topigments nearly as quickly as the cones.[2] On the other hand, the cones are sensitive to colors, assuming that at least two different cone types are present (Table 8-2).

3. The ratio of photoreceptors to interconnecting cells varies from the central to the peripheral retina. Vision

TABLE 8-1
A Tabular Description of the Histologic and Cellular Makeup of the Human Retina and the Three Functional Layers that Correspond to the Cellular and Histologic Components

Functional Layer Correlates	Retinal Histologic Correlates	Cellular Correlates
Receiving layer	Retinal pigment epithelium	Retinal pigment epithelium
	Photoreceptor layer (rod and cone layer)	Rods and cones
	External limiting membrane	Footplates of Mueller cells
Interconnecting layer	Outer plexiform layer	Horizontal cells
	Outer cellular layer	Bipolar cell nuclei
	Inner plexiform layer	Amacrine cells
	Inner nuclear layer	Amacrine ganglion connections
Transmitting layer	Ganglion cell layer	Ganglion cells
	Nerve fiber layer	Axon from ganglion cell to optic nerve
	Internal limiting membrane	Internal limiting membrane

TABLE 8-2

The Physiologic Differences Between Rods and Cones

Photoreceptor Function	Rods	Cones
Sensitivity	To dim light	To bright light
Spatial resolution	Course visual acuity	Fine acuity
Temporal modulation	Only slow flicker (<10/sec)	Follow fast flicker (up to 30/sec)
Maximal spectral sensitivity	Blue-green (500 nm)	Greenish-yellow (560 nm)
Rate of dark adaptation	Slow	Fast
Color vision	Absent	Present (requires at least two cone types)

Source: Reprinted with permission from RE Carr, IM Siegel. Electrodiagnostic Testing of the Visual System: A Clinical Guide (2nd ed). Philadelphia: FA Davis, 1990;5.

is more sensitive in the central retina, where the interconnections approximate a one-to-one ratio, and less sensitive in the periphery, where the ratio decreases to approximately 300 to one.[1]

The retina contains approximately 126 million photoreceptors.[1] The rods are the predominant cell type, numbering approximately 110–125 million, whereas there are only about 6.3–6.5 million cones in the human retina. The cone concentration is greatest in the fovea, reaching a maximum concentration of 145,000/mm^2, while at 10 degrees from the fovea, the cone concentration drops to 10,000/mm^2. The rod concentration is 0 at the center of the fovea and increases to approximately 135,000/mm^2 at 18 degrees from fixation.

Physiology of the Receptive Fields

The retinal electrical hierarchy is arranged in such a manner that isolated areas of the retina act as separate visual recognition loci. These areas and their corresponding visual field location are termed *receptive fields*. Each receptive field can be stimulated by a very precise stimulus. Examples of different types of stimuli include lines at a certain orientation, colored stimuli, checkerboard patterns, and white light. What they tell us is that the retina not only responds to light but also responds to these different stimuli in a very unique way. A patient's receptive fields are smaller in the center of vision than in the periphery, and the limits of these receptive fields are defined by where the receptive field stimulus no longer causes ganglion cell firing or inhibition. Receptive fields can be "turned off" by certain stimuli as well as "turned on." The importance of receptive fields in visual field testing is that usually larger stimuli are needed to stimulate the more peripheral retina.[1]

Architecture of the Visual Pathway

The visual pathway extends from the photoreceptors in the retina to the visual recognition cells located in the occipital cortex. The visual pathway is composed of the retina, optic nerve, optic chiasm, optic tract, lateral geniculate body, and optic radiations (temporal, parietal, and occipital, also called the *geniculocalcarine tract*) ending in Brodmann's areas 17, 18, and 19 of the visual cortex (Figure 8-5). The visual pathway can be classified anatomically into the prechiasmal pathway, the chiasm, and the

FIGURE 8-5 ▶

A schematic representation of the visual pathway. Here, the pathway begins with the ganglion cell nuclei, which discharge after light stimulates the left retina of each eye from the right visual field (A). The signal is transmitted to the optic nerve (B). At the chiasm (C), the signal from the left half of the right retina crosses to the left side and the temporal fibers from the left retina stay ipsilateral. The fibers corresponding to the right visual field then move through the optic tract (D) to synapse at the lateral geniculate body (E). After the synapse the fibers move anterior through the temporal lobe (F). From there they pass through the parietal lobe (G), and end at the occipital lobe (H). Lesions at different locations along the visual pathway cause characteristic localizing visual field defects. 1. Total loss of the ipsilateral eye from an optic nerve lesion. The unilaterality of the field loss defines it as a prechiasmal defect. 2. Total loss of one eye with a left hemianopsia of the left visual field in the left eye is characteristic of a junction scotoma at the anterior knee of Wilbrand. This lesion also can present as a left-eyed quadrantanopsia suggesting a progressing lesion. 3. A bitemporal defect representative of chiasmal damage. The lesion affects the crossing fibers of each eye only. This damage is suggestive of a pituitary adenoma. 4. An optic tract lesion. An incongruous left homonymous hemianopsia with macular splitting. 5. A left-eyed left hemianopsia with a right-eyed left superior quadrantanopsia. Temporal lobe lesions typically have "pie in the sky" defects and may present as bilateral incongruous quadrantanopsias. 6. A left homonymous hemianopsia; "pie on the floor" defects may also occur with lesions of the parietal lobe. 7. A left homonymous hemianopsia with macular sparing, typical of occipital lobe lesions. 8. A temporal wedge defect of the anterior lip of the calcarine fissure. 9. A right homonymous macular hemianopsia with macular splitting.

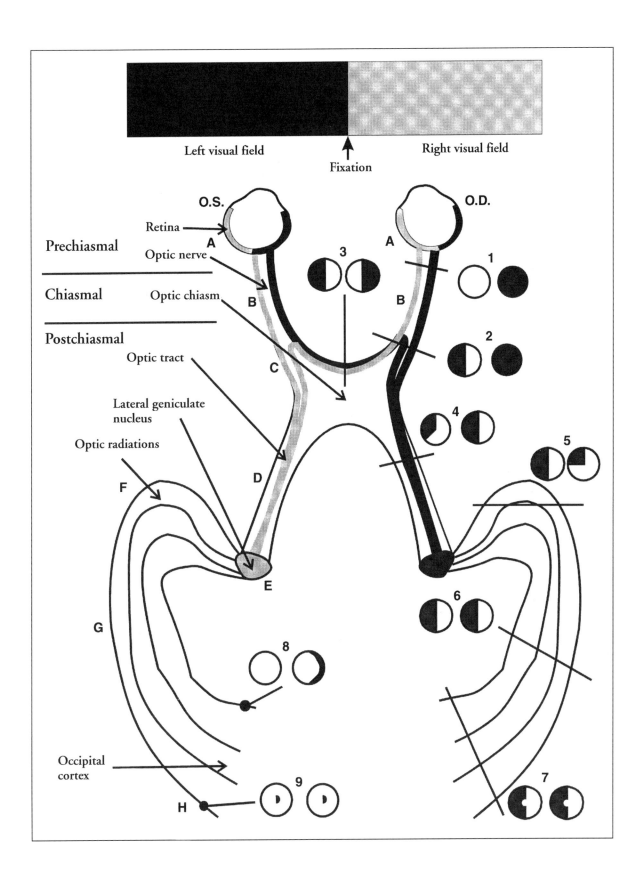

Left visual field

Right visual field

Fixation

O.S.

O.D.

Retina

Prechiasmal

Optic nerve

Chiasmal

Optic chiasm

Postchiasmal

Optic tract

Lateral geniculate nucleus

Optic radiations

Occipital cortex

postchiasmal pathway. The prechiasmal pathway consists of the retina and the optic nerve. The chiasm is the area where the fibers from the right and left eyes cross. As seen in Figure 8-5, the temporal retinal fibers from each eye stay ipsilateral in the chiasm, whereas nasal retinal fibers cross in the chiasm to go to the contralateral optic tract. The crossing fibers in the chiasm actually make a slight bend into the contralateral optic nerve, forming the anterior knee (genu) of Wilbrand.

Lesions at different locations along the visual pathway cause characteristic localizing visual field defects:

1. Total loss of the ipsilateral eye's vision from an optic nerve lesion. The unilaterality of the field loss defines it as a prechiasmal defect.

2. Total loss of one eye's vision with a left hemianopsia of the left eye is characteristic of a junction scotoma at the anterior knee of Wilbrand. This lesion also can present as a quadrantanopsia of the left eye suggesting a progressing lesion.

3. A bitemporal defect representative of chiasmal damage. The lesion affects the crossing fibers of each eye only. This damage is extremely suggestive of a pituitary adenoma.

4. An optic tract lesion. An incongruous left homonymous hemianopsia with macular splitting.

5. A left hemianopsia of the left eye with a left superior quadrantanopsia of the right eye. Temporal lobe lesions typically have "pie in the sky" defects and may present as bilateral incongruous quadrantanopsias.

6. A left homonymous hemianopsia. "Pie on the floor" defects often occur with lesions of the parietal lobe.

7. A left homonymous hemianopsia with macular sparing is typical of occipital lobe lesions.

8. A peripheral temporal defect is caused by a lesion at the anterior tip of the calcarine fissure.

9. A right homonymous macular hemianopsia with macular splitting.

The ipsilateral temporal fibers from one optic nerve and the contralateral optic nerve's nasal fibers enter the optic tract together from the chiasm and terminate in the lateral geniculate body. A synapse is made in the lateral geniculate body, and the fibers then spread out into the optic radiations. The optic radiations course anteriorly through the temporal lobe (Meyer's loop), through the parietal lobe, and finally to the occipital cortex, where they terminate in Brodmann's areas 17, 18, and 19.

Understanding the topography of the visual pathway is extremely helpful in that a cortically located lesion will often cause a corresponding visual field deficit that reveals the location of the lesion, which allows better localization for imaging and possible surgical intervention.

Note that the visual pathway is organized in a way such that an image in the patient's right visual field will eventually stimulate cells in the left occipital cortex and vice versa. Figure 8-5 illustrates that any postchiasmal lesion will cause bilateral visual field defects, whereas prechiasmal lesions will cause unilateral defects. Also, the visual pathway is divided vertically through the fovea, not the optic nerve.

LUMINANCE

Luminosity and Clinical Conventions for Visual Field Testing

In its most basic form, perimetry is an attempt to determine exactly what luminance of light falling on the retina is necessary to make the patient respond that he or she "sees" the stimulus. Classifying this light has been a monumental problem throughout the history of perimetry. From a physicist's point of view, light is merely that part of the electromagnetic spectrum that humans are able to see. It is simple, then, to classify this electromagnetic energy with the unit of power (watts) divided by the area on which this energy is falling—e.g., watts per square meter. Unfortunately these units have not been practical because of the complicated relationships of color, brightness, saturation, and hue, which tend to create a subjectively confusing stimulus when classified with the physicist's power per area nomenclature. For example, a color with more saturation may actually appear brighter even though the wattage per area may be less. Numerous classification schemes, some subjective and others objective, have been derived. None of these is totally accepted.

Physiologic optics researchers use the radiometric system because there is no subjective interpretation involved in assessing the brightness of a light. Brightness in the radiometric system is termed *radiance*. The amount of brightness falling on an object is termed *irradiance*.[1]

Brightness in the luminance system is termed *luminance*. Luminance involves the subjective interpretation that a light has a certain amount of brightness. In this system, illumination is defined as the amount of light falling on a target. The standard unit for illuminance in this system is the NIT (candela per square meter) as recommended by the Commission Internationale de L'Eclairage (CIE). Other units of luminance include the apostilb (asb), lambert, foot-lambert, candela per square foot, candela per square inch, and the stilb or candela per square centimeter. All of these

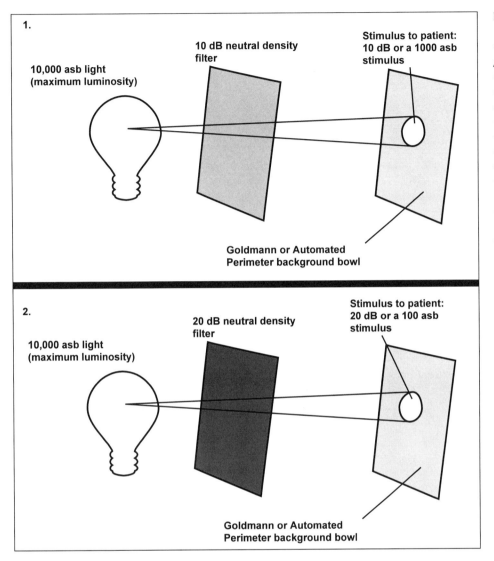

FIGURE 8-6

The production of a stimulus by a Goldmann bowl or automated perimeter. As the maximal luminosity light passes through a neutral density filter, the stimulus is dimmed by a logarithmic factor. (1) A decibel is one tenth of a log unit, therefore the 10-dB neutral density filter dims the 10,000-asb maximal luminosity light source by one log unit (i.e., the stimulus becomes 1000 asb). (2) A 20-dB neutral density filter dims the light source by two log units, yielding a stimulus of 100 asb.

units measure subjective brightness and can be interconverted by a constant. For example, an apostilb is:

$$\pi \times NIT \ (candela/m^2) = asb$$

Because luminance (brightness) values vary so much in magnitude, it is more convenient to refer to the logarithm base 10 of luminance units rather than actual units. A second reason for switching to a logarithmic scale is that the subjective interpretation of brightness is more related to the ratios of intensity than to the scale itself.[3] For example, a light that is 10 asb in brightness appears half as bright as a light 20 asb in brightness, and a light 100 asb in brightness appears approximately half as bright as a light 200 asb in brightness, even though the differences between the values differ greatly.

To add more accuracy to the discussion, it is useful to divide the log base 10 numbers into tenths. One tenth of a log unit is known as a decibel.[3] The decibel has become a confusing term in health care. It is possible to convert any number system to a logarithmic scale whether it be noise level, luminance level, or some other level. The important detail is knowing what numbers are being converted to the logarithmic scale. In clinical perimetry the apostilb unit is the popular choice for the classification of luminance.

In perimetry, decibels, which are commonly noted to classify the stimulus, actually label the neutral density filter in front of the projection stimulus bulb and not the bulb itself. For example, a 10-dB stimulus is brighter than a 20-dB stimulus. In other words, if a perimeter has a maximum stimulus of 10,000 asb and a 1.0-log unit (10-dB) filter is placed in front of that light, the resulting brightness of the light the patient sees will be 1000 asb. A 2.0-log unit filter (20 dB) will have an intensity of 100 asb (Figure 8-6).

TABLE 8-3
The Goldmann Classification of Stimulus Size by Roman Numerals*

Goldmann Stimulus Size	Area of Stimulus	Approximate Change
0	0.0625 mm^2	
I	0.25 mm^2	+5 dB (0.5 log unit) from the size 0
II	1 mm^2	+5 dB (0.5 log unit) from size I
III	4 mm^2	+5 dB (0.5 log unit) from size II
IV	16 mm^2	+5 dB (0.5 log unit) from size III
V	64 mm^2	+5 dB (0.5 log unit) from size IV

*The system is based on the physiologic perception that a doubling of the radius (4¥ the area) creates a change in perceived brightness of approximately 0.5 log units.

It should be noted that a 10-dB stimulus on one perimeter may not be a 10-dB stimulus on another perimeter because of differences in maximal stimulus intensity created by the bulb behind the neutral density filter.

The stimulus of a Goldmann bowl is actually the summation of the background stimulus and the projected stimulus. For example, a 100-asb (20-dB filter with a 10,000 asb bulb) stimulus presented against a 32-asb background actually has a total brightness of 132 asb (100 asb + 32 asb) and a relative brightness of 100 [total brightness (132) – surrounding brightness (32)] apostilbs. It is conventional to classify this stimulus as a 100-asb (20-dB) stimulus because the background remains constant.

Weber's Law

The human retina can exist in three states: a scotopic or dark-adapted state, a photopic or light-adapted state, and an in-between mesopic state. In the scotopic state the rods are responsible for vision, and this is generally accepted to range in luminance from 10^{-5} asb (just perceptible light) to the sum of the stimulus and background light being less than 0.003 asb.[1] When the stimulus and background light range from 0.003 asb to 3 asb, light levels are in the mesopic level of retinal adaptation. The rods and cones are both considered responsible for vision at these levels. Above 3 asb is considered to be within the photopic range, and the cones primarily contribute to vision at these levels.

A unique characteristic of the human eye is that under photopic conditions, it obeys Weber's law. Weber's law states that a just-noticeable change in stimulus divided by the stimulus is a constant—i.e., $dL/L = C$. If the background luminance of a bowl perimeter (L) is considered the stimulus and the projected light of the stimulus is considered the change in stimulus (dL), then the relative difference between the stimulus and background is what is most important as far as characterizing the stimulus and the patient's threshold; the absolute values of the background and the stimulus are not as critical.

Goldmann Luminance Levels

The Goldmann bowl, shown in Figure 8-3, was designed to accurately define the luminance levels used to create a stimulus. The precursor to the Goldmann bowl, the tangent screen, lacked any significant control of stimulus luminosity, and the need for accurate categorizing of stimuli was obvious. The simple but elegant system of the Goldmann bowl for categorizing the size and luminance of stimuli is still widely used today.

As mentioned, the Goldmann bowl has a single stimulus light providing the brightest stimulus possible for the instrument. All of the other stimuli produced by the Goldmann bowl have less intensity than the maximal stimulus and are incrementally dimmed through the use of neutral density filters. The sum of these neutral density filters is the designation given the stimulus (i.e., a 10-dB stimulus). As stated previously, a 10-dB stimulus is actually a 10-dB neutral density filter placed in front of the maximal stimulus light (see Figure 8-6).

Goldmann categorized his stimulus values by size as well as by intensity. For the size of the stimulus he used a Roman numeral system shown in Table 8-3. Note that with each increase in Roman numeral, the area is quadrupled (doubling the radius). This increase in size approximates a 0.5-log unit (5-dB) increase in stimulus intensity.

Goldmann categorized the stimulus intensity levels using a system of 0.5- and 0.1-log unit neutral density filters and labeled them with Arabic numbers (1–4) for 0.5-log unit (5-dB) changes and lowercase letters (a–e) for 0.1-log unit (1-dB) changes (Table 8-4).

For example, a Goldmann stimulus could be characterized as a I-3c. The I ("one") means the stimulus is 0.25 mm^2 in size. The 3 means that there is one 0.5-log unit (5-dB) neutral density filter in front of the stimulus light, and the c means that there is a 0.2-log unit (2-dB) neutral density filter in front of the stimulus creating a 0.7-log unit (7-dB) intensity stimulus 0.25 mm^2 in size (Figure 8-7). Gold-

TABLE 8-4
The Organization of the Goldmann Stimulus Intensity Classification Scheme *

0.5 Log Unit Neutral Density Filter Label	Value of the Neutral Density Filter	0.1 Log Unit Neutral Density Filter Label	Value of the Neutral Density Filter
4	No filter	e	No filter
3	0.5 log unit (5 dB)	d	0.1 log unit (1 dB)
2	1.0 log unit (10 dB)	c	0.2 log unit (2 dB)
1	1.5 log unit (15 dB)	b	0.3 log unit (3 dB)
		a	0.4 log unit (4 dB)

*Correlating intensity levels are currently used on many automated perimeters.

mann's classification system resulted in easily producing a large variety of accurately characterized stimuli.

Standardization

From a theoretical and practical point of view, visual field examinations should be performed under precisely controlled conditions. The function of a perimetric examination is to detect defects in the visual field, to help discover the causes of these defects, and to measure the rates at which the defects progress. If standard test conditions are not maintained, the visual field data cannot be compared with previous test results, nor can a standard result be determined for any given examination.

Many components of the examination can influence the measured extent of the visual field and of the blind spot. The major external considerations—that is, factors not related to patient or examiner—include the angular size, luminance, and color of the test object; luminance of the background; and contrast between the target and the background.

Large variations in visual field data may be caused by differences in testing instrumentation. The contrast between a target and its background has a great influence on the extent of the plotted defect and should always be

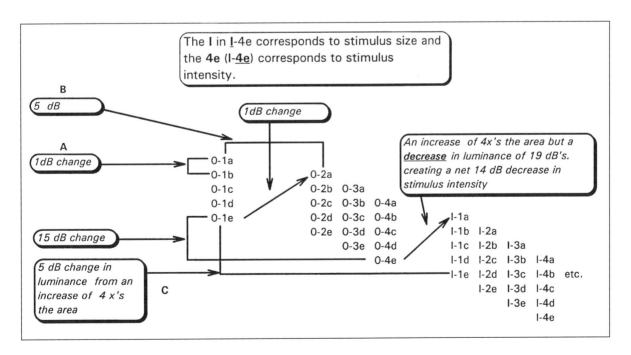

FIGURE 8-7
The step increases in Goldmann stimuli. A. Each change in lowercase letter causes a 1-dB (0.1 log unit) change in luminance. B. Each change in Arabic numeral causes a 5-dB (0.5 log unit) change in luminance. C. Increasing the Roman numeral by one unit quadruples the area, which approximates a 5-dB (0.5 log unit) change in luminance.

TABLE 8-5
Standard Stimulus Conditions for Visual Field Testing

Instrument	Test Object Size (diameter)	Testing Distance	Angular Size of Test Object (degrees)	Test Object Luminance	Background Luminance	Contrast	O.D.[b] Horizontal	O.D. Vertical	O.S. Horizontal	O.S. Vertical
Tangent screen	1.0 mm	1,000 mm	0.057	21.58 cd/m²	0.46 cd/m²	45.91	5.76	8.07	5.67	8.06
Goldmann Bowl	0.56 mm[a] or 4 mm²	300 mm	0.108	100 asb	31.5 asb	3.17	7.23	9.39	7.29	9.56
Humphrey automated perimeter (model 640)	0.56 mm[a] or 4 mm²	300 mm	0.108	100 asb	31.5 asb	3.17				
Octopus automated perimeter	0.56 mm[a] or 4 mm²	300 mm	0.108	10 asb	4 asb	2.50				

[a]Goldmann size III stimulus.
[b]Values in the last four columns are a comparison of different blind spot sizes measured on the tangent screen and a Goldmann bowl.
Source: Modified from JP Schoessler. The influence of visual field testing procedures on blind spot size. J Am Optom Assoc 1976;47:898.

considered when comparing visual fields from different or even similar instruments (Table 8-5). It is highly suggested not to interchange testing instruments unless absolutely necessary; the interinstrument variability causes serial analysis to be practically impossible.

Tangent screens lack control over screen reflectance and target luminance; therefore, exact testing conditions cannot be known. Historically, the standards for tangent screen visual field testing were expressed in terms of illuminance on the testing surface, with 7 foot-candles being the accepted value. However, this does not take into account the reflectance of this light from the background screen or from the test object to the eye. The student of perimetry must be aware that to eliminate stimulus and background variables as a source of inconsistency in visual field measurements, instruments that contain a means of calibration for a known set of testing conditions should be used. A light meter should be used to determine ambient lighting conditions of the tangent screen, and test objects should be kept clean to provide maximum reflectance.

The Goldmann bowl has a light meter to determine that the background luminance is exactly 31.5 asb. Once the background is set, all of the other stimuli created by the bowl are known to be accurate because of its use of neutral density filters to create different stimulus intensities.

When using a Goldmann bowl or automated perimeter, room lighting must always be kept constant. Many practitioners recommend testing in a totally darkened room to decrease ambient light shadowing. Some manufacturers recommend a small amount of ambient light during the test to allow the perimetrist to move easily while the test is being performed.[4] Some automated instruments will automatically adjust their background lighting depending on the ambient room conditions.

Goldmann Bowl Luminosity Standardization

The Goldmann bowl is designed to be a clinical tool. It uses a photopic level of background luminance (31.5 asb) because the retina obeys Weber's law when photopically adapted and photopic conditions allow for rapid clinical testing. These were the standards set by the International Perimetric Society in 1979,[4] mainly because they work so well in the clinical setting. Most manufacturers of automated perimeters have adopted this level of background luminance.

THE VISUAL FIELD CONCEPT AND ITS RELATION TO MODERN PERIMETRY

Traquair has likened the visual field to a three-dimensional "island or hill of vision."[5] This is a useful concept, because it portrays not only the extent (X and Y axes) of the visual field but also the sensitivity (Z axis) of the field for different locations in the peripheral vision (Figure 8-8). The analogy is such that all of the "air" above the hill of vision represents light so dim that it is imperceptible to the patient and all of the "land" below the hill represents sensitivity levels that the patient can see. An isolated point located on the hill of vision represents the luminance and location of the threshold stimulus nec-

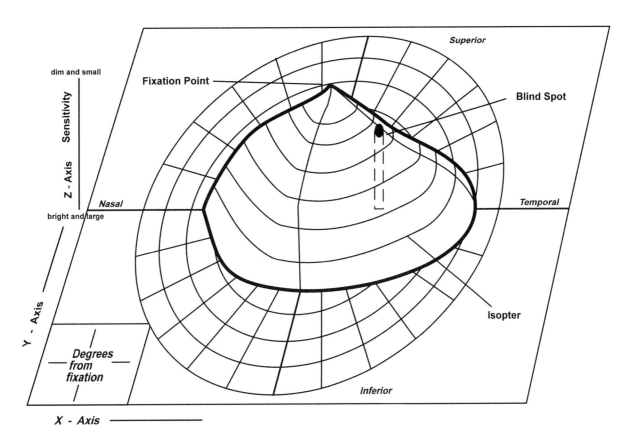

FIGURE 8-8

Traquair's island or hill of vision. The X and Y axes represent the distance from fixation the visual sensitivity is tested. The Z axis represents the sensitivity of vision. Note that the fixation point is the most sensitive locus in the visual field and that the blind spot is an absolute scotoma with the "hole" extending all the way to the floor of the hill of vision.

essary to elicit a patient response 50% of the time under photopic (Goldmann) background luminance.[3] This concept is widely used today on automated visual field printouts. The printouts give numerical representations of the sensitivity of the patient's field at different statically tested points. If the clinician thinks of these values as analogous to a topographic map, then reading the visual field and correlating these values to a hill of vision is quite simple.

If a perimetrist determines the threshold for retinal locations along the same meridian or axis, a "profile" of that meridian can be developed (Figure 8-9). The retinal threshold sensitivity changes as fixation is approached from the periphery, a stronger stimulus being required peripherally and a dimmer stimulus closer to fixation. When all of the threshold points along one meridian are connected, a profile plot for that meridian is accomplished. With the joining of several meridians, a model of the island of

vision can be constructed (see Figure 8-8). Plotting the threshold in this manner is called *profile*, or *light-sense* (as opposed to form-sense, which is also called visual acuity) perimetry and is very useful for early detection of visual loss. With the advent of automated projection perimetry, profile perimetry has become a routine method of analyzing the visual field.

The visual field may be tested with either isopter (kinetic) perimetry or static perimetry. Isopter perimetry is a method of visual field testing in which a constant stimulus is moved from the periphery toward fixation until it is perceived. The kinetically presented target is projected in different meridians, producing a series of points that are connected to form an isopter (Figure 8-10). Static perimetry is the method of testing the visual field in which a stimulus is briefly flashed at a particular locus within the visual field. For screening modalities a single, constant stimulus may be presented throughout the field, or

FIGURE 8-9
Profile perimetry. A profile of the hill of vision along one meridian showing both the extent and sensitivity of the visual field for this meridian.

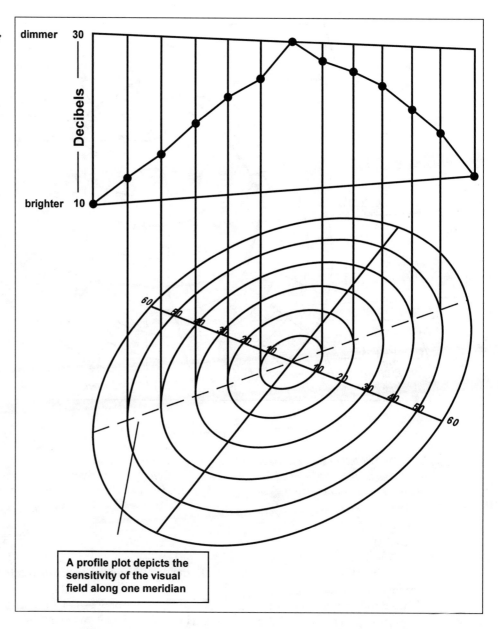

A profile plot depicts the sensitivity of the visual field along one meridian

for detailed testing, static stimuli of varying brightnesses may be presented to determine the threshold of vision.

THE NORMAL VISUAL FIELD

As mentioned, the visual field is a combination of dimensions and sensitivity. Its extent is illustrated in Figure 8-1. The visual field of the human eye extends approximately 95 degrees temporally and 60 degrees nasally. The vertical dimension of the visual field is limited by the patient's brow and averages 60 degrees superior and about 75 degrees inferior to the line of sight.

There are several terms used to characterize visual field. Their use depends on what type of testing was performed. The first is the isopter. An isopter is the boundary line formed by the connection of a group of kinetically tested points that share the same threshold value. This boundary line normally approximates a circle. By definition, the vision inside (closer to fixation) an isopter will be sensitive enough to detect the stimulus and the vision outside the isopter will not detect the stimulus.

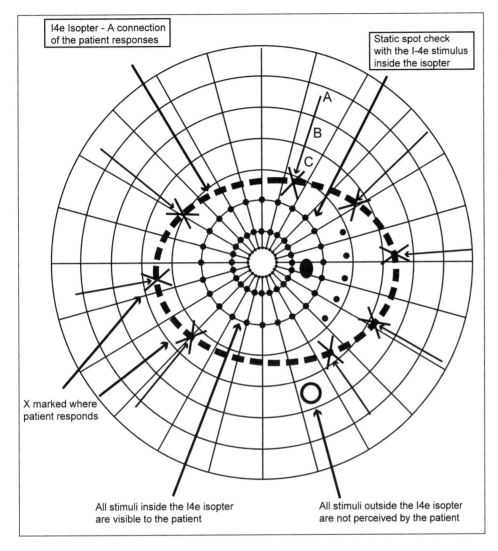

Text boxes within the figure:

I4e Isopter - A connection of the patient responses

Static spot check with the I-4e stimulus inside the isopter

X marked where patient responds

All stimuli inside the I4e isopter are visible to the patient

All stimuli outside the I4e isopter are not perceived by the patient

FIGURE 8-10

Kinetic and static perimetry. The perimetrist chooses a stimulus at the 25-degree locus. The patient is then tested kinetically by moving the chosen stimulus from position A at a rate of 3–4 degrees per second towards position B and C until the stimulus is seen. The perimetrist connects the responses for that stimulus at different meridians to form an isopter. By definition, all vision inside the isopter (closer to fixation) is sensitive enough to see the stimulus, but outside the isopter the stimulus is imperceptible. After the isopters have been determined, the area inside the isopter is statically spot-checked with the same stimulus.

In theory, the isopter is a line representing the threshold of the patient's vision, whereas in reality the line represents the center of an area of uncertainty (Figure 8-11). Isopters can only be determined by using a kinetically presented stimulus.

A scotoma is defined as an area of decreased sensitivity within an area of greater sensitivity. Scotomata have boundary lines that delineate their size. The boundary line of a scotoma is different from an isopter in that the area inside the boundary line is not sensitive to the characterizing stimulus, whereas the area inside an isopter is sensitive to the identifying stimulus.

There are several types of commonly occurring scotomata named specifically for their location within the visual field (Figure 8-12). A central scotoma encompasses the fixation point. A cecocentral scotoma is a scotoma that encompasses both the blind spot and fixation. An altitudinal defect respects the horizontal midline. A paracentral scotoma is located off fixation within the central 30 degrees of fixation. An arcuate scotoma radiates from the blind spot into the paracentral area. This is also sometimes referred to as a Bjerrum scotoma. A ring scotoma leaves the central vision intact and is usually located in the midperiphery.

On an automated numeric printout, an isolated scotoma will show a decrease in decibel sensitivity (smaller numbers) when compared with the statically tested points around it (Figure 8-13).

A depression refers to decreased sensitivity within the visual field. A generalized depression involves the entire visual field and may be caused by media opacities or inappropriate refractive correction during testing. General-

FIGURE 8-11

Every isopter has a zone of uncertainty associated with it. The zone transitions from usually seeing the stimulus near the inside edge of the zone to barely seeing the stimulus on the outside edge.

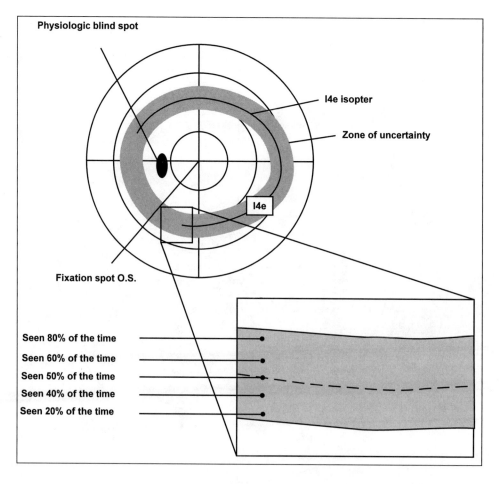

ized depressions cause the hill of vision to decrease in altitude toward the X axis.

Localized depressions can also occur, and they result in a decrease in sensitivity in a localized area. When referring to a Goldmann visual field plot, localized depressions are represented by an isopter bowing that points toward fixation (Figure 8-14). Isolated scotomata are often preceded by localized isopter depressions. On a profile plot a localized depression reveals itself as a steepening of the hill of vision, but not worsening to the point that the surrounding area is actually more sensitive than the depression. When the surrounding visual field becomes more sensitive than the area in question, a scotoma has become evident.

A contraction is defined as the contraction of all of the isopters toward the center of vision. It differs from a depression in that with a depression the maximal stimulus isopter (usually the V-4e on the Goldmann bowl) is still as large as in the normal population, but with a contraction of the visual field, the maximal stimulus isopter decreases in size (Figure 8-15).

GENERAL CONSIDERATIONS FOR THE VISUAL FIELD EXAMINATION

There are guidelines that can be applied to most perimetric tests to achieve a proper assessment of the patient's visual field. The creation of optimal conditions for testing should always be attempted, but keep in mind that they cannot always be attained. Sometimes the clinician has to be inventive to obtain reliable visual field test results.

At the beginning of a visual field examination, the patient should be seated comfortably without any unnatural tilting of the head or back. If a chin rest or headrest is part of the instrumentation, proper adjustments should be made so that there is no discomfort during the testing period. The patient should not have to hunch or stretch to reach the chin rest.

If a tangent screen is used, the seat should be adjusted so that the eye is approximately on the same level as the fixation point. Visual field testing should be performed in a room where there are no distracting noises or other

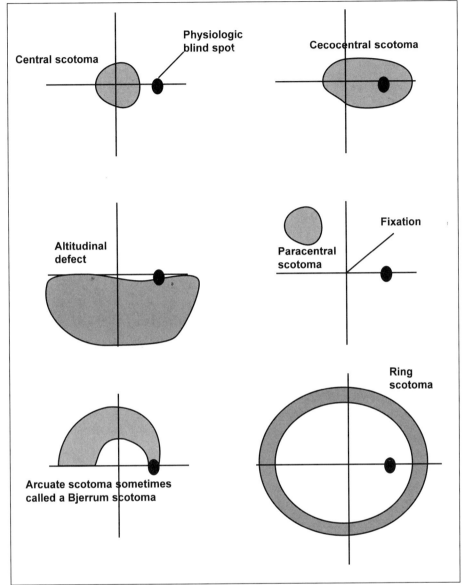

FIGURE 8-12

A central scotoma, a cecocentral scotoma, an altitudinal defect, a paracentral scotoma, an arcuate scotoma (a Bjerrum scotoma), and a ring scotoma.

stimuli that may cause confusion during the testing procedure. The room lighting and instrument background conditions should be constant and repeatable from examination to examination. The examiner should also accurately measure the testing distance if using a tangent screen.

In most instances of tangent screen testing, a patient may be able to hold a rigid occluder in front of the eye not being tested. If an eye patch occluder is used, fresh gauze or tissue should be placed between the eye and the patch to prevent the patient from seeing around the edge of the patch. The patch should be loosely tied so that excessive pressure is not exerted on the globe.

The patient should understand the purpose and nature of the test and, in particular, the way he or she is to respond. In tangent screen testing, the use of a clicker, buzzer, or coin tapped on a table keeps responses simple, speeds the test, and eliminates lengthy verbal responses. Response buttons for the patient to press are usually provided on Goldmann and automated perimeters. The patient must understand that the responses refer to the test stimulus only and not to the fixation point, test object carrier, hand, or arm.

When central 30-degree visual field testing is being performed on a tangent screen, the patient should wear

FIGURE 8-13

An automated perimetry numeric printout from the Humphrey Visual Field Analyzer of the hill of vision. Although the numerals represent decibel levels, they can be thought of as representations of a topographic map with the higher numerals representing a higher altitude on the hill of vision. The lower decibel values (brighter stimuli) correlate to areas of decreased sensitivity (arrow). A scotomatous point is represented on this printout as a locus exhibiting at least a 6-dB difference relative to the values for immediately surrounding areas.

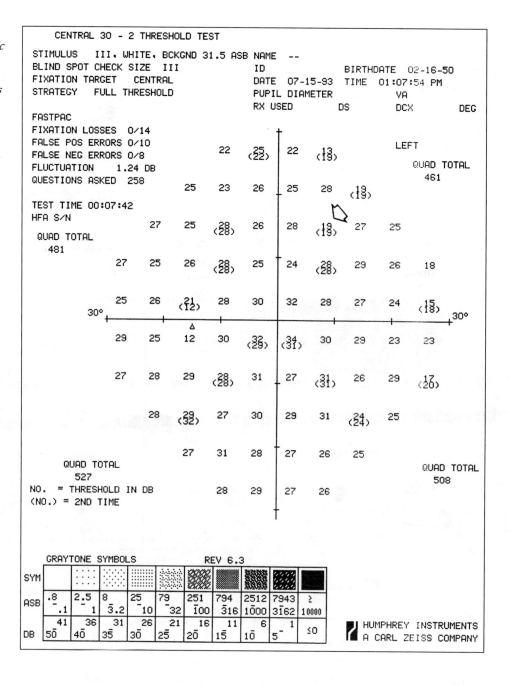

the proper vision correction for the test distance (1 meter) to eliminate field defects caused by an uncorrected refractive error. The patient's own spectacles should not be used for visual field testing. Instead, it is best to use a newly refracted correction in a trial frame. Depending on the patient's refraction, accommodative status, and instrument requirements, a nearpoint or "working distance lens" may need to be added to the distance correction. The vertex distance should be reduced as much as possible to eliminate any interference from the trial frame or lenses. The larger trial frame lenses with a silver metal band around the edge work very well to eliminate any peripheral involvement by the frame. The wider framing of some corrected curve trial lenses can obstruct peripheral vision and are not ideal for visual field testing. Peripheral field testing outside 30 degrees from fixation should be performed without spectacle correction. Correction of refractive error with a contact lens may be necessary if the amount is exceedingly high.

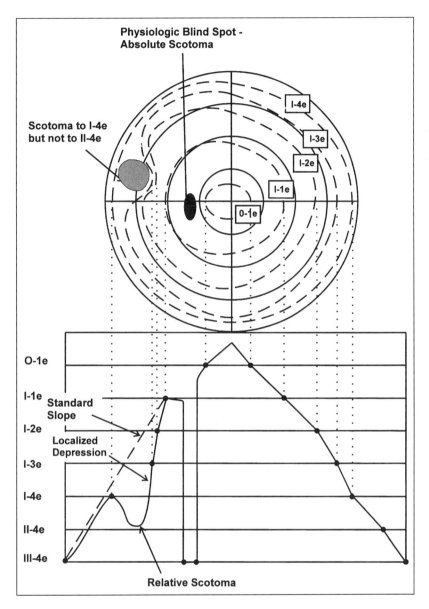

Physiologic Blind Spot - Absolute Scotoma

Scotoma to I-4e but not to II-4e

I-4e
I-3e
I-2e
I-1e
0-1e

O-1e
I-1e **Standard Slope**
I-2e
Localized Depression
I-3e
I-4e
II-4e
III-4e

Relative Scotoma

FIGURE 8-14

A localized depression shown in Goldmann and profile plots associated with a relative scotoma. The depression (an inward shift and closing together of the isopters in the superior temporal field) causes an increase in the slope of the hill of vision (profile plot). An isolated scotoma often occurs adjacent to the isoptoral depression. The depth of this scotoma is not to the abscissa and therefore this is a relative and not an absolute scotoma.

If hand-held test objects are used during tangent screen testing, the examiner should hold the test object wand back far enough so that the hand and arm do not become a distraction to the patient. Test object carriers should match the background as closely as possible to minimize distraction.

The perimetrist should be as efficient as possible with testing to avoid the effects of fatigue. The examination of one eye should optimally not take longer than 10 minutes. In addition, the examiner should constantly monitor patient fixation and attention and should watch for consistent data, especially when plotting a defect. If contradictions in responses are encountered, the field should be retested after a short rest period. Likewise, the perimetrist should be alert for malingering (a patient trying to create a defect that does not really exist).

When using the Goldmann bowl or the automated perimeters, the test should be properly explained to the patient to allow familiarization with the instrumentation. The patient should go through a learning process before the actual test is started. Many automated perimeters incorporate this feature into their testing options. The patient should be made aware that he or she is to respond only after the stimulus appears and that the light will quickly extinguish whether or not he or she responds.

FIGURE 8-15
A contraction of the visual field retains sensitive central acuity but more peripheral vision becomes less sensitive to bright stimuli. The diameter of the peripheral isopters is decreased, resulting in a "contracted" appearance of the visual field plot.

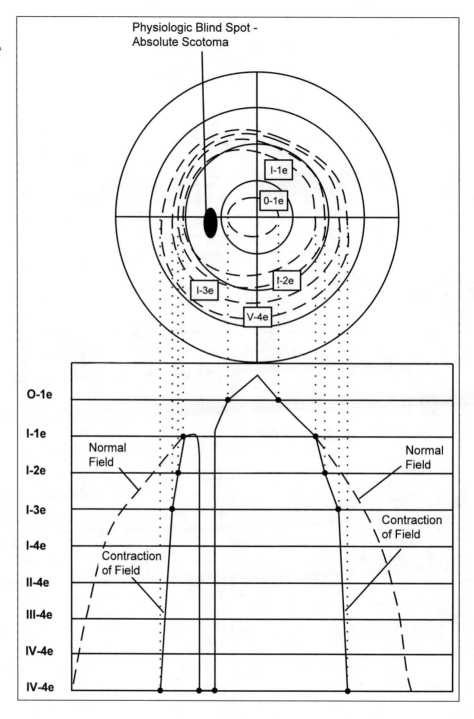

Patient fixation should be monitored with the observation techniques available on the different machines. Even with the use of automated perimeters, the perimetrist should remain by the patient at all times giving support and instructions.

All information regarding the visual field test must be recorded. The visual field record will be less useful for future reference, interpretation, or comparison if testing conditions have not been recorded accurately. The following information should be recorded:

Patient's name
Date
Instrument used

Test conditions (target size and luminance, background luminance, test distance)

The spectacle or contact lens prescription in place for the test

Clearly marked isopters in the case of Goldmann bowl testing (with colored pencils to differentiate isopters)

Pupil size

Examiner's name

Remarks about patient cooperation and reliability

Glaucomatous Field Loss

Because glaucoma encompasses such a prevalent group of diseases and because a majority of the central and peripheral visual field tests that are performed today are for evaluating glaucomatous visual field loss, a review of the disease process and how it affects the visual field will be given before discussing techniques of central visual field testing.

Glaucoma is defined as "an ocular disease, occurring in many forms, having as its primary characteristic an unstable or a sustained increase in the intraocular pressure which the eye cannot withstand without damage to its structure or impairment of its function."[6] Glaucoma can ultimately be considered an optic nerve disease. The optic nerve is the location of axonal cell death, which is the eventual cause of field loss and blindness. The exact pathogenesis of glaucoma has been deliberated for many years. A widely held opinion is that axonal transport and nerve fiber cell death occur secondary to either mechanical blockage or poor vascular perfusion to the optic nerve head.[7] There are problems with both theories, but the vascular theory of nerve damage is supported by significant experimental evidence consisting of histopathologic studies that show a severe reduction in the number and size of peripapillary choroidal vessels around the optic nerve head of glaucoma patients.[8-10] Also, the occlusion of either the short posterior ciliary arteries or the central retinal artery can obstruct axonal transport.[11-14] There is experimental evidence from fluorescein angiography studies that there is a decrease in intraocular blood flow as a result of elevated intraocular pressure.[15-17] Because of such important but still circumstantial evidence, many clinicians choose to believe that poor vascular perfusion to the optic nerve eventually results in optic nerve dysfunction.

Glaucoma is highly correlated with the clinical finding of increased intraocular pressure (IOP). However, the mechanism by which an increase in IOP results in nerve fiber cell death is the key question in understanding the etiology of this difficult disease.

The pattern in which nerve fibers course through the retina to enter the optic nerve is schematically represented in Figure 8-16. The papillomacular bundle carries the macular fibers directly to the optic nerve. The temporal retinal fibers must go around the macula and the papillomacular bundle in an arcuate fashion. The horizontal raphe divides the temporal fibers into an upper and lower region. Any fiber originating above the raphe will traverse superior to the papillomacular bundle and any fiber originating inferior to the horizontal raphe will travel below the papillomacular bundle. The nasal retinal fibers take a relatively direct route from their beginning to the optic nerve.

The projection of these fibers into the patient's visual field is exactly opposite from their retinal location— i.e., the superior retina projects to the patient's inferior field, the nasal retina projects to the temporal field, the inferior arcuate bundle projects to the superior field in an arcuate fashion, etc. Also, the optic nerve head, located 13–18 degrees nasally[3] from the macula, projects 13–18 degrees temporal from fixation and causes the physiologic blind spot.

The arcuate fibers from the temporal retina are long, thin, and very susceptible to pressure or anoxia. They are commonly the first fibers/axons affected in the glaucomatous process. The site of glaucomatous damage is actually at the optic nerve (see Figure 8-16), but the effects are transmitted to the peripheral field. If only one or two axons correlating to an area in the visual field are damaged, the defect will not be clinically observed as a visual field deficit. In fact, it has been proposed that 50% of the axons in an area correlated with a visual field defect must be damaged before any visual field deficit is demonstrable.[18]

Scotomata and Depressions

The first observable signs of glaucomatous field damage are isolated scotomata.[19] A scotoma, as already noted, is an area of decreased sensitivity surrounded by an area of normal or greater sensitivity.[6] Scotomata may be caused by a wide variety of disease processes. In glaucoma, these early scotomata are associated with the arcuate bundles that project about 20 degrees above and below fixation.[19] This paracentral region is commonly referred to as the Bjerrum region. Arcuate, or comet-shaped, scotomata within this area are often referred to as Bjerrum scotomata.

A scotoma looks like a "dip" in the profile plot (Figure 8-17). Scotomata can and should be classified by the depth and steepness of their margins. When a scotoma plunges all the way to the X-axis of a profile plot (max-

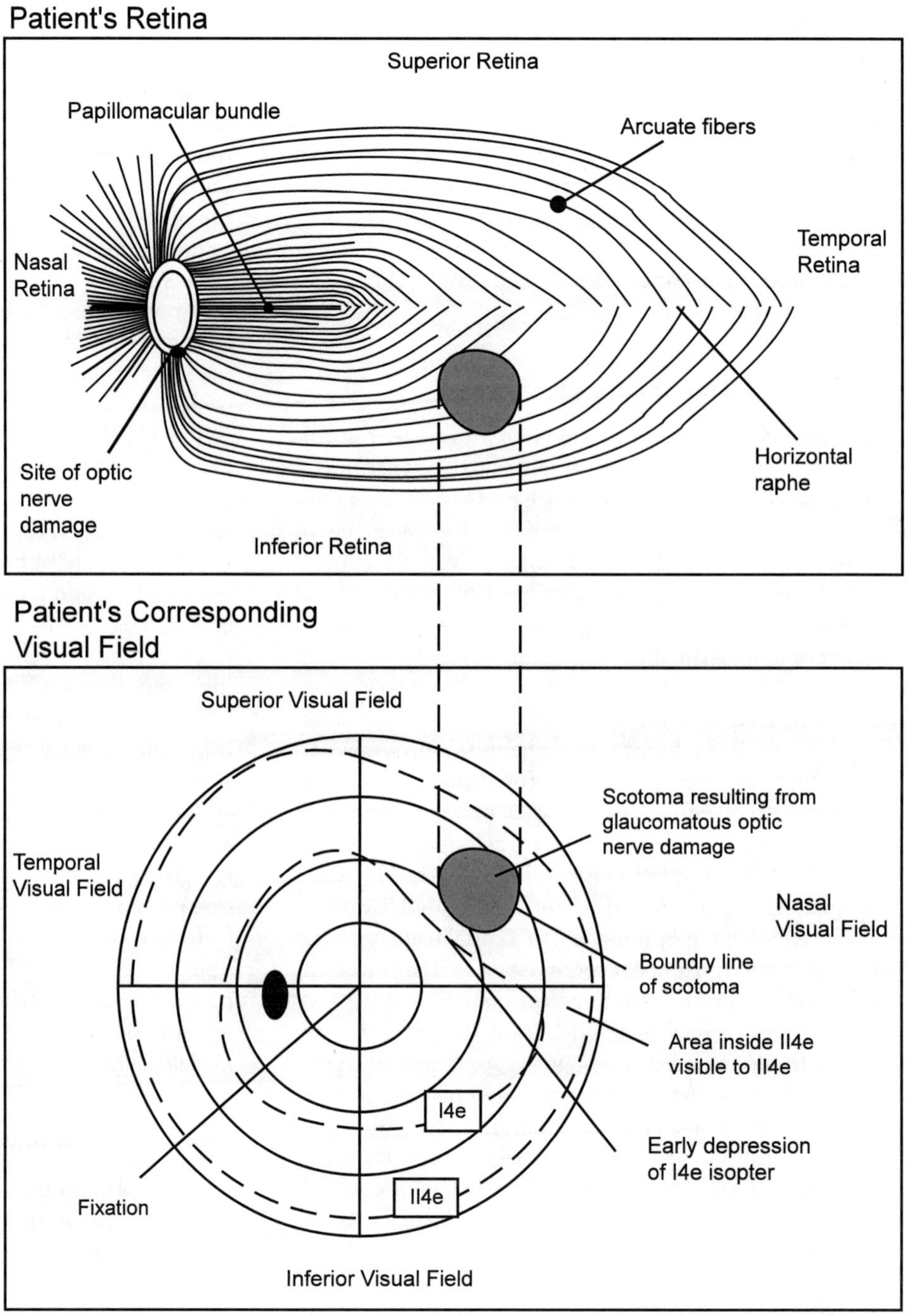

FIGURE 8-16

Glaucoma and visual field defects. The optic nerve head damage site transmits its functional damage early in the process to the long temporal retinal fibers, which results in early scotomatous damage to the paracentral visual field.

Patient's Retina

Superior Retina

Papillomacular bundle

Arcuate fibers

Nasal Retina

Temporal Retina

Site of optic nerve damage

Horizontal raphe

Inferior Retina

Patient's Corresponding Visual Field

Superior Visual Field

Scotoma resulting from glaucomatous optic nerve damage

Temporal Visual Field

Nasal Visual Field

Boundry line of scotoma

Area inside II4e visible to II4e

I4e

Early depression of I4e isopter

II4e

Fixation

Inferior Visual Field

imal stimulus), it is said to be an absolute or maximal luminosity scotoma. In theory there is a difference between a maximal luminosity scotoma and an absolute scotoma, but clinically there is no difference. In most clinics if the strongest stimulus available on the field machine does not evoke a patient response, then the term *absolute* should be used to describe the scotoma, even though the correct term should be a *maximal luminosity* scotoma. Obviously, if different machines have different maximal intensities of stimuli, then maximal luminosity scotomata cannot be compared from one machine to another.

If the dip of the profile plot representing a scotoma does not reach the abscissa, the defect is referred to as a rela-

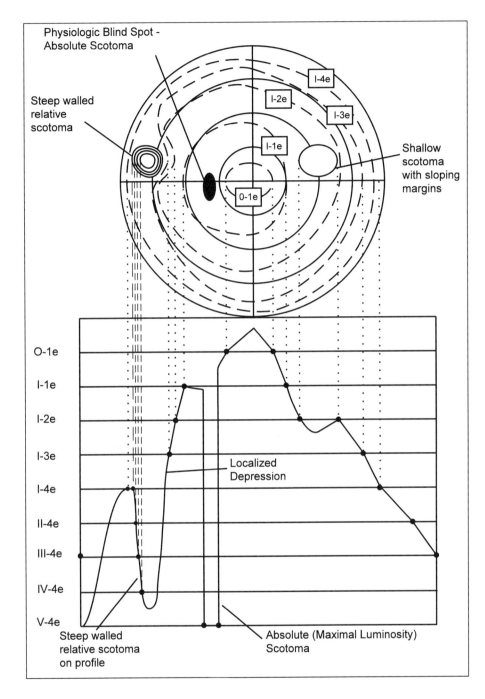

Physiologic Blind Spot - Absolute Scotoma

Steep walled relative scotoma

Shallow scotoma with sloping margins

I-4e
I-2e
I-3e
I-1e
0-1e

O-1e
I-1e
I-2e
I-3e
I-4e
II-4e
III-4e
IV-4e
V-4e

Localized Depression

Steep walled relative scotoma on profile

Absolute (Maximal Luminosity) Scotoma

FIGURE 8-17

Two examples of scotomata on profile and Goldmann visual field printouts. Steep-walled scotomas have boundary lines very close to each other and delineate more advanced disease. The shallow scotomas with sloping margins indicate earlier stages of a disease. Early scotomas are usually more difficult to find and verify.

tive scotoma. Here, stimuli above threshold sensitivity (brighter) will be detected and stimuli dimmer than threshold sensitivity will not be detected.

If the walls of the scotoma are close to vertical, the scotoma is referred to as a steep-walled scotoma or a scotoma with steep borders. If the sides of the scotoma are approaching horizontal or are less vertically steep on a profile plot, the scotoma is referred to as having sloping borders. From Figure 8-17 it can be seen that a steep-walled scotoma has a very small distance between its characterizing boundary lines. In general, a steep-walled scotoma is older and more stable than a shallow-walled scotoma. Thus, the presence of a shallow-walled scotoma may imply that a more active disease process exists. Old, steep-walled scotomata may result from previous vascular infarction along the visual pathway, whereas shallow-walled scotomata may be caused by a slowly progressive compressive lesion.

In clinical practice the terms "positive" or "negative" may be used to describe a type of scotoma. A positive scotoma refers to a defect that is perceived by the patient, whereas a negative scotoma is not perceived by the patient. The physiologic blind spot is an example of an absolute negative scotoma.

The progression of visual field deficits as determined with a Goldmann bowl is shown in Figure 8-18. Note the contraction and decreasing sensitivity associated with advanced glaucomatous damage.

The progression of glaucomatous visual field defects on single-field analysis printouts from a Humphrey Visual Field Analyzer appear in Figures 8-19 and 8-20. Note how the sensitivity of the retina decreases with increasing glaucomatous damage when comparing Figure 8-19 and Figure 8-20.

CLINICAL VISUAL FIELD TESTING STRATEGY AND PRACTICE

The central field of vision can be explored kinetically or statically with a tangent screen, a Goldmann manual perimeter, or an automated perimeter. Static testing is currently the chosen form of testing with the marked increase in use of automated perimetry. Automated perimeters can much more easily conduct a statically driven test than a kinetic one for the simple reason that it is much easier and more economical to manufacture a static machine than a kinetic one.

The two strategies used to explore the field of vision are threshold-related testing and screening-related testing. By definition, all kinetic testing is threshold testing because each isopter represents the threshold at which the patient just barely perceives the stimulus, but static testing can either be threshold related or screening related.

Static thresholding is a method of testing the visual field to determine within certain accuracy limits (usually 2 dB) the sensitivity of the retina at a specific location. Static screening for visual field deficits involves testing a point two or three times to determine a less exact estimation of the visual function at that locus. This type of testing makes clinical sense only when trying to rule out gross visual defects. It should be kept in mind that subtle defects can easily be missed with static screening.

With clinical perimetry, central visual field testing is most commonly performed, whereby the central 50–60

degrees (25–30 degrees radial from fixation) of the field is explored. This is the area of the visual field where most defects are found. In the clinical setting, this is referred to as the central 30 degrees.

Black Felt Tangent Screen

The tangent screen is the classical way of testing the central visual field. The standard tangent screen (see Figure 8-2) still offers some benefits that none of the other types of visual field instruments can offer. The black felt tangent screen is less intimidating than the bowl instruments, and patients generally understand the test fairly easily. The tangent screen is still an excellent tool for evaluation of malingerers because it is so easy to change test distances, thereby confusing the patient in his or her attempt to determine an accurate field size. Patients with absolute central scotomata can be tested with the tangent screen by placing two white strips of tape on the tangent screen that intersect at the center and having the patient fixate where he or she expects the two pieces of tape to cross.

The black felt tangent screen also offers low cost and versatility, whereas a projection-type tangent screen has the advantages of a projected target that eliminates distraction and pantographically records data. With either instrument, the standard testing procedure devised by Sloan[20] is recommended. This procedure is described in the following section:

1. The testing distance should be 1 meter.

2. The proper vision correction should be worn, and if the patient has good correctable acuity (20/30 or better), a test object 1 or 2 mm in diameter should be used. A black test object carrier or wand about 2.5 feet long is recommended. If the patient has decreased correctable acuity (e.g., due to cloudy media), then larger test objects should be used to adjust for the reduction in acuity. There are two reasons for using a small (1 or 2 mm) test object. First, early scotomata are usually small and have a greater chance of going undetected with a larger stimulus. Second, the peripheral visible limit for a 1 or 2 mm target at a 1-m distance is about 25 degrees, which allows the isopter to be plotted within the screen (30 degrees in radius at a 1-m testing distance) and its shape to be analyzed.

3. The blind spot should be plotted at six to eight locations ("1" in Figure 8-21). The most useful aspect of plotting the blind spot is its role in familiarizing the patient with the test. The patient quickly learns the routine of not seeing and then seeing the stimulus as the basis of visual field testing. In plotting this physiologic absolute scotoma,

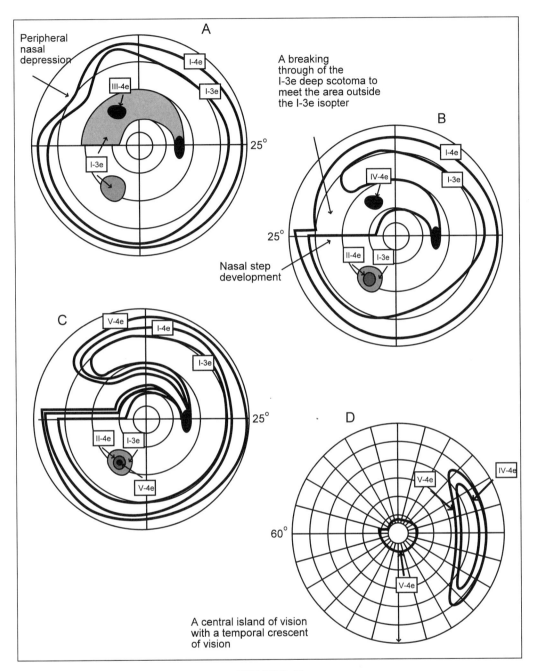

FIGURE 8-18

Progression of the glaucomatous process diagrammed with the Goldmann bowl. The nasal steps become prominent from A to B with the paracentral defects steepening and deepening. Eventually an entire quadrant becomes amaurotic (C) and finally almost all nasal vision is lost, leaving a temporal island of vision with central tunnel vision (D). (Adapted from DR Anderson. Perimetry With and Without Automation. St. Louis: Mosby, 1987.)

FIGURE 8-19

Printout from a Humphrey Visual Analyzer Model 640 of a moderately advanced glaucomatous visual field. The numerals in the top visual field plot located to the left of the grayscale depict the threshold of vision in decibels at that locus in the visual field with a "0" being a maximal luminosity scotoma.

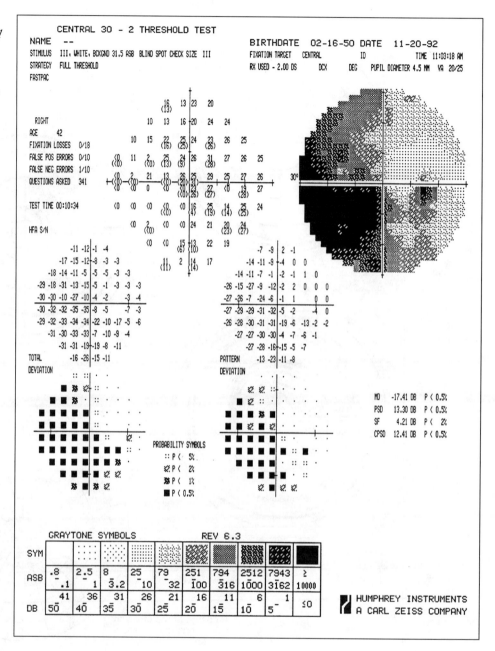

the clinician or technician is able to check on the patient's responses and reliability. Slight enlargement of the blind spot on tangent screen testing can have so many extraneous causes that, unless correlated with ophthalmoscopic appearance at the nerve head (e.g., papilledema), it is often felt to have no diagnostic importance. A Seidel scotoma, which is a small, comma-shaped, upward or downward prolongation of the blind spot occurring in glaucoma, is very difficult to find clinically and is not well accepted today as a significant test result.

4. The limit of the field (always plotted kinetically as nonseeing to seeing) can be plotted at 12 points around the periphery ("2" in Figure 8-21). The shape of the isopter is established by this procedure. The isopter is established on both sides of the horizontal and vertical meridians, rather than on the meridians themselves, since it is along these meridians that the borders of hemianopsias (see Defect Characteristics) and quadrantanopsias are frequently encountered.

5. After the plotting of a peripheral isopter, it is recommended that the same stimulus be moved in a zigzag pat-

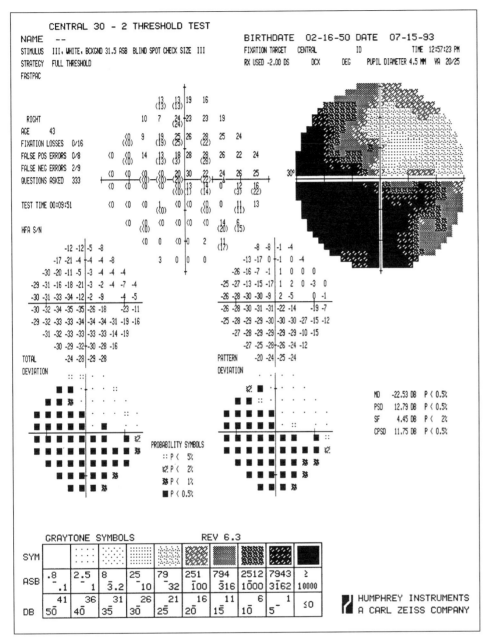

FIGURE 8-20

A more advanced glaucomatous defect 9 months later from the same patient whose visual field plot is shown in Figure 8-19. Progression of the scotomas is noticeable.

tern throughout the central 20 degrees at a speed of about 3–4 degrees/second ("3" in Figure 8-21). The beginning perimetrist generally moves the wand too quickly, and early scotomata may be missed. It should be noted that the conduct of the test has now changed. Now the patient is being asked to detect when the stimulus disappears instead of appears. Because of reaction time, real scotomata will appear smaller in size or go undetected with this procedure.

A static spot check of the area works just as well (Figure 8-22). The spot check on the tangent screen is carried out

by merely rotating the wand so that the stimulus either faces the tangent screen or the patient. Because the perimetrist is now asking the patient to detect stimulus appearance rather than disappearance, the patient responses are thought to be more reliable. It is recommended in the Armaly-Drance technique that at least 76 points be spot checked before the presence of a visual field defect is ruled out.[3]

6. If defects are encountered, they must be plotted in the same manner as the blind spot (i.e., from the depressed area to the seeing area). This has the effect of making a

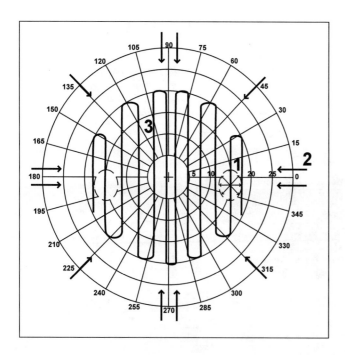

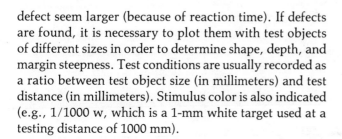

FIGURE 8-21

Procedure for central visual field examination with the tangent screen. 1. Plot the blind spot at six to eight locations. 2. Plot the isopter at a minimum of 12 locations around the field as illustrated. 3. Zigzag the test target throughout the central 20 degrees at a rate of 3–4 degrees per second.

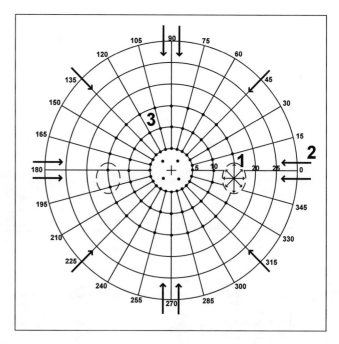

FIGURE 8-22

Combined method of isopter and static perimetry on the tangent screen. 1. Determination of the blind spot. 2. Isopter determination in at least 12 meridians. 3. Static spot-check of the central 15 degrees with 76 points.

defect seem larger (because of reaction time). If defects are found, it is necessary to plot them with test objects of different sizes in order to determine shape, depth, and margin steepness. Test conditions are usually recorded as a ratio between test object size (in millimeters) and test distance (in millimeters). Stimulus color is also indicated (e.g., 1/1000 w, which is a 1-mm white target used at a testing distance of 1000 mm).

Defects are recorded by transferring the information on the screen to a recording sheet consisting of a pattern that corresponds to the sewn-in markings on the screen. Figure 8-23 is an example of how to record the results of a traditional tangent screen examination using two different sizes of test objects to plot the scotoma. The second boundary line of an inner scotoma is usually filled in with a different pattern to easily demarcate it as a different level of visual loss.

The Goldmann Bowl

The Goldmann bowl grew into popularity as the standard clinical tool for testing visual fields in the middle

and late 1970s. The advantages of the Goldmann bowl over the tangent screen are controlled luminance levels of both the stimulus and background environment, magnified monitoring of the patient's fixation, and the ability to test the central and peripheral fields during one sitting. Also, better monitoring of the patient's disease progression can be maintained with the standardized background and stimulus values provided by the Goldmann bowl.

The Goldmann bowl is designed to effectively illuminate all retinal points equally and get rid of interoffice ambient lighting variability. The system was never designed to become a standard, but through sound engineering and office practicality it became the standard visual field testing apparatus. For a discussion of the luminance classification scheme used by Goldmann, see the previous section on luminance.

Setup Procedure for Goldmann Bowl Testing

When testing the visual field with a Goldmann projection perimeter, the patient should initially be instructed about the basis of the test, how the test will be administered, and what is expected of the patient.

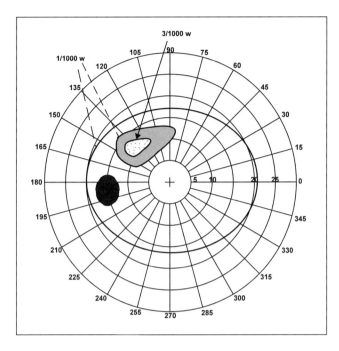

FIGURE 8-23

Plotting a paracentral scotoma with the tangent screen. All boundary lines are labeled according to the stimulus variables (stimulus diameter/distance in millimeters to screen and color), and the delineated zones are usually shaded with a pattern for easier identification.

1. The patient should be comfortably seated, with his or her head against the forehead rest and chin in the chin rest. The chin should be all the way forward for proper patient alignment. If the patient's head is tilted too far one way or the other, it will affect the size of the patient's field. For proper alignment and monitoring, the patient should be comfortably lined up with the reticule in the observation scope.

2. If the central 30 degrees is to be tested, a proper corrective lens that takes into consideration the patient's refractive error, age, and 30-cm near working distance should be used. Testing of the peripheral field does not require a corrective lens, and even if used the edges of a trial lens or its holder may cause falsely scotomatous areas to appear. When a corrective lens is used for central field testing, the lens holder must be placed as close to the patient's eye as possible without touching the brow or eyelashes.

If a patient is cyclopleged, the full 30-cm working distance prescription must be given for central visual field testing. If the patient's pupils are dilated for the initial visual field examination, then the patient's pupils should

be dilated for every examination after that. Likewise, if the initial visual field test was done with the pupils undilated, then the patient's follow-up visual field testing should be done in a similar manner. If the patient has less than a 4-mm pupil, or if he or she has lens or other media opacities, then dilation is recommended.

Goldmann Testing Procedure

The Goldmann bowl testing procedure for an initial visual field examination consists of three parts:

1. Testing the central visual field kinetically and plotting two or three isopters. The central 30 degrees of vision should always be tested first because this is the area where most visual field defects occur (especially with glaucoma), and the patient will be more alert at the beginning of the examination than near the end of the examination.
2. Statically testing the central visual field to determine if any isolated scotomata are present.
3. Kinetically testing the peripheral field, plotting two or three isopters, and looking for any abnormalities inside any isopter that may warrant further investigation.

To begin the examination, the correct stimulus value should be chosen for the 25- to 30-degree isopter. This can be accomplished either kinetically or statically. To statically determine the correct stimulus, four spots (one in each quadrant) are spot-checked about 30 degrees from fixation and thresholded to within 2 dB. The standard stimulus at this point for the normal eye with no pathologic entities is the I-4e.

To kinetically check for the proper spot size, the test begins with an assumed stimulus intensity that should create a response at approximately 25 degrees as the stimulus is moved in from the periphery. If the patient responds before the 25-degree desired spot, then the luminance of the stimulus is decreased. Likewise, if a response occurs too late (at 10 or 15 degrees), then the luminance of the stimulus is increased. The test should then be started at the resultant stimulus intensity. Preferably two or three different stimuli are used to plot isopters within the central 30 degrees using the kinetic method.

A monocularly occluded patient should be instructed that when he or she first sees the stimulus he or she should respond by either tapping a coin or pressing the response button (verbal responses should not be encouraged because head movement can result). After the patient responds, the perimetrist immediately extinguishes the stimulus by using the button on the side of

FIGURE 8-24
A closer view of the Goldmann procedure in the central 30 degrees. Each area between the isopters is examined statically with the stimulus used to establish the isopter just peripheral to the testing region.

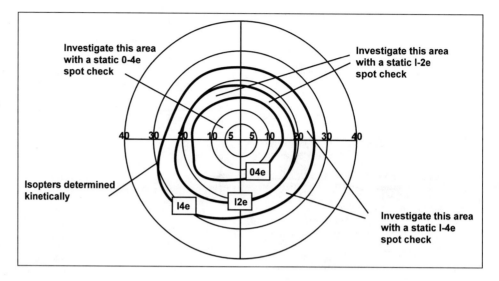

the machine. As with tangent screen testing, approximately three or four meridians per quadrant (12–16 total points per isopter) are recommended for an initial visual field examination.

The second part of a Goldmann bowl visual field examination involves statically spot-checking the central 30 degrees. As discussed, static (implying a nonmoving stimulus) testing involves choosing a spot in the field, turning the stimulus silently on at that point, waiting a second or two, and then turning it off again. The stimulus is characterized by a certain size, intensity (luminance), and duration. With Goldmann perimeters, the duration, size, and intensity of the stimulus are all chosen by the tester. In testing for glaucoma, the central 30 degrees of the visual field should be statically checked with approximately 76 test points. This was originally recommended by Armaly and Drance.[3]

After the initial isopters have been determined, the area between each isopter should be statically checked with a stimulus consistent with the more peripheral isopter line (Figure 8-24).

The choice of stimulus duration is very important. If it is too short, the patient (especially elderly patients) may not have time to respond. In the ideal situation, the stimulus duration should be about 0.5 sec[3] to ensure that the retina is fully stimulated (i.e., temporal summation of the retina is allowed to reach its maximum) without giving the patient enough time to turn his or her eye and look where he or she thought the stimulus appeared.

If a scotoma is found, it should be investigated from nonseeing to seeing to determine its maximum size. Also, it should be classified with at least two stimuli to determine the depth, shape, and steepness of its margins.

Before the peripheral isopters can be determined, the corrective trial lens must be removed and the stimuli should be adjusted (brightened). The patient should be informed that the peripheral visual field will be tested in the same manner as the central vision was tested.

The results of the Goldmann bowl testing are placed on the visual field recording paper supplied with the machine. All of the information previously recommended for inclusion on the tangent screen test should be included on the Goldmann recording sheet as well. It is usually advantageous to indicate the isopters with different colored pencils for easier interpretation. If a scotoma is found, lightly coloring the area of the scotoma aids in its identification.

Automated Perimeters

Automated perimetry is currently the predominant form of visual field testing. The need for repeatable and verifiable examinations without intertechnician variability, as well as the need for the clinician to be less involved with the actual gathering of data, has increased the popularity of automated visual field machines.[4]

It became apparent in Goldmann bowl testing that the perimetrist could significantly influence the outcome of the testing procedure. The recommended technique for investigating the central 30 degrees involves statically testing 76 points according to the Armaly-Drance method. It is almost certain that most perimetrists do not investigate all of these points and do not threshold them because of the tediousness of the process. Computerized automation is well suited to performing this routine task.

The ideal automated visual field machine would have the patient sit in a chair and would measure the patient's full field of vision with no loss of fixation, no patient fatigue, and absolute values on the patient's hill of vision at every point within 0.2 degrees of each other. It has been calculated that it would take 240 hours to complete this task.[1] Therefore, carefully choosing the areas of the visual field to be tested is extremely important in gaining the greatest amount of information in the least amount of time. Most automated perimeters give the clinician a large variety of well-conceived point selections that allow for very specific testing modalities that concentrate on visual field regions most likely to exhibit anomalous results.

Automated perimeters come in two forms based on their stimulus type: projection perimeters and light-emitting diode (LED) perimeters. The projection perimeters project a stimulus from an apparatus similar to the Goldmann bowl arm. The LED systems have numerous light-emitting diodes placed in small holes throughout the entire bowl. Projection perimeters are generally more expensive because they have more moving parts, but they usually have a wider range of luminance values for their stimuli and the size of their stimuli can be varied, which is not possible with the LED systems.

Some of the common characteristics of automated perimeters can be compared and contrasted. These include test type, stimulus type, number of test spots, stimulus characteristics, time limits for running standard screening and full threshold tests, types of fixation monitoring, and computer hardware and software.

Test Type

There are many types of test menus available on the wide variety of automated perimeters on the market. These menus differ based on the manufacturer's approach to testing (i.e., whether the examination should be a central, peripheral, or full-field test and whether it should either be a screening test or a threshold-related test). These menus can be further divided based on test strategy: If it is a screening test, how many times and in what form should each point be tested? If it is a threshold-related test, how accurately should each point be quantified? Most automated perimeters also have a variety of specialized tests for glaucoma, neurologic deficits, and other commonly occurring field defects.

Stimulus Type

The three most common types of stimuli are projection, light-emitting diode (LED), and LED with moving fixation. Projection systems similar to the Goldmann bowl system project a white stimulus onto a white bowl. The stimuli are scaled in different luminosity steps by placing neutral density filters in front of a maximal luminosity bulb (see Figure 8-6).

In the LED machines, a LED about 4 mm^2 in size is inserted in a slightly larger hole and a white translucent screen is placed in front of it. The various LEDs are placed at a number of different locations in the patient's visual field. This is a direct rather than an indirect stimulus, and the intensity of the stimuli is adjusted by changing the voltage applied to the LED. The LEDs are placed in strategic locations throughout the visual field to gain the most amount of information in the least amount of time.

Number of Test Spots

Each perimeter tests a different number of test spots within the central 30 degrees and in the periphery for both screening and threshold testing. A large number of test spots will fatigue the patient, but too few may leave large gaps in the tested field, allowing a depression or scotoma to go undetected. When testing the central 30 degrees, most static automated perimeters have an interspot distance between 6.0 and 8.5 degrees. This interspot distance has been shown to be larger than the average size variability of a kinetically tested isopter with the stimulus moving at 3–4 degrees/second.[1] Many automated perimeters use an overlay characteristic in which two different tests can be overlaid to create an interspot distance of approximately 4 degrees (e.g., the 30-1 and 30-2 test patterns of the Humphrey Visual Field Analyzer, Humphrey Instruments, Inc., San Leandro, CA).

Stimulus Characteristics

Stimuli are characterized by their size, range of luminosity, duration, background lighting conditions, interstimulus time, and color. Stimulus intensity is the only variable that needs to be changed for the large majority of patients being tested. The size III Goldmann stimulus used on many automated perimeters subtends 0.43 degrees, which is small enough to detect very small scotomata[21] and is relatively unaffected by residual refractive error.[22] Most perimeters have larger stimulus sizes, but they are rarely needed. Simultaneously changing both size and intensity leads to interpretive problems, and such changes are not needed to make clinically significant variations in the stimulus.

Stimulus size is limited in that a stimulus that is too large may trigger more than one receptive field in the retina and may also interfere with proper blind spot monitoring if the Heijl-Krakau method is used to check fixation (see Types of Fixation Monitoring). The early stages of various disease processes may not be detected with a stimulus that is too large. Likewise, it may be difficult for elderly patients to perceive a stimulus that is too small. One case in which the Goldmann size V stimulus is needed is when a perimetric examination for a low vision patient is required and the size III stimulus is not large enough. If a stimulus larger than a Goldmann size V is needed, then the best instrument for testing the visual field is the tangent screen using "large disc stimuli."

The stimulus duration of automated perimeters differs between various instruments. Two factors enter into determining the appropriate duration of the stimulus. First, temporal summation of the retina dictates that up to a point (approximately 0.5 second), the longer a stimulus is left on, the more likely it will be detected. After 0.5 second, temporal summation begins to gradually fade, thereby having a lessened effect on stimulus identification. Bleaching of the retina can occur if the stimulus is left on for an extended period, causing a retested point to have a different threshold. The algorithms of most programs do not allow a missed point to be tested again until the retinal locus has had time to readapt to the background conditions (approximately 2 seconds). This pattern of stimulus presentation is termed *randomization* and uniquely lends itself to computer programming when the visual field is being statically tested.

The second issue affecting stimulus duration is the length of time it will take the patient to turn his or her eye to see a statically presented point. A stimulus lasting 0.25 second cannot be detected by a saccade to the stimulus location because the eye will not have time to move to the eccentric point before the stimulus is extinguished. Many perimeters therefore do not allow a stimulus to last longer than 0.25 second.[3,4]

Background lighting conditions also vary among different perimeters. A large majority of automated perimeters use the standard luminance of 31.5 asb, which was established by Goldmann's manual perimeter. A few manufacturers use a 4-asb background, contending that the 31.5-asb background causes falsely abnormal results.

Most automated perimeters either have white stimuli or green stimuli (LED systems). The ability to test with different colors has lost popularity because of the lack of significant results indicating that the use of colored stimuli is advantageous over white or single wavelength green stimuli. The use of green stimuli in LED systems is founded on the idea that the green wavelength is in the middle of the visual spectrum and will closely match peak spectral sensitivity. Recent research indicates that blue stimuli on a yellow background may detect early glaucomatous defects before white-on-white perimetry.[23] The recently introduced testing method is termed *short wavelength automated perimetry* (SWAP).

Time Limits for Standard Screening and Full Threshold Tests

A basic goal of visual field testing in a busy office (in the interest of examiner availability and patient fatigue) is to gather the most information in the shortest period of time. Different manufacturers take different approaches to this problem. One method of reducing the time required for a test is to save the findings of the first test and then compare future examination results with the original results. Every test after the first one does not have to start out thresholding the field of vision at the 25-degree locus in all four quadrants. Instead, subsequent visual field tests can start at a level slightly above threshold values found on the preceding examination.

Types of Fixation Monitoring

The three types of fixation monitoring include the Heijl-Krakau blind spot monitor, computer eye observation, and perimetrist observation of the patient's eye through a television system.

The Heijl-Krakau method of fixation monitoring involves determining the location of the blind spot and loading it into the computer's memory. Periodically throughout the test, a stimulus will be presented in the blind spot. If the patient responds to the stimulus, it indicates that there has been a fixation loss at that moment of testing. In the clinical setting, 20% is considered to be the upper limit of acceptability for fixation losses.[24] If the rate of fixation losses is above this value, the reliability of the test should be questioned. It has been shown that the most common cause for unreliable visual field test results is a high percentage of fixation losses.[25-27]

A second and more expensive technique for monitoring fixation is the use of a television projection system. In this system a camera fixates on the patient's pupil. Any time the patient loses fixation, the computer detects the change in contrast between the pupil and the iris and the computer signals the patient to look at the fixation target. Dark irides may occasionally cause unreliable monitoring with this system due to reduced iris-pupil contrast.

The third and most effective way to monitor fixation is for the perimetrist to monitor the patient throughout the entire examination to get a reliable estimate of the patient's fixational ability and to correlate the questionable test points with fixation losses. To observe the general conduct of a patient as well as to provide encouragement during an automated perimetry examination, the patient should never be left alone during testing.

Computer Hardware

Some systems use a light pen input system and an internal computer. Others use a standard personal computer linked to the perimeter. There are many variations in the use of computer hardware. The basic function of the computer is to retrieve, store, analyze, and make available the data for future reference. Most of the computer-driven systems on the market can retrieve and store data relatively well. The differences are in the ability of the software (the program running the computer) to analyze the data effectively and give the clinician the information needed to properly treat the patient.

Computer Software

The computer software is the "brain" of the computer that defines the capabilities of the automated perimeter. The software should have the ability to perform statistical analysis on the raw data (i.e., calculating both the patient reliability indices as well as the visual field indices, described in a later section).

One advantage of a computer-driven system is that a standard hill of vision can be stored in the memory of the computer and the visual field examination results for a patient can be compared with a "normal" age-corrected visual field and discrepancies noted. The Octopus system software (Interzeag AG, Schlieren, Switzerland) uses a Gaussian model of the hill of vision, whereas the Humphrey STATPAC software uses an empirically derived hill of vision.

The Gaussian model assumes that each point in the visual field will have the same variability of 2.4 dB (1 SD).[28,29] The second assumption is that each point on the hill of vision will decrease in sensitivity by 0.1 dB per decade of life. When deriving a hill of vision, these hypotheses have not proved to be totally accurate.

The empirically derived "normal" field of vision for the Humphrey automated perimeter showed that points in the visual field do not generate a Gaussian curve with the same standard deviation. It was determined that the more peripheral the point, the more the distribution becomes non-Gaussian, with there being an increase in the range (variability)[30] of normal values. Points closer to fixation (the central 5–15 degrees) resemble a Gaussian distribution and have a smaller standard deviation.[28]

It has become common to accept a 5-dB range in clinical testing as the standard variability in the normal population. What has been determined from the empirically derived hill of vision is that points close to fixation approximate this 5-dB variability rule very well, but as the periphery is approached, the 5-dB rule loses significance.[31] Therefore an 11-dB defect at 30 degrees may not be as significant as a 6-dB defect near fixation. Also, each quadrant of the visual field shows a different variability: The superior field loses sensitivity faster than the inferior field.[28] This concept should be taken into account whenever mirror image comparisons of the top-to-bottom field is performed. The empirical model also found that different points on the hill of vision progressively lose sensitivity at different rates.[32] In general, the Gaussian model and the empirical model

agree within 15 degrees of fixation, but the discrepancies increase further from fixation.[33]

Automated Perimeter Test Strategy and Procedure

Automated perimeters almost exclusively use a static rather than kinetic testing strategy. Humphrey Instruments, Inc., has produced a kinetic automated perimeter test strategy available on some of its instrument models. The two most common algorithms (a sequential set of logical instructions) used on automated perimeters are the static screening method and the static threshold method.

Static Screening Strategies

A screening test is designed to quickly test the patient's hill of vision and determine if more accurate threshold testing is needed. The goal is not to accurately define the hill of vision but to get a quick estimate of the patient's field.

The Humphrey Instruments' computer-derived testing strategies are available on all models. The screening strategies are divided into four levels: threshold-related, three-zone, quantify defects, and single intensity.

Threshold-Related Screening Strategy A threshold-related screening strategy is based on an initial four-point thresholding in each of the four quadrants 25 degrees from fixation. This is similar to the Goldmann bowl technique. The second most sensitive stimulus of the four loci tested is chosen as the selected sensitivity to predict the patient's hill of vision.[33]

All of the tested points in this strategy are initially tested at 6 dB brighter than the expected hill of vision. If a point is missed once, it is retested, and if it is missed a second time the point is termed a defect known to be at least 6 dB deep but the exact depth is not determined (Table 8-6).

Three-Zone Screening Strategy The three-zone screening strategy takes the threshold-related strategy one step further. It does this by testing a twice-missed point (6 dB brighter than expected stimulus) a third time with a maximal luminosity stimulus. This strategy will quantify a defective point as a relative defect of at least 6 dB, or a maximal luminosity scotoma. The test will not quantify the defect any further because it is still considered a screening test.

Quantify Defects Screening Strategy The quantify defects screening strategy will threshold all the points at which the 6 dB brighter than expected stimulus is missed twice. It classifies the defect by its distance from the expected value. The points are thresholded to within 2 dB using the standard 4-2 algorithm (see algorithm in Automated Perimetry, Figure 8-25).

TABLE 8-6

Results of Four Screening Strategies and What They Would Tell the Practitioner When, For Example, the Patient Actually Had a 10-dB Scotoma*

Screening Strategy	How Each Screening Strategy Would Classify a 10-dB Scotoma	Time Scale (1 = shortest; 4 = longest)
Threshold-related	A scotoma is present and it is at least 6 dB in depth.	2
Three-zone	A scotoma is present that is greater than 6 dB in depth but is not a maximal luminosity scotoma.	3
Quantify defects	A scotoma is present that is 10 dB in depth.	4
Single intensity	A scotoma is present relative to the chosen single intensity.	1

*The "threshold-related" screening strategy would indicate the presence of a scotoma of at least 6 dB in depth (in this example it is 10 dB). The "three-zone" strategy would indicate the scotoma is somewhere between 6 dB from expected and an absolute defect. The "quantify defects" strategy would indicate the defect is actually 10 dB deep. This strategy is the most accurate but takes the most time. The "single intensity" strategy may or may not determine there is a defect, depending on what level of intensity the perimetrist chooses. The practitioner must decide that if a screening test is to be performed, exactly how much information is required and how lengthy a test can the patient withstand and still give accurate readings.

FIGURE 8-25

How a specific locus in the visual field is thresholded. The first stimulus (1) is calculated by the computer from the expected hill of vision to be 6 dB brighter than threshold. After the patient responds to (1), the next stimulus presented (2) is 4 dB dimmer and again the patient has responded. A third test at 16 dB (3) reveals no response by the patient, so the computer brightens the stimulus but just 2 dB. The patient responds (4), causing the subsequent stimulus to be 2 dB dimmer. The patient does not respond, implying the threshold at this locus is 15 dB (5).

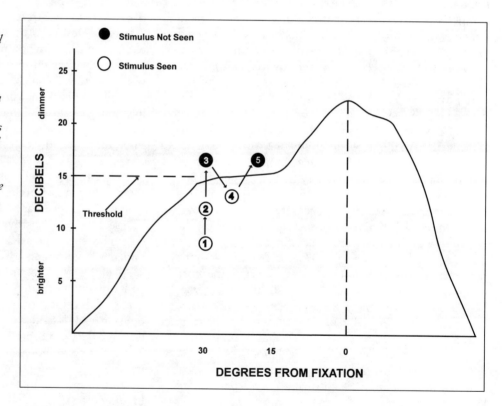

Single-Intensity Screening Strategy   The single-intensity screening strategy presents stimuli of only one intensity at every point in the visual field. Twenty-four decibels is the default stimulus intensity, but it can be adjusted from 0 to 50 dB. Points are either labeled as seen (checked twice if missed once) or missed. This strategy does not realize the hill of vision and will not follow the contour of the hill of vision. Although limited information is provided, this screening strategy may be used for disability testing or to determine if a person meets certain functional visual requirements for various activities such as driving.

These different strategies can be used with a wide variety of test patterns as seen in Table 8-7.

Static Threshold Strategies

Threshold testing determines the exact hill of vision to within 2 dB. The sensitivity at each point is accurately determined and these values are then compared with the "normal" data stored in the computer's memory. Threshold testing is the recommended visual field strategy for monitoring change in the glaucomatous population.[33]

TABLE 8-7

Test Strategies Available on the Humphrey Field Analyzer for Screening Test Patterns and the Strategy that can be Used with Each Pattern

Test Pattern	Threshold-Related	Three-Zone	Quantify Defects	Single Intensity	Application
Glaucoma tests					
Armaly central	*	*	*	*	Glaucoma
Armaly full field	*	*	*	*	Glaucoma
Nasal step	*	*	*	*	Glaucoma
Central 30-degree tests					
Central 40 point	*	*	*	*	General
(Central 64 point)[a]	*	*	*	*	Glaucoma
Central 76 point	*	*	*	*	General, glaucoma, neurologic
Central 80 point	*	*	*	*	General, glaucoma, neurologic
Central 166 point[b]	*	*	*	*	General, glaucoma, neurologic
Peripheral tests					
Full field 81 point	*	*	*	*	General, retinal, glaucoma, neurologic
Full field 120 point	*	*	*	*	General, retinal, glaucoma, neurologic
(Full field 135 point)[a]	*	*	*	*	General, retinal, glaucoma, neurologic
Full field 246 point	*	*	*	*	General, retinal, glaucoma, neurologic
Peripheral 68 (60) point[c]	*	*	*	*	General, neurologic, with central exam, retinal, glaucoma
Custom tests	Points can be added to any test pattern or used alone				
Automatic diagnostic		*			General

[a]Parentheses indicate test patterns available on newer instrumentation, the Humphrey Field Analyzer II (HFA II).
[b]Eliminated on the HFA II.
[c]Modified to 60 points for the HFA II.
Source: The Humphrey Field Analyzer Owner's Manual, Humphrey Instruments, San Leandro, CA, 1991.

The threshold strategies are divided into three levels in the Humphrey Instruments machine: Full threshold, full threshold from prior data, and fast threshold. Most automated machines have some variations on these basic routines. These testing strategies can be applied to many different test patterns (Table 8-8).

Full Threshold For the full threshold strategy, the examination is initiated similar to that in the screening strategy in that four points equidistant from fixation are statically thresholded to within 2 dB. From that information, neighboring points are thresholded and from that information the process continues until all the predetermined points have produced a threshold value. This test gives the most accurate information but also takes the most time and causes the most patient fatigue.

Full Threshold from Prior Data The full threshold from prior data method for thresholding the patient's field of vision uses data from the patient's previous examination as a starting point for the current examination, thereby reducing the testing time. This is very helpful with older patients or with patients with known field defects. For any locus, the initial stimulus is 2 dB brighter than the last examination's finding at that point. For newer Humphrey instrumentation and software, improved methods on this type of strategy are being developed.

Fast Threshold The fast threshold strategy is a variation of the full threshold from prior data algorithm. The difference is that if the patient responds to a stimulus that is 2 dB brighter than threshold, it is assumed that the point has not changed and it is not thresholded. The only points that are thresholded in this strategy are the points that are missed twice with the 2 dB greater than last threshold value. This strategy will not show improvement in the hill of vision. This strategy should not be used if a condition that may show improvement, such as pseudotumor cerebri, is being monitored.

Algorithms in Automated Perimetry

An algorithm is a software-driven decision-making process that tells the perimeter how to test the patient. Computers typically use a 4-2 algorithm to test patients. These numbers represent the change in decibels of the step levels as the algorithm converges on the threshold of vision at a certain point in the visual field. These algorithms

TABLE 8-8

Threshold Test Patterns Available on the Humphrey Field Analyzer[a]

Test Pattern	Point Density (Degrees)[b]	Number of Points Tested	Average Test Time (Minutes Per Eye)[c]	Application
Central tests				
24-1[d]	6	56	10–12	Glaucoma, general
24-2	6	54	10–12	Glaucoma, neurologic, general
30-1[d]	6	71	12–15	Glaucoma, neurologic, retinal, general
30-2	6	76	12–15	Glaucoma, neurologic, retinal, general
Peripheral tests				
Peripheral 30/60-1	12	63	12–15	Retinal, glaucoma
Peripheral 30/60-2	12	68	12–15	Retinal, glaucoma
Nasal step	—	14	2–3	Glaucoma
Temporal crescent	8.5	37	3–4	Retinal, neurologic, advanced glaucoma
Specialty tests				
Neurologic 20[d]	—	16 (tested 2×)	5–6	Hemianopsia
Neurologic 50[d]	—	16 (tested 2×)	8–9	Hemianopsia
Central 10-2	2	68	10–12	Macular, retina, neurologic, advanced glaucoma
Macula	2	16	8–10	Macular, retina, advanced glaucoma

[a]A custom test function to allow the examiner to design his or her own test pattern if necessary is also available.
[b]Point density is the distance between each point.
[c]For an eye with no pathologic processes.
[d]Eliminated on newer instrumentation, the Humphrey Field Analyzer II (HFA II).
Source: The Humphrey Field Analyzer Owner's Manual, Humphrey Instruments, San Leandro, CA, 1991.

are based on the concept that the computer can easily remember the luminosity of the stimulus presented as well as whether or not the patient responded.

The 4-2 algorithm (Figure 8-25) starts out testing a spot using a relatively bright stimulus. If the patient responds to the stimulus as expected, then the stimulus is adjusted 4 dB dimmer (that is, a higher decibel number) and the spot is rechecked. The sequence continues in this fashion until the patient does not respond to the stimulus. When the patient fails to respond (reversal) to the stimulus, the subsequent stimulus is 2 dB brighter than the level at the last response. If the patient responds to the stimulus, then the algorithm is concluded and the threshold of vision is determined. The 4-2-2 algorithm takes this process one step further and does one more 2-dB reversal.

The FASTPAC option (only available for static threshold strategies) of the Humphrey Instruments' visual field machine uses an algorithm designed to decrease the testing time and still gain as much information as possible. The algorithm uses a 3-dB step instead of a 2-dB step around fixation and only crosses the threshold once before threshold is determined. This decreases the testing time by approximately 40%.[33]

A dilemma is created for the practitioner when he or she must decide whether to use the FASTPAC option for testing a patient. In its favor, it will test patients 40% faster, alleviating significant fatigue and thereby yielding more reliable results. A negative factor associated with

using FASTPAC is that the patient's hill of vision is not as accurately determined, leaving the clinician with a less precise representation of the visual field.

One strategy to alleviate the problem is to use the FASTPAC option on the first visual field because this initial visual field gives very little accurate information. Subsequent examinations are then performed with a full threshold from prior data strategy to make use of the glaucoma change probability printout but to keep patient testing time to a minimum.

Frequency of Seeing Curve

Any determination of threshold must consider the "frequency of seeing curve." This curve illustrates that a threshold value is very difficult to determine. What threshold actually means is that the patient will respond to a certain stimulus 50% of the time.[3] In visual field testing there is a stimulus at locus X to which the patient will always respond (100% frequency of seeing) and there is a stimulus level that will never elicit a response (0% frequency of seeing). The threshold for a locus in the visual field is 50% frequency of seeing as shown graphically in Figure 8-26. The steeper the slope of the frequency of seeing curve, the easier it is to determine the patient's threshold. The opposite is true for a flatter slope. Due to false-positive and false-negative responses in clinical testing, the top and bottom limits of the frequency of seeing curve do not actually reach the 100% and 0% frequency of seeing.

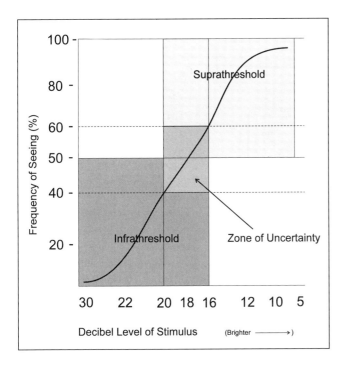

FIGURE 8-26
The frequency of seeing curve shows that on a statically presented stimulus, threshold is defined as 50% frequency of seeing and the zone of uncertainty around threshold (40–60% frequency of seeing) characterizes the segment of the visual spectrum that may or may not be seen. As the stimulus gets brighter, the chance of a response increases.

An area of uncertainty is created by the frequency of seeing curve that is defined as being in the range of 40–60% frequency of seeing.[1] Usually this area of uncertainty does not extend more than 5 dB in the very center of vision, but disease processes such as glaucoma cause a widening of the area of uncertainty and lead to large fluctuations in testing results before a defect is actually determined. This should be kept in mind when evaluating a patient with early stage glaucoma whose visual field results show a large fluctuation in a point tested numerous times.

Humphrey 30-2 Threshold Test Printout and Interpretation

The Humphrey Instruments' threshold test printout can print visual field results in four different formats: numeric, defect depth, grayscale, and profile. The numeric printout gives the absolute decibel value of each thresholded point. The defect depth printout shows how far (plus or minus) from the expected value (in decibels) the statically determined values deviated. The grayscale printout incorporates a scale of varying degrees of gray that darken in areas of lower visual field sensitivity and lighten in areas of greater sensitivity. The rings of gray approximate isopters but should not be confused with an isopter. The grayscale plot should only be used to aid the clinician in identifying possible areas of decreased sensitivity. The grayscale can sometimes be misleading and any area of darkening on the grayscale should cause the clinician to investigate the absolute decibel values of the corresponding points to determine if a defect is truly present. Finally, the profile plot will print the hill of vision for any meridian the clinician chooses (similar to Figure 8-9). This option is only available on some perimeter models.

Figure 8-27 shows a frequently used combination printout that includes data from the STATPAC statistical analysis program. At the top of the printout is the demographic information as well as the stimulus type, the strategy used for this test, the spectacle correction used, the time and date the test was run, pupil size, and the type of fixation. The next section shows the eye tested and the age of the patient. The amount of testing time is printed just under the indices of reliability (described in the next section). Just to the right of the indices of reliability is the numeric printout in decibels for this patient. Note that some points were tested more than once and those results are in parentheses. Just to the right of the numeric printout is the grayscale printout with decreasing areas of sensitivity showing up as darker gray areas. A scale correlating the shades of gray to apostilbs and decibels is given at the bottom of the page. The next row below the numeric printout and to the left shows the defect depth of each point compared with an age-corrected normal.

The field to the right of the defect depth shows the pattern deviation within the field. The pattern deviation plot first raises the hill of vision to where it is expected to be. The results are then analyzed to see if there are any focal defects (bumps) within the visual field. In other words, if there is a generalized depression along with isolated scotomata, the entire hill of vision is "raised" to its normal value, then the deviations from the expected hill of vision are indicated. Cataracts and miosis are felt to be the two most common causes for a generalized depression in the hill of vision.[33] The pattern deviation analysis is designed to discard the decreased sensitivity from these complications and to merely evaluate the pattern deviation and how it differs from normal.[34] The clinical benefit of the pattern deviation plot is that if, for instance, a patient's cataracts worsen, his or her glaucoma can still be evaluated. When a patient reaches end-stage glaucoma and only has a small central island of vision remaining, the pattern deviation plot will improve to show no defects. This is because the hill of vision has been raised from amaurotic to normal

FIGURE 8-27
A Humphrey Visual Field Analyzer STATPAC single field analysis.

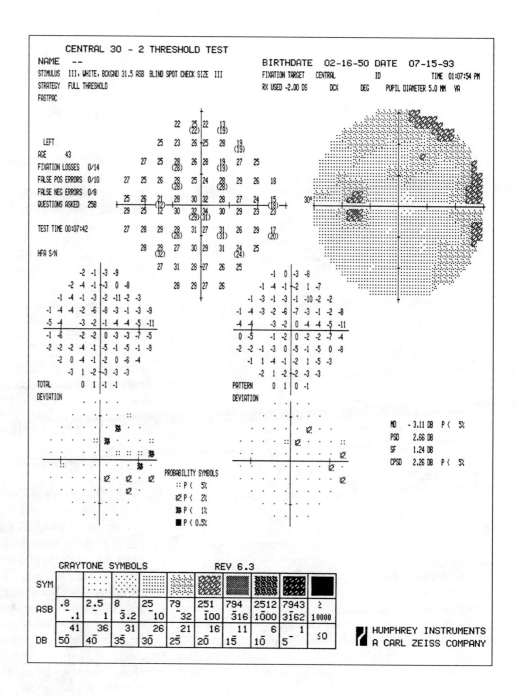

with no focal variations in the hill of vision. Therefore, pattern deviation plots are best used on moderately glaucomatous patients who have developed mild cataracts. Severe cataracts and mild glaucoma can cause the same "normal" pattern deviation plot, and it is up to the clinician to determine which is occurring.

Below the total deviation and pattern deviation decibel printouts are the probability symbol values. Their purpose is to inform the clinician how statistically significant

a defect is from normal. For example, a totally blackened check correlates to a point that has a *P* value of less than 0.5%. This means that the frequency of this level of sensitivity occurring in normal patients is less than 0.5%. To the right of the probability printouts are the global indices (to be described later).

Indices of the Reliability of the Test In many clinics the patient is not actually tested by the doctor. The indices of the patient's reliability are recorded by the computer to aid the clinician in deciding how well the patient performed and how much "weight" should be placed on the visual field to influence the management of the patient. The patient's reliability is assessed by four variables: fixation losses, false-positive responses, false-negative responses, and short-term fluctuation.

FIXATION LOSSES The fixation losses as described earlier are monitored by the Heijl-Krakau method on the Humphrey Visual Field Analyzer and indicate whether the patient is fixating properly. This is an indirect measurement of patient reliability. A high-fixation loss rate (>20%) may occur because there is either poor patient fixation or the patient's blind spot was not plotted correctly at the initiation of the test.

With the more recent versions of software, the blind spot is presumed to be at a certain location. If early in the examination the patient responds to the blind spot check, the perimeter will halt the test and replot the blind spot. If a good perimetrist is carefully observing the test, he or she may pause the test and replot the blind spot before the perimeter software determines that this should be done.

The Humphrey Visual Field Analyzer will test the blind spot more frequently early in the visual field test to determine whether the patient is fixating properly. Over the course of an entire examination, fixation checks will occupy about 5% (10% with older software) of all the stimuli that are presented.

FALSE-POSITIVE RESPONSES False-positive and false-negative responses are an indication that the patient is responding inappropriately. A false-positive response occurs when the patient presses the response button when no stimulus has been presented. For example, the patient may interpret the tempo of the stimuli generated by the perimeter to appear in a rhythmical pattern and will subsequently press the response button even though a stimulus has not been presented. In some instances the patient is merely nervous and afraid that he or she is going to miss a stimulus. If the perimetrist explains that there will be stimuli that will not be detectable and encourages the patient throughout the test, a reduction in false-positive response errors may occur. A high false-positive response rate (above 33%) characterizes a "trigger happy" patient. A visual field printout with a false-positive response rate this high should be rejected.

FALSE-NEGATIVE RESPONSES A false-negative response occurs when a patient initially responds to a stimulus but later does not respond to a much stronger (9 dB brighter) stimulus. Of 33 stimulus presentations, one will be a false-positive test (no stimulus presented) and one will be a false-negative test (brighter stimulus presented). A high false-negative response rate may indicate a fatigued or inattentive patient.[4] If the false-negative response rate exceeds 33%, the index is marked with an X. If all of the other reliability indices are normal, then a high false-negative rate may be an indicator of actual disease. It has been shown that glaucoma patients have higher false-negative response rates than normal subjects.[35] It is recommended that the visual field be considered abnormal when the repeat examination again shows a high false-negative response rate and point values in the "good" areas of the field are within 2 dB of each other.[33]

Global Indices

MEAN DEVIATION The mean deviation (MD) is the mean elevation or depression of the patient's overall field compared with the normal reference field.[4] A significantly low MD implies that the patient either has a generalized depression in the field of vision or a large localized scotoma. The mean deviation may be artifactually depressed from miosis or cataracts. The clinician is given probability values next to each global index to assist in determining how significantly an index deviates from normal.

PATTERN STANDARD DEVIATION The pattern standard deviation (PSD) value is "calculated" by first raising or lowering the hill of vision to the STATPAC expected hill of vision and then calculating the difference between the tested and expected points. Because the hill of vision is adjusted, this global index just examines how the pattern of the tested field varies from normal. A low PSD indicates a smooth hill of vision and a high PSD indicates an irregular hill. The intention is to identify focal visual field defects. Just as the pattern deviation plot may not show any irregularity when a severe cataract or end-stage glaucoma is present, the PSD index may not indicate irregularity as well. These pathologic entities can significantly lower the hill of vision without causing much irregularity in the hill of vision, which will cause the PSD to appear within normal limits. In the absence of severe cataracts and end-stage glaucoma, the PSD has proven to be a useful indicator of an abnormal field when the PSD index P value is 5% or less in reliable patients.[36]

SHORT-TERM FLUCTUATION Short-term fluctuation (SF) is a measure of the intra-test variability the patient shows. It is an indicator of the patient's reliability and consistency of responses. The SF is calculated by retesting the thresholds at 10 points within the visual field and then comparing the second threshold values with the values from the first test. The mathematical calculation of the SF is performed by taking the square root of the mean of the squared difference between the readings (RMS). In determining this global indice, as well as others, the Humphrey software more heavily weights points closer to fixation than the periphery (i.e., the index is "center-weighted"). If the fluctuation rate is high, it may indicate the first signs of glaucomatous visual field loss. High fluctuation values are also associated with established field loss in reliable test subjects. A third possibility for a high fluctuation value is that the patient is inattentive or does not understand the test properly.[4] The computer software will indicate on the printout those SF values that are outside normal limits.

CORRECTED PATTERN STANDARD DEVIATION   The corrected pattern standard deviation (CPSD) is similar to the pattern standard deviation (PSD) in that it is a measure of the irregularity of the hill of vision. The CPSD value is related to the PSD but is modified so that intra-test variability (SF) is taken into consideration. The theory behind subtracting the SF from the PSD is that the patient's hill of vision may differ from expected either because the patient is giving unreliable responses or the patient may have actual field loss. By subtracting out the SF, the CPSD eliminates the patient's unreliability (SF) and just measures the actual variability of the visual field.

GLAUCOMA HEMIFIELD TEST   Glaucoma hemifield analysis has become recognized as an excellent way of determining if the visual field is glaucomatous.[37] Because the superior and inferior visual fields rarely progress evenly in glaucoma, it makes sense to compare the two halves of the field to each other to look for discrepancies. An advantage of this analysis is that the patient is being compared against himself or herself and not against "normal" data, which alleviates complex statistical analysis and also compensates for the testing effects of small pupils and cataracts (since these artifacts are thought to affect each half of the field equally).

The glaucoma hemifield test (GHT) has computerized mirror image analysis that automatically scores each of five pairs of zones in the visual field based on the patient's pattern deviation probability map and then evaluates these scenes based on the frequency with which the values are found in normal individuals (Figure 8-28). After the hemispheres are compared, the computer will print out one of five results (Table 8-9). These five possible GHT results are outside normal limits, borderline, general reduction in sensitivity, abnormally high sensitivity, or within normal limits.[33]

STATPAC   STATPAC is the name Humphrey Instruments gives its database and statistical analysis software. The database was empirically designed by testing a large number of normal patients ranging in age from 20 to 80

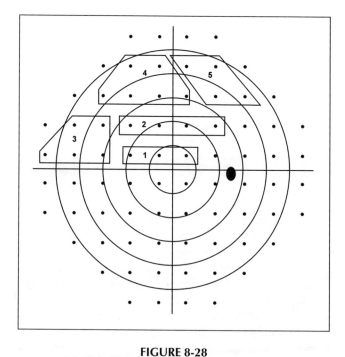

FIGURE 8-28
The glaucoma hemifield test zones for the superior visual field are compared with the correlating inferior visual field to detect mirror image defects. (Adapted from the Humphrey Visual Field Owner's Manual. Humphrey Instruments, San Leandro CA, 1991.)

years and determining an age-corrected "normal" visual field. The patients under age 65 years had to have a visual acuity of 20/20 without cataracts or miosis and for those between 65 and 80 years the visual acuity had to be no worse than 20/30. The visual field had to obey the reliability indices recommended as upper limits for a single visual field (fixation losses less than 20% and false-positive and false-negative responses less than 33%). The field tests were performed three times with the first result being discarded because of its expected increased variability.[33]

After the data were defined for each point in the visual field, the results were stored in the computer memory as the age-corrected visual field. Most visual fields run on the Humphrey Instruments machine are compared with the age-corrected data, but in a few sophisticated analyses, the patient's field is compared with his or her own personal data.

OVERVIEW ANALYSIS   Very important to glaucoma management is determining how a patient's visual field is changing over time, and it is very helpful to be able to quickly compare perimetric performance over multiple examinations. The problem with single field analysis is

TABLE 8-9
Synopsis of Glaucoma Hemifield Test (GHT) Results

Possible Results	Description
Outside normal limits	A score is assigned to each member of the pair of matched zones (Figure 8-28) on either side of the horizonal midline based on the percentile deviation from normal. The "outside normal limits" message will appear when one of two conditions is met: First, if one of the zone pairs yields a score that is found in less than 1% of normal subjects, it is considered outside of normal limits. Second, if both zones in a pair have scores that individually are outside the 0.5% level of probability, "outside nomal limits" will also appear.[33]
Borderline	If one of the matched zones is at 3% *P* level or the paired zones are at the 1% level the borderline message will appear. A borderline GHT can result from unreliable or inexperienced patients and the field test results should be scrutinized closely to determine if they are dependable or if another field test should be run.
General reduction of sensitivity	This message will identify patients with end-stage glaucoma and/or significant cataracts that have depressions that are equal above and below the horizontal midline.
Abnormally high sensitivity	This message occurs whenever the patient's responses are higher than those occurring in 0.5% of the age-corrected population. This response can occur from a high number of false-positive response errors.
Within normal limits	This message appears whenever none of the above conditions is met. A shallow paracentral defect may go unnoticed with this result, and the field should be watched for consistency in subtle defects.

Source: The Humphrey Field Analyzer Owner's Manual. Humphrey Instruments, Inc., San Leandro, CA, 1991.

that it is very difficult to distinguish whether a defective point is either a normal fluctuation in sensitivity or actually a defective point resulting from disease. The overview printout will print up to 16 perimetric examinations to allow the clinician to analyze defective points over time and determine if they are repeatable. Pathologic defects will be repeatable, whereas normal fluctuations for a normal patient will constantly vacillate between improved and deteriorated responses (Figure 8-29). The overview printout includes the grayscale, numeric, total deviation, pattern deviation, GHT results, reliability indices, and global indices.

CHANGE ANALYSIS   The change analysis printout is a graphical representation of change in the global indices over time. The printout consists of four plots at the bottom half of the page showing short-term fluctuation, pattern standard deviation, mean deviation, and corrected pattern standard deviation and a box plot at the top of the page (Figure 8-30). Each graph is plotted as decibels versus time. The probability of normal values (*P* values) is shown as horizontal lines based on the age-corrected normal values for that patient. The type of visual field done (e.g., threshold-related) for each point graphed is indicated in the legend to the left of the plots.

Above the global indices plots is the box plot. Each box plot represents the range of values found relative to age normal for a specific examination. The box itself corre-

lates to the central 70% distribution of results with the central horizontal bar in the middle of the box indicating the median of all threshold values determined for that specific examination.

The upper arm attached to the box correlates to the range in the top 15% of the threshold values and the lower arm correlates to the range in the lowest 15% of the threshold values found for that examination. The examination date is printed beside each box. If the values in the box continue to decline over time, it is an indication that the hill of vision is declining. The most common clinical cause is an increase in the density of a cataract. Early in the glaucomatous process the increased variability associated with a visual field will increase the vertical size of the box plot. New scotomata or an increase in old scotomata will cause the inferior arm to extend while the upper arm stays at the same decibel level.

GLAUCOMA CHANGE PROBABILITY   The glaucoma change probability printout (Figure 8-31) is designed to ascertain if a glaucomatous visual field is progressing. Because a glaucoma patient is no longer "normal," the data for that patient should not be compared with normal test results. The Humphrey Corporation determined how a stable glaucomatous hill of vision appears and what kind of fluctuation it has by evaluating a large number of glaucoma patients over a short period of time. Patients with diagnosed glaucoma were given four visual field examinations

FIGURE 8-29
Overview analysis plot of a glaucoma patient showing worsening of the visual field over time. (Courtesy of Michael A. Chaglasian, O.D.)

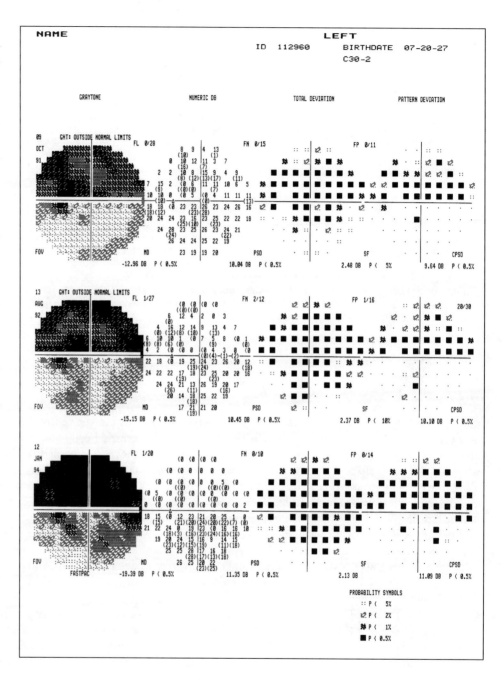

over a 1-month period and the information was entered into the STATPAC II database.

The glaucoma change probability printout is an attempt to determine if the observed visual field changes exceed the normal inter-test variability that occurs with stable glaucoma patients.

Two visual field tests are required before the glaucoma change probability can be produced, although three is more desirable. The first two (or three) fields are averaged into one baseline and the succeeding fields are measured against this patient-defined baseline. If the results of one of the baseline tests are judged to be significantly different from the results of all of the patient's other tests, the perimetrist can discard these test results and use the results of the next two chronological tests as the baseline data.

The printout for the glaucoma change probability has a grayscale plot, the mean deviation graphed over time,

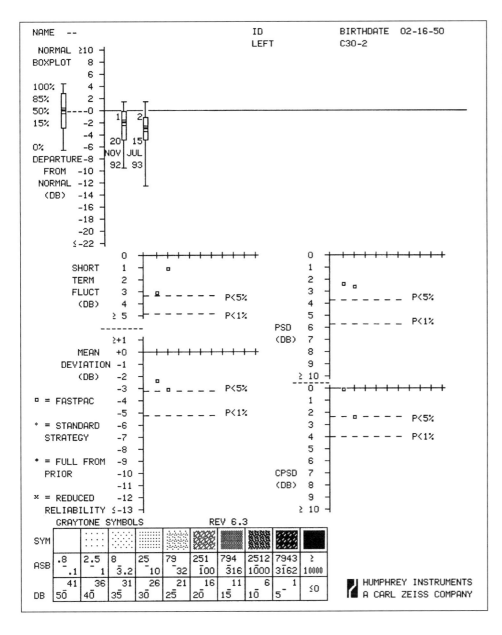

FIGURE 8-30
Change analysis plot showing the trends of the global indices over time. Each index is measured in decibels. The "0" value is considered the age-matched normal for the patient and the P values are represented as horizontal lines. The lower the position of the value on the graph, the worse the reading.

total deviation probability plot, an absolute value of the deviation (total deviation from patient-defined baseline plot), and the glaucoma change probability plot.

The grayscale is determined from the absolute value of the raw data and should be used as a generalized summary to tell the clinician where the defective areas may be located. The mean deviation plot over time is similar to the mean deviation plot seen in the change analysis printout (see previous section). It is an indication of the changes in the entire hill of vision. The total deviation probability plot is a measure of how the current field compares with the patient-defined baseline depth. The

corresponding probability plot is calculated by comparing the total deviation raw data to the computer's glaucoma patient data and determining appropriate probability levels.

The glaucoma change probability plot is seen in the bottom right of Figure 8-31 and it shows the *P* values (represented by black triangles or open triangles) for the defect values seen in the total deviation value plot. The defects for the glaucoma change probability plot are represented by a black triangle, indicating a change from baseline occurring in less than 5% of glaucomatous patients, or an open triangle, indicating a sensitivity

FIGURE 8-31

Glaucoma change probability plot showing the grayscale, mean deviation graphed over time, total deviation probability plot, total deviation from the patient-defined database, and glaucoma change probability plots. No significant change is evident in this example. (Courtesy of Michael A. Chaglasian, O.D.)

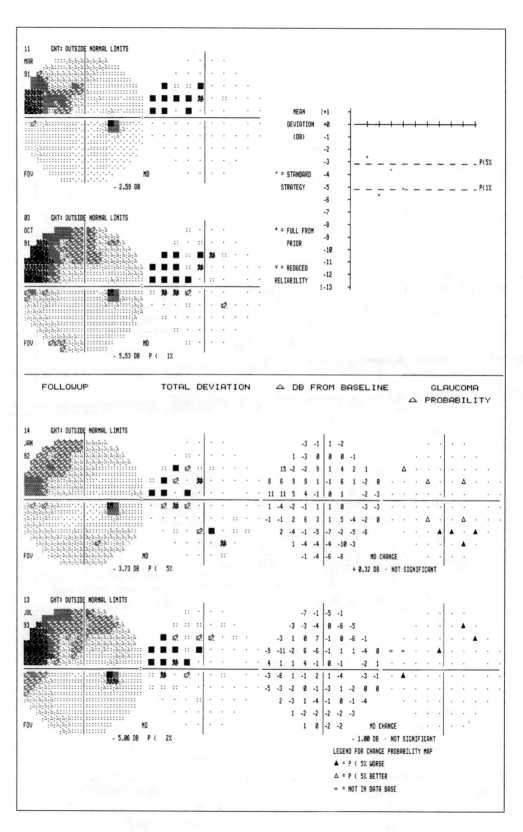

that is better than for all but 5% of glaucoma patients. If an X appears on the glaucoma probability plot, it indicates a value that is outside the level of evaluation for the STATPAC II database (–15 dB) and cannot be assessed by the computer.

Glaucoma change probability analysis should be done with caution. The patient-determined baseline may be erroneously elevated or depressed, making comparisons difficult. This is especially true if the baseline is determined from the patient's first few automated perimetry experiences, because the learning curve and subsequent improvement of perimetric results could significantly flaw the analysis. Also the effects of cataract progression or increased miosis from pharmacologic treatment are not taken into account with each successive field test. Because of these changes over time, the baseline should constantly be upgraded to allow only inter-test (long-term fluctuation) and intra-test (short-term fluctuation) variability to remain. As always, if consistent defects in the hill of vision are observed over time, it is likely that the defect is caused by a pathologic process and is not a normal fluctuation.

ALTERNATIVE METHODS FOR TESTING THE VISUAL FIELD

Because perimetry can be a tedious and time-consuming procedure, many practitioners use procedures other than the usual bowl or tangent screen apparatuses for detection of visual field anomalies. These techniques can range from very simple tests such as confrontation tests to sensitive procedures employing expensive instrumentation.

Confrontation Field Testing

Confrontation field testing is the most expedient way to test the field of vision. Although it will not quantify the visual field, it can yield significant information about the integrity of the visual pathway. The expeditious nature of confrontation field testing allows it to be part of every routine eye examination. For some patients, it is the only form of visual field testing that is possible.

A confrontation test using fingers is usually too insensitive to detect a pathologic process that is not already well advanced, although the test still has merit as a basic screening tool. Confrontations using spherical test objects or a dimmed ophthalmoscope light improve the usefulness of the test. Although confrontation testing is only a screening modality, it is advantageous in that it can be performed on large numbers of patients by ancillary personnel.

Two suggested confrontation techniques deserve discussion. The first involves a central field screening procedure; the second, a peripheral isopter field test. A simple way to screen the central field of the patient is by comparison with the examiner's field. The basic procedure is illustrated in Figure 8-32.

Confrontation testing is performed as follows:

1. The examiner should be seated directly opposite the patient at a distance of 2–3 feet. It is helpful if the background behind the examiner is uniform (such as a blank, evenly lit wall).
2. If the right eye is to be tested first, the patient's left eye must be occluded, and the patient can be instructed to fixate on the examiner's left eye.
3. The test object should be a 3-mm spherical white object or other suitable target.
4. While performing the test, the examiner should close his or her right eye so that his or her own left eye's field of vision and blind spot can be compared with responses that are given for the visual field of the patient's right eye.
5. The test target should be held midway between the patient and examiner as if on an imaginary tangent screen in that plane. The blind spot, isopter boundary, and interior of the field can be quickly explored.

Using a slightly different procedure, the peripheral extent of the field can be explored and estimated by performing perimetry on an imaginary perimeter arc:

1. The patient should be seated comfortably, and the eye not under testing should be occluded.
2. The patient can look at the examiner's finger or a suitable object across the room.
3. The examiner should bring the test object in from the periphery at eye level along an imaginary arc with a radius of about 1 foot, with the patient's eye being the center of curvature.
4. The test should be performed in at least eight meridians.
5. Departures from average limits (60 degrees nasally, 60 degrees superiorly, 100 degrees temporally, 70 degrees inferiorly) are easily estimated and should be noted.

This procedure can also be performed on infants. Here, a parent or a continuously running cartoon is used as a fixation point, and a familiar toy or light is used as the test object. Head or eye movements toward the stimulus

FIGURE 8-32

The standard setup for confrontation field testing with the perimetrist situated directly across from the patient and asking the patient to determine when the stimulus is first perceived. The perimetrist opens his eye, which is directly across from the patient's open eye to determine if the responses approximately match his own. A. Simultaneous finger presentation looking for the extinction phenomenon. B. Simultaneous hand presentation confrontation fields, checking for vertical midline discrepancies. C. A red cap confrontation field to check for more subtle neurologic transmission deficits. D. Confrontation fields on an imaginary perimeter arc.

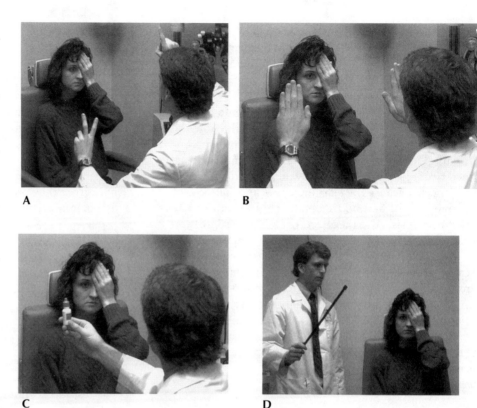

indicate the object is seen. The limit of the field can then be estimated, and gross abnormalities, such as hemianopsia or quadrantanopsia, can be noted.

Finger Counting Method of Confrontation Field Testing

The finger counting method is used mainly because of its ease of administration. The technique is similar to the method described above. The patient is seated 2–3 feet away from the examiner and covers the eye that is not being tested with the palm. The examiner closes his or her corresponding eye so that his or her field matches that of the patient's. The examiner then will show one, two, or five fingers in each quadrant and ask the patient to count the fingers while fixating on the examiner's eye or nose. It is difficult to distinguish three and four fingers, so using them in confrontation testing is not recommended.

If the patient has trouble fixating, the examiner can hold up both hands and tell the patient to total the fingers in both hands. Each hand is presented simultaneously, and the fingers should only be shown for a short time, thereby not giving the patient enough time to look at both

hands. A variation on this technique is to only display fingers from one hand at a time, varying the hand that is the stimulus.

One advantage of using the simultaneous presentation of two hands is that the extinction phenomenon can be tested for. Patients who exhibit the extinction phenomenon will not be able to see both stimuli at the same time even though the patient will respond properly to each stimulus when presented individually in either quadrant. This phenomenon is indicative of neurologic disease and a more thorough visual field and neurologic work-up is advised.

Comparison Techniques

Comparison confrontation field tests can be useful in defining a hemianopsia. The technique involves using the red caps from mydriasis solution bottles or merely the examiner's two hands and presenting them to a monocularly occluded patient on either side of the midline of vision. If the patient has a hemianopsia, one of the caps will not be visible or it may appear dimmer on one side relative to the other. To confirm a defect, one of the caps can be moved

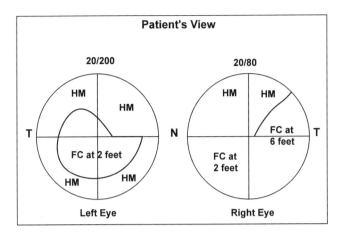

FIGURE 8-33
The proper method for diagramming a confrontation field. The fields are from the patient's point of view and not from the examiner's, as is common with many confrontation field diagrams. FC = finger counting; HM = hand motion; N = nasal; T = temporal.

across the visual field to see if the patient can detect a change in its appearance as it crosses the vertical midline.

If the patient is asked to compare the "brightness" of each hand, care should be taken that each hand is equally illuminated; otherwise artifactual defects may occur.

Diagramming Confrontation Fields

The recommended technique for diagramming confrontation fields is shown in Figure 8-33. This technique[3] is not always honored in clinical practice. The field should be recorded as though the patient were looking at it, but it is customary for many examiners to diagram the confrontation fields from the doctor's view instead of the patient's view. It is recommended that whichever way the field is diagrammed, the viewpoint should be written on the chart to aid in later interpretation of the confrontation field.

The Facial Amsler

Facial Amsler testing is another way to quickly screen the patient's visual field. The patient is asked to close one eye and fixate on the examiner's nose. The patient is then asked if the examiner's facial features, including the forehead, eyes, ears, and chin, are fully visible. If the patient can see the examiner's features without contrast differences or metamorphopsia, then the central field is considered grossly normal.

Although the word *Amsler* is associated with this confrontation test, this evaluation method is more a test of the gross visual field than it is of macular function. Macular function is best tested with the Amsler charts.

The Amsler Charts

The Amsler charts are a series of seven finely ruled charts that are used to analyze disturbances of central visual function. The primary chart that is used is shown at the top left of Figure 8-34. When held at a distance of about 29 cm from the eye, each square of the chart subtends an angle of 1 degree, and the entire chart will correspond with an area of the retina that is 10 degrees in radius from the center of the fovea. The primary goal of the test is to locate distortions (metamorphopsia, micropsia, or macropsia), depressed areas, or missing areas that may indicate dysfunction. The examination procedure follows this outline:

1. The patient should be seated comfortably and must have proper refractive correction for a 29-cm viewing distance. It is preferable to use a trial frame correction instead of a bifocal, because the bifocal may not fit properly and may interfere with the line of sight to the Amsler chart. The patient's eyes should not be dilated nor should they have just undergone procedures such as tonometry, gonioscopy, or ophthalmoscopy.
2. The eye not being tested should be occluded.
3. The chart should be evenly illuminated and placed at the 29-cm test distance.
4. The patient should fixate on the center white dot and, while concentrating on this point, notice the whole of the chart and its grid pattern.
5. The patient should point out distortions, blurs, missing areas, shining areas, disruptions, vibrations, or other defects in the network of the grid.
6. The patient observations should be recorded as accurately as possible on a black-on-white recording form, which is a replica of the standard Amsler grid pattern.

In addition to the standard Amsler chart, there are several additional charts that may be used, including a chart with diagonal lines to aid in fixation when the patient has a central defect and cannot see the white dot, a chart with dots to help reveal scotomata, and a chart with parallel lines (white on black) to be held horizontally and vertically to reveal metamorphopsia (distortions in the grid pattern). Also available is a chart with parallel lines (black on white) for minute examination for distortion along reading lines, a standard red-on-black chart to be used for detecting subtle color scotomata, and a chart more finely subdivided in the center for more detailed examination and for use in high myopia, where the chart can be held at the punctum remotum of the uncorrected eye.

The Amsler grid is a very good supplemental test to the regular visual field examination. It is especially useful for

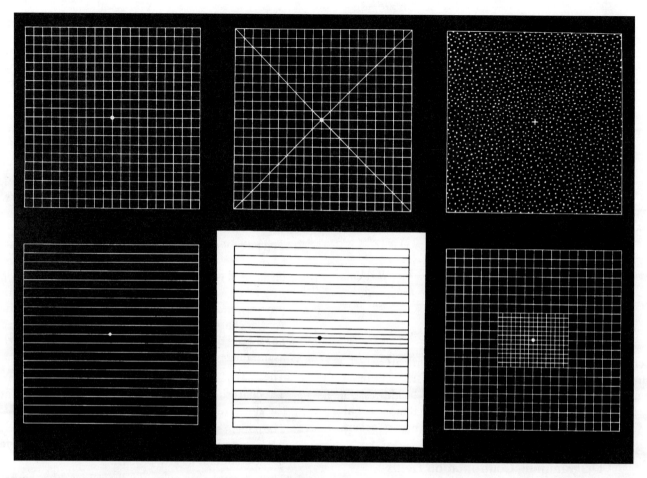

FIGURE 8-34

The Amsler charts. (Top left) The primary grid. (Top center) Chart used to plot central scotomata. (Top right) Dot chart to reveal scotomata. (Bottom left) Line chart to reveal horizontal or vertical distortions. (Bottom center) Chart to reveal distortions in a simulated reading situation. (Bottom right) Chart with more finely ruled central area and for use at the punctum remotum of the eye in high myopia. Not shown is a chart ruled in red for the detection of color scotomata.

evaluating older patients and those in whom retinal edema is a possibility. Often, disturbances indicated by the Amsler grid are only barely discernible with direct evaluation of the macula. Positive findings on an Amsler grid test should be followed by a fundus lens examination and possibly fluorescein angiography to aid in the diagnosis of macular disease. It should be noted, however, that optic nerve disease or lesions located elsewhere in the visual pathway may also cause central visual defects that are detectable with the Amsler grid.

DEFECT CHARACTERISTICS

It is important to understand that the shape of a defect and other characteristics revealed by multiple isopter test-

ing contribute greatly to the interpretation of a visual field test result. The vast majority of visual field defects are not totally blind areas but are areas of partial visual loss. Therefore, testing with different sizes and intensities of test objects will reveal different sizes for the defect. Thus, the size and depth of the defect will be helpful in the eventual diagnosis of the problem.

Shape and Location

The shape and location of a defect are very significant. Defects that roughly split the field with vertical or horizontal boundaries are called hemianopsias, and the location is given usually as right, left, superior, or inferior. Bilateral hemianopsias that occur on the same side of the field for both eyes are homonymous defects (see Figure 8-5); if they are in opposing fields, they are heteronymous defects (binasal or bitemporal). Quadrantanopsias are defects that occupy a quadrant of the visual field. A half field defect with a horizontal boundary is called an altitudinal defect. Any defect that is approximately defined by two radii of the visual field may be classified as a sector defect. Any type of defect, such as a hemianopsia, that passes through the center of fixation causes macular splitting. Defects that extend up to but do not involve central fixation yield macular sparing. With homonymous defects it is necessary to note whether or not the shapes of the defects are nearly identical, that is, congruent (see Figure 8-5 [6]), or whether the shapes are clearly different, that is, incongruent (see Figure 8-5 [4]). As a general rule, the more congruent a visual field defect, the closer the lesion is positioned to the occipital cortex. An overall shrinkage for all isopters is referred to as general depression of the visual field and commonly is the result of small pupils, cloudy media, or uncorrected refractive error. Figure 8-12 shows some common scotomata, classified according to shape and position. These characteristics of a visual field defect are of great diagnostic importance.

Density

The density of a visual field defect is related to the loss of vision within the defective area. Thus, total blindness (an absolute defect) is an area of the highest density. The normal blind spot is a good example of an absolute defect illustrating high density. Only multiple isopter testing or automated threshold perimetry will reveal the density of a defect. The greater the visual loss (density), the greater the pathway interference (destruction) and generally the poorer the prognosis for recovery. The area of greatest density in a defect generally is indicative of the initial and most long-standing pathway interference.

Margins

As a general rule, if a lesion is still active, multiple isopter testing will show large variations in the size and shape of the defect (see Figure 8-17). In such cases the margins are said to be sloping. In many nonprogressive lesions, the margins of the plotted deficit overlap one another or are close together and are called steep. Steep margins occur with defects of higher density.

INTERPRETATION OF FIELD DEFECTS

For proper interpretation of any test result in perimetry, a thorough understanding of the anatomy and function of the neural visual pathway and its relationship to surrounding

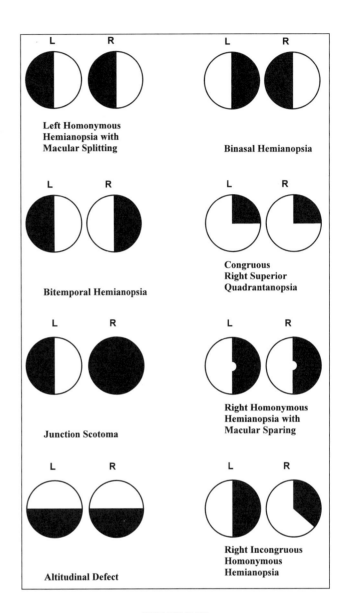

FIGURE 8-35
Commonly occurring visual field deficits and their proper nomenclature. Note that the junction scotoma schematic shows complete loss of vision in the right eye. A scotoma involving the central visual field with relative sparing of the peripheral field is commonly the presentation.

structures is necessary. Figures 8-5 and 8-35 and Table 8-10 are included to summarize the relationships between lesions and resulting field loss. The following is a list of general rules regarding interpretation of test results in perimetry:

1. Sudden visual loss or onset of a field deficit generally indicates a vascular lesion or inflammation.

TABLE 8-10

Summary of Components of the Visual Pathways, Their Respective Blood Supplies, and the Types of Field Defects Produced by the Common Pathologies Affecting Them

Visual Pathway	Blood Supply	Common Lesions	Defect Characteristics
Retina	Choriocapillaris Central retinal artery	Uveitis Neoplasms Retinal detachment Vascular Diabetic Toxic Degenerative	Round, oval, or irregular scotomata Nerve fiber bundle defects Local depression
Optic nerve	Prepapillary choroid Vessels from posterior ciliary arteries Ophthalmic artery Anterior circle of Willis	Papilledema Optic neuritis Tumors Vascular	Enlarged blind spot Central scotoma Altitudinal hemianopsia Blindness in one eye and temporal defect in the other
Chiasm	Circle of Willis Middle cerebral artery	Aneurysm Inflammation Pituitary adenoma	Nasal or binasal defects Bizarre shape Bitemporal defects Junction defects
Optic tract	Posterior communicating artery Middle cerebral artery Anterior choroidal artery Posterior cerebral artery	Vascular Tumors	Incongruent homonymous hemianopsia with macular splitting
Optic radiations	Middle cerebral artery Anterior choroidal artery Posterior cerebral artery	Vascular Tumors	Homonymous quadrantanopsia or hemianopsia Anterior lesions produce incongruency and macular splitting Posterior lesions produce congruency and macular sparing
Visual cortex	Posterior cerebral artery Middle cerebral artery	Vascular Tumors Trauma	Homonymous quadrantanopsia or hemianopsia congruent and with macular sparing Double homonymous hemianopsia Homonymous hemianopic scotomata

Source: The Humphrey Field Analyzer Owner's Manual. Humphrey Instruments, Inc., San Leandro, CA, 1991.

2. Slow onset of a field deficit indicates conditions such as glaucoma, tumors, and chronic toxic or systemic disorders.

3. Except for the region of the posterior optic tract and lateral geniculate nucleus, lesions affecting the superior neural visual pathway produce defects in the lower visual field, and lesions affecting the inferior portion of the visual pathway produce defects in the upper visual field. Thus, the dense superior defect noted in Figure 8-5 (4) was produced by a lesion (pituitary tumor) initially disrupting the lower fibers of the optic chiasm.

4. Postchiasmal lesions produce contralateral field defects in each eye.

5. Unilateral defects are generally caused by prechiasmal lesions (retina or optic nerve).

6. Defects produced by chiasmal lesions are often unusual in shape and usually bitemporal [Figure 8-5 (3)] in appearance.

7. Defects with low density and sloping margins indicate minimal visual pathway destruction or the early stages of a progressive lesion.

8. Dense defects indicate severe pathway destruction and may indicate long-standing disease.

9. The characteristics of hemianopsia and partial hemianopsia visual field loss resulting from postchiasmal pathway disruption are: (a) tract lesions produce defects that are incongruent and have a tendency toward macular splitting; (b) optic radiation involvement from temporal lobe lesions produces superior quadrantanopsias with a tendency toward splitting of fixation; (c) optic radiation involvement from parietal lobe lesions produces contralateral inferior quadrantanopsias with a tendency toward sparing of fixation and toward congruency; (d) other neurologic signs (e.g., paresis) accompany optic radiation lesions and the asso-

ciated homonymous hemianopsias; (e) neurologic signs or symptoms (other than vision) are not likely to accompany occipital lobe lesions, and resulting hemianopsias are likely to show macular sparing and congruency.

10. A good case history will often give clues to the nature of a lesion producing visual loss.

11. Steep margins of a defect may indicate an old or nonprogressing lesion.

12. Psychogenic defects do not resemble defects produced by an organic disease and often manifest as constricted 5- to 10-degree fields for all test objects. Isopters are occasionally interlaced.

In interpreting field defects, the apparent defects that can be caused by conditions other than those affecting the visual pathway must be kept in mind. The following are common causes of general isopter depression or other field defects that are not related to the neural visual pathway:

1. Small pupils
2. Uncorrected refractive error
3. Cloudy media
4. Psychogenic causes
5. Distortions from high spectacle prescriptions
6. Malingering
7. Slow reaction time
8. Anatomic restrictions such as a drooping lid or a large prominent nasal bridge

EVALUATION OF VISUAL FIELD LOSS

In medicolegal cases, it sometimes becomes necessary to quantify visual field loss. Although further development of methods of evaluation are needed, two methods in particular have emerged and have commonly been used for such evaluation.

American Medical Association Method

For evaluation of visual efficiency, the American Medical Association (AMA) has adopted a system in which three visual functions are mathematically coordinated: visual acuity, visual fields, and ocular motility.[38] The percentages of efficiency for these three areas are multiplied together to give the total visual efficiency (VE) for one eye. The total binocular visual efficiency (BVE) is given by the following formula:

TABLE 8-11

*The table shows how the sum of the visual field adds to 500 degrees**

Temporal	85 degress
Superior and temporal	55 degrees
Superior	45 degrees
Superior and nasal	55 degrees
Nasal	60 degrees
Inferior and nasal	50 degrees
Inferior	65 degrees
Inferior and temporal	85 degrees
Total	500 degrees

*The percent visual field efficiency is given by the following equation: Percent efficiency = [(sum of field extent in 8 meridians) × 100]/500.

$$BVE = [3 \times (\% \text{ VE of better eye}) + \text{VE of worse eye}]/4$$

The percentage of visual acuity loss is determined from a table based on best correctable Snellen acuity for distance and on Jaeger type for near. The percentage of motility efficiency is based on the extent of diplopia in various directions of gaze.

The percentage of visual field loss is determined by plotting the extent of the visual field for a 3-mm white test object using a standard perimeter arc under 7 foot-candles of illumination. Eight half meridians are tested and the limits are determined for each meridian. The minimum normal field for the eight meridians that sums to 500 degrees is listed in Table 8-11.

Scoring Grid

A second method of determining visual field loss has been developed by Esterman.[39,40] Grids for scoring the central visual field and the peripheral visual field are shown in Figure 8-36. The central grid is used for the tangent screen, using a 2-mm white target under 7 foot-candles of illumination at a 1-m test distance. The peripheral scoring grid is used to evaluate the peripheral field as plotted with a 3-mm white target on the standard perimeter arc under 7 foot-candles of illumination. The grids are divided into 100 units (representing 1% of the functional field) of unequal area based on the functional importance to the patient. This system is different from the AMA system in that it is not based on area alone but considers certain parts of the field as functionally more important than others. Some automated visual field machines have this grid programmed into their testing sequence. The grids can be photographically adjusted to be compatible with any visual field recording chart. The visual field chart is overlaid on the grid, and dots falling within a scotomatous area

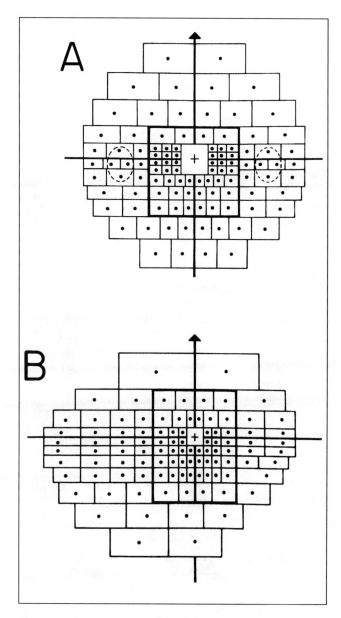

FIGURE 8-36
The Esterman scoring grids (A) for the central field and (B) for the peripheral field. (Adapted from B Esterman. Grid for scoring visual fields: I. Tangent screen. Arch Ophthalmol 1967;77:780; and B Esterman. Grid for scoring visual fields: II. Perimeter. Arch Ophthalmol 1968;79:400.)

or outside the isopter are counted and correlated with a percentage of field loss. This scoring system improves on the AMA system by providing a more realistic evaluation of functional visual loss.

REFERENCES

1. Lynn JR, Fellman RL, Starita RJ. Exploring the Normal Visual Field. In R Ritch, MB Shields, T Krupin (eds), The Glaucomas (Vol. 1). St. Louis: Mosby, 1989;361–79.
2. Carr RE, Siegel IM. Electrodiagnostic Testing of the Visual System: A Clinical Guide (2nd ed). Philadelphia: FA Davis, 1990;5–6.
3. Anderson DR. Perimetry With and Without Automation. St. Louis: Mosby, 1987;32, 419.
4. The Visual Field Primer. San Leandro: Allergan Humphrey, 1987:1, 134.
5. Traquair HM. An Introduction to Clinical Perimetry (5th ed). St. Louis: Mosby, 1946.
6. Cline D, Hofstetter HW, Griffin JR. Dictionary of Visual Science (4th ed). Radnor, PA: Chilton, 1989;556.
7. Lewis TL, Chronister CL. Etiology and Pathophysiology of Primary Open-Angle Glaucoma. In TL Lewis, M Fingeret (eds), Primary Care of the Glaucomas. Norwalk, CT: Appleton & Lange, 1993:74–5.
8. Minckler DS, Spaeth GL. Optic nerve damage in glaucoma. Surv Ophthalmol 1981;26:128–48.
9. Jonas JB, Naumann GOH. Parapapillary retinal vessel diameter in normal and glaucomatous eyes. II. Correlations. Invest Ophthalmol Vis Sci 1989;30:1604–11.
10. Hayreh SS. Pathogenesis of optic nerve head changes in glaucoma. Semin Ophthalmol 1986;1:1–13.
11. Levy NS, Adams CK. Slow axonal protein transport and visual function following retinal and optic nerve ischemia. Invest Ophthalmol Vis Sci 1975;14:91–7.
12. Levy NS. The effect of interruption of the short posterior ciliary arteries on slow axoplasmic transport and histology within the optic nerve of the rhesus monkey. Invest Ophthalmol 1976;15:495–9.
13. Radius RL. Optic nerve fast axonal transport abnormalities in primates. Occurrence after short posterior ciliary artery occlusion. Arch Ophthalmol 1980;98:2018–22.
14. Radius RL, Anderson DR. Morphology of axonal transport abnormalities in primate eyes. Br J Ophthalmol 1981;65:767–77.
15. Radius RL. Anatomy of the optic nerve head and glaucomatous optic neuropathy. Surv Ophthalmol 1987;32:35–44.
16. Nanba K, Schwartz B. Nerve fiber layer and optic disc fluorescein defects in glaucoma and ocular hypertension. Ophthalmology 1988;95:1227–33.
17. Shaffer RN. Nerve fiber loss and disparity of disc and field changes in glaucoma. Symposium on the laser in ophthalmology and glaucoma update. Trans New Orleans Acad Ophthalmol 1985;129–33.
18. Quigley HA, Adicks EM, Green WR. Optic nerve damage in human glaucoma. III. Quantitative correlation of nerve fiber loss and visual field defect in glaucoma, ischemic neuropathy, papilledema, and toxic neuropathy. Arch Ophthalmol 1982;100:135–46.
19. Werner EB, Drance SM. Early visual field disturbances in glaucoma. Arch Ophthalmol 1977;95:1173–5.

20. Sloan PG. Perimetric screening for glaucoma. Am J Optom Arch Am Acad Optom 1960;37:388–94.

21. Flammer JE, Eppler, Niesel P. Quantitative perimetry in the glaucoma patient without local viual field defects. Graefes Arch Clin Exp Ophthalmol 1982;219:92–4.

22. Benedetto MD, Cyrlin MN. The effect of blur upon static perimetric thresholds. Doc Ophthalmol Proc Ser 1985;42:563–7.

23. Johnson CA, Adams AJ, Casson EJ, Brandt JD. Progression of early glaucomatous visual field loss as detected by blue-on-yellow and standard white-on-white automated perimetry. Arch Ophthalmol 1993;111:651–6.

24. Humphrey A. Field Analyzer Owner's Manual. San Leandro: Allergan Humphrey, 1991:5–25.

25. Katz J, Sommer A. Reliability indices of automated perimetric tests. Arch Ophthalmol 1988;106:1252–4.

26. Katz J, Sommer A, Witt K. Reliability of visual field results over repeated testing. Ophthalmology 1991;98:70–5.

27. Sanabria O, Feuer WJ, Anderson DR. Pseudo-loss of fixation in automated perimetry. Ophthalmology 1991;98:76–8.

28. Bebie H. Computerized Techniques of Visual Field Analysis. In SM Drance, DR Anderson (eds), Automatic Perimetry in Glaucoma. A Practical Guide. Orlando: Grune & Stratton, 1985:148–85.

29. Heijl A, Lindgren G, Olsson J. A package for the statistical analysis of visual fields. Doc Ophthalmol Proc Ser 1987; 49:153–68.

30. Katz J, Sommer A. Asymmetry and variation in the normal hill of vision. Arch Ophthalmol 1986;104:65–8.

31. Heijl A, Lindgren G, Olsson J, Asman P. Visual field interpretation with empiric probability maps. Arch Ophthalmol 1989;107:204–8.

32. Young WO, Stewart WC, Hunt H, Crosswell H. Static threshold variability in the peripheral visual field in normal subjects. Graefes Arch Clin Exp Ophthalmol 1990; 228:454–7.

33. Lalle PA. Visual fields. In TL Lewis, M Fingeret (eds), Primary Care of the Glaucomas. Norwalk, CT: Appleton & Lange, 1993:164–84.

34. Lam BL, Alward WLM, Kolder HE. Effect of cataract on automated perimetry. Ophthalmology 1991;98:1066–70.

35. Heijl A, Lindgren G, Olson J. Reliability parameters in computerized perimetry. Doc Ophthalmol Proc Ser 1987; 49:593–600.

36. Enger C, Sommer A. Recognizing glaucomatous field loss with the Humphrey STATPAC. Arch Ophthalmol 1987; 105:1355–7.

37. Sommer A, Enger C, Witt K. Screening for glaucomatous visual field loss with automated threshold perimetry. Am J Ophthalmol 1989;107:199–203.

38. Committee on Rating of Mental and Physical Impairment. JAMA 1958;168:475–8.

39. Esterman B. Grid for scoring visual fields: I. Tangent screen. Arch Ophthalmol 1967;77:780–6.

40. Esterman B. Grid for scoring visual fields: II. Perimeter. Arch Ophthalmol 1968;79:400–6.

9

Evaluation of Pupillary Disorders

RUTH A. TRACHIMOWICZ AND JOHN E. CONTO

The ability to recognize abnormal pupil conditions requires a working knowledge of both the neural circuitry of the pupillary light reflex, the parasympathetic and sympathetic pathways controlling pupil size, and the anatomic relationships among these pathways. In addition, the clinical evaluation of the pupil is an integral part of the ophthalmic examination and can provide valuable insight into the functioning and effects of various disorders of the visual pathways. This chapter has been separated into several sections, beginning with an overview of the anatomy, blood supply, and innervation of the iris, followed by a methodical approach to pupil testing. The third section outlines commonly encountered pupillary disorders, their clinical presentation and etiologies, and the diagnostic tests available to assess the disorders.

ANATOMY, FUNCTION, AND INNERVATION OF THE PUPIL

Anatomy and Function

The pupil is a round opening near the center of the iris, the circular muscular diaphragm that divides the anterior segment of the eye into the anterior and posterior chambers. The pupil has several functions including the regulation of light reaching the retina, control of the depth of focus, and the reduction of spherical and chromatic aberration. These actions are achieved by altering the size of the pupil, which is governed by the sphincter and dilator muscles of the iris. The pupil also provides a passage for the aqueous humor to flow from the posterior chamber into the anterior chamber of the eye.[1]

The average diameter of the iris is about 12 mm. The collarette marks the division of the anterior surface of the iris into two distinct zones. The pupillary zone appears relatively smooth and flat, while the surface of the wider ciliary zone is irregular from numerous central contraction furrows, crypts (of Fuchs), and occasional iris processes near the iris root[1] (Figure 9-1).

The iris is composed of four layers: (1) the anterior border layer, (2) the iris stroma, (3) the anterior pigmented epithelium, and (4) the posterior pigmented epithelium. The anterior border layer is a discontinuous sheet of fibroblasts and melanocytes, whereas the underlying iris stroma is composed of highly vascularized connective tissue containing melanocytes. The smooth muscle fibers of the sphincter muscle, which are arranged in a circular fashion, lie within the iris stroma at the pupillary margin. Two epithelial layers, the anterior and posterior pigmented epithelium, line the posterior surface of the iris. The dilator muscle is composed of smooth muscle arranged in a radial fashion, located within the base of the anterior pigmented epithelial cells. The dilator muscle extends from the peripheral border of the sphincter muscle to the iris root[1] (Figure 9-2).

Iris color is mainly determined by the amount of pigment granules in the stromal melanocytes, with fewer pigment granules in the melanocytes of blue irides than in dark brown irides. Formation of pigment granules by the stromal melanocytes is largely under control of the sympathetic nervous system. If sympathetic innervation to the eye is disrupted early in development, the melanocytes in the affected iris will not produce pigment granules, and the iris will appear to be lighter in the involved eye.[2] This occurs in congenital Horner's syndrome, which is discussed in a later section.

The iris is supplied by blood from the major arterial circle of the iris, which is located near the iris root in the ciliary body stroma. The major arterial circle is formed by the anterior ciliary and the long posterior ciliary arteries and has branches that extend radially into the iris stro-

FIGURE 9-1

Composite diagram of the iris showing a surface view of the iris on the left and the distribution of the iris vasculature on the right. The pupillary zone (A) and the ciliary zone (B) are separated by the iris collarette (=). Crypts of Fuchs (C) are seen in both the pupillary and ciliary portions of the iris. Circular contraction furrows (D) are seen in the ciliary zone. The iris vessels are shown beginning at the major arterial circle (E), which is located in the ciliary body. Radial branches extend toward the pupillary zone, and at the collarette the arteries form an incomplete minor arterial circle (F). Branches of the minor circle form capillary arcades in the pupillary zone.

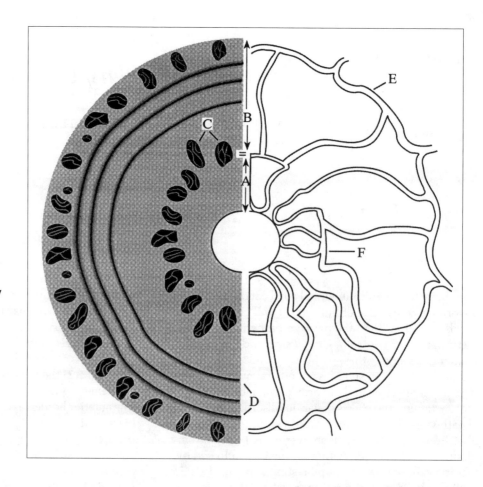

ma. At the collarette, the radial branches anastomose to form the incomplete minor arterial circle. Offshoot vessels of the minor circle create the capillary arcades in the pupillary portion of the iris[1] (see Figure 9-1).

Sensory innervation to the iris is provided by branches of the ophthalmic division of the trigeminal nerve carried in the long and short posterior ciliary nerves. Motor innervation to the sphincter muscle is served by parasympathetic fibers carried in the short posterior ciliary nerves, whereas the dilator muscle is innervated by sympathetic fibers that are carried within the long posterior ciliary nerves.[1]

Pupillary Light Reflex

When light is directed into either eye under normal conditions, the pupils constrict. The reaction that occurs in the illuminated eye is referred to as the "direct light response," and the reaction occurring in the opposite, non-illuminated eye is referred to as the "consensual light response." The afferent limb of this light reflex originates within the retinal ganglion cells, whose axons contain pupillomotor information in addition to visual information.[1] The pupillary fibers course through the optic nerve and decussate in the optic chiasm in the same manner as the nerve fibers that carry the visual information. Since about 53% of the axons cross, each optic tract contains pupillary fibers from the ipsilateral temporal retina and contralateral nasal retina.[3] Research suggests that the axons in the optic tract have collateral branches that send pupillary information to the pretectal area, while the visual information is relayed to the lateral geniculate nucleus.[1] The pupillary fibers exit at the posterior portion of the optic tract and enter the dorsal aspect of the midbrain through the brachium of the superior colliculus.[4] The fibers synapse on cells in the ipsilateral pretectal nucleus, which then hemidecussate by passing ventrally in the periaqueductal gray matter to terminate in the ipsilateral Edinger-Westphal (EW) nucleus, and dorsally through the posterior commissure to synapse in the contralateral EW nucleus.[4] This pathway provides equal bilateral retinal input to the EW nuclei.[1]

The efferent limb of the pupillary light reflex begins in the EW nuclei.[5,6] Preganglionic parasympathetic fibers from the EW nuclei join the third cranial nerve (oculomotor nerve) in a superficial position just beneath the

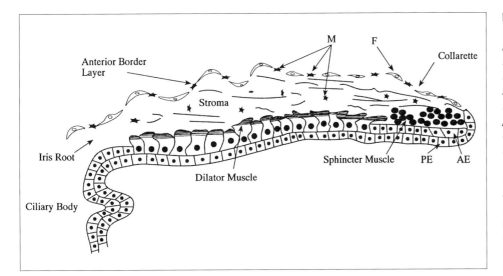

FIGURE 9-2
Cross-section of the iris showing all four layers. Fibroblasts (F) and melanocytes (M) form the anterior border layer. Melanocytes are also seen in the vascular loose connective tissue of the iris stroma. The posterior surface of the iris is covered by an anterior (AE) and posterior (PE) pigmented epithelium. The sphincter muscle lies free in the stroma near the pupil, but the dilator muscle lies in the base of the anterior pigmented epithelial cells. The dilator muscle is considered a myoepithelium because the muscle fibers lie in the cytoplasm of the epithelial cells.

epineurium, the connective tissue covering the nerve. The preganglionic parasympathetic fibers lie in the superior, dorsomedial portion of the third nerve.[7] As they exit the midbrain, the third nerve fibers traverse the red nucleus and corticospinal tracts. They then course forward toward the cavernous sinus, passing between the superior cerebellar and posterior cerebral arteries, and traveling between the free and attached margins of the tentorium cerebelli. The oculomotor nerve fibers pass lateral to the posterior communicating artery before entering the wall of the cavernous sinus and then are located superior to the fourth cranial nerve (trochlear nerve) within the wall.[8] The pupillomotor fibers are medially located within the third nerve as it exits the subarachnoid space and eventually move to a more inferior position. The pupillary fibers enter the orbit through the superior orbital fissure, traveling in the inferior division of the third nerve and in the inferior division's branch to the inferior oblique muscle. The fibers synapse in the ciliary ganglion.[7] In the past it was believed that the oculomotor nerve divided into superior and inferior divisions either in the cavernous sinus, at the entrance into the orbit, or in the orbit proper. However, recent clinical evidence suggests that the bifurcation may occur more proximal, at the level where the oculomotor fascicles pass through the midbrain.[9]

The postganglionic parasympathetic fibers exit the ciliary ganglion as the short posterior ciliary nerves and enter the globe by piercing the back of the eyeball in a circular distribution around the optic nerve. They travel forward in the suprachoroidal space to innervate the sphincter and ciliary body muscles.[1] The ratio of neurons in the ciliary ganglion that innervate the sphincter muscle compared with those that innervate the ciliary body is approximately

1 to 30. Recent studies offer evidence that a direct pathway from the midbrain to the intrinsic muscles of the eye exists in monkeys and rabbits. This direct pathway bypasses the ciliary ganglion, and either does not have an intermediate synapse, or synapses in or near the intrinsic muscles.[10,11] Several clinical cases of patients with unilateral preganglionic third nerve palsy and associated pupillary mydriasis show a preganglionic supersensitivity to low concentrations (0.1%, 0.125%) of pilocarpine, which implies that this direct pathway may also exist in humans[12,13] (Figure 9-3).

Near Reflex and Accommodation

A different afferent pathway, involving the occipital lobe, is used for pupillary constriction during accommodation. This pathway is poorly understood, but along with the visual information tract, selected retinal fibers provide input to the striate cortex. Striate cortex fibers project to visual association areas, which in turn project fibers to the EW nuclei.[1,14] These nuclei can be divided into three functionally different regions. The rostral part is concerned with accommodation, whereas stimulation of the middle section results in accommodation and pupil constriction. The caudal part controls pupil constriction. Visual association areas are presumed to project fibers to the middle region of the EW nuclei to initiate pupil constriction during accommodation.[6] Because the EW nuclei are located more ventrally in the midbrain compared with the pretectal nuclei concerned with the pupillary light reflex, they are unaffected by dorsal midbrain lesions (disrupting the pretectal nuclei, posterior commissure, or afferent pupillary light reflex fibers), which would result

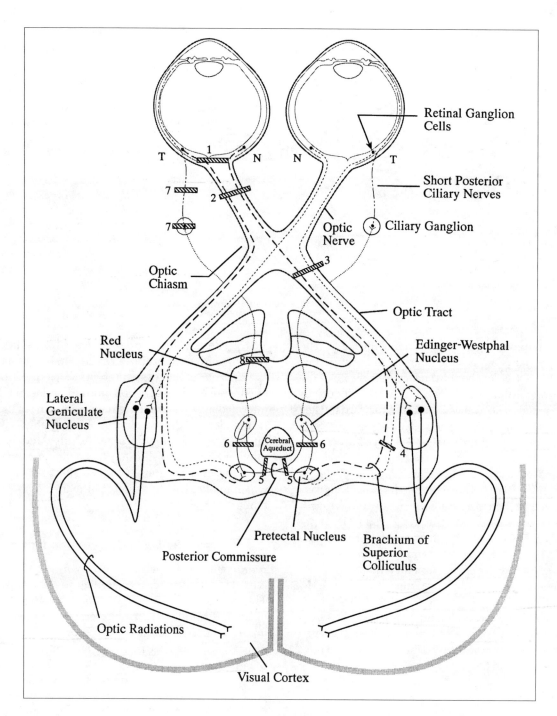

FIGURE 9-3

Schematic of the pupillary light reflex pathway. Pupillary disorders can result from interruption of this pathway anywhere along the afferent or efferent limbs. Possible sites of damage leading to some of the more common pupillary disorders are shown. An afferent pupillary defect in the ipsilateral eye can be caused by a lesion in the ipsilateral retina or macula (1), ipsilateral optic nerve (2), contralateral optic tract (3), or contralateral brachium of the superior colliculus (4). Midbrain pupils can be caused by lesions in the posterior commissure or pretectal nuclei (5). Argyll Robertson pupils can be caused by a lesion in the periaqueductal gray matter (6). Adie's tonic pupils can be caused by damage to the ciliary ganglion or short posterior ciliary nerves (7). Third nerve palsy can be caused by a lesion along the third nerve pathway (8).

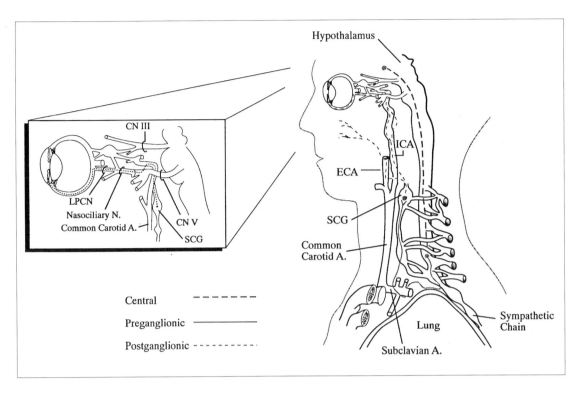

FIGURE 9-4

Diagram of the oculosympathetic pathway illustrating the course of the central, preganglionic, and postganglionic sympathetic fibers in the head and neck. The inset shows in more detail the pathway of the postganglionic sympathetic fibers to the eye. The postganglionic sympathetic fibers originate in the superior cervical sympathetic ganglion (SCG) and travel into the head on the internal carotid artery (ICA). Some postganglionic fibers branch and follow the distribution of the external carotid artery (ECA). In the orbit, the postganglionic sympathetic fibers join the nasociliary nerve and then travel with the long posterior ciliary nerve (LPCN) to be distributed to the iris dilator muscle.

in pupils that constrict to a near target but not to light. The situation of intact near constriction when there is absent light reaction is known as light-near dissociation.[1]

Oculosympathetic Pathway

The pathway for sympathetic innervation to the iris dilator muscle consists of three neurons: (1) the central or first order neuron; (2) the preganglionic, or second order neuron; and (3) the postganglionic, or third order neuron (Figure 9-4). Cell bodies of the central (first order) neuron lie in the posterolateral part of the hypothalamus. Their axons descend ipsilaterally through the tegmentum of the midbrain and pons to the medulla, where the fibers occupy a lateral position. The central neurons synapse in the ciliospinal center of Budge, which is located in the intermediate gray horn of the spinal cord at the vertebral levels C8–T2.[1]

Most of the preganglionic sympathetic (second order neuron) fibers leave the spinal cord through the ventral root at the T1 vertebral level, but some exit through the C8 or T2 ventral roots. The fibers enter the sympathetic chain via the white ramus communicans, ascend through either the first thoracic ganglion or the stellate ganglion (the first thoracic and inferior cervical ganglion combined) and pass across the apex of the lung. The fibers then loop around the subclavian artery in the anterior part of the ansa subclavia, which connects the inferior cervical or stellate ganglion to the middle cervical ganglion. At the base of the skull, the preganglionic pathway synapses in the superior cervical ganglion.[1]

The postganglionic sympathetic (third order neuron) fibers emerge from the superior aspect of the sympathetic chain and travel on the common carotid artery. At the bifurcation of the common carotid artery, the postganglionic sympathetic fibers divide and follow either the external or internal carotid artery. The sympathetic fibers traveling on the external carotid artery and its branches innervate sweat glands in the skin of the face (with the exception of a patch of skin on the forehead above the orbit). Sympathetic fibers to the eye pass through the carotid canal with the internal carotid artery and enter the middle cranial fossa. At the opening of the canal, some sympathetic fibers join the tympanic branch of the ninth cranial nerve (glossopharyngeal nerve) to form the tympanic plexus in the middle ear cavity.[1] These sympathetic fibers later rejoin the internal carotid plexus in the carotid canal and follow the internal carotid artery into the cavernous sinus, where they briefly course with the sixth cranial nerve (abducens nerve). They then follow the ophthalmic division of the fifth cranial nerve (trigeminal nerve) and enter the orbit through the superior orbital fissure.[15,16] Within the orbit, branches of the postganglionic sympathetic fibers are distributed along branches of the ophthalmic artery and the ophthalmic division of the fifth cranial nerve. The sympathetics innervating the dilator muscle travel with the nasociliary nerve and couple with the long posterior ciliary nerves. After they enter the eyeball, the fibers travel through the suprachoroidal space to finally synapse on the dilator muscle. Sympathetic fibers innervating sweat glands on the forehead course with the supraorbital nerve, which is a branch of the ophthalmic division of the fifth cranial nerve. Other sympathetic fibers that innervate the Müller's muscle of the eyelid follow the branches of the ophthalmic artery.[1]

GENERAL METHODS OF TESTING

The evaluation of pupil function is an essential part of any eye examination, especially in those patients suspected of having a number of different pathologic ocular conditions. While providing important objective information regarding the afferent and efferent visual systems, the pupillary assessment requires minimal additional equipment. A light source with a strong, adjustable, focused beam is an absolute necessity. Many practitioners prefer to use either a transilluminator or the binocular indirect ophthalmoscope. Disposable penlights should be avoided because they tend to provide an uneven beam and are often too dim to detect subtle pupil abnormalities. A device for measuring the pupil size, such as a pupillary distance ruler or a pupillary size gauge, is also required equipment. The device should have the ability to measure in 0.5-mm increments. Gauges that are calibrated for area rather than a linear measurement are considered to be more accurate. The examination room should be at least 10 feet in length

with a fixation target at distance, and have overhead lights that permit alteration of the background illumination. A Burton lamp or a biomicroscope should be available for magnified inspection of the iris and the pupillary area. Finally, topical pharmaceutical agents, such as hydroxyamphetamine, cocaine, phenylephrine, and pilocarpine, are also important tools used in diagnosing various pupillary disorders.

A methodical and step approach in the clinical testing of pupillary function allows for the accurate assessment of any pupillary disorder. Pupillary size and shape, the reaction to light and near targets, and the testing for an afferent pupillary defect are critical elements.

Pupil Size and Shape

Determination of pupil size and shape is often the first step in the evaluation of the pupils. Because pupil size varies and depends on factors including ambient light levels and accommodation, it is important to control room illumination and to have the patient fixate on a distant target. The room illumination should be adequate for visualization of the pupils but not so bright as to cause unnecessary miosis. Anisocoria, a size difference between the pupils, is usually easier to detect when the pupils are moderate in size. In patients with dark irides, the examiner may need to hold an ancillary light source underneath the patient's chin to appreciate the appearance of the pupils. The light source should be directed from below the chin to prevent corneal reflections from interfering with observing the pupillary reaction, and away from the line of sight to prevent stimulation of a near response. The light source should initially be only as bright as necessary to see the pupil and should be placed in a position that evenly illuminates both eyes. In patients with dark irides, a Burton lamp may help to visualize the pupils, especially in dim illumination.

If anisocoria is present, the pupil size should be measured in both bright and dim illumination. Pupil disorders resulting from sympathetic (dilator) disturbances, such as Horner's syndrome, will produce an anisocoria that is greater in dim illumination. Parasympathetic (sphincter) anomalies will demonstrate an anisocoria that is greater in bright illumination. Pupils that maintain the relative size difference in various lighting situations are usually designated as having physiologic, or essential, anisocoria (Figure 9-5). It should be noted that retinal or optic nerve disorders that cause an afferent pupillary defect do not cause anisocoria. This is because the midbrain input from the optic nerves is equally distributed to each EW nucleus, thereby resulting in equal direct and consensual pupillary response.[17]

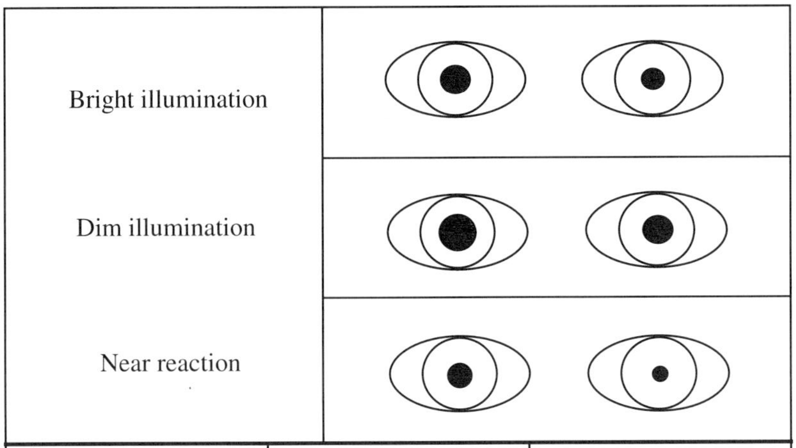

Bright illumination		
Dim illumination		
Near reaction		

Signs and Symptoms	Etiologies	Diagnostic Tests
No difference in anisocoria in either bright or dim light Normal pupillary reaction to near No lid ptosis	Physiological	None

FIGURE 9-5

Essential anisocoria. Anisocoria is a difference in size between the two pupils. With essential (physiologic) anisocoria, the relative size difference remains the same in both bright and dim illumination. This is in contrast to sympathetic disorders (e.g., Horner's syndrome), which show an anisocoria that is greater in dim illumination, and parasympathetic disorders (e.g., third nerve palsy), which show an anisocoria that is greater in bright illumination.

Light Reflex

The direct pupillary light response is usually tested after the evaluation of pupil size and shape. The normal pupillary reaction to light is brisk constriction that is equal between the direct and consensual response. As previously discussed, a moderately illuminated light source should be positioned below and out of the line of sight. Initially, the light is directed toward the eye to induce pupillary constriction, then withdrawn to allow the pupil to redilate to its prior posture. This procedure is repeated several times so the examiner may observe both the consensual and direct response in each eye.

The pupillary light reflex may become diminished from a number of disorders, including sphincter muscle dysfunction, third cranial nerve palsy, and tonic pupil. Depending on the disease process, one or both pupils may be involved, and both the direct and consensual light reflex may be affected.

Near Reflex

Both pupils normally constrict during fixation on a near target. The near reaction is tested by having the patient alternate his or her fixation between a distant and near target several times, with room illumination sufficient to observe the pupillary movement. The near response can be reduced in tonic pupils and in third cranial nerve palsy, but is intact in light-near dissociated conditions, such as an Argyll Robertson pupil, tonic pupil, or midbrain pupil. Tonic pupils may also exhibit light-near dissociation.

Alternate Light Test

Direct Afferent Testing

An afferent defect can be effectively observed by using the alternate light test. This test should be performed with a bright stimulus, such as a transilluminator or a binocular indirect ophthalmoscope, in a dimly lighted room.[18] Under dim lighting the pupils will be more dilated at the beginning of the test, and the amplitude of pupil movement will be greater, thus allowing easier detection of an afferent pupillary defect (APD). Although a bright stimulus is necessary, if it is too bright, the pupil may remain relatively constricted for several seconds, thereby obscuring the pupillary dilation of the affected eye.[19-21] A setting of 6 V on a binocular indirect biomicroscope is considered to be a standardized light level.[22] The patient must look at a distant target to avoid an accommodative pupil constriction.[20,21] The test light should be directed into each eye from slightly below the visual axis. This positioning of the light source prevents corneal reflections from interfering with the observed response and leaves the other eye in the shadow produced by the nose.[19,20] Initially, the light should be held in front of one eye for 1–3 seconds to allow stabilization of the pupils and then quickly switched to the other eye.[21] It is important that the light be held in front of each eye an equal amount of time. This process should be repeated several times.[19–21] It must be emphasized that the light source be moved quickly from one eye to the other; otherwise, pupil dilation may occur before the light stimulates the other eye, thereby masking an APD.[21]

When an afferent pupillary defect is present, both pupils exhibit a brisk constriction to light that is directed into the normal eye. However, as the light is quickly moved to illuminate the affected eye, both pupils will initially dilate. This reflex dilation occurs because the affected eye senses less entering light compared with the normal eye. As the light is switched back to the normal eye, both pupils will again constrict. The amplitude of the pupil dilation seen in the affected eye is a function of the severity of the light conduction deficit.[2,22]

An APD can be quantified by placing neutral density filters (0.3, 0.6, 0.9, 1.2 log unit filters) over the unaffected eye. The alternate light test is repeated, and additional filters are added until the responses of the pupils are balanced, thereby effectively eliminating the APD response. The density of the filters over the unaffected eye should be increased until a paradoxical APD is induced in that eye. The filter density should then be reduced again to the point of balancing pupillary responses. This will ensure an accurate measurement. To prevent overbleaching the retina of the affected eye, the examiner should remove the filters after every three cycles and repeatedly shine the light in both eyes to equalize the retinal illumination.[19,20] Otherwise, the magnitude of the APD will be overestimated because of increased retinal bleaching in the affected eye, which is not shaded by the filter. In other words, the affected eye is more light adapted, leading to increased pupillary dilation as the light source is switched to it.[20]

If the results of quantifying the APD are equivocal, the defect asymmetry can be further exaggerated by placing a neutral density filter over the suspected eye. Then pupillary dilation in the affected eye will be easier to detect.[19,20]

Anisocoria of less than 1 mm in bright light should not affect the results of the alternate light test. However, if anisocoria is 2 mm or greater, the smaller pupil may exhibit a false APD, because the larger pupil allows the entrance of a significantly greater amount of light. Neutral density filters should be placed over the larger pupil (0.1 log units for each millimeter of anisocoria) to compensate for this effect.[19,20]

Monocular patching may produce a clinically significant APD in the opposite, unpatched eye. Here the patched eye becomes dark adapted, which causes an increased retinal light sensitivity compared with the unpatched eye. The resultant effect during the alternate light test is a pseudo-APD in the unpatched eye. Therefore, the alternate light test should not be performed on a patient immediately after a patch is removed. Instead, it is best to wait at least 10 minutes, giving both eyes ample time to equally adjust to the existing ambient lighting.[23]

Reverse Afferent Testing

If one pupil is unreactive to light because of trauma, mydriatics, oculomotor nerve palsy, or synechia formation, the presence of an APD can still be assessed with the alternate light test by comparing the direct and consensual responses of the reactive pupil. If the reactive pupil constricts to direct light but immediately dilates when light is switched to the eye with the unreactive pupil, then the eye with the unreactive pupil has an afferent defect.[2,20,22]

PUPILLARY DISORDERS

Pupillary disorders can be classified into three main categories: (1) anisocoria, (2) bilateral abnormal pupillary responses to light, with or without light-near dissociation, and (3) afferent pupillary defects.

Tonic Pupils

Damage to the ciliary ganglion or the short posterior ciliary nerves (SPCNs) can result in a pupil with an impaired ability to constrict. A pupil with this absent or sluggish response is ascribed as being tonic. Tonic pupils can be categorized as local, neuropathic, or idiopathic (Adie's), with the idiopathic form being the most common.[24] Tonic pupils have one or more characteristics, which can include a poor or absent pupillary light reflex, an accommodative paresis, a reduced constriction response to a near target, or a slow redilation after switching from near to distant fixation. At onset, tonic pupils show mydriasis in bright illumination. They also demonstrate a supersensitivity to cholinergic agents such as pilocarpine.[2,17,25]

Local tonic pupils result from focal injury to the ciliary ganglion or the SPCNs, which can be caused by orbital or choroidal tumors and ocular and orbital inflammations or infections, such as herpes zoster, measles, scarlet fever, syphilis, and sarcoidosis.[2,24,26] Local tonic pupils can also occur secondary to ocular or orbital trauma or surgery, especially if the inferior oblique or inferior rectus muscles are involved. Similar to the parasympathetic pupillomotor fibers, axons innervating these muscles travel within the inferior division of the third cranial nerve; therefore traction on the third nerve's inferior division may disrupt the ciliary ganglion, causing pupillary dysfunction as well as motility disturbance. Localized compression of the SPCNs in the suprachoroidal space after scleral buckle surgery for retinal detachment can cause a tonic pupil characterized by segmental iris sphincter palsy corresponding to the location of buckle placement. Tonic pupils may also develop after a retrobulbar injection or from ischemia of the ciliary ganglion associated with giant cell arteritis.[2,17,27]

Neuropathic tonic pupils are associated with a generalized or peripheral autonomic nervous system dysfunction that also affects the ciliary ganglion or SPCNs.[24] Common disorders that can produce neuropathic tonic pupils include syphilis, diabetes mellitus, chronic alcoholism, and neurotrophic viruses such as varicella.[2,17,24,26]

Adie's tonic pupil is a benign disorder of sudden onset and unknown etiology, although neurotrophic viral infection or traumatic injury to the ciliary ganglion have been implicated as possible causes. Whereas the sudden onset and progression of symptoms over time suggest a viral cause, the lack of significant elevation of serum viral antibodies in Adie's patients compared with normal individuals questions such a cause.[24] In addition, histopathologic examination of the ciliary ganglion reveals neuronal degeneration rather than inflammatory scarring.[28] An individual with Adie's tonic pupil is otherwise healthy and has no other associated neurologic deficits, with the occasional exception of impaired deep tendon reflexes.[24]

Patients with Adie's tonic pupil are between 20 and 50 years of age at onset. Women are affected twice as often as men. In 80% of the cases the condition is unilateral. If a patient has bilateral tonic pupils, syphilis should be suspected. On initial examination, the affected pupil is larger relative to the opposite pupil and reacts poorly to light when either the direct or consensual response is tested (Figure 9-6). The near response is also affected, but usually of lesser magnitude than the light reaction. When switching from near to distant fixation, the pupil redilates slowly and may require several minutes to return to the original size. Thus, after near work (before redilation is completed), an Adie's pupil may actually appear relatively miotic compared with the normal pupil.[2,24]

The most common complaints are of an anisocoria causing a cosmetic concern and photophobia. Retinal bleaching from inadequate pupillary constriction results in delayed dark adaptation. Browache with attempted near work or blurred distance vision in the involved eye after prolonged near tasks is caused by decreased accommodative ability, ciliary spasm, or induced astigmatism from sector paralysis of the ciliary body muscle. Near-to-distant fixation blur may last for several seconds while the sluggish accommodative response releases.[2,24]

Segmental paralysis of the iris sphincter muscle occurs in Adie's pupils and results from the loss of postganglionic parasympathetic innervation to certain muscle segments while innervation is preserved in other segments.[2,24] The paralysis is randomly distributed in the iris sphincter muscle. The vermiform movements of the iris sphincter, seen on biomicroscopy, are thought to be from the physiologic unrest of iris segments whose light reflex pathways are still intact.[24] Corneal sensation usually is mildly decreased in the affected eye, which could be a result of damage to the sensory fibers of the long or short posterior ciliary nerves, nasociliary nerves, or fibers passing through the ciliary ganglion. Eighty or ninety percent of patients with Adie's tonic pupils also have decreased or absent deep tendon reflexes. The muscle stretch reflexes of the upper and lower limbs are impaired with equal frequency, but the reflexes of the ankle and triceps muscle are usually the most severely affected.[24]

The light-near pupillary dissociation in Adie's pupils is explained by the anatomy of the ciliary ganglion. The ciliary ganglion contains 30 times more postganglionic parasympathetic neurons, which innervate the ciliary body, compared with the iris sphincter.[5] When the ciliary ganglion is damaged, the chances of survival are greater for the neurons innervating accommodation compared with neurons innervating the iris sphincter. This results in the initial presentation of a dilated, fixed pupil that does not demonstrate cholinergic supersensitivity and may even fail to constrict to 1% pilocarpine. This appearance may mimic a pharmacologically blocked pupil. The near response is reduced, but to a lesser extent than the light response. With time, the ciliary body and the iris are reinnervated by regenerating damaged axons and collateral sprouts from surviving neurons in the ciliary ganglion.[29] Because the postganglionic pathway consists of a 30-to-1 ratio of accommodative fibers to pupillary light reflex fibers, the sphincter muscle is usually reinnervated by misdirected accommodative fibers rather than by the original light reflex fibers. After this aberrant regeneration, the new fibers may innervate both the ciliary body muscle and the iris sphincter, so that the near reaction may become even greater compared with the light response.[29,30]

Abnormalities associated with Adie's tonic pupils tend to progress with time. The pupillary light reaction

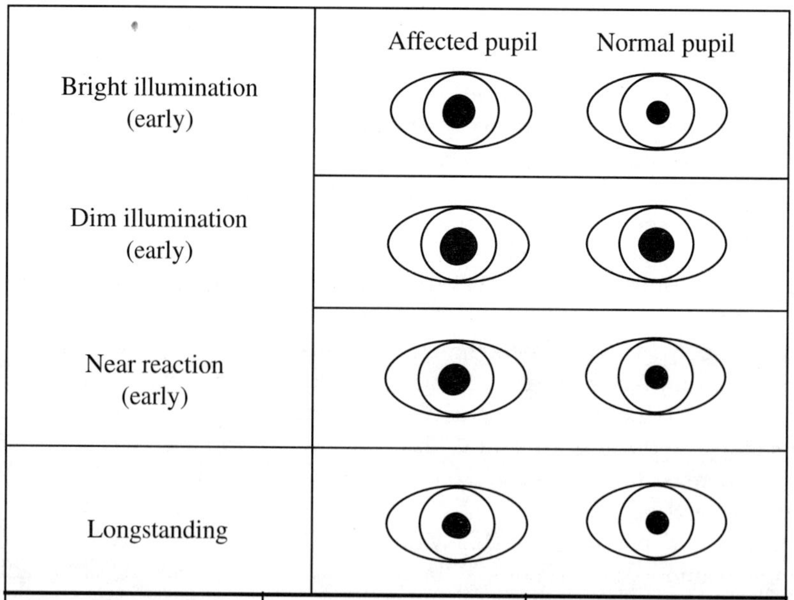

FIGURE 9-6

Adie's tonic pupil. At the onset, the affected pupil classically appears larger compared with the fellow eye in normal room illumination and reacts poorly to light. The near response is likewise reduced, but to a lesser extent. After prolonged near work, the Adie's pupil redilates slowly when switching to distance fixation. Also, vision at distance and near may blur because of sectoral paralysis of the ciliary body, which causes accommodative paresis and tonicity. The Adie's pupil is typically irregular because of segmental paralysis of the iris sphincter muscle, and it exhibits movement of inactive pupillary zones toward active pupillary zones in a circumferential fashion (vermiform movement) when the eye is illuminated by a bright light. Longstanding Adie's pupils tend to become smaller over time. Adie's pupils demonstrate supersensitivity to cholinergic agents such as 0.125% pilocarpine. Greater pupil constriction in the affected eye compared with the normal eye with this weak miotic is diagnostic of Adie's tonic pupil. (SPCN = short posterior ciliary nerve.)

	Affected pupil	Normal pupil
Bright illumination (early)		
Dim illumination (early)		
Near reaction (early)		
Longstanding		

Signs and Symptoms	Etiologies	Diagnostic Tests
Poor or absent light reflex	Unknown	0.125% pilocarpine
Initial mydriasis in bright illumination	Suspected (viral or trauma) damage to SPCNs or ciliary ganglion	Affected pupil will constrict
Accommodative paresis		Normal pupil does not constrict
Intact, slow response to near targets		
Decreased deep tendon reflex		
Cholinergic super-sensitivity		

usually declines and does not recover. Increased hyporeflexia occurs from progressive impairment of deep tendon reflexes. Accommodation, however, tends to recover because of the greater reinnervation of the ciliary body. Initially, the Adie's pupil is larger than normal but gradually becomes smaller, causing a less marked anisocoria over time. A larger pupil in bright illumination compared with the fellow eye implies a recent onset, whereas a miotic Adie's pupil suggests a more longstanding condition.

Involvement of the second eye occurs at the rate of about 4% per year during the first decade of the disease, and after 10 years, the rate increases to 50% per year. Most cases of Adie's pupils eventually become bilateral.[2,24]

Pharmacologic Testing

The majority of Adie's pupils exhibit denervation supersensitivity to weak cholinergic agents.[24,30–32] Whereas Adie's tonic pupils can often be diagnosed from other clinical findings alone, the demonstration of denervation supersensitivity can be helpful. The pupils may be tested by instilling one drop of a weak cholinergic agonist, such as 0.125% pilocarpine, in each eye, followed by a second drop 1 minute later. The test must be performed on an untouched cornea (i.e., before applanation tonometry, corneal sensitivity testing, or prior drop instillation) because any manipulation of the epithelium may lead to unequal drug penetration between the eyes and false results. The size of the pupils are remeasured 45 minutes

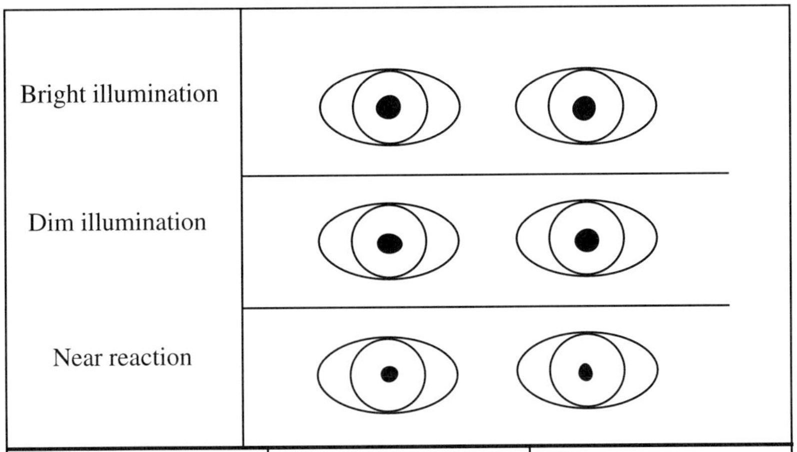

Bright illumination		
Dim illumination		
Near reaction		

Signs and Symptoms	Etiologies	Diagnostic Tests
Small pupils Fail to dilate in dim illumination Poor constriction in bright illumination Constriction to near	Neurosyphilis Sarcoidosis Lyme disease Diabetes mellitus Midbrain lesion	FTA-ABS VDRL RPR ACE Chest films/MRI of chest, gallium scan Lyme IFA Lyme ELISA Blood glucose levels MRI

FIGURE 9-7

Argyll Robertson pupil. Argyll Robertson pupils are small, irregularly shaped pupils that react poorly or not at all to light stimulation but constrict more briskly to a near target (light-near dissociation). Their miotic appearance is most striking in dim illumination because they fail to dilate. The irregular shape of Argyll Robertson pupils is caused by damage to the iris. Atrophy of the iris stroma may be seen in some patients. Classically, they appear oval or teardrop-shaped. Pupil involvement is usually bilateral, although asymmetric and unilateral presentations can occur. The lesion site for Argyll Robertson pupils is in the periaqueductal gray matter of the midbrain at the level of the superior colliculus. Pupillary light reflex fibers and central sympathetic inhibitory fibers are interrupted by this lesion.

later. Pupillary constriction that is greater in the affected eye by 1 mm or more compared with the normal eye is diagnostic of Adie's tonic pupil.[17,25,32]

Management

Management of Adie's tonic pupils is usually conservative and limited to supportive measures. The patient should be reassured that the condition is benign, and that the mydriasis will typically resolve in a few months, and usually within 1 to 2 years.[24] For those patients especially concerned with the cosmetic appearance of one dilated pupil, or accompanying photophobia, tinted spectacles or contact lenses may offer relief. Because ciliary body spasm may be pharmacologically induced, the topical use of miotics such as pilocarpine and eserine are generally discouraged.[33,34]

In the early course of the disease, headaches and asthenopia associated with prolonged near work might develop from accommodative paresis or induced astigmatism in the affected eye. Relief may be provided by plus lenses at near to equalize accommodation or occlusion of the affected eye while reading.[2,35]

Argyll Robertson Pupil

Argyll Robertson (AR) pupils are small, irregularly shaped pupils that have poor or no reaction to light stimulation but constrict to a near target (light-near dissociation) (Figure 9-7). An impaired rather than an absent pupillary light reaction is more common. Argyll Robertson pupils fail to dilate in the dark, making the miotic appearance of the pupils more striking in dim illumination.[2,36,37] The pupil irregularity is from damage to the iris, appearing as an oval or tear-drop–shaped pupil that is horizontally or vertically oriented. The pupil may appear to be eccentrically located. Atrophy of the iris stroma, with loss of the iris crypts of Fuchs, may also be noted in some AR patients.[2] Argyll Robertson pupils usually develop over months to years, and pupillary reactivity to light progressively changes from a sluggish response to a complete loss of constriction. As mentioned, the near response is spared.[2,36] Pupil involvement is usually bilateral, although it can be asymmetric or strictly unilateral.[2]

The lesion site for AR pupils, which has been demonstrated by magnetic resonance imaging (MRI), is located in the periaqueductal gray matter of the midbrain at the level of the superior colliculus.[2,36-38] The pupillary light reflex fibers are presumed to descend from the pretectal area to the Edinger-Westphal nuclei through the periaqueductal gray matter. The central sympathetic inhibitory fibers also terminate in the EW nuclei. Both pathways are interrupted by this lesion.[2,36] Loss of the sympathetic inhibitory fibers results in increased parasympathetic outflow from the EW nuclei, which leads to pupillary constriction.[39] The fibers for accommodation-induced pupillary constriction are spared because these fibers travel more ventrally, bypassing the periaqueductal gray matter.[2,36]

Argyll Robertson pupils have been classically associated with neurosyphilis (tertiary syphilis), but they have also been reported to occur in patients with diabetes mellitus, multiple sclerosis, sarcoidosis, alcoholism, Lyme disease, Wernicke's encephalopathy, and midbrain tumors involving the area of the superior colliculus.[36-38,40,41] Therefore, if a patient has AR pupils, the initial work-up may include the following tests to help in the differential diagnosis: fluorescent treponemal antibody (FTA-AbS), serum VDRL, and rapid plasma reagin (RPR) for neurosyphilis; angiotensin-converting enzyme (ACE), gallium scans, chest x-ray films, and possibly MRI of the chest to rule out sarcoidosis; Lyme IFA and Lyme ELISA titers for Lyme disease; blood glucose testing to rule out diabetes; and MRI to rule out midbrain lesions.

Midbrain Pupils

Rostral midbrain lesions in the region of the pretectal nuclei interrupt the pupillary light reflex but may spare the pupillary response to near, producing a light-near dissociation.[42] Affected pupils, known as midbrain pupils, appear round and are either in midposition or slightly dilated. They do not react well to light stimulation but do constrict with near fixation (Figure 9-8).

If the posterior commissure is affected, the resultant pupillary light-near dissociation is part of Parinaud's (dorsal midbrain) syndrome. This disorder is characterized by paralysis of upgaze and eyelid retraction on attempted upgaze (Collier's sign). Convergence-retraction nys-

tagmus on attempted upgaze may occur, especially with vertical saccades directed superiorly. This may be elicited by rotating an optokinetic drum or tape downward in front of the patient. Vertical saccades, directed inferiorly below the horizontal meridian, may also be slowed. Possible impairment of vergences may be evident. In the acute phase, the eyes may be tonically deviated downward ("setting sun sign").[2,43] The most common cause of the dorsal midbrain syndrome is a pinealoma, but additional causes include aqueductal stenosis, infiltrative gliomas, vascular lesions, trauma, and sarcoidosis.[2]

Mesencephalic lesions that involve the oculomotor nuclei usually damage both the central sympathetic fibers descending through the midbrain to the ciliospinal center of Budge, and the parasympathetic fibers to the eye. Affected pupils in these circumstances become fixed and partially dilated, irregular in shape, unequal in size, and nonreactive to light.[2] Fixed, partially dilated pupils are most commonly caused by transtentorial herniation of the temporal lobe uncus, which compresses and damages the mesencephalon. Other causes include neoplasms, hemorrhages, infarcts, or granulomatous damage in the midbrain.[2,44] If the fixed, dilated pupil is associated with a complete third nerve palsy, then the lesion is located ventrally in the midbrain by the oculomotor fascicles. These midbrain lesions are usually bilateral, which helps to distinguish them from peripheral third nerve palsies, which are predominantly unilateral.[2]

Afferent Pupillary Defect

If there is significant unilateral or asymmetric retinal or optic nerve disease, the pupillary response to direct light stimulation will differ between the two eyes. On direct stimulation, the pupil of the affected eye will respond with a less brisk, subnormal constriction compared with the pupil of the normal eye. However, when light is directed into the normal eye, the affected pupil constricts more extensively. This difference between the direct and consensual response to light of the affected pupil constitutes the afferent pupillary defect (APD).[22,45]

An APD is an objective finding that indicates the presence of a conduction deficit anywhere along the afferent visual pathway from the retina to the lateral geniculate nucleus.[2,20,25] This sign does not indicate a specific disease. The differential diagnosis for conditions causing an afferent pupillary defect includes lesions in the macula, retina, optic nerve, optic chiasm, or optic tract.[20,25]

Most often, an APD is caused by unilateral or asymmetric optic neuropathy.[25] Here, the magnitude of the APD correlates closely with the amount of visual field loss and not the reduction in visual acuity.[46] Afferent

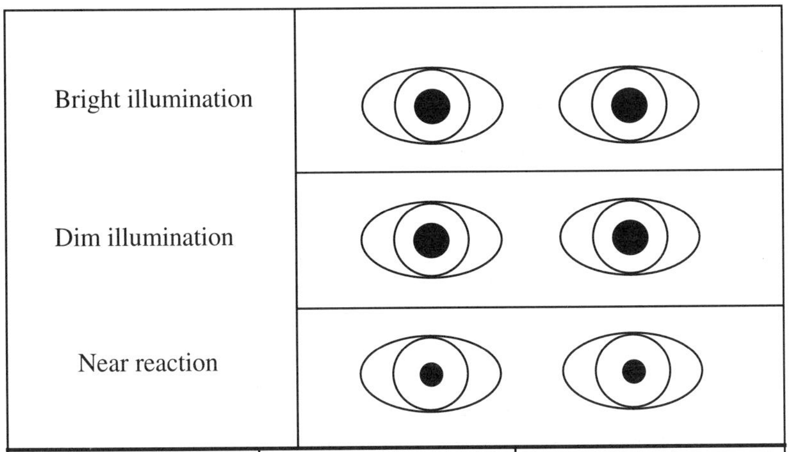

Bright illumination		
Dim illumination		
Near reaction		

Signs and Symptoms	Etiologies	Diagnostic Tests
Bilateral	Transtentorial uncal herniation	MRI
Do not react to light		
Constrict to near target	Pinealoma (Parinaud's)	MRI
Parinaud's signs: Upgaze paralysis Eyelid retraction on attempted upgaze Convergence-retraction nystagmus	Midbrain infarcts, neoplasms, or hemorrhages	MRI
	Sarcoidosis	ACE Chest films/MRI of chest, gallium scan

FIGURE 9-8

Midbrain pupils. Lesions in the region of the pretectal nuclei of the midbrain produce "midbrain pupils." The affected pupils appear round and are either in midposition or slightly dilated. They react poorly to light and exhibit a more brisk constriction with near fixation (light-near dissociation). If the posterior commissure is affected (e.g., by a pinealoma, aqueductal stenosis, vascular lesions, or sarcoidosis) Parinaud's syndrome (dorsal midbrain syndrome) results, which is characterized by upgaze paralysis and eyelid retraction and convergence–retraction nystagmus on attempted upgaze. Likewise, mesencephalic lesions (especially transtentorial herniation) can simultaneously affect both the oculomotor nuclei and associated parasympathetic fibers as well as central preganglionic sympathetic fibers descending through the midbrain from the hypothalamus. This results in fixed, mid-dilated pupils that are unreactive to light.

defects are often caused by ischemic, compressive, or inflammatory optic nerve disease.[22,25,47] Demyelination or asymmetric glaucoma can also cause an APD.[22,25,48–52] If a patient has clinically apparent unilateral optic neuritis, but no APD can be elicited, further evaluation should be performed for subclinical optic neuritis in the fellow eye or a compressive optic neuropathy that affects both optic nerves or the optic chiasm.[48] Chiasmal lesions located anteriorly are more likely to cause an APD.[45]

Because the optic tract is composed of slightly more crossed nasal retinal fibers than ipsilateral temporal fibers, a complete optic tract lesion will produce a modest APD

in the contralateral eye.[53,54] An afferent defect can also be created in the contralateral eye from unilateral lesions affecting the brachium of the superior colliculus. Here, pupillary fibers coming from the ipsilateral optic tract are damaged.[55,56]

Homonymous hemianopsias resulting from lesions or compression of the optic radiations do not have an associated APD because pupillary fibers are not involved. This is because pupillary fibers leave the posterior one third of the optic tract and enter the midbrain via the brachium of the superior colliculus.[17]

Afferent pupillary defects associated with retinal disease may be secondary to various conditions including

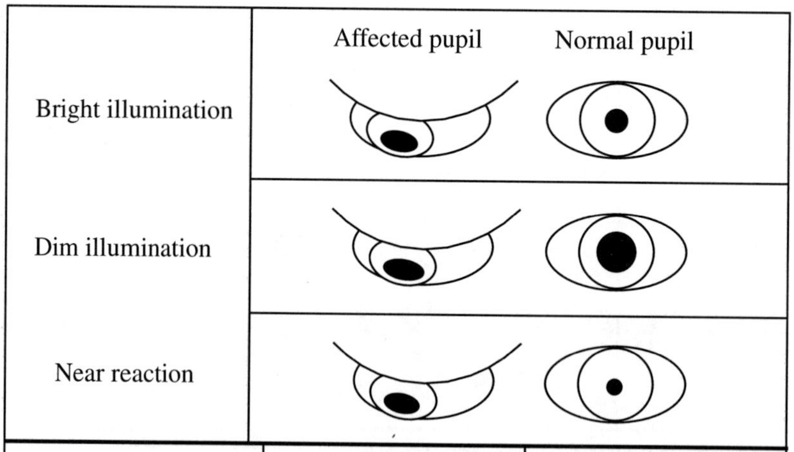

FIGURE 9-9

Third cranial nerve palsy. The clinical signs of a complete third nerve palsy include ptosis, an eye that is positioned down and out, loss of accommodation, and a dilated pupil that does not constrict to light or near. Anisocoria is greater in bright illumination. Third nerve palsies with or without pupil involvement can result from lesions anywhere along the course of the nerve between the midbrain and ciliary ganglion. Pupil involvement suggests the presence of an aneurysm or lesion compressing the superficially located pupillomotor fibers. Sparing of the pupil suggests either ischemia of the third nerve from a vascular disorder, such as diabetes, or an aneurysm in the basilar artery or intracavernous portion of the internal carotid artery, which would compress portions of the oculomotor nerve but miss the pupillomotor fibers.

	Affected pupil	Normal pupil
Bright illumination		
Dim illumination		
Near reaction		

Signs and Symptoms	Etiologies	Diagnostic Tests
Marked ptosis	Intracranial tumor aneurysm	MRI
Eye positioned down and out		
Fixed or little response to light or near targets of affected pupil	Diabetes mellitus	Fasting blood glucose
Anisocoria greater in bright than dim illumination		

extensive retinal detachments, retinoschisis, branch and central retinal vessel occlusions, and unilateral or asymmetric retinitis pigmentosa.[20,22,45,57-59] The APD associated with macular disease is usually less profound than defects seen with optic nerve disease.[20] Macular lesions causing an APD, such as macular toxoplasmosis, histoplasmosis, and disciform degeneration, are usually obvious and severe.[2,20,45,60,61]

Although uncommon, deep strabismic or anisometropic amblyopia may cause a modest afferent defect.[20,62,63] Conditions with vision loss that do not produce an APD include macular drusen and isolated vitreous hemorrhages.[2,64] Cataracts are not associated with APDs.[2,20,65,66]

Third Cranial Nerve Palsy

A complete oculomotor nerve palsy produces ptosis, an eye positioned down and out, a loss of accommodation, and a dilated pupil that does not constrict to light or near (Figure 9-9). Third cranial nerve palsies with pupil involve-

ment can result from a lesion anywhere along the course of the nerve between the midbrain and ciliary ganglion. Infarcts, tumors, demyelination, and infections are common lesions associated with third cranial nerve palsies.[67]

The fibers of the third nerve fan out in separate fascicles after emerging from the oculomotor nuclei in the midbrain tegmentum and then assemble into a single nerve trunk shortly after exiting from the brain stem.[68] Pupillomotor fibers are located in the most medial aspect of the third nerve fascicles, followed successively (in a lateral direction) by the fibers innervating the inferior rectus, levator palpebrae superioris, medial rectus, and superior rectus. The fibers to the inferior oblique muscle are the most lateral in the fascicle. A small lesion or infarct in the midbrain tegmentum at the level of the fascicles could cause an isolated muscle palsy or a partial third nerve palsy. Pupil involvement is dependent on the site of the infarct.[69]

Ventrally, the fibers of the third cranial nerve pass through the red nucleus and the portion of the cerebral peduncles carrying the corticospinal and corticobulbar tracts. A lesion in this area would result in a complete ipsilateral third nerve palsy associated with other neurologic signs. A lesion involving the third nerve and the red nucleus (Benedikt's syndrome) is characterized by a complete ipsilateral third nerve palsy with contralateral ataxia and arm tremor. Damage to third nerve fibers passing through the cerebral peduncles (Weber's syndrome) causes symptoms of complete ipsilateral third nerve palsy and associated contralateral paralysis of the body, tongue, and lower face.[67]

As the third nerve passes toward the cavernous sinus in the subarachnoid space, it becomes vulnerable to compression in several locations. If the medial aspect of the nerve is compressed, there will be associated pupil involvement. A supratentorial space-occupying mass, such as a tumor, and an epidural or subdural hematoma, can displace the brain stem caudally, causing compression of the third nerves. Aneurysms in either the posterior cerebral or superior cerebellar arteries can compress the third cranial nerve because it travels between the arteries after emerging from the brain stem. Herniation of the temporal lobe uncus over the free edge of the tentorium cerebelli can compress the third nerve against the posterior clinoid process. In all of these instances, the dorsomedial pupillomotor fibers are affected. Finally, an aneurysm in the posterior communicating artery can first compress the medial aspect of the third nerve, leading to pupillary involvement.[67]

In adults, the two most common causes of an isolated third cranial nerve palsy are aneurysms (20%), ruptured or unruptured, of the basilar or posterior communicating artery, and ischemic vascular disorders (20%), which include diabetes, hypertension, and atherosclerosis.[67,70-72] Aneurysms most commonly occur at the junction of the internal carotid and posterior communicating arteries.[67,72] Third nerve palsies secondary to microinfarction of the nerve fibers are also seen in patients with cardiovascular disease risk factors such as hypercholesterolemia, smoking, advanced age, and a family history of vascular disease.[73,74] Trauma and parasellar tumors (pituitary adenomas, meningiomas, craniopharyngiomas, metastatic tumors, and primary brain stem tumors) each account for 10–15% of third nerve palsies.[67,70] Third nerve palsies are also associated with inflammatory disorders, such as herpes zoster, systemic lupus erythematosus, sinusitis, temporal arteritis, and syphilis.[67,70,74]

The presence or absence of pupil involvement in an isolated third cranial nerve palsy is an important diagnostic sign in identifying the cause. Involvement of the pupil suggests the presence of an aneurysm or a lesion compressing the superficially located pupillomotor fibers. In these cases, neuroimaging or angiography is indicated.

Sparing of the pupil suggests ischemia of the third nerve from a vascular disorder or a midbrain infarct.[69-71,75,76] In microvascular diseases, the ischemia is either caused by occlusion of the nutrient arteries or by hyalinization of arterioles in the center of the oculomotor nerve. As a result of ischemia, demyelination and axonal necrosis of centrally located neurons occurs, whereas superficial pupillomotor fibers are spared.[72,77,78] Management includes determining the systemic cause of the ischemia and careful observation for late (within 1 week after the acute presentation of the third nerve palsy) pupillary involvement. If the pupil remains responsive in a third nerve palsy, an aneurysm is unlikely as the cause.[67,72,73]

Although the general rules regarding pupil involvement are typically accurate, it has been demonstrated that aneurysms may produce a pupil-sparing partial third nerve palsy.[67,72,74,79,80] Such cases have occurred with an aneurysm of the intracavernous internal carotid artery. In these instances, the inferior division of the third nerve, where the pupillomotor fibers are carried, may be spared.[70,72] A precavernous aneurysm, originating at the apex of the basilar artery, can also cause a pupil-sparing third nerve palsy. Basilar apex aneurysms probably compress the inferior aspect of the third nerve, which allows the dorsomedial pupillary fibers to escape damage.[79] In contrast, the dorsomedial pupillomotor fibers can become compressed by aneurysms located laterally at the junction of the internal carotid artery and the posterior communicating artery, resulting in a third nerve palsy with pupillary involvement.[67,74]

Third cranial nerve palsies caused by intracranial aneurysms are almost always associated with severe ocular or periorbital pain, especially with junction aneurysms of the internal carotid and posterior communicating arteries. However, basilar artery aneurysms are painless; therefore the absence of pain on initial examination should not eliminate an aneurysm as a possible cause of the third nerve palsy.[72,74,79,80]

Management of patients with third nerve palsies, regardless of pain or pupillary involvement, should include neuroimaging to exclude intracranial lesions.[72,74,81] If radioimaging studies produce negative results, investigation for a related systemic cause, as well as careful observation over several months for progression, is indicated. Improvement usually occurs within 3 months with palsies caused by ischemia. If a palsy has not begun to resolve during this time period, cerebral angiography is indicated to rule out an aneurysm.[72-74,79,82,83] When patients have a third nerve palsy from a midbrain ischemic infarct and a history of cardiovascular disease, echocardiography and carotid studies should be performed to search for embolic sources.[76]

Pupil abnormalities can also occur secondary to aberrant regeneration after a third nerve palsy. Aberrant regeneration is characterized by the misdirection of regenerating axons, leading to the new pattern of innervation to incorrect muscles. One sign (Czarnecki's) of aberrant third nerve regeneration is pupillary constriction occurring when a patient attempts to look into the field of action of an extraocular muscle innervated by the third nerve.[84] Here, fibers designated for the extraocular muscle have been misdirected to innervate the pupillary sphincter muscle. Segmental constriction of the pupil during light stimulation may also be an indication of aberrant regeneration.[17] When selected segments of the iris sphincter are innervated by misdirected fibers, detection of aberrant regeneration may be difficult unless the iris is carefully examined with a biomicroscope. The presence of eyelid elevation on attempted adduction, upgaze, or downgaze (pseudo–von Graefe's sign) may also indicate aberrant regeneration of the third nerve. Here, third nerve fibers intended for the medial rectus, superior rectus, or inferior oblique muscles have been misdirected to innervate the levator palpebrae superioris.

Aberrant regeneration may be seen after oculomotor nerve palsies because of compressive lesions, infectious disorders such as syphilis, or congenital third nerve palsies, but not after ischemia, because the direction of the regenerating axoplasm has not been disrupted.[17,25] A patient with signs of aberrant third nerve regeneration and no prior history of a third nerve palsy should be evaluated for compressive lesions including cavernous sinus meningioma or intracavernous aneurysm.[85]

If a third nerve palsy is caused by a lesion in the cavernous sinus, oculosympathetic fibers may be simultaneously impaired. In this case, the pupil may be fixed because of the simultaneous paresis of the dilator muscle. Pharmacologic testing would be initiated to confirm sympathetic denervation, and when combined with a third nerve paralysis, would localize the lesion to the cavernous sinus.[17]

A dilated, unreactive pupil with no other signs of third nerve dysfunction is rarely caused by third nerve paresis. Such patients should be further evaluated for possible signs of ocular trauma, Adie's syndrome, or pharmacologic blockade.

Unlike the situation in adults, third nerve palsies in children are very often congenital (43–47%), with many of these exhibiting aberrant regeneration. Birth trauma is the probable cause for most congenital third nerve palsies. Other forms of trauma account for 13–23%, while tumors account for 10%. Intracranial aneurysms are responsible for only 7% of third nerve palsies in children.[86]

Horner's Syndrome

Lesions or compressions anywhere along the course of the oculosympathetic pathway, from the hypothalamus to the dilator muscle, can lead to an ipsilateral Horner's syndrome. The clinical manifestations of Horner's syndrome include a partial ptosis of the upper eyelid from paresis of Müller's muscle, and anisocoria, with the affected pupil exhibiting a smaller diameter (Figure 9-10). The anisocoria is more marked in dim illumination than in bright illumination. Pupillary reaction to light and near stimuli is normal. The interpalpebral fissure is narrowed from a ptotic upper eyelid and concurrent elevation of the lower eyelid (reverse ptosis), giving the eye a pseudo-enophthalmic appearance. The pupils will have a dilation lag, a sluggish redilation when illumination is reduced or when fixation is changed from a near to a distant target. Because the Horner's pupil dilates more slowly than normal, requiring 10–15 seconds to dilate fully, the anisocoria will be greater after 5 seconds of darkness than after 15 seconds.

If sympathetic fibers are damaged or compressed anywhere along the oculosympathetic pathway before the common carotid artery bifurcation, a complete ipsilateral facial anhidrosis (decreased facial sweating) can occur. If only the sympathetic fibers along the distribution of the internal carotid artery are involved, decreased sweating is limited to the skin of the forehead above the orbit. When the sympathetic fibers along the external carotid artery are affected, facial sweating is absent except on the forehead. In the acute stage, transient vasodilation can cause increased facial skin temperature, conjunctival hyperemia, and facial flush. Decreased intraocular pressure and increased amplitudes of accommodation may also be seen early in the disease. Iris heterochromia is usually seen with congenital Horner's syndrome, with the lighter colored iris on the affected side. This pigmentation change occurs because the formation of pigment granules by melanocytes in the iris stroma is under sympathetic control. If this sympathetic innervation is disrupted early in life, no pigment is formed on the affected side. Iris depigmentation is rare with adult-onset sympathetic denervation.[2]

Acquired Horner's syndrome can be classified as central, preganglionic, or postganglionic. Central Horner's syndrome results from damage to the first order neuron of the sympathetic pathway. The incidence of central Horner's syndrome has been reported to be as low as 3–13% of Horner's syndrome cases to as high as 63% of cases.[87-89] The majority are caused by vascular disease.[2,22] Patients with cerebral and hypothalamic infarction may have an ipsilateral Horner's syndrome, a contralateral hemiplegia, and, occasionally, homonymous hemianopsia and aphasia. Infarction of the brain stem, especially

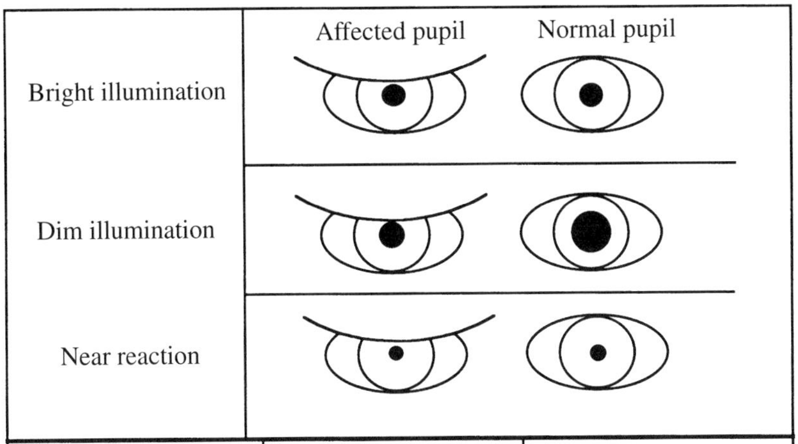

	Affected pupil	Normal pupil
Bright illumination		
Dim illumination		
Near reaction		

Signs and Symptoms	Etiologies	Diagnostic Tests

Slight ptosis
 	
Miosis of affected eye
 	
Anisocoria greater in dim than bright light
 	
Dilation lag
 	
Ipsilateral facial anhidrosis
 	
Iris heterochromia in congenital Horner's
	Central:
	Cerebral infarct
	Cerebral hemorrhage
	Intracranial/spinal mass
	Brain stem infarct
	Demyelination
	Trauma
	
	Preganglionic:
	Pancoast's tumor
	Breast carcinoma
	Neuroblastoma
	Lymphadenopathy
	  from Hodgkin's
	  disease, leukemia,
	  tuberculosis
	Trauma
	Thoracic aneurysms
	Mediastinal tumors
	
	Postganglionic:
	Aneurysm
	Cavernous sinus
	  syndrome
	Migraine
	Cluster headaches
	Inflammation
	Trauma
		10% cocaine test
		
		No dilation of the affected pupil in central, pre-, or postganglionic lesions
		
		1% hydroxyamphet-amine test
		
		Dilation of the affected pupil in central lesion or preganglionic lesion
		No dilation of affected pupil in postganglionic lesion
		
		Chest x-rays
		
		MRI

FIGURE 9-10

Horner's syndrome. The classic clinical signs of Horner's syndrome include partial ptosis of the upper eyelid, a miotic pupil, and facial anhidrosis on the affected side. Anisocoria is greater in dim illumination. The pupils react to both light and near stimuli; however, the affected pupil redilates slowly when illumination is reduced or when fixation is changed from near to distance. This phenomenon is called dilation lag. The interpalpebral fissure is narrowed as a result of concurrent ptosis of the upper eyelid and elevation (reverse ptosis) of the lower eyelid, giving the involved eye a pseudoenophthalmic appearance. Iris heterochromia is usually an additional ocular sign seen in congenital Horner's syndrome, with the affected side having the lighter colored iris. A suspected Horner's syndrome is confirmed with pharmacologic testing using 10% cocaine, which will dilate the normal eye but not the abnormal eye. One percent hydroxyamphetamine localizes the lesion to either a central or preganglionic site (affected pupil dilates) versus a postganglionic site (affected pupil does not dilate).

from occlusion of the posterior inferior cerebellar artery, may result in Wallenberg's lateral medullary syndrome. Accompanying ipsilateral neurologic deficits include impaired pain and temperature sensation on the face and Horner's syndrome. Contralateral deficits include impaired pain and temperature sensation on the trunk and limbs. Cerebellar ataxia, dysphagia, dysarthria, and rotary nystagmus may also occur. Other causes of central Horner's syndrome include cerebral hemorrhage, intracranial and intraspinal tumors, trauma, and multiple sclerosis.[2,22]

Preganglionic Horner's syndrome can result from interruption of the second order neuron at spinal cord levels C8–T2 as the sympathetic chain passes in close proximity to the apex of the lung and great vessels in the superior or posterior mediastinum or as the sympathetic fibers ascend in the neck to terminate in the superior cervical ganglion. The incidence of preganglionic Horner's syndrome varies from 21% to 67% of cases.[2,87–89] The principal causes are tumors and trauma.[2] When the cervical sympathetic outflow is interrupted in the lower neck, a complete Horner's syndrome is likely to be present, but if pathway disruption occurs in the spinal cord, a partial presentation may be evident.[2,22]

A leading cause of preganglionic Horner's syndrome is bronchogenic carcinoma, or Pancoast's tumor, which interrupts the cervical sympathetic chain at the apex of the lung. Associated pain in the ipsilateral shoulder and arm suggests that the tumor has extended beyond the pleural cavity. Preganglionic Horner's syndrome may also be produced by breast carcinomas or sarcomas that spread into the mediastinum by the apex of the lungs, and by tumors of the meninges or vertebral column that affect the proximal portions of the preganglionic sympathetic fibers or their cell bodies. Traumatic causes include injury to the brachial plexus and cervical spinal cord, and surgical or procedural neck trauma such as radical thyroid surgery, arteriography, spinal fusions, and epidural anesthesia.

Patients suspected of having central or preganglionic lesions require chest films, including lordotic views, mediastinal computed tomographic or magnetic resonance scanning, cervical radiologic studies of the spine, and angiography.[2,22]

Postganglionic Horner's syndrome develops when the third order sympathetic neurons are damaged as they ascend in the neck in association with the carotid arteries. This can occur because of trauma, either blunt or penetrating, and basal skull fractures. Other causes include tumors, enlarged lymph nodes, carotid thrombosis, and carotid aneurysm. When a lesion occurs at the base of the skull, in the carotid canal, or in the cavernous sinus, the postganglionic Horner's syndrome often has associated cranial nerve neuropathies that are helpful in localizing the lesion.[2,22] Simultaneous Horner's syndrome and ipsilateral abducens nerve palsy suggest a cavernous sinus lesion.[90,91] If sympathetics of the tympanic plexus are damaged, the Horner's syndrome may be associated with a middle ear infection. In adults, most isolated postganglionic syndromes have a benign cause, such as neck trauma or neck surgery (endarterectomy). Another cause is vascular disorders, including cluster headaches and migraines, where vasodilation of the internal carotid artery leads to compression of the sympathetic plexus during passage through the carotid canal. Atherosclerosis of the internal carotid artery may also produce a benign postganglionic Horner's syndrome, as well as occlusion of the vascular supply to the superior cervical sympathetic ganglion.[2,22,92,93]

Horner's syndrome needs to be differentiated from Raeder's syndrome, which has a similar presentation of ptosis and miosis, but also has associated unilateral headache or facial pain along the distribution of the trigeminal nerve. The headache pain is mild to severe and persistent rather than episodic and excruciating as in a cluster headache. Raeder's syndrome has a male predilection and is characterized by recurrent attacks of transient ptosis and miosis, usually occurring before the onset of the headache. With repeated episodes, the associated ptosis and miosis may become permanent.[94]

Pediatric Horner's syndrome is frequently associated with severe underlying diseases, including neuroblastomas, spinal cord and infiltrative tumors, metastases, leukemia, lymphomas, aneurysms, birth trauma, and cardiothoracic trauma.[95–97] If preganglionic Horner's syndrome occurs in a child with no history of trauma or surgery, a complete neurologic and systemic evaluation is warranted to rule out neoplasms. The evaluation should include chest films, radiologic imaging of the head and neck, and a catecholamine assay.[2,22]

Congenital Horner's syndrome is an uncommon disorder characterized by ptosis, miosis, anhidrosis, and a lighter-colored iris on the affected side. Surgical or obstetric injury to either the preganglionic sympathetic fibers or to the postganglionic sympathetic fibers traveling with the internal carotid artery in the neck can cause a congenital Horner's syndrome. Many cases are caused by injury to the lower brachial plexus during birth. This results in a congenital Horner's syndrome with associated paralysis of the hand and wrist (Klumpke's palsy) on the ipsilateral side. Other causes include congenital tumors and viral infections.[2,22]

Pharmacologic Testing

A suspected Horner's pupil should be confirmed with pharmacologic testing. Ipsilateral miosis and ptosis may be produced by separate, unrelated disorders mimicking true Horner's syndrome (pseudo-Horner's syndrome). A patient may have simple anisocoria and a ptotic upper eyelid from congenital ptosis, asymmetric senile ptosis, blepharochalasis, or myasthenia gravis.[2]

When pharmacologic testing for sympathetic denervation, eyedrops should be instilled in each eye, so that the reaction of the normal pupil can act as a control. Any procedure that can disrupt the corneal epithelium should not be performed before the instillation of the eyedrops. Light irides have a better response to pharmacologic testing than dark irides because increased pigmentation may bind the drugs, producing false-positive results.[96,98]

The cocaine test confirms the presence of a true Horner's syndrome regardless of the lesion site. Ten percent cocaine dilates the normal pupil by blocking the reuptake of norepinephrine released by the postganglionic neurons. The resulting mydriasis is caused by accumulation of norepinephrine at the receptor sites of the dilator muscle. If the oculosympathetic pathway is completely interrupted anywhere along its course, administration of 10% cocaine eyedrops will not cause pupillary dilation because norepinephrine is not released into the postsynaptic space and therefore cannot accumulate. Mild mydriasis may be noted when partial disruption of the pathway exists. All sympathetically denervated pupils will show poor or no dilation after administration of 10% cocaine compared with the pupil of the normal eye.

To perform the test, one drop of 10% cocaine solution is placed in each eye, followed by instillation of a second set of drops 5 minutes later. The responses of the normal and abnormal pupils are compared after 50–60 minutes.[99] The cocaine test is positive if anisocoria greater than 1 mm results, with the normal pupil becoming larger compared with the sympathetically denervated pupil.[100,101] As previously mentioned, the cocaine test may not be appropriate in the diagnosis of Horner's syndrome in patients with heavily pigmented irides because of the poor dilation characteristically seen in such cases.[98] If performed on a patient with dark irides, 2–3 hours may be required before dilation occurs. If dilation is not noted after 45 minutes, more cocaine should be instilled in each eye. The pupils should then be observed again for a longer period of time.[102]

Hydroxyamphetamine localizes the lesion to either a central or preganglionic site versus a postganglionic site. This agent causes pupillary dilation by enhancing the release of norepinephrine from the nerve terminals of the postganglionic sympathetic neurons.[99] If a lesion destroys the postganglionic sympathetic neurons, there will be no norepinephrine stored in the postganglionic nerve terminals to be released, and the pupil will not dilate when 1% hydroxyamphetamine is instilled into the eye.[102–104] If the postganglionic neurons are only partially damaged, the pupil of the affected eye poorly dilates compared with the normal pupil.[102] If there is a central or preganglionic sympathetic neuron lesion, 1% hydroxyamphetamine causes pupil dilation because the postganglionic neurons are still intact and the nerve fiber endings still contain stores of norepinephrine.[102–104] This pupil dilation may be exaggerated in the affected eye either because of an enhanced receptor sensitivity at the dilator muscle or increased accumulation of norepinephrine in the postsynaptic nerve endings.[104]

Pupil testing with 1% hydroxyamphetamine is performed by instilling one drop of the solution into each eye, followed in 5 minutes by a second set of drops. The pupils are evaluated in a darkened room after 45 minutes. Pretreatment with cocaine interferes with the action of hydroxyamphetamine, so if the cocaine test has been performed, the hydroxyamphetamine test should not be performed for at least 48 hours.[99]

It should be noted that failure of the affected pupil to dilate accurately localizes the lesion to the postganglionic neuron in only 84% of cases.[87] However, an exaggerated pupillary dilation in the affected eye resulting in anisocoria greater than 1 mm confirms the presence of a central or preganglionic lesion.[87,103] Central and preganglionic lesions must be further differentiated on the basis of symptoms and signs that accompany the Horner's syndrome, since there are no pharmacologic tests currently available to distinguish between central and preganglionic lesions.[99]

REFERENCES

1. Miller NR. The Pupil: Embryology, Anatomy, Innervation, and Reflex Movements of the Iris. In NR Miller (ed), Walsh and Hoyt's Clinical Neuro-ophthalmology (4th ed). Vol 2. Baltimore: Williams & Wilkins, 1985;400–41.
2. Miller NR. Disorders of Pupillary Function, Accommodation, and Lacrimation. In NR Miller (ed), Walsh and Hoyt's Clinical Neuro-ophthalmology (4th ed). Vol 2. Baltimore: Williams & Wilkins, 1985;469–556.
3. Kupfer C, Chumbley L, Downer J. Quantitative histology of optic nerve, optic tract, and lateral geniculate nucleus of man. J Anat 1967;101:393–401.
4. Carpenter MB, Pierson RJ. Pretectal region and the pupillary light reflex. An anatomical analysis in the monkey. J Comp Neurol 1973;149:271–300.
5. Warwick R. The ocular parasympathetic nerve supply and its mesencephalic sources. J Anat 1954;88:71–93.
6. Jampel RS, Mindel J. The nucleus for accommodation in the midbrain of the macaque. Invest Ophthalmol 1967;6:40–50.
7. Kerr FWL, Hollowell OW. Location of pupillomotor and accommodation fibres in the oculomotor nerve: experimental observations on paralytic mydriasis. J Neurol Neurosurg Psychiatry 1964;27:473–81.
8. Miller NR. Embryology and Anatomy of the Ocular Motor System. In NR Miller (ed), Walsh and Hoyt's Clinical Neuro-ophthalmology (4th ed). Vol 2. Baltimore: Williams & Wilkins, 1985;559–607.
9. Hriso E, Masdeu JC, Miller A. Monocular elevation weakness and ptosis: an oculomotor fascicular syndrome? J Clin Neuro-ophthalmol 1991;11:111–3.
10. Jaeger RJ, Benevento LA. A horseradish peroxidase study of the innervation of the internal structures of the eye. Invest Ophthalmol 1980;19:575–83.
11. Parelmann JJ, Fay MT, Burde RM. Confirmatory evidence for a direct parasympathetic pathway to internal eye structures. Trans Am Ophthalmol Soc 1985;84:371–80.
12. Ponsford JR, Bannister R, Paul EA. Methacholine pupillary responses in third nerve palsy and Adie's syndrome. Brain 1982;105:583–97.
13. Slamovits TL, Miller RN, Burde NR. Intracranial oculomotor nerve paresis with anisocoria and pupillary parasympathetic hypersensitivity. Am J Ophthalmol 1987;104:401–6.

14. Miller NR. Accommodation: Embryology, Anatomy, Innervation and Normal Function. In NR Miller (ed), Walsh and Hoyt's Clinical Neuro-ophthalmology (4th ed). Vol 2. Baltimore: Williams & Wilkins, 1985;442–57.

15. Parkinson D, Johnston J, Chaudhuri A. Sympathetic connections to the fifth and sixth cranial nerves. Anat Rec 1978;191:221–6.

16. Parkinson D. Further observations on the sympathetic pathway to the pupil. Anat Rec 1988;220:108–9.

17. Weinstein JM. Pupillary disorders. Curr Opin Ophthalmol 1990;1:453–62.

18. Johnson LN. The effect of light intensity on measurement of the relative afferent pupillary defect. Am J Ophthalmol 1990;109:481–2.

19. Thompson HS, Corbett JJ, Cox TA. How to measure the relative afferent pupillary defect. Surv Ophthalmol 1981;26:39–42.

20. Thompson HS, Corbett JJ. Asymmetry of pupillomotor input. Eye 1991;5:36–9.

21. Thompson HS. Pupillary signs in the diagnosis of optic nerve disease. Trans Ophthalmol Soc UK 1976;96:377–81.

22. Slamovits TL, Glaser JS. The Pupils and Accommodation. In W Tasman, EA Jaeger (eds), Duane's Clinical Ophthalmology. Vol 2. Philadelphia: Lippincott, 1992;1–24.

23. Lam BL, Thompson HS. Relative afferent pupillary defect induced by patching. Am J Ophthalmol 1989;107:305–6.

24. Thompson HS. Adie's syndrome: some new observations. Trans Am Ophthalmol Soc 1977;75:587–626.

25. Slamovits TL. The pupil in neuro-ophthalmology: abnormal pupillary reactions and anisocoria. Semin Ophthalmol 1987;2:209–28.

26. Fletcher WA, Sharpe JA. Tonic pupils in neurosyphilis. Neurology 1986;36:188–92.

27. Currie J, Lessell S. Tonic pupil with giant cell arteritis. Br J Ophthalmol 1984;68:135–8.

28. Harriman DGF, Garland H. The pathology of Adie's syndrome. Brain 1968;91:401–18.

29. Loewenfeld IE, Thompson HS. The tonic pupil: a re-evaluation. Am J Ophthalmol 1967;63:46–87.

30. Loewenfeld IE, Thompson HS. Mechanism of tonic pupil. Ann Neurol 1981;10:275–6.

31. Pilley SFJ, Thompson HS. Cholinergic supersensitivity in Adie's syndrome: pilocarpine vs. mecholyl. Am J Ophthalmol 1975;80:955.

32. Bourgon P, Pilley SFJ, Thompson HS. Cholinergic supersensitivity of the iris sphincter in Adie's tonic pupil. Am J Ophthalmol 1978;85:373–7.

33. Bell RA, Thompson HS. Ciliary muscle dysfunction in Adie's syndrome. Arch Ophthalmol 1978;96:638–42.

34. Wirtschafter JD, Herman WK. Low concentration eserine therapy for the tonic pupil (Adie) syndrome. Ophthalmology 1980;87:1037–43.

35. Rouse MN, Polte L. Accommodative involvement with Adie's pupil. Am J Optom Physiol Opt 1984;61:54–5.

36. Loewenfeld IE. The Argyll Robertson pupil, 1869–1969. A critical survey of the literature. Surv Ophthalmol 1969;14:199–299.

37. Dacso CC, Bortz DL. Significance of the Argyll Robertson pupil in clinical medicine. Am J Med 1989;86:199–202.

38. Poole CJM. Argyll Robertson pupils due to neurosarcoidosis: evidence for site of lesion. Br Med J 1984;289:356.

39. Sears ML. The cause of the Argyll Robertson pupil. Am J Ophthalmol 1971;72:488–9.

40. Kirkham TH, Kline LB. Monocular elevator paresis, Argyll Robertson pupils and sarcoidosis. Can J Ophthalmol 1976;11:330–5.

41. Koudstaal PJ, Vermeulen M, Wokke JHJ. Argyll Robertson pupils in lymphocytic meningoradiculitis (Bannworth's syndrome). J Neurol Neurosurg Psychiatry 1987;50:363–5.

42. Thompson HS. Pupillary light-near dissociation. A classification. Surv Ophthalmol 1975;19:290–2.

43. Seybold ME, Yoss RE, Hollenhorst RW, Moyer NJ. Pupillary abnormalities associated with tumors of the pineal region. Neurology 1971;21:232–7.

44. Shuaib A, Israelian G, Lee MA. Mesencephalic hemorrhage and unilateral pupillary deficit. J Clin Neuro-ophthalmol 1989;9:47–9.

45. Levatin P. Pupillary escape in disease of the retina or optic nerve. Arch Ophthalmol 1959;62:768–79.

46. Thompson HS, Montague P, Cox TA, Corbett JJ. The relationship between visual acuity, pupillary defect, and visual field loss. Am J Ophthalmol 1982;93:681–8.

47. Hayreh SS. Anterior ischemic optic neuropathy. Arch Neurol 1981;38:675–8.

48. Cox TA. Relative afferent pupillary defects in multiple sclerosis. Can J Ophthalmol 1989;24:207–10.

49. Brown RH, Zilis JD, Lynch MG, Sanborn GE. The afferent pupillary defect in asymmetric glaucoma. Arch Ophthalmol 1987;105:1540–3.

50. Kohn AN, Moss AP, Podos SM. Relative afferent pupillary defects in glaucoma without characteristic field loss. Arch Ophthalmol 1979;97:294–6.

51. Prywes AS. Unilateral afferent pupillary defects in asymmetric glaucoma. Arch Ophthalmol 1976;94:1286–8.

52. Quigley HA, Addicks EM, Green WR. Optic nerve damage in human glaucoma: III. Quantitative correlation of nerve fiber loss and visual field defect in glaucoma, ischemic optic neuropathy, papilledema and toxic neuropathy. Arch Ophthalmol 1982;100:135–46.

53. Newman SA, Miller NR. Optic tract syndrome: neuro-ophthalmologic considerations. Arch Ophthalmol 1983;101:1241–50.

54. O'Connor PS, Kasdon D, Tredici TJ, Ivan DJ. The Marcus Gunn pupil in experimental tract lesions. Ophthalmology 1982;89:160–4.

55. Ellis CJK. Afferent pupillary defect in pineal region tumour. J Neurol Neurosurg Psychiatry 1984;47:739–41.

56. Johnson RE, Bell RA. Relative afferent pupillary defect in a lesion of the pretectal afferent pupillary pathway. Can J Ophthalmol 1987;22:282–4.

57. Folk JC, Thompson HS, Farmer SG, et al. Relative afferent pupillary defect in eyes with retinal detachment. Ophthal Surg 1987;18:757–9.

58. Servais GE, Thompson HS, Hayreh SS. Relative afferent pupillary defect in central retinal vein occlusion. Ophthalmology 1986;93:301–3.

59. Jiang MQ, Thompson HS. Pupillary defects in retinitis pigmentosa. Am J Ophthalmol 1985;99:607–8.

60. Thompson HS, Watsky RC, Weinstein JM. Pupillary dysfunction and macular disease. Trans Am Ophthalmol Soc 1980;78:311–7.

61. Newsome DA, Milton RC, Gass JDM. Afferent pupillary defect in macular degeneration. Am J Ophthalmol 1981; 92:396–402.

62. Portnoy JZ, Thompson HS, Lennarson L, Corbett JJ. Pupillary defects in amblyopia. Am J Ophthalmol 1983;96:609–14.

63. Greenwald MJ, Folk ER. Afferent pupillary defects in amblyopia. J Pediatr Ophthalmol Strabismus 1983;20:63–7.

64. Folk JC, Thompson HS, Han DP, Brown CK. Visual function abnormalities in central serous retinopathy. Arch Ophthalmol 1984;102:1299–1302.

65. Sadun AA, Bassi CJ, Lessell S. Why cataracts do not produce afferent pupillary defects. Am J Ophthalmol 1990; 110:712–4.

66. Thompson HS. Do cataracts influence pupillary responses? Int Ophthalmol Clin 1978;18:109–11.

67. Miller NR. Topical Diagnosis of Neuropathic Ocular Motility Disorders. In NR Miller (ed), Walsh and Hoyt's Clinical Neuro-ophthalmology (4th ed). Vol 2. Baltimore: Williams & Wilkins, 1985;652–82.

68. Miller NR. Embryology and Anatomy of the Ocular Motor System. In NR Miller (ed), Walsh and Hoyt's Clinical Neuro-ophthalmology (4th ed). Vol 2. Baltimore: Williams & Wilkins, 1985;568–79.

69. Castro O, Johnson LN, Mamourian AC. Isolated inferior oblique paresis from brain-stem infarction. Perspective on oculomotor fascicular organization in the ventral midbrain tegmentum. Arch Neurol 1990;47:235–7.

70. Rucker CW. The causes of paralysis of the third, fourth, and sixth cranial nerves. Am J Ophthalmol 1966;61:1293–8.

71. Rucker CW. Paralysis of the third, fourth and sixth cranial nerves. Am J Ophthalmol 1958;46:787–94.

72. Kissel JT, Burde RM, Klingele TG, Zeiger HE. Pupil-sparing oculomotor palsies with internal carotid-posterior communicating artery aneurysms. Ann Neurol 1983;13: 149–54.

73. Trobe JD. Third nerve palsy and the pupil. Arch Ophthalmol 1988;106:601–2.

74. Moreland RP. Asymptomatic third nerve palsy secondary to intracranial aneurysm. South J Optom 1993;11: 27–30.

75. Breen LA, Hopf HC, Farris BK, Gutmann L. Pupil-sparing oculomotor nerve palsy due to midbrain infarction. Arch Neurol 1991;48:105–6.

76. Kumar P, Ahmed I. Pupil-sparing oculomotor palsy due to midbrain infarction. Arch Neurol 1992;49:348.

77. Dreyfus PM, Hakim S, Adam RD. Diabetic ophthalmoplegia: report of a case, with post-mortem study and comments on vascular supply of human oculomotor nerve. Arch Neurol Psychiatry 1957;77:337–49.

78. Asbury AK, Aldredge H, Hershberg R, Fisher CM. Oculomotor palsy in diabetes mellitus: a clinico-pathological study. Brain 1970;93:555–66.

79. Lustbader JM, Miller NR. Painless, pupil-sparing but otherwise complete oculomotor nerve paresis caused by basilar artery aneurysm. Arch Ophthalmol 1988;106:583–4.

80. O'Connor PS, Tredici TJ, Green RP. Pupil-sparing third nerve palsies caused by aneurysm. Am J Ophthalmol 1983;95:395–400.

81. Terry JE, Stout T. A pupil-sparing oculomotor palsy from a contralateral giant intracavernous carotid aneurysm. J Am Optom Assoc 1990;61:640–5.

82. Tomsak RL, Masaryk TJ, Bates JH. Magnetic resonance angiography (MRA) of isolated aneurysmal third nerve palsy. J Clin Neuro-ophthalmol 1991;11:16–8.

83. Trobe JD, Glaser JS, Post JD. Meningiomas and aneurysms of the cavernous sinus. Arch Ophthalmol 1978;96:457–67.

84. Czarnecki JSC, Thompson HS. The iris sphincter in aberrant regeneration of the third nerve. Arch Ophthalmol 1978;96:1606–10.

85. Schatz NJ, Savino PJ, Corbett JJ. Primary aberrant oculomotor regeneration. Arch Neurol 1977;34:29–32.

86. Burde RM, Savino PJ, Trobe JD. Clinical Decisions in Neuro-ophthalmology. St. Louis: Mosby, 1985;147–95.

87. Maloney WF, Younge BR, Moyer NJ. Evaluation of the causes and accuracy of pharmacologic localization in Horner's syndrome. Am J Ophthalmol 1980;90:394–402.

88. Keane JR. Oculosympathetic paresis: analysis of 100 hospitalized patients. Arch Neurol 1979;36:13–5.

89. Giles CL, Henderson JW. Horner's syndrome: an analysis of 216 cases. Am J Ophthalmol 1958;46:289–96.

90. Parkinson D, Bernard M. Horner's syndrome and others? Surg Neurol 1979;11:221–3.

91. Hartmann B, Kremer I, Gutman I, et al. Cavernous sinus infection manifested by Horner's syndrome and ipsilateral sixth nerve palsy. J Clin Neuro-ophthalmol 1987;7:223–6.

92. Sears ML, Kier EL, Chavis RM. Horner's syndrome caused by occlusion of the vascular supply to sympathetic ganglia. Am J Ophthalmol 1974;77:717–24.

93. Fields CR, Barker FM. Review of Horner's syndrome and a case report. Optom Vis Sci 1992;69:481–5.

94. Grimson BS, Thompson HS. Raeder's syndrome: a clinical review. Surv Ophthalmol 1980;24:199–210.

95. Saure C, Levinsohn MW. Horner's syndrome in childhood. Neurology 1976;26:216–30.

96. Motameni M, Jaanus SD. Pediatric Horner's syndrome. Clin Eye Vision Care 1992;4:103–7.

97. Musarella MA, Chan HSL, deBoer G, Gallie BL. Ocular involvement in neuroblastoma: prognostic implications. Ophthalmology 1984;91:936–40.

98. Friedman JR, Whiting DW, Kosmorsky GS, Burde RM. The cocaine test in normal patients. Am J Ophthalmol 1984;98:808–10.

99. Alexander LJ, Skorin L, Bartlett JD. Neuro-Ophthalmic Disorders. In JD Bartlett, SD Jaanus (eds), Clinical Ocular Pharmacology (3rd ed). Boston: Butterworth-Heinemann, 1995;515–59.

100. VanderWeil HL, VanGijn J. The diagnosis of Horner's syndrome: use and limitations of the cocaine test. J Neurol Sci 1986;73:311–6.

101. Kardon RH, Denison CE, Brown CK, Thompson HS. Critical evaluation of the cocaine test in the diagnosis of Horner's syndrome. Arch Ophthalmol 1990;108:384–7.

102. Thompson HS, Mensher JH. Adrenergic mydriasis in Horner's syndrome: hydroxyamphetamine test for diagnosis of postganglionic defects. Am J Ophthalmol 1971;72:472–80.

103. Cremer SA, Thompson HS, Digre KB, Kardon RH. Hydroxyamphetamine mydriasis in Horner's syndrome. Am J Ophthalmol 1990;110:71–6.

104. Burde RM, Thompson HS. Hydroxyamphetamine: a good drug lost? Am J Ophthalmol 1991;111:100–2.

10

Evaluation of Disorders of Ocular Alignment and Motility

Leland W. Carr

Alignment, stability, motility, and single binocular vision are miraculous functions that reveal much about the health of a patient. Clinical findings that include "normal, steady, central, monocular fixation" suggest healthy brain stem centers and good integration of inputs from the vestibular system. Normal horizontal and vertical gaze without diplopia or suppression signifies that motility centers, interconnecting neurologic pathways, and extraocular muscles are all functioning appropriately. A brisk near triad including convergence, accommodation, and pupillary constriction reveals that supranuclear midbrain centers, oculomotor subnuclei, third nerve pathways, and effector muscles are all performing adequately. It is the purpose of this chapter to (1) review the basic anatomy and physiology of ocular motility, (2) suggest a systematic protocol for assessing the ocular motility system, and (3) emphasize the significance of the more common clinical causes of abnormal alignment and disorders of movement.

EYE MOVEMENTS

Saccadic Eye Movements

Eye movements can be classified as either fast or slow. Fast eye movements include saccades to pick up fixation, as well as the rapid jerk phase of certain forms of nystagmus. Slow movements include smooth pursuits as used in maintaining foveal imaging of moving targets, convergence, and divergence. The endolymph-driven components of the vestibular ocular reflex, and the pursuit portion of the optokinetic reflex are also slow eye movements.[1]

Saccadic eye movements, as well as other types of eye movements, are initiated through distinct supranuclear mechanisms. Their initiation arises within the cortical hemispheres and perhaps within certain subcortical areas

as well. Neurologic information from these regions descends into the brain stem via the internal capsule. Significant processing occurs within the brain stem before specific cranial nerves are stimulated to control the extraocular muscles.

The saccadic system is responsible for all fast eye movements.[2] The frontal lobe eye fields (FEFs) appear vital in the generation of voluntary saccades ("look up, look down, look left, look right").[3] Involuntary saccades, including perception-driven movements to fixate a new sight or to look toward a new sound, are generated from within the occipital, parietal, and temporal lobes.[4]

The superior colliculi are important in generating involuntary reflex saccades. They are critical in the production of rapid jerk movements associated with many forms of nystagmus. It is not clear if the superior colliculi function purely as integration centers, or if they have the potential to actually initiate saccades by themselves.[5]

Saccades are initiated by cortical activity that occurs contralateral to the direction of the resulting fast eye movement. Thus, the right frontal cortex directs a saccade toward the left, whereas the left frontal lobe generates a saccade toward the right. Interestingly, in cases of hemispheric disease the intact, contralateral frontal lobe is often able to assume control over voluntary saccades in both directions.[6] In similar fashion, the right brain's cortical confluence (junction of occipital, parietal, and temporal lobes) seems to be important in generating visually dependent saccades toward the left. The left confluence produces visually driven saccades toward the right.[7]

It appears that voluntary vertical saccades result from simultaneous and equivalent activity within both frontal lobes.[8] Initiation of involuntary vertical saccades is less clearly understood.

Cortical and subcortical saccadic centers communicate with immediate prenuclear gaze centers in the brain stem.

Horizontal gaze centers lie within the pons. Vertical gaze centers are within the midbrain. Axons descend from the initiation centers and cross over (decussate) to terminate within the contralateral paramedian pontine reticular formation (PPRF).

The PPRF can be thought of as the horizontal gaze center. It has immediate communications with two populations of neurons within the adjacent abducens nuclear complex. One group of neurons sends its axons forward within cranial nerve VI to reach the ipsilateral lateral rectus muscle. The other neuron group conveys horizontal saccadic information to the contralateral medial rectus subnucleus by way of the medial longitudinal fasciculus (MLF) (Figure 10-1).

It appears that the prenuclear saccadic vertical gaze center lies within the pretectal region of the midbrain. This neuronal cluster is referred to as the rostral interstitial nucleus of the medial longitudinal fasciculus (riMLF).[9,10] Input and output from the riMLF is poorly understood but probably involves intercommunication between the PPRF, the vestibular nuclei, and the cerebellum.[10]

The cerebellum is clearly involved in fast eye movements and serves as a refining, smoothing, and adjusting center. It suppresses unwanted movements and works with the vestibular nuclei in coordinating eye movements with head rotations. Disease processes that affect the cerebellum often result in either weakened or disrupted fast eye movements. Slow eye movements may also be affected simultaneously.[11]

Saccadic system dysfunction typically manifests as absent, slow, or inaccurate fast eye movements. Hypometric saccades are those with insufficient amplitude, and hypermetric saccades are those exhibiting excessive amplitude or overshoots. At times, saccadic system dysfunction leads to erratic, disruptive movements. Nystagmus or ocular oscillations also occur with saccadic system disorders.

Pursuit Eye Movements

The smooth pursuit system allows the eyes to follow a moving object of interest and is activated during head movements. Accurate pursuits can achieve a maximum tracking velocity of approximately 60 degrees per second. If a retinal image slides off the fovea, a fast correctional saccade is normally generated to recapture the target.

Both cerebral hemispheres appear to be involved in initiating smooth pursuits in either direction, although the ipsilateral cortex may play the predominant role. The occipital, temporal, and parietal lobes are all involved. The frontal lobe eye fields may also play a role. Motion sensing cells within the retina and visual cortex are also vital.[8,12]

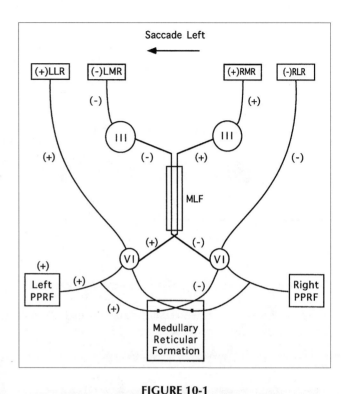

FIGURE 10-1
Neural pathways relevant to the PPRF and MLF. In the diagram, stimulation (+) of the left PPRF causes a saccade to the left. Inhibitory impulses (–) allow relaxation of opposing muscles. (Courtesy of Daniel K. Roberts, O.D.)

From the cerebral cortex, pursuit projections descend via pathways including the posterior limb of the internal capsule to reach the dorsal lateral pontine nuclei (DLPN). It has been suggested that the DLPN functions as a pursuit horizontal gaze center.[13] Projections continue from the DLPN, descending to the flocculus, paraflocculus, and vermis of the cerebellum. The flocculus communicates with the ipsilateral vestibular nuclear complex in the pons. Information then traverses the MLF, passing through the PPRF (saccadic horizontal gaze center) and eventually reaching the nuclei of the third, fourth, and sixth cranial nerves. It is unclear whether the PPRF plays a major role in pursuit eye movements or simply serves in projecting the information forward.

Clinically speaking, smooth pursuits are never completely abolished by disease that leaves saccades intact. Both systems are affected. The resulting eye movements are "cogwheel" and erratic, with jerky pursuits that are frequently interrupted by refixation attempts. Cerebral, cerebellar, or brain stem disease can produce abnormal pursuits, and so too can inattention, fatigue, sedation, or drug overdose.[14,15]

Vergence Eye Movements

Convergence and divergence represent directionally opposite movements of the eyes. These vergence movements are used to achieve and maintain bilateral imaging of "closer" or "farther" objects. Although the anatomic and physiologic basis of vergence eye movements remains poorly understood, the cortical confluence appears vital for convergence. This area where the occipital, parietal, and temporal lobes join together probably controls divergence as well. The pretectal midbrain, midbrain tegmentum, and the paramedian pontine tegmentum also play key roles in vergence movements. Small populations of convergence and divergence "burst cells" exist within the midbrain. They probably serve an immediate prenuclear function and help initiate vergence movements via their input to the oculomotor nuclear complex.[16]

Specific lesions have not been associated with isolated convergence or divergence anomalies. Instead, most pathologic conditions of the brain stem that have an impact on the vergence system also disrupt horizontal or vertical conjugate movements.[17,18]

Vestibular Reflexes

Vestibular reflexes allow the visual system to maintain foveal imaging in spite of head movement. Grossly simplified, this reflex originates within the "balance organs," the semicircular canals of the inner ears. When stimulated by a head movement, they signal the vestibular nuclei, which through reflex pathways will cause a counterrotation of the eyes away from the direction of the head movement. The complex vestibular reflex actually involves the cerebellum, numerous brain stem centers, the ocular cranial nerves, and the muscles of motility. Just as the reflex can be triggered by head or body movements, it can also be stimulated by injection of warm or cold water into the outer ear canal (see caloric testing, Chapter 19).

The value of vestibular testing is that intactness of a normal response demonstrates that neurologic pathways from the brain stem to the eyes are functioning normally. Caloric testing may be performed even on the unconscious patient.

Optokinetic Reflex

The optokinetic reflex is used to override the vestibular reflex when it becomes disruptive. For example, an individual is observing an object moving from the left toward the right. As the head rotates from the left toward the right in a pursuing fashion, the vestibular reflex will counterrotate the eyes back toward the left. This would quickly result in the eyes "falling behind" the object if the optoki-

netic reflex did not become active, thus allowing the eyes to continue pursuing the object toward the right as the head moves. The optokinetic reflex is dependent on visual input. It allows the eyes to maintain position within the orbit even if the eyes and body are rotating.

Optokinetic reflexes are assessed clinically by simulating a rotation of the visual environment. If a series of vertical bars or patterned contours are passed before the eyes, a visually induced nystagmus results. For example, a strip consisting of alternate light and dark vertical bars is moved from left to right before the eyes. A jerk nystagmus will result. Here, a slow movement from left toward right occurs, which is interrupted by a fast saccade back toward the left. This, by definition, is a left-beating, jerk nystagmus. The slow phase of this nystagmus, toward the right, is equivalent to the slow phase of an optokinetic response generated in response to rotation of the head toward the right. Optokinetic nystagmus (OKN) testing affords a means for assessing basic visual intactness, the mechanisms of reflex processing, and the functional integrity of the neurologic pathways and muscles that move the eyes.

EXTRAOCULAR MUSCLES

Each globe is controlled by six extraocular muscles (Figure 10-2). Five of them originate from the posterior orbital apex. The sixth arises from the nasal orbital floor. These muscles are driven by input from the third, fourth, and sixth cranial nerves. Respective innervation is illustrated in Table 10-1.

Each extraocular muscle is "yoked" with a corresponding muscle in the opposite eye. More precisely, yoked muscle groups are those muscles in the two eyes that collectively act to rotate both eyes in the same direction (conjugate eye movements). For simplicity, the innervational signal to one muscle in one eye can be thought of as being matched precisely by a signal to an equivalent muscle in the opposite eye. Thus, a signal to the right eye to rotate X degrees toward the right would be matched precisely by a signal to the left eye to also rotate X degrees toward the right.

The yoked muscle arrangement results in equal strength innervational signals going to paired muscle groups in the two eyes and is the basis of Hering's law of equal innervation (Figure 10-3). Different yoked muscle arrangements exist for movements of both eyes in the same direction versus convergence and divergence.

Another law used in explaining eye movements is Sherrington's law of reciprocal innervation. It is based on the principle that the innervation to any muscle is accompanied by an equivalent inhibitory impulse to the antago-

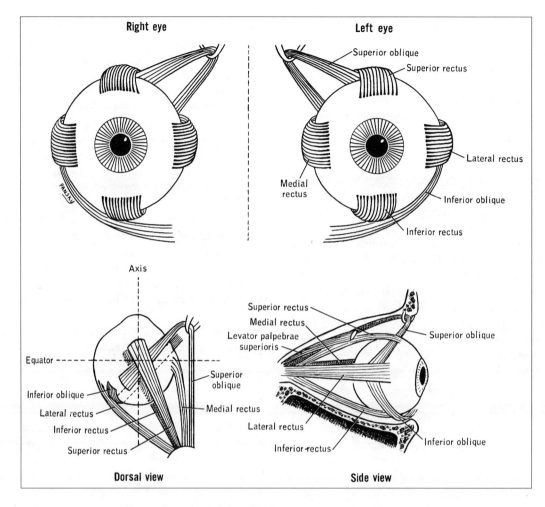

FIGURE 10-2

The extraocular muscles. (Reprinted with permission from EL House, B Pansky. A Functional Approach to Neuroanatomy [2nd ed]. New York: McGraw-Hill, 1967;265.)

nist muscle (Figure 10-4). For example, if the right eye's medial rectus is stimulated to adduct the eye, the right lateral rectus is simultaneously inhibited by an equal amount. The end result is adduction of the eye.

Hering's and Sherrington's laws are particularly helpful in the evaluation of neurologic motility deficits, and they can be used in identifying the paretic nerve, muscle, or muscle group.

Just as an evaluation of pupil responsiveness and facial sensitivity can provide insights into lesion localization in cases of acquired strabismus, a thorough eyelid examination may provide invaluable information. Since the third cranial nerve innervates the superior levator muscle, a clinical presentation of unilateral acquired ptosis, mydriasis, and motility disturbance indicates a palsy of

TABLE 10-1

Innervation to the Extraocular Muscles

Oculomotor nerve (III)
  Superior division
    Levator palpebrae superioris
    Superior rectus

  Inferior division
    Medial rectus
    Inferior rectus
    Inferior oblique

Trochlear nerve (IV)
  Superior oblique

Abducens nerve (VI)
  Lateral rectus

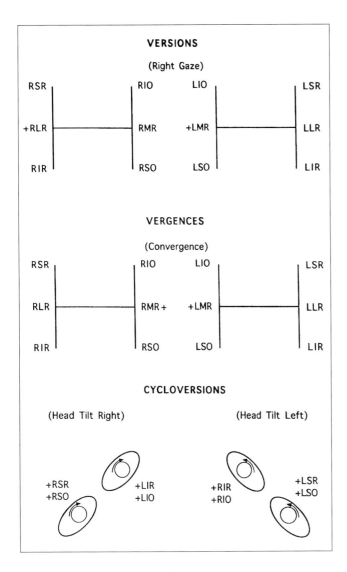

FIGURE 10-3

Hering's law of equal innervation. Yoked muscle arrangements allow for equal strength innervational signals to paired muscle groups during versions, vergences, and cycloversions. + = stimulation; R = right; L = left; SR = superior rectus; LR = lateral rectus; IR = inferior rectus; IO = inferior oblique; MR = medial rectus; SO = superior oblique. (Courtesy of Daniel K. Roberts, O.D.)

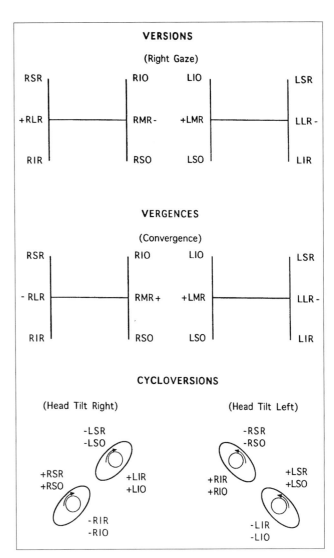

FIGURE 10-4

Sherrington's law. Innervation to any muscle is accompanied by an equivalent inhibitory signal to the antagonistic muscle. + = stimulation; – = inhibition; R = right; L = left; SR = superior rectus; LR = lateral rectus; IR = inferior rectus; IO = inferior oblique; MR = medial rectus; SO = superior oblique. (Courtesy of Daniel K. Roberts, O.D.)

this nerve. Müller's muscles retract the upper and lower lids on adrenergic stimulation via the oculosympathetic pathways. Thus, a patient with an acquired third, fourth, or sixth nerve palsy accompanied by a mild ptosis of recent onset probably has a lesion located within the cavernous sinus or orbital apex where the relevant pathways run in closest proximity to one another.

Müller's muscles are susceptible to inflammation and fibrosis, as often occurs in cases of dysthyroid disease.[19] A

patient with eyelid retraction combined with impaired motility may thus be manifesting signs of ocular Graves' disease.

The seventh nerve contributes to eyelid closure through its stimulation of the orbicularis muscle. Within the pons the seventh nerve fibers follow a course across the surface of the sixth nerve nucleus. Thus, a patient who has an acquired adduction deficit combined with poor lid closure, loss of facial expression, facial droop, etc., is likely to have a pontine lesion.

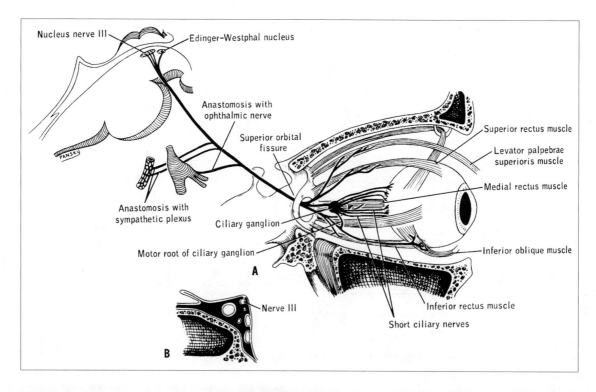

FIGURE 10-5

The oculomotor nerve (cranial nerve III). A. Course, distribution, and relationship to other structures. B. Its relationship to other structures within the cavernous sinus. (Reprinted with permission from EL House, B Pansky. A Functional Approach to Neuroanatomy [2nd ed]. New York: McGraw-Hill, 1967;326.)

The orbicularis is often involved in neuromuscular junction disease. A clinical presentation of variable lid closure weakness, variable ptosis, and variable diplopia, especially if exaggerated by fatigue or illness, could be an indicator of myasthenia gravis.[20]

OCULAR CRANIAL NERVES AND NEUROPARALYTIC STRABISMUS

The cranial nerve nuclei that drive the extraocular muscles lie within the brain stem. Nuclei governing the third and fourth cranial nerves occupy the dorsal midbrain. The sixth nerve's abducens nucleus is located within the pons. Also important is the vestibular nucleus associated with the eighth cranial nerve. It lies near the junction of the pons and the medulla. Extensive intercommunication occurs between all of these nuclei. The MLF is the pathway providing this linkage.

Oculomotor Nerve (Cranial Nerve III) Palsy

As with all cranial nerves, the number of disease processes that can have an impact on the third nerve are numerous. Any lesion that compresses or otherwise disrupts the nerve or its vascular supply can disrupt neuronal impulses at virtually any point from the brain stem to the target muscles (Figure 10-5). A complete palsy of the third nerve would be expected to present as an eye deviated down and out with a fixed and dilated pupil but covered by a ptotic upper lid. This would be the result of loss of innervation to the levator, the superior rectus, the inferior oblique, the medial rectus, the inferior rectus, and the pupillary sphincter.

Once a third nerve palsy is identified, it becomes essential to assess the site and significance of the responsible lesion. Is the lesion in the brain stem? Is it within the subarachnoid space? The cavernous sinus? The orbit? After localization of a lesion is considered, an attempt must be made to identify the specific type of pathologic condition responsible.

A palsy of the oculomotor nerve may present in various ways. For example, the third nerve may be affected in isolation. The resulting dysfunction would be isolated to the distribution of that nerve. On the other hand, if there are signs that additional cranial nerves are affected—pathways to the arms and legs are involved, cognitive deficits are present, the palsy is accompanied by intensifying pain, etc.—the threat to the patient may be much greater. Consequently, no cranial nerve palsy should be considered an isolated problem until proven so. The work-up must include extensive review of both neuro-ocular and general neurologic health.

Most third nerve palsies affect adduction, whereby the eye shows limited ability to rotate in toward the nose. Upper lid ptosis is almost always present. While ischemic causes of third nerve palsy often leave efferent pupil signals intact, nonischemic, compressive lesions typically impair pupil constriction, with both light and near responses being abnormal.

Nuclear Lesions
Third nerve palsy resulting from an isolated lesion within the oculomotor nuclear complex is probably an academic concept. Clinically speaking, lesions within the neurologically "busy" midbrain almost always show more generalized signs of impaired function. Theoretically, the patient would have bilateral ptosis, because there is a single subnucleus that controls elevation of both upper lids. The patient would also demonstrate an ipsilateral adductional paresis, a nonconstricting (light or near) pupil, and a down-and-out ocular deviation. The contralateral eye would show evidence of superior rectus palsy in addition to the lid droop. This is because each superior rectus is controlled by a contralaterally located subnucleus.

Fascicular Lesions
Lesions of the third nerve fascicles (axonal pathway within the brain stem) in their course within the midbrain will produce a third nerve palsy accompanied by neurologic signs involving the arms and legs. Lesions in the region of the superior cerebellar peduncles will produce unilateral third nerve deficits along with cerebellar ataxia. Lesions near the red nucleus will exhibit ipsilateral third nerve weakness with contralateral hemiparesis. These fascicular territory lesions are most often related to stroke or tumor.

Subarachnoid Lesions
Statistically, an aneurysm of the posterior communicating artery is the most likely cause of subarachnoid compression of the third nerve. Acute bleeding from the aneurysm is the event that usually precipitates the signs and symptoms.[21] Affected patients show obvious evidence of severe brain impairment, because they are in the process of developing subarachnoid intracranial hemorrhage. Many are unconscious immediately or within minutes. Others are severely obtunded. Pain, when described, is excruciating and characterized by an explosive onset and rapid build-up.[22]

Uncal herniation syndrome arises in many patients who develop large space-occupying lesions within the supratentorial region. These masses produce pressure, forcing the brain downward toward the base of the skull. This squeezes the third nerve against the firm tentorial edge, producing a compressive palsy. Clinical presentation includes significant impairment of consciousness, a dilated and nonresponsive pupil, ptosis, and adductional palsy. At this point, the life of the patient is in jeopardy.

Ischemic infarction of the third nerve often occurs within the subarachnoid space. If nonperfusion affects the central vascular supply of the nerve, innervation to the lids and extraocular muscles is affected. In these cases, pupillary efferent fibers are often spared. This results from the peripheral location of pupillary fibers within the nerve throughout its subarachnoid course. A redundant meningeal arterial supply provides sufficient support for these outer pupillary fibers to remain functional.[23]

Cavernous Sinus Lesions
Lesions affecting the third nerve in its course through the cavernous sinus almost always have an impact on other nervous pathways at the same time. The sixth, fifth, and fourth cranial nerves, as well as the oculosympathetic fibers, are all vulnerable in this territory. Cavernous sinus disease often affects the third nerve axonal bundles asymmetrically. Thus, some patients retain normal or near normal pupillary responses in spite of progressive ptosis and adductional weakness. Additionally, slowly evolving compression, as is often associated with a tumor or aneurysm, may lead to axonal injury followed by aberrant regeneration of fibers. The resulting misdirected innervation can produce bizarre and unnatural co-contractions by ocular territory muscles. Lid/gaze and pupil/gaze dyskinesias are most typical. Aberrant third nerve regeneration is virtually never seen in ischemic palsies and should be considered clinical evidence of compression in all cases.[22-24]

Tolosa-Hunt syndrome involves the acute onset of unrelenting orbital region pain accompanied by progressive ophthalmoplegia. In essence, an idiopathic inflammatory response occurs in the locality of the anterior cavernous sinus and superior orbital fissure. Sensory fibers carried by the fifth nerve are affected, and in addition, the sixth, third, and fourth nerves are susceptible to progressive impairment at different rates and in various combinations.

Diagnosis is dependent on thin-section imaging studies, including enhanced magnetic resonance imaging (MRI).[22]

Superior Orbital Fissure and Orbital Lesions

Orbital involvement of the third nerve may selectively affect the superior rectus and levator muscles, while leaving other third nerve driven muscles functional. The reverse situation is also true. This is because of the separation of the nerve into a superior and an inferior division before it passes through the superior orbital fissure. Thus, one division can be impaired by a disease process that leaves the other division intact. In most cases of orbital disease, however, the patient acquires multiple pathway dysfunction, and isolated third nerve impairment with involvement limited to a single division is rare in clinical practice.[22]

In most cases of orbital disease the patient demonstrates signs affecting the globe, lid, and periorbital tissue. Hyperemia, edema, and vasocongestion result from interference with normal blood flow into and out of the orbit.

Isolated Third Nerve Palsy

Most cases of isolated third nerve palsy are ischemic in origin.[22,24] Pupillary sparing occurs in over 80% of these cases.[25] Most often the affected patient experiences an acute onset after a day or two of orbital region pain. As the neurologic dysfunction begins to manifest itself, the pain often starts to subside. Function typically begins to return within 2–4 weeks. Full recovery, without evidence of aberrant regeneration, is typically achieved within 3–6 months. A thorough systemic health evaluation is usually advised in managing these patients. Diabetes, hypertension, arteritis, systemic lupus, and other disorders associated with vascular insufficiency and microvascular occlusions need to be ruled out. Patients may require temporary occlusion to help them deal with diplopia.

Trochlear Nerve (Cranial Nerve IV) Palsy

As with the third nerve, the fourth cranial nerve follows a long and rather complicated course as it projects from the brain stem to the muscle it innervates, the superior oblique. Almost any disease process along this route can lead to partial or complete paralysis of the associated muscle (Figure 10-6). This is the only cranial nerve to exit from the dorsal aspect of the brain stem. It is also the only cranial nerve to immediately cross-over (decussate) to travel within the opposite side of the cranial vault and to innervate a muscle within the contralateral orbit. Although isolated fourth nerve palsies may occur, additional neurologic dysfunction is often present[25] because of the large number of pathways passing in close proximity.

Axial trauma affecting the head and spine is the most common cause of acquired fourth nerve palsy, and fourth nerve palsy is the most common neurologic cause of acquired vertical diplopia.[25] Typically, patients attempt to minimize vertical and torsional misalignment through head tilts and face turns. Most often, head tilt opposite from the affected eye is used to minimize misalignment in primary gaze. As a rule, diplopia is exaggerated during efforts to look down and in—the field of action of the superior oblique muscle. Thus, Park's procedure is useful in pinpointing dysfunction of the fourth nerve and the superior oblique (see discussion that follows).

Nuclear and Fascicular Lesions

Midbrain infarctions and demyelinating disease are the most common causes of nuclear and fascicular territory fourth nerve palsy.[26] Usually other neurologic pathways are also affected, such as the descending oculosympathetic pathway, resulting in an associated contralateral Horner's syndrome.

Subarachnoid Space Lesions

The subarachnoid territory is the most common location for lesions causing acquired fourth nerve palsy.[27] The nerve is particularly vulnerable immediately after it emerges from the dorsal surface of the brain stem. In this region contrecoup forces conveyed during injury of the skull or spinal column can traumatize axons as they cross over the free tentorial edge. Trauma is therefore the leading cause of fourth nerve dysfunction arising from lesions within its subarachnoid course.[26,27]

Cavernous Sinus Lesions

In almost every case of fourth nerve palsy associated with cavernous sinus disease, additional ocular cranial nerves are compromised, and the fourth nerve is the least likely of all neuro-ocular pathways to be involved in an isolated fashion by pathologic conditions of the cavernous sinus.[26] Aneurysmal compression, invasion by parasellar tumors, inflammation, and infection represent the cavernous sinus disorders most often implicated.

Superior Orbital Fissure and Orbital Lesions

The fourth cranial nerve also is unlikely to be impaired in isolation in the region of the superior orbital fissure. Other neurologic pathways are almost always affected. Orbital trauma, tumors, infiltrations, and inflammations are likely to affect the fourth nerve along with the oculosympathetic pathway, the third nerve, the fifth nerve, and the sixth cranial nerve. Various combinations and various levels of dysfunction have been reported.[27] In addition, proptosis, chemosis, and hyperemia of the globe, lids, and periorbital tissues usually arise.

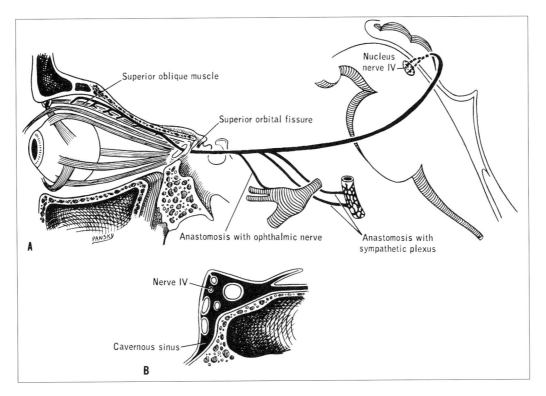

FIGURE 10-6

The trochlear nerve (cranial nerve IV). A. Course, distribution, and relationship to other structures. B. Its relationship to other structures within the cavernous sinus. (Reprinted with permission from EL House, B Pansky. A Functional Approach to Neuroanatomy [2nd ed]. New York: McGraw-Hill, 1967;327.)

Isolated Fourth Nerve Palsy

Isolated fourth nerve palsy is most often congenital. The frequent causes include various forms of birth trauma or fetal injury. Affected babies rapidly acquire compensatory head tilts and may develop very large compensatory vertical fusion amplitudes (10–15 prism diopters in some cases). On occasion these compensatory mechanisms breakdown in adulthood, and the patient begins to experience vertical diplopia. In these cases a review of childhood photographs is helpful in confirming the palsy as a longstanding condition through identification of pre-existing head tilts.

Acquired isolated fourth nerve palsy is most often seen in cases involving jarring injury to the head or spine. The case history becomes critical in arriving at the appropriate diagnosis.

Less often, vascular ischemia or compression by a neoplasm or aneurysm is found to underlie the condition.[28] The typical clinical presentation has already been described, which universally includes head tilts and face turns that reduce the angle of deviation. Imaging studies are usually warranted, especially in those cases exhibiting additional signs of evolving neurologic compromise.

Abducens Nerve (Cranial Nerve VI) Palsy

The sixth cranial nerve also follows a complex pathway between the brain stem and the orbit (Figure 10-7), and a wide variety of disease processes can affect it. Acquired sixth nerve palsies are relatively common and characteristically present as an acquired abductional weakness. Because of difficulty moving the affected eye outward, the patient develops an esophoric or esotropic posture. This is associated with intermittent or constant horizontal diplopia. Image separation becomes more pronounced during distance fixation and especially during gaze toward the affected side.

Nuclear and Fascicular Lesions

The abducens nuclear complexes are located within the pons in close proximity to the oculosympathetic path-

FIGURE 10-7

The abducens nerve (cranial nerve VI). A. Course, distribution, and relationship to other structures. B. Its relationship to other structures within the cavernous sinus. (Reprinted with permission from EL House, B Pansky. A Functional Approach to Neuroanatomy [2nd ed]. New York: McGraw-Hill, 1967;329.)

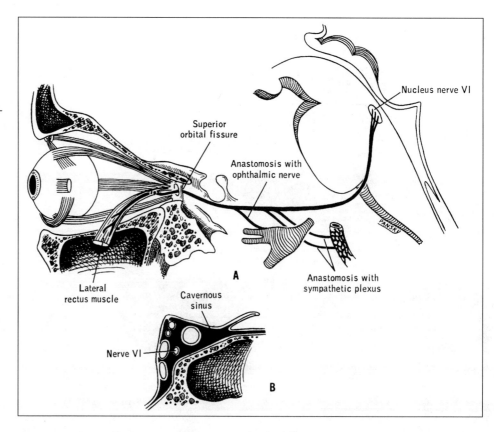

way's first order neuron. Also nearby is the ipsilateral horizontal gaze center (PPRF). Axons of the seventh cranial nerve (facial nerve) course directly across the sixth nerve nucleus on their way to the ipsilateral facial muscles. These associations result in multiple neurologic signs when this region of the brain stem becomes diseased. Patients usually have some combination of acquired ipsilateral abduction weakness, ipsilateral Horner's syndrome, ipsilateral horizontal gaze palsy, ipsilateral internuclear ophthalmoplegia, contralateral hemiparesis, and facial nerve palsy. Pontine infarction is the most common cause of nuclear sixth nerve palsy.[29]

Subarachnoid Space Lesions

In its course toward the cavernous sinus, the sixth nerve remains vulnerable to ischemic vascular disease, compression, inflammation, and infection. After severe infection of the inner ear, an abscess may produce inflammation of the petrous apex of the temporal bone. This can spread to directly involve the sixth nerve as it courses across the bone's surface. Thus, an inner ear infection can lead to Gradenigo's syndrome, consisting of sixth nerve palsy, ipsilateral hearing loss, facial pain, and facial muscle weakness.

Elevated intracranial pressure can produce downward pressure on the brain stem. This may stretch the sixth nerve as it exits from the pons or at its entry site into Dorello's canal in the parasellar region. Thus, an acquired abduction palsy may be an indication of intracranial hemorrhaging, inflammation, tumor, or other space-occupying disease. Papilledema often accompanies the motility disorder in these cases.

Disease processes associated with small vessel occlusion—e.g., diabetes mellitus, hypertension, systemic lupus, cranial arteritis, or syphilis—can produce an ischemic sixth nerve palsy. Patients typically complain of ipsilateral retro-orbital headache, which begins to subside as diplopia becomes established. This is not usually the excruciating pain of a subarachnoid hemorrhage or aneurysmal compression but is almost always noted by the patient. In all cases of ischemic cranial nerve palsy, it is advisable that a thorough systemic health evaluation be obtained.

Other sources of acquired sixth nerve palsy associated with lesions within the subarachnoid space include subarachnoid hemorrhage (the patient will be in severe pain and mentally obtunded or, more commonly, unconscious); viral, bacterial, or fungal meningitis; sarcoid inflammation; leukemic infiltration; and tumorous compression. Aneurysmal compression here is quite rare.[29,30]

Cavernous Sinus Lesions

The sixth nerve is the ocular motor nerve most susceptible to disease within the cavernous sinus.[30] It lies in a relatively unprotected location within the spongy matrix of this venous sinus, adjacent to the internal carotid artery. Vascular disease, including arteriovenous malformations and aneurysms, may impinge on the nerve here. Neoplasms and invasive carcinomas are other causes of sixth nerve palsy arising inside the cavernous sinus, as are inflammatory or ischemic processes.

Superior Orbital Fissure and Orbital Lesions

Orbital tumors, pseudotumors, infiltrates, inflammations, and trauma may affect the sixth nerve in the region of the superior orbital fissure. Proptosis and anterior segment congestion are commonly present. Other neuro-ocular pathways are routinely affected as well.[22]

Isolated Sixth Nerve Palsy

The sixth nerve is the ocular cranial nerve most likely to be affected in isolation.[31,32] Ischemic vascular disease should be suspected in these cases, and evaluation performed to rule out treatable systemic disorders.

In younger patients, a sudden onset of isolated sixth nerve palsy should alert the clinician of a potential tumor of the brain stem. Whereas most children suffering an acute unilateral abductional palsy are victims of post-viral inflammation,[32] some studies suggest that up to 50% of such presentations actually herald the presence of neoplasm. Imaging studies therefore are probably warranted in all pediatric cases.[32]

Medial Longitudinal Fasciculus

The medial longitudinal fasciculus (MLF) is a major axonal tract permitting communication between the third, fourth, sixth, and eighth cranial nerve nuclei. It extends from the rostral midbrain above the oculomotor complex, all the way to the midthoracic level of the spinal cord. Function of the MLF is vitally important for accomplishing smooth, coordinated horizontal and vertical gaze movements. It is probably not vital for convergence.[33]

Lesions of the MLF result in weakness or complete paralysis of one or both eyes. This is most apparent during rapid versional eye movements. Both voluntary and involuntary saccades are affected, and tests emphasizing large-amplitude, rapid velocity movements tend to accentuate the motility impairment. Most commonly an adductional paresis is demonstrated during horizontal gaze testing.

The most common disorder involving the MLF is internuclear ophthalmoplegia (INO).[34,35] Here lesions block gaze information passing between the pontine horizontal gaze center and the contralateral third nerve nuclear complex. This causes degradation of the horizontal gaze information reaching the contralateral medial rectus subnucleus. A slowed and weakened adductional ability results.

By convention, the sidedness of internuclear ophthalmoplegia is determined by the eye suffering the adductional deficit during horizontal gaze. Convergence adduction is usually normal. Thus, a classic right INO would be demonstrated by a patient with a normal ability to look toward the right and normal convergence. On efforts to gaze toward the left, however, the left eye would be seen to abduct while the right eye would be slowed or unable to achieve an adducted position. Typically it is also possible to detect an endpoint jerk nystagmus in the abducted left eye. This results from relative overstimulation of the left lateral rectus created as the left horizontal gaze center steps up its output in an effort to drive the affected right medial rectus to contract more strongly.

Internuclear ophthalmoplegia arising in an older patient is almost always unilateral and is typically the result of a brain stem infarction associated with small vessel disease.[36] Unilateral and bilateral internuclear ophthalmoplegia arising in middle age most often suggests demyelination and is therefore a common presenting sign in multiple sclerosis.[23]

Orbital and Cavernous Sinus Considerations

The orbit is a conical funnel with a flattened side toward the nose. It is formed by seven bones of the skull and contains the lacrimal gland, globe, ophthalmic veins, ophthalmic artery, and the cranial nerves associated with sensation, sight, and ocular motility. The orbital apex is especially crowded with vascular and neurologic tissues. Thus, orbital apex disease usually manifests itself with numerous signs and symptoms.[37]

Orbital bones contain numerous holes, spaces, and pathways that communicate directly with the paranasal sinuses. This provides a source and a route for infection to reach the orbit. Sinus carcinoma and mucocele can also enter quite readily. Orbital tissues behind the globe include fat, muscle, blood vessels, fibrous connective tissue sheets, and periosteal membranes. This material is prone to entrapment or herniation through orbital floor fractures. It may become inflamed or infiltrated by various disease processes. Metastatic cancers may seed to the region because of the extensive intraorbital vascular network. All of these diseases have the capacity to displace the eye, reduce vision, and impair motility.

The superior orbital fissure conducts into the orbit cranial nerves III, IV, and VI, along with the ophthalmic division of cranial nerve V and those oculosympathetic fibers destined for the dilator muscle of the iris. The optic nerve, ophthalmic artery, and additional oculosympathetic fibers enter through the more medially located optic foramen. This is therefore a very "busy" neuro-ocular area. Disease usually affects multiple pathways.

Aneurysms, nasopharyngeal carcinoma, meningioma, metastatic tumors, and inflammation are the most common disorders to affect the superior orbital fissure.[38] These are the same processes that most often affect the cavernous sinus.

Because venous drainage from the orbit, globe, and periorbital tissue is dependent on passage through the orbital apex, superior orbital fissure, and cavernous sinus, disease here is often associated with outflow obstruction. A congested, proptosed globe may result. The lids and conjunctiva may become edematous, congested, or discolored with venous blood, the episcleral venous plexuses are likely to be engorged, and the retina may show evidence of venous stasis retinopathy.[39] These ocular signs are likely to accompany motility deficits associated with pathologic processes of the orbit, superior orbital fissure, or anterior cavernous sinus. They should be looked for and ruled out in every case involving eye movement abnormalities.

CLINICAL EVALUATION OF MOTILITY DISORDERS

History and General Considerations

Obtaining a history is a critical first step in evaluation of motility disorders. In addition to general information pertaining to past ocular and systemic medical history, specific questions should be asked relative to exact symptomatology (e.g., diplopia, blurred vision, pain, peripheral numbness). The time of onset, frequency, duration, and course (improvement or worsening) all warrant specific investigation. Because motility disturbances are often not isolated events, it is critical to inquire about other neurologic signs and symptoms including "new" headaches, paresthesias, paresis, aphasia, tinnitus, ataxia, confusion, and personality shifts. The general neurologic history and workup pertinent to in-office optometric examinations is discussed in detail in Chapter 19.

Other components of the history should be added as needed. For instance, in a patient exhibiting proptosis and motility deficits consistent with Graves' disease, it would be important to ask about general symptoms of hyperthyroidism such as weight loss, heat intolerance, heart palpitations, nervousness, anxiety, and insomnia in spite of fatigue.

In a patient complaining of double vision, it is important to inquire whether the diplopia is horizontal (abductional or adductional), vertical (elevator or depressor problem), or oblique (combination) in nature. It is helpful to know if the image separation increases on a particular direction of gaze (right, left, up, down), and if the images move closer in a particular gaze. Determination of whether the diplopia is worse with distance vision (divergence or abductional problem) or near vision (convergence or adductional problem) is also useful. As an example, a patient with purely horizontal diplopia that is worse at distance than near and with gaze right, very likely exhibits a problem with the right lateral rectus (or its innervation—i.e., right abducens nerve palsy). This conclusion may be tentatively drawn because greater stimulation of the lateral rectus is required with gaze at distance than during convergence at near and because the field of action of the right lateral rectus is toward gaze right. Other tests would be needed to confirm this, however.

Careful observation of the patient should begin even before the case history. Often, features are more apparent during an initial questioning than during artificial testing. For example, a relaxed individual may exhibit a head tilt or face turn, yet on intensive questioning, the tilt may be masked by a more rigid posture assumed by the patient "under pressure." Patients with neurologic or muscular weaknesses often use head positioning to minimize their use of paretic muscles. They keep their eyes positioned in an opposite field of gaze, looking away from the weakened gaze. An example is provided by a patient with a paretic right lateral rectus. The patient may turn the face toward the right, thus reducing or eliminating the need for contraction of that muscle.

Other characteristics that should be noticed include gait, coordination, speech, memory, personality, and general appearance. Look for abnormalities including unusual head movements, nystagmus, lid droop, lid retraction, conjunctival or episcleral injection, proptosis, exophthalmus, or pupillary disorders. The presence of ptosis can indicate a number of problems including third nerve disease, oculosympathetic pathway palsies, or myasthenia gravis. Likewise, lid retraction may be significant and can be a sign of Graves' disease or a lesion affecting the midbrain. Progressive proptosis can be associated with Graves' disease, or it may indicate the presence of an orbital mass.

Conjunctival or episcleral injection could be an indicator of an orbital space-occupying lesion, cavernous sinus disease, and even seventh nerve impairment (resulting from exposure keratoconjunctivitis in association with poor orbicularis function).

Pupil Assessment

A careful pupillary evaluation should always be a component of the motility evaluation. A patient who does not dilate normally to dimness may have an oculosympathetic pathway impairment. When combined with ophthalmic motor nerve palsies, this finding strongly suggests the presence of an orbital apex or cavernous sinus lesion.

Oculosympathetic palsy may arise with ipsilateral abduction weakness, ipsilateral gaze palsy (both eyes affected), and a seventh nerve palsy producing ipsilateral facial muscle droop. At times contralateral hemiparesis also occurs. These dysfunctions occur in various combinations, according to the precise pathways affected. Caused by pontine lesions, the Millard-Gubler syndrome and Foville's syndrome delineate specific clinical manifestations.

A sluggish or fixed-dilated pupil accompanied by ptosis, severe pain, adductional weakness, or upgaze palsy suggests third nerve compression within the subarachnoid space. This can occur with aneurysms of the circle of Willis, most commonly arising off the posterior communicating artery. Aneurysms in the region are usually asymptomatic until hemorrhaging begins. The patient therefore is likely to exhibit clinical signs of acute subarachnoid hemorrhage, including severe impairment of consciousness.[21]

Fixation

Pathologic ocular instability is usually apparent when the eyes are in the primary gaze position. Brain stem disease from the medulla-cervical spinal cord to the dorsal midbrain can produce pathologic nystagmus, as can vestibular disease at either the peripheral (end-organ, inner ear) level, or centrally within the pons.

Often pathologic instability will present with some degree of asymmetry. Detection requires close comparison of the two eyes. There may be disconjugate movements including converging or diverging nystagmus, or see-saw movements with one eye deviating upward as the opposite eye deviates down. Typically, patients will complain of dizziness, "swimming" of the visual environment, ringing in the ears, or nausea.[8,22,25]

Diplopia Assessment

In addition to general symptoms surrounding a diplopia complaint—e.g., onset duration, frequency, direction—it is important to quickly establish whether diplopia is monocular or binocular in nature. If present at the time of examination, this can be determined by occluding first one eye and then the other. When monocular in nature, image-doubling will be present when the causative eye is viewing, but will disappear when that eye is covered. If binocular, the diplopia will be alleviated with occlusion of either eye.

Monocular diplopia most often results from uncorrected refractive error, an irregular corneal surface, or media opacities such as cataracts. Rarely, it may occur in cases of retinal or central nervous system disease.[19]

Cover Test

The cover test is one of the first objective tests performed on a patient with binocular diplopia. Both unilateral and alternating cover tests should be performed. Usually the patient's spectacle correction, if any, is left in place and the test is performed at both distance and near. With this technique any significant misalignment can usually be detected and quantified through neutralization with loose prisms.

To characterize a deviation further, several gazes can be evaluated with cover testing. With head or fixation target repositioning, the patient is tested in gaze right, left, up, down, and oblique positions as deemed appropriate.

Red Lens and Maddox Rod Tests

Although objective, cover testing can, at times, be difficult to interpret. A subjective method for qualifying and quantifying ocular deviations involves red lens or Maddox rod testing. Red lens testing is performed by simply placing a red lens in front of the patient's right eye and then having the patient fixate on a white muscle light or transilluminator. The patient is asked to describe the relative positions of the white and red images he or she perceives. Test distances and gaze directions can be altered to assess for variability in the angle of deviation. Quantification is relatively simple and can be accomplished by using hand held, loose or adjustable Risley prisms.

A variation of the red lens test is the Maddox rod test. This is performed by placing a red Maddox rod over the right eye with the ridges oriented either horizontally or vertically. The patient is asked to look at a bright white fixation target. Depending on the orientation of the Maddox rod, the patient will perceive a horizontal (ridges oriented vertically) or vertical (ridges oriented horizontally) red line with the right eye. The left eye will see a white light. The patient is asked whether the red line is seen above or below the light when testing vertical deviations. Again, prisms can be used to neutralize the angle. The patient is asked whether the red line is to the right or left of the light when testing horizontal deviations.

Versions and Ductions

Versional testing involves observing eye movements of a patient as he or she binocularly attempts to pursue a target being moved into the various diagnostic gaze positions. The examiner should look for speed, accuracy, and extent of movement. Asymmetry should be noted.

Ductional testing is performed by repeating this same procedure, except now observations are made of one eye with the contralateral eye occluded. An eye that appears slower, limited in the extent of its excursions, or somehow "weaker" than its fellow eye during versional testing needs an especially careful assessment of its ductional abilities. When versions are abnormal yet ductions appear intact, a cranial nerve palsy should be suspected. If the eye shows impaired motility during both binocular and monocular movements, then a restrictive, myopathic, or neuromuscular junction problem is more likely to exist.

Convergence

In any case of adductional weakness noted during versional and ductional testing, convergence adduction should be carefully examined. An eye that adducts slowly or incompletely during horizontal gaze assessment but that shows normal adductional ability during convergence is likely to have a lesion affecting the MLF.

Forced Ductions

Whenever restrictive myopathy is suspected (e.g., orbital floor fracture, Graves' disease), the clinician should perform a forced duction test to look for evidence of extraocular muscle entrapment or inelasticity. This will be revealed as an inability to "force" the globe to rotate into a position it is unable to attain on its own. The examiner detects mechanical restriction as the patient and examiner both seek to move the eye. Forced duction testing involves the administration of a drop of topical anesthetic, followed by placement of a pledget presoaked in 10% cocaine onto the conjunctiva overlying the anterior aspect of a rectus muscle insertion or posterior to the limbus. A blunt-tipped forceps is then used to grasp the conjunctiva at the anesthetized site, and an attempt made to pull the eye into its paretic field. At the same time, the patient is told to look in that direction. If the clinician is unable to easily rotate the globe in the direction of reduced motility, then restriction most likely exists. A simpler (and less painful) version of the forced duction test makes use of topical anesthetic and a moistened cotton-tipped applicator. Again, the patient is instructed to look in the paretic gaze direction. This time, however, the examiner uses the applicator in an attempt to gently "push" the globe into the paretic field.

Examination for Fatigability

Myasthenia gravis is often associated with variable motility impairments, variable misalignments, and intermittent diplopia. It is therefore essential to consider neuromuscular disease in all cases of acquired diplopia. Although variations of the edrophonium chloride (Tensilon) test are generally required to diagnose myasthenia, suggestive clues can often be obtained through use of noninvasive tests including prolonged upgaze. Here the patient is asked to sustain an upgaze position for 1 minute and 30 seconds. Within this timeframe the myasthenic will often become fatigued, and a significant, asymmetric lid droop will become obvious. Typically there is not a perception of "tiredness" associated with the muscular fatigue, yet the patient is unable to maintain an upper lid elevation.

Once the lid has been rendered ptotic, the Cogan's lid twitch sign can be evaluated. After upgaze, the patient is instructed to look downward in the reading gaze position. Then, after several seconds, the patient quickly refixates into primary gaze. The myasthenic will often have an initially normal lid elevation, followed quickly by a downward floating movement back into a ptotic posture.

It is much easier to demonstrate fatigability of the levator muscle than of the orbicularis or extraocular muscles, yet they also reveal the phenomenon. On occasion the clinician can also observe progressive lid closure weakening by having the myasthenic forcibly open, then tightly close the lids.

The Tensilon test provides laboratory support for a definitive diagnosis of myasthenia gravis. To perform this test, it is clinically useful to first induce an exaggerated ptosis by having the patient maintain upgaze until the levator demonstrates fatigue. Meanwhile, 1 ml of Tensilon is drawn into a small-caliber syringe, and a small-gauge butterfly needle is placed intravenously. An initial injection of 0.1–0.2 ml is given as the lids are observed closely. If the lid strength improves, or if "jittery" muscle fasciculations become apparent, the test result is considered positive. If no improvement is noted at the end of 1 minute, the remainder of the 1-ml syringe load is slowly injected over 30–45 seconds. The lid is continuously watched for evidence of strengthened lid elevation.[40] In similar fashion, ocular alignment and motility can be assessed under the influence of Tensilon. However, it is often difficult to make these observations, and best results involve documenting muscle strength through electrophysiologic recordings made during the test.

Isolation of the Paretic Muscle or Nerve

Once restrictive causes and neuromuscular junction diseases have been ruled out, the clinician must concentrate on identifying the muscle or nerve responsible for impaired motility. This information can then be assessed relative to the accompanying signs and symptoms, and a specific lesion can be predicted. The site of pathologic involve-

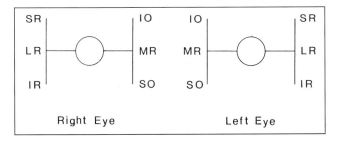

FIGURE 10-8
The diagnostic gaze positions.

ment is then assessed relative to the patient's age, health, and specific history. A list of the more probable clinical syndromes is generated. This leads, in turn, to development of a logical plan for additional testing.

The underlying principle used in identification of a paretic extraocular muscle is that the dysfunction of the muscle (or of its associated cranial nerve) will become most apparent when that muscle is required to produce a maximal effort. Figure 10-8 illustrates the diagnostic positions of gaze. Notice that a single muscle can be identified as primarily responsible for rotating and maintaining the eye in any of the specified directions of gaze. Understanding this relationship is essential in the process of isolating a paretic muscle. For example, if the patient has acquired a left esotropia from palsy affecting the left sixth nerve, the angle of deviation will be greatest when the patient attempts to gaze toward the left—the field of action of the paretic left lateral rectus. Similarly, if the patient has acquired vertical diplopia, is left hypertrophic in primary gaze, and is maximally diplopic on gaze down and right, the functionally weakened muscle can be identified as the left superior oblique (indicating possible left fourth nerve palsy).

Paretic Horizontal Rectus Assessment

Maintaining the eyes in primary gaze requires appropriately balanced contraction by all twelve extraocular muscles controlling the two eyes. However, it is primarily the balanced contractions of the medial recti and lateral recti that affect the horizontal alignment. If a lateral rectus muscle becomes impaired, the resulting muscular imbalance produces an esodeviation that is greater on distance fixation than it is during near fixation. The esodeviation can be further exaggerated by asking the patient to look toward the side with the affected lateral rectus muscle. For example, a patient acquires a right sixth nerve palsy, which effectively weakens the right lateral rectus. The patient would be expected to experience horizontal diplopia. The right eye would see the image to the right and the left eye would see the image to the left (uncrossed diplopia). The esodeviation, and thus

the image separation, will be greater with distance fixation than with near fixation. It will be further accentuated if the patient is asked to fixate on a target in right gaze.

A patient with acquired medial rectus paresis as the result of third nerve compression would be expected to notice horizontal diplopia with the right eye perceiving the left image and the left eye perceiving the right image (crossed diplopia). This is associated with an exodeviation. The exodeviation is exaggerated in this case by fixations that place heaviest demands on the weak medial rectus muscle. Thus, the exodeviation is greatest during convergence and during gaze toward the side opposite the affected eye. For example, a right third nerve palsy produces horizontal crossed diplopia, with image separation that is greater at near than at distance and that is especially noticeable during left gaze.

Vertical Paresis: Park's Procedure and the Bielschowsky Head Tilt Test

The head tilt test is incorporated into Park's procedure and assists in the isolation of a paretic muscle in cases of acquired vertical diplopia. The procedure is most appropriate for cases of acquired vertical neuroparalytic misalignment. It is not used in assessing horizontal diplopia and is of no value in workups of restrictive or neuromyopathic strabismus. Furthermore, test results become extremely confusing when the patient has had extraocular muscle surgery.

Park's procedure relies, again, on the concept of primary fields of muscle action. It uses the scheme illustrated in Table 10-2.

TABLE 10-2
The Park's Three-Step Test for Isolation of the Paretic Vertical Muscle. The Possible Muscles for Each of the Steps Are Shown.

Hyper eye in primary gaze

Right Eye	Left Eye
RSO } *depresses*	LSO
RIR	LIR
LSR } *elevators*	RSR
LIO	RIO

Hyper greater with gaze...

Right	Left	Right	Left
RIR	RSO	LSO	RIO
LIO	LSR	RSR	LIR

Hyper greater with head tilt to the...

Right	Left	Right	Left	Right	Left	Right	Left
LIO	RIR	RSO	LSR	RSR	LSO	LIR	RIO

R = right; L = left; SR = superior rectus; IR = inferior rectus; LR = lateral rectus; MR = medial rectus; SO = superior oblique; IO = inferior oblique.

FIGURE 10-9

A right superior oblique palsy diagnosed with the Park's three-step test. The box in the upper right corner illustrates a method of recording during clinical testing. (LIO = left inferior oblique; LIR = left inferior rectus; LSO = left superior oblique; LSR = left superior rectus; RH = right hyper; RIO = right inferior oblique; RIR = right inferior rectus; RSO = right superior oblique; RSR = right superior rectus.) (Courtesy of Daniel K. Roberts, O.D.)

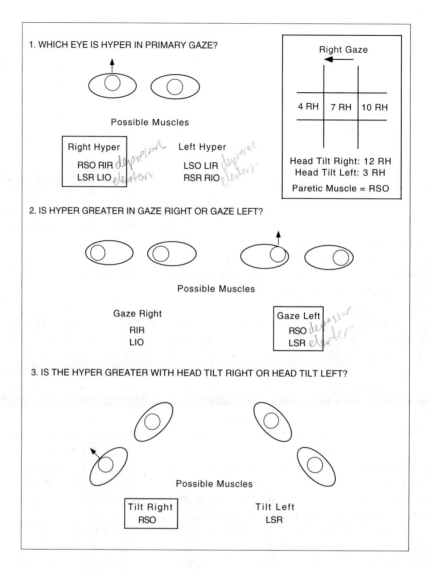

Step 1 involves identification of the eye that is hyperdeviated in primary gaze. This reduces the number of potentially paretic muscles to four. Either one of the depressor muscles in the hyperdeviated eye is paretic, or one of the elevators in the hypodeviated eye is paretic.

Step 2 involves determining whether the vertical deviation is greater during gaze left or during gaze right. This reduces the number of potentially responsible muscles to two.

Step 3 involves tilting the head toward the right and then toward the left shoulder. This is the Bielschowsky head tilt test. The amount of vertical misalignment is assessed. The greatest misalignment will occur when the paretic muscle is stimulated to counterrotate the eyes via the vestibular reflex. For example, if a right superior oblique palsy exists, hyperdeviation is greater with head tilt to the right side (Figure 10-9). Here, the weakened right superior oblique is stimulated to produce intorsion of the globe. Because of its inefficiency, the right superior rectus, which also produces intorsion, is stimulated. This in effect also produces further elevation of the right eye. Table 10-3 summarizes the effect of head tilts on stimulation and inhibition of the extraocular muscles.

A final step sometimes used in confirming the results of Park's procedure involves having the patient look toward the side that exaggerates the vertical misalignment. Next the patient is asked to look up and then down, while maintaining that side-gaze direction. When the paretic muscle is asked to work maximally, the vertical diplopia will become most pronounced. This helps confirm the paretic muscle previously identified by the three-step method.

TABLE 10-3
Effect of Head Tilts on the Extraocular Muscles

Head tilt toward right shoulder
1. Stimulates clockwise ocular counter rolling through vestibular stimulation
2. Right eye
    Stimulates right superior oblique
    Stimulates right superior rectus
    Inhibits right inferior oblique
    Inhibits right inferior rectus
3. Left eye
    Stimulates left inferior oblique
    Stimulates left inferior rectus
    Inhibits left superior oblique
    Inhibits left superior rectus
4. Right eye principal elevator becomes: Right superior rectus
    Right eye principal depressor becomes: Right superior oblique
5. Left eye principal elevator becomes: Left inferior oblique
    Left eye principal depressor becomes: Left inferior rectus

Head tilt toward left shoulder
1. Stimulates clockwise ocular counter rolling through vestibular stimulation
2. Right eye
    Stimulates right inferior oblique
    Stimulates right inferior rectus
    Inhibits right superior oblique
    Inhibits right superior rectus
3. Left eye
    Stimulates left superior oblique
    Stimulates left superior rectus
    Inhibits left inferior oblique
    Inhibits left inferior rectus
4. Right eye principal elevator becomes: Right inferior oblique
    Right eye principal depressor becomes: Right inferior rectus
5. Left eye principal elevator becomes: Left superior rectus
    Left eye principal depressor becomes: Left superior oblique

COMMON CONDITIONS THAT SIMULATE NEUROPARALYTIC STRABISMUS

Common causes of acquired motility disorders include inflammatory/infiltrative muscular disease, myasthenia gravis, cranial nerve palsy, and lesions affecting the MLF.[41] Less frequent causes include orbital apex or cavernous sinus disease, cortical lesions, and descending pathway or cerebellar disease. The discussion to follow will emphasize two frequently encountered entities affecting ocular motility.

Ocular Graves' Disease

Ocular Graves' disease, with its restrictive myopathy, is the single most common cause of sudden-onset diplopia arising in the adult patient group.[22,25] The classic presentation is that of a middle-aged to elderly patient with a congested orbit and asymmetric, slowly progressing, painless exophthalmus. Vertical diplopia experienced during upgaze is a feature in many cases. Lid edema is often present and causes a "rolled fold" of tissue adjacent to the orbital rim. This may look much like the age-related tissue bulge associated with dermatochalasis. The classic Graves' disease patient is described as demonstrating gross lid retraction with exposure of sclera along the superior and inferior limbal regions. The upper lid lags behind the globe as it rotates down into the reading position. Signs and symptoms of mild to moderate exposure keratoconjunctivitis are often present. Conjunctival and episcleral vessel injection is commonly found and is particularly visible within the interpalpebral region. The horizontal rectus muscle insertions may appear thick and congested. With more pronounced infiltration of the muscles, the insertions take on a purple-pink coloration, and the associated vessels may become prominent.

The classic Graves' disease patient has a health history that includes a prior diagnosis of hyperthyroidism. Systemic involvement is apparent, with symptoms including weight loss despite increased appetite, irritability, nervousness, emotional instability, heat intolerance, and heart palpitations.[42]

Many Graves' disease patients do not present such a clear picture, however. They have no systemic symptoms, and their eyes may appear remarkably quiet and normal. Evidence of ocular involvement may be as subtle as a slightly depressed blink rate or a mild tendency to staring. Although laboratory investigations may be helpful in confirming the diagnosis, often they are not. Serologic evidence of dysthyroid disease may be apparent initially, or it may develop months to years after initial development of eye signs. A serologically abnormal patient with no ocular involvement may be returned to a normal (euthyroid) state after treatment for hyperthyroidism, only to develop ocular Graves' disease many months later.

The best approach is to consider the diagnosis of Graves' disease in all cases of acquired motility impairment. Definitive diagnosis of Graves' restrictive myopathy is based on orbital sonography, orbital CT scanning, or magnetic resonance imaging. These studies will reveal swollen, congested extraocular muscles. In most cases, the tendinous insertions of the extraocular muscles into the sclera are not inflamed, and infiltration is limited to the muscle tissue itself. This helps differentiate ocular Graves' disease from other forms of extraocular muscle inflammation.[43]

Myasthenia Gravis

Myasthenia gravis is another great imposter of neurologic disease and paralytic strabismus. This autoimmune disorder can affect any of the extraocular muscles and tends to present with variable ptosis, with or without diplopia. Pathogenesis appears to involve production of antibodies specific for acetylcholine receptors on skeletal muscles.[20] The impact on function is that the muscle responds as if it were receiving insufficient transmitter (as though reduced amounts of acetylcholine were being released). This manifests as skeletal muscle weakness that is variable and that can be exaggerated by prolonged or repeated contraction. Characteristically, muscle strength varies from minute to minute, day to day, and week to week. Fatigue, exhaustion, stress, and illness can cause exacerbations of weakness.

Like Graves' ophthalmolopathy, ocular myasthenia is often misdiagnosed. Generally, any acquired motility disorder in which the pupils are normal should be considered potential myasthenia, and an appropriate evaluation made.

Myasthenia can occur at any age. Myasthenics younger than 40 years are most likely to be female. Beyond middle age, men and women are equally affected. Over 90% of myasthenics will have ocular muscle involvement and over 75% have ptosis or diplopia as their initial concern.[22] Thus, myasthenics often are seen initially by eye and vision care providers.

While 20–50% of myasthenia patients have disease that remains localized to the ocular skeletal muscles, many will develop more generalized systemic involvement. Nonocular manifestations typically become apparent within 2 years after the onset of eye signs. The likelihood of generalized systemic involvement decreases with the passage of each additional year. Treatment may consist of oral pyridostigmine bromide (Mestinon), which is an anticholinesterase drug that decreases muscle weakness by inhibiting the destruction of acetylcholine at the neuromuscular junction.

Myasthenia gravis is an autoimmune disease, and many affected patients show clinical evidence of additional autoimmune problems. Thus, myasthenics should be evaluated for dysthyroid disease, lupus, rheumatoid disease, and other connective tissue disorders. Because approximately 10% of myasthenics harbor tumors or hyperplasias of the thymus gland, standard practice should include radiologic assessment for thymoma.[44]

REFERENCES

1. Leigh RJ, Zee DS. The Neurology of Eye Movements. Philadelphia: FA Davis, 1983;2.
2. Daroff RB, Troost BT, Leigh RJ. Supranuclear Disorders of Eye Movements. In JS Glaser (ed), Neuro-ophthalmology (2nd ed). Philadelphia: Lippincott, 1990;299–323.
3. Fox PT, Fox JM, Raichle ME, Burde RM. The role of cerebral cortex in the generation of voluntary saccades: A positron emission tomographic study. J Neurophysiol 1985;54:348–69.
4. Pierrot-Deseilligny C, Gray F, Brunet P. Infarcts of both inferior parietal lobules with impairment of visually guided eye movements, peripheral inattention and optic ataxia. Brain 1986;109:81–97.
5. Burde RM, Savino PJ. Gaze Disturbances. In RM Burde, PJ Savino, JD Trobe (eds), Clinical Decisions in Neuro-ophthalmology. St Louis: Mosby-Year Book, 1993;208.
6. Steiner I, Melamed E. Conjugate eye deviation after acute hemispheric stroke. Ann Neurol 1984;16:509.
7. Pierrot-Deseilligny C, Rivaud S, Penet C, Rigolet MH. Latencies of visually guided saccades in unilateral hemispheric cerebral lesions. Ann Neurol 1987;21:138–48.
8. Newman NM. Supranuclear Eye Movement Systems and Their Substrates. In NM Newman (ed), Neuro-ophthalmology: A Practical Text. Norwalk, CT: Appleton & Lange, 1992;171–80.
9. Bogousslavsky J, Meienberg O. Eye movement disorders in brain-stem and cerebellar stroke. Arch Neurol 1987;44:141–8.
10. Buttner-Ennever JA, Buttner U, Cohen B, Baumgartner G. Vertical gaze paralysis and the rostral interstitial nucleus of the medial longitudinal fasciculus. Brain 1982;105:125–49.
11. Optican LM, Robinson DA. Cerebellar-dependent adaptive control of primate saccadic system. J Neurophysiol 1980;44:1058–76.
12. Tusa RJ, Zee DS. Cerebral Control of Smooth Pursuit and Optokinetic Nystagmus. In S Lessell, JTW Van Dalen (eds), Current Neuro-ophthalmology (Vol 2). Chicago: Mosby-Year Book, 1989;115–46.
13. Glickstein M, Cohen JL, Dixon B, et al. Corticopontine visual projections in macaque monkeys. J Comp Neurol 1980;190:209–29.
14. Henn V, Lang W, Hepp K, Reisine H. Experimental gaze palsies in monkeys and their relation to human pathology. Brain 1984;107:619–36.
15. Troost BT, Abel LA. Pursuit Disorders. In G Lennerstrand, DS Zee, EL Keller (eds), Functional Basis of Ocular Motility Disorders. New York: Pergamon, 1982;511–7.
16. Mays LE, Porter JD, Gamlin PDR, Tello CA. Neural control of vergence eye movements: neurons encoding vergence velocity. J Neurophysiol 1986;56:1007–21.
17. Mays LE. Neural control of vergence eye movements: convergence and divergence neurons in midbrain. J Neurophysiol 1984;51:1091–108.
18. Roper-Hall G, Burde RM. Diagnosis and management of divergence paresis. Am Orthop J 1987;37:113–21.
19. Glaser JS. Neuro-ophthalmologic examination: general considerations and special techniques. In JS Glaser (ed), Neuro-ophthalmology (2nd ed). Philadelphia: Lippincott, 1990;37–60.
20. Seybold ME. Myasthenia gravis: a clinical and basic science review. JAMA 1983;250:2516–24.
21. Hyland HH, Barnett HJM. The pathogenesis of cranial nerve palsies associated with intracranial aneurysms. Proc Royal Soc Med 1956;47:141–3.

22. Glaser JS, Bachynski B. Infranuclear Disorders of Eye Movement. In JS Glaser (ed), Neuro-ophthalmology (2nd ed). Philadelphia: Lippincott, 1990;361–418.
23. Bajandas FJ, Kline LB. Neuro-ophthalmology Review Manual (2nd ed). Thorofare, NJ: Slack, 1987;43–66, 87–96.
24. Weber RB, Daroff RB, Mackey EA. Pathology of oculomotor nerve palsy in diabetics. Neurology 1970;20:835–8.
25. Newman NM. Nuclear and Infranuclear Control of Eye Movements. In NM Newman (ed), Neuro-ophthalmology: A Practical Text. Norwalk, CT: Appleton & Lange, 1992;197–216.
26. Younge BR, Sutula F. Analysis of trochlear nerve palsies: diagnosis, etiology, and treatment. Mayo Clin Proc 1977;52:11–2.
27. Khawam E, Scott AB, Jampolsky A. Acquired superior oblique palsy. Arch Ophthalmol 1967;77:761–8.
28. Miller MT, Urist MJ, Folk ER, Chapman LI. Superior oblique palsy presenting in late childhood. Am J Ophthalmol 1970;70:212–4.
29. Rush JA, Younge BR. Paralysis of cranial nerves III, IV, and VI: cause and prognosis in 1,000 cases. Arch Ophthalmol 1981;99:76–9.
30. O'Connor PS, Glaser JS. Intracavernous Aneurysms and Isolated Sixth Nerve Palsy. In JL Smith (ed), Neuro-Ophthalmology Focus. New York: Masson, 1980;155.
31. Asbury AK, Aldredge H, Hershberg R, Fisher CM. Oculomotor palsy in diabetes mellitus: a clinico-pathological study. Brain 1970;93:555–66.
32. Harley RD. Paralytic strabismus in children. Etiologic incidence and management of the third, fourth, and sixth nerve palsies. Ophthalmology 1980;87:24–43.
33. Hoyt WF, Daroff RB. Supranuclear Disorders of Ocular Control Systems in Man: Clinical, Anatomical, and Physiological Correlations. In P Bach-y-Rita, CC Collins, JE Hyde (eds), The Control of Eye Movements. New York: Academic, 1971;175–235.
34. Zee DS, Hain TC, Carl JR. Abduction nystagmus and internuclear ophthalmoplegia. Ann Neurol 1982;21:383–6.
35. Kirkham TH, Katsarkas A. An electrooculographic study of internuclear ophthalmoplegia. Ann Neurol 1977;2:385–9.
36. Gonyea EF. Bilateral internuclear ophthalmoplegia: association with occlusive cerebrovascular disease. Arch Neurol 1974;31:168–73.
37. Burde RM, Savino PJ, Trobe JD. Proptosis and Adnexal Masses. In RM Burde, PJ Savino, JD Trobe (eds), Clinical Decisions in Neuro-ophthalmology. St. Louis: Mosby-Year Book, 1993;379–416.
38. Trobe JD, Glaser JS, Post JD. Meningiomas and aneurysms of the cavernous sinus: neuro-ophthalmologic features. Arch Ophthalmol 1978;96:457–67.
39. Barrow DL, Spector RH, Braun IF. Classification and treatment of spontaneous carotid-cavernous sinus fistulas. J Neurosurg 1985;62:248–56.
40. Seybold ME, Daroff RB. The office tensilon test for ocular myasthenia. Arch Neurol 1986;43;842–9.
41. Gray LG. Paralytic strabismus. In JE Terry (ed), Ocular Disease: Detection, Diagnosis, and Treatment. Springfield, IL: Charles C Thomas, 1984;314–48.
42. Fries PD, Char DH. Hyperthyroidism and Hypothyroidism. In DH Gold, Weingeist TA (eds), The Eye in Systemic Disease. Philadelphia: Lippincott, 1990;86–8.
43. Leib ML, Michalos P. Orbital Computed Tomography. In S Lessell, JTW Van Dalen (eds), Current Neuro-ophthalmology (Vol 3). St. Louis: Mosby-Year Book, 1991;377–88.
44. Sweeney PJ, O'Donovan PB. Myasthenia gravis, Thymoma, and the Anterior Junction Line. In JL Smith (ed), Neuro-ophthalmology Now. New York: Field, Rich, and Assoc., 1986;239–44.

11

Evaluation of the Lacrimal System

Gerald G. Melore

Disorders of the lacrimal system are frequently encountered in ophthalmic practice. Entities that fall within this category of ocular disease actually result from a number of different pathologic processes affecting various components of the lacrimal system. Included are disorders affecting tear secretion (quality and quantity), tear distribution, and tear drainage. Patients with lacrimal system diseases, however, commonly have similar symptoms, despite very different physiologic processes accounting for their complaints. An example of this is a patient complaining of epiphora (i.e., tearing that spills onto the outer lid or cheek). This could be attributed to excess tear production or to a reduction in tear outflow, two very different causes for a similar end result. In addition, there are a number of possible causes for each of these basic problems. For example, excess tear production can be the result of tumors or inflammation affecting the lacrimal gland or its neuronal supply, conjunctival or corneal irritation secondary to dryness, foreign body or trauma, systemic disease such as hypothyroidism, and, finally, psychogenic influences associated with emotional states. A reduction in tear outflow can also result from several different causes, including congenital punctal stenosis, traumatic or surgical disruption of the lacrimal drainage route, dacryocystitis (inflammation within the lacrimal sac), or age-related stenosis of the lacrimal duct.

During the evaluation of a patient with a suspected lacrimal system disorder, it is necessary to approach the problem systematically to sort out the basic type of defect (i.e., a problem with tear production [secretory system], surface disease, or tear drainage [excretory system]).

LACRIMAL SYSTEM ANATOMY

Secretory System: Anatomy and Physiology of the Tear Film

The tear film has several functions and is necessary for the normal health and integrity of the corneal and conjunctival surfaces. It smooths out the irregular surface of the cornea, yielding better refraction of light. It also provides oxygen to the avascular corneal tissue and the conjunctiva and provides lubrication during the action of blinking. In addition, the tear layer contains a number of substances that function to provide immunity and nutrition.

The tear film has three basic anatomic components: (1) an outer or superficial lipid layer, (2) a middle aqueous layer, and (3) an inner mucin layer (Figure 11-1). Each of these layers originates from different secretory structures within the ocular adnexa, and each has a unique physiologic role in the maintenance of the anterior ocular surface.

Lipid Layer

The most superficial component of the tear film is the lipid layer. This is an oily layer that inhibits evaporation of fluid from the thick aqueous layer. Secretions that constitute the lipid layer primarily arise from the meibomian glands, which are large, linear glands situated side-by-side within the tarsal plates of the upper and lower lids (Figure 11-2). The glands are oriented perpendicular to the lid margins. There are approximately 30–40 of these glands within the upper tarsus and 20–30 in the lower. Also contributing in part to the lipid layer are the glands of Zeis, which are small modified sebaceous glands connected with the lash follicles at the eyelid margins.

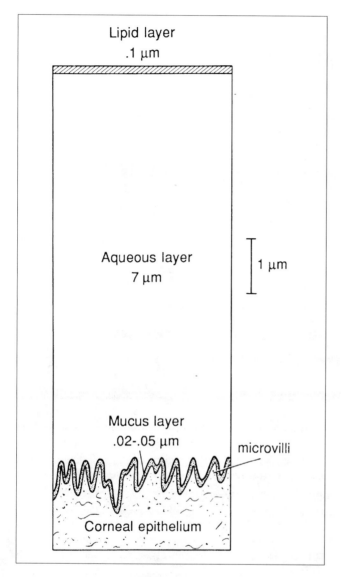

FIGURE 11-1
The components of the tear film.

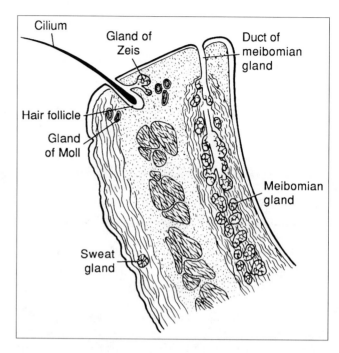

FIGURE 11-2
Cross section of the eyelid illustrating some of its glandular components. The meibomian glands and the glands of Zeis provide lipid secretions to the tear film. The glands of Moll located near the base of the lashes are modified sweat glands.

substantia propria of the conjunctiva (Figure 11-3). There are approximately 20 of these glands located within the upper conjunctival fornix and six to eight within the lower. The glands of Wolfring are located along the upper border of the tarsal plate. The plica and the caruncle are histologically the same glandular tissue as the glands of Krause and Wolfring, and it has been surmised that this tissue may also contribute to basal secretion of the aqueous layer.

The main lacrimal gland primarily contributes aqueous tears under different circumstances. These circumstances may include instances of ocular surface irritation or psychogenic stimuli. Neuronal control to the main lacrimal gland is not completely understood; however, the autonomic nervous system clearly plays a major role.[1] Primary control is through the parasympathetic system. Any sympathetic contribution is controversial.

Mucin Layer

The mucin layer is the thinnest and innermost layer of the tear film. It provides a thin hydrophilic covering to the normally hydrophobic corneal epithelium. This allows for an even spreading of the other tear film components

Aqueous Layer

The middle layer of the tear film consists of an aqueous layer, which constitutes the vast majority of the tear film thickness. Its composition is approximately 98% water. Other components include proteins, organic salts, glucose, metabolites, and electrolytes. Providing functions such as lubrication, nutrition, and immunity, the aqueous layer also cleanses the ocular surface by flushing away debris.

Under usual circumstances, the aqueous layer is secreted by the accessory lacrimal glands of Krause and Wolfring. The glands of Krause are embedded within the

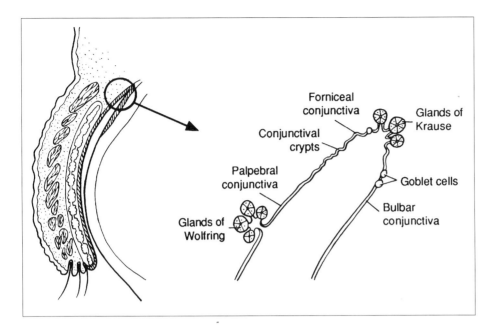

FIGURE 11-3
Accessory lacrimal glands of Krause and Wolfring. The glands of Krause are embedded within the conjunctival substantia propria in the upper fornix. The glands of Wolfring are located near the upper border of the tarsal plate. Also shown are goblet cells, which secrete mucin.

over the ocular surface. Mucin is produced by the goblet cells, which are contained within the conjunctiva (see Figure 11-3).

Excretory System

Bony Conduit

Within the nasofrontal process of the maxilla and the anterior nasal portion of the orbit is the lacrimal fossa, a depression in which lies the nasolacrimal sac. From there the nasolacrimal canal, which contains the nasolacrimal duct, extends downward inside the lateral wall of the nose and opens into the meatus (space) under the inferior turbinate bone (Figure 11-4). The inferior turbinate is situated on the outer wall of the nasal passageway. It consists of a layer of thin spongy bone, curved on itself like a scroll. It is covered by the mucosal membrane lining the nose, and it articulates by its margins with the groove on the back of the nasal process of the superior maxillary, and thus contributes to the formation of the canal for the nasolacrimal duct. The inferior turbinate bone therefore is an eave-like structure under which the nasolacrimal duct opens.

The nasolacrimal canal is about 16 mm posterior from the anterior tip of the turbinate and is located between the anterior third and middle third of the meatus of the turbinate.[2] The nasolacrimal duct is 16–18 mm above the floor of the nose laterally. Individual anatomic differences and alterations can extend the canal further downward, resulting in varying positions of the duct opening in the lateral wall of the nose.

Membranous Conduit

Contained within the bony conduit and the nasal portion of the eyelids is the epithelium-lined tear apparatus through which the tears pass from the eyelids into the nose. The openings for this membranous conduit in the eyelids consist of an upper and lower puncta. Both are located on the lid margin about 6 mm from the inner canthus and point backward toward and in contact with the globe. The puncta fit into a groove formed by the plica semilunaris and the globe, and tears are directed along this groove into the puncta. The puncta are approximately 0.3 mm in diameter and are surrounded by a ring of connective tissue. When the eyelids are closed, both the upper and lower puncta are directly opposed and in contact with each other.[3]

The punctum opens up into the canalicular portion of the drainage apparatus. The canaliculus lies within the eyelid margin and consists of a 2-mm vertical component and an 8-mm horizontal, nasally oriented component (see Figure 11-4). The junction of the vertical and horizontal component of the canaliculus is called the ampulla and is about 2 mm in diameter. The linear diameter of the canaliculus varies during blinking. When the eyelids are closed during each blink, tears are drawn into the excretory system, and the lumen diameter increases in size under the force of the pumped tears. Nasal to the inner canthus, the upper and lower canaliculi join to form a common canaliculus emptying into the lateral wall of the nasolacrimal sac at the junction of the upper one third and lower two thirds of the sac. At their joining is a small dila-

FIGURE 11-4

The lacrimal drainage apparatus, or excretory system, consists of the canaliculi, the nasolacrimal sac, and the nasolacrimal duct. The nasolacrimal duct empties into the inferior meatus located under the inferior turbinate bone of the nasal passageway.

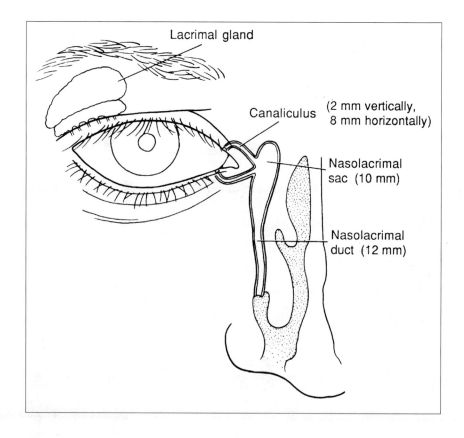

Lacrimal gland

Canaliculus

(2 mm vertically, 8 mm horizontally)

Nasolacrimal sac (10 mm)

Nasolacrimal duct (12 mm)

tion called the ampulla of Maier. This common opening forms an internal punctum, which is slitlike with folds of tissue surrounding it. These folds act as a valve to prevent the retrograde flow of tears back into the canalicular system.

The nasolacrimal sac is approximately 10 mm in length along its vertical dimension, and is located in the bony lacrimal fossa on the anterior aspect of the medial wall of the orbit. For the most part, the lumen of the sac is collapsed and is slitlike when the eyelids are open, but the lumen balloons out and fills with tears when the eyelids close during blinking.[2] The nasolacrimal duct, an extension of the nasolacrimal sac, travels about 12 mm through the nasolacrimal canal and then terminates in the inferior meatus under the inferior turbinate bone. At the end of the nasolacrimal duct is the valve of Hasner (plica lacrimalis), which is a mucous membrane fold that serves to prevent the retrograde flow of air or nasal secretions. The opening of the duct is about 3–4 cm posterior from the external naris of the nose.[4]

Dynamics of Tear Flow

The process of the elimination of tears is not passive and is not the result of gravity; rather, it is a result of a pumping mechanism induced by the action of the orbicularis oculi muscle.[5] The route of the tears on entering the lacrimal system is as follows: Tear molecules flow across the surface of the globe and eyelids, and each blink pushes fluid with the meniscus along the lower lid margin (the River of Norn) nasally, where it drains into the puncta (Figure 11-5). On passing through the punctal opening, the tears traverse the canaliculi, and then enter the common canaliculus and inner punctum before draining into the lacrimal sac. Once inside the sac, tears flow downward through the sac and into the nasolacrimal duct. Once through the duct, the tears drain to the floor of the nose, which is sloped backward, causing the tears to flow into the throat where they are swallowed.

Jones[6] has summarized the dynamics of tear flow further by stating that a negative pressure is created within the drainage system as the eyelids relax after each blink. Tears are thus pulled from the lacrimal lake and through the punctal opening. When the eyelids are open, the lacrimal sac is normally collapsed; however, as the eyelids close, tears are squeezed into the sac. Negative pressure within the lacrimal sac helps prevent the retrograde flow of tears back into the canalicular system. Also preventing retrograde flow of tears are membranous valves within the lacrimal sac and duct.

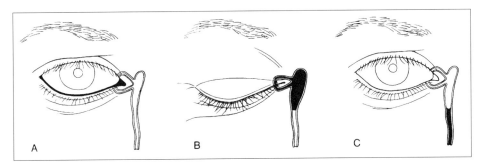

FIGURE 11-5

Dynamics of tear flow. A. Tears collect predominantly within the tear meniscus along the lower lid margin and then flow toward the punctal opening. B. After reaching the punctal openings, tears flow through the canalicular system and into the nasolacrimal sac. Because of gravity and the accumulation of most tear fluid along the lower tear meniscus, only a small percentage of tears drain through the upper canalicular channel. C. Once inside the nasolacrimal sac, tears flow downward through the nasolacrimal duct and into the inferior meatal space of the nasal passageway. (Adapted with permission from JJ Kanski. Clinical Ophthalmology [3rd ed]. London: Butterworth-Heinemann, 1994.)

DISEASES OF THE LACRIMAL SYSTEM

Diseases of the Secretory System

Dry Eye Syndrome

Dry eye syndrome is a common disorder seen in everyday practice, particularly among the elderly. There are several different potential causes. A deficiency in the outermost lipid layer of the tear film will result in poor quality tears that will be subject to excessive evaporation, leading to dry eyes. Similarly, if there is a deficiency in the middle aqueous layer of the tear film, the quantity of tears will be reduced, which also may cause dry eyes. Corneal irregularities or irregularities along the lid margin—e.g., blepharitis, lid lesions, and notches, can cause dry eyes because of the uneven spread of tears over the globe by the blinking lids.

Patients with dry eyes of different causes usually have similar complaints. The symptoms include burning, stinging, aching, foreign body sensation, a feeling of dryness sometimes followed by tearing, and an accumulation of debris in the conjunctival sac. The degree of symptoms varies from patient to patient, and ocular surface changes can be mild to severe. The syndrome at all levels is characterized not only by a reduction in tear formation, quality, or quantity, but also by conjunctival or corneal changes, which may be demonstrated with clinical testing. The potential causes of dry eye syndrome are quite extensive. Table 11-1 provides a listing of these according to the layer of the tear film that is affected.

Lipid Deficiency   Lipid deficiency of the tear film is usually the result of chronic blepharitis of the eyelids. Here, bacteria cause the breakdown of meibomian secretions into free fatty acids, which causes instability of the tear film leading to dry spot formation. In addition, any condition that adversely affects meibomian gland function can potentially lead to an inadequate lipid layer. An example is trauma leading to destruction of the meibomian glands or scarring of the meibomian gland orifices. Chronic meibomianitis may also potentially alter the quantity or quality of the lipid layer.

Aqueous Deficiency   Aqueous deficiency may be caused by many different conditions that result in a partial or complete deficiency in aqueous tear production, and the resultant clinical condition is referred to as keratoconjunctivitis sicca (KCS). It may exist as an isolated condition or in conjunction with certain systemic disorders, particularly connective tissue vascular disease.

The clinical signs of KCS include a scanty tear meniscus along the lower lid, excessive debris in the tear film, large mucous threads in the tear film, or any combination of these signs. Punctate staining with rose bengal and fluorescein is commonly present within the interpalpebral zone of the cornea and conjunctiva. In more severe cases, filaments of dried mucin and sheets of desquamating corneal epithelial cells adhere to the desiccated areas of the cornea. These devitalized cells and mucin readily retain rose bengal stain. Secondary infection is more likely with KCS than with other causes of dry eye, in part because the lack of aqueous results in lower amounts of lysozyme compromising the host defense mechanism. Staphylococcal

TABLE 11-1
Conditions Affecting the Layers of the Tear Film

Lipid layer
    Blepharitis (staphylococcal, seborrheic, mixed)
    Meibomianitis
    Rosacea
    Trauma
Aqueous layer
    Age-related atrophy of the lacrimal gland
    Collagen vascular disease (e.g., rheumatoid arthritis,
        systemic lupus erythematosis, scleroderma, polyarteritis)
    Sarcoidosis
    Lymphoma
    Congenital causes (Riley-Day syndrome, anhidrotic
        ectodermal dysplasia, congenital hypoplasia of the
        lacrimal gland)
    Dacryoadenitis
    Neurologic causes (tumors or other lesions affecting the
        innervational pathway of the lacrimal gland)
    Trauma
    Tumors of the lacrimal gland
Mucin layer
    Hypovitaminosis A
    Ocular pemphigoid
    Stevens-Johnson syndrome
    Trauma
    Trachoma

blepharitis and keratoconjunctivitis are commonly seen in patients with KCS. Keratoconjunctivitis sicca commonly manifests as a component of an autoimmune disorder known as Sjögren's syndrome, which is characterized by the triad of KCS, dry mouth (xerostomia), and a connective tissue disease.[7] At least two components of the triad must be present for the diagnosis to be made. Sjögren's syndrome may actually be divided into primary and secondary disease categories. Primary Sjögren's syndrome is characterized by the sicca complex (KCS and xerostomia) without recognizable evidence of an associated connective tissue disease. In secondary Sjögren's syndrome, at least one of the sicca components is present in addition to a recognizable connective tissue disease. Some reported systemic associations with KCS are listed in Table 11-1.

Mucin Deficiency Mucin deficiency disorders are not common. The main cause of a mucin deficiency is hypovitaminosis A. Vitamin A deficiency produces uneven wetting of the corneal surface, resulting in an unstable tear film. Any condition that causes inflammation of the conjunctiva and destruction of the goblet cells may also cause a mucin-deficient tear film. These conditions include ocular pemphigoid, Stevens-Johnson syndrome, trachoma, and chemical burns. The main clinical diagnostic sign of this type of dry eye is an unstable tear film manifested by an abnormally rapid break-up time.

Diagnostic Tests for Dry Eye

FLUORESCEIN DYE TEST Fluorescein dye will stain the corneal or conjunctival surface any time epithelial integrity is compromised. Hence, its use may be helpful in the diagnosis of dry eye disorders. Although fluorescein dye does not stain epithelial cells themselves, it pools within intercellular defects, thus highlighting punctate epithelial erosions characteristic of dry eye disorders. Although fluorescein staining is relatively nonspecific, occurring with any condition affecting epithelial integrity, characteristic staining patterns can be helpful in the diagnosis of a patient with dry eye syndrome. For example, in the aqueous-deficient patient, staining is interpalpebral and may be especially prominent along the inferior corneal and conjunctival surface. In someone with exposure keratitis secondary to nocturnal lagophthalmos or Bell's palsy, staining may occur exclusively inferiorly. Areas of "negative staining," whereby fluorescein is repelled from the corneal surface, may occur in mucin-deficient situations. Fluorescein staining of the ocular surface is best observed with the aid of a blue light.

ROSE BENGAL DYE TEST Rose bengal is a water-soluble dye that is customarily considered to stain dead or devitalized cells. The staining color of rose bengal is bright red and is observed with white light. The rose bengal dye test yields a direct evaluation of epithelial cell damage and an indirect measurement of tear volume deficiency. Rose bengal also stains mucus, which is often a prominent finding in dry eye conditions. Rose bengal can be applied to the ocular surface in two ways. One involves wetting the tip of a commercially available rose bengal strip with sterile saline, followed by brief application of the strip to the conjunctival surface. A 1% rose bengal solution may also be used and applied to the ocular surface in drop form. The liquid rose bengal seems to yield better results than the rose bengal strip but may be more irritating on instillation. This is probably related to the concentration of dye reaching the eye. For the application of two dyes at the same time, a drop of rose bengal solution can be placed onto the tip of a fluorescein strip.

As with fluorescein dye, the staining pattern with rose bengal tends to be interpalpebral in a patient with dry eye syndrome. Staining may be more pronounced inferiorly, and the overall staining pattern of the cornea and conjunctiva may be more evident on spreading the eyelids wide apart (Figure 11-6). The conjunctival staining pattern consists of characteristic triangle-shaped zones with their bases on either side of the cornea.

SCHIRMER I TEST The Schirmer I test can be helpful in determining decreased lacrimal secretion. However, it is a gross test at best, and the diagnosis of dry eye cannot be made on the basis of Schirmer results alone. Schirmer testing is described in detail later in this chapter.

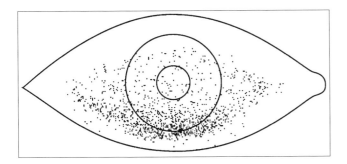

FIGURE 11-6
Schematic representation of interpalpebral staining pattern secondary to keratoconjunctivitis sicca (KCS). (Courtesy of Daniel K. Roberts, O.D.)

TEAR BREAKUP TIME The tear breakup time (TBUT) test is commonly used to assess the wetting quality of the tear film. The TBUT is defined as the time interval between a complete blink and the initial development of a random dry spot on the corneal surface. Dry spot function is typically visualized with the aid of fluorescein dye. In clinical practice the TBUT is often erroneously thought to exclusively indicate a measure of the quantity or quality of the aqueous layer of the tear film. In actuality, the mechanics of tear breakup are quite complex and are dependent on many variables affecting the tear film stability. For example, a deficiency in the mucin layer can lead to dry spot function because of the inability of the aqueous layer to spread over the normally hydrophobic epithelial surface. Additionally, a scant lipid layer may lead to quicker evaporation of the aqueous layer and subsequent dry spot formation as detected during the TBUT test. Therefore, it is false to conclude that a reduced TBUT is always an indication of aqueous deficiency; rather, it is a sign of overall tear film instability, the cause of which needs further evaluation. Whereas some patients with aqueous deficiency do indeed exhibit a decreased TBUT, some may not.

The TBUT test is performed by placing plain fluorescein dye into the conjunctival cul-de-sac, followed by visualization of the precorneal tear film with the aid of the blue slit lamp filter. The patient should keep his or her eyes fully open after providing an initial complete blink. Afterward the examiner begins counting in seconds until the first appearance of a random spot within the diffusely spread dye. Typically, less than 10 seconds is considered indicative of an unstable tear film and 10–15 seconds is considered borderline.[8]

OTHER TESTS Although there have been many attempts at development of additional testing procedures to aid in the evaluation of patients with dry eyes, none has gained widespread clinical acceptance because of questions regarding their validity as well as practicality in the office setting. Included is the determination of lysozyme and lactoferrin concentrations in the tear film. Both of these proteins are produced by the lacrimal gland and are present in reduced concentrations in KCS, perhaps even before aqueous production is abnormal.[9-11] One method used to determine lysozyme concentration is referred to as the agar diffusion lysozyme test.[12] Here, a tear-saturated Schirmer strip is placed on an agar medium inoculated with a suspension of *Micrococcus lysodeikticus* bacteria. Lysozyme, a bacteriolytic enzyme, will then cause a zone of lysis around the strip, which is correlated with lysozyme concentration. Evaluation of lactoferrin concentration has been marketed with a commercially available assay called the Lactoplate test (Eagle Vision, Inc., Memphis, TN). With this test, a small disc of tear-wetted filter paper is placed on an agar surface for 72 hours, followed by measurement of a precipitation ring, which is correlated with lactoferrin concentration.

Additional tests include the microscopic evaluation of epithelial cell changes characteristic of dry eye disorders. Samples have been obtained through either routine conjunctival scraping or via a technique referred to as impression cytology. Impression cytology is a technique whereby a specimen one to three cell layers thick is collected through the application of circular discs of cellulose acetate filter material onto the ocular surface.[13] Cellular morphology may be thoroughly examined for goblet cell density, squamous metaplasia, and the presence of inflammatory cells. Tear film osmolarity, which has been determined to be higher in patients with KCS, has also been inconsistently used in the evaluation of the dry eye patient.[14]

Treatment for Dry Eye
REPLACEMENT OF TEARS Artificial tears remain the mainstay in the treatment of dry eye syndromes. In recent years there have been several different types of preparations manufactured for routine use. Ideally an artificial tear solution has relatively low viscosity yet exhibits a good retention time within the eye. It is also compatible with the surface physiology of the eye, nontoxic, and comfortable on instillation. Although various attempts have been made to improve these qualities, the ideal tear supplement has yet to become available. Usually, improvement in one area leads to compromise in another—e.g., improved retention time at the expense of higher viscosity. Nevertheless, overall improvements have been made in current preparations, and artificial tears are relatively effective for the relief of symptoms in many patients.

The major problem with most solutions is the rate at which the drops dissipate from the eye. Consequently, tear supplements often must be instilled into the eye numerous times daily. Exact usage is dependent on the severity of the disease and the patient's symptoms.

The most basic tear preparation consists of an isotonic sodium chloride solution. Over the years, numerous polymers have been added to increase efficiency of the solution. Although there are several different types of tear supplements currently being marketed as well as several being studied, selection of the most appropriate solution is often an uncertain task for an individual patient. On the recommendation of a particular supplement, the patient should be monitored for his or her response. If results are unsatisfactory, then a substitute can be prescribed.

In addition to artificial tear solutions, bland lubricating ointments are also prescribed for dry eye conditions. Because of their high viscosity, retention is very good, but their use during the day is usually not tolerated because of their blurring effects on vision. Consequently, ointment preparations are usually prescribed for use at bedtime. The usual dose is a 0.5- to 1.0-inch ribbon in the lower cul-de-sac. Ointments are very beneficial in instances of exposure, such as may occur in nocturnal lagophthalmos or proptosis secondary to thyroid eye disease.

Timed-release artificial tear inserts consisting of 5 mm hydroxypropyl cellulose rods (Lacriserts, Merck, Sharp, and Dohme Co., West Point, PA) are available for severe cases of dry eye or in situations where it is difficult or impractical for the patient to repeatedly instill drops. The rods are placed in the inferior cul-de-sac and then allowed to slowly dissolve, which may take up to 12 hours after insertion. Cellulosic inserts are relatively expensive and can cause blurred vision, especially during nearpoint tasks. A rather fine degree of manual dexterity is required for insertion, so assistance from a family member or caregiver may be necessary for some patients. If the dry eye is severe and hydration is minimal, Lacriserts need to be used in conjunction with an artificial tear solution to promote dissolution of the rod.

PRESERVATION OF EXISTING TEARS   Moist chamber shields for use with spectacles provide a relatively air-tight chamber around the eyes. Evaporated tears then remain trapped within the enclosed spaces surrounding the eyes. This provides a moist atmosphere and helps retard further evaporation of tears.

Soft hydrophilic bandage contact lenses can be used to relieve the discomfort of dry eye by providing a moisture reservoir as well as by preventing the constant friction between the upper lid and cornea. Generally, their use is limited to more severe cases or when filamentary keratitis is present.[15] Bandage contacts are used in conjunction with artificial tears so they do not dry out. Frequent replacement of these lenses is necessary because deposits develop quickly. In addition, secondary infections are more prone to occur with bandage contact lenses because of an immunologically compromised tear film as well as stagnation of the tears beneath the lenses. Therefore, the prudent use of bandage contact lenses is necessary. A prophylactic antibiotic may be prescribed concurrently in some instances.[15]

A common method for preserving existing tears involves punctal occlusion. The puncta may be occluded temporarily or permanently. The decision to proceed with permanent punctal occlusion should be made with caution, however, because keratoconjunctivitis sicca tends to have a waxing and waning course. If the puncta are permanently occluded and tear production subsequently increases, epiphora may result. An alternative to permanent occlusion is the use of temporary intracanalicular collagen implants or removable silicone plugs. Because of the reversibility of the occlusion, either of these devices can be used as a trial to evaluate those patients who might benefit from more permanent occlusion. Collagen plugs are small, water-soluble rods that gradually dissolve within about 1 week after their insertion into the upper and lower canalicular channels (Figure 11-7). Silicone plugs are more permanent devices used for punctal occlusion, yet the occlusion is still reversible. They are relatively easy to install and can be removed if necessary with forceps (Figure 11-8).

When permanent punctal occlusion is deemed necessary in more severe cases of dry eye, surgical intervention can be employed. Typically, this form of occlusion is performed via electrocautery or laser photocoagulation applied to the punctal orifice.

STIMULATION OF TEARS   The stimulation of tear production through pharmacologic therapy is an expanding area of study. Thus far, however, success has been very limited. Although aqueous tear production is at least partially regulated by the autonomic nervous system, very little is known regarding the complexity of the tear production process. Cholinergic agents (e.g., pilocarpine) are known to increase tear production. However, undesirable side effects are typically encountered. Locally, these include accommodative spasm and miosis, and systemically, cardiovascular and gastrointestinal disturbances occur. Other drugs that have been or are currently being studied include bromhexine hydrochloride,[16] eloisin,[17] estrogens,[18] and cyclosporine.[19-21]

SURGICAL MEASURES   Surgical intervention aside from electrocautery or laser photocoagulation for punctal closure is limited and is usually reserved for the most severe cases of dry eye. Furthermore, the use of argon laser has been shown to be ineffective for long-term punctal occlusion.[22] Typically, surgery is limited to creation of a partial tarsorrhaphy, whereby the palpebral aperture is

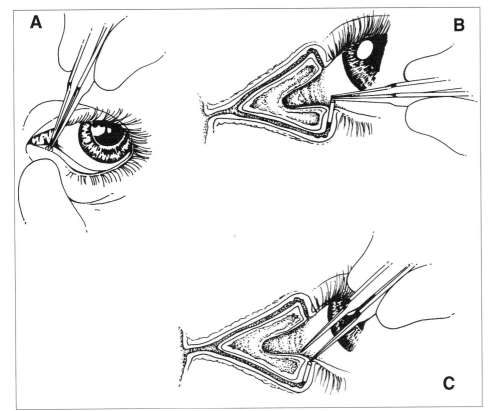

FIGURE 11-7
Insertion of temporary intra-canalicular collagen implants. A. Forceps are used to grasp the implant and then place it into the punctal opening. B, C. The tip of the forceps is then used to force the plug further into the canalicular system. (Redrawn with permission of Eagle Vision, Inc., Memphis, TN.)

reduced by joining the lateral aspects of the upper and lower lids. This allows for retention of central vision while decreasing evaporation from the ocular surface.

Dacryoadenitis

Dacryoadenitis is characterized by inflammatory enlargement of the main lacrimal gland, the causes of which include trauma, infection, and granulomatous disease such as sarcoidosis and Sjögren's syndrome. It is a rare condition that is acute or chronic and unilateral or bilateral. Typically, an S-shaped curvature to the upper eyelid is produced. There is a variable degree of tenderness, edema, and erythema. Either one or both sections of the gland (palpebral vs. orbital) may be affected.

The acute form is usually unilateral and is characterized by the S-shaped lid at the onset. Mild swelling and tenderness of the upper lid is present initially but later may develop into a preseptal cellulitis. Acute dacryoadenitis may be secondary to a systemic infection. If bacterial in nature, common causative organisms include *Staphylococcus aureus, Streptococcus* species, *Gonococcus,* and *Pneumococcus* organisms.[23] If viral in origin, mononucleosis and mumps are commonly implicated.[24] Acute dacryoadenitis is usually self-limiting, resolving in

4–8 weeks. Nevertheless, medical consultation may be indicated to rule out systemic associations.

Symptomatic relief for viral forms include ice packs for mild pain. Strong analgesics may be necessary if pain is severe. Cultures and smears of tear discharge are helpful in determining a specific etiologic agent in instances of bacteria-related disease. Oral and possibly intravenous antibiotics are necessary when bacterial infection is present.

The chronic form of dacryoadenitis is more difficult to diagnose. If it follows an acute episode, it may gradually resolve over months with slow regression of the swollen gland. If the enlargement persists or increases in size, a biopsy is necessary to rule out tumor formation.

Diseases of the Excretory System

Upper Excretory System

If the examiner can see the patient's punctum without touching the lids, the punctum is out of position. Similarly, if the examiner can see the lower punctum when the patient looks up while keeping the head in the primary position, the punctum's position during blinking may not be adequate for normal tear elimination.[25] Often in aging patients the lower punctum may become everted as a result

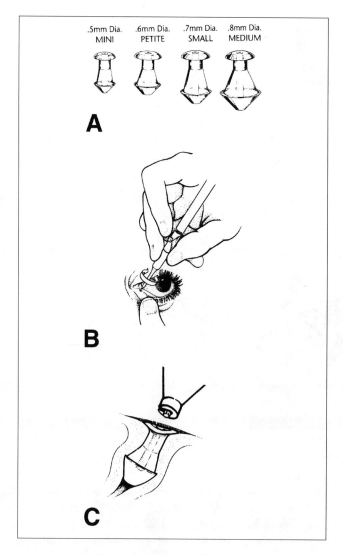

FIGURE 11-8

*Silicone punctal plugs for the treatment of aqueous deficiency.
A. The different sizes of plugs provided by Eagle Vision, Inc.
B. After punctal dilation, this type of silicone plug is inserted
with a slight rolling motion using a specialized preloaded device
provided by the manufacturer. C. After the plug is inserted to
the base of the dome head, it is released from the applicator
device. (Redrawn with permission of Eagle Vision, Inc., Memphis, TN.)*

of senile ectropion. The extent of the eversion can vary
from slight to severe. When the punctum is out of position
for any reason, tear drainage is most likely affected.

If the punctum is mildly displaced secondary to a lid
problem (e.g., a lid growth) treatment of the underlying
condition may place the punctum in its normal position.
If mild punctal eversion is caused by an early state of

involutional senile ectropion, the patient may be counseled
to wipe the teary eye with a clean tissue or handkerchief
in an "up and in" motion of the lower inner
canthus. This will place the flaccid skin of the lower lid
with the punctum into its normal position. If this is
unsuccessful in the symptomatic patient, surgical correction
may be required.[26] If the punctum has a partially
closed or stenosed orifice, careful dilation with a
punctal dilator may reestablish the punctum's patency.
If the punctum is completely stenosed, a surgical
"one or three snip procedure" may be necessary to create
an opening into the lacrimal drainage system.[27]

If the canaliculus develops stenosis, or canaliculitis
results in cicatricial shrinkage of the lumen, silicone rubber
tubing may be threaded continuously through the
upper and lower canaliculi and left in place for 3–4 months
while the canalicular wall heals around it.[28]

Lower Excretory System

Dacryocystitis   Dacryocystitis is an infection or inflammation
of the lacrimal sac. There are two types: chronic
and acute. In the chronic form, if an obstruction exists high
up in the sac, or in the canaliculus, epiphora may be the
only symptom; however, if the obstruction is in the sac
proper or in the nasolacrimal duct, there may be epiphora
with some degree of infection.[29] The sac becomes a stagnant
pool of tear film debris and infectious agents. The sac
may or may not be tender depending on the degree of infection
or inflammation. If the examiner applies digital pressure
externally over the area of the sac, the patient may
feel tenderness, and pus may be expressed out of the lower
punctum (Figure 11-9). The latter sign is pathognomonic
of dacryocystitis. The most common organisms in the adult
chronic from of dacryocystitis are *Staphylococcus, Streptococcus,*
and *Pneumococcus* species. *Haemophilus influenzae*
is the usual organism in children.[29]

Treatment of chronic dacryocystitis consists of lacrimal
sac drainage, which is performed by external massage and
irrigation in conjunction with the use of topical and systemic
antibiotics. Daily external massage over the sac will
help to empty the sac, as will daily irrigation of the sac
with an appropriate topical antibiotic ophthalmic solution.
Once the dacryocystitis quiets down, a dacryocystorhinostomy
(DCR) may be necessary if lacrimal drainage
is not adequate. A DCR is a surgical procedure characterized
by the creation of an alternative tear drainage route
into the nasal cavity.

The acute form of dacryocystitis is quite painful. A distal
obstruction in the sac or duct results in a distended sac
filled with infectious material. The infection often spreads
from the sac to the surrounding tissue, causing edema, erythema,
and pain in the medial canthal region (Figure 11-10).

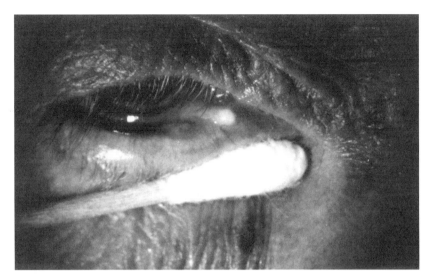

FIGURE 11-9
Expression of pus from the lower punctum secondary to chronic dacryocystitis.

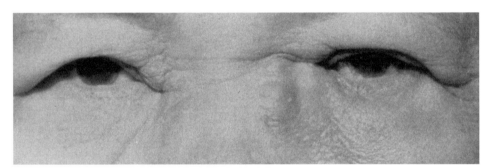

FIGURE 11-10
Acute staphylococcal dacryocystitis on the patient's left side. (Courtesy of Stephanie S. Messner, O.D.)

If an abscess is formed, the sac may need to be lanced from the skin side to evacuate its contents. Immediate attention is necessary or the sac may form a fistula and drain on its own. The bacterial infection needs to be controlled with topical and systemic antibiotics as well as daily irrigations with antibiotics. If cultures are performed, specific antibiotic therapy against identified infectious organisms may be initiated. In mild cases, treatment can be given on an outpatient basis. In severe cases, hospitalization requiring intravenous antibiotics and narcotic pain control may be needed. Again, drainage of the sac is necessary to relieve the pain and to reduce the infection. When the acute episode resolves, a DCR may be necessary if lacrimal drainage is impaired.

Miscellaneous Obstructions Obstructions in the lacrimal drainage system can lead to epiphora and dacryocystitis. Lacrimal system dacryoliths are fairly common, having an incidence of 10–30% in patients with chronic dacryocystitis. Obstructions of the nasolacrimal system in adults are often idiopathic in nature. Most likely, many occur because of an underlying anatomic predisposition. Foreign bodies of the canaliculus or sac often are a major cause of obstruction. The foreign bodies may consist of cilia, seeds, grit, insect parts, bristles, vegetable debris, paper dust, sawdust, or any other airborne materials that may find their way into the tear film.[30-32]

Lacrimal stones or casts can form in the lacrimal sac or duct as a result of fungal infections, organized blood clot, or mucus plugs. Almost all canalicular and sac obstructions resulting from mycotic infections occur in areas of fairly high seasonal temperatures. The most common organisms to cause this type of obstruction are *Actinomyces israelii* and *Candida albicans*.[33] Stones and casts are most common in heavy smokers and in people under 20 years old.

Nasal disease is also a major cause of obstruction. Swollen mucosa of the inferior turbinate resulting from nasal infection, heavy smoking, or chronic overuse of nasal sprays can lead to distal obstruction, which closes off the nasolacrimal duct.

Sometimes the casts or stones may pass through the system on their own, or irrigation of the system can force them out. Often the turbulence of the irrigation may only temporarily dislodge the cast so that the lacrimal system becomes patent. The patient may not experience epiphora for an indeterminate amount of time until the cast again works its way into a position to cause partial or complete obstruction of tear flow. Eventually these patients may need a DCR.

Finally, nasal or midfacial fractures are common causes of stenosis of the nasolacrimal canal. Tumors in the lacrimal sac area may also cause partial or complete occlusion of the nasolacrimal passage.

Dacryostenosis Dacryostenosis is a rather common condition in which the most distal portion of the nasolacrimal duct beneath the inferior turbinate fails to complete its canalization during the newborn period. Normally, the small membrane covering the opening to the nasolacrimal duct will spontaneously resolve 2–4 months after birth. In some instances, however, this process is delayed (or does not occur at all), resulting in acute dacryostenosis and possibly chronic epiphora. The use of topical antibiotics and regular digital massage over the sac will prevent symptoms and acute infection in 60–70% of cases. It is generally accepted that probing of the nasolacrimal system should only be done if the condition does not resolve in 3–4 months.[34]

DIAGNOSIS IN THE PATIENT WITH EPIPHORA

Epiphora may result from many causes and is the most common symptom in lacrimal system disorders. It may result from blockage or malfunction occurring anywhere along the drainage system or may be secondary to the production of a high volume of tears that cannot be normally drained away. Hence, many people who complain of epiphora do not have lacrimal obstruction. It is often helpful during initial questioning of patients to determine whether tearing is occurring unilaterally or bilaterally. Unilateral tearing is more likely a sign of inadequate tear drainage, whereas bilateral tearing may signal reflex tearing secondary to external influences such as dry eye syndrome.

External examination of a patient complaining of epiphora should be carefully performed and certain characteristics should be noted, including the blink rate and the extent of closure of the lids. Normally the blink rate should be frequent and characterized by full closure in order for the lacrimal pump to operate effectively. This observation should be made without the patient being aware of it. The position of the punctum should be noted. It should be pointing toward the globe into the lacrimal lake and should not be visible without slight eversion of the lid. The punctum should be open and not stenotic. Caution should be taken not to manipulate the lids before the punctum is evaluated. Slight manipulation can alter the usual position of the punctum, particularly in elderly patients with excessive and flaccid skin. The lid margins, especially the lower lid, should be observed for irregularities that may impede the flow of tears toward the punctum. Other external diseases should be noted that could cause hypersecretion secondary to reflex tearing (e.g., keratitis, infection, foreign body, and trichiasis). Dry eye syndrome should always be ruled out, since it commonly produces intermittent reflex tearing.

The clinician should apply external digital pressure over the lacrimal sac in an attempt to regurgitate pus through the punctal opening. Any discharge is indicative of dacryocystitis and obstruction in the nasolacrimal sac or duct.

The systematic evaluation of the lacrimal system is performed in two parts. The first involves testing the secretory system; the second, testing the excretory system. Schirmer tests are used to evaluate the secretory system, and Jones testing is used to evaluate the excretory system. Since the secretory system is made up of two parts, the basic secretors and the reflex secretors, the clinician must be able to distinguish the contribution made to total tear output by each secretory component. The basic secretors provide a basal level of moisture to the ocular surface during normal situations, whereas the reflex secretors provide tears under abnormal circumstances. The reflex secretors may be stimulated by emotional factors or by irritation of the fifth cranial nerve such as occurs in keratitis, sinusitis, or rhinitis.

Schirmer Tear Tests

Schirmer I Test

The Schirmer I test, also known as the standard Schirmer test, is ideally done before manipulation of the lids, refraction, tonometry, or instillation of any eyedrops, since all of these may stimulate reflex tearing (Table 11-2). Commonly used for this technique is a standardized strip of filter paper, which usually is bent and placed over the lower eyelid margin at the junction of the lateral and middle thirds (Figure 11-11). The test is done on both eyes with the patient in a sitting position and the lights dimmed. The patient is instructed to keep both eyes open but to blink normally. Gaze should be fixed slightly upward to help avoid corneal irritation and subsequent reflex tearing. After 5 minutes the strips are gently removed and the

TABLE 11-2
Schirmer Tear Tests

Schirmer I test (standard Schirmer test)
A standardized strip of filter paper is placed over the lower eyelid margin. The length of wetting is measured after 5 minutes. No topical anesthetic is used.

Basic secretion Schirmer test
The test is performed in the same manner as the Schirmer I test except that a topical anesthetic is placed in the eye, and the lower cul-de-sac is swabbed before testing.

Schirmer II test
The test can be performed to further evaluate lacrimal function if minimal wetting occurs with the Schirmer I test. The strip used for Schirmer I testing is left in place and a cotton-tipped applicator is used to stimulate the nasal mucosa. Minimal or no additional wetting may occur when reflex secretion is impaired because of severe lacrimal gland dysfunction.

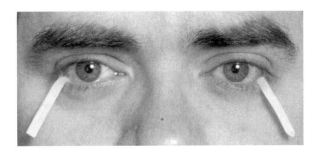

FIGURE 11-11
Schirmer testing for tear production level is performed with a standardized strip of filter paper, which is bent on its end and placed over the lower eyelid margin.

extent of wetness on the strip is measured in millimeters from the point at which the strip was bent for placement over the lid margin.

The Schirmer I test measures both the basic and reflex tear secretions, although the technique just described attempts to minimize the degree of reflex secretion. Results with this test can be highly variable and should therefore not be taken as conclusive evidence of the presence or absence of an aqueous deficiency. Although normative valves are subject to controversy in the literature, readings less than 10 mm are commonly considered significant and those between 10 mm and 15 mm are considered borderline.[35-37]

Basic Secretion Schirmer Test

The "basic secretion" test is performed by placing an anesthetic in the eye before testing. This procedure is often performed when results without anesthetic are normal. The technique is performed in the same manner as the Schirmer I tear test, except that the lower cul-de-sac is swabbed with a cotton-tipped applicator to dry any excess moisture. Otherwise, false wetting of the strip can occur from fluid present before the actual test is done. Similar to the Schirmer I test, abnormal values are again subject to controversy. Because of the addition of an anesthetic and subsequent reduction in reflex tearing, abnormal values should be lower when compared with those of the Schirmer I test. With the basic secretion test, abnormal values indicative of an aqueous deficiency have been considered to be as low as 0–3 mm.[38]

Schirmer II Test

If there is minimal wetting on the Schirmer I test, the Schirmer II test can be performed to further evaluate

lacrimal function (i.e., fatigue of the reflex secretors can be distinguished from a complete lack of function). Complete loss of function of the secretory system may be caused by diseases which lead to the destruction of the glandular elements, such as Stevens-Johnson disease, pemphigus, and sarcoidosis.[33]

The Schirmer II test may be done immediately after the Schirmer I test without removing the Schirmer strips. A cotton-tipped applicator is placed far enough in the nostril to touch its back wall and moved back and forth for several seconds. If there is a fatigue block, the Schirmer strip may be significantly wetted beyond the original wetting from the Schirmer I test. If there is no additional wetting or a minimal increase in wetting, then reflex secretion may be impaired secondary to lacrimal gland dysfunction.

If normal wetting is found with both the Schirmer I and the basic secretion tests, then the lacrimal excretory system must be evaluated to find the cause of tearing.

Jones Testing

The Jones primary and secondary dye tests are important fundamental tests used for evaluation of lacrimal obstruction in the office setting (Table 11-3). Instrumentation used for Jones testing and evaluation of the lacrimal drainage system is shown in Figure 11-12.

Jones No. 1 Test (Primary Dye Test)

The Jones No. 1 test measures the ability of tears to pass through the lacrimal channels under normal physiologic conditions. Only one eye should be tested at a time. Ideally, one or two drops of 2% liquid sodium fluorescein is instilled into the lower cul-de-sac of the eye being tested. If sodium fluorescein solution is unavailable, fluorescein strips can be used. The patient is instructed to sit

TABLE 11-3
Jones Testing

Jones No. 1 test (primary dye test)

2% liquid sodium fluorescein is placed into the lower cul-de-sac. The test is positive (lacrimal patency exists) if dye is detected via direct observation of the back of the throat, by inspection of mucus blown from the nose or cleared from the throat, or through probing of the inferior meatus of the nose.

Jones No. 2 Test (secondary dye test)

The test is performed if the Jones No. 1 test result is negative. After anesthetization and dilation of the lower punctum, irrigation of the nasolacrimal drainage system is performed with a 23-gauge cannula attached to a syringe filled with sterile normal saline. Fluid that drains from the nose is then inspected for fluorescein dye.

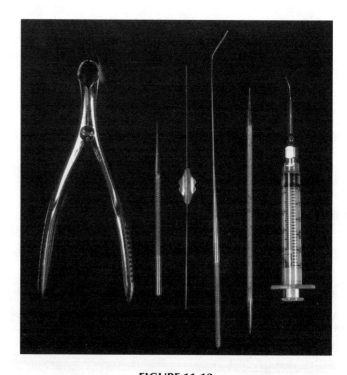

FIGURE 11-12
Instruments used for evaluation of the lacrimal drainage system. From left to right: nasal speculum, fine-tapered punctal dilator, Bowman probe, Dean applicator, combination medium- and wide-tapered punctal dilator, 23-gauge cannula and syringe.

upright with the head held straight and the eyes open. Normal blinking should be maintained and the patient should be discouraged from tightly squeezing the lids together. After 5 minutes the clinician notes whether the amount of fluorescein in the eye has lessened or if dye has spilled onto the patient's cheek. If there is minimal or no evidence of dye remaining within the tear layer or meniscus, then it can be assumed that lacrimal drainage has occurred. If a significant amount of dye is noted, then normal tear drainage may not be present. This can occur for several reasons. Among these are poor apposition between the lower punctum and globe, and any obstruction involving any component of the lacrimal drainage route. An inadequate lacrimal pump mechanism can also contribute in some cases. This may happen when a patient has an incomplete blink.

After the ocular surface has been evaluated for dye disappearance, the clinician may then perform a few other measures to determine if dyed tears have traversed the drainage route. First, the back of the throat can be checked for the presence of fluorescein. The floor of the nose is sloped back toward the throat in such a manner that tears passing into the inferior meatus through the lacrimal duct flow into the throat, where they are swallowed. If fluorescein is observed in the throat, then the lacrimal system is patent and the findings on the Jones No. 1 test are positive. The clinician may find it helpful to view the throat through a Burton lamp or some other blue light source so that visibility of the fluorescein is enhanced. The dye is usually also observed with white light, however. Use of a tongue depressor to more clearly visualize the back of the throat is often helpful.

If no fluorescein is observed on the back of the throat, then the patient may next be instructed to create positive pressure in the nasal passageway by blowing the nose into a clean white tissue while the nostril not being tested is

occluded. If fluorescein is present on the tissue then the findings of the Jones No. 1 test are positive and the lacrimal system is deemed patent. If no dye is found, then the patient can be instructed to withdraw mucus from the nasopharynx area by strongly sniffing out its contents backward into the mouth by exerting negative pressure. The mucus is then spat onto a clean white tissue, and again the specimen is examined for the presence or absence of dye. As before, if dye is present, the system is patent and the test result is positive.

If no dye is found on this third step, then probing of the meatus under the inferior turbinate may be performed. The literature is replete with incorrect descriptions of this step. The usual reference states that the meatus beneath the inferior turbinate is probed by inserting a cotton-tipped applicator into the nose. It may be possible to retrieve dye on a cotton-tipped applicator by inserting it into the nostril of the patient, but if this is the case it is not because the meatus of the inferior turbinate bone was entered. It results from that fact that the lacrimal system is so open that tears and fluorescein freely enter the nose. This being the case, probing the meatus of the inferior turbinate would be unnecessary because dye would have

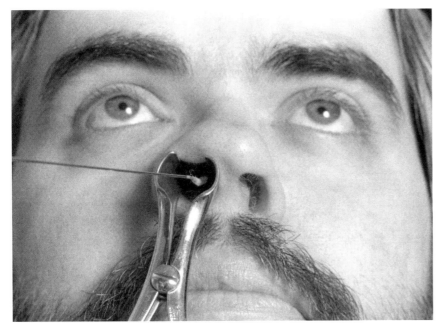

FIGURE 11-13
Procedure for probing the meatus of the inferior turbinate. A malleable wire (Dean applicator) is used with a wisp of cotton tightly twisted on its end, and the naris of the nostril is held widely open with a nasal speculum.

shown up somewhere on the previous three steps, most assuredly on the back of the throat.

According to Jones, to probe the meatus of the inferior turbinate, a malleable wire with a wisp of cotton tightly twisted on its end is necessary (Figure 11-13). The cotton wisp must be small in size so that it may pass freely into the inferior meatus and it should be attached firmly enough so that it does not come free in the nostril. The wire is bent about 1 inch from the cotton-tipped end at an angle of about 30 degrees. The patient should be seated with the head and body upright, not tilted backward. The naris of the nostril to be probed should be held open with a nasal speculum to expose the meatus of the inferior turbinate. The examiner should wear a head mirror to direct bright light into the patient's nostril. A bright illumination source such as a gooseneck lamp or a binocular indirect ophthalmoscope can also be used. Before the cotton-tipped wire is inserted, the cotton should be soaked in 4% xylocaine. Probing may be mildly uncomfortable until the anesthetic becomes effective.

The actual probing procedure is a "blind" technique based on "feel" and knowledge of nasal anatomy. The bent wire is held by the examiner in such a manner that the bent end with the cotton wisp is directed straight into the meatus under the inferior turbinate. To do this, the long end of the wire by which it is held is angled out about 30 degrees from the sagittal plane of the patient's face. When the bent end is completely inserted into the meatus, the end of the wire held by the examiner is angled 30

degrees toward the sagittal facial plane. This causes the bent end to rotate 30 degrees under the inferior turbinate. Now the wire is further inserted into the nostril, causing the cotton wisp to come in contact with the opening of the nasolacrimal duct. The wire is left in the nostril for a few seconds, during which time it is gently rotated back and forth. It is then withdrawn from the nostril and the cotton inspected for dye. If dye is seen, the system is patent.

Jones No. 2 Test (Secondary Dye Test)
If the Jones No. 1 procedure produces negative results at all four steps, then the Jones No. 2 procedure is indicated. With this technique, a cotton-tipped applicator is first soaked in 4% xylocaine and applied to the lower punctum. This pledget of anesthetic is held against the punctum for 30–60 seconds to desensitize the punctal area and canaliculus. The patient remains in a seated, upright position with the head erect throughout this procedure. The lower lid is pulled slightly away from the globe and then gently stretched laterally. This will put tension on the lid and allow for easier penetration of the punctum with a dilator. The patient is instructed to look superotemporally to place the cornea away from the area in which the procedure is performed. This will lessen the likelihood of injury. The clinician must respect the anatomy of the lacrimal drainage system. The dilator is inserted vertically into the punctum to a depth of about 2 mm (Figure 11-14A). The dilator is gently rolled between the fingers while it is entering the punctum. This facilitates penetra-

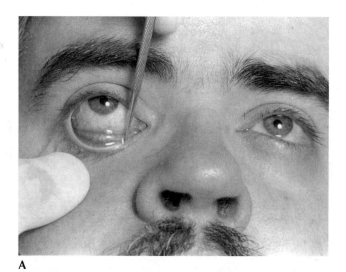
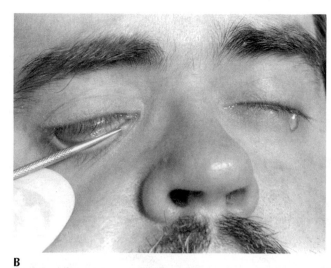

A   **B**

FIGURE 11-14

Punctal dilation. The dilator is inserted vertically into the punctum to a depth of 2 mm (A) and is then rotated laterally before it is inserted further into the canaliculus horizontally (B).

tion. Once the dilator is 2 mm into the punctum, the top of the dilator is rotated laterally and downward about 90 degrees and then further inserted into the canaliculus horizontally (Figure 11-14B). At this point, the clinician should observe a whitening of the tissue surrounding the punctum. This blanching is evidence that dilation is being effected. The dilator is removed and an irrigation cannula is placed (Figure 11-15A) into the punctum and canaliculus.

Irrigation is performed with a 23-gauge cannula mounted on a 3- to 5-ml disposable syringe filled with sterile normal saline. The cannula is threaded into the drainage system in a similar manner as was the dilator. Once the cannula is in place, the patient is instructed to tilt his or her head forward in the "silent prayer" position. This places the chin against the chest. The patient also holds a white basin or a kidney-shaped basin lined with white tissue under the chin (Figure 11-15B). Pressure can now be applied to the syringe plunger so that fluid is forced into the lacrimal system. One of the following events should result:

1. No fluid comes out of the nose, which is evidence that a complete obstruction exists.
2. The fluid comes out of the nose with fluorescein stain, which is a positive result with the Jones No. 2 test. This indicates that the lacrimal pump and canaliculi are functioning and the sac fills. The obstruction is in the nasolacrimal duct but is not complete. The dye-stained tears pass through the upper excretory system and enter the sac but cannot exit under normal conditions because of partial obstruction. With forced

pressure on the syringe, the obstruction is overcome and the dye-stained tears pass into the nose.
3. The fluid comes out of the nose clear. The secondary test results are negative. An obstruction exists between the punctum and the sac. Dye was unable to get into the sac because of a punctal stenosis, a punctal ectropion, a partial or complete canalicular obstruction, or a weakness of the orbicularis oculi pump. Treatment of the problem should be directed to the lids, puncta, lacrimal pump, or canaliculi.

If dye appears on the Jones No. 2 test but not the Jones No. 1 test, there is an obstruction of the lower nasolacrimal sac or nasolacrimal duct. This is often the case, and DCR may be necessary to correct the condition.

Jones testing attempts to determine the patency of the nasolacrimal system by tracing fluorescein dye as it works its way, via the tears, through the system. Two factors cannot be accurately determined, however. If dye is retrieved, the amount of dye that is observed cannot be ascertained relative to the known amount that was initially introduced into the eye. It cannot be known if all the dye that entered the system actually exited the system. The second factor difficult to evaluate is the amount of time it takes the dye to pass through the system. The passage time depends on several things: the individual anatomy of the patient's nasolacrimal system, possible partial obstruction or constriction within the system, and the volume of tears being produced by the patient.

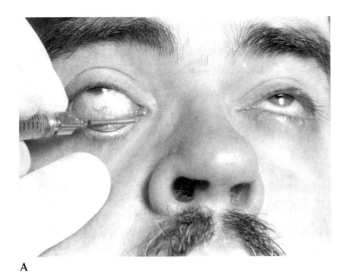

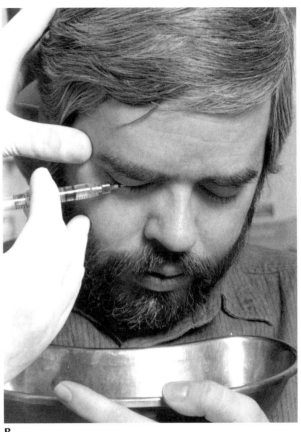

FIGURE 11-15
Lacrimal irrigation. A. Immediately after punctal dilation, a 23-gauge cannula is fully inserted into the lower canaliculus in the same manner as the punctal dilator. B. Once the cannula is in place, the patient tilts his head forward and holds a basin to collect the fluid that drains from the nostril.

REFERENCES

1. Miller NR. Anatomy, Physiology, and Testing of Normal Lacrimal Secretion. In Walsh and Hoyt's Clinical Neuro-ophthalmology (4th ed). Vol 2. Baltimore: Williams & Wilkins, 1985;458–68.
2. Tanenbaum M, McCord CD. The Lacrimal Drainage System. In TD Duane (ed), Clinical Ophthalmology. Vol 4. Philadelphia: Lippincott, 1991;1–25.
3. Werb A. The Anatomy of the Lacrimal System. In B Milder, BA Weil (eds), The Lacrimal System. Norwalk, CT: Appleton-Century-Crofts, 1983;23–32.
4. Hect SD. Evaluation of the lacrimal drainage system. Ophthalmology 1978;85:1250–8.
5. Hill JC, Bethell W, Smiraul HJ. Lacrimal drainage—a dynamic evaluation. Part I. Mechanisms of tear transport. Can J Ophthalmol 1974;9:411–6.
6. Jones LT. The cure of epiphora due to canailicular disorders, trauma, and surgical failures of the lacrimal passages. Trans Am Acad Ophthalmol Otolaryngol 1962;66:506–25.
7. Sjögren H, Bloch KJ. Keratoconjunctivitis sicca and the Sjögren syndrome. Surv Ophthalmol 1971;16:145–59.
8. Lemp MA, Hamill Jr. Factors affecting tear film breakup in normal eyes. Arch Ophthalmol 1973;89:103–5.
9. Boersma HGM, van Bijsterveld OP. The lactoferrin test for the diagnosis of keratoconjunctivitis sicca in clinical practice. Ann Ophthalmol 1987;19:152–4.
10. McEwan WK, Kimura SJ. Filter paper electrophoresis of tears: I. Lysozyme and its correlation with keratoconjunctivitis sicca. Am J Ophthalmol 1955;39:200–2.
11. Janssen PT, van Bijsterveld OP. Comparison of electrophoretic techniques for the analysis of human tear fluid proteins. Clin Chim Acta 1981;114:207–18.
12. Bonavida B, Sapse AT. Human tear lysozyme: II. Quantitative determination with standard Schirmer strips. Am J Ophthalmol 1968;66:70–6.
13. Nelson JD. Impression cytology. Cornea 1988;7:71–81.
14. Lucca JA, Nunez JN, Farris RL. A comparison of diagnostic tests for keratoconjunctivitis sicca; lactoplate, Schirmer, and tear osmolarity. CLAO J 1990;16:109–12.
15. Holly FJ, Lemp MA. Tear physiology and dry eyes. Surv Ophthalmol 1977; 22:69–87.
16. Avisar R, Savir H. Our further experience with bromhexine in keratoconjunctivitis sicca. Ann Ophthalmol 1988; 20:382.
17. Giunta G, Boresellino F, Tamborin A, Criscito M. Eloisin in the treatment of lacrimal hyposecretion. Ann Ottal 1977;103:223–30.

18. Lemp MA. General measures in the management of the dry eye. Int Ophthalmol Clin 1987;27:36–43.
19. Laibovitz RA, Solch S, Andriano K, et al. Pilot trial of cyclosporine 1% ophthalmic ointment in the treatment of keratoconjunctivitis sicca. Cornea 1993;12:315–23.
20. Liegner JT, Yee RW, Wild, JH. Topical cyclosporine therapy for ulcerative keratitis associated with rheumatoid arthritis. Am J Ophthalmol 1990;109:610–2.
21. Kaswan RL, Salisbury MA, Ward DA. Spontaneous canine keratoconjunctivitis sicca. A useful model for human keratoconjunctivitis sicca: treatment with cyclosporine eye drops. Arch Ophthalmol 1989;107:1210–6.
22. Benson DR, Hemmady PB, Snyder RW. Efficacy of laser punctal occlusion. Ophthalmology 1992;99:618–21.
23. Milder B. Diseases of the Lacrimal Gland. In B Milder, BA Weil (eds), The Lacrimal System. Norwalk, CT: Appleton-Century-Crofts, 1983;105–10.
24. Charamis J, Koliopoulos J, Palimeris G, Magogritsas N. Management of the obstruction of the lacrimal passages. Eye, Ear, Nose, and Throat Monthly 1972;51:116–21.
25. Milder B. Physiology of Lacrimal Excretion. In B Milder, BA Weil (eds), The Lacrimal System. Norwalk, CT: Appleton-Century-Crofts, 1983;55–62.
26. Putterman AM. Basic Oculoplastic Surgery. In GA Peyman, DR Sanders, MF Goldberg (eds), Principles and Practice of Ophthalmology. Vol III. Philadelphia: Saunders, 1980;2246–333.
27. Silver B. Involutional Changes and the Lacrimal System. In B Milder, BA Weil (eds), The Lacrimal System. Norwalk, CT: Appleton-Century-Crofts, 1983;165–75.
28. Hurwitz JJ, Archer KF. Canaliculodacryocystrohinostomy. In JV Linberg (ed), Contemporary Issues in Ophthalmology. Lacrimal Surgery. Vol 5. New York: Churchill Livingstone, 1988;263–80.
29. Lindberg JV. Disorders of the Lower Excretory System. In B Milder, BA Weil (eds), The Lacrimal System. Norwalk, CT: Appleton-Century-Crofts, 1983;133–43.
30. Berlin AJ, Rath R, Rich L. Lacrimal system dacryoliths. Ophthalmic Surg 1980;11:435–6.
31. Daxecker F, Philipp W, Müller-Holzner E, Tessadri R. Analysis of a dacryolith. Ophthalmologica 1987;195:125–7.
32. Wilkins RB, Pressly JP. Diagnosis and incidence of lacrimal calculi. Ophthalmic Surg 1980;11:787–9.
33. Jakobiec FA, Jones IS. Orbital Inflammations. In TD Duane (ed), Clinical Ophthalmology. Vol 2. Philadelphia: Lippincott, 1990;1–75.
34. Semes L, Melore GG. Dilation and diagnostic irrigation of the lacrimal drainage system. J Am Optom Assoc 1986; 57:518–25.
35. Shapiro A, Merin S. Schirmer test and breakup time of tear film in normal subjects. Am J Ophthalmol 1979;88:752–7.
36. van Bijsterveld OP. Diagnostic tests in the sicca syndrome. Arch Ophthalmol 1969;82:10–4.
37. Clinch TE, Benedetto DA, Felberg NT, Laibson PR. Schirmer's test: a closer look. Arch Ophthalmol 1983; 101:1383–6.
38. Lamberts DW, Foster CS, Perry HD. Schirmer test after topical anesthesia and the tear meniscus height in normal eyes. Arch Ophthalmol 1979;97:1082–5.

12

Carotid Artery Disease and Ophthalmodynamometry

NEIL A. PENCE

Cerebral ischemia and stroke are major causes of disability, illness, and death. The etiologic factors for cerebral ischemia and stroke fall into three general categories. The first category is cardiac-related disorders, including long-standing systemic hypertension, and hypotension resulting from conditions such as cardiac arrhythmias or myocardial infarction. The second category consists of blood disorders, which encompasses hypercoagulation problems (e.g., polycythemia, oral contraceptives), hyperviscosity syndromes, and various anemias. Arterial disease is the third category, with the major form being atherosclerosis. Other arterial disorders such as anomalous vessel formations, unusual collateral circulation, and inflammatory vascular disease (e.g., collagen diseases, syphilis, Takayasu's disease, phlebitis) can also be implicated.

Disorders of the carotid circulation cause approximately 20–25% of all strokes. The most commonly involved site of atherosclerotic disease within the carotid system is the internal carotid artery (ICA).[1] It has been reported that over 90% of ICA obstructions occur below the origin of the ophthalmic artery, usually just distal to the bifurcation of the internal and external carotid arteries.[2] Therefore, blood flow in the ophthalmic artery would be expected to be affected in the majority of cases of ICA occlusion or significant stenosis. In fact, in those patients with symptomatic carotid insufficiency, 75–85% will have ocular symptoms.[3,4] Of these symptomatic patients, 30–35% will suffer a serious stroke if left untreated.[3,5,6] Therefore, by being alert to the symptoms and signs of carotid artery insufficiency, the primary eye care practitioner can play an important role in the prevention of stroke.

ATHEROSCLEROTIC DISEASE

Atherosclerosis is primarily a disease of the intima of the vessel wall. Its development initially consists of focal accumulations of foam cells. Foam cells are derived from an interaction between oxidized low-density lipoprotein (LDL)–cholesterol and blood-derived monocytes, which leads to the formation of lipid-laden macrophages. Accumulated foam cells form yellowish fatty-streak lesions. Plaques progressively increase in collagen, which begins to narrow the vessel lumen. Increasing invasion, or accumulation, of lipids, lipoproteins, and dead endothelial cells causes the plaque to further impinge on the lumen.

Serious consequences result from either a significant reduction in blood flow or embolization. Embolization occurs when a region of atheromatous plaque "ulcerates." Ulceration, which may be related to calcification or possibly intraplaque hemorrhage, exposes the atheromatous material (e.g., cholesterol crystals, cellular debris) to the vessel lumen and allows fragments to break off. These emboli can then precipitate occlusion elsewhere in the vascular system. The irregularity of the roughened, ulcerated surface and the characteristics of the plaque material itself tend to attract platelet fibrin aggregates.[7] These form on the surface of the plaque and serve as another source of emboli but are less likely to cause occlusion.

A transient ischemic attack (TIA) is the predominant symptom of carotid artery disease. This event, which occurs secondary to temporary embolic occlusion of the cerebral vasculature, typically lasts from 2 to 30 minutes (but can last hours) and leaves no permanent disability. Transient ischemic attacks caused by carotid insufficiency include hemiparesis, sensory loss (such as numbness or tingling of the lower face, arm, or hand on one side), and aphasia. The most common symptom, however, is amaurosis fugax.[4] Amaurosis fugax is a sudden, painless, monocular transient loss of vision. It may be described as a dimming, darkness, or blackness of vision. Sectoral or altitudinal visual field loss may occur, giving the effect of a curtain falling and rising. Amaurosis fugax is nearly always an indication of atheromatous disease. It is caused by microemboli loosening from the ulcerated atherosclerotic plaque (usually located at the bifurcation of the ipsilateral common carotid or in the extracranial portion of the internal carotid artery) and being swept through the ICA circulation and lodging in either the ophthalmic artery, one of the posterior ciliary arteries, or somewhere in the retinal circulation. The embolus either fragments into small pieces, or the vessel dilates and allows it to dislodge, thus ending the TIA.

SIGNS AND SYMPTOMS OF CAROTID ARTERY DISEASE

Although amaurosis fugax is the most likely ocular symptom of carotid artery insufficiency, there are a number of other ocular effects. Understanding their relationship to carotid artery disease is very important if the eye care practitioner is to play an effective role in the prevention of stroke.

Cholesterol Emboli

Small, bright yellow plaques lodged at bifurcations of small- and medium-sized retinal arterioles are cholesterol emboli. These may be detected during ophthalmoscopy and are indicative of atherosclerotic disease of the carotid system or possibly the aorta. When an atherosclerotic plaque ulcerates, material containing cholesterol is exposed, which then may break off into small fragments. When originating from the carotid system, these small bodies are carried to the eye, the brain, or both. These bright, sometimes multiple, yellow retinal emboli are often referred to as Hollenhorst plaques.[4,8] Depending on how they become lodged at the bifurcations of retinal arterioles, cholesterol emboli can cause significant obstructions, although most do not. They will move distally in the vessel and fragment in days to weeks. It is unusual for them to be visible months later.

Even in the absence of significant obstruction, there may be a localized inflammatory reaction in the involved vessel, leading to perivascular sheathing at the site of the cholesterol embolus. Therefore, the presence of any localized vessel sheathing may be indicative of a previous Hol-

lenhorst plaque at that location. This vessel sheathing may be highlighted during fluoroscein angiography as a focal staining.[9,10]

Platelet Emboli

Other types of emboli may be visible in the eye as well. Platelet emboli are white or dirty white plugs that may become lodged within a vessel lumen for a period of time, but they tend to fragment easily and move distally in the bloodstream. Platelet emboli may cause frequent, brief attacks, are unlikely to be witnessed by the eye care practitioner, and leave no residual effect. They are often indicative of an ulcerative lesion in the carotid system, as this is where they tend to originate.

Calcific Emboli

Larger, more chalky white emboli that sometimes lodge at or near the disc are calcific emboli. These tend to lodge permanently and cause central or branch retinal artery occlusions. Calcific emboli originate from heart valves or occasionally the aorta.

Thrombotic Emboli

The heart can also be the source of thrombotic emboli, which are rarely visible in the eye because they are usually too large to enter the ophthalmic artery. If present in the eye, the appearance can range from a dirty white to dark red, depending on the number of red blood cells trapped in the fibrin network of the thrombus. The typical size of these emboli makes vessel occlusion likely. The presence of thrombotic emboli usually indicates the need for long-term anticoagulation therapy.[9]

Venous Stasis Retinopathy

When there is significant reduction of the blood flow to the ophthalmic artery and/or central retinal artery, retinal hypoperfusion can result. Classically, due to this hypoperfusion, scattered microaneurysms and dot and blot hemorrhages occur in the mid-peripheral retina. The posterior pole may also be involved, however, which may resemble background diabetic retinopathy. The retinal veins are usually dilated and may be irregular in caliber or segmented. The constellation of retinal changes associated with ipsilateral hypoperfusion is referred to as venous stasis retinopathy.[11] In most instances of venous stasis retinopathy, the ICA is found to be severely stenotic,[12] over 95% occluded in most cases.[13] Rapid resolution of the venous stasis retinopathy is often seen after bypass and endarterectomy surgery, which is further indication that nonperfusion is the cause of venous stasis retinopathy.[14,15]

Ocular Pain

Occasionally the vascular insufficiency caused by carotid occlusive disease can cause eye pain. This is not a common effect of carotid occlusion, but perhaps 5% of the patients with symptoms of carotid occlusion will have the complaint of ocular pain in or over the orbit. This ischemic pain (unrelated to secondary neovascular glaucoma) may be transient in nature and has been demonstrated to disappear after bypass surgery.[16]

Retinal Vascular Occlusion

Cholesterol emboli that result from carotid atherosclerosis, as previously discussed, can cause both branch and central retinal artery occlusions. They can also occlude a short posterior ciliary artery, which is responsible for the blood supply to the optic nerve at the level of the lamina, resulting in ischemic optic neuropathy. Therefore, in cases of retinal vascular occlusion and ischemic optic neuropathy, carotid occlusive disease must be recognized as a possible underlying mechanism.

Aside from embolic obstruction, central retinal artery occlusion can also result from severe carotid stenosis causing mean blood pressure to drop below the intraocular pressure. Here, the perfusion pressure is not adequate to maintain blood flow in the central retinal artery. A second ischemic mechanism responsible for central retinal artery occlusion may occur with the development of anterior segment neovascularization. In this situation, a resultant secondary neovascular glaucoma can lead to elevated intraocular pressure and subsequent compression of the central retinal artery. Hayreh and Podhajsky[17] reported that in the vast majority of cases where central retinal artery occlusion and neovascular glaucoma are present concurrently, the secondary glaucoma resulting from chronic ischemia occurred first, and that this caused the central retinal artery occlusion. They noted that in two-thirds of the cases of central retinal artery occlusion studied, carotid artery disease was responsible. Therefore, in the presence of central retinal artery occlusion or neovascular glaucoma, complete carotid artery evaluation is necessary.

Ocular Ischemic Syndrome

Carotid insufficiency can lead to chronic anterior or posterior segment ischemia and can cause a constellation of ophthalmic signs and symptoms denoted as the ocular ischemic syndrome.[18-20] Hypoperfusion in the choroid and retina, as well as retinal neovascularization, may occur. Anterior segment complications can include uveitis, corneal edema, neovascularization of the iris and angle, and secondary glaucoma. Two common components of the ocular ischemic syndrome, venous stasis retinopathy and ischemic orbital pain, were individually discussed in previous sections.[20]

Unilateral Retinopathy

Hypertensive or diabetic retinopathy that is significantly less pronounced in one eye may be indicative of ICA disease on the side of the less involved eye. Less retinopathy is present because of the impaired blood flow to that side, which apparently has the effect of somewhat sparing the retinal vessels from damage.[3,20]

EVALUATION OF THE CAROTID VASCULAR SYSTEM

Several tests that fall in the general category of physical diagnosis testing are useful in the evaluation of patients suspected of having carotid disease. These are quick, inexpensive, in-office procedures that can easily be performed by the ophthalmic practitioner.

Carotid Auscultation

Auscultation of the carotid artery may detect the presence of a bruit. Bruits are caused by turbulent blood flow. A bruit found high in the neck, just below the angle of the jaw is usually caused by stenosis at the carotid bifurcation.[21] Bruits found lower in the neck may have common carotid or subclavian origins or may be transmitted aortic and heart sounds. The Framingham Study[22] found neck bruits in 7% of the population aged 65–79 years. Of patients with neck bruits, 86% in one study were found to have vascular abnormalities or lesions.[23] Bruits have been found in 88% of carotid arteries with stenosis greater than 50%.[23] Thus, the bruit may be a significant sign of ICA occlusive disease and may be found in many asymptomatic patients. The absence of a bruit, however, cannot be taken as a sign that significant stenosis is not present.[23] When there is total occlusion present, for example, no bruit will be heard because of the lack of any blood flow. Therefore, the presence of a bruit signifies a narrowed but open vessel.

To listen for a bruit, the diaphragm or bell end of the stethoscope chest piece is placed high on the neck, between the mandibular bone and the sternomastoid muscle, or below the angle of the jaw (Figure 12-1). Care must be taken

FIGURE 12-1
Auscultation of the carotid artery to detect the presence of a bruit. The diaphragm end of the stethoscope may help distribute pressure more evenly so that an artificial murmur is not created, but the bell side is more sensitive to low-pitched sounds, which are typical of carotid bruits. (Reprinted with permission from NA Pence. Ophthalmodynamometry. J Am Optom Assoc 1980;51:49.)

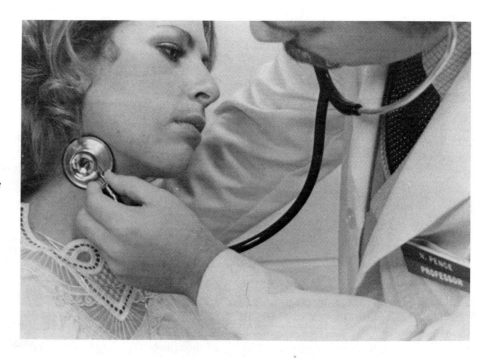

to place the stethoscope lightly over this area because pressure may compress the artery and cause an artificial murmur to be heard.[24] In one respect, the round, flat diaphragm end is better than the bell side, since its greater surface area distributes pressure more evenly. However, the bell end is more sensitive to low-pitched sounds such as the carotid murmur, or bruit. The diaphragm is more sensitive to high-pitched sounds. The patient is asked to cease inhaling and exhaling momentarily so that those sounds will not muffle any subtle murmurs. The carotid bruit is a rushing or low blowing sound, somewhat like the breathing sounds heard just before the patient holds his or her breath. It will pulse or gush in spurts corresponding to cardiac systole.[23] The carotid bruit may be more evident with the patient's head turned to the opposite side.

Carotid Palpation

The carotid pulse should be palpated and its strength gauged. The area over the carotid artery on both sides is alternately lightly palpated (Figure 12-2). The strength of the pulse is rated on a scale of 0–4 and the results for the two sides are compared. A weaker pulse or increased firmness occurring unilaterally is a sign of carotid disease. A thrill is a vibration, or fremitus, felt by the fingertips of the examiner and is caused by the same flow eddies in the carotid bloodstream that result in a bruit and are created by blood passing through areas of vessel constriction or irregularity.[25] The amount or intensity of the thrill increas-

es as the obstruction increases. A thrill felt high in the neck is most commonly caused by carotid constrictions, whereas one felt low in the neck may be transmitted from a diseased aortic arch or a cardiac valve impairment.[24,25] A thrill can be roughly simulated by palpating one's own upper neck and very lightly humming.

Noninvasive Carotid Testing

There are a number of noninvasive tests that can aid in the detection of carotid vascular problems. Most of these are basically screening tests and are used to determine if more expensive and more invasive tests are warranted. Two general categories of noninvasive tests exists: direct and indirect. Indirect types attempt to evaluate the flow of blood distal to any occlusion. These include ophthalmodynamometry (ODM), oculoplethysmography (OPG), oculopneumoplethysmography (OPPG, or OPG-Gee), and, to a very small extent, fundus fluorescein angiography. Direct noninvasive tests attempt to image the carotid bifurcation area to actually show the obstruction or lesion. Direct imaging tests include B-scan ultrasonography, Doppler imaging, duplex scanning, and magnetic resonance imaging (MRI).

Indirect Noninvasive Tests
Ophthalmodynamometry Ophthalmodynamometry (ODM) may be the most commonly performed indirect noninvasive test. Advantages of this procedure are that oph-

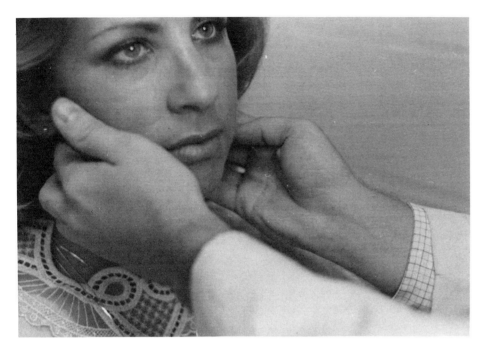

FIGURE 12-2
The area over the carotid arteries is palpated to compare the strength of the pulse and the rigidity of the two sides. (Reprinted with permission from NA Pence. Ophthalmodynamometry. J Am Optom Assoc 1980;51:49.)

thalmodynamometers are fairly inexpensive, the procedure is relatively quick, patients experience only minor discomfort, it is safe, and it can be done in the eye care practitioner's office. ODM was introduced by Paul Baillart in 1917[26] as a method of gauging the perfusion pressure of the central retinal artery pressure. This measurement is performed by initially raising the intraocular pressure through external force applied to the sclera or cornea and simultaneously observing when arterial pulsations are induced in vessels at the optic nerve head. The pressure is then increased until the central retinal artery completely collapses. As a vessel begins to close, it is supplied with a greater flow of blood by its next most proximal segment, and its pressure is raised very nearly to the pressure in that vessel.[27,28] Relative to the central retinal artery, that vessel would be the ophthalmic artery. Vander Werff[27] found that the systolic values as determined by ODM were 14–17 mm Hg higher than the central retinal artery pressures themselves and that they corresponded to the pressure at some point in the ophthalmic artery. Therefore, ODM is best defined as a measure of the relative ophthalmic artery pressures and not the central retinal artery pressure. Only relative values are obtained because the measurement is affected by such factors as IOP, scleral rigidity, elasticity of the vessels, and length of time that external pressure is applied to the globe.[1] The ODM procedure and its interpretation will be discussed in more detail later in this chapter.

As a screening test for carotid disease, ODM has several good features and one major weakness. First of all,

there is usually a very low false-positive rate with ODM, so that an abnormal finding is usually highly diagnostic.[1,29,30] It is fairly good at detecting severe stenosis (i.e., where stenosis is greater than 85–90%).[30,31] The major drawback of ODM is that it is not very sensitive for obstructions of less than 75%. ODM, like other indirect tests, is generally only capable of detecting a stenosis of greater than 75–80%, and some stenoses at this level of blockage will not be detected. Experimental studies in fluid dynamics show that a significant drop in pressure distal to an obstruction is not expected until the lumen is narrowed past a critical stenosis of about 80%, so ODM and other indirect measures are not good at detecting less severe obstructions.[32] Therefore, ODM is a useful in-office test, since abnormal findings signify serious carotid artery problems, but ODM is not as accurate as other procedures.

Oculoplethysmography OPG is a test that measures pulse arrival time for comparison between the two eyes. If an obstruction to flow exists, the length of time it takes for blood to travel from the heart to the origin of the internal carotid will be longer on the side of the stenosis. OPG devices can use fluid or air manometers. Like ODM, the stenosis must be greater than 80% before it will be detected, and bilateral stenosis is not well detected. Other tests are generally accepted as superior to OPG.

Oculopneumoplethysmography OPPG (or OPG-Gee) involves applying suction to the eye, thus raising the pressure past the point where the central retinal artery is closed and the pulse is stopped, and then lowering the pressure until the pulse reappears. The test was developed by William Gee and is felt to be capable of detecting stenoses greater than 60%.[33,34] Although roughly comparable with ODM, patients may experience slightly more discomfort with OPPG. The test also requires considerably more elaborate equipment and is therefore more costly.

Fundus Fluorescein Angiography   Although typically not thought of as a test for carotid blood flow, fundus fluorescein angiography can sometimes serve as an indirect measure of carotid circulation. At least some patients with carotid occlusive disease will have retinal ischemic and neovascular problems that warrant fluorescein angiographic studies. If an occlusion exists, the arm-to-retina circulation time may be delayed. Therefore, attention should be paid to the timing of fluorescein arrival. A significant delay indicates a monocular circulation problem, but not specifically a carotid problem. Nevertheless, this delay should be noted and fundus fluorescein angiography recognized as another type of indirect test in cases of suspected carotid disease.

Direct Noninvasive Tests

B-Scan Ultrasonography   B-scan ultrasonography can be used to directly image the carotid bifurcation area. Somewhat ironically, this test is more accurate for small occlusions than for large ones.[35] For detecting ulcerated plaques, ultrasound may in some instances detect smaller pathologic changes than arteriography.[35,36] Therefore, when ulceration is suspected but arteriography reveals a low-grade stenosis only, B-scan ultrasonography may be warranted to detect potentially dangerous ulcerations.

Doppler Imaging   The Doppler signal can be used to image the carotids. Although standard or continuous-wave Doppler is not sensitive enough, a pulsed Doppler with frequency spectrum analysis significantly enhances sensitivity. The Doppler with frequency analysis technique compares the peak systolic velocity in the internal carotid to the end-diastolic velocity in the common carotid to detect stenosis.[37] Therefore, it works by imaging the blood flow rather than the obstruction.

Duplex Scanning   The most significant application of the Doppler frequency analysis technique is in a procedure called duplex scanning. A duplex scanner entails the simultaneous use of a B-scan ultrasound signal to image the carotid artery while a pulsed Doppler scanner samples and analyzes the frequencies at various positions within the blood column. Studies have demonstrated an accuracy for duplex scanning ranging from 92% to 97% in detecting stenoses as small as 10%. Such results establish the duplex scanner as the most accurate of all noninvasive tests in determining the status of the carotid system.[38,39]

Magnetic Resonance Imaging   MRI can be used to produce images of large and medium-sized vessels; the technique is sometimes termed "MR angiography."[40] By obtaining sequences of images, it can be used to assess blood flow in a manner similar to Doppler ultrasonography. MRI also has the potential to directly image the carotid artery, rather than to indirectly assess blood flow. Therefore the same information as carotid angiography could be obtained but via a noninvasive test. As better imaging technology develops, however, this may prove to be a very important tool.[41-43] Use of MRI in conjunction with other components or testing procedures may offer more complete analysis than is presently available with any single technique.

Invasive Carotid Evaluation

The best test for evaluating the extent of disease in the carotid arteries is arteriography. The standard by which all other tests are judged is selective four-vessel carotid arteriography. The procedure uses an arterial injection of contrast material. Although the morbidity and mortality rates are now very low, there is some risk associated with the procedure.[44] Neurologic complications such as stroke occur 0.5–3.0% of the time.[45] This risk, combined with the expense involved, make arteriography warranted only in the workup of patients who are candidates for surgery. In the cases of patients who are poor surgical candidates or who refuse surgery, noninvasive tests should be used to evaluate the need for medical treatment. Because of the greater amount of information gained and the risk of surgical complications, arteriograms are probably desirable before surgery even when noninvasive testing has been diagnostic.

Less invasive are the digital subtraction angiographic techniques. Intravenous digital subtraction angiography is essentially noninvasive compared with conventional arteriography but yields less information and images that are somewhat lower in quality. Intra-arterial selective contrast angiography with digital subtraction, however, can produce high-quality images faster, with less contrast material, and is safer than normal arteriography. If surgery is to be done, however, most surgeons prefer to have conventional arteriograms as a matter of course.[46]

OPHTHALMODYNAMOMETRY TECHNIQUES

There are two methods of ODM: compression and suction. Compression ODM is performed using a spring-loaded cylinder to apply the external force to the globe. In suction ODM, a suction cup device with a syringe-like plunger connected to it is used to create a vacuum. With this in place against the sclera, the negative pressure applied externally distorts the globe, causing the intraocular pressure to rise.[25] Only compression ODM will be discussed in this chapter, because its use is more widespread in clinical practice, it is simpler to perform, and it is less expensive.

Compression Ophthalmodynamometry

Compression ODM is accomplished by applying pressure against the sclera or the cornea. The two conventional types of scleral compression dynamometers are linear devices and dial devices (Figure 12-3). As pressure is applied with a linear dynamometer, a central post with graduated markings is exposed from within its outer sleeve. The typical dial dynamometer has a scale on a dial with one "drive" arrow, or pointer, connected to the spring, and a second "passenger" arrow. The passenger arrow is carried along as pressure is increased; when pressure is reduced it remains stationary at the highest pressure attained.

Two other compression instruments are also available. The MacKay-Marg tonometer may be used for ODM by switching the recording mode to the "4X" setting and using it as a spring-type scleral compression dynamometer.[47] An ophthalmodynamometer attachment that can be used with a slit lamp is also available. This is a corneal compression instrument.

Scleral Compression Technique
A topical anesthetic is instilled in the eye just before ODM is performed. Wide dilation of the pupil is also necessary for adequate visualization of the disc. The patient is instructed to fixate on a specific point in an upward and nasal direction during the procedure. Room illumination is kept high enough to allow the dial to be read easily. The footplate of the ophthalmodynamometer is then placed lateral to the limbus, approximately at the globe's temporal equator (Figure 12-4). The footplate surface should be exactly tangential to the sclera, and the shaft of the dynamometer *must* be kept perpendicular to the sclera as pressure is exerted. The examiner locates the optic nerve head clearly with the ophthalmoscope and begins exerting pressure with the ophthalmodynamometer (Figure 12-5). During the procedure, it will be necessary for the examiner to change his or her angle of observation slightly to keep the disc in view, since the globe will be displaced nasally a small amount as pressure is exerted temporally. Both direct and indirect ophthalmoscopy may initially be utilized so the examiner can determine which method he or she prefers. As the ODM technique is begun

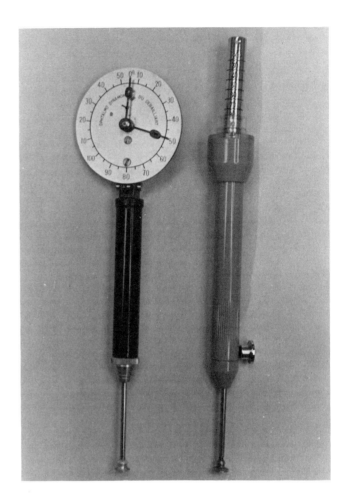

FIGURE 12-3
The dial-type ophthalmodynamometer (left) shows that the passenger arrow has been pushed to 50 g, where it remains, whereas the drive arrow has returned back to 0. A linear ODM (right) is shown with its reading of 90 g. (Reprinted with permission from NA Pence. Ophthalmodynamometry. J Am Optom Assoc 1980;51:49.)

and intraocular pressure increases very slightly, the veins will pulsate and then quickly collapse. The disc artery that the examiner is observing will begin to pulsate at a higher pressure. This point of initial arterial pulsation is noted as the diastolic pressure. The pressure is increased quickly until the artery ceases pulsating and collapses. This is the systolic pressure reading. The dynamometer is then quickly removed. It is important to increase the pressure rapidly up to systole, because prolonged pressure forces fluid from the globe and reduces the IOP. Therefore, a falsely elevated reading would be obtained, since it would be necessary to apply extra force externally to account for the lower IOP.

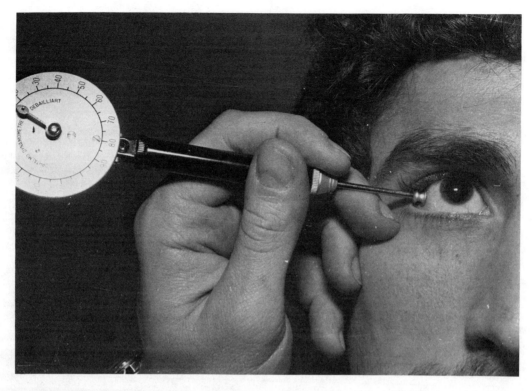

FIGURE 12-4

To perform compression ophthalmodynamometry, the instrument's footplate is correctly positioned perpendicular to the temporal aspect of the globe while the patient looks slightly upward and nasally. (Reprinted with permission from JE Terry. Ophthalmodynamometry. In JE Terry (ed), Ocular Disease: Detection, Diagnosis, and Treatment. Springfield IL: Thomas, 1984;597–610.)

If available, an assistant can note the diastolic pressure on the dial when the examiner verbally indicates arterial pulsation has begun. With or without an assistant, the passenger arrow will mark the systolic pressure. The systolic end point may at first be difficult to identify. As pressure is raised past the point of central retinal artery collapse, the IOP may decrease enough, because of the fluid being forced out, to cause the artery to begin pulsating again in a few seconds.[39] This makes it very difficult to visualize the systolic pressure end point until the examiner becomes adept at noting when the artery first collapses. It may be easier to raise the pressure quickly to a point above the expected systole and then reduce the pressure until the first pulsation is seen. This pressure would also represent the systolic pressure. It may be helpful when first developing procedural skill to have an assistant read aloud the pressures as force is applied. In this way, the examiner develops a better feeling for how much pressure is being exerted as well as the application rate.

If no assistant is available, the examiner can try to first note the diastolic pressure and then proceed to systole, or

proceed first to the systolic pressure (which the passenger arrow will record) and then go back down until the last pulsation is seen. The examiner can then note this pressure on the dial (as the instrument is still held in place) as the diastolic reading. The various methods correspond well, and the latter method is similar to the technique used in taking systemic blood pressure.

Diastolic measurements can be quickly and easily repeated several times in a bracketing manner without affecting accuracy.[48] Several minutes must elapse, however, before systolic measurements are repeated to allow for the replenishment of fluid forced out of the globe. This allows the IOP to stabilize to its normal level. Because of this problem, it is best to alternate systolic pressure measurements between the two eyes rather than taking repeated readings on one eye. The speed with which the pressure is raised should be kept nearly constant for both eyes. Repeated readings are important because if the footplate is tilted even a small amount, the line of force will no longer be toward the center of the globe, and an erroneously high reading will result. Three readings are desir-

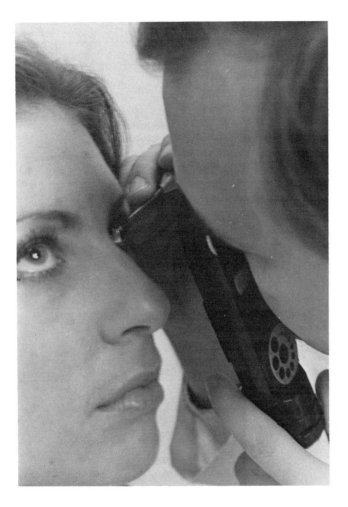

FIGURE 12-5

During ophthalmodynamometry, the examiner observes the disc arteries with the ophthalmoscope as pressure is applied to the globe with the instrument's footplate. (Reprinted with permission from NA Pence. Ophthalmodynamometry. J Am Optom Assoc 1980;51:49.)

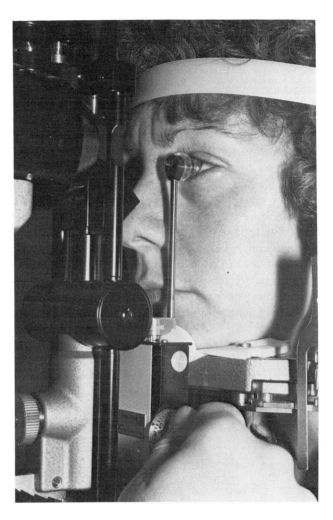

FIGURE 12-6

The fundus lens of the Dynopter is brought into contact with the cornea by moving the joystick until the disc is clearly focused. (Reprinted with permission from JE Terry. Ophthalmodynamometry. In JE Terry (ed), Ocular Disease: Detection, Diagnosis, and Treatment. Springfield IL: Thomas, 1984;597–610.)

able and should be averaged. However, readings widely disparate from the others (especially those on the high side, since procedural errors generally result in higher readings) should be discarded.

Corneal Compression Technique

An ophthalmodynamometer manufactured by American Optical, known as the Dynoptor, was invented by H. A. Sisler in 1972. This instrument allows the examiner to observe the disc arteries biomicroscopically with an acrylic fundus lens that also acts as a contact piece. This lens allows a graded pressure to be applied along a precise radial axis of the globe, coincident with the examiner's axis of visualization of the optic disc (Figure 12-6).

The slit lamp beam should be placed in a paracentral or paraxial position as is normally done for fundus viewing. The magnification is set at approximately 10×. ODM may be performed with normal or slightly reduced room illumination. The measuring dial is set at the lowest setting that does not cause forward tilting of the arm, which would blur the image of the disc. The fundus lens is then positioned very close to the cornea, allowing the examiner to visualize the fundus through the lens. The patient is instructed to fixate with the opposite eye, and the fixation target is slowly moved until the optic disc is seen by the examiner. The joystick is slowly brought forward until the fundus lens contacts the cornea and the fundus image becomes sharply focused and bright. The examiner then increases the pressure by turning the dial, and watches the central retinal artery to observe the onset of arterial pulsation and then the cessation of pulsation with increasing pressure.

Indirect Ophthalmodynamometry

If the patient has a miotic pupil that for some reason cannot be dilated (e.g., posterior synechiae, iris-fixed intraocular lens implant) or if the fundus cannot be viewed clearly (cornea or crystalline lens opacity), then indirect ODM should be attempted.[49] In indirect ODM, the opposite eye is occluded, and the pressure is increased with the ophthalmodynamometer until the patient reports peripheral vision beginning to fade out or darken. The amount of pressure needed to reach this point corresponds to the ophthalmic artery diastolic pressure. Likewise, the pressure at which the central vision begins to fade corresponds to the systolic pressure.[49] In comparing direct and indirect ODM, it has been reported that the diastolic measurement in indirect ODM is consistently slightly higher than that found in direct ODM.[50] This difference may not be important, however, since abnormal results of ODM are detected by comparing the findings between the two eyes. Therefore, absolute values have less meaning.[51]

Contraindications to Ophthalmodynamometry

Any patient with a history of retinal detachment or any condition that strongly predisposes the patient to the development of a detachment is generally not considered a candidate for ODM.[2] Patients with iris or retinal neovascularization or those who are in some other way prone to retinal bleeding are best handled with caution, and systolic measurements are not generally recommended.[52] Some practitioners may have reservations about performing ODM on patients with Hollenhorst plaques or branch retinal occlusions for fear of further complicating the problem, but these have not been viewed as contraindications by many experts.[52] Although there have been no reported instances of problems, caution would certainly be indicated in patients who have intraocular lens implants. One final contraindication according to at least one source is glaucoma.[2] However, it is questionable whether raising the intraocular pressure for the very brief period needed to perform ODM is really dangerous. It has been listed as a contraindication probably because of those cases in which there is a large difference in IOP between the eyes and in which the values cannot be used directly. In most glaucoma cases, the IOP differ-

ence will not be relatively large (less than 10 mm Hg), and ODM can still be performed. Even when there is a large IOP difference, approximate corrections can be made. The measurements determined for a given eye while a patient maintains different postures can be compared as well, which would require no adjustment for IOP.

INTERPRETATION OF OPHTHALMODYNAMOMETRY RESULTS

In either the direct or indirect methods, the difference in pressure between the readings from the two eyes should be less than 15% in individuals with normal ICA circulation.[1-3,53] Most of the time the difference is no greater than 5% in normal subjects.[3] Several investigators state that any difference greater than 10% between the diastolic pressures or 15% between the systolic pressures is suspect,[2,3,54] and nearly all studies agree that differences greater than 20% between the two eyes represent a definite reduction in ICA blood flow.[2,4,48,53,54] When the examiner has achieved skill in performing ODM, differences of 10% may be diagnostic. When the patient is hypertensive, there must be a greater difference between the two eyes before it is significant,[3,54] and 20% should be the minimal difference considered diagnostic of ICA disease in such cases.

Using the 20% minimum difference criterion, most studies indicate that ODM detects about 70–75% of patients who have ICA occlusive disease.[1-3,23] False-positive rates are very low,[1,29] making abnormal ODM findings highly diagnostic. A normal ODM finding, however, does not rule out the possibility of ICA occlusive disease, since the presence of collateral circulation may mask the abnormality in 25–30% of patients. Furthermore, for abnormal ODM readings to occur, there usually must be at least a 50% stenosis.[2,31,55] Hence, milder vascular stenosis is not usually detected with ODM.[55] Thus, those patients with abnormal ODM findings are generally those with serious carotid artery obstruction who are in need of further vascular evaluation.

Postural ODM, which consists of taking measurements with the patient both sitting and supine, can be used to increase the sensitivity of testing. Smith and Cogan[56] were the first to point out the effect of posture on ophthalmodynamometric values. They found that changes in posture had little or no effect on normal subjects, whereas in those patients with known carotid occlusive disease, a large number (85%) had a difference of greater than 20% between the pressures found with the two postures on the occluded side. Calderon[57] further found that postural

ODM was very important in cases of bilateral ICA obstruction. He found little difference among normal subjects (except in one patient with known, pronounced hypotension) but concurred that in patients with known ICA obstructions, 65% showed differences of greater that 20% between the pressures obtained in the supine and sitting postures for the eye on the affected side. More important, he found patients who had no abnormal pressure differences between the two eyes in any single posture, but who were correctly detected as having ICA disease solely because of significant differences between the measurements obtained with the patient in the supine and sitting postures.[57] Therefore, if ODM is performed on a seated patient and the results are normal, it should be repeated with the patient in a supine position to increase the sensitivity of the procedure. Examination in two postures is especially important if the readings in both eyes in the seated posture are low. This will allow the detection of some cases of bilateral ICA insufficiency. Also, if the patient reports any symptoms, such as amaurosis fugax, that seem to be related to changes in posture, postural ODM should be performed.

The ophthalmodynamometer may not be accurate in the range below 20 on the dial, so a larger percentage difference may be needed to show a significant difference between the two eyes. Readings in this range, however, are significant in themselves for being so low. The ophthalmic and brachial artery pressures may be compared in order to further evaluate ODM values that may be low on both sides. The dynamometer is designed to measure in grams, while sphygmomanometry measures in millimeters of mercury. Conversion tables are available that convert grams to millimeters of mercury for ODM, but because the readings are generally compared with themselves, values obtained through ODM are usually recorded without designating any units. If the ODM findings are compared directly with the brachial artery pressures (ignoring all units), it is found that the diastolic pressure determined with ODM is approximately two-thirds that of the brachial diastolic pressure.[54] The ODM systolic pressure is typically three-fourths that of the brachial artery systolic pressure.[54] In hypertensive patients, the vessels become more rigid, and the pressures in the different parts of the vascular system tend to become more equal. Thus, in patients with hypertension the ophthalmic artery pressure should represent a higher percentage of the brachial artery pressure than the normal two-thirds and three-fourths values. Whenever the ODM value is less than 50% of the corresponding brachial artery value, ICA disease should be suspected.[54] The lower the percentage, the more diagnostic it is of ICA stenosis or occlusion.

MANAGEMENT OF CAROTID OCCLUSIVE DISEASE

The management of carotid occlusive disease is an area of great controversy. As with all therapies, the benefit of treatment must outweigh the risks of that treatment. There is no agreement on nor are the benefits and risks clearly known for both medical and surgical management of carotid vascular problems. Therefore, continued studies involving longer follow-up periods, better designs, and increasing numbers of patients will be needed to determine the optimal treatment of various levels of carotid artery disease.

Medical Management

Medical therapies for carotid occlusive disease have involved the use of platelet antiaggregants and anticoagulants. Although not conclusive in all studies, aspirin has been shown to be significantly effective in reducing the risk of stroke in a number of investigations. The Canadian Study Group[58] found that in men who had suffered TIAs, 325 mg of aspirin four times a day reduced the risk for stroke and death by nearly 50%. This and other studies that have looked at the effectiveness of aspirin in women and at other platelet aggregation inhibitors such as dipyridamole and sulfinpyrazone have produced results that are somewhat inconclusive.[58-61] Dipyridamole does appear to have a significant role to play in the prevention of platelet aggregation in cardiac conditions and may be useful in carotid problems as well.[60,62]

Studies on the use of anticoagulants in patients with carotid artery disease have failed to demonstrate a significant reduction in stroke. Furthermore, when used in elderly patients, anticoagulants increase the risk of intracerebral hemorrhage.[63-65] The primary effectiveness of anticoagulants in preventing stroke appears to be more with emboli of cardiac origin rather than carotid origin. In patients with rheumatic heart disease and myocardial infarction, long-term anticoagulant therapy significantly reduces the risk of cerebral embolism.[66,67]

Surgical Management

Surgical management of carotid disease has been extremely controversial. Carotid endarterectomy is a surgical procedure that removes fatty deposits from within the carotid artery. It is performed as an attempt to reduce the risk of stroke or death in patients with known carotid artery disease. There remains considerable debate over its effectiveness in achieving this goal and the accompanying risks.[68-70] There is a risk of both stroke or death during the surgery and postoperatively with endarterectomy. Most studies have reported surgical and 30-day postoperative rates of stroke or death on the order of 3–5%.[71-74] Many centers not involved in these investigations will have higher rates. To accept such risks, the value of the surgery for all types of cases needs to be established. Despite the lack of certainty concerning its efficacy, the number of carotid endarterectomies increased in the United States from about 15,000 in 1971 to over 100,000 in 1986.[75,76]

An extensive retrospective look at carotid endarterectomy was conducted by the Rand/UCLA Health Services Utilization Study.[77] After reviewing over 1,300 procedures performed in three separate geographic locations, this study determined that 32% were not appropriate. Another 30–35% of the procedures were rated as equivocal, meaning there was no strong agreement whether they were appropriate. The study also reported a morbidity rate of 3.4% and a mortality rate of 6.4%. This combined complication rate of 9.8% must be compared with the fact that there is probably a 10% annual risk of death or stroke when there is no treatment.[78] There is no clear agreement on how much medical treatment such as aspirin therapy reduces this rate, but it is believed to reduce the risk of stroke by at least 25%.[79] Therefore, even for those procedures deemed appropriate, the study states that they are appropriate only if the major complication rate of the surgeon or center is less than 8%, and ideally it should be at the 3–4% level.[77]

Rated as most appropriate were surgical procedures performed on patients who were symptomatic for TIAs of carotid origin, especially multiple or crescendo TIAs. These patients should have a carotid stenosis in the range of 70–99%, be a low to medium surgical risk patient only, and have mainly ipsilateral carotid problems. Patients with 50–70% occlusions may be candidates if ulcerations are present. Asymptomatic patients, even with 70–99% stenosis, are rated as equivocal at best. There is sound evidence that carotid endarterectomy is not appropriate in cases of complete occlusion, a stroke less than 3 weeks previously, or when there is stenosis less than 50%. Endarterectomy was also generally felt to be less appropriate in those cases of high surgical risk, or for those patients who had suffered a stroke or who are suffering a stroke-in-evolution.[77,78]

The efficacy of endarterectomy in symptomatic patients with high-grade carotid stenosis has been confirmed in a number of well-designed studies.[73,74,80] Foremost among these are the randomized clinical trials performed in the North American Symptomatic Carotid Endarterectomy Trial (NASCET), and the European Carotid Surgery Trial (ECST).[73,74] The NASCET study found surgery to be clearly beneficial when the stenosis was 70% or greater, and when there had been recent episodes of TIAs or a nondisabling stroke. Likewise, the ECST study found benefit for symptomatic patients with stenosis from 70–99% but concluded that the risk of surgery outweighs the benefits for milder stenosis, even in symptomatic patients.

A number of studies have looked at the use of endarterectomy in asymptomatic patients. The Carotid Artery Stenosis with Asymptomatic Narrowing Study[81] found no benefit in the surgically treated group compared with the aspirin-treated group. A Mayo Clinic comparison[82] was terminated early because of excessive complications in the surgically treated group compared with the aspirin-treated group. A third study looking at the same question concluded that in patients with stenosis of 75–99% but no symptoms, surgery resulted in less neurologic complications compared with a group treated with daily aspirin.[71] There was no benefit of surgery, however, in decreasing the occurrence of the most important neurologic complications—stroke and death.[71]

At this point, the best recommendations are to institute medical therapy in all patients with carotid occlusive disease, whether symptomatic or not. In addition to aspirin therapy, these persons should be advised not to smoke and to maintain good control of any existing hypertension. When stenosis of greater than 70% is detected and the patient has been recently symptomatic and is a good surgical risk patient, endarterectomy is indicated. For milder levels of stenosis in symptomatic persons, and for all levels in asymptomatic persons, the value of surgery has yet to be established.

Carotid endarterectomy has probably been over-performed and its use should be at least somewhat curtailed. In those cases where it seems appropriate, the complication rate needs to be sufficiently low to justify surgical intervention.[77,78] As further advances are made in both medical therapies and surgical procedures, the comparative risks and benefits of each will need to be continually recalculated.

REFERENCES

1. Wood FA, Toole JF. Carotid artery occlusion and its diagnosis by ophthalmodynamometry. JAMA 1957;165:1254–70.
2. Toole JF, Patel AN. Cerebrovascular Disorders (2nd ed). New York: McGraw-Hill, 1974;92–8.
3. Hollenhorst RW. Carotid and vertebral-basilar arterial stenosis and occlusion: Neuro-ophthalmologic considerations. Trans Am Acad Ophthalmol Otolaryngol 1962;66:166–80.
4. Hollenhorst RW. Ocular manifestations of insufficiency or thrombosis of the internal carotid artery. Am J Ophthalmol 1959;47:753–67.

5. Muuronen A, Kaste M. Outcome of 314 patients with transient ischemic attacks. Stroke 1982;13:24–31.
6. Goldner J, Wisnant JP, Taylor WF. Long-term prognosis of transient cerebral ischemic attacks. Stroke 1971;2:160–7.
7. Imparato AM, Riles TS, Mintzer R, et al. The importance of hemorrhage in the relationship between gross morphologic characteristics and cerebral symptoms in 376 carotid artery plaques. Ann Surg 1983;197:195–203.
8. Hollenhorst RW. Vascular status of patients who have cholesterol emboli in the retina. Am J Ophthalmol 1966;61:1159–65.
9. Arruga J, Sanders MD. Ophthalmologic findings in 70 patients with evidence of retinal embolism. Ophthalmology 1982;89:1136–47.
10. Pfaffenbach DD, Hollenhorst RW. Morbidity and survivorship of patients with embolic cholesterol crystals in the ocular fundus. Am J Ophthalmol 1973;75:66–72.
11. Kearns T, Hollenhorst, LR. Venous stasis retinopathy of occlusive disease of the carotid artery. Proc Mayo Clin 1963;38:304–312.
12. Berguer R, Weiss H (eds). The Carotid and the Eye. New York: Praeger, 1985.
13. Hedges TR. Ophthalmoscopic findings in internal carotid artery occlusion. Bull Johns Hopkins Hosp 1962;111:89–97.
14. Neupert JR, Brubaker RF, Kearns TP, Sundt TM. Rapid resolution of venous stasis retinopathy after carotid endarterectomy. Am J Ophthalmol 1976;81:600–2.
15. Kearns TP, Younge BR, Piepgras DG. Resolution of venous stasis retinopathy after carotid artery bypass surgery. Mayo Clin Proc 1980;55:342–6.
16. Sundt TM Jr, Siekert RG, Piepgras DG et al. Bypass surgery for vascular disease of the carotid system. Mayo Clin Proc 1976;51:677–92.
17. Hayreh SS, Podhajsky P. Ocular neovascularization with retinal vascular occlusion II. Occurrence in central and branch retinal artery occlusion. Arch Ophthalmol 1982;100:1585–96.
18. Brown GC, Magargal EE, Simeone FA, et al. Arterial obstruction and ocular neovascularization. Ophthalmology 1982;89:139–46.
19. Gonder JR, et al. The ocular ischemic syndrome. An indication for neovascular surgery. Ann Royal Coll Surg (Canada) 1983;16:447–53.
20. Brown GC, Magargal LE. The ocular ischemic syndrome: Clinical fluorescein angiographic and carotid angiographic features. Int Ophthalmol 1988;11:239–51.
21. Riles TS, Liebman A, Kopelman I, Imparato AM. Symptoms, stenosis, and bruit. Inter-relationships in carotid artery diseases. Arch Surg 1981;116:218–20.
22. Wolf PA, Kannel WB, Sorlie P, McNamara P. Asymptomatic carotid bruit and the risk of stroke: The Framingham Study. JAMA 1981;245:1442–5.
23. David TE, Humphries A, Young J, Beven E. A correlation of neck bruits and arteriosclerotic carotid arteries. Arch Surg 1973;107:729–31.
24. Abramson DI. Vascular Disorders of the Extremities (2nd ed). Hagerstown, MD: Harper & Row, 1974.
25. Keeney AH. Ocular Examination: Basis and Technique. St. Louis: Mosby, 1970:213–8.
26. Bailiart P. La pression artérielle dans les branches de l'artère centrale de la rétine; nouvelle technique pour la déterminer. Ann Oculist (Paris) 1917;154:648–66.
27. Vander Werff TJ. The pressure measured in ophthalmodynamometry. Arch Ophthalmol 1972;87:290–2.
28. Duke-Elder S. The ocular circulation: Its normal pressure relationships and their physiological significance. Br J Ophthalmol 1926;10:513–572.
29. Yuson CP, Toole JF. Bruits, ophthalmodynamometry and rectilinear scanning on transient ischemic attacks. Stroke 1976;7:541–5.
30. Samples JR, Trautman JC, Sundt TM. Interpretation of results of compression ODM. Stroke 1982;13:655–9.
31. Cohen DN, Wangelin R. A comparison of the sensitivity of carotid tonography with ophthalmodynamometry in the diagnosis of internal carotid artery occlusive disease. Trans Am Acad Ophthalmol Otolaryngol 1976;81:882–92.
32. May AG, DeWeese JA, Rob CG. Hemodynamic effects of arterial stenosis. Surgery 1963;53:513–24.
33. Gee W. Carotid physiology with ocular pneumoplethysmography. Stroke 1982;13:666–73.
34. Marck KW, Ong KH, Andhyiswara T, Yo TI. A comparison of angiography with oculopneumoplethysmography in carotid artery disease. Neth J Surg 1982;34:104–8.
35. Comerota AS, Cranley JJ, Cook SE. Real-time b-mode carotid imaging in diagnosis of cerebrovascular disease. Surgery 1981;89:718–29.
36. Zweibel WJ. High resolution carotid sonography. Semin Ultrasound 1981;2:316–32.
37. Bendick PJ, Glover JL. Detection of subcritical stenosis by Doppler spectrum analysis. Surgery 1981;91:707–11.
38. Fell G, Breslau P, Knox RA, et al. Importance of non-invasive ultrasonic-Doppler testing in the evaluation of patients with symptomatic carotid bruits. Am Heart J 1982;102:221–6.
39. Clark WM, Hatten HP. Noninvasive screening of extracranial carotid disease: Duplex sonography with angiographic correlation. AJNR 1981;2:443–7.
40. Higgins CB. The potential role of magnetic resonance imaging in ischemic vascular disease. (Editorial.) N Engl J Med 1992;326:1624–6.
41. Owen RS, Carpenter JP, Baum RA, et al. Magnetic resonance imaging of angiographically occult runoff vessels in peripheral arterial occlusive disease. N Engl J Med 1992;326:1577–81.
42. Ross JS, Masaryk TJ, Modic MT, et al. Magnetic resonance angiography of the extracranial carotid arteries and intracranial vessels: A review. Neurology 1989;39:1369–76.
43. Litt AW, Eidelman EM, Pinto RS, et al. Diagnosis of carotid artery stenosis: Comparison of 2DFT time-of-flight MR angiography with contrast angiography in 50 patients. AJNR 1991;12:149–54.
44. Faught E, Trader SD, Hanna GR et al. Cerebral complications of angiography for transient ischemia and stroke: Prediction of risk. Neurology 1979;29:4–15.
45. Hankey GJ, Warlow CP, Sellar RJ. Cerebral angiographic risk in mild cerebrovascular disease. Stroke 1990;21:209–22.

46. Brody WR, Enzmann DR, Miller DC et al. Intravenous arteriography using digital subtraction techniques. JAMA 1982:248:671–4.

47. Biotronics Inc. MacKay-Marg Tonometer Model 12 Instruction Manual, p. 13.

48. Spalter HF. Ophthalmodynamometry and carotid artery thrombosis. Am J Ophthalmol 1959;47:453–67.

49. Toole JF. Ophthalmodynamometry: A simplified method. Arch Intern Med 1963;112:981–93.

50. Pence NA. Indirect ophthalmodynamometry: Its comparison with direct ophthalmodynamometry in the detection of carotid artery occlusive disease. Am J Optom Physiol Opt 1980;57:724–8.

51. Holladay JT, Arnoult JB, Ruiz RS. Comparative evaluation of current ophthalmodynamometers. Am J Ophthalmol 1979;87:665–74.

52. Taylor J. Idiopathic ischemic optic neuritis. Ophthalmology Tape 22 (Vol. 16). Glendale, CA: Audio Digest Foundation, 1978.

53. Conn HL, Horowitz O. Cardiac and Vascular Diseases (Vol 2). Philadelphia: Lea & Febiger, 1974.

54. Smith JL. Ophthalmodynamometry and cerebrovascular disease. Neuro-Ophthalmology Tape 7. Miami: Audio Digest Foundation, 1978.

55. Machleder H, Barker W. Non-invasive methods for evaluation of extracranial cerebrovascular disease. Arch Surg 1977;112:944–6.

56. Smith JL, Cogan DG. The ophthalmodynamometric posture test. Am J Ophthalmol 1959;48:735–40.

57. Calderon RG. Postural ophthalmodynamometry in carotid artery occlusive disease. JAMA 1963;185:826–30.

58. Canadian Cooperative Study Group. A randomized trial of aspirin and sulfinpyrazone in treated stroke. N Engl J Med 1978;299:53–9.

59. Bousser MG, Eschwege E, Haguenau M, et al. "AICLA" controlled trial of aspirin and dipyridamole in the secondary prevention of athero-thrombotic cerebral ischemia. Stroke 1983;14:5–14.

60. The Persantine-Aspirin Reinfarction Study Research Group. Persantine and aspirin in coronary heart disease. Circulation 1980;62:449–61.

61. Sorensen PS, Pederson H, Marquardsen J, et al. Acetylsalicylic acid in the prevention of stroke in patients with reversible cerebral ischemic attacks: A Danish cooperative study. Stroke 1983;14:15–22.

62. Aspirin Myocardial Infarction Study Research Group. A randomized controlled trial of aspirin in persons recovered from myocardial infarction. JAMA 1980;243:661–9.

63. Whisnant JP, Cartlidge NEF, Elveback LR. Carotid and vertebral-basilar transient ischemic attacks: Effect of anticoagulants, hypertension, and cardiac disorders on survival and stroke occurrence—a population study. Ann Neurol 1978;3:107–15.

64. Millikan CH. Reassessment of anticoagulant therapy in various types of occlusive cerebrovascular diseases. Stroke 1971;2:201–8.

65. Olsson JE, Muller R, Berneli S. Long-term anticoagulant therapy for TIAs and minor strokes with minimum residuum. Stroke 1976;7:444–5.

66. Easton JD, Sherman DG. Management of cerebral embolism of cardiac origin. Stroke 1980;11:433–42.

67. Adams GF, Merritt JD, Hutchinson WM, Pollock AM. Cerebral embolism and mitral stenosis: Survival with and without anticoagulants. J Neurol Neurosurg Psychiatry 1974;37:378–83.

68. Chassin MR, Brook RH, Park RE, et al. Variations in the use of medical and surgical services by the Medicare population. N Engl J Med 1986;314:285–90.

69. Shaw DA, Venables GS, Cartlidge NEF, et al. Carotid endarterectomy in patients with transient cerebral ischemia. J Neurol Sci 1984;65:45–53.

70. Fields W, Maslenikov V, Meyer J, et al. Joint study of extracranial arterial occlusions: Progress report of prognosis following surgery or non-surgical treatment for TIAs and cervical carotid artery lesions. JAMA 1970;211:1993–2003.

71. Hobson RW II, Weiss DG, Fields WS, et al. Efficacy of carotid endarterectomy for asymptomatic carotid stenosis. N Engl J Med 1993;328:221–7.

72. Norris JW, Zhu CZ, Bornstein NM, Chambers BR. Vascular risks of asymptomatic carotid stenosis. Stroke 1991;22:1485–90.

73. North American Symptomatic Carotid Endarterectomy Trial Collaborators. Beneficial effect of carotid endarterectomy in symptomatic patients with high-grade carotid stenosis. N Engl J Med 1991;325:445–53.

74. European Carotid Surgery Trialists' Collaborative Group. MRC European Carotid Surgery Trial. Interim results for symptomatic patients with severe (70–99 percent) or with mild (0–29 percent) carotid stenosis. Lancet 1991;337:1235–43.

75. Dyken ML. Carotid endarterectomy studies: A glimmering of science. Stroke 1986;17:355–8.

76. Dyken ML, Pokras R. The performance of endarterectomy for disease of the extracranial arteries of the head. Stroke 1984;15:948–50.

77. Chassin MR, Koescoff J, Park RE, et al. The appropriateness of selected medical and surgical procedures. Publication R-3204-CWF/PMT/HF/RWJ. Philadelphia: The Rand Corporation, 1989.

78. Merrick NJ, Fink A, Brook RH, et al. A review of the literature and ratings for the appropriateness of indication for selected medical and surgical procedures: Carotid endarterectomy. Publication R-3204/6-CWF/PMT/HF/RWJ. Philadelphia: The Rand Corporation, May 1986.

79. Warlow C. Secondary prevention of stroke. Lancet 1992;339:24–9.

80. Mayberg MR. Wilson SE, Yatsu F, et al. Carotid edarterectomy and prevention of cerebral ischemia in symptomatic carotid stenosis. JAMA 1991;266:3289–94.

81. The CASANOVA Study Group. Carotid surgery versus medical therapy in asymptomatic carotid stenosis. Stroke 1991;22:1229–35.

82. Mayo Asymptomatic Carotid Endarterectomy Study Group. Effectiveness of carotid endarterectomy for asymptomatic carotid stenosis: Design of a clinical trial. Mayo Clin Proc 1989;64:897–904.

13

Electrodiagnosis

JEROME SHERMAN AND SHERRY J. BASS

Although there are many useful chairside tests to aid the practitioner in making certain decisions, most of these tests require subjective responses and therefore pose their own inherent problems. In addition, some of these tests may not provide the necessary information for arriving at a differential diagnosis. For example, a patient with reduced visual acuity may have a retinal or visual pathway problem, and traditional tests often will not reveal the site of involvement. Electrodiagnostic tests, however, may objectively reveal sensory information unobtainable by any other means.

Electrodiagnostic testing has been available for at least two decades, but even today too few clinicians consider providing these services. With the recent introduction of compact, easy-to-use, and easy-to-interpret systems, however, in-office electrodiagnostic testing has become more routine.

This chapter discusses three electrodiagnostic procedures—the visual evoked potential, electroretinography, and electro-oculography—and the applications of these procedures in the differential diagnosis of ocular disease.

THE VISUAL EVOKED POTENTIAL

The visual evoked potential (VEP) is an objective measurement of visual function monitored at the level of the occipital cortex using scalp electrodes. An evoked potential is actually the electrical activity of the brain in response to sensory (in this case, visual) stimulation. The patient is treated as a "black box," whose eyes receive a stimulus and whose brain then elicits a response or potential, which

is measured. Verbal responses are not necessary from patients in order to assess their ability to see, both qualitatively and quantitatively.

Current optometric applications for VEP testing include objective estimates of refractive error, visual acuity, binocular function, accommodation, stereopsis, prognostic assessment of amblyopia, and detection of retinal (macular) and optic nerve dysfunction in the absence of observable pathologic conditions and visual symptoms.

The objective nature of VEP testing makes it extremely useful to the clinician confronted with a nonverbal child or a malingering adult patient. Patients with autism, Down's syndrome, Alzheimer's disease, and cerebral palsy have had their visual function successfully assessed with VEP testing. Psychogenic problems (such as hysteria and malingering) resulting in reduced subjective visual acuity also can be successfully exposed using the VEP. Demyelinating disease (such as multiple sclerosis) can be detected and diagnosed early with the aid of the VEP.

Other VEP applications include the presurgical prediction of postsurgical visual function in patients with media opacities, objective visual field measurements, assessment of optic nerve damage in glaucoma, objective color vision analysis, investigation of migraine headaches, early detection of poisoning, optic pathway misrouting in albinism, prognostic evaluation of traumatic brain injury, and objective determination of neurologic development.

The theoretical aspects and technical considerations of the VEP have been greatly minimized in the subsequent discussion. Additional information is available in two excellent comprehensive sources.[1,2]

Portions of this chapter were modified with permission from J Sherman, VG Sutija. Visual-Evoked Potentials. In JB Eskridge, JF Amos, JD Bartlett (eds), Clinical Procedures in Optometry. Philadelphia: Lippincott, 1991;514–29.

About a century ago, Richard Caton first reported on both spontaneous brain rhythms and evoked potentials.[3] Spontaneous brain rhythms, or intrinsic brain rhythms, are merely the random fluctuations of electrical activity that can be recorded from the scalp with surface electrodes. Evoked potentials, although having certain characteristics similar to intrinsic brain rhythms, are not spontaneous but result from specific sensory stimulation. For example, the VEP is the electrical activity that can be elicited from the occipital cortex by visual stimuli. Even though evoked potentials exist in other sensory modalities (e.g., the auditory evoked potential and somatosensory evoked potential), the discussion here will be limited to the visual system.

Basic Concepts of the Visual Evoked Potential

The VEP, as typically recorded, is a cortical response originating primarily from the central retinal cones. A surface electrode attached to the scalp slightly above the inion (or external occipital protuberance) monitors and transmits the response.

The finding that the central retinal cones dominate the response can be readily explained by considering two aspects of the visual system. First, the central 5 degrees of the retina comprising the macula project onto about half of the occipital cortex. Thus, a disproportionately large cortical area corresponds to a rather small retinal area. This is because the relationship between the central retinal cones and the corresponding bipolar and ganglion cells is approximately one to one. In contrast, large numbers of peripheral photoreceptors funnel into a small number of ganglionic cells. The high spatial resolution (i.e., good visual acuity) found in the central retina and the poor spatial resolution found in the periphery are a direct consequence of these neural connections.

The second aspect of visual system anatomy that explains why the central retinal cones dominate the response is that the macula projects most posteriorly onto the occipital cortex and is therefore close to the recording electrodes. In view of the anatomy of the visual system and the position of the recording electrode, the VEP, recorded under standard conditions, is presumed to reflect macular function primarily.

Electrophysiology

Each visual stimulation initiates a chain of electrochemical events, which are transmitted to the occipital cortex. However, a single response to a single stimulus is generally too small in magnitude to be consistently measured.

This is because of the inherent and spontaneous "noisiness" of the underlying cortex. For example, the response to a single flash of light, when measured at the inion (Figure 13-1), is usually about 10 microvolts (μV) in amplitude, whereas the intrinsic overall brain activity, as seen in an electroencephalogram (EEG), might be larger than 100 μV. Thus, the small ripples of the VEP are overshadowed by the large waves of the EEG. Therefore, the amplitude of the VEP must be enhanced or amplified. This is accomplished by repeating the visual stimulus many times. Since each response occurs at a fixed time interval after each stimulus, the response is said to be "time-locked" to the stimulus. By using a computer to average the responses to repetitive stimuli, the individual VEP signals are electronically superimposed and enhanced. At the same time, background brain activity, or "noise," which is not time-locked to the visual stimulus, is averaged out by the use of analog or digital filters built into the computer. Figure 13-2 graphically depicts this process. The instrument capable of averaging responses to a repetitive stimulus is known as a computer of average transience or CAT for short. Preliminary VEP research did not ensue until the advent of the CAT.

During VEP testing, there are recordable potentials evoked or generated by sources other than the brain, such as muscle fiber activity, eye movements, tongue and facial movement, and the heart beat. These high-amplitude "artifacts" are eliminated by the software of most commercially available systems.

The electrical activity recorded during VEP testing is collected through the use of electrodes, which most commonly consist of metal disks or cups, which act as conductors, connected to a lead wire and a plug for insertion into the computer. The surface of these disks is typically made of gold, chlorided silver, or similar materials that do not interact with the skin. When VEP testing is performed, an electrode is usually attached to both earlobes (a reference electrode and a ground electrode) and to the scalp at a point just above the inion (the electrode that records the visual evoked response).

Modes of Stimulation

A VEP is generated by a visual stimulus, which is either presented repetitively or altered repetitively. Two major VEPs occur depending on the rate of stimulus presentation or alteration. A transient VEP is the result of an isolated abrupt change in some stimulus parameter.[1] It occurs when the repetition rate is relatively slow (i.e., one stimulus per second) such that a distinct response is attributable to a physiologically distinct stimulus. In contrast, a steady-state VEP is evoked by a stimulus of sufficiently high repetition frequency, which results in an overlap of

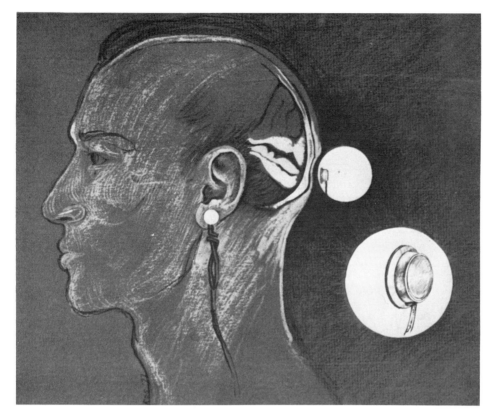

FIGURE 13-1
Schematic representation of the active electrode placed slightly above the inion. Note the proximity of the occipital cortex and the surface electrode. An ear clip electrode is also shown, which may be either a reference electrode or ground electrode.

the responses so that no individual response cycle can be related to any particular stimulus cycle.[1] The point at which a VEP is no longer a transient response but becomes a steady-state response depends not only on the repetition rate but also on the type of stimulus used.

The checkerboard pattern is presently the most common stimulus used in clinical VEP investigations. This consists of an array of black and white squares. An evoked potential is generated when each of the squares repeatedly changes from black to white or white to black (known as "pattern reversal"). An advantage of a pattern reversal stimulus is that the average luminance remains constant. If the aspects of form vision (e.g., visual acuity, refractive error) are being investigated, the investigator is looking for a response to a pattern and not to large changes in luminance (known as a "luminance response"). The rate at which the squares reverse can be slow, resulting in a transient VEP, or fast, yielding a steady-state VEP.

Some clinical researchers prefer testing at a slow rate, whereas others feel a faster rate uncovers subtle abnormalities not evident at a slower rate. Some suggest that testing includes a slow rate, resulting in a transient VEP, and also a faster rate, so that a steady-state VEP is also

generated. Testing at various rates and also with checks or bars of different sizes appears to stimulate somewhat different channels in the visual pathway and hence may yield additional information.

Figure 13-3 depicts a transient and a steady-state VEP. The steady-state VEP resulted from the pattern reversal of the individual small checks of a large checkerboard. The pattern reversal rate was 3.75 Hz (7.5 reversals per second) and the major responses can be observed to be a series of sine-like waves occurring 7.5 times per second (1 Hz = 2 reversals per second). The repetitive wave is actually the linear sum of elementary sinusoidal terms known as Fourier components. The fundamental component (or first harmonic) occurs at the tested frequency rate. In this example, the fundamental is at 7.5 Hz because the pattern reversal rate was 7.5 reversals per second. The second harmonic component is at double the pattern reversal rate, or 15 Hz. The third harmonic component is at triple the pattern reversal rate, or 22.5 Hz, and so on. A mathematical manipulation can be performed to measure the amplitude of the harmonic components. For the purposes of this discussion, it is sufficient to consider only the fundamental or first harmonic component.

FIGURE 13-2
A. Each stimulus of the stimulus train results in an isolated response, but noise is ever present. Clinically, the stimuli response plus the noise are recorded simultaneously. B. By averaging the response plus noise complexes as shown, the noise averages out, thus unmasking the response.

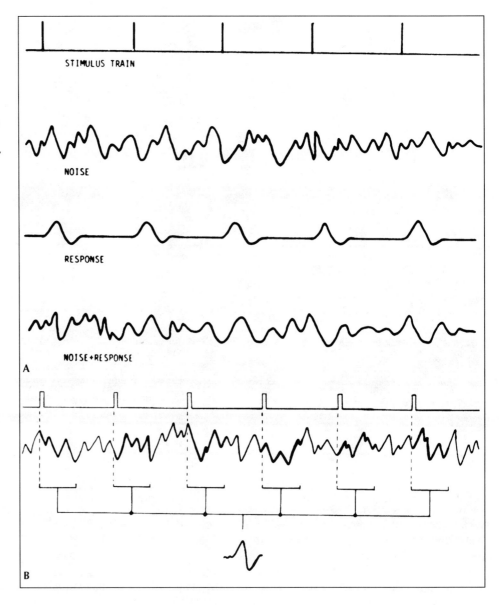

Reversal rates of 7.5 or 15 reversals/second are clinically useful because these rates avoid the alpha rhythm, generally the largest of the intrinsic brain patterns. The alpha rhythm, which has a frequency of 8 and 13 cycles/second, may sometimes contaminate the response.

VEPs also may be obtained using a nonpatterned photic or bright flashing light. This is useful when evaluating the integrity of the visual system in patients with media opacities, such as cataracts, corneal scarring, or vitreal hemorrhage. However, this technique provides only qualitative, not quantitative, information about the visual system, since the stimulus is not patterned.

Other modes of presentation include pattern onset-off-set, or appearance and disappearance, and sweep VEPs. Because of the limited scope of this chapter, the reader should refer to more detailed information on these techniques elsewhere.[1] VEPs can be performed simultaneously with electroretinography (ERG). Simultaneous recording of electrical activity from the retina (ERG) as well as the brain (VEP) could be of great clinical value in differentiating retinal from visual pathway dysfunction. However, this technique currently suffers from lack of standardization that limits its usefulness. In addition, the origin of the pattern ERG is still somewhat controversial.

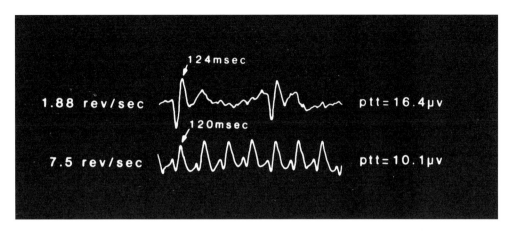

FIGURE 13-3

The stimulus in this example was a checkerboard composed of 14 minutes-of-arc checks, and the analysis time was 1,000 msec, or 1 sec. The checks were pattern reversed at a slow rate (1.88 reversals/second), which resulted in a transient VEP, as shown with the top recording. The lower recording is a steady-state VEP that resulted from a pattern reversal rate of 7.5 reversals/second. Since this represents 1,000 msec, or 1 sec, of cortical activity, 7.5 sine-like waves are expected to result when the pattern reversal rate is 7.5. A positive deflection is indicated by an upward pointing spike. Amplitudes of individual responses are measured from peak to trough (ptt). The first positive peak occurred at 124 msec and 120 msec in the upper and lower traces, respectively. Under the conditions of these tests, the amplitudes and latencies (peak times) are within normal limits.

FIGURE 13-4

The Tomey PE-410 portable electrophysiology system is capable of performing both VEPs and ERGs. The tabletop screen with the checkerboard pattern is viewed during VEP examinations. Three surface electrodes are affixed to the patient during testing, and the signal, after amplification, is transmitted to the system hardware, which also fits onto a tabletop. (Courtesy of Tomey Technology, Cambridge, MA.)

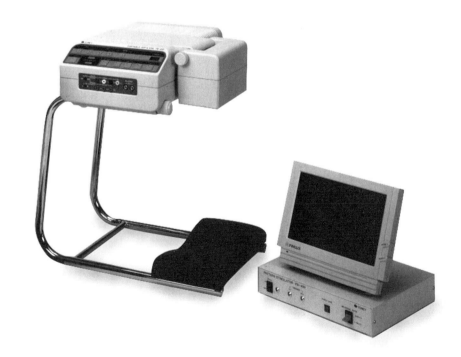

Visual Evoked Potential Testing

If a patient's visual system can resolve the squares on the checkerboard, then a normal VEP will result. The patient need not verbalize what is seen, and acuity is objectively confirmed.

Figure 13-4 portrays commercially available clinical VEP equipment. A VEP apparatus contains three basic components: (1) the visual stimulator; (2) an apparatus that is capable of recording electrical brain wave activity, including amplification, filtering, and averaging; and (3) the means to analyze and present data. Usually three surface electrodes are used for monitoring and transmitting the induced voltage change or potential occurring at the visual cortex. The active electrode is placed just above the inion, the reference electrode may be attached to one ear, and the ground electrode is attached to the other ear.

One typical pattern VEP protocol includes monocular testing at four different check sizes (e.g., 42, 21, 14, and 7 minutes of arc) at a reversal rate of 11.0 reversals/second. Sometimes a slower rate of 3.0 reversals/second is used for obtaining a transient response. Typical waveforms produced at these reversal rates are depicted in Figure 13-5. Contrast and mean luminance are generally held constant throughout testing. The responses are analyzed with respect to amplitude and latency (implicit time) of the waveforms.

Commercially available VEP systems run the gamut from systems that are compact, inexpensive, easy to operate, and easy to interpret to systems that are expensive, remarkably sophisticated, and complex. A system that may have appeal to eye care practitioners in smaller office settings is the Tomey PE-410 electrodiagnostic apparatus (Tomey Technology, Cambridge, MA), which is the size of a bread box, weighs less than 15 lbs, and can generate ERGs or VEPs in less than 15 minutes. The clinician should be able to obtain ERGs and VEPs after about 1 hour of in-service instruction. The printout is obtained about 2 seconds after a test is complete and includes the waveform and all the necessary amplitude and latency measurements. Electroretinographic testing can be performed on both eyes simultaneously, but only single channel VEP recordings are possible. This is not usually a drawback in most clinical situations.

Neuro Scan has introduced the Electric Signal Imaging 128 (ESI-128) (Neuro Scan, Herndon, VA), which can obtain VEPs from 128 sites simultaneously. Attaching one scalp electrode for a one-channel recording may take a minute but placing the 128 scalp electrodes used in the Neuro Scan system requires considerably more time.

Other systems use 16 active electrodes and then display the responses in a topographic or VEP mapping display. Such systems are expensive and testing requires a major time commitment. However, research endeavors are better served with the more elaborate systems now available.

Clinical Applications

Refractive Error

Harter and White,[4] using a transient stimulus, were the first to report a systematic relationship between retinal image clarity and the amplitude of the VEP. In 1972, Ludlum and Meyers[5] extended the research of Harter

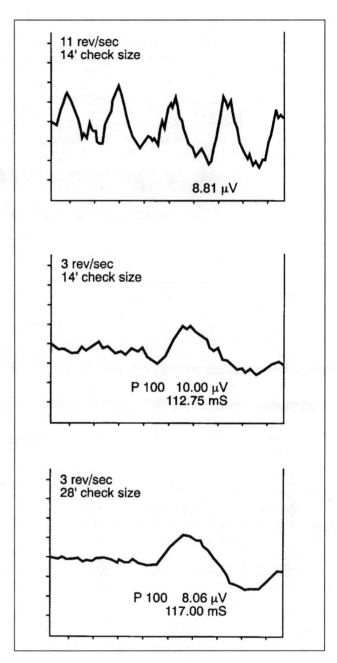

FIGURE 13-5

VEP waveforms produced by the PE-400 (Tomey Technology, Cambridge, MA) at a fast, steady-state reversal rate (11.0 reversals/second) and a slower, transient reversal rate (3.0 reversals/second). In the transient VEP waveforms, the "P100" refers to the main positive deflection, which should occur in a normal eye at approximately 100 ms from the onset of the stimulus. This is the point at which the amplitude and latency are measured.

and White and made objective refractive error assessments clinically feasible for the first time. Regan[6] later developed a system that is reported to approximate the spherocylindrical refractive error to within 0.50 D in less than 1 minute.

Visual Acuity

A quick and accurate objective method of assessing visual acuity is still a highly coveted goal of both vision researchers and ophthalmic clinicians. As a general rule, patients with normal visual acuity and no ocular disease usually generate the largest amplitude VEP with checks of intermediate size (e.g., 10–15 minutes of arc). Smaller or larger checks generally result in smaller amplitudes. This "tuning" of the check size versus VEP amplitude function, which peaks at an intermediate check size, is likely related to receptive field size and to the concept of "channels" within the visual system. Since 20/20 acuity corresponds to 1 minute of arc, a response to this size check would theoretically indicate 20/20 acuity. However, it is technically difficult to generate 1-minute-of-arc checks, and if done, the potentials generated are immeasurable. Hence, direct measurements of visual acuity are not easily attainable. Still, by using various size checks as a stimulus and plotting the amplitude of the evoked potential versus check size, visual acuity can be estimated.[7]

Tyler and associates[8] used an electronic spatial frequency or sweep technique to measure VEPs to various spatial frequencies. The Enfant 4010 system (NeuroScientific Corp., Farmingdale, NY) is a commercially available system capable of rapid sweep techniques and appears to be capable of estimating visual acuity in as little as 10 seconds. The system rapidly changes the bar size (e.g., spatial frequency) of a vertical sinusoidal luminance grating through 16 values and then allows contrast reversal VEPs to be collected and analyzed. This type of VEP apparatus allows VEPs to be obtained from patients with short attention spans such as infants.

Using commercially available equipment, patients with acuities of 20/15 to 20/25 typically generate the largest responses to the 14-minutes-of-arc checks but also generate a smaller but repeatable response to the 7-minute checks. When acuity falls to the level of 20/30 to 20/40, usually no response can be recorded to the 7-minute checks, and the amplitude is reduced to 14-minute checks. When visual acuity is 20/50 or worse, no response is recordable to the 7- or 14-minutes-of-arc checks, although responses are still present to 28- and 56-minute checks. Generally, the visual acuity is at the 20/200 level or less when no response to these four check sizes is recordable. Although these typical

findings can be used only for visual acuity estimates, these approximations are often the only objective assessment available and are of major clinical importance. In some patients, however, as will be discussed later, the correlation between visual acuity and VEP amplitude breaks down.

Evaluation of small children is a challenge because a child's attention must be maintained during testing in order to obtain a VEP. In addition, stable application of the electrode may be difficult. Although the VEP exam is objective in nature, fixation of the visual stimulus by the patient is essential to generate a response. Regan[1] has used a movie cartoon superimposed on the checkerboard which, although quite visible, minimally affected VEP amplitude. Such cartoons combined with rapid sweep techniques can allow VEPs to be generated from even difficult patients.

Prognosis of Amblyopia

The VEP can be used in the assessment of the prognosis for visual acuity improvement following amblyopia therapy. For unilateral amblyopia, monocular VEPs can be recorded and compared. Although not common, some amblyopic eyes generate essentially normal VEPs to small checks when compared with the normal eye. These patients have a relatively normal sensory pathway and have a good prognosis for visual acuity improvement. On the other hand, if no response can be elicited from an "amblyopic" eye with checks of any size, the logical assumption is that significant organic dysfunction exists and that improvement in acuity is highly unlikely.

If the pattern VEP is flat, a flash stimulus should be used. A reduced, delayed, or extinguished response to a flash stimulus is suggestive of macular or optic nerve dysfunction. Amblyopic eyes will have normal responses to flash stimulation.

VEPs can be used to monitor occlusion therapy in infants and toddlers. Improvement in VEP amplitude in an amblyopic eye indicates that occlusion of the normal eye may be effective. In addition, a reduced VEP in the occluded eye can be used as a warning sign that the occlusion schedule needs to be modified in order to prevent amblyopic development.

Binocular Vision Assessment

Bartlett et al.,[9] using unpatterned light flashes, demonstrated that the amplitude of the VEP was substantially larger with binocular stimulation than with monocular stimulation. The degree of summation was not the same in each patient. A decade later, Srebro[10] demonstrated that the binocular VEP amplitude is 25–30% larger than the sum of the monocular VEP amplitudes (binocular facil-

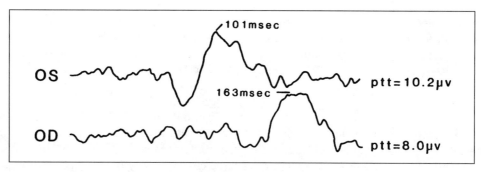

FIGURE 13-6

VEPs in a patient with retrobulbar optic neuritis in the right eye. The stimulus in this episode was a pattern-reversed checkerboard composed of 14-minutes-of-arc checks. The pattern was reversed at 1.88 reversals/second resulting in a transient VEP. The amplitudes of the first positive wave are within normal limits in both eyes. However, the implicit time (measured from the stimulus onset to the peak of the response) is markedly delayed in the right eye but normal in the left eye. Under the conditions tested, any response occurring later than 130 msec is abnormal. The implicit time of the response of the left eye is 101 msec, well within the normal limits. The implicit time of 163 msec in the right eye represents a very significant transmission delay.

itation). In addition, he showed that "facilitation" did not occur in small-angle esotropia, nor did it occur in normal patients whose binocularity was interrupted using a vertical prism. Amigo et al.[11] further demonstrated binocular facilitation even in the earliest period of life. VEPs also have been recorded using depth stimuli and random-dot stereograms.

Macular Disease

Since the VEP reflects the integrity of the macular projection pathways, it can be used for the objective assessment of macular function. The amplitude of the VEP will typically be reduced in macular disease. Evidence suggests that the latency of the VEP response can be delayed in macular disease (e.g., central serous choroidopathy).[12,13]

Optic Nerve Involvement in Multiple Sclerosis

The VEP can indicate both slowing and attenuation of the visual signal transmitted from the eye to the brain. Multiple sclerosis (MS) is a disseminated disease affecting the myelin covering of the nerves throughout the body. Myelin is responsible for the fast transmission of impulses in the central nervous system. Hence, myelin disorders, such as MS, can slow the speed of conduction. Scores of researchers have demonstrated that the VEP is a sensitive technique to measure this effect of demyelinating disease. A delayed VEP in a patient without visual symptoms, but with other symptoms such as increased frequency of urination, paresthesias, or unilateral paresis, supports the diagnosis of MS.[14]

The following case of atypical retrobulbar neuritis exemplifies the sensitivity of VEP testing. A 26-year-old woman complained of blurred vision in the left eye, accompanied by some pain on eye movement. Although the Snellen visual acuity measured 20/15 in each eye on three different occasions, she consistently complained of "blur" in the left eye. Pupillary response, color vision, and visual field test results and ophthalmoscopic findings were all normal. Her pattern VEPs were normal in amplitude in each eye but were significantly delayed in the left eye (Figure 13-6). A normal amplitude, but delayed VEP, may indicate a demyelinating process that has not resulted in axonal death. If and when axonal death occurs, the amplitude of the VEP will be reduced, along with visual acuity, visual fields, or both. After an episode of optic neuritis, the visual acuity often returns to normal but the VEP may still exhibit an increased latency of response.

Other Optic Nerve Disorders

In addition to optic neuritis secondary to MS, the VEP appears to be affected by other disorders of the optic nerve head as well. In a study of 10 patients exhibiting a tilted or oblique entrance of the optic nerve head, 70% of the eyes undergoing VEP testing showed a delayed response. Delays occurred even in eyes with 20/20 visual acuity.[15]

In ischemic optic neuropathy (ION), which may cause a sudden onset of decreased vision in one eye due to vascular occlusion involving the optic nerve, a reduction in amplitude of the VEP may occur with only a minor increase in the latency. This finding can be helpful in differentiating ION from visual pathway dysfunction due

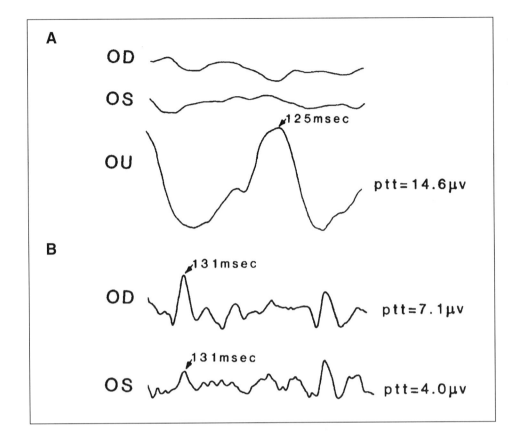

FIGURE 13-7
A. Visual evoked potentials generated from the right eye, left eye, and both eyes of a patient with subtle latent nystagmus and amblyopia in the left eye. The check size was 14 minutes of arc, the reversal rate was 7.5 reversals/second, and the analysis time was 200 msec. Although the monocular acuity was 20/20 OD and 20/30 OS, the monocular VEPs are grossly abnormal. The binocular VEP is within normal limits. B. VEPs generated from the right eye and left eye of the same patient in A using a stimulus rate of 1.88 reversals/second and resulting in transient evoked potentials. The analysis time here was 800 ms. As depicted, the monocular transient VEPs are superior to the monocular steady-state VEPs shown in A.

to MS. In addition, neoplasms that compress the visual pathways are expected to result in abnormal VEPs. Halliday et al.[16] reported abnormal waveforms and reduction in amplitude as the most marked VEP findings in compressive lesions of the anterior visual pathways. The literature concerning VEPs in glaucoma is quite extensive but a discussion of VEPs and glaucoma is beyond the scope of this chapter.

Orbital Disease

Little attention has been given to the study of VEPs in orbital disease. However, Millman et al.[17] have obtained pattern VEPs on 54 patients with orbital disease. A standard eye examination including visual field and color vision studies was performed, as well as computed tomographic (CT) or magnetic resonance imaging (MRI) scans of the orbit and brain. The most consistent finding in patients with reduced visual acuity and abnormal central visual fields was a reduction in the amplitude of the VEP to 14-minutes-of-arc checks at 7.5 reversals/second. Some patients had markedly reduced amplitudes even with good visual acuity and normal threshold visual fields. This so-called "dissociation" (see the next section) was found in 16% of patients with Graves' disease,

67% of patients with cavernous sinus fistulas, and 40% of patients with pseudotumors.

Dissociation of the Visual Evoked Potential from Visual Acuity (Paradoxical VEP)

In the great majority of patients, there is good agreement between the VEP findings and visual acuity. However, there are some cases where there is a "dissociation" of the VEP findings from visual acuity (i.e., the visual acuity is relatively normal compared to the VEP result). This may indicate a subtle abnormality or deficit in the visual pathway. The patient whose VEPs are depicted in Figure 13-7A had monocular visual acuities of 20/20 OD and 20/30 OS. Binocular acuity was 20/20. Note the abnormal monocular VEPs but normal binocular VEPs. Careful evaluation of eye movements under monocular and binocular fixation revealed the presence of subtle latent nystagmus, which was previously undetected. When VEPs were repeated at a slower reversal rate (1.88 reversals/second), the monocular VEPs were nearly normal (Figure 13-7B). Thus, a fast, steady-state VEP might be more sensitive in the detection of a subtle abnormality than a slower, transient VEP, especially in cases of nystagmus or other fixation abnormalities.

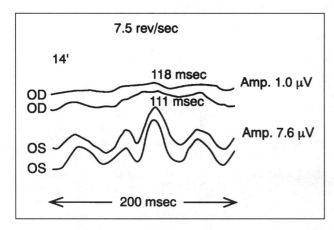

FIGURE 13-8

Visual evoked potentials from a 58-year-old man with a progressive, painless proptosis, as well as deep injection of the right eye of 4 months' duration. Although visual acuity was 20/20 and threshold visual fields were normal, the VEPs from the right eye were flat. Angiography demonstrated a carotid-cavernous sinus fistula. (Modified and reprinted with permission from J Sherman, VG Sutija. Visual-Evoked Potentials. In JB Eskridge, J Amos, JD Bartlett [eds], Clinical Procedures in Optometry. Philadelphia: Lippincott, 1991;514–29.)

Abnormal VEPs with normal visual acuity also may be indicative of impending visual compromise. Figure 13-8 depicts the VEPs from a 58-year-old man with progressive, painless proptosis and deep injection in the right eye of 4 months duration.[18] Visual acuities were 20/20 in each eye and threshold visual fields were normal; however, the VEPs were nearly flat. Angiography demonstrated a carotid-cavernous sinus fistula. The visual acuity dropped to 20/50, and the patient was treated with an embolization procedure to occlude the fistula. After surgery, visual acuity improved to 20/30+.

The patient whose VEPs are depicted in Figure 13-9 complained of reduced vision in the left eye for 2 weeks. Visual acuity in that eye was 20/50. VEPs from the left eye were flat. Although 20/50 visual acuity corresponds to 2.5 minutes of arc, the VEPs were flat, even to 112-minutes-of-arc checks. The diagnosis was nonarteritic ischemic optic neuropathy. Two weeks later, the visual acuity dropped to light perception in that eye, as "predicted" by the flat VEPs. The ability of the VEP to "predict" enables this test to play a role in early disease detection.

A second type of dissociation is one in which the visual acuity is reduced but the VEP is normal. Although this can certainly occur in a malingerer (to be discussed later), it has been reported to occur in cases where there is damage to Brodmann's areas 18 and 19. Bodis-Wollner et al.[19] reported the presence of near normal pattern VEPs

in a behaviorally blind young child. A CT scan revealed a normal Brodmann's area 17, which explained the normal VEP, but areas 18 and 19 were adversely affected, which explained the reduced visual acuity.

Presurgical Prediction of Postsurgical Visual Acuity in Patients with Media Opacities

When patients have clear ocular media, a checkerboard or grating stimulus can be used to estimate visual acuity, refractive error, and so forth. However, the checkerboard pattern is inappropriate when the patient has media opacities that preclude a clear focus on the retina. In such cases, information about visual function can be obtained using a nonpatterned, bright, flashing light.

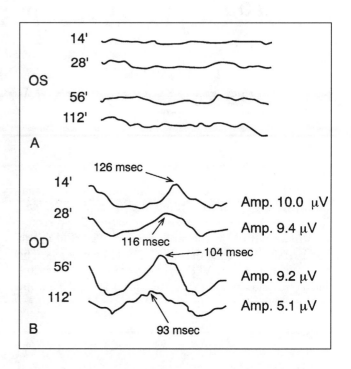

FIGURE 13-9

A. The ability of the VEP to predict the eventual loss of vision is demonstrated in this example of a patient who complained of reduced vision in the left eye of 2 weeks onset. Although the visual acuity was 20/50 in the left eye, the VEPs were flat to all check sizes, which is typical of much poorer vision. The diagnosis was nonarteritic ischemic optic neuropathy. Two weeks later, the acuity dropped to light perception, as "predicted" by the VEP. B. The VEPs were normal in the right eye, which had a 20/20 visual acuity. (Modified and reprinted with permission from J Sherman, VG Sutija. Visual-Evoked Potentials. In JB Eskridge, J Amos, JD Bartlett [eds], Clinical Procedures in Optometry. Philadelphia: Lippincott, 1991;514–29.)

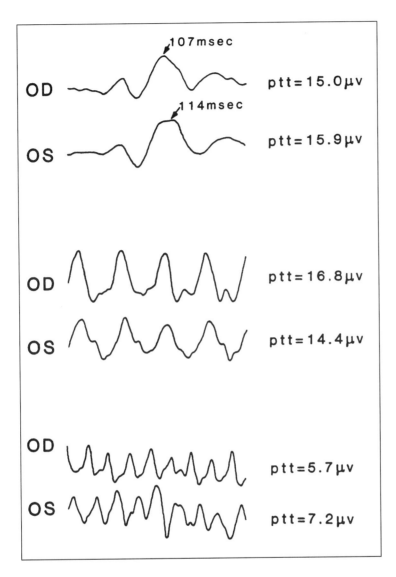

FIGURE 13-10
The patient whose VEPs are shown had a dense cataract in the right eye with visual acuity of 3/300. The left eye had a mild cataract with visual acuity of 20/40. The VEPs to a nonpatterned, bright, flashing light were recorded at 1 Hz, 10 Hz, and 20 Hz (top, middle, and bottom, respectively) in each eye. The responses are similar under the three conditions, suggesting a good prognosis for visual acuity in the right eye after cataract extraction.

The light is presented at varying temporal frequencies and qualitative but not quantitative information concerning vision can be obtained. Temporal frequencies such as 1 Hz, 6 Hz, 10 Hz, and 20 Hz may be used. Typical responses to flash VEPs performed on a normal eye with cataracts are depicted in Figure 13-10. The effects of aging, pupil dilation, and iris pigmentation in normal subjects with simulated cataracts has been studied and normative data have been established.[20] Special attention is paid to the double-peaked 10-Hz response, which, according to Weinstein,[21] is thought to be associated with macular function. The 20-Hz response (as well as higher frequencies) is believed to indicate normal optic nerve function.[22]

At the present level of knowledge, a normal VEP to a bright light flash does not guarantee foveal functioning or potential 20/20 visual acuity, although it does sug-gest a favorable prognosis for good vision after the surgical removal of the media opacity. On the other hand, an abnormal response to flash stimulation would indicate a poor prognosis.

Differential Diagnosis of Macular Disease from Optic Nerve Disease

Patients complaining of reduced visual acuity in the absence of a clear-cut diagnosis present a challenge to the clinician. Often, the differential diagnosis is narrowed to either macular or optic nerve disease; obviously the differentiation between these two can have significant implications regarding prognosis and management. Table 13-1 lists several tests that are quite useful in helping to make the differential diagnosis, especially when there is a more normal eye for comparison. In addition to some

TABLE 13-1

Differentiation of Macular and Optic Nerve Disease

Test	Early Macular or Retinal Disease	Early Optic Nerve Disease
Amsler grid	Metamorphopsia	Scotomas
Color vision testing	Typically blue-yellow defects	Typically red-green defects
Color comparison test (unilateral cases)	Usually minimal differences between the two eyes in color perception	Usually gross differences between the two eyes in color perception
Pupillary reflexes (unilateral cases)	Normal or nearly normal responses	Positive Marcus Gunn pupil
Pupil cycle time	Normal	Longer than normal
Light-brightness comparison test (unilateral cases)	Little difference, if any, between perceived brightness; equal responses on the "dollar" test	Gross difference in perceived brightness between eyes
Macular dazzle	Prolonged recovery times	Normal or near normal recovery times
Fluorescein angiography	Leakage or "window" defects in the macular area	Usually normal but possibility of leakage of disc vessels; possible microaneurysms of disc vessels
VEP to checks	Frequently delayed or reduced in amplitude	Frequently delayed or reduced in amplitude
VEP to gratings	No orientational asymmetry	Frequent orientation asymmetry
Simultaneous VEP and ERG to pattern	Both VEP and ERG reduced in amplitude: may or may not be delayed	VEP reduced in amplitude and frequently delayed, but not always; ERG probably normal

Source: Reprinted with permission from J Sherman, VG Sutija. Visual-Evoked Potentials. In JB Eskridge, JF Amos, JD Bartlett (eds), Clinical Procedures in Optometry. Philadelphia: Lippincott, 1991;514–29.

simple chairside tests, electrodiagnostic evaluation, including VEP testing, can be helpful.

Since VEPs to checks may be delayed or reduced in amplitude in both macular disease and optic nerve/visual pathway disease, VEP testing cannot be used in isolation from other tests for the differential diagnosis. Macular disease must first be ruled out with other examination procedures to conclude that abnormal responses are due to an optic nerve/visual pathway disorder. While abnormal VEPs to checks are not specific to either macula or optic nerve/visual pathway disease, delays in VEPs to gratings of one orientation but not to another have been reported in multiple sclerosis[23] and retrobulbar neuritis.[24] Although this "orientational asymmetry" has not been reported in macular disease,[25] larger numbers of patients need to be tested.

Simultaneous Electroretinography and Visual Evoked Potential Testing

While the VEP is not usually delayed in macular disease, it may be, and although the VEP is usually delayed in optic nerve disease, it is not always. To help localize the lesion site in various visual disorders, there is a modification of the VEP technique that involves performing simultaneous pattern reversal VEP testing and an ERG. Vaughan and Katzman[26] reported almost three decades ago that ERGs and VEPs could be recorded simultaneously. Additional electrodes are applied to obtain an ERG response at the same time as a VEP response is obtained.

The VEP is obtained by applying electrodes as discussed previously. To record the ERG, a gold foil electrode is inserted beneath the lower lid. This technique of recording an ERG using a patterned stimulus is known as a pattern ERG or PERG (Figure 13-11).

Although the origins of the VEP and ERG responses are well known, the origin of the PERG response remains controversial. Sherman[27] reported that several patients with total optic nerve atrophy had normal PERG responses, suggesting that the PERG response must be generated from preganglionic structures. In contrast, Maffei and Fiorentini[28] believe the origin of the PERG response to be ganglion cells. Since these early studies, there has been a plethora of literature concerning the PERG response and its source. A few studies have appeared more recently that suggest the first positive component of the PERG response, the P50, is a result of preganglionic elements but that the negative response, the N90, is a result of ganglion cell activity. It is therefore possible that careful analysis of the PERG might yield information of both retinal and optic nerve function.

Sherman et al.[29] suggested simultaneous PERG and VEP testing for the differential diagnosis of retinal disease from optic nerve disease, but they assumed the source of the PERG to be preganglionic elements. If this is the case, then patients with macular disease would generate reduced VEP and ERG responses, whereas patients with optic nerve disease would generate a reduced or absent VEP response but a normal PERG response.

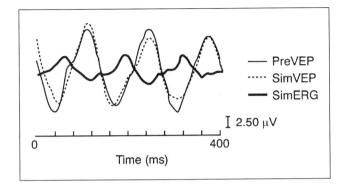

FIGURE 13-11
Simultaneous pattern reversal VEP and ERG testing. In this example, VEP responses were first recorded under standard conditions (14-minutes-of-arc checks, 7.4 reversals/second) from a normal eye (PreVEP). Then simultaneous ERG and VEP responses (SimVEP, SimERG) were recorded under the same conditions. The VEP traces show good reliability. The "pattern ERG" (PERG) occurs first, but is smaller in amplitude, as depicted. (Modified and reprinted with permission from J Sherman, VG Sutija. Visual-Evoked Potentials. In JB Eskridge, J Amos, JD Bartlett [eds], Clinical Procedures in Optometry. Philadelphia: Lippincott, 1991;514–29)

Celesia and Kaufman[30] have also recorded simultaneous PERGs and VEPs for differential diagnostic purposes. They added the measurement of the "retino-cortical time," or the transit time between the activation of the retinal structures and the arrival of the signal in the visual cortex. The preliminary findings of Celesia and Kaufman suggest that the retino-cortical time is normal in maculopathies but prolonged in optic nerve demyelination.

Although the origin of the PERG response is in question, there is agreement that the PERG response appears to be abnormal in early macular disease and is probably normal in early optic nerve disease. Once the origin of the PERG response is determined, simultaneous pattern VEPs and ERGs may have significant clinical applications.

Psychogenic Disorders
Occasionally a patient will have distressing visual symptoms such as reduced visual acuity but will fail to demonstrate any refractive, accommodative, or organic signs to explain the symptoms. Such a patient is always a challenge to the concerned clinician. If the patient's chief complaint is reduced visual acuity and the patient fails to elicit any abnormalities on any testing procedure, then the pattern VEP can be a very useful test to rule out hysteria or malingering. A normal VEP strongly suggests normal macular function and normal visual pathway func-

tioning to Brodmann's area 17 (occipital cortex). Therefore, a normal VEP response with a subjective complaint of poor visual acuity may provide substantial evidence of a psychogenic disorder.

The patient suffering from hysteria is often unaware of the unconscious and deeply rooted emotional conflict responsible for the lowered visual acuity. In contrast, the malingerer is purposely and consciously trying to deceive the practitioner, usually for personal gain, such as in cases of accident litigation or disability determination. Although the VEP cannot conclusively prove a patient is hysterical or malingering, it makes the presumed diagnosis highly likely. If classic tubular or spiral visual fields are also demonstrated in a patient, the diagnosis is confirmed.

Ophthalmic clinicians frequently encounter patients whose visual symptoms are distressing yet who exhibit no overt disease process. The possibility that these symptoms are psychogenic in origin (or of organic cortical origin in some cases) is often entertained. Before a psychogenic diagnosis can be assumed, however, other disease entities must be considered. Table 13-2 lists nine such conditions and the test results used in the differential diagnosis. These conditions and test results are discussed in greater detail elsewhere.[31] This list is by no means exhaustive, but it does provide a systematic approach in which the patient is objectively evaluated by means of various examination procedures, including electrodiagnostic testing, to confirm either the presence or absence of specific disease entities.

Other Applications
Additional applications of VEP testing include the assessment of the developmental growth and maturation of the visual system in newborns, infants, and young children. In addition, VEP testing has been used to rule out blindness in infants with congenital ocular motor apraxia.[32] VEPs have also been used as an index of visual recovery in behaviorally blind patients. Gittinger and Sokol[32] have shown that VEPs can anticipate and parallel the progressive return of useful vision.

ELECTRORETINOGRAPHY

The single objective test that best reflects overall retinal function is the standard, full-field flash electroretinogram. The electroretinogram (ERG) is the summed electrical response from the retina that is the consequence of light energy stimulating the different types of retinal cells. Although the ERG was discovered in 1865 by the Swedish physiologist Holmgrem, recordings in humans first became popular in 1941 when Riggs introduced a practical record-

TABLE 13-2
Differential Diagnosis for Psychogenic Disorders and Disease Entities

Condition	Visual Acuity	External Observation	Ophthalmoscopy	Visual Fields	Color Vision	Dark Adaptometry	Flash ERG	EOG	Pattern Visual Evoked Response	Fluorescein Angiography	Mode of Inheritance
Stargardt's macular degeneration	20/25–20/400	Negative	Normal to "beaten bronze" appearance with pigmentary changes and yellow flecks	Central scotomas with sloping margins	Subtle shift toward red (Rayleigh equation); otherwise normal	Normal	Normal	Variable	Abnormal to small checks or gratings	Abnormal (pigment epithelial abnormality)	Autosomal recessive
Leber's congenital amaurosis	Decreased (20/80–20/400)	Nystagmus: possible keratoconus, keratoglobus, enophthalmos	Normal to an appearance resembling retinitis pigmentosa	Normal peripheral fields (?)	Variable	Probable elevated final thresholds	Abnormal	Abnormal	Abnormal	Possible pigment epithelial changes	Autosomal recessive
Albinism and ocular albinism	20/30–20/200	Iris transillumination; nystagmus of varying degrees	Pigmentary abnormality may be subtle; foveal hypoplasia	Normal (?)	Normal	Normal	Normal or supranormal	Normal	Abnormal to small checks or gratings; hemispheric asymmetry	Abnormal macular pigment	Oculocutaneous albinism is usually autosomal recessive; ocular albinism is usually X-linked
Isolated foveal hypoplasia	20/60 or worse	Nystagmus	Foveal hypoplasia	Normal (?)	Normal	Normal	Normal	Normal	Abnormal to small checks or gratings	Abnormal macular pigment	Uncertain: might be a variant of albinism
Rod monochromatism	20/100–20/200	Nystagmus of varying degrees	Normal or subtle macular changes	Possible central scotoma	Markedly abnormal	No cone threshold; rapid adaptation	Abnormal photopic response; abnormal flicker response	Normal	Abnormal	Possible macular pigment epithelial changes	Autosomal recessive
Retinitis pigmentosa sine pigmento	Usually normal	Usually normal	Possible arteriolar constriction	Possible retinitis pigmentosa-type field defects	Usually normal	Elevated final thresholds	Abnormal	Abnormal	Usually normal if visual acuity is normal	Pigment epithelial changes	Autosomal dominant, autosomal recessive, or X-linked
Retrobulbar optic neuritis	Decreased, usually monocular	Often a Marcus Gunn pupil	Normal	Variable; central scotoma	Variable color defects;	Variable	Normal	Normal	Abnormal; usually delayed	Normal	Dependent on systemic cause;

			poor red discrimination	to large field defects						usually not inherited
									Normal	usually not inherited
Amblyopia	Decreased, usually monocular	Strabismus or aniso-metropia	Normal	poor red discrimi-nation	Displaced blind spot; eccentric fixation; normal peripheral fields	Possible higher cone thresholds	Normal	Normal	Usually abnormal to small checks or gratings	Normal	Usually not inherited
Psychogenic problems	Decreased, may be monocular	Normal	Normal	Normal or abnormal	Normal or spiral defect or tubular field	Normal or exhaustion phenomenon; possibly elevated thresholds	Normal	Normal	Normal	Normal	Usually not inherited

Source: Reprinted with permission from J Sherman, SJ Richter, A Epstein. The differential diagnosis of visual disorders in patients presenting with marked symptoms but no observable ocular abnormality. Am J Optom Physiol Opt 1980;57:516–22.

ing contact electrode. In the late 1940s, Granit,[33] working with cats, demonstrated that the ERG consists of three processes (i.e., PI, PII, and PIII) in the order of their disappearance under ether anesthesia.

After a light flash, three major deflections occur in the ERG recording. The first is a negative deflection, traditionally called the a-wave, which coincides in time with Granit's PIII process. This is followed by a large positive deflection, the b-wave, which corresponds in time with Granit's PII process. The c-wave, a later positive deflection, corresponds to Granit's PI process.

Our present knowledge of the cellular origin of the various ERG components has resulted from numerous research endeavors. These include microelectrode studies of individual retinal layers, destruction of selective retinal cells with specific tissue toxins, ERG component analysis under various testing conditions, and comparative study of retinas that are predominantly rod and retinas that are composed of predominantly rods or cones.[34]

Based on these methods, it is believed that the a-wave is generated by the photoreceptors, the b-wave reflects activity of the inner nuclear layer and appears to be generated primarily by the Müller cells of the inner nuclear layer,[35] and the c-wave appears to have its origin in the retinal pigment epithelium.

Clinically, the a-wave and b-wave are relatively easy to obtain, but the c-wave requires special procedures and equipment. For this reason, the electro-oculogram, to be discussed in the next section, is more appropriate for evaluating the retinal pigment epithelium. In addition to these three components, there is an early receptor potential (ERP), a d-wave, as well as oscillatory potentials, which may all be recorded under the appropriate testing conditions. The ERP, occurring earlier than the a-wave, is thought to reflect molecular events within the photoreceptor outer segments. The d-wave occurs just as the light flash goes off and is sometimes referred to as the "off" response. Oscillatory potentials are high-frequency components that occur on the ascending arm of the b-wave under dark-adapted conditions when a bright stimulus is used. Oscillatory potentials possibly reflect the activity of amacrine and bipolar cells.[36,37] These potentials have been reported to decrease in amplitude in early stages of diabetic retinopathy.[38–40] No ERG component reflects ganglionic cell activity; therefore the ERG is normal in optic nerve disease, because it is made up of the axons of the ganglion cells.

Recording the Clinical Electroretinogram

The development of clinical ERGs was initially promoted by Karpe (1945) in Europe[41] and Riggs (1941) in the United States, who developed the first electrode embedded in a contact lens.[42] To perform an ERG, a bright flashing light source is needed. The most frequently used light source is the Grass photostimulator with adjustable flash rate and intensity. Other devices also incorporate color filters as well. The ideal stimulus source for performing an ERG includes a full dome of diffuse light produced by a bowl-like apparatus called the Ganzfeld.

The color and intensity of the light source can be modified to separate rod function from cone function. Bright stimuli, especially red, presented to a light-adapted retina, produce mainly cone responses. Dim stimuli, especially blue, presented to a dark-adapted retina, produce mainly rod responses. In addition, high-frequency rates of presentation (i.e., 30 flashes/second) affect the cone system, since the rod system cannot respond to stimulus rates faster than about 18–20 flashes/second. Figure 13-12 depicts typical ERGs to a bright white stimulus under light-adapted (photopic) and dark-adapted (scotopic) conditions.

In addition to a light source, a contact lens or corneal electrode is required to monitor and transmit the induced voltage change that occurs across the retina because of light stimulation. When a recording of a pattern ERG or an ERG from a localized area, such as the macula, is desired, a gold foil electrode is needed. Other components of the ERG testing system include an amplifier to enlarge the signal and a recording device to store the response.

Figure 13-13 shows a patient prepared for a standard ERG examination. The pupils are dilated and a contact lens electrode is placed on each cornea. A reference electrode is placed directly on the skin in the middle of the forehead, and an ear clip electrode is attached to serve as a ground. The International Society for Clinical Electrophysiology of Vision (ISCEV) has established a standardized protocol for performing a full-flash ERG. See Marmor et al.[43] for a detailed description of this protocol.

Once an ERG is recorded, the examiner analyzes the amplitude and the implicit time of the response. There are several factors that affect the ERG response. Over a wide range of stimuli, as the intensity is increased, the amplitude of the ERG increases and the implicit time decreases. Although media opacities such as cataracts diffuse the light reaching the retina, they do not decrease the amplitude of the ERG. An exception to this is a dense vitreal hemorrhage.[44]

The ERG recorded during dark adaptation is larger in amplitude and longer in implicit time compared with the light-adapted response because the rods outnumber the cones by 20 to 1 and because the rod system responds more slowly than the cone system. Both increasing age and increasing refractive error minimally affect the ERG response. However, in high myopia, the ERG response

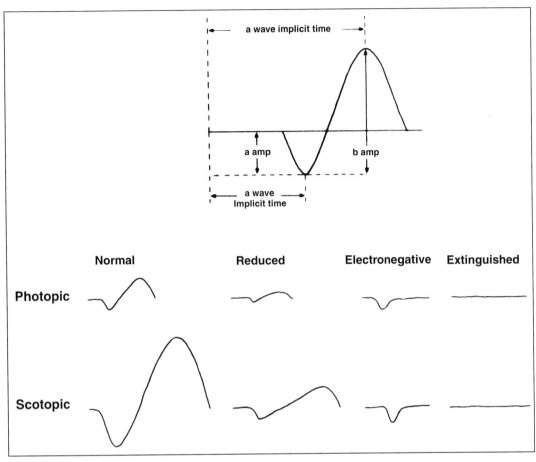

FIGURE 13-12

Example ERGs to a bright white stimulus under light-adapted (photopic) and dark-adapted (scotopic) conditions. The peak latency, or implicit time, is measured from the stimulus onset to the peak of the response. Peak latency of the a-wave and of the b-wave are usually measured. In clinical ERGs the amplitude of the b-wave is measured from the bottom of the a-wave to the top of the b-wave. Scotopic responses are normally larger and slower than photopic responses. Reduced ERG responses, the electronegative ERG response (looking at the b-wave), and extinguished ERG responses are contrasted to normal responses.

can be considerably reduced in amplitude, which suggests large areas of retinal dysfunction that would be observable with ophthalmoscopic evaluation.

Clinical Use of the Full-Field Flash Electroretinogram

Retinitis Pigmentosa

The disease that best exemplifies the importance of electroretinography is retinitis pigmentosa (RP). In all three genetic patterns of RP (autosomal dominant, autosomal recessive, and X-linked recessive), the ERG abnormality can precede both visual symptoms and ophthalmoscopic signs. The most prominent abnormality of the ERG response in RP is a significantly reduced amplitude or an extinguished scotopic (dark-adapted) ERG resulting from a generalized degeneration of the photoreceptors, with the rods preceding the cones. Photopic, or light-adapted, reductions in ERG amplitude as well as b-wave implicit time delays are also encountered.

In most cases of autosomal recessive RP and X-linked RP, the ERG response is extinguished early in the course of the disease. In the autosomal dominant variety of RP, a recordable but reduced ERG response reflects the later onset, less rapid progression, and milder nature of the disease process with a better prognosis.

Marmor[45] has reported a group of patients with RP (12 of a group of 70 who were studied) who demonstrated relatively large scotopic ERG amplitudes (greater than 100 μV) and normal b-wave implicit times to flicker (less than 32 ms). Marmor believes that this group of patients

FIGURE 13-13

To perform an ERG, a corneal electrode is placed on the eye, a reference electrode is attached to middle of the forehead, and an ear clip electrode is attached to serve as a ground. Current ERG systems allow for simultaneous testing; therefore corneal electrodes are placed on both eyes at the same time. A Ganzfeld stimulator is also shown (Nicolet Biomedical, Madison, WI).

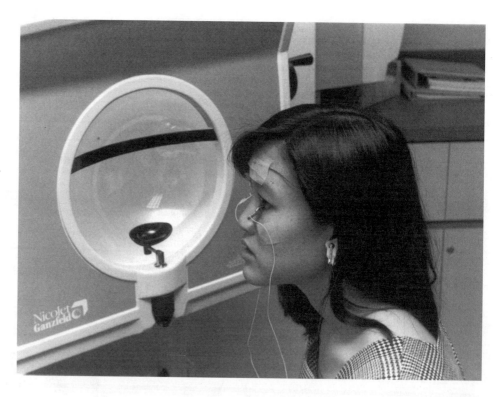

constitutes a subgroup of RP that is characterized by a milder disease process that causes less severe functional symptoms and carries a good visual prognosis.

Pseudoretinitis Pigmentosa

When a patient has night vision or peripheral vision complaints and the fundus demonstrates obvious signs of RP, such as bone spicule pigment deposition and attenuated arterioles, the ERG is not an essential procedure. However, every practitioner has, at one time or another, examined a patient who bitterly complains of reduced night vision, but whose examination findings and visual fields are inconclusive. In these cases, an ERG is an essential diagnostic tool.

The term *pseudoretinitis pigmentosa* is often used to describe a group of diverse conditions, the common feature being a pigment hyperplasia that resembles, to a variable extent, the classic fundus findings in RP. In contrast to RP, those conditions falling into the category of pseudoretinitis pigmentosa are not inheritable and do not progress. Some of the established causes of pseudoretinitis pigmentosa include trauma, chorioretinitis (syphilis and rubella), drugs (phenothiazines and chloroquine), and ophthalmic artery occlusion.[46] Normal or near normal ERG results suggest pseudoretinitis pigmentosa. However, the ERG may occasionally be extinguished in some of these conditions, causing difficulty in the differential

diagnosis. The few reported cases of unilateral RP are probably pseudoretinitis pigmentosa[46] when the ERG result is normal in the other eye. If the ERG is abnormal in the fellow eye, then RP, more advanced in one eye, is the probable diagnosis.

Leber's Congenital Amaurosis

Leber's congenital amaurosis deserves special consideration because it often goes undiagnosed by many knowledgeable clinicians who have had no firsthand experience with clinical ERGs. Patients with this disorder typically have nystagmus and reduced vision, which became apparent shortly after birth. The fundus evaluation can be completely normal, although mildly attenuated arterioles and subtle pigment abnormalities may be evident. The diagnosis of Leber's congenital amaurosis in a young child with nystagmus and reduced visual function is confirmed when the ERG response is extinguished or severely reduced, even if the fundus is normal. This disorder is not uncommon, as evidenced by reports that nearly 20% of the blind children studied have this disease.[47,48]

Leber's congenital amaurosis is characterized by an overall retinal dysfunction, which is sometimes loosely classified as a variant of RP. However, unlike RP, it is present at birth, initially affects both central and peripheral vision, causes minimal or no fundus abnormalities, and is generally nonprogressive. Sometimes mental retardation, gen-

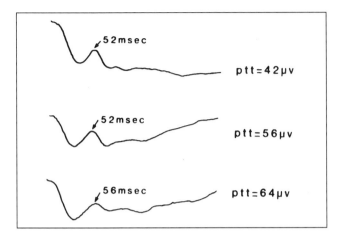

FIGURE 13-14

Light-adapted (top) and two dark-adapted (middle and bottom) ERGs from a patient with congenital stationary night blindness (CSNB). The b-wave is very reduced and does not reach the baseline, resulting in an electronegative response. The implicit time of the light-adapted and dark-adapted b-waves is nearly equal. Both of these findings are characteristic of one type of CSNB.

eralized neuromuscular problems, keratoglobus, and keratoconus may be associated with this disorder.[48]

Congenital Stationary Night Blindness

One type of night blindness, congenital stationary night blindness (CSNB), is present at birth, does not progress, and may be inherited as an autosomal dominant, autosomal recessive, or X-linked trait. All hereditary types of CSNB are characterized by a normal fundus, normal daylight visual fields, and the absence of rod-mediated dark adaptation. Visual acuity is usually normal; however it is sometimes reduced in the autosomal recessive and X-linked varieties.

The diagnosis of CSNB is confirmed when the ERG demonstrates two characteristic findings. First, the peak times (implicit times) of the light-adapted and dark-adapted responses are nearly identical (normally the dark-adapted b-wave occurs at almost double the implicit time of the light-adapted b-wave).[49] Second, the scotopic (and sometimes photopic) b-wave is very reduced in amplitude, resulting in what is termed an electronegative response. The a-wave, which is the electronegative component, is usually normal and predominates the ERG (Figure 13-14). Since the a-wave reflects the activity of the photoreceptors, these neural cells are not implicated in CSNB. The abnormal b-wave suggests a deficit in the transmission from the photoreceptors to the bipolar cells or the bipolar cell layer. In addition to the ERG abnor-

malities, patients with CSNB have dark-adaptation curves that do not reveal a rod component.

Syndromes

The ERG is helpful in establishing the diagnosis of some syndromes in which a tapetoretinal degeneration (degeneration of neurosensory retina along with the RPE) is a typical component. In Usher's, Refsum's, Laurence-Moon, and Bassen-Kornzweig syndromes, the extinguished or very reduced ERG response reflects severe overall retinal dysfunction. Of particular interest is that parenteral, water-soluble vitamin A supplements appear to increase the electrical activity of the photoreceptors in some patients with Bassen-Kornzweig syndrome,[50] where very low serum levels of vitamin A exist. In addition, vitamin A supplements (15,000 IU/day) in the palmitate form have been shown to slow the progression of loss of the cone ERG amplitude in patients with common forms of retinitis pigmentosa.[51] However, the relative overall benefit to the visual function of RP patients is controversial. Deutman has enumerated scores of other syndromes that are associated with a pigmentary retinopathy.[52]

Vascular Occlusion

It is well known that the retina has a dual blood supply. The central retinal artery supplies the inner half of the retina, including the inner nuclear layer, and the choriocapillaris supplies the outer half of the retina up to and including the outer plexiform layer. Closure of the central retinal artery will result in a normal a-wave but a reduced or absent b-wave. The a-wave is normal because the photoreceptors still have a normal blood supply from the choriocapillaris. The b-wave is diminished because the central retinal artery supplies the inner nuclear layer from which the b-wave originates. Branch artery or vein occlusions will also cause a reduction in the b-wave amplitude, but to a lesser degree. In contrast, closure of the ophthalmic artery will result in a very reduced or extinguished a-wave and b-wave, because the ophthalmic artery supplies the short posterior ciliary arteries (supplying the choriocapillaris) as well as the central retinal artery. As previously mentioned, an occlusion of the ophthalmic artery might mimic unilateral RP, since pigment changes result when the nutritional supply to the retinal pigment epithelium is impaired.

Although b-wave abnormalities can be present with a normal a-wave, the opposite situation is not encountered. An abnormal a-wave reflects photoreceptor impairment, in which the normal propagation of the neural impulses to the bipolar cell layer cannot occur. Hence, an a-wave abnormality is always accompanied by an abnormal b-wave.

Macular Versus Optic Nerve Disease

The standard full-field ERG results from electrical activity of the entire retina. Therefore, it does not reflect activity from small retinal areas such as the macula. If a patient with observable macular disease has an extinguished or very reduced ERG response, the macular involvement represents only a small part of the overall retinal dysfunction. Such is the case in cone degeneration, cone-rod degeneration, and inverse RP, which are all generally considered variants of RP in which cone dysfunction or central retinal involvement occur initially.[53] As previously mentioned, special techniques are available for monitoring retinal activity predominantly from the macula. These include presenting a bright-red stimulus to a light-adapted retina as well as using higher frequency rates of stimulation.

Since no ERG component reflects activity of the ganglion cells, the ERG will be normal in optic nerve disease. Patients with 20/1000 vision resulting from age-related macular degeneration or patients with light perception vision caused by advanced glaucoma will generate normal full-field ERGs. In the electrodiagnosis of these visual problems, the VEP is most appropriate.

The Enhanced S Cone Syndrome

Marmor et al.[54] studied eight patients who had night blindness, cystoid maculopathy, and an unusual ERG. These patients showed no response when dark-adapted to low-intensity stimuli, but exhibited supernormal, slow responses to high-intensity stimuli that persisted during light adaptation. The sensitivity of this response was much greater to short wavelength stimuli than to long wavelength stimuli. Because this disease demonstrates a hypersensitivity of the short (blue) wavelength cones as seen in the ERG, Marmor proposed that this slowly progressive disease be called the enhanced S cone syndrome.

Miscellaneous

There are many other conditions in which the ERG is useful. Certain drugs, such as thioridazine (Mellaril),[55] can be toxic to the retina and can cause a fundus picture that may mimic RP. Here, the ERG response can be abnormal even in the absence of any symptoms or fundus signs.

The ERG is useful in ascertaining the health of the retina before the removal of a media opacity, such as a cataract or opacified cornea, where visualization of the fundus may not be possible. A normal ERG in these cases does not, however, rule out the presence of a maculopathy or optic nerve disorder. The flash VEP is a more appropriate test in these cases since the results will be abnormal in gross maculopathies and in optic nerve disease.

The ERG also has applications in instances of retained intraocular foreign bodies. Specifically, in patients with retained iron intraocular foreign bodies, retinal changes may occur, which include a peripheral retinal pigmentary degeneration (siderosis bulbi).[56] The earliest ERG changes in these patients may be a transient supernormal response.[56] Eventually, an electronegative pattern may appear, followed by a nondetectable response as the condition progresses.

Some clinical researchers find that the ERG is helpful in differentiating ischemic from nonischemic central retinal vein occlusion. The poorer that some aspects of the ERG response are, the higher the probability that the eye in question with central retinal vein occlusion will develop rubeosis.

ELECTRO-OCULOGRAPHY

The term *electro-oculogram* (EOG) was introduced by Marg in 1951.[57] It has been defined by Arden as "the clinical test using electro-oculography to monitor saccadic eye movements of 34.5 degrees during periods of dark and light."[58] The test is performed by placing skin electrodes near the lateral and medial canthus of the eye, as well as an electrode on the forehead to serve as a ground (Figure 13-15). The patient then places his or her head in a diffusing sphere that contains one central fixation point and two other points 30 degrees apart. After undergoing a standard period of light adaptation, the patient makes 30-degree saccadic movements between the two fixation points, followed by measurements in the shift in the corneal-retinal potential (Figure 13-16). These measurements serve as a baseline. The lights are subsequently turned off and samples of these potential shifts during the 30-degree saccadic movements are taken at 1-minute intervals. These samples are taken for 15 minutes as dark adaptation occurs. The lights are then turned on, and the procedure is repeated for 15 minutes under light-adapted conditions.

The resultant potential shifts measured are mass responses,[58] which are clinically useful in assessing the integrity of the retinal pigment epithelium. Less simplistically, however, the normal EOG depends on functioning photoreceptors, functioning pigment epithelial cells, contact between the neurosensory and pigment epithelial layers, and an adequate choroidal blood supply.[58]

The responses decrease as the patient adapts to the dark and reach a minimum value in 8–12 minutes. When the lights come on again, the responses increase, reaching a maximum value in 6–9 minutes (Figure 13-17). A ratio of the maximum value during the period of light adaptation (the light peak, or LP) to the minimum value obtained during dark adaptation (the dark trough, or DT) is then taken. This ratio, LP/DT, is known as the Arden ratio

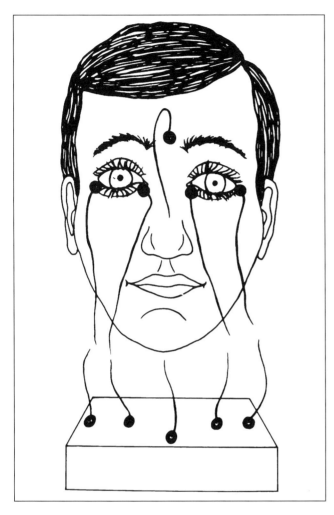

FIGURE 13-15
Schematic representation of electrode placement for recording the EOG. The forehead electrode is the ground. (Modified with permission from SJ Richter, J Sherman. Electro-oculography, dark adaptometry, and laser interferometry. J Am Optom Assoc 1979;50:101–4.)

and has a normal value of 1.8 or greater.[59] An Arden ratio of less than 1.65 is considered evidence of a widespread disorder affecting the retinal pigment epithelium.[34] Ratios of 1.65–1.80 are considered borderline.

Electro-oculography is not used as widely as the ERG in the differential diagnosis of retinal disease. However, in Best's vitelliform macular dystrophy, the EOG can be used to identify both affected patients as well as carriers of this dominantly inherited disease, even in the absence of visual and fundus changes. The EOG can be abnormal in flecked retinal syndromes, choroidal dystrophies, and tapetoretinal degenerations. It is normal in optic nerve disease and is affected variably by inflammatory retinal

changes, depending on the extent of the lesions. In the majority of cases, overall retinal integrity is better assessed using the ERG. A disadvantage of the EOG is that it requires some fixation ability and patient cooperation.

EXEMPLARY CASES (TABLE 13-3)

Case 1

A 19-year-old man had a 2-year history of intermittent hazy vision in his right eye only. His vision only became hazy after 30 minutes of vigorous exercise. General health was reported as perfect and he had no other symptoms. Visual acuity was 20/15 in each eye. Evaluation of motility, pupils, threshold visual fields, and color vision produced normal findings, as did a dilated fundus evaluation. The pattern VEPs exhibited delays of about 30 ms under all conditions tested in each eye (Figure 13-18). A MRI study revealed bilateral periventricular plaques strongly suggestive of focal demyelination secondary to MS. Although his complaints were only uniocular, the bilateral VEP and bilateral MRI abnormalities confirmed dysfunction and structural involvement within both halves of the brain.

Case 2

A 46-year-old, asymptomatic man was seen for an evaluation because his 47-year-old brother was diagnosed with optic neuropathy thought to be caused by a mitochondrial mutation. Both brothers had point mutations at nucleotide sites 4216 and 4917. Visual acuity was 20/15 in each eye and pupils were normal, as was color vision and 30-degree central threshold visual fields. A dilated fundus evaluation revealed normal discs. However, pattern VEPs to small checks were reduced in amplitude in the left eye only.

Thus, the patient was exhibiting a subclinical hereditary optic neuropathy.

Case 3

A 19-year-old woman had a history of legal blindness since early childhood. Three previous clinicians had diagnosed optic atrophy, diffuse retinal degeneration, and cortical blindness, respectively. Visual acuity was 20/200 in each eye but pupil evaluation, motility, slit lamp evaluation, and fundus examination results were normal. VEPs to patterns of various sizes were normal under all conditions tested. Psychotherapy eventually revealed that the patient was sexually abused by her father, and subsequently developed hysterical blindness and multiple personalities.

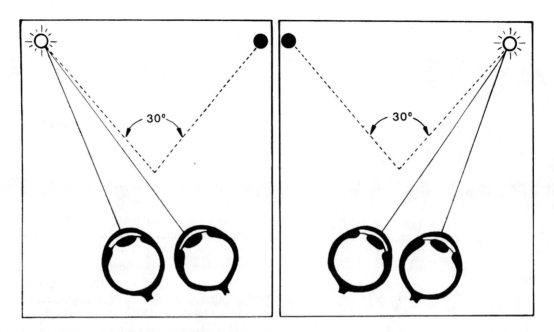

FIGURE 13-16

During EOG testing, the patient is required to make 30-degree eye movements, first during light adaptation and then at regular intervals during a period of dark adaptation. Measurements in the shift in the corneal-retinal potential are recorded. (Modified with permission from SJ Richter, J Sherman. Electrooculography, dark adaptometry, and laser interferometry. J Am Optom Assoc 1979;50:101–4.)

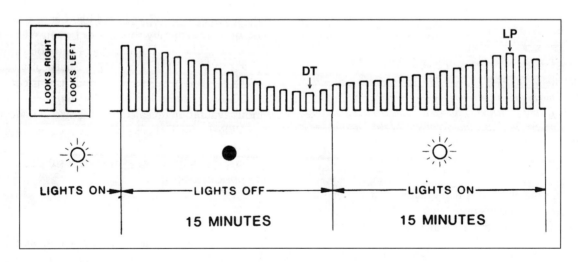

FIGURE 13-17

As a patient performs the 30-degree eye movements during periods of dark adaptation and light adaptation, shifts in corneal-retinal potential gradually occur, which are represented in the diagram. The Arden ratio is determined by dividing the light peak (LP) value by the dark trough (DT) value (LP/DT). An Arden ratio value of 1.8 or greater is considered normal. (Modified with permission from SJ Richter, J Sherman. Electro-oculography, dark adaptometry, and laser interferometry. J Am Optom Assoc 1979;50:101–4.)

TABLE 13-3
Clinical Electrodiagnosis at a Glance

Flash ERG	The best objective test of overall retinal function.
	Can be used to confirm or deny the presence of an overall retinal dysfunction regardless of the retinal appearance.
	Normal or near normal results in macular disease.
	Normal or near normal results in optic nerve disease.
	Supernormal ERG amplitudes may occur in albinism initially and in some optic nerve disorders.
Pattern ERG	Abnormal results in macular disease. Certain components of the pattern ERG perhaps abnormal in optic nerve disease. (Site of origin still controversial.)
Flash VEP	Abnormal results in gross macular and optic nerve disorders. Not as sensitive to dysfunction as the pattern VEP but useful with opaque media.
Pattern VEP	Generally reduced in amplitude in most types of macular degeneration. Delayed in wet macular involvement, especially in central serous. Abnormal results nearly always with optic nerve dysfunction, especially when the axial portion of the nerve is involved. Delayed in optic neuritis even with visual acuity of 20/20.
	Reduced in amplitude when the axons of the optic nerve are involved such as in toxic-nutritional amblyopia. Amplitude reductions generally correspond to visual acuity reductions.
	VEP delays to checks cannot be used, in isolation of other tests, in the differential diagnosis of macular versus optic nerve disease.
EOG	The best objective test of overall retinal pigment epithelial function. Abnormal in Best's disease.

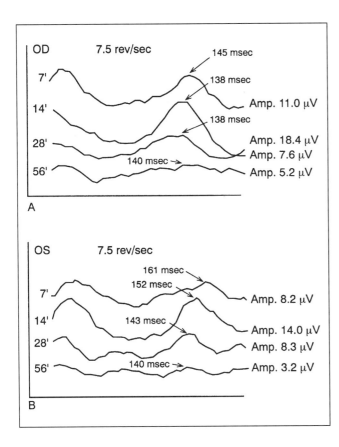

FIGURE 13-18

Case 1. The pattern VEPs of a 19-year-old man with a 2-year history of hazy vision in the right eye after vigorous exercise. The first major positive deflection (P100) should occur around 100 ms. This patient exhibited delays of about 30 ms under all conditions tested in each eye. The patient was diagnosed with multiple sclerosis.

Case 4

A 23-year-old male optometry student was examined by a fellow classmate, who observed pigment proliferation around venules in all quadrants of both eyes (Figure 13-19). The patient denied any visual symptoms, had no family history of night blindness, and had no atypical health or eye history. Visual acuity was 20/20 in both eyes, peripheral visual fields were full, and the ERG and EOG results were normal. The diagnosis was pigmented paravenous retinochoroidal atrophy, and the visual prognosis of this rather benign fundus disorder was quite good.[60] Disorders such as this (i.e., pseudoretinitis pigmentosa) must be differentiated from true retinitis pigmentosa.

Case 5

An asymptomatic, 40-year-old woman was seen for a routine eye examination. Visual acuity was 20/20 in each eye, but visual fields exhibited a mild nerve fiber layer defect in both eyes. The fundus examination revealed attenuation of the pigment epithelium and bone spicule pigment clumping superior and inferior to each disc (Figure 13-20). The ERG was in the low normal range. The diagnosis was peripapillary pigmentary retinal degeneration,[61] which is a nonprogressive or slowly progressive disorder with a good visual prognosis.

Case 6

A 31-year-old man had a complaint of progressive loss of vision over a period of about 10 years. Best-corrected visual acuity was 20/100 OD and 20/200 OS, and the fundus evaluation revealed a macular degeneration in both

286

FIGURE 13-19

Case 4. Pigmented paravenous retinochoroidal atrophy. This patient had no complaints, exhibited a 20/20 visual acuity in each eye, had normal visual fields, and had normal ERGs and EOGs.

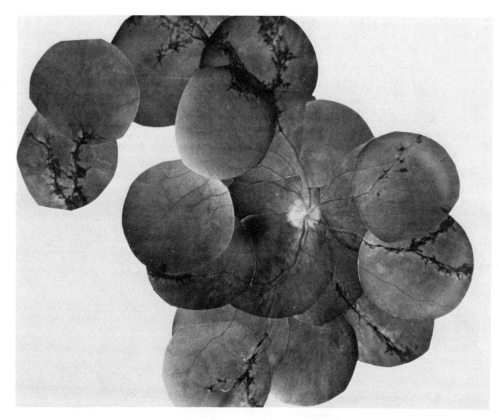

FIGURE 13-20

Case 5. Peripapillary pigmentary retinal degeneration. This 40-year-old, asymptomatic patient exhibited 20/20 visual acuity in each eye, mild relative visual field defects corresponding to areas of bone spicule pigment clumping superior and inferior to the discs, and normal ERGs.

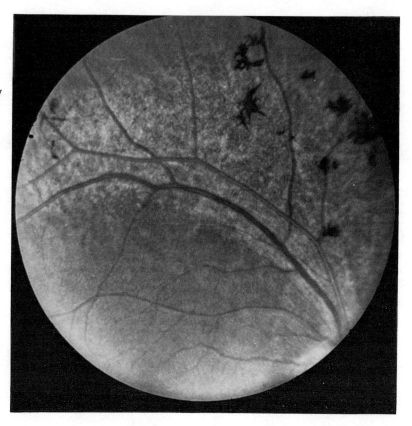

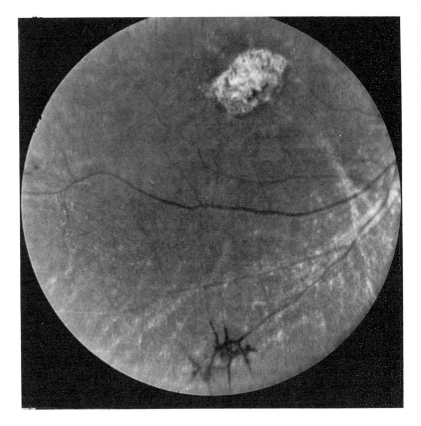

FIGURE 13-21

Case 6. This patient with retinitis pigmentosa with associated macular degeneration exhibited a ring scotoma on visual field testing as well as a markedly abnormal ERG response. Bone spicule pigmentary changes were minimal in the fundus periphery.

eyes. Visual fields demonstrated a ring scotoma and a central scotoma in each eye. The ERG responses were very reduced. Repeat funduscopy revealed a few areas of bone spicule formation in the periphery (Figure 13-21). The diagnosis was retinitis pigmentosa with associated degeneration of the macula.

Case 7
A 20-year-old man had a diagnosis of congenital nystagmus. Best-corrected visual acuities were 20/100 OD and 20/200 OS. The fundus evaluation was essentially normal, but the nystagmus precluded detailed examination. The ERG response was severely reduced in both eyes. Based on the reduced vision, the nystagmus from birth, and the reduced ERG response, a diagnosis of Leber's congenital amaurosis was made.

Case 8
A precocious 10-year-old boy had complaints of poor vision at night. His best-corrected visual acuities through a myopic correction were 20/30 OD and 20/80 OS. The

fundus of each eye appeared normal. The ERGs demonstrated an electronegative response under both photopic and scotopic conditions. The a-wave and b-wave implicit times were also similar under photopic and scotopic conditions. The diagnosis was congenital stationary night blindness. This disease when associated with myopia is characterized by reduced visual acuities.

Case 9
A 34-year-old asymptomatic woman was referred from a vision screening because of diffuse white spots in the posterior pole of each eye (Figure 13-22). Best corrected visual acuities were 20/20 in each eye. When carefully questioned, she did report some difficulty seeing at night. The ERG was significantly reduced both under photopic and scotopic conditions. One eye was patched for 3 hours so that the patient could dark adapt for a prolonged period, and the ERG was repeated. After 3 hours of dark adaptation, the ERG response was normal (Figure 13-23). The patient was diagnosed with fundus albipunctatus, which increases the dark adaptation time necessary to reach a normal ERG amplitude.

FIGURE 13-22
Case 9. A 34-year-old woman exhibited diffusely scattered white spots in the posterior pole of each eye. Careful questioning revealed mild reduced night vision, and ERG testing confirmed a diagnosis of fundus albipunctatus.

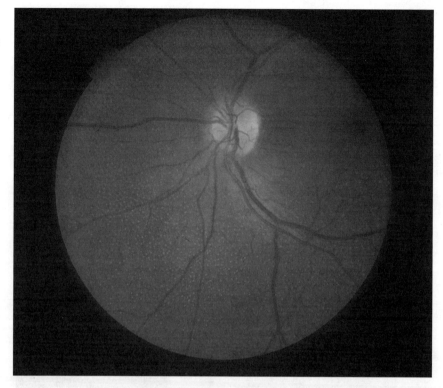

FIGURE 13-23
Case 9. The ERGs under photopic and scotopic conditions of the patient with fundus albipunctatus in Figure 13-22. The ERG amplitude is reduced in both situations but becomes normal after prolonged dark adaptation. Visual acuity was 20/20 in each eye, and the patient reported mildly reduced night vision.

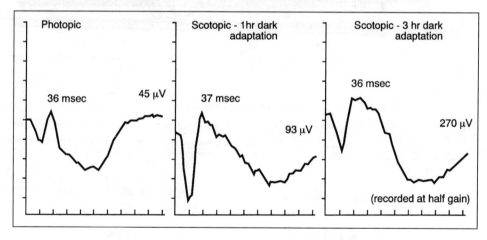

Case 10

A 19-year-old woman had reduced vision in the left eye for the preceding year. Best-corrected visual acuities were 20/20 OD and 20/50 OS. The fundus evaluation revealed a cyst-like lesion with a diffuse pigment abnormality in the macula of the right eye (Figure 13-24, top). The left macula exhibited a whitish scar of irregular shape (Figure 13-24, bottom). The retinal vessels and periphery were normal. The ERG response in each eye was normal. However, the Arden ratio of the EOG was 1.40 OD and 1.35 OS. The abnormal EOG ratios reflect a widespread func-

tional abnormality of the pigment epithelium in both eyes. This case was a classic presentation of Best's vitelliform macular dystrophy.

Case 11

A 5-year-old boy had signs of nystagmus, first noted by his parents 7 months earlier. Night vision seemed to be fine. Best corrected visual acuities were 20/100 in each eye. Ophthalmoscopy revealed normal fundi except that the foveal reflexes were not well defined. Color vision

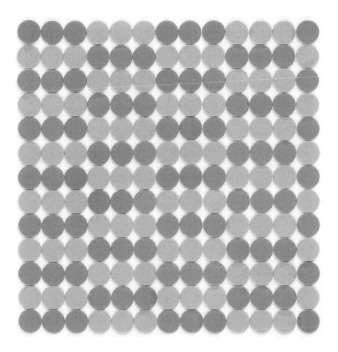

PLATE 7-I

Farnsworth F2 Plate. Two overlapping squares, one yellow-green and one blue, are presented on a purple background. Normal trichromats will see both squares with the yellow-green square being more distinct. Tritan defectives will fail to see the yellow-green square (severe) or will report the blue square as more distinct (mild). Congenital red-green defectives fail to see the blue square.

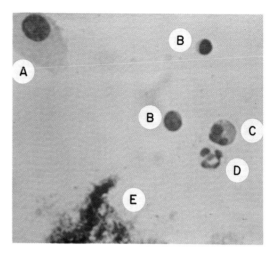

PLATE 17-I

Cytologic features revealed by Diff-Quik stain. A. Epithelial cell. B. Mononuclear cell. C. Eosinophil. D. Polymorphonuclear leukocyte. E. Fibrin.

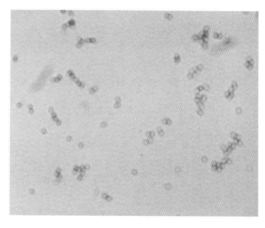

PLATE 17-II

Neisseria gonorrhoeae. *Note the kidney-bean-shaped diplococci. (Gram's stain; original magnification 250×.) (Reproduced with permission from JD Bartlett. Clinical Ocular Microbiology and Cytology. In JE Terry [ed], Ocular Disease: Detection, Diagnosis, and Treatment. Springfield: Thomas, 1984;395–435.)*

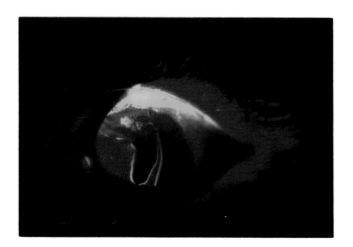

PLATE 15-I

Seidel's sign indicating wound dehiscence. The sodium fluorescein highlights the leading edge of the leaking aqueous, allowing detection of wound gap. (Courtesy of Jane Bachman, O.D.)

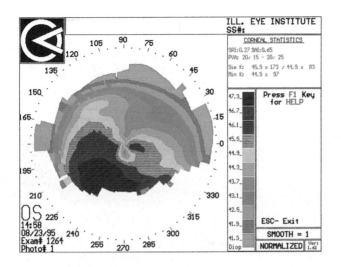

FIGURE 22-I

Computerized corneal topographic analysis of pellucid marginal degeneration. The region of greatest corneal curvature is shown in dark red inferior and peripherally. The central cornea is flatter and exhibits against-the-rule astigmatism. The keratoscopic photograph of the same eye is shown in Figure 22-15. (Courtesy of Daniel K. Roberts, O.D., and Pamela J. Boyce, O.D.)

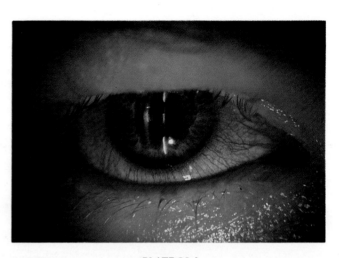

PLATE 23-I

Circumlimbal injection associated with anterior uveitis.

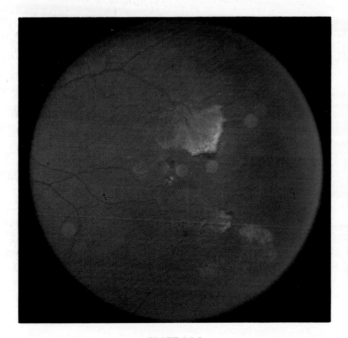

PLATE 24-I

Peripheral neovascularization, "sea fans," associated with proliferative sickle cell retinopathy.

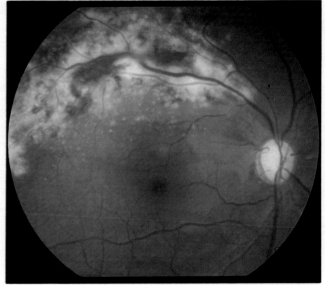

PLATE 24-II

Cytomegalovirus retinitis associated with AIDS. (Courtesy of Sara L. Penner, O.D.).

FIGURE 13-24

Case 10. Best's vitelliform macular dystrophy. The right eye (top) exhibited a cyst-like lesion in the macula and a 20/20 visual acuity. The left eye (bottom) exhibited an irregular scar and a 20/50 visual acuity. The Arden ratio of the EOG was reduced in each eye, confirming the diagnosis.

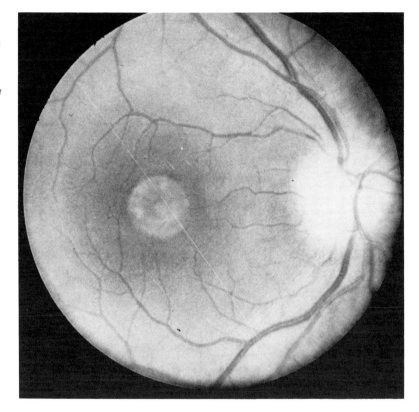

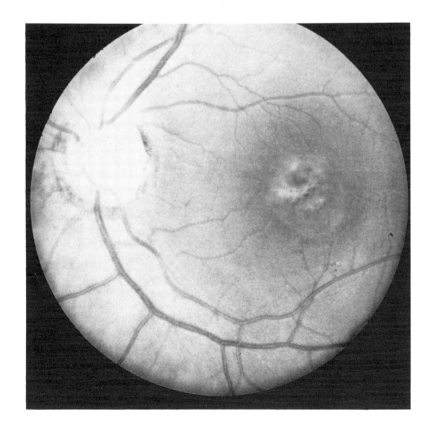

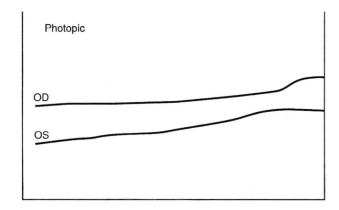

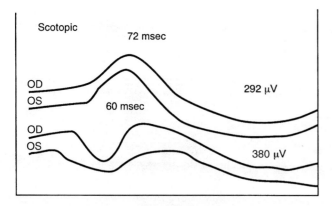

FIGURE 13-25

Case 11. ERG testing results in a patient with rod monochromatism. The photopic ERG in each eye is flat, indicating absence of cone function. Scotopic ERGs are normal as tested with two different stimuli (low-intensity blue and high-intensity white) in each eye. This indicates normal functioning rods. The ERGs tested with the low-intensity blue stimulus characteristically do not exhibit an a-wave (the upper scotopic tracings in the diagram). Visual acuity was 20/200 in each eye, and the patient reported better vision at night than during the day. (Modified and reprinted from J Sherman. The theory of relativity. Optometric Management 1993;Jan:84–5.)

testing results were unreliable. An ERG was attempted, but the child was uncooperative. Therefore an ERG and color vision testing was performed on his 33-year-old uncle who also had reduced vision and nystagmus. Color vision testing was abnormal. The photopic ERG was flat but the scotopic ERG response was normal (Figure 13-25). Reduced acuity, nystagmus, poor color vision, and an absent photopic with normal scotopic ERG responses are all indicative of the condition known as rod monochromatism. Rod monochromats have functioning rods but minimal or no functioning cones.

REFERENCES

1. Regan D. Human Brain Electrophysiology. In D Regan (ed), Evoked Potentials and Evoked Magnetic Fields in Science and Medicine. New York: Elsevier, 1989.
2. Sokol S. Visually evoked potentials: theory, techniques and clinical applications. Surv Ophthalmol 1976;21:18–44.
3. Caton R. The electric currents of the brain. Br Med J 1875;2:278.
4. Harter MR, White CT. Effects of contour sharpness and check size on visually evoked cortical potentials. Vision Res 1968;8:701–11.
5. Ludlum WM, Meyers RR. The use of visual evoked responses in objective refraction. Trans NY Acad Sci 1972;34:154–70.
6. Regan D. Rapid objective refraction using evoked brain potentials. Invest Ophthalmol 1973;12:669–79.
7. Sokol S, Dobson V. Pattern reversal visually evoked potentials in infants. Invest Ophthalmol 1976;15:150–3.
8. Tyler CW, Apkarian P, Levi D, Nakayama K. Rapid assessment of visual function: An electronic sweep technique for the pattern visual evoked potential. Invest Ophthalmol 1979;18:703–13.
9. Bartlett NR, Eason RG, White CT. Binocular summation in the evoked cortical potential. Percept and Psychophysics 1968;3:75–6.
10. Srebro R. The visually evoked response. Arch Ophthalmol 1978;96:839–44.
11. Amigo G, Fiorentini A, Pirchio M, Spinelli D. Binocular vision tested with visual evoked potentials in children and infants. Invest Ophthalmol 1978;17:910–5.
12. Bass SJ, Sherman J, Bodis-Wollner I, Noble K. VEPs in macular disease. Invest Ophthalmol Visual Sci 1985;26:1071–4.
13. Sherman J, Bass SJ, Noble KG, et al. Visual evoked potential (VEP) delays in central serous choroidopathy. Invest Ophthalmol Visual Sci 1986;27:214–21.
14. McAlpine D, Lumsden CE, Acheson ED. Multiple Sclerosis: A Reappraisal. Edinburgh: Churchill Livingstone, 1972.
15. Bass SJ, Sherman J. Visual evoked potential (VEP) delays in tilted and/or oblique entrance of the optic nerve head. Neuro-ophthalmology 1988;8:109–22.
16. Halliday AM, Halliday E, Kriss A, et al. The pattern evoked potential in compression of the anterior visual pathways. Brain 1976;99:357–74.
17. Millman A, Sherman J, Della Rocca RC, Eichler J. Pattern visual evoked potentials in orbital disease. Invest Ophthalmol Visual Sci 1988;29(ARVO Suppl):433.
18. Sherman J. The case of the not-so-simple red eye. Optom Man 1991;26:46–7.
19. Bodis-Wollner I, Atkin A, Raab E, Wolkstein M. Visual association cortex and vision in man: Pattern evoked occipital potentials in a blind boy. Science 1977;198:629–31.
20. Davis ET, Schnider CM, Sherman J. Normative data and control studies of flash VEPs for comparison to a clinical population. Am J Optom Physiol Opt 1987;64:579–92.
21. Weinstein GW. Clinical aspects of the visually evoked potential. Ophthalmic Surg 1978;9:956–65.

22. Huber C. Amplitude vs. frequency of VEP to sine modulated light in optic nerve disease. Proc ISCERG Symp, 1976:13.

23. Camisa J, Mylin LN, Bodis-Wollner I. The effect of stimulus orientation of the visual evoked potential in multiple sclerosis. Ann Neurol 1981;10:532–9.

24. Kupersmith MJ, Seiple WH, Nelson JI. Retrobulbar neuritis: Loss of cortically mediated function. Invest Ophthalmol Visual Sci 1984;25(ARVO Suppl):312.

25. Bass SJ, Sherman J, Davis B. Effect of stimulus orientation on the VEP in macular disease. Invest Ophthalmol Visual Sci 1985;32(ARVO Suppl).

26. Vaughan HG, Katzman R. Evoked responses in visual disorders. Ann NY Acad Sci 1964;112:305–19.

27. Sherman J. Simultaneous pattern-reversal electroretinograms and visual evoked potentials in diseases of the macula and optic nerve. Ann NY Acad Sci 1982;382:214–25.

28. Maffei L, Fiorentini A. Electroretinographic responses to alternating gratings before and after section of the optic nerve. Science 1981:211:953–5.

29. Sherman J, Bass SJ, Richardson V. The differential diagnosis of retinal disease from optic nerve disease. J Am Optom Assoc 1981;52:933–9.

30. Celesia GG, Kaufman D. Pattern ERGs and visual evoked potentials in maculopathies and optic nerve diseases. Invest Ophthalmol Visual Sci 1985;26:726–35.

31. Sherman J, Richter SJ, Epstein A. The differential diagnosis of visual disorders in patients presenting with marked symptoms but with no observable ocular abnormality. Am J Optom Physiol Opt 1980;57:516–22.

32. Gittinger JW Jr, Sokol S. The visual evoked potential in the diagnosis of congenital ocular motor apraxia. Am J Ophthalmol 1982;93:700–3.

33. Granit R. Sensory Mechanisms of the Retina. London: Oxford University Press, 1947.

34. Fishman, GA. The Electroretinogram and Electro-oculogram in Retinal and Choroidal Disease. Rochester, MN: American Academy of Ophthalmology and Otolaryngology, 1975:9.

35. Dowling JE. Organization of vertebrate retinas. Invest Ophthalmol 1970;9:655–80.

36. Ogden TE. The oscillatory waves of the primate electroretinogram. Vision Res 1973;13:1059–74.

37. Genest AA: Oscillatory potentials in the electroretinogram of the normal human eye. Vision Res 1964;4:595–604.

38. Yonemura D, Aoki T, Tsuzuki K. Electroretinogram in diabetic retinopathy. Arch Ophthalmol 1962;68:19–24.

39. Simonsen SE. ERG in Diabetics. In J Francois (ed), The Clinical Value of Electroretinography VI. ESCERG Symposium, Ghent, 1966. New York: Karger, 1968:403–12.

40. Ohtsubo S. Clinical and experimental study of electroretinogram in diabetic state. Jpn J Ophthalmol 1970;14:278–90.

41. Karpe G. The basis of clinical electroretinography. Acta Ophthalmol 1945;24(Suppl):1–118.

42. Riggs LA. Continuous and reproducible recordings of the electrical activity of the human retina. Proc Soc Exp Biol 1941;48:204–7.

43. Marmor MF, Arden GB, Nilsson SEG, Zrenner E (International Standardization Committee). Standard for clinical electroretinography. Arch Ophthalmol 1989;107:816–9.

44. Kinghton RW, Blankenship GW. Electrophysiological Evaluation of Eyes with Opaque Media. In S Sokol (ed), Electrophysiology and Psychophysics: Their Use in Ophthalmic Diagnosis. Int Ophthalmol Clin 1980;20(1).

45. Marmor MF. The electroretinogram in retinitis pigmentosa. Arch Ophthalmol 1979;97:1300–4.

46. Carr RE, Heckenlively JR. Primary Retinal Degenerations. In T Duane (ed), Clinical Ophthalmology (Vol 4). Hagerstown MD: Harper & Row, 1986;21.

47. Schappert-Kimmijser J, Henkes HE, van den Bosch J. Amaurosis congenita (Leber). Arch Ophthalmol 1959;61:211–8.

48. Alstrom CH, Olson O. Heredo-retinopathio congenitalis myohydrida recessive autosomalis. Hereditas 1957;43:1–10.

49. Krill AE. Congenital Stationary Night Blindness. In AE Krill (ed), Hereditary Retinal and Choroidal Diseases (Vol 2). Hagerstown, MD: Harper & Row, 1977;391–420.

50. Sperling MS, Hiles DA, Kennerdell JS. Electroretinographic responses following vitamin A therapy in A-beta-lipoproteinemia. Am J Ophthalmol 1972;73:342–51.

51. Berson EL, Rosner B, Sandberg MA, et al. A randomized trial of vitamin A and vitamin E supplementation for retinitis pigmentosa. Arch Ophthalmol 1993;111:761–72.

52. Deutman AF. Rod-Cone Dystrophy: Primary, Hereditary, Pigmentary Retinopathy, Retinitis Pigmentosa. In AE Krill (ed), Hereditary Retinal and Choroidal Diseases (Vol 2). Hagerstown, MD: Harper & Row, 1977;479–576.

53. Krill AE. Cone Degenerations. In AE Krill (ed), Hereditary Retinal and Choroidal Diseases (Vol 2). Hagerstown, MD: Harper & Row, 1977;421–78.

54. Marmor MF, Jacobson SG, Foerster MH, et al. Diagnostic clinical findings of a new syndrome with night blindness, maculopathy, and enhanced S cone sensitivity. Am J Ophthalmol 1990;110:124–34.

55. Henkind P, Carr RE, Siegel IM. Early chloroquine retinopathy: Clinical and functional findings. Arch Ophthalmol 1964;71:157–65.

56. Fishman GA, Sokol S. Electrophysiologic Testing in Disorders of the Retina, Optic Nerve and Visual Pathway. Ophthalmology Monographs, Vol 2. San Francisco: American Academy of Ophthalmology, 1990.

57. Marg E. Development of electro-oculography. Arch Ophthalmol 1951;45:169–85.

58. Afanador AJ. The EOG ratio and its evaluation of retinal function. J Am Optom Assoc 1977;48:1149–56.

59. Arden GB, Fojas MR. Electrophysiological abnormalities in pigmentary degenerations of the retina. Arch Ophthalmol 1962;68:369–89.

60. Brooks DN, Potter JW, Bartlett JD, Nowakowski R. Pigmented paravenous retinochoroidal atrophy. J Am Optom Assoc 1980;51:1097–101.

61. Noble KG, Carr RE. Peripapillary pigmentary retinal degeneration. Am J Ophthalmol 1978;86:65–75.

14

Ophthalmic Ultrasonography

JEROME SHERMAN

The clinical use of ophthalmic ultrasonography has increased dramatically over the past few decades and is universally regarded as an essential means for examining the soft tissues of the eye and orbit.[1] In selected cases, the traditional clinical examination can be supplemented, refined, and extended by the inclusion of ophthalmic ultrasonography. An understanding of the limitations of ophthalmic ultrasonography is just as important as being familiar with its uses. Ultrasonography yields information that is limited to the *structural* integrity of the eye and orbit. Objective tests that provide information on the *functional* integrity of the visual system include electroretinography and the visual evoked potential (see Chapter 13).

Sound waves can be used advantageously as an alternative to light in the examination of the eye under two major conditions.[2] First, when the tissues are translucent or opaque to light (e.g., in the presence of dense cataract or vitreous hemorrhage), sound can easily penetrate and reflect a visual representation of the ocular structures. Second, the relatively slow speed of sound can be used for obtaining distance and thickness measurements. The measurement of intraocular distances, or ocular biometry, is routinely used for calculating the power of intraocular lenses.

PRINCIPLES OF ULTRASONOGRAPHY

Ultrasound is an acoustic wave in which compressions and rarefactions occur because of changes in density within fluid and solid substances.[1] An ultrasonic wave differs from a sonic wave in that the former exhibits frequencies above 20 kHz (1 kHz equals 1,000 cycles per second) and is thus not audible to humans. Like light waves, ultrasonic waves can be directed, focused, and reflected according to established principles. In ophthalmic ultrasonography, high frequencies (about 10 MHz, or 10 million cycles per second) and small wavelengths make detailed resolution of ocular structures possible. The resolution of images formed by reflected sound waves is related to frequency in the same way that the frequency or the wavelength of the light used in a microscope places a limit on the resolution of the instrument as a result of diffraction and interference effects.

Sound travels in biological tissue at a rate of approximately 1,500 meters per second, and for most purposes the speed in a tissue may be considered independent of frequency. The time required for sound to travel to the rear of the eye and return is only about 33 microseconds (1 microsecond equals 1 millionth of a second). The cathode ray tube (the face of which resembles a small TV screen) provides a suitable means for displaying and measuring such short time intervals.

In exactly the same way that one might shout "ho ho" against a mountain and record the time required for the echo to return to estimate the distance to the mountain, one can direct a small pulse of sound into the eye and measure the time for the echoes to return.[3] Intraocular distances can then be measured through application of the formula: distance = velocity × time. In ophthalmic ultrasonography, the application of an electrical pulse to a piezoelectric crystal generates a short pulse of ultrasonic energy, which traverses a known path in the eye at a known speed. The piezoelectric crystal expands and contracts rapidly as the applied voltage is varied in polarity, and ultrasonic vibrations result. The crystal acts as a transducer, because electrical energy is converted into sound energy. The ultrasonic pulse undergoes partial reflection at various tissue boundaries because of abrupt changes in the acoustic properties of the tissues. When the reflected sound energy returns to the crystal, it is

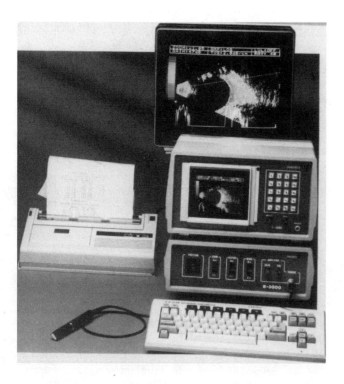

FIGURE 14-1
Ophthalmic ultrasound unit. The instrumentation allows for reflected sound from ocular tissues to be graphically displayed on a screen.

transformed back into electrical energy. The same crystal can transmit and then receive back the sound wave because the duration of a pulse is very small compared with the time between pulses.

Methods Of Display

After the electrical energy is converted into sound energy and then reconverted into electrical energy by the crystal, the echoes can be displayed in graphic form (Figure 14-1). The three types of display are A-mode, B-mode, and M-mode. Each of these presents structural information in a unique display format.

A-Mode Systems

Tissue boundaries or interfaces are graphically displayed as a function of distance along any selected axis. The amplitudes of the returned echoes on the display are proportional to the sound energy reflected at the corresponding tissue boundaries. A-mode systems were the first to be used in ophthalmology and are now widely used because they are ideal for biometric applications, primarily for axial length determination in intraocular lens calculations (Figure 14-2). Time-amplitude ultrasonog-

raphy, as A-mode is sometimes called, only provides a unidimensional display, and therefore it is not useful for the creation of a detailed ophthalmic image. During A-mode ultrasonography, the corneal apex may be lightly applanated in a technique similar to Goldmann tonometry (Figure 14-3).

B-Mode Systems

Transducer scanning and electronic processing are incorporated into a basic ultrasonic system to produce cross-sectional images of the eye and orbit (Figure 14-4). Whereas in A-mode the transducer is fixed in position, resulting in a unidimensional display, in B-mode the transducer undergoes a sweeping or scanning motion in any selected plane, and the resulting display is two-dimensional. (Although the word "scan" is loosely used in the terms A-scan and B-scan, it is inappropriate to describe A-mode as a scan because no scanning motion of the transducer takes place.) The resultant two-dimensional image is composed of numerous spots, and the brightness of each spot is proportional to the sound energy reflected by the corresponding tissue boundary. This type of B-mode is also known as intensity modulated ultrasonography, and the term *gray-scale* is often used to describe the relative brightness of the displayed tissue echoes. A system that incorporates a gray-scale with many steps or gradations of gray, ranging from black to white, is quite desirable since the relative brightness of a displayed echo helps the examiner identify the corresponding tissue.

In A-mode ultrasonography, the reflections displayed at any one time are those produced by directing the probe in a particular direction, and the examiner, from his or her knowledge of anatomy and pathology, must mentally assemble a three-dimensional percept from the systematic movement of the probe. This requires considerable and continuing practice, and those who have acquired the requisite level of expertise are inclined to favor this method. It is far easier mentally to assemble the two-dimensional images obtained from B-mode ultrasonography into the three-dimensional percept than to remember all the unidimensional images obtained from A-mode and perform the complex mental manipulation required to create the three-dimensional representation.

M-Mode Systems

In cardiology, M (motion)-mode ultrasonography and TM (time-motion)-mode ultrasonography are ideal systems for monitoring dilations and constrictions of blood vessels. As time progresses, tissue structures that are stationary produce a display of a series of parallel lines. If tissue positions fluctuate with time, corresponding variations occur in the distance between these lines so that a

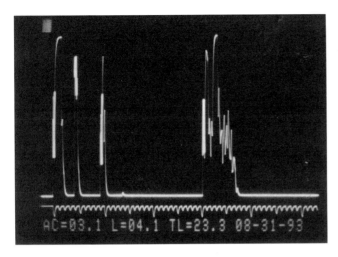

FIGURE 14-2

Typical A-mode display acquired during axial length determination. The amplitudes of the echoes are proportional to the sound energy reflected at the corresponding tissue. (C = cornea; ALS = anterior lens surface; PLS = posterior lens surface; R = retina; OF = orbital fat; AC = anterior chamber; L = lens, TL = total length, in millimeters.)

complete time history of tissue position is portrayed.[1] M-mode systems are infrequently applied to ocular studies.

EXAMINATION PROCEDURE

The typical B-mode ultrasound examination is remarkably simple for the clinician and the patient alike. If no abnormalities are uncovered, the procedure can be completed in a minute or two. After the patient is comfortably situated in either a lying or sitting position with the eyelids closed, a coupling agent, such as gonioscopic methylcellulose, is applied to the end of the probe or the closed lid. Sound waves of very high frequency such as those used in ophthalmic ultrasonography are not transmitted through air, and thus the probe must be coupled with the closed lid with the gel-like coupling agent.

The examination is dynamic, and the examiner must move the scanning head over the closed lid in all directions to ensure that representative cross sections of the globe are obtained (Figure 14-5). A Polaroid camera or printer attachment is used to document any desired cross section, although

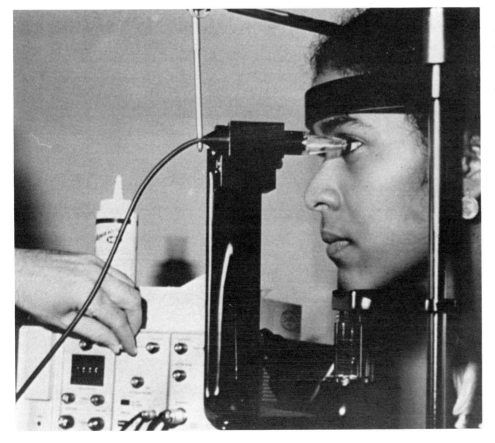

FIGURE 14-3

During axial length determination, the A-scan probe may be used in a manner similar to the Goldmann tonometer during applanation tonometry.

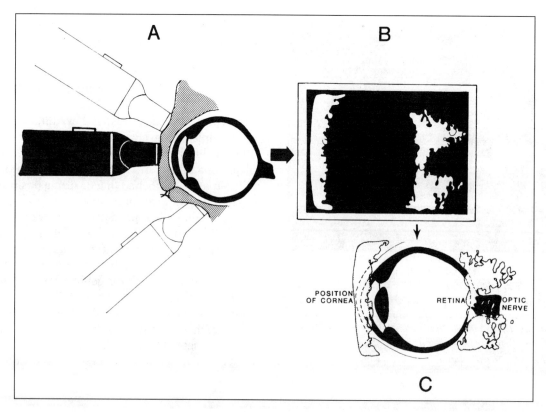

FIGURE 14-4

A. Diagrammatic representation of a B-scan probe in contact with the closed lid. Movement of the probe results in different cross sections. B. Resultant B-mode ultrasonogram. The cornea and closed lid are not visualized well, but their position is represented at the extreme left of the image. The retina-choroid-sclera complex is displayed to the right. Note the sonolucent (echo free) vitreous and the sonolucent horizontal V-shaped optic nerve. C. An artist's conception of the globe and ultrasonogram that is depicted in B.

FIGURE 14-5

During a typical B-mode ultrasound examination the probe is placed against the closed lid and then pivoted in various directions to obtain different cross sections of the globe. A coupling agent is placed on the lid surface to aid in the transmission of sound waves from the probe to the lid and globe.

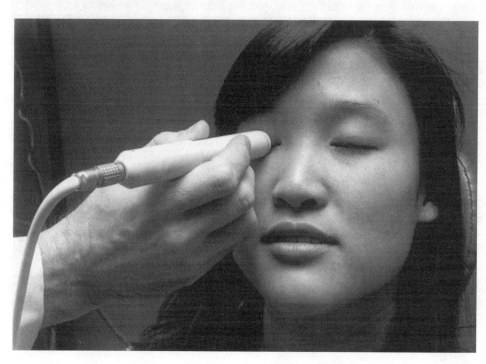

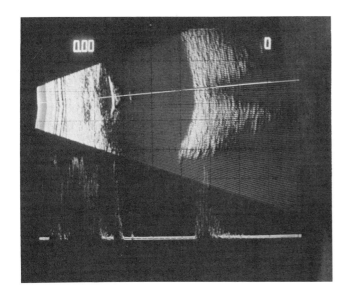

FIGURE 14-6

Normal B-mode (with simultaneous A-mode) ultrasonogram. The horizontal line through the B-mode display is the vector scan used to select the axis of imaging that is displayed in the A-mode below. The vector scan clearly traverses through the crystalline lens on the left (crescent-shaped B-mode echo) and the optic nerve on the right (V-shaped echo-free region).

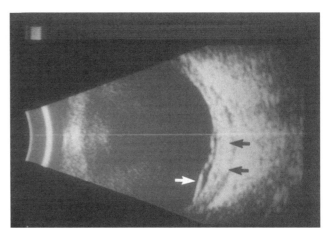

FIGURE 14-7

Ophthalmic ultrasonogram demonstrating a thickened choroid (dark arrows) and a localized retinal detachment (white arrow).

static photographic representations are never as useful as the actual dynamic scan. Various recording systems are available so that each photograph can be labeled as to which of the infinite cross sections it represents.[4]

In addition to moving the position of the probe during the examination, the sensitivity control should be varied. The sensitivity control allows the examiner to estimate the relative acoustic densities of various tissues. As mentioned earlier, the brightness of each individual spot that composes a B-mode ultrasonogram is proportional to the sound energy reflected by the corresponding tissue boundary. Initial B-mode examination is performed at high sensitivity so that even weak echoes will be detected.

In a typical contact B-mode examination, the anterior portion of the eye is not visualized well. However, the posterior lens capsule is typically noted behind the position of the cornea and closed lid, which is at the extreme left of the screen (Figure 14-6). Normal vitreous does not reflect sound well, and such poorly reflecting structures are termed *sonolucent*. The echo free, or *anechoic* areas appear black as opposed to structures that reflect sound well, which appear white or shades of gray. Similarly, the optic nerve is sonolucent and appears black. The black horizontal V-shaped optic nerve is an important landmark in B-mode ultrasonography. In the normal eye, the retina appears as

a smooth, concave surface with a sharp acoustic boundary on the right of the ultrasonogram, which disappears later as sensitivity is reduced. This acoustically opaque concave surface results from echoes arising from the vitreoretinal interface and is inseparable from the echoes emanating from the choroid and sclera. However, a thickened choroid in select disorders is usually obvious. These include Harada's disease, choroidal effusion syndrome, and posterior scleritis (Figure 14-7). If a sheet-like membrane is observed in the vitreous, the sensitivity should be reduced to estimate its relative acoustic density. If the echo persists at low sensitivity, then the membrane is likely retina, whereas if it disappears early, a vitreal membrane is the more likely diagnosis.

CLINICAL APPLICATIONS

The following section discusses the ultrasonographic characteristics of several ophthalmic disorders. The clinician should realize that ultrasonography is not an essential technique in the diagnosis and management of many of these conditions. Indications for ultrasonography as summarized by Koplin et al.[5] are given in Table 14-1. Situations in which ultrasonography provides minimal helpful information include (1) resolving lesions elevated less than 1 mm from the retina/choroid; (2) detecting lesions in the orbital apex or lesions placoid in nature and adhering to the bony orbit; (3) differentiating old hemorrhage from amyloid or old inflammatory debris in vitreous; and (4) evaluating very small lesions in the angle of the anterior chamber or along the ciliary body.

TABLE 14-1
Indications for Ophthalmic Ultrasonography

Opaque media
Tumor differentiation: defining elevated lesions
Membrane differentiation: retina versus organized membranes versus choroidal separation
Ocular trauma/foreign body evaluation
Endophthalmitis evaluation
Orbital tumors and extraocular muscle evaluation
Axial length determination

Retinal Detachment

In total retinal detachment, the appearance of the ultrasonogram is usually unmistakable. The retina can be viewed extending back to the optic nerve, which is the only part of the posterior aspect of the globe where the retina is attached. In the ultrasonogram in Figure 14-8, the patient had a dense cataract of the right eye that precluded examination of the fundus by ophthalmoscopy. Ultrasonography was performed and yielded a presumed diagnosis of total retinal detachment since the displayed membrane extended back to the optic nerve and was present at low sensitivity levels. In view of a history of trauma to that eye 5 years previously and a total retinal detachment as observed with ultrasonography, the patient was advised not to undergo a cataract extraction.

Even in the case of total retinal detachment, only those cross sections through the optic nerve will show the classical configuration whereby a funnel-shaped membrane tapers toward and attaches to the optic nerve. Other cross sections may appear like the one depicted at the bottom of Figure 14-8. As mentioned previously, ultrasonography is a dynamic procedure, and the clinician must use many cross sections to assemble the three-dimensional percept mentally. Blood on the interface of a detached posterior vitreous face can usually be distinguished from retinal detachment by lowering the sensitivity of the ultrasound instrument. Echoes from blood disappear earlier than echoes from retinal tissue. In recent retinal detachments, movement of the patient's eye will result in slow undulation of the sheet-like membrane. Long-standing retinal detachments with fibrous tissue proliferation move relatively little.

On rare occasions, a dense vitreal membrane characterized by blood adhering to a detached posterior hyaloid face might appear remarkably similar to a total detachment on ultrasonic examination.[6] However, when the patient looks from side to side, undulation of the membrane is greater for a posterior vitreal detachment than a retinal detachment. Moreover, lack of an afferent pupillary defect and the presence of normal or near-normal

results on bright flash ERG and VEP rule out a total retinal detachment and support the diagnosis of a dense vitreal membrane with a normal underlying retina.

Shallow retinal detachments are more difficult to detect with ophthalmoscopy, but ultrasonography can confirm the diagnosis (Figure 14-9). Proliferative fibrovascular membranes are relatively common in diabetics (Figure 14-10). In advanced stages, it is often extremely difficult to differentiate between large, acoustically dense membranes and tractional retinal detachments.

Pathologic Conditions of the Vitreous

In addition to fibrovascular vitreal membranes discussed previously, abnormal granular or globular vitreous opacities of varied acoustic densities are clinically encountered. With the use of the ultrasonographic gray-scale, the whitest reflections, which disappear late as instrument sensitivity is decreased, represent acoustically dense opacities, whereas those that are dimmer and that disappear early are less dense acoustically. The degree of vitreal pathologic involvement can be estimated by the extent and the acoustic density of the displayed echoes.

Vitreal hemorrhages cannot be differentiated from inflammatory debris with ultrasonography.[4] Asteroid hyalosis, which is an accumulation of calcium soaps dispersed throughout the vitreous, also has a similar appearance to a vitreal hemorrhage (Figure 14-11). However, calcium reflects sound extremely well, and the calcium soaps will typically reflect sound better at low sensitivity than hemorrhages. In addition, movement of the globe will reveal that asteroid particles move in a smooth flowing motion; however, in long-standing vitreal hemorrhages, debris is usually somewhat fixed in position. Intraocular foreign bodies, which result in vitreal hemorrhages or inflammatory debris, are often associated with fibrous membrane formation, and in such cases the interpretation is often more difficult.

Intraocular Tumors

The ultrasonic evaluation of an eye with a suspected tumor can be diagnostically helpful but is generally difficult and challenging. Usually ultrasonography cannot be solely relied on when evaluating intraocular tumors. In many cases it is necessary to perform additional tests such as fluorescein angiography, radioactive P_{32} analysis, transillumination, and visual fields to help form an overall diagnostic picture. In visually opaque globes suspected of harboring a tumor, ultrasonography becomes vital and provides information about the size, shape, position, and tissue density of any detected mass.

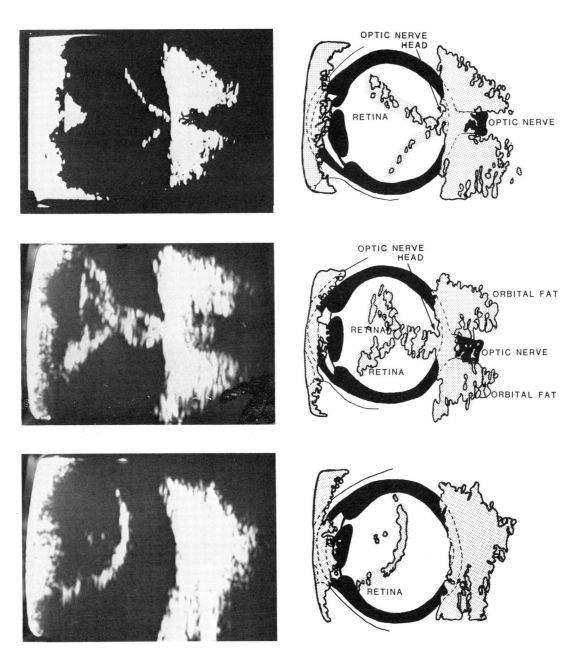

FIGURE 14-8

Sonograms from an eye with total retinal detachment. Cross sections through the optic nerve demonstrating attachment to the funnel-shaped retinal membrane (top, center). Cross section remote from the optic nerve whereby no attachment of the retina to the rear of the eye is seen (bottom).

In tumors extending into the vitreous, the initial echoes are very strong because of the abrupt change in acoustic impedance from the normal vitreous to the tumor. Dense tumors absorb a great amount of sound energy and often result in an acoustically quiet zone at the base of the mass itself or shadowing of the normal orbital fat pattern. Decreasing the sensitivity of the instrument results in a more marked attenuation of the signal as it passes through the mass. As a result, the shadowing effect becomes more obvious.

Retinoblastoma
The most common malignant intraocular tumor of childhood is retinoblastoma, and success in its treatment is

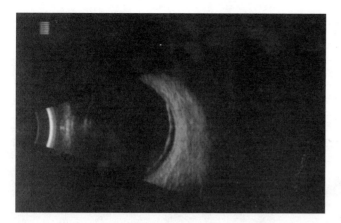

FIGURE 14-9

Ultrasonographic demonstration of a shallow retinal detachment that was missed on ophthalmoscopic examination by two examiners.

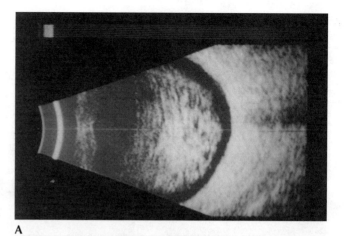

A

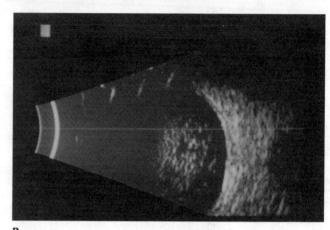

B

FIGURE 14-11

B-mode ultrasonographic sections of an eye with asteroid hyalosis. A. The opacities, which result from the accumulation of calcium soaps within the vitreous cavity, yield pronounced echoes at standard instrument sensitivity (gain = 76). B. At a reduced sensitivity (gain = 59), the echoes persist.

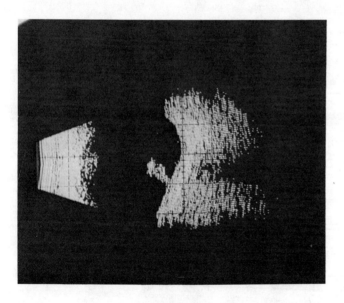

FIGURE 14-10

A proliferative fibrovascular membrane originating inferior to the disc in a patient with diabetic retinopathy. In this case, the retina was attached. In advanced cases with fibroproliferation, large, acoustically dense membranes might mimic tractional retinal detachments.

related to early diagnosis. Ultrasonography is especially useful when retinoblastoma is suspected in an eye with a vitreal hemorrhage, retinal detachment, or inflammatory reaction. Two retinoblastoma configurations have been described: solid and cystic.[7] The ultrasonic display in the cystic type is virtually indistinguishable from that of a massive, organized vitreous hemorrhage.[1] The differential diagnosis of retinoblastoma from other tumors is, at

best, difficult. In general, the ultrasonic differential diagnosis of intraocular tumors requires a level of expertise attained by very few examiners.

Choroidal Melanoma

Although the diagnosis of choroidal melanoma is generally made by an experienced clinician using a binocular indirect ophthalmoscope, modern day ophthalmic ultrasonography is quite valuable in the differential diagnosis of melanoma from other choroidal masses such as metastatic carcinoma, hemangioma, and organized subretinal hemorrhage. In recent decades, accuracy in the diagnosis of choroidal melanoma has increased from 80% (in a study of over 500 eyes in the mid-1960s) to over 99% (in the initial reports of the collaborative Ocular Melanoma

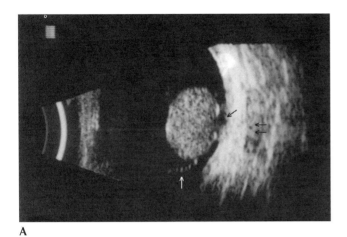

A

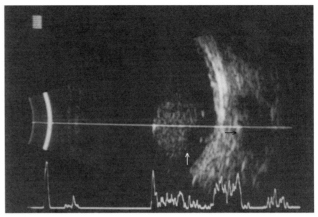

B

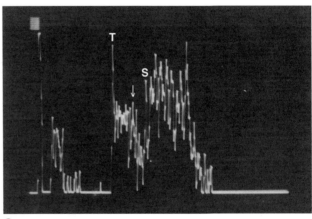

C

FIGURE 14-12

*Ultrasonograms of a malignant melanoma. A. The lesion is near-
ly spherical and has caused a secondary retinal detachment (white
arrow). Choroidal excavation (black arrow) and orbital shadowing (double arrows) are also demonstrated. B. Orbital shadowing (black arrow) caused by absorption of sound by the lesion
is demonstrated better at lower sensitivity—i.e., gain = 64.
Acoustic hollowing at the base of the tumor is also evident
here (white arrow). This results partially from greater homo-
geneity of the tumor in this region. C. A-mode image illustrating the acoustic profile of the lesion, which is characteristic of
a malignant melanoma. Because of a homogenous cellular architecture, low to medium internal reflectivity is exhibited by the
tumor (arrow). (T = tumor surface echo; S = scleral echo.)*

Study of more than 400 eyes reported in 1989).[8] The extensive use of modern combined A-mode and B-mode systems undoubtedly contributed to the improved accuracy with which this tumor is diagnosed.

Malignant melanomas, like metastatic carcinoma, can
range in size from a small localized mass to a tumor filling the entire globe. Melanomas may be placoid, oval,
mushroom-shaped, or diffuse lesions. The mushroom-
shaped or "collar-button" appearance results from the
tumor penetrating Bruch's membrane. This configuration
exhibits a markedly elevated mass relative to its width
and is very characteristic if not pathognomonic of
choroidal melanoma.

Ultrasonography, complemented by fundus photography, is an ideal procedure for documenting changes in the
size of a lesion. A small lesion can be followed for evidence
of growth; a large lesion being treated with irradiation can
be followed to document regression. Ultrasonography is
also useful in determining whether a reduction in visual
acuity and visual fields in a patient with a melanoma is the
result of an increase in the size of the lesion or the spread
of overlying retinal detachment.

Figure 14-12 shows an ultrasonogram of a 55-year-old
man with a 2-month history of blurred vision in the right
eye and an increasing right-sided field defect secondary to
a malignant melanoma. The visual acuity was 20/100 in the
right eye and 20/20 in the left eye. The lesion occupied greater
than one "lens field" using a binocular indirect ophthalmoscope with a standard 20 D lens. With a 2.2 Volk lens, which
has a field of view of approximately 52 degrees, the entire
lesion could almost be viewed in one lens field, thereby giving an estimate of the lesion's size at about 60 degrees. An
overlying retinal detachment extended inferonasal to the
lesion. The color of the lesion varied from cream to slate
gray, depending on the type of illumination.

Ultrasonography, as shown in the figure, reveals a
nearly spherical solid mass whose epicenter was nasal
to the disc. It measured approximately 10 mm by 10 mm
by 10 mm. In a case such as this, serial tomographic sections should be performed to trace the source of the mass
as one emanating from the choroid. During ultrasonographic examination, sensitivity should be varied to
reveal expected findings such as shadowing. Use of a
simultaneous A-mode and B-mode or of an A-mode sys-

FIGURE 14-13
A large juxtapapillary, plaque-like, slightly elevated, cream-colored fundus lesion. The appearance and position suggest an osseous choristoma of the choroid (choroidal osteoma).

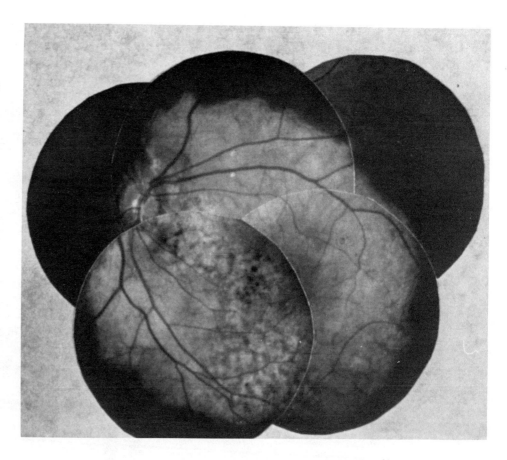

tem is advisable to assess the acoustic profile (which includes the height of the leading echo, the loss of sound energy as it is transmitted through the mass, and the characteristics of internal reflecting surfaces within the tumor) of the mass (Figure 14-12C). When comparing the amplitude of the retinal and scleral echoes to reflections arising within the tumor using A-mode, the retinal/scleral amplitudes are usually 2.5–10.0 times greater than those within the tumor.

Choroidal Hemangioma

As mentioned in the previous section, the differential diagnosis of melanoma includes choroidal hemangioma. Unlike melanoma, a choroidal hemangioma is generally flat, demonstrates minimal sound attenuation, high internal reflectivity (90–100%), and absence of growth over time. However, the differential diagnosis is not always easy because there are similarities such as choroidal location, regular acoustic structure, solid consistency, and the presence of vascularity. Vascularity can be observed with ultrasonography as distinct spontaneous movements within the lesion.

Metastatic Choroidal Carcinoma

Metastatic choroidal carcinoma can usually be differentiated from melanoma by its diffuse shape, medium sound attenuation, variable acoustic structure, high internal reflectivity, slow growth, and lack of spontaneous movements related to vascularity.

Osseous Choristoma of the Choroid

Although a bone tumor of the choroid is a rare clinical entity, when it is suspected, B-mode ultrasonography is the procedure of choice to confirm the diagnosis. Figure 14-13 depicts the left eye of an 11-year-old girl with a suspected osseous choristoma of the choroid (choroidal osteoma). The visual acuity was 20/25 in the left eye, and visual fields displayed a mild relative scotoma roughly corresponding to the observable lesion. This plaque-like, slightly elevated, cream-colored lesion with well-defined edges was thought to be an osseous choristoma because of its appearance and juxtapapillary position. However, a diagnosis of an amelanotic malignant melanoma was also entertained. Contact B-mode ultrasonography revealed a flat, acoustically dense lesion at the level of the

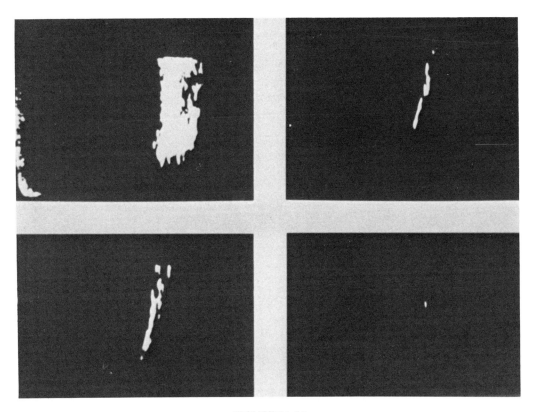

FIGURE 14-14

Contact B-mode ultrasonogram reveals an acoustically dense, flat lesion at the level of the choroid, which is shown to persist at progressively lower sensitivity levels, thus confirming the diagnosis of the suspected choroidal osteoma depicted in Figure 14-13.

choroid that persisted at low sensitivity levels (Figure 14-14), findings which are characteristic of a choroidal osteoma.[9] The presence of echoes at very low sensitivity levels should suggest certain diagnoses, such as a metallic intraocular foreign body or bone tissue, as in this case.

Melanocytoma of the Optic Disc

An ultrasonic display of a protrusion of the optic nerve head into the vitreous may be encountered in papilledema, papillitis, and disc drusen. Melanocytoma of the optic disc is a benign tumor composed of melanocytes that may also cause nerve head elevation.[10] The lesions are gray to black masses that are often located eccentrically over the edge of the disc. Often, choroidal pigmentation is present contiguous with the lesion. An afferent pupillary defect may be present in some cases, presumably because of nerve fiber compression.[11] Visual acuity is usually normal nonetheless. Melanocytomas are probably congenital in nature and occur most frequently in blacks and other dark-complexioned people. These tumors may grow very slowly over several years, but malignant transformation is rare.[12] They almost always occur unilaterally. Figure

14-15 is a fundus photo of a melanocytoma in the right eye of an asymptomatic 30-year-old black woman with a 20/20 visual acuity. The ultrasonogram (Figure 14-16) graphically displays the elevation and extent of this lesion, which does not appear to invade into deeper tissue.

Dislocated Lens

Ultrasonography is useful in the detection of intraocular foreign bodies. In a similar fashion, it might aid in the detection of normal but displaced ocular structures. Figure 14-17 shows two ultrasonographic sections of a patient's right eye. The patient's chief complaint was a sudden loss of vision in the right eye. Visual acuity was reduced to 4/400. Retinoscopy and subjective examination yielded a high plus refractive error and acuity was correctable to 20/25. Biomicroscopy failed to reveal a crystalline lens in the right eye, but the patient denied having undergone cataract extraction. The large stature of the patient, his long spider-like fingers, and the observation of a high arched palate and an excavated chest all contributed to the diagnosis of Marfan's syndrome. A

FIGURE 14-15
Fundus photograph of the right eye of an asymptomatic 30-year-old black woman. The visual acuity in this eye is 20/20, and the diagnosis is melanocytoma of the disc.

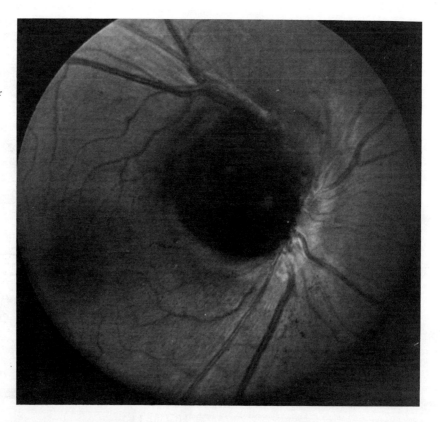

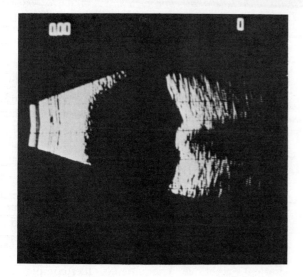 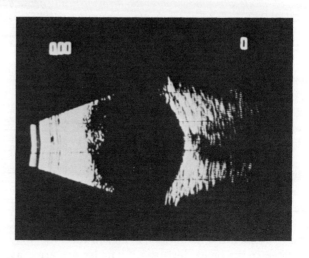

FIGURE 14-16
B-mode ultrasonogram displaying the elevation and extent of the lesion (left) shown in Figure 14-15. The lesion does not appear to invade deeper tissue. Note the normal fellow eye for comparison (right).

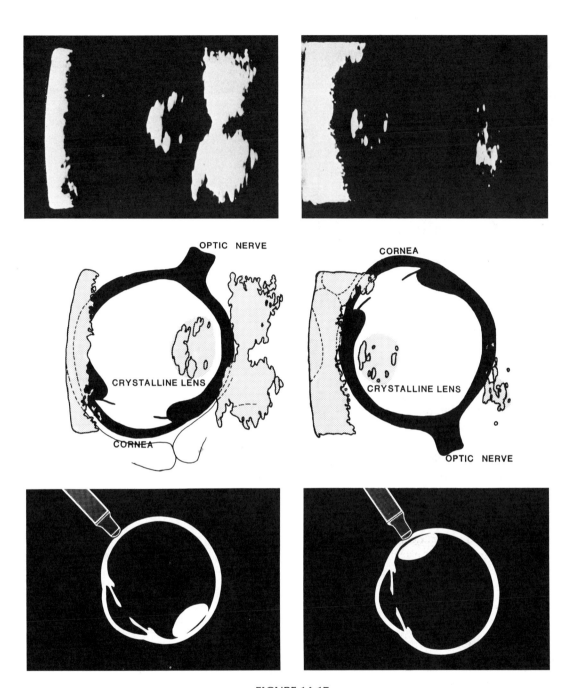

FIGURE 14-17

Two ultrasonograms of an eye with the crystalline lens dislocated inferiorly in the vitreous. The patient is looking down in the figures on the left; the patient is looking up in the figures on the right. The importance of knowing the position of the probe relative to the eye is illustrated.

common finding in this connective tissue disorder is dislocation of the lens. In the figures shown on the left in Figure 14-17, the patient was instructed to look down, and the B-scan probe was placed somewhat superiorly, yielding a cross section with the lens to the right in the ultrasonogram. In the figures on the right in Figure 14-

17, the patient was asked to look up, the probe was introduced from below, and the lens was displayed to the left in the ultrasonogram. To interpret these two ultrasonograms correctly, it is imperative to consider the relative position of the probe to the eye in each. When the patient's pupil was fully dilated, the lens was observable

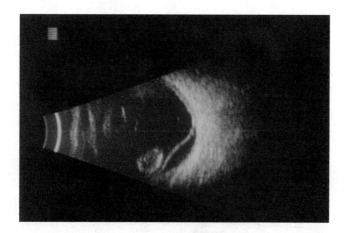

FIGURE 14-18

B-mode ultrasonogram of a Marfan's syndrome patient with a retinal detachment and dislocation of the crystalline lens into the inferior vitreous.

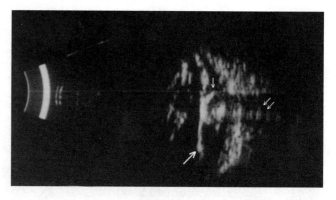

FIGURE 14-19

A BB pellet (small arrow) causing a retinal detachment (large arrow) and vitreal hemorrhage. Reduplication echoes appear to the right of the foreign body signal (double arrows). These echoes are caused by the reverberation of sound within the spherical pellet, resulting in delayed and intermittent reflectance of sound back to the transducer.

inferiorly near the equator when viewed with a binocular indirect ophthalmoscope.

In addition to subluxated or dislocated lenses, patients with Marfan's syndrome often have myopic eyes with peripheral retinal degeneration. The ultrasonogram in Figure 14-18 is of a 20-year-old woman with Marfan's syndrome and bilateral lens dislocation. She developed a retinal detachment 5 years previously in the right eye that was surgically repaired with a scleral buckle. At that time she underwent prophylactic cryopexy for numerous small tears within areas of lattice in the left eye. Despite the therapy, she later developed a retinal detachment in her left eye. A cross section inferiorly demonstrates the crystalline lens anterior to the retinal detachment. The patient did well after a triple procedure of lensectomy, vitrectomy, and scleral buckling.

Foreign Bodies

Ophthalmic ultrasonography can be extremely useful in the identification and evaluation of intraocular or orbital foreign bodies. Depending on the type of material and its precise location, ultrasonography may even be more useful than other examination methods such as ophthalmoscopy, computed tomographic scanning, or radiography.

Because the variety of foreign bodies within the eye or orbit is potentially limitless, echographic characteristics may also vary widely. Certain types of foreign bodies do have consistent characteristics that can be helpful in their identification. For example, with B-mode ultrasonography, spherical metallic foreign bodies exhibit a chain of

multiple echoes immediately behind the actual foreign body signal. These reduplication echoes are brightest directly behind the true foreign body signal and gradually decrease in intensity (Figure 14-19). Their formation is caused by reverberation of sound within the object itself, which results in delayed, intermittent reflectance of sound back to the transducer.

Because of the high reflectivity of the orbital soft tissues and bony orbital walls, orbital foreign bodies are more difficult to detect and evaluate than intraocular foreign bodies. In general, orbital foreign bodies that are spherical or located more anteriorly are more easy to detect than those that are irregular or more posterior in location.

Drusen of the Disc

An important differential diagnosis is papilledema from pseudopapilledema. A patient with blurred disc margins may have elevated intracranial pressure (caused by a space-occupying lesion) or buried drusen in the optic nerve head. Calcified drusen reflect sound more effectively than do retinal and optic nerve tissue. Figure 14-20 shows cross sections through the optic nerve at two different sensitivity levels in a patient with blurred disc borders. At high sensitivity, a slight elevation at the optic nerve head is noted. At lower sensitivity, all typical reflections have disappeared except for a localized nerve head echo, probably indicating buried drusen. In questionable cases, fluorescein angiography can be performed. Leakage of fluorescein at the disc is typical in papilledema but not in

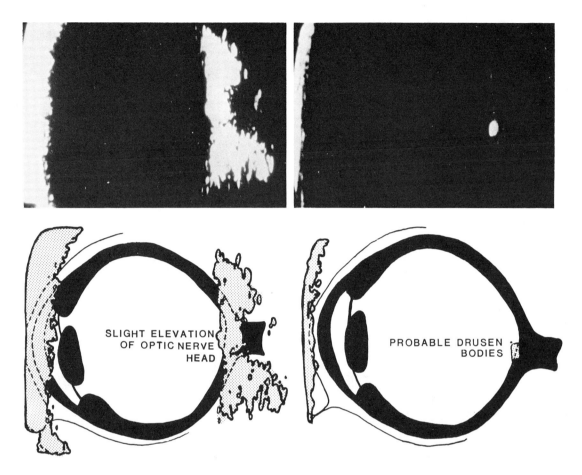

FIGURE 14-20

Two cross sections through the optic nerve head in a patient with blurred disc borders. At high sensitivity a slight elevation at the optic nerve head is noted (left). At lower sensitivity all typical reflections have disappeared except for a localized echo in the region of the nerve head (right). Drusen of the disc is the presumed diagnosis.

pseudopapilledema. Prior to angiography, one can also examine the optic nerve head for autofluorescence, a characteristic common to buried drusen. To check for this, the exciter and barrier filters used for angiography (see Chapter 5) are inserted in the fundus camera and the nerve head is examined. A subtle irregular fluorescence may be detected without the injection of any dye.

Variations in the Size and Shape of the Globe

Although accurate axial length measurements are best obtained with A-mode ultrasonography, gross deviations in contour of the globe can be dramatically displayed with contact B-mode ultrasound evaluation. A common finding is a posterior staphyloma in eyes with high myopia (Figure 14-21). A 5-mm increase in axial length due to the posterior pole accounts for approx-

imately 15 D of myopia (1 mm represents approximately 3 D).

Ultrasonography is a valuable tool in the evaluation of patients with unusual disc abnormalities and other contiguous lesions. An ultrasonic evaluation of such a patient revealed a remarkable dumbbell-shaped excavation inferior to and including the optic disc (Figure 14-22), which represented an atypical coloboma.

A short axial length is graphically displayed in the condition referred to as microphthalmia (Figure 14-23). Also of diagnostic significance is the identification of a patient with phthisis bulbi. Figure 14-24 is a simultaneous B-mode and A-mode ultrasonogram of an eye with an opaque cornea. Accurate Goldmann readings were impossible, but the intraocular pressure was estimated to be low by digital examination. Ultrasound evaluation demonstrates a very short axial length, suggesting shrink-

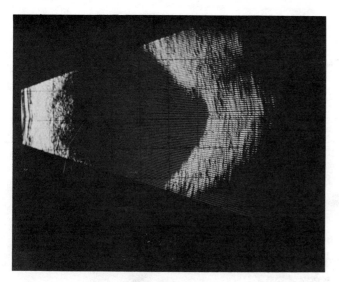

FIGURE 14-21
B-mode ultrasonogram of a posterior staphyloma in a 25 D myopic patient.

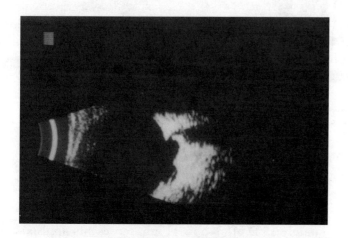

FIGURE 14-22
A patient with an unusual appearing disc and a larger contiguous lesion inferiorly underwent ultrasonography, which revealed a remarkable dumbbell-shaped excavation inferior to and including the optic disc. This represents an atypical coloboma.

age of the globe. Additional findings in phthisis bulbi include a disorganization of normal architecture and choroidal thickening. In this case the echoes from the vitreous might represent an old retinal detachment and secondary fibrous tissue proliferation. Surgical intervention would not be helpful in such an eye.

FIGURE 14-23
B-mode ultrasonogram of a patient with microphthalmia (top). A gross difference in axial length is noted when compared to the patient's contralateral eye (bottom).

Orbital Ultrasonography

Ultrasonic diagnosis of the orbit is difficult but may be very useful in the evaluation of orbital disease. Although the mechanical aspects of the examination are the same for the orbit as for the globe, the interpretation is more difficult. Ultrasound evaluation of the normal orbit reveals the sonolucent optic nerve, the sonolucent extraocular muscles, and the acoustically dense orbital fat (Figure 14-25). Depending on the equipment used, the orbital walls may or may not be discernible. Most abnormalities of the orbit are displayed as dark or black defects surrounded by the acoustically dense orbital fat. This is in direct con-

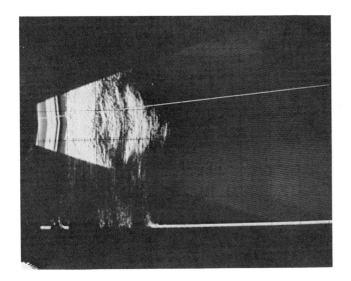

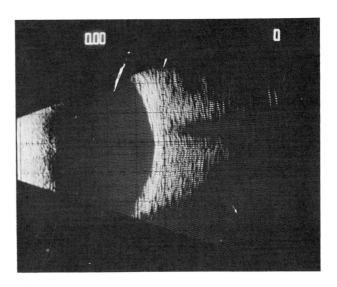

FIGURE 14-24

The history of this patient revealed normal visual acuity 15 years earlier in this eye, which now exhibits an opaque cornea. The simultaneous B-mode and A-mode ultrasonogram indicates shrinkage of the globe and dense echoes from the vitreous. Intraocular pressure was very low as demonstrated by digital evaluation. The diagnosis is phthisis bulbi, possibly secondary to long-standing retinal detachment.

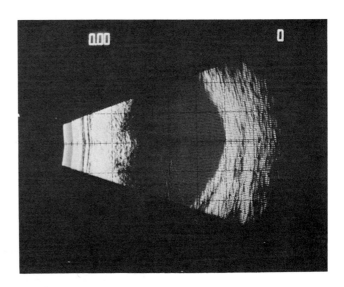

FIGURE 14-25

In the normal orbit, the sonolucent V-shaped optic nerve (top) and extraocular muscles (bottom), which appear dark (arrows), are surrounded by the acoustically dense orbital fat.

trast to abnormal findings in the globe, which appear white or gray against a black background.

Orbital tumors may be characterized ultrasonically in terms of their location, size, and configuration.[13] An expert ultrasonographer, using the best available instrument, can usually differentiate orbital mass lesions into the following major categories: rounded cystic tumors (mucocele, dermoid); rounded solid tumors (glioma, meningioma); irregular angiomatous tumors (diffuse hemangioma, lymphangioma); and irregular infiltrative tumors (lymphoma, metastatic carcinoma).[1]

An example of a rounded cystic tumor is depicted in Figure 14-26. The patient was a 7-year-old boy with a best-corrected visual acuity of 7/140 in the left eye and 20/40 in the right eye. The left eye was nearly 3 mm shorter than the right and also exhibited microcornea and an optic pit. An afferent pupillary defect was present in the left eye. Although the ultrasonic examination revealed a rounded cystic tumor with some evidence of compression of the globe, no proptosis, choroidal folds, or retinal striae were observed.

A computed tomographic (CT) scan (Figure 14-27) was obtained to complement the orbital ultrasonograms. In this case the ultrasonograms strongly suggested a rounded cystic mass, which is typically benign. The CT scan, which is limited in differentiating between cystic and solid masses, provided minimal information concerning the cause. The diagnosis was microphthalmos and an orbital cyst based on the ultrasound examination findings.

Another major application of orbital ultrasonography is in the evaluation of a patient with unilateral or bilateral exophthalmos who is suspected of having orbital Graves' disease. Standard laboratory test results are sometimes normal in such a patient. The ultrasonic findings that strongly support the diagnosis of orbital Graves' dis-

FIGURE 14-26
B-mode ultrasonogram of the retrobulbar orbital region. Note the large rounded sonolucent mass behind the left globe (shown below) as contrasted to the normal right orbit (shown above). Such a sonolucent mass is likely a cystic tumor such as a mucocele or a dermoid.

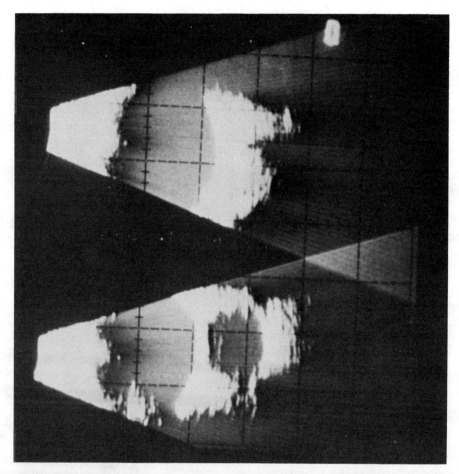

FIGURE 14-27
The orbital mass that is depicted in Figure 14-26 is sonolucent to sound but is opaque to x-rays, as shown in this CT scan.

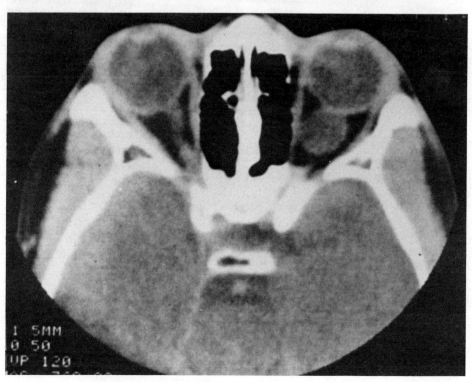

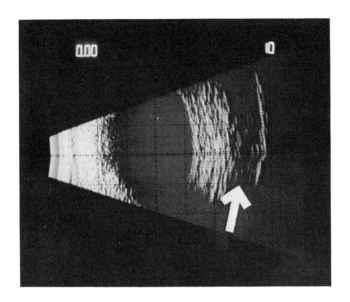

FIGURE 14-28

In a patient with orbital Graves' disease, the ultrasonogram reveals an accentuation of the orbital walls and enlargement of the extraocular muscles (arrow). This diagnosis usually requires an experienced ultrasonographer.

ease are the accentuation of the orbital walls and the enlargement of the extraocular muscles. The orbital wall is outlined more clearly than normal in these cases, presumably because tissue is compressed against it, creating a better reflecting surface.[1] Since the extraocular muscles are sonolucent, the enlargement of the muscles will appear as a generalized widening of the echo-free area between the retrobulbar fat pad and the orbital wall (Figure 14-28).[1]

REFERENCES

1. Coleman DJ, Lizzi FL, Jack RL. Ultrasonography of the Eye and Orbit. Philadelphia: Lea & Febiger, 1977.
2. Giglio E, Sherman J. Ophthalmic ultrasound as a diagnostic tool. J Am Optom Assoc 1979;50:73-8.
3. Giglio E. Diagnostic Ultrasound Application of A-scan to the Eye. In J Sherman (ed), Advanced Diagnostic Procedures. Ducan, OK: Optometric Extension Foundation, 1976:23-7.
4. Bronson NR, Fisher YL, Pickering NC, Trayner EM. Ophthalmic Contact B-scan Ultrasonography for the Clinician. Westport, CT: Intercontinental Publications, 1976:27.
5. Koplin RS, Gersten M, Hodes B. Real Time Ophthalmic Ultrasonography and Biometry: A Handbook of Clinical Diagnosis. Thorofare, NJ: Slack, 1985.
6. Knighton RW, Blankenship GW. Electrophysiological Evaluation of Eyes with Opaque Media. In S Sokol (ed). Electrophysiology and Psychophysics: Their Use in Ophthalmic Diagnosis. Int Ophthalmol Clin 1980;20:1-19.
7. Sterns GK, Coleman DJ, Ellsworth RM. The ultrasonographic characteristics of retinoblastoma. Am J Ophthalmol 1974:78:606-11.
8. Mackley TA, Teed RW. Unsuspected intraocular malignant melanomas. Arch Ophthalmol 1979;11:1849-51.
9. Baum MD, Pilkerton AR, Berler DK, Kramer KK. Choroidal osteoma. Ann Ophthalmol 1979;11:1849-51.
10. Naumann G, Yanoff M, Zimmerman LE. Histogenesis of malignant melanoma of the uvea. I. Histopathologic characteristics of nevi of the choroid and ciliary body. Arch Ophthalmol 1966;76:784-96.
11. Osher RH, Shields JA, Layman PR. Pupillary and visual field evaluation in patients with melanocytoma of the optic disc. Arch Ophthalmol 1979;97:1096-9.
12. Apple DJ, Craythorn JM, Reidy JJ, et al. Malignant transformation of an optic nerve melanocytoma. Can J Ophthalmol 1984;19:320-5.
13. Coleman DJ, Dallow RL. Orbital Ultrasonography. In IS Jones, FA Jackobiec (eds), Diseases of the Orbit. Hagerstown, MD: Harper & Row, 1979:91.

15

Evaluation and Postoperative Management of the Cataract Patient

JOHN E. CONTO

As the mean age of the population rises every year, the number of patients requiring cataract surgery also increases. With an estimated 1.4 million cataract extractions annually in the United States, cataract surgery is one of the most frequently performed procedures in patients over the age of 65 years.[1,2] Along with the changing demographics, the upsurge in the number of cataract operations can also be attributed to a refinement in microsurgical techniques and the development of intraocular lenses. Because of these advances, the majority of cataract extractions can be done as outpatient procedures, with a postoperative recovery period that is typically 6 weeks or less. Patients who may have previously delayed surgery because of the associated hospital stay or the disturbing adaptive effects of optical correction of aphakia are now able to restore their vision with minimal overall impact to their lifestyle.

The delivery of care to cataract patients has become increasingly multidisciplinary and includes anesthesiology, internal medicine, ophthalmology, and optometry. Ancillary personnel, such as nurses, opticians, and ophthalmic technicians, assist in various capacities during the course of care. Coordination between each of these specialists is critical to avoid any errors that may affect the overall visual outcome for the patient. Since optometrists often provide the ophthalmic care before and after the surgery, they must be familiar with the examination techniques and procedures used in the management of cataract patients.

PREOPERATIVE EVALUATION

Patients with symptoms consistent with cataracts should receive a complete eye examination that includes a care-ful review of the ocular and medical history, measurement of visual function, pupillary responses, keratometry, refraction, biomicroscopy, tonometry, and ophthalmoscopy. When the vision loss does not correlate with the appearance of the cataract, or the integrity of the posterior segment structures cannot be determined, supplemental testing, such as appreciation of entoptic phenomenon, ophthalmic ultrasonography, or electrodiagnostic tests may be necessary. A comprehensive preoperative evaluation should detect any predisposing conditions that may reduce the chance of a favorable visual result. About 5–10% of cataract patients will not demonstrate improvement in vision after surgery because of preexisting ocular conditions.[3]

The management options should be considered on analysis of the examination findings and presented to the patient for further discussion. Although cataract surgery is highly successful in restoring vision in the majority of cases, there is an inherent risk of complications that could have an impact on the patient's visual rehabilitation. Because cataract surgery is an elective procedure in most instances, the final decision of whether or not to have cataract surgery should be made by an informed patient. Some patients, depending on their lifestyle and health, may elect to be managed in a conservative fashion with spectacles or low vision devices.

Ocular History

Since the decrease in vision associated with cataract development often produces a certain degree of anxiety for the patient, the initial interview should be conducted in a sensitive and skillful manner that will provide insight into the cause of the vision loss. A comprehensive history cannot be obtained by untrained ancillary personnel or a cursory checklist. In addition to investigating the nature of the decrease in vision, the examiner should also question the patient about previous diagnoses of diabetic retinopathy, glaucoma, retinal detachment, trauma, or uveitis, conditions that are associated with the development of cataracts. Any previous ophthalmic surgical procedures should also be noted. If obtainable, records from prior examinations may be helpful in documenting past ocular conditions. Specific questions include the following[4]:

1. *Is the vision loss gradual or sudden?* A patient with a developing cataract will usually have a chief complaint of gradual progressive loss of vision. In isolation, cataracts never cause sudden vision loss, although a patient may occasionally have a sudden awareness of decreased vision, particularly when unilateral cataract formation occurs in the nondominant eye. Sudden vision loss usually implies a vascular cause, and the ocular examination should investigate causes other than a cataract.

2. *When did you first notice the vision loss?* Inquiring about the onset of the vision decrease can help determine the type of cataract. Posterior subcapsular cataracts usually progress more rapidly than nuclear or cortical opacities and disturb vision earlier because of their location on the visual axis. They tend to develop in younger patients. It is also important to ascertain the time period between the onset of the vision decrease and the seeking of care, which can give a sense for the degree of intolerance to the loss of vision and the likelihood that the patient may desire surgical intervention. Whereas cataracts usually are bilateral, they tend to be asymmetric. If the decision is made to operate, the cataract in the eye with a greater loss of vision is usually extracted first.

3. *When is your vision most affected?* The patient may report that the vision loss is more noticeable in certain lighting conditions or while performing particular tasks. Decreased vision while reading or problems with glare in bright sunlight are characteristic of posterior subcapsular cataracts. Nuclear opacities can also cause a vision decrease in bright light environments. Difficulty driving at night, because of glare produced by approaching headlights, may be seen with either nuclear or posterior subcapsular cataracts. If it occurs to a significant degree, the myopic shift caused by progressive nuclear sclerosis may cause a "second sight," allowing the patient to read without his or her habitual near correction. The effects of cortical opacities are usually most pronounced in dim illumination, when pupillary dilation permits peripheral spoking to produce a glare effect.

4. *Do you ever see double?* When a patient with cataracts has a complaint of diplopia, the clinician must determine if the diplopia is monocular or binocular and if it is related to the developing cataract. Monocular diplopia can be caused when the refractive index differs between the various layers of a cataractous lens. This effect may be described by the patient as a "ghost image" occurring alongside objects that are viewed. Distinct image doubling may also occur. A pinhole aperture may reduce or eliminate the diplopia, particularly if it is related to an uncorrected myopic refractive shift from increasing nuclear sclerosis. Other lenticular causes of monocular diplopia include fluid clefts, cortical spokes, and water vacuoles. When refractive shift is markedly asymmetric between the eyes, the induced anisometropia may cause binocular diplopia, especially when the patient attempts to read. Unequal near adds or slab-off prism may be become necessary in these cases.

5. *Have you noticed any pain, discomfort, or redness?* Cataracts do not cause symptoms of pain or injection unless a secondary lens-induced uveitis, glaucoma, or both are present. Any cataract patient with these symptoms should be examined for concurrent ocular surface disease, intraocular inflammation, or angle closure. Occasionally, a patient may complain of photophobia or discomfort from glare induced by a cataract.

6. *Do you notice any part of your vision missing?* Patients with cataracts often are found to have a generalized depression of the visual field. A focal defect is unlikely to be related to a cataract, and retinal or optic nerve disease should suspected. Lesions of the visual pathway will also produce characteristic focal loss of the visual field. Macular disorders may cause distortion or metamorphopsia of the central visual field.

7. *Have you ever been told that you had an eyeturn or lazy eye?* Patients should be questioned regarding possible strabismus or amblyopia. Whereas cataract surgery in these patients may not be contraindicated, the patient must be aware of the postoperative visual expectations.

8. *What impact has the vision loss had on your activities?* The ocular history should be concluded with an open-ended question regarding the effect that a cataract has had on the patient's daily activities. Review of these considerations together with the results of the ocular examination will help the examiner properly counsel the patient and allow him or her to make an informed decision regarding surgical intervention.

Medical History

Since many systemic diseases or medications (Table 15-1) can cause cataract formation, the patient's general medical history must be reviewed. The clinician should also inquire about any existing conditions that may be aggravated by the surgery or increase the risk of complications.

TABLE 15-1
Medications and Conditions Associated with Cataract Formation

Cataract Type	Medications	Conditions
Anterior subcapsular	Naphthalene Phenothiazines Topical miotics	Atopic dermatitis Chronic iritis Diabetes mellitus Electrical shock Myotonic dystrophy Trauma Wilson's disease
Nuclear	Paradichlorobenzene	Congenital rubella Diabetes mellitus Trauma
Cortical	—	Galactosemia Hypoparathyroidism Hypothyroidism
Posterior subcapsular	Corticosteroids Alcohol abuse	Diabetes mellitus Intraocular tumor Ionizing radiation Myotonic dystrophy Neurofibromatosis Posterior uveitis Retinal detachment
Nonspecific	Allopurinol Psoralens compounds Retinoids	—

Diabetics may exhibit poor wound healing. Marked hypertension may increase the chance of hemorrhage. Patients with chronic obstructive pulmonary disease (COPD) should be questioned about whether they can lie supine for an hour or more to have surgery because some with advanced disease states must keep their head and torso elevated. Constant use of oxygen may also be required. Situations such as this obviously are a significant consideration when evaluating surgical risks. Patients with pulmonary disease may have difficulty with possible postoperative medications, such as beta blockers. Similarly, carbonic anhydrase inhibitors are contraindicated in patients with a history of renal calculi. Cataract surgery usually causes some degree of stress, and patients with chronic depression or anxiety disorders may deteriorate after the procedure. Supportive nursing care may be required during the postoperative period for patients with physical or mental limitations. Current or recent medications should be listed (especially aspirin, warfarin, or the nonsteroidal anti-inflammatory drugs), and any previous drug reactions or allergies should be documented.

All patients anticipating cataract surgery are required to undergo a preoperative physical examination, which is usually done by an internist. The preoperative examination should be performed within a month before the surgery. The general medical condition of the patient is determined, with emphasis on the state of the cardiopulmonary system. Routine screening blood tests, electrocardiography, thoracic radiologic studies, and urinalysis are also conducted.[5]

Measurement of Visual Function

Quantifying the degree of vision loss and predicting postoperative acuity are two important considerations when evaluating the visual function of a patient with a cataract. Unfortunately, many of the clinical testing methods are designed to measure only one aspect of visual function. A basic understanding of these testing methods and instruments is necessary to avoid improper test selection in the evaluation of the patient's visual complaints.

Snellen Visual Acuity Chart

The Snellen acuity chart is the traditional entry method of measuring the level of vision. However, because the optotypes on the chart are high-contrast targets, the Snellen chart does not accurately measure the patient's ability to discern objects that are of low or medium contrast. This can result in an overestimation of the patient's functional ability. The Snellen visual acuity should be recorded for each eye at distance in both dim and bright lighting conditions. Using sufficient overhead illumination, a reduced Snellen chart should be used to measure near vision. Nuclear sclerosis tends to more adversely affect distance vision compared with near vision, whereas posterior subcapsular cataracts may have a greater impact on near vision. Nuclear cataracts and posterior subcapsular opacities can cause a relative reduction in vision under bright illumination because of their location on the visual axis in combination with pupillary constriction.

Pinhole Aperture Acuity

If Snellen visual acuity is reduced, a pinhole aperture may be helpful in distinguishing between vision loss from uncorrected refractive error and an ocular pathologic condition. The pinhole aperture helps eliminate the light-scattering effect that occurs with cataracts and increases the depth of focus. The optimal aperture device has multiple pinholes that are not smaller than 1 mm in diameter.[3] Smaller pinholes tend to decrease the illumination and cause aberrations from a diffraction effect. If vision improves with pinhole testing, uncorrected refractive error or a media opacity that causes scattering may be present. If vision loss is secondary to some other ocular condition, the pinhole aperture will generally not improve acuity. The aperture is placed over the habitual spectacle prescription, and the pinhole acuity is measured monocularly by viewing the distance Snellen acuity chart. The opposite eye should be occluded during testing. The patient may have to adjust the aperture device to properly align the pinholes with the visual axis. Although the pinhole aperture is generally simple to use, many patients will have a poor subjective response. Dense cataracts can cause a false-negative response.

Contralight Acuity Test

The contralight acuity test attempts to simulate the effect that daylight conditions have on vision by placing a distance Snellen acuity chart on a window that is exposed to outside light.[4,6,7] The test should be conducted before pupillary dilation. Although the contralight test provides only qualitative information, it is an attractive method because it is relatively inexpensive and simple to perform. A similar effect can also be achieved in the examination room by directing a moderate light source, such as a transilluminator or penlight, into the eye from below the visual axis. This causes pupillary constriction and can provide an estimation of the effect that a centrally located opacity will have on vision in bright lighting situations.

Interferometry

Laser or white light interferometry is a useful clinical method for measuring the potential postoperative visual acuity. Interferometers project coherent light directly onto the retina, producing a grating, or fringe, pattern on the retina.[6,8] Since interferometry does not depend on the optics of the eye, the pattern is relatively unaffected by refractive error or media opacities. The grating pattern is adjusted to finer separations (higher frequencies) until the patient reports a negative response, which can then be converted to Snellen equivalent visual acuity. The orientation of the grating pattern can also be varied to prevent false-positive results. There are several interferometers that are used clinically, including the Acuiometer and IRAS white light interferometer (both manufactured by Randwal Instruments, Southbridge, MA), Lotmar Visometer (Haag-Streit Service, Waldwick, NJ), and the Retinometer (Coburn Optical Industries, Muskogee, OK).[6,9–11] The Acuiometer is tabled-mounted, whereas the Retinometer and the Visometer are designed to be attached to a slit lamp biomicroscope. The IRAS white light interferometer is a hand-held instrument (see Figure 1-12). While the IRAS interferometer and the Visometer use a white incandescent light, the others use a red helium laser as the light source.

Interferometry has been reported to be 50–90% accurate in predicting an improvement in postoperative vision in cataract patients, which is comparable with other methods for determining potential acuity.[6,12–16] The predictive value of interferometers appears to be directly related to the density of the cataract, with more reliable results achieved with mild to moderate opacities. Overestimation of the postoperative acuity by interferometers can occur when certain preexisting conditions are present, including amblyopia, cystoid macular edema, geographic atrophy of the retinal pigment epithelium of the macula, macular hole or cyst, serous detachment of the sensory retina in the macula, recently reattached retinal detachment, and visual field defects involving fixation.[6,13]

Potential Acuity Meter

The Guyton-Minkowski Potential Acuity Meter (PAM) (Mentor Ophthalmics, Norwell, MA) is another instrument used to predict potential visual acuity after cataract surgery.[6,11] The instrument attaches to a slit lamp biomicroscope. It measures the potential acuity by projecting a reduced image of a Snellen acuity chart through the lens onto the retina. The image is projected through relative clear zones if the lens is passable. Unlike interferometry, the PAM does not rely on an interference grating, and therefore defocusing of the projected image occurs due to uncorrected refractive error. To account for this, the instrument contains a bank of spherical lenses that can be adjusted to a desired refractive correction that will focus the light beam appropriately. The patient's pupils are usually dilated for testing. The smallest Snellen line that the patient can discern is recorded as the potential visual acuity. The PAM chart best penetrates mild to moderate lenticular opacities. It will often underestimate postoperative visual acuity when a cataract is particularly dense.

The PAM is accurate to within two lines of postoperative acuity in 75–90% of cases and to within three lines in 85% of cases.[6,17] In a study of patients where the PAM-predicted acuity was inaccurate by three lines or greater, about 20% had better postoperative vision and 5% had a visual acuity that was worse than expected.[17] Although the PAM appears to be less able to penetrate denser opacities compared with interferometers, the Snellen acuity chart is a more familiar target to patients than a grating pattern. False-positive results can occur in the same conditions as with interferometry but apparently do not occur as frequently.[6,13] However, false-negative results are more common with the PAM and are often related to decreased brightness or poor alignment of the beam.[6]

Blue Field Entoptoscopy

Blue field entoptoscopy (BFE) subjectively measures the visual function in patients with media opacities. This qualitative method uses a blue luminous field to help the patient visualize the entoptic effect of Scheerer's flying corpuscles.[6,18] A patient with an intact macular retinal circulation should be able to appreciate movement of his or her own white blood cells as they course through the capillary circulation in an arcuate-like fashion. When there is good visual acuity, 20–40 white blood cells may be appreciated at the same time. The MIRA (Medical Instrument Research Associates, Waltham, MA) blue field entoptoscope was found to be 94% accurate in predicting a 20/40 or better visual acuity.[6,19] It also demonstrated a 75% accuracy rate in identifying poor macular function of 20/50 visual acuity or worse. However, other studies have shown that patients with dense nuclear cataracts may not be able to sufficiently appreciate the blue background, causing false-negative responses; false-positive responses have also been shown to occur when macular disease is present.[6,20] Blue field entoptoscopy tends to be difficult for some patients to understand, which reduces the overall reliability of this technique.

Contrast Sensitivity Tests

Many patients will complain of difficulty performing certain tasks but demonstrate relatively normal Snellen visual acuities. Although Snellen charts are designed to measure the ability of the eye to resolve a critically sized, high-contrast object, they tend to be very poor indicators of the effect that luminance has on functional vision. Contrast sensitivity testing expands the basis of Snellen visual acuity and determines the minimum contrast level at which an observer can discern targets of different sizes.[21] Cataracts, especially nuclear sclerosis, may significantly reduce vision in low- to medium-contrast situations, and contrast sensitivity testing may more accurately measure the patient's ability to function in certain lighting environments.

There are several commercially available charts that measure contrast sensitivity.[22,23] The Vistech Vision Contrast Test System (Vistech Consultants, Dayton, OH) uses sine wave grating targets of alternating light and dark linear stripes. The patterns are oriented in a vertical, horizontal, or oblique direction. The chart has five rows of targets, and each row exhibits a different separation (spatial frequency) of the grating stripes. Each successive target within a row has a lower contrast than the preceding target. There are nine targets on a row. For each row of targets the patient reports the orientation of the grating patterns until a negative response occurs (see Figure 1-10). A contrast sensitivity function curve can then be determined for different contrast levels. The Pelli-Robson Letter Sensitivity Chart (Clement Clarke International Ltd., London) consists of lines of letters that are arranged in decreasing contrast.[24,25]

Glare Sensitivity Testing

Most patients with cataracts suffer from the disabling effects of glare, which can affect visual acuity, contrast sensitiv-

ity, and the overall visual field. Glare is defined as the degradation of the retinal image by irregularly scattered light.[21] Cataracts produce veiling glare by scattering light from a bright source, such as a headlight or the sun.

Glare is produced in varying degrees by the different types of lens opacities. Posterior subcapsular cataracts are the most noteworthy in producing glare, particularly in bright sunlight when pupillary constriction occurs. Nuclear sclerosis seems to cause more symptoms with night vision when the opacification causes both light scattering and light filtration. Peripheral lenticular changes, such as cortical cataracts, cause glare problems in dim illumination when the pupil dilates.

Glare testing devices are available either as self-contained table-top units, combined together with autorefractors, or as hand-held devices.[2,21] These tests generally rely on subjective responses and suffer from lack of standardization.[26] All methods are done before pupillary dilation and use a bright light source to simulate the effect of glare on the vision.

A commonly used glare tester is the Brightness Acuity Tester (BAT) (Mentor Ophthalmics, Norwell, MA).[2,27] The BAT is a hand-held instrument that contains a bright light source within a small white hemispheric bowl (see Figure 1-11). The patient looks through the bowl at a distant Snellen acuity chart while the illumination of the BAT light source is increased. The illumination settings of low, medium, and high correspond to indoor, partly sunny, and bright sunny lighting conditions, respectively. The medium setting is considered to reflect the effect of outside glare most accurately.[26] The BAT has demonstrated an 84% correlation with outdoor Snellen visual acuities.[27]

Mature Cataract Evaluation

Visual Discrimination Tests

Because tests of visual discrimination tend to measure extrafoveal retinal function rather than foveal ability, they are generally considered to be of secondary importance in predicting vision after cataract surgery.[2–4,6,28,29] However, they can provide useful qualitative information about gross retinal or optic nerve function when a dense cataract prevents adequate visualization of the posterior segment.

Although the accuracy of other potential acuity methods are significantly affected by dense cataracts, the ability to detect a bright light source should not be impaired. A negative response to a transilluminator held in front of the patient indicates a poor prognosis for good vision after surgery. Although opaque media can cause significant diffusion of the light source, the loss of light projection in one quadrant only may indicate a condition such as a retinal detachment or glaucoma.

Two-light discrimination by a patient implies more sensitive retinal function than light projection and should be performed with two transilluminators of equal intensity held adjacent to each other. Again, cloudy media may cause the two lights to appear fused, producing a false-negative result.

A transilluminator with a red or green filter held in front of the light source may be used to test color perception, which, if intact, usually indicates gross macular or optic nerve function. The visual prognosis is poor if a patient cannot perceive a colored target. However, because some cone receptors are present in the retinal periphery as well as the macular region, this test is not considered to be the most reliable measure of foveal function. In addition, conditions such as dry age-related macular degeneration seldom affect color perception. The other eye must also be tested to rule out congenital color deficiency to avoid false-negative responses.

Perception of the Purkinje entoptic phenomenon suggests that gross retinal anatomy and function are relatively intact. A transilluminator is gently pressed against a closed upper eyelid while the patient directs his or her gaze upward. When the light is moved in a horizontal sweeping motion across the eyelid, a branching pattern corresponding to the retinal vascular tree should be appreciated by the patient. This phenomenon is not specific for foveal function, and the absence of the pattern is considered to be significant only if the other eye can detect the pattern. The diagnostic reliability of this test decreases if localized macular disease is present.

A Maddox rod can be used to test for gross retinal function. The patient fixates on a transilluminator held at 16 inches while a red Maddox rod is placed in front of the eye to be tested. A red line should be seen in either the horizontal or vertical meridian depending on the orientation of the rod. A break or distortion in the center may indicate a macular problem. The rod should also be rotated to test the oblique meridians. A partial loss in any direction may indicate a retinal detachment or other conditions that may produce a field defect.

Electrophysiologic Tests

Electrophysiologic tests such as the electroretinogram (ERG) or the visual evoked potential (VEP) indirectly measure visual function.[3,6,29,30] Because of the expense and complexity of the instrumentation, these tests are not frequently used in the presurgical evaluation of cataracts. Since the VEP reflects macular and visual pathway function and the ERG measures the total activity of the retinal photoreceptors, these tests should be used in combination to obtain the best predictability. Both the ERG and VEP examinations should yield normal results to indicate a good visu-

al prognosis following surgery. These tests do not, however, correlate well with final visual acuity in the presence of localized macular disease such as amblyopia or macular degeneration.

Ultrasonography

B-scan ultrasonography is a very useful technique for evaluating the eye when a dense media opacity prevents an adequate view of the posterior pole. The high-frequency sound waves can easily penetrate opaque tissue, providing a two-dimensional or cross-sectional view of the structures in the posterior globe. Ultrasonography can detect many conditions that may indicate poor visual prognosis after cataract surgery, including retinal detachment, vitreous hemorrhage, intraocular tumors, or end-stage glaucoma (see Chapter 14).

Entrance Tests

Pupillary Responses

In the absence of gross retinal or optic nerve disease, the afferent pupillary response in a cataract patient should be normal. This is especially useful information when a dense cataract prevents an adequate view of the posterior segment. The presence of an afferent pupillary defect in an eye is highly suggestive of asymmetric optic nerve or severe retinal disease, and the prognosis for postsurgical improvement in vision should be considered to be guarded. Although there have been anecdotal case reports of mild afferent defects resolving after cataract extraction, it is generally believed that even dense cataracts alone will not produce an afferent conduction defect. Most cataracts are thought to decrease the transmission of light to the retinal elements, but because this process is gradual, the retinal ganglion cells adapt and respond in a normal manner.[31]

It is also important to evaluate the ability of the pupil to dilate before a surgery is planned. Certain procedures, such as phacoemulsification, require a large pupil to remove the cataract or to properly position the intraocular lens implant. Prior knowledge of a poorly reactive pupil will allow the surgeon to alter surgical technique or to include a pupil-enlarging step in the operation.

Cover Test and Extraocular Motilities

A cover test and extraocular motilities should be performed to detect any existing tropias or restrictions in gaze. Although patients with a congenital squint will usually continue to suppress after surgery, a patient with an acquired strabismus may report diplopia upon restoration of vision. Prisms or secondary muscle procedures may provide relief, but the results are often disappointing, especially in long-standing cases. In these instances, patient education before surgery is extremely important. With congenital tropias, the possibility of preexisting reduction in vision secondary to amblyopia should be considered.

Visual Field Testing

Cataracts tend to cause a uniform depression in the sensitivity of the visual field rather than focal defects, such as nasal steps, quadrantanopsias, or hemianopsias.[32] The visual field of each eye should be tested monocularly by the confrontation method whether or not cataracts are present. If no gross defects are found in any quadrant of either eye, then formal threshold testing is usually not necessary but certainly may give more evidence that no abnormality exists.

Keratometry and Refraction

Keratometry

Keratometry readings may be necessary to perform an accurate refraction, especially when an opacity significantly degrades the retinoscopy reflex. The degree of corneal toricity is also crucial for the calculation of intraocular lens implant power. At least three consistent readings should be obtained and then averaged. For implant power, the average corneal curvature is calculated by combining the measured vertical and horizontal corneal power and dividing by a factor of two. Keratometry measurements should be taken before A-mode ultrasonography is performed, since biometry may cause corneal distortion.

Refraction

Retinoscopy provides information on the degree of ametropia and the quality of the ocular media. With many older patients who have miotic pupils, it may be difficult to observe the retinoscopy reflex, especially when a central or dense opacity is present. In these cases, retinoscopy should be attempted after pupillary dilation, which may greatly improve the perceived reflex. With mature cataracts, the reflex may be absent, and radical retinoscopy (performed at a close distance) may be necessary. A subjective refraction may prove to be difficult, since many patients are unable to respond to small lens increments; bracketing in larger dioptric should be attempted in these cases. Although many patients show an improvement in visual acuity after a careful refraction, some patients may not be able to adapt to large changes in the spectacle prescription. Trial framing is advisable in these cases in an attempt to detect any possible adaption difficulties.

Ocular Health Assessment

Biomicroscopy

Inspection of the ocular adnexa and anterior segment is an integral part of the presurgical cataract evaluation, and any disorder that may have an impact on the overall surgical success should be treated preoperatively. The lids and lashes should be examined for any sign of blepharitis or other infections and the appropriate antimicrobial therapy initiated. The eyelids should be in good apposition to the globe without ectropion or entropion. Loss of lid apposition can lead to ocular surface problems, such as trichiasis, exposure keratitis, or corneal ulceration. The tear film should be adequate to prevent desiccation of the corneal epithelium. Patients with decreased tear function are more prone to develop ocular infections, and topical lubricants may be necessary preoperatively. Any conjunctival infections must be resolved before surgery. It is very important to carefully examine the cornea and to assess its integrity since preexisting conditions such as endothelial guttata, keratoconus, or central scarring can have a direct impact on the postoperative visual result.

The anterior chamber and iris should be evaluated for any sign of current or previous intraocular infection or inflammation. Corneal endothelial keratic precipitates or pigment deposition may also be an indication of present or past intraocular inflammation. The anterior chamber angle should be open without signs of angle closure. The presence of pigment deposition in the angle may contribute to elevated postoperative intraocular pressure, and neovascularization, loss of sphincter muscle tone, dilator muscle damage, atrophy, or posterior synechiae of the iris require further investigation for associated causes. Anterior chamber structures, especially the anterior lens capsule, should be examined for exfoliative material since the pseudoexfoliation syndrome may cause weakening of the lens zonules. Weakened lens zonules may cause technical difficulty during extracapsular surgical procedures. The condition of the anterior vitreous should also be determined with the biomicroscope.

Intraocular Pressure

It is mandatory to measure intraocular pressure preoperatively to screen for undiagnosed high-tension glaucoma. Goldmann applanation tonometry is generally preferred over other methods unless there is a contraindication for its use. An intumescent lens may cause relative pupillary block and narrowing or even closure of the anterior chamber angle. In cases of chronic or acute angle closure glaucoma, measures including a laser peripheral iridotomy may need to be performed before cataract surgery can be performed. Although less common, leaking proteins from a hypermature lens may initiate an inflammatory response with a secondary rise in intraocular pressure (phacolytic glaucoma). Removal of the lens is usually necessary to fully resolve the inflammatory reaction and to return the intraocular pressure to normal. Glaucomas that may be aggravated by cataract surgery include pseudoexfoliative glaucoma and pigmentary glaucoma.

Ophthalmoscopy

A dilated fundus examination is mandatory for all patients with cataracts, and the clinician must be adept with the techniques that are used to visualize the posterior segment, including direct ophthalmoscopy, indirect slit lamp biomicroscopy, and binocular indirect ophthalmoscopy. Each method has limitations and advantages. Although the view of the posterior segment with a direct ophthalmoscope is often impaired by lenticular opacities, useful information is obtained regarding the position of the cataract and the effect on vision. Binocular indirect ophthalmoscopy can penetrate most opacities and may provide an excellent view of the retinal periphery. However, it lacks the magnification necessary to detect subtle macular or optic nerve changes. Indirect slit lamp biomicroscopy can provide a highly magnified view of the posterior pole, but inspection of the retinal periphery may be limited.

While performing the dilated fundus examination, the examiner should determine whether or not the ophthalmoscopic view through a cataract correlates with the decrease in the patient's vision. If other concurrent posterior segment conditions are discovered, their effect on vision should be estimated. The peripheral retina and vitreous, especially in secondary intraocular lens implant candidates, must be evaluated for any predisposing conditions that would increase the risk of postoperative retinal detachment. If cystoid macular edema is suspected in a secondary implant candidate, fluorescein angiography should be performed. Consultation with a retinal specialist may be indicated before surgery when certain forms of retinal disease are present.

Dilated Cataract Evaluation

The crystalline lens can be more thoroughly examined when the pupil is fully dilated. As mentioned above, retinoscopy should be repeated if the reflex was difficult to observe because of a miotic pupil or central lens opacity. The reflex may appear to be irregular or diminished, and central lenticular changes, such as a posterior subcapsular opacification or an outlining of the nucleus (nuclear button) due to index of refraction alterations can be seen. The direct ophthalmoscope, set at about +10 D,

can be used to evaluate the red fundus reflex for extent, size, and position of cortical spikes, vacuoles, or posterior capsular changes. The lens should also be evaluated with the slit lamp biomicroscope. The depth and position of cortical spokes may be delineated with an optic section, whereas retroillumination of the lens often demonstrates subtle water vacuoles or granular posterior subcapsular changes. Direct illumination can be used to inspect the anterior lens capsule for signs of exfoliation. Nuclear sclerosis is best observed by optic section and may appear as a prominence of the nuclear zone with loss of clarity. The nucleus may appear light yellow in mild nuclear sclerosis and brownish-orange in moderate cases. Advanced nuclear sclerosis will be brown or brunescent in appearance. Posterior subcapsular cataracts may appear in direct illumination as an irregular film with ridges and crevices. They may exhibit a crater-like appearance.

There have been many attempts to grade cataractous changes for both clinical and research applications.[33-36] Most classification schemes endeavor to categorize the lens appearance either by inspection with the biomicroscope or by lens photography. Unfortunately, no classification system has been developed that can reliably correlate vision loss with the degree of opacification. Most practitioners will rate lens changes on an ascending numerical scale of 0 to 4+ that is based on individual clinical experience. A clear lens is rated as 0, and a grade of 4+ indicates a very dense cataract. This method of grading lens opacities lacks interobserver reliability and does not consider the visual function of the patient. Other clinicians grade lenticular changes according to the degree of vision loss. This system may be consistent with lenticular opacities that have a direct impact on vision as they form, such as nuclear or posterior subcapsular cataracts, but it demonstrates poor correlation with cortical cataracts, which are usually moderately advanced before vision is affected.

Some patients may complain of vision loss that is inconsistent with the appearance of the lens. If no posterior segment disorders are detected, these patients may be suffering from decreased contrast sensitivity. One method of objectively assessing this is the lenticular blue light test, which is based on the absorption of blue light emitted from a slit lamp beam by developing nuclear sclerosis.[4] The blue slit lamp beam will transmit through the entire thickness of a normal lens, whereas it may not extend all the way through a lens with significant nuclear sclerosis. To perform this test, the pupil should be dilated and the slit lamp illumination set at maximum. An optic section of white light from a 45-degree angle is focused on the lens and the degree (depth within the lens) of penetration by the white light is estimated, which is usually 100% even

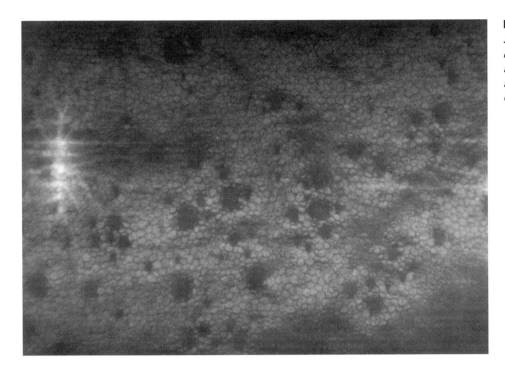

FIGURE 15-1
Specular photomicrograph of a cornea exhibiting endothelial guttata associated with Fuchs' dystrophy. (Courtesy of David Lee, O.D., Ph.D.)

with dense opacities. The blue filter is then rotated into place on the slit lamp, and the degree of blue light transmission is noted. If the blue light penetrates three-fourths of the distance into the lens compared to white light, the blue light test result would be recorded as 75%.

Endothelial Cell Count

Depending on the surgical technique and the skill level of the surgeon, about 5–10% of the endothelial cell layer may be permanently destroyed during cataract surgery.[37] A preoperative assessment of the corneal endothelium may be indicated to determine the risk of development of persistent postoperative corneal edema. Corneal endothelial cell analysis can determine regional endothelial cell density and morphology and should be performed when a patient has a history of previous intraocular surgery, chronic uveitis, or if signs of poor endothelial integrity such as corneal edema, guttata, or advanced endothelial dystrophy are present.

The simplest technique for analyzing the endothelium uses a biomicroscope with a modified ocular of 25× that contains a 1-mm^2 estimation grid. The biomicroscope is adjusted for specular reflection, and endothelial cell counts of the superior, central, and inferior cornea are estimated. The size and shape of the corneal endothelial cells are also noted. Counting the endothelial cells by this method is imprecise, and endothelial cell contact photography (Figure 15-1) may be indicated when a more thorough assessment of the cell layer is appropriate. The average endothelial cell density between the ages of 40 and 90 years is 2,400–3,000 cells/mm^2.[37] Patients with densities under 2,000 cells/mm^2 are considered to be at moderate risk for persistent postoperative corneal edema, whereas those with a density of 1,000 cells/mm^2 or less represent the highest risk.[37]

MANAGEMENT OPTIONS

If examination results indicate that a patient's visual complaints are related to cataract formation, the management options should be reviewed with the patient. Because cataract surgery is a procedure with an inherent risk of complications, the final decision rests with the patient. In most instances, cataract surgery remains an elective procedure, although the personal views of the practitioner are undoubtedly a major deciding factor in many cases. Surgical counseling should ideally include written and verbal information about the surgical process, which can be reviewed by the patient and his or her family.[38] The prime consideration for surgical intervention should be that the cataract has a significant negative impact on the ability of the patient to perform essential daily activities or avocations. Other indications for cataract removal possibly include lens-induced disease, such as phacogenic angle closure glaucoma or lens-induced uveitis, and when opacification prevents adequate examination and/or therapy to treat significant posterior segment disorders.

If surgery is declined, an attempt can be made to improve the patient's vision by modifying either the patient's current spectacles or living environment. Addressing task-specific needs is usually more successful than attempting to improve overall visual function. Improved lighting, large-letter print, and high add powers may help with reading or near activities, whereas glare disability may be controlled with sunglasses or short-wavelength filters. Patients with cataracts may note a subjective improvement in vision with Corning CPF filters (Corning Inc., Marion, VA), particularly the 511-nm and 527-nm filters.[39] Although these filters do not seem to improve Snellen visual acuity, they can reduce light scattering and increase contrast sensitivity.

Optical Correction of Aphakia

If a patient elects to have cataract surgery, there are several refractive options for managing aphakia. Deciding factors include the age of the patient and coexistent ocular disorders. Although the surgical technique to remove the cataract may make certain options more advantageous than others, aphakic spectacles, contact lenses, or intraocular implants may be used in conjunction with any of the surgical procedures to correct the patient's postoperative vision.

Aphakic spectacles are considered to be the least desirable option for correcting aphakia because of the innate optical problems of high-plus lenses, which include spatial distortion of images, spherical and chromatic aberrations, and a reduced peripheral visual field. High-plus lenses can cause objects to be magnified up to 33%, which causes adaptation difficulty for many patients, particularly those with monocular aphakia.[40-43] The peripheral vision appears to be blurred because 8–12% of the visual field remains peripheral to the edges of the lenses and is refractively uncorrected.[40-43] Additionally, high-plus lenses create a considerable base-in prismatic effect, causing the peripheral light rays to not enter the pupil. Aphakic lenses produce a ring scotoma 50–60 degrees from fixation that constantly moves as the eye rotates.[40-43] This causes objects to suddenly appear and disappear from the field of view and is referred to as the "jack-in-the-box effect."

Many of the optical concerns with aphakic high-plus lenses can be reduced by careful spectacle lens selection.[42-44] Patients are often concerned about the cosmetic appearance of aphakic spectacle lenses, and high index material may be helpful to decrease the thickness and weight. The choice of a lens is also dependent on the patient's needs. A lenticular lens design will give the best acuity but can reduce the field of view. A patient with limited mobility might benefit from this type of lens. Full-field lenses with greater asphericity give a wider field of view but create more distortion and blurring of vision. These lens designs might better serve a patient who has moderate near requirements but is highly mobile. The add power of aphakic lenses might be less than expected because of the high magnification induced by these types of lenses.

The type of spectacle frame can help to minimize the optical effects of aphakic high-plus lenses. In general, the frame should be light, sturdy, and easily adjustable.[42-44] The eye size should be small, and the distance between the lens similar to the patient's pupillary distance. This minimizes the need to decenter the lenses, reducing the induced prismatic effects. Lighter and thinner lenses will also result. The vertex distance should be kept to a minimum, which will help to reduce induced magnification, and the pantoscopic angle should not be excessive to help minimize unwanted cylinder. Education is highly important, and patients should be instructed on how to use new aphakic spectacles. They should be told to slowly turn their head instead of their eyes to view objects. Wearing the spectacles part-time may be necessary during the adaptive period, with a gradual increase to full-time wear. In an aphakic prescription, the bifocal segment should be set higher, close to the typical level of a trifocal. This will reduce the prismatic effect from the carrier-to-bifocal junction. If the patient has significant difficulty adjusting to a bifocal lens, separate spectacles for distance and near may be indicated.

A variety of contact lenses, including extended-wear hydrophilic, daily wear hydrophilic, and daily wear rigid, have been used to correct aphakia. Contact lenses magnify objects by about 7%, which is certainly more tolerable than spectacles to patients, especially those with monocular aphakia.[40,43-45] To minimize the image size difference in monocular aphakic patients, the power of the contact lens can be adjusted to make the aphakic eye slightly less hyperopic, or more myopic, than the phakic eye. Aphakic contact lenses do not limit the peripheral field, create spatial distortion, or produce the ring scotoma, which are drawbacks associated with aphakic spectacles.

Aphakic contact lenses present certain problems that have limited their acceptance. Many aphakic patients have difficulty inserting and removing a daily wear lens either because of decreased dexterity or the uncorrected high hyperopia. If the patient is not able to remove the lens, a family member or a friend can be trained to assist. Prescribing a hydrophilic lens on an extended-wear basis may partially address the handling concern. However, even extended-wear soft lenses must be removed for cleaning

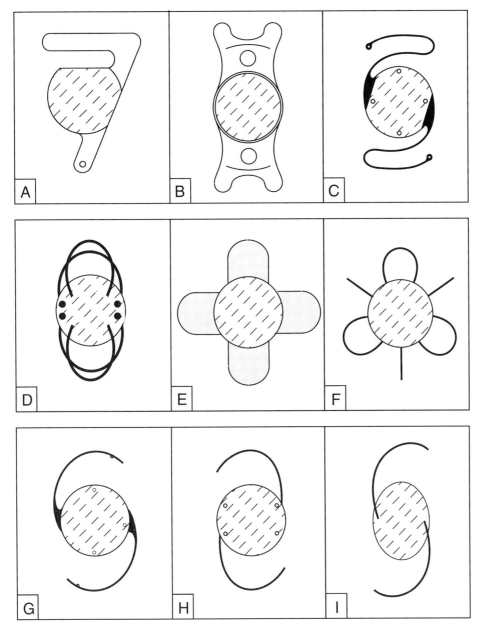

FIGURE 15-2
Various intraocular lens implants. A. Three-point fixation rigid anterior chamber IOL. B. Four-point fixation rigid anterior chamber IOL. C. Semiflexible anterior chamber IOL. D. Iris support IOL. E. Collar-stud iris support IOL. F. Iris clip IOL. G. One-piece PMMA posterior chamber IOL. H. Short C-loop posterior chamber IOL. I. Oval haptic posterior chamber IOL.

and disinfection, and many patients must rely on frequent office visits to have the lens removed, cleaned, and reinserted by the practitioner or a member of the office staff. This is often a significant inconvenience to patients, particular those with mobility concerns, and can lead to poor compliance or complications from overwear. Aphakic contact lenses have been associated with an increase in ocular infections, particularly the extended-wear hydrophilic lenses. Elderly patients often have coexisting ocular surface disorders that would contraindicate the

wearing of a contact lens, such as dry eye syndrome, lagophthalmus, and blepharitis.

Improvements in designs and materials have made intraocular lens (IOL) implants the preferred method of correcting aphakia (Figure 15-2). Magnification is reduced to 2–4%, and the visual field is not noticeably affected.[40,41,44] The handling difficulties and increased risk of ocular surface infection that occur with contact lenses are also eliminated with IOL implants. Although these factors have made implants attractive, severe complications unique to intraocular lenses can still occur, including chronic intraocular inflammation, iris and ciliary body erosion, and glaucoma. The majority of intraocular lenses currently being implanted are designed to be placed in the posterior chamber (PCIOL). Anterior chamber (ACIOL) and iris-fixated (IFIOL) lenses exist, but have an increased risk of complications. Intraocular lenses can be made from a variety of materials, including polymethyl methacrylate (PMMA), polypropylene, hydrogel, and silicon. They can be rigid, semiflexible, or foldable in form.

As the amount of data supporting the biocompatibility of intraocular implants has grown, the contraindications to implanting an IOL have decreased. Although it is still relatively uncommon to use an IOL in a patient younger than 20 years of age, most surgeons consider patients in other age groups to be acceptable candidates. Implants are generally tolerated by patients with previous retinal detachment, primary glaucoma, and nonproliferative diabetic retinopathy, but careful monitoring of these conditions postoperatively is indicated. Intraocular lens implants are contraindicated in patients with active chronic uveitis or neovascular glaucoma.

Calculation of Intraocular Lens Power

There are several methods available to calculate the dioptric power of the implant, including previous spectacle prescription, theoretical formulas, and linear regression formulas. Before the development of modern biometric techniques, the IOL power was estimated by using the previous spectacle prescription. This method frequently resulted in large residual refractive errors. Theoretical formulas are generally based on geometric optics with certain theoretical constants developed from schematic eyes. Although the newer generation theoretical formulas have added correction factors to improve the overall reliability, they still tend to be less popular than linear regression formulas.[40,41,46,47] Linear regression formulas predict the lens implant power by analyzing the relationship between the refracting components of the eye, including corneal curvature, anterior chamber depth, and the axial length.[40,41,46-49] They were developed by comparing the postsurgical refractive results with the presurgical findings in a large series of cases.

The SRK (Sanders, Retzlaff, and Kraff) formula, a widely used linear formula for predicting the postoperative refractive error, combines dependent variables or coefficients with independent or prediction variables for corneal curvature, lens implant power, and axial length.[40,41,46-49] The SRK formula is

$$P = A - 2.5L - 0.9K$$

where P = the implant power needed to produce emmetropia in diopters, A = the specific constant derived for each lens type and manufacturer, L = the axial length, and K = the average keratometer readings in diopters.

The A constant is specified by the different manufacturers for each type of IOL; however, a modification of the original formula, the SRK II formula, allows the A constant to be "surgeon specific" for a given surgical technique and lens implant. This correction factor has improved the predictability of the formula to 80% of eyes being within 1 D of the predicted refractive error, and less than 1% having a 3 D or greater error from the preoperative estimation.[47] The SRK II also demonstrates an improved performance over the original formula in short (≤ 22 mm) and long (≥ 25 mm) eyes. Despite the relative accuracy of the SRK formula, there can be sources of error when using it, with the majority attributed to inaccurate preoperative measurements. An error of 1 mm in the preoperative axial length measurement can result in a 2 D error in implant power, whereas a measurement error of 0.25 D in the average corneal keratometry reading produces a postoperative error of 0.50 D.[41,50]

Estimation of Postoperative Refraction

Although the optimum postoperative refractive error is still debated, most practitioners agree that reducing the refractive error toward emmetropia is desirable. The postoperative refractive error is also dependent on the refractive status of the second, untreated eye, especially in the case of a monocular cataract.

When the corrected vision in the second, untreated eye is 20/50 or better, the postoperative refraction must be no more than 2 D different toward emmetropia to avoid significant anisometropia.[51] It is particularly important to maintain this difference in the vertical meridian because of the spectacle-induced differential vertical prism encountered during up-gaze and down-gaze. If significant anisometropia does exist in the vertical meridian, slab-off prism, asymmetric adds, or separate spectacles for distance and near may need to be prescribed. Aniseikonic problems can be treated by modifying the spectacle lens base curve, thickness, or vertex distance.

If bilateral cataracts are present and the second eye is likely to be operated on within 6 months, the goal for the postoperative prescription for the first eye should be set between emmetropia and low myopia.[51] Residual hyperopia is never desirable, since patients cannot accommodate after cataract surgery. A prediction for low myopia allows for inaccuracies in the preoperative measurements or surgical technique and also permits the patient to retain reasonable distance and near vision without the use of spectacles if necessary.

As mentioned, the postoperative prescription for the second eye must be within 2 D of the refractive error of the first eye to avoid significant effects of anisometropia. Errors in predicting the postoperative refraction are often related to inaccurate preoperative measurements, mainly axial length.[2,52,53] If both eyes had a similar preoperative refractive error, an implant power for the second eye that is greater than the implant power for the same predicted postoperative refractive error in the first eye should be suspected as being inaccurate, and biometry and keratometry measurements should be retaken.

There are several instances in which, despite repeated preoperative measurements, the predicted IOL power that will result in emmetropia of the second eye does not correspond closely with that of the first eye, resulting in undesired anisometropia. In the first situation, the power of the implant for the first eye was accurately predicted, but the predicted power of the implant for the second eye is greater by more than 1 D. In this case, a power for the lens of the second eye should be chosen that is intermediate between the predicted powers of the two implants.[52] Another situation occurs when the predicted power for the implant was inaccurate in the first eye, but the predicted power for the implant for the second eye is in close agreement with that for the first eye. The predicted power for the implant for the second eye should be used in this circumstance.[52]

A-Mode Ultrasonography

A-mode ultrasonography is used to measure the axial length of the eye (ocular biometry), which is a necessary variable in calculating the power of the intraocular lens implant.[2,41,53] The A-mode ultrasound device transmits weak, high-frequency sound wave pulses into the eye, creating echographic signatures of the ocular structures. The time it takes these echoes to travel through the eye and reflect back to the ultrasound probe is recorded and used to determine the axial length. To measure true axial length the probe must be properly aligned. This is accomplished by positioning the probe so that the four major echographic spikes, representing the cornea, the anterior lens and posterior lens surfaces, and the retina, are obtained on the oscilloscope screen (Figure 15-3). If the probe is properly aligned for axial length measurement, the corneal and retinal spikes will be approximately equal in height. A convenient feature on some biometers is pattern recognition, which will record a reading automatically when the probe is approximately aligned. Several similar readings are ideally obtained and then averaged

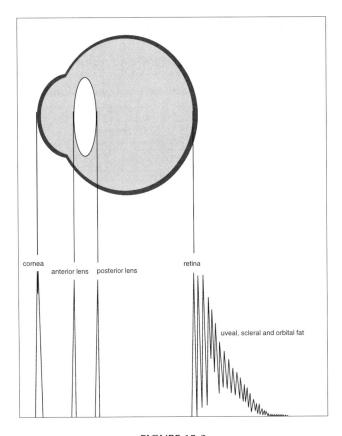

FIGURE 15-3

Schematic demonstrating the major echographic spikes obtained with A-mode ultrasonography during axial length determination.

for the final axial length determination. Any measurement error is usually a result of the technique of the biometrist. Other errors can result from increased retinal thickness and indentation of the cornea.

Most human eyes have an axial length between 20 and 26 mm, with the majority between 22 and 24 mm.[54] Axial lengths typically do not differ greater than 0.3 mm between the eyes.[54] If the difference in axial length is not consistent with the refractive error, the biometric measurements should be repeated. An eye with a smaller than expected anterior chamber depth may have been excessively applanated.

A local anesthetic is instilled into the eye, and the patient is instructed to fixate at a distant target. The probe is brought lightly into contact with the cornea and the axial length is recorded. The axial lengths of both eyes should be recorded for comparison and accuracy with the other portions of the preoperative examination. For further discussion of ophthalmic ultrasonography, see Chapter 14.

GENERAL SURGICAL PROCEDURES

Improvements in modern cataract surgery occur rapidly, with techniques and materials commonly becoming obsolete within a few years. Because many of the postoperative complications that arise are directly related to the surgical procedure, it is essential that the participants responsible for the postoperative care be aware of all the surgical aspects for a particular case. Personal communication with the surgeon is highly recommended in all cases that are comanaged. Vital surgical information is also contained in the surgical report, which should always be forwarded before the postoperative examination. The surgical report provides information on the preoperative preparation and sedation, surgical instrumentation and materials, anesthesia, extraction technique, intraocular implant, and details of the intraoperative course, including complications.

Preoperative Medications

Topical broad-spectrum antibiotics, anti-inflammatory agents, or antiglaucoma medications may be used if necessary for several days before the operation. Oral carbonic anhydrase inhibitors or osmotics may also be prescribed to lower the intraocular pressure preoperatively. In most cases, mydriatic drops for pupillary dilation are given immediately before the operation. Whenever possible, cataract surgery is performed under local or topical anesthesia. Preoperative sedation is often required, and the patient may receive either an oral or intramuscular tranquilizer before surgery. In addition to sedation, tranquilizers provide an antiemetic effect and muscle relaxation. During surgery, an intravenous tranquilizer may be given to maintain sedation.

Anesthesia

Most surgeons prefer to conduct cataract surgery with the patient under local anesthesia, which decreases the likelihood of cardiac, respiratory, or CNS complications. Local anesthesia, performed either by retrobulbar or peribulbar injection, also has the additional advantage of reducing the degree of postoperative pain. Retrobulbar injection delivers a bolus of anesthetic that reaches the region of the muscle cone, thereby blocking ciliary nerve fiber conduction. These fibers normally provide sensation to the conjunctiva, cornea, and uvea; therefore, anesthesia of these structures occurs. Akinesia of the extraocular muscles is also produced by the retrobulbar injection, due to blockade of the third, fourth, and sixth cranial nerves. A facial nerve block, if performed, will prevent ble-

pharospasm of the orbicularis oculi muscle. Complications that can occur from a retrobulbar injection include globe perforation, retrobulbar hemorrhage, optic nerve trauma, and CNS toxicity. An alternative local anesthesia technique is the peribulbar injection.[55] This method is thought to be safer than a retrobulbar injection because it delivers the anesthetic farther away from vital ocular structures and is technically easier to perform.[56,57] However, a greater amount of time is necessary for anesthesia to occur with a peribulbar injection because the anesthetic must diffuse further through the orbital tissue. General anesthesia is useful when a patient has difficulty remaining still or is extremely anxious about surgery.

Global Pressure

After injection of the local anesthetic, direct pressure is applied to the globe. This compresses any blood vessels that may have been nicked by the needle, lowers the intraocular pressure, and reduces the vitreous volume. Firm, steady pressure for 20-second intervals over 3–10 minutes may be applied either by hand or with specially designed mechanical devices such as a mercury bag, a rubber ball, or a pneumatic balloon.[40,41] The intraocular pressure should be reduced to 5 mm Hg or less before proceeding with surgery.

Preparation of the Surgical Field

The field is then prepared and disinfected for surgery. The patient's face is scrubbed with a mild surgical soap or detergent that contains a disinfectant such as iodine or hexachlorophene. Although the eyelashes and eyebrows are no longer shaved, the eyelid margins are cleaned with cotton-tipped applicators moistened with a disinfectant that does not irritate ocular surface tissues. The globe and cul-de-sac are irrigated with a sterile saline solution, and the surgical field is then demarcated by the application of an adhesive fenestrated surgical drape. The lids are positioned away from the surgical field by inserting an eyelid speculum or applying adhesive tape. Some surgeons prefer to place a superior rectus bridle suture to immobilize the globe during surgery.

Intracapsular Cataract Extraction

Intracapsular cataract extraction (ICCE) removes the entire lens, including the complete capsule, via cryoextraction (Figure 15-4). Intracapsular cataract extraction is most likely to be used to remove dislocated or subluxated lenses.

The ICCE procedure requires a large limbal incision that is 10–14 mm in size.[40,41] A knife is used first to create a par-

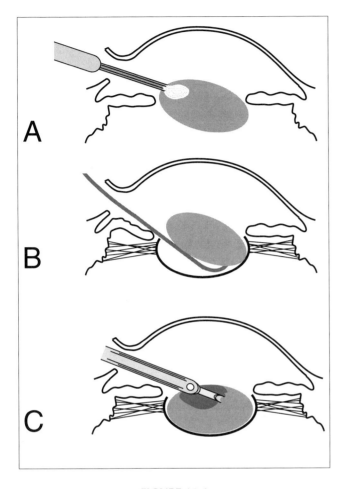

FIGURE 15-4
Cataract extraction techniques. A. Cryoextraction (ICCE). B. Expression (ECCE). C. Phacoemulsification (ECCE).

tial-thickness scleral groove and then to enter the anterior chamber. The wound is enlarged with scissors. Once the zonules are enzymatically dissolved with alpha-chymotrypsin, a cryoprobe is used to remove the lens from the eye. Depending on the case, an anterior chamber intraocular lens may be implanted. The incision is typically closed with five or more interrupted radial sutures, which can induce a moderate amount of corneal astigmatism.

Extracapsular Cataract Extraction

Extracapsular cataract extraction (ECCE) removes the anterior lens capsule, the cortex, and the nucleus of the lens. The posterior capsule is left intact (see Figure 15-4). The posterior capsule is believed to provide more stability and to decrease the likelihood of postoperative complications such as retinal detachment. Many surgeons also

prefer to use an ECCE procedure when significant nuclear brunescence is present or when an increased risk of endothelial dysfunction or damage exists.

The incision in planned ECCE procedures is 9–12 mm in length and placed posterior to the limbus.[40,41] This helps reduce the amount of induced astigmatism and promotes quicker wound healing. Viscoelastics may be placed into the anterior chamber to protect the corneal endothelium and other intraocular structures. An anterior capsulotomy is performed, followed by nuclear expression. The remaining cortical material is then aspirated, and the posterior capsule polished to remove any residual cortex. A posterior chamber intraocular lens is typically implanted either in the capsular bag or in the ciliary sulcus. If the posterior capsule is ruptured or torn during surgery, preventing PCIOL placement, an anterior chamber lens can be inserted. The incision is closed with several interrupted radial sutures or a single continuous running suture.

Phacoemulsification

Phacoemulsification is a variant of extracapsular surgery, which, by using a smaller incision, expedites healing and induces less corneal astigmatism than other extraction procedures (see Figure 15-4). Contraindications to phacoemulsification include brunescent cataracts, dislocated or subluxated lenses, a shallow anterior chamber, a miotic pupil, and advanced endothelial disease.

Phacoemulsification is performed through an incision that is 3.5–4.0 mm, which can be located either in the posterior limbal area or temporal peripheral cornea.[40,41,56,57] These incisions are relatively astigmatically neutral. When a limbal incision is used, the surgeon creates a scleral pocket or tunnel to enter the anterior chamber. These incisions are self-sealing and often do not require sutures. Conservative surgeons may use a single horizontal or radial suture to close the wound.

After the anterior chamber is entered, an anterior capsulotomy or a continuous curvilinear capsulorhexis (CCC) is performed.[56,57] Viscoelastics are also instilled to protect the corneal endothelium. If a traditional capsulotomy has been done, the lens nucleus is delivered into the anterior chamber or pupillary plane for emulsification. With the development of the capsulorhexis, hydrodissection (a technique in which viscoelastic substance is injected beneath the lens capsule, which separates the capsule from the cortical tissue) and emulsification of the nucleus can be done within the capsular bag.[58] This is thought to cause less overall trauma to the corneal endothelium. After removal of the nucleus, the remaining cortical material is aspirated and the posterior capsule polished.

TABLE 15-2
Typical Postoperative Examination Schedule

Postoperative Examination	First (1 day)	Second (1–2 Weeks)	Third (3–5 Weeks)	Fourth (6–8 Weeks)	Fifth (3 Months)
History	Yes	Yes	Yes	Yes	Yes
Visual acuity	Yes	Yes	Yes	Yes	Yes
Pupils	No	Yes	Yes	Yes	Yes
Keratometry	No	Yes	Yes	Yes	Yes
Refraction	No	Yes	Yes	Yes	Yes
Biomicroscopy	Yes	Yes	Yes	Yes	Yes
Tonometry	Yes	Yes	Yes	Yes	Yes
Ophthalmoscopy	Yes	Yes	Yes	Yes	Yes
Dilation	If visual acuity does not correlate with anterior segment appearance	Yes	Optional	Optional	Yes

POSTOPERATIVE EVALUATION

The postoperative recovery period depends on the type of procedure, the individual healing characteristics of the patient, and whether intraoperative or postoperative complications occur. Most patients are closely monitored on a variable basis for at least 3 months, the critical period during which the majority of postoperative complications will manifest themselves. Because it is difficult to predict an individual patient's rate of recovery, it is advantageous to develop a generalized examination scheme that not only provides a framework for the postoperative period but also allows for variation if any complications should arise (Table 15-2).

Since the majority of cataract extractions can be performed as outpatient procedures, patients are released from the surgical center on the same day unless the patient has certain health limitations or intraoperative complications that require careful monitoring. The patient should receive general instructions regarding postoperative care before being discharged (Figure 15-5). All patients are examined the following day.

The advantage of the smaller incision is partially lost when a standard-sized posterior chamber IOL is used, because the wound must be enlarged to 6–8 mm to insert the implant. Silicon acrylic or hydrogel foldable lenses may be used to preserve the smaller incision. Oval PMMA lenses may also be used in conjunction with small incisions. The ideal location for a PCIOL is within the capsular bag. This provides greater stability and reduces the likelihood of intraocular tissue disruption from the implant.

One-Day Postoperative Examination (First Follow-Up)

Patients typically come to the one-day postoperative visit with the eye dressed and covered by a protective metal or plastic shield. Despite the advances in small-incision surgery and self-sealing wounds, the shield offers an added measure of protection against trauma and should be used until the incision has sufficiently healed. The patient also tends to be more comfortable with the eye occluded, since there is usually some photophobia from postoperative intraocular inflammation or localized irritation from the incision. The patient should be interviewed regarding any eye discomfort or pain or if he or she experienced any noticeable side effects from the medications or anesthetics used during surgery. Analgesics that do not contain aspirin are usually prescribed for any pain. The patient may have also received medication to control postoperative intraocular pressure, including acetazolamide tablets or topical antiglaucoma drops. A postoperative care kit may have been issued at the time of discharge that contains any needed medications or supplies. The protective shield and dressing are gently removed and the eye irrigated with a sterile saline wash to remove any accumulated debris, mucus, or blood. Gross inspection of the ocular adnexa may demonstrate a varying degree of edema and ecchymosis to the surrounding periocular region.

The uncorrected distance Snellen visual acuity should correlate with the anticipated residual refractive error but may be reduced beyond this because of transient corneal edema or intraocular inflammation. When due to residual refractive error, a pinhole aperture may demonstrate

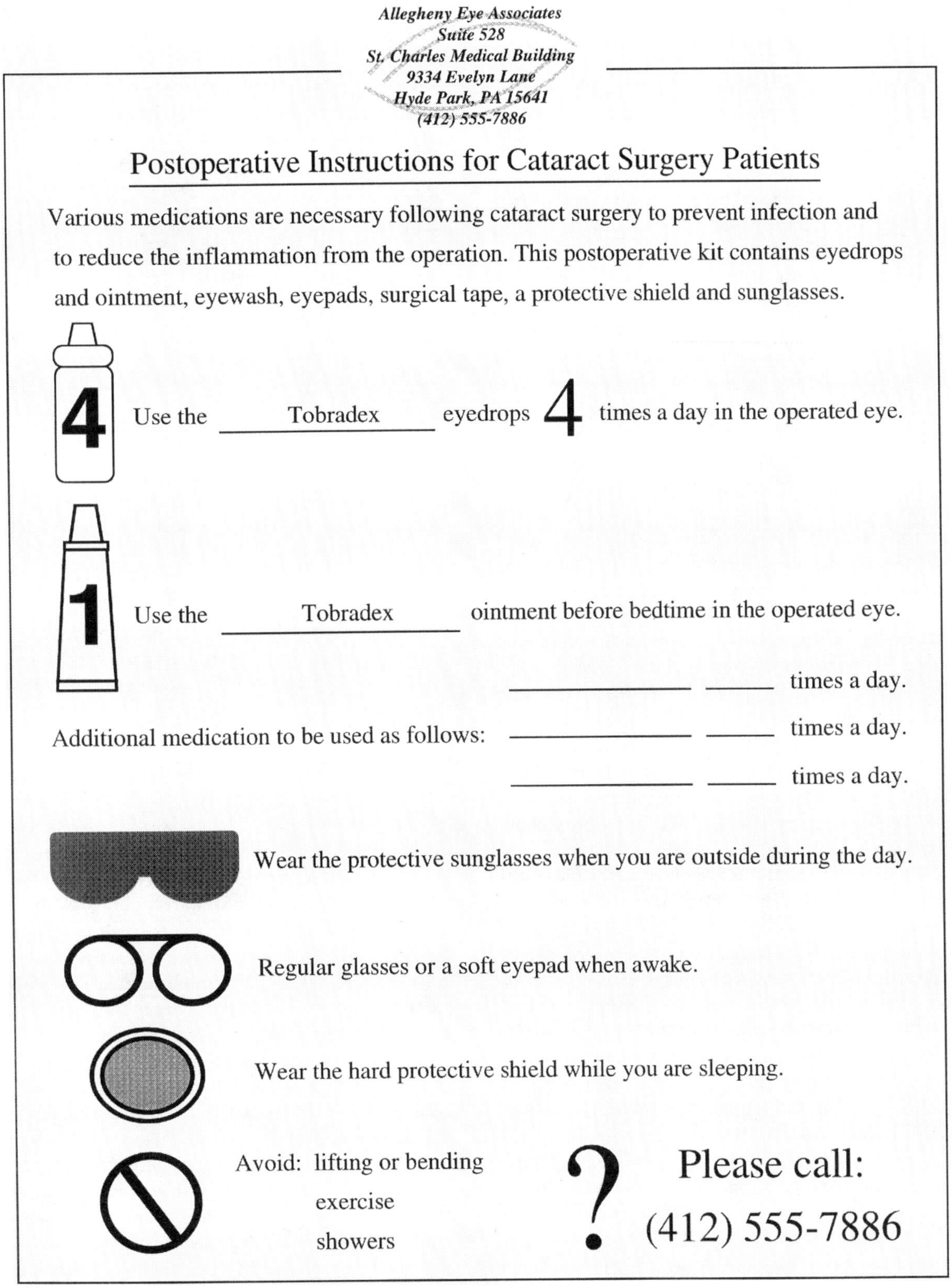

Allegheny Eye Associates
Suite 528
St. Charles Medical Building
9334 Evelyn Lane
Hyde Park, PA 15641
(412) 555-7886

Postoperative Instructions for Cataract Surgery Patients

Various medications are necessary following cataract surgery to prevent infection and to reduce the inflammation from the operation. This postoperative kit contains eyedrops and ointment, eyewash, eyepads, surgical tape, a protective shield and sunglasses.

Use the _____Tobradex_____ eyedrops **4** times a day in the operated eye.

Use the _____Tobradex_____ ointment before bedtime in the operated eye.

Additional medication to be used as follows:

_____ _____ times a day.

_____ _____ times a day.

_____ _____ times a day.

Wear the protective sunglasses when you are outside during the day.

Regular glasses or a soft eyepad when awake.

Wear the hard protective shield while you are sleeping.

Avoid: lifting or bending
exercise
showers

? Please call:
(412) 555-7886

FIGURE 15-5

Postoperative instructions for cataract surgery patients.

improvement in the reduced acuity. When acuity loss is due to another cause, the pinhole will not yield improvement in the vision. The pupillary reactions of the operated eye may be sluggish from the pharmacologic agents used during surgery, but the afferent pathway may still be tested by observing the pupillary responses of the other eye (reverse afferent pupillary testing during the swinging flashlight test). Extraocular muscle motilities should be full in range, and confrontation visual fields should not demonstrate any defects.

Biomicroscopic examination of the incision site should reveal good edge apposition, with no gaping of the wound. A variable degree of subconjunctival hemorrhage can be expected. If present, sutures should ideally be buried and covered by the conjunctiva. The cornea may be edematous, with posterior corneal folds evident. The anterior chamber inflammatory reaction is graded, with the condition of the iris and pupil noted (e.g., dyscoria, correctopia). The anterior chamber should be deep, without any sign of hyphema. If an intraocular lens implant was used, its condition and position should be evaluated. The integrity of the posterior capsule (e.g., opacified, torn) is assessed when an extracapsular or phacoemulsification procedure was used. The anterior vitreous face should be intact without prolapse into the pupillary zone or anterior chamber. Intraocular pressure is measured, with Goldmann applanation tonometry preferred over noncontact methods. The posterior segment is inspected with at least direct ophthalmoscopy. If vision is substantially reduced and the reduction cannot be ascribed to any apparent finding, then the pupil should be dilated and the posterior segment fully examined for further investigation of the unexplained vision loss.

If no unusual complications are present, the patient is typically prescribed topical corticosteroid drops, such as prednisolone acetate, to be used every 2–4 hours to reduce the postoperative inflammation. Topical broad-spectrum antibiotic drops are also given to be used four times a day to prevent infection. Gentamicin and tobramycin are effective antibiotics for this purpose. A corresponding antibiotic ointment may be used to provide antimicrobial protection during the night. Combination antibiotic/steroid topical drops are an excellent alternative to the standard regimen, and commonly are used four to six times a day in the early postoperative period. A combination ointment may also be used at bedtime. To protect the eye against mechanical injury, patients are instructed to use either the protective shield or their habitual glasses during the day and the eyeshield during periods of sleep (Figure 15-6). Wrap-around sunglasses that provide ultraviolet light protection should be used when the patient is outside. Analgesics that do not contain aspirin

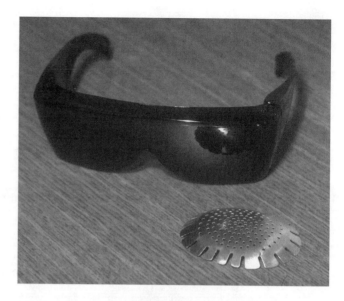

FIGURE 15-6
Protective metal shield and wrap-around sunglasses used during the postoperative recovery period.

may be prescribed for pain. The patient is asked to restrict his or her physical activities, particularly bending and lifting, and to return for a follow-up examination in about one week.

One-Week Postoperative Examination (Second Follow-Up)

At the one-week postoperative visit, the patient should report a subjective improvement in vision and have decreasing complaints of photophobia and foreign body sensation. The uncorrected distance visual acuity should be obtained and keratometry measurements and a preliminary refraction performed to measure the residual refractive error. The pupillary responses should demonstrate a return to the preoperative state.

Biomicroscopy of the anterior segment should show an improvement in the overall appearance, with decreasing subconjunctival hemorrhage, corneal edema, and intraocular inflammation. The wound site should be secure without evidence of leakage (i.e., negative Seidel's sign; Color Plate 15-1). There should not be any iris adhesions to the intraocular lens, and pigment deposition on the implant should be minimal. The posterior capsule should be clear without opacification or significant wrinkling. Goldmann applanation tonometry should again be performed at this visit. Direct ophthalmoscopy of the posterior pole should reveal the preoperative state of the optic nerve and macular region. Dilation is usually performed, especially if there is unexplained reduced visual acuity or if there was excessive intraocular manipulation at the time of surgery or capsular disruption has occurred.

The broad-spectrum antibiotic can be discontinued or its frequency of instillation decreased if there are no signs of infection. If the degree of intraocular inflammation is minimal, then the topical steroid drops can be tapered and used four times a day. The patient may continue to wear the protective shield at night and to limit physical activity as appropriate. Lifting heavy objects and bending over should be avoided. Patients who have had intracapsular and extracapsular surgery can return for follow-up care 2 weeks after this visit, whereas most patients with uncomplicated phacoemulsification are usually released for 3 weeks.

Three- to Four-Week Postoperative Examination (Third Follow-Up)

Patients returning for the third postoperative visit are given an examination similar to that performed one week after surgery. A careful refraction is done at this time, including keratometry and retinoscopy. The anterior segment should show minimal signs of inflammation. A dilated fundus examination is often performed to inspect the posterior pole and retinal periphery.

The time it takes for the postoperative refraction to stabilize is usually 3–8 weeks and depends on the size and location of the incision, the use of topical steroids, and the type of suture material. Postoperative retinoscopy may be difficult, especially in aphakic patients, in whom the reflex is dim and irregular astigmatism is common. Reflections from the intraocular lens implant may make the retinoscopy reflex difficult to interpret in pseudophakics. Postoperative keratometry readings and automated refraction readings may be helpful in obtaining refractive data, especially if retinoscopy is of limited value.

The patient usually remains on topical steroids but may taper the drops further if residual inflammation is minor. The patient may discontinue wear of the protective shield during sleep. A return to limited activities may be permitted, but caution should be used with tasks that require heavy lifting, straining, or bending. The patient can be scheduled to return in several weeks for a repeat refraction and evaluation.

Subsequent Postoperative Examinations

The next visit occurs usually 4–6 weeks postoperatively, depending on the surgical procedure and rate of individual recovery. Most patients who have had small-incision surgery with phacoemulsification are stable within a month after the operation, whereas patients who have undergone large-incision procedures usually require a longer time period for the eye to sufficiently heal.

Subsequent postoperative visits repeat many aspects of previous testing, and when the eye is normal in appearance with no signs of inflammation, final spectacle prescription may be determined. The patient may discontinue all topical ocular medications that were initially prescribed during the immediate postoperative period. The protective shield is no longer needed beyond 8 weeks in most cases and can often be discarded after 2–3 weeks in patients with small incisions. Usually, the patient can return to normal activities at this time.

In the absence of significant complications, the next scheduled postoperative examination should occur approximately 3 months after surgery. The patient is then seen at the 6-month and 12-month postoperative intervals. If no complications arise, the patient may be seen on a yearly basis thereafter.

POSTOPERATIVE COMPLICATIONS

Early and late postoperative complications involving the various structures of the eye are listed in Table 15-3.

Allergic Dermatitis or Conjunctivitis

Allergic dermatitis or conjunctivitis can be caused by any topical medication that is used in the postoperative period, particularly compounds containing neomycin.[59] Patients may also develop a contact allergic reaction to the surgical tape. The initial symptoms include red, itchy eyes, with swollen, erythematous lids. The bulbar conjunctiva may appear to be edematous with superficial injection. The palpebral conjunctiva may demonstrate a mild to marked papillary reaction. Treatment consists of discontinuing the offending topical medication and applying cold compresses every hour. A 0.5% hydrocortisone or 0.025% triamcinolone cream may be used to reduce the lid inflammation. Most allergic reactions are self-limited, but severe cases need to be managed with topical corticosteroids and oral antihistamines.

Induced Corneal Astigmatism

Induced corneal astigmatism can result from any cataract surgical procedure, particularly when the incision is large and close to the cornea. The type of suture and the method of incisional closure may also contribute to postoperative

TABLE 15-3
Postoperative Complications of Cataract Surgery

Area of Eye	Early Complications	Delayed Complications
Eyelids/adnexa	Allergic dermatitis Ecchymosis Ptosis	Ptosis
Conjunctiva/sclera	Allergic conjunctivitis Subconjunctival hemorrhage Wound dehiscence Exposed suture	Wound dehiscence Exposed suture Wound fistula
Cornea	Induced astigmatism Keratitis Transient corneal edema Dellen	Epithelial down-growth Bullous keratopathy Dellen
Anterior chamber	Hyphema Transient inflammation Endophthalmitis	Persistent hyphema Chronic inflammation Endophthalmitis
Iris/uvea	Pupillary block Iris tuck Atonic pupil	Pupillary block Iris chafing
IOL/posterior capsule	Pupillary capture IOL dislocation Capsular tear Windshield wiper syndrome	Capsular opacification
Vitreous/retina	Vitreous prolapse Vitreous wick Vitreous detachment Ischemic optic neuropathy Cystoid macular edema Retinal detachment	Vitreous detachment Cystoid macular edema Retinal detachment

IOL = intraocular lens.

cylinder. Intracapsular techniques usually induce against-the-rule (ATR) cylinder because the anchoring suture is placed in the horizontal meridian. The superior limbal placement of sutures in extracapsular procedures causes steepening of the vertical meridian with resultant with-the-rule (WTR) astigmatism. Surgically induced astigmatism may continue to change in direction and magnitude toward the preoperative level for at least 2 years after surgery.[60] A 0.50 to 1.00 D reduction in WTR astigmatism is seen during the immediate postoperative period in extracapsular surgical extractions.[61,62]

The incision size and location are both factors contributing to the development of postoperative astigmatism, and the amount of induced cylinder is directly proportional to the cube of the length of the incision and inversely proportional to the distance of the incision from the limbus.[63] Therefore, a funnel-shaped zone is effectively present in which the potential for inducing astigmatism is minimal. Ideally, the incision should be placed in this zone (Figure 15-7). When used, a longer incision should be placed farther from the cornea, whereas a smaller incision can be placed closer. Phacoemulsification procedures

are more technically difficult when a long posterior incision is used because the instruments are restricted in their maneuverability. A frown incision that curves away from the limbus is advantageous because it remains close to the cornea to facilitate phacoemulsification but stays relatively posterior within the astigmatic neutral area.

The incision in standard extracapsular procedures is closed by either a radial running suture or multiple radial interrupted sutures in the limbal region. If the suture is excessively tight, wound compression occurs. This causes flattening of the limbal curvature with secondary steepening of the central corneal curvature (Figure 15-8).[64] The induced astigmatism results along the plus cylinder axis of the tightest suture or at the combined vector of several tight sutures. Greater wound compression occurs with long suture bites than with short bites. Nonabsorbable sutures, such as nylon or polypropylene, will maintain wound compression longer.[64]

To reduce postoperative astigmatism caused by incisional closure, newer techniques use either a horizontal suture or smaller tunnel incisions. Radial interrupted or

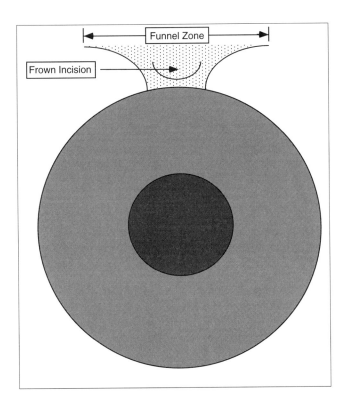

FIGURE 15-7

An incision placed within this funnel-shaped zone is less likely to induce significant astigmatism. The frown incision (surgeon's view) allows close limbal placement to facilitate phacoemulsification without inducing excessive cylinder power.

running sutures close the scleral incision gap, which causes wound compression and flattening at the limbus.[63] Horizontal sutures close the wound at the scleral tunnel, which produces less limbal wound compression. No-stitch cataract procedures combine a scleral tunnel with a short distance of intracorneal lamellar dissection. The incision is watertight and not compressed, resulting in minimal induced astigmatism.[65]

Inadequate incisional closure or poor wound apposition in extracapsular procedures may cause wound dehiscence and induce ATR cylinder. Excessive scarring of the wound can also be a source of induced postsurgical astigmatism.

Mild to moderate amounts of postoperative astigmatism can be corrected with spectacles or contact lenses. However, if the induced cylinder is in excess of 3 D, one or more sutures may need to be cut.[60,62] The optimal time to cut a suture depends on the type of suture and the rate of wound healing. Because of the small reduction in WTR cylinder during the early postoperative period, premature cutting of sutures may result in overcorrection. Generally, radial sutures can be cut at about 6 weeks postopera-

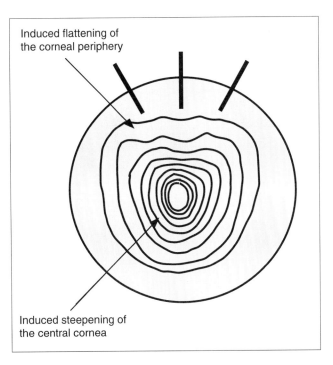

FIGURE 15-8

Diagram demonstrating the induced cylinder produced by limbal radial sutures. While the peripheral cornea flattens, the central cornea becomes steeper.

tively, whereas a continuous running suture should not be cut until 8–10 weeks after surgery.[64] This time period ensures that adequate wound healing has occurred. The number of sutures to be cut is based on the amount of induced astigmatism, and a single tight suture is identified by the axis of the plus refractive cylinder and the axis of the higher keratometry reading. The cylinder axis may also be the vector result of two or more tight sutures, and keratoscopy or corneal topography may be useful in identifying which sutures to cut.

A radial interrupted suture should be cut with a blade where the bite exits closer to the cornea. Often the cut ends will retract into the wound. If a portion of the suture remains exposed, it may need to be removed with jeweler's forceps to prevent irritation or inflammation. The entire portion of a running suture should be removed, because retained suture fragments may precipitate wound infection or endophthalmitis.

Postoperative Corneal Edema

One of the surgical goals during cataract extraction is to minimize the damage to intraocular structures, particularly the corneal endothelium. Phacoemulsification in the

FIGURE 15-9
Postoperative bullous keratopathy in a patient with an anterior chamber IOL. (Courtesy of Sara L. Penner, O.D.)

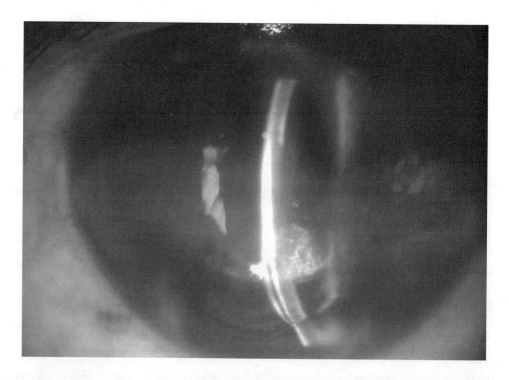

iris plane or posterior chamber, the use of viscoelastics during surgery, and placement of the implant in the capsular bag are thought to reduce the likelihood of trauma to corneal endothelium. Despite these preventative measures, some endothelial cell loss does occur in 65–85% of all cataract extractions, whether or not an intraocular lens has been implanted.[66] Severe endothelial cell loss greater than 1,200 cells/mm^2 occurs in 1% of intracapsular cataract extractions, 4% of planned extracapsular cataract extractions, 13% of posterior chamber phacoemulsifications, and 17% of the anterior chamber phacoemulsifications.[66] Phacoemulsification procedures result in a mean decrease of endothelial cell density of 17–20% compared with 11% in standard extracapsular or intracapsular extractions.[66]

Minor trauma to the endothelium will result in mild corneal edema that typically resolves within the first several weeks after surgery. This appears as a slight thickening of the superior and central corneal stroma. Folds in the posterior corneal layers may be present. Hypertonics are usually not necessary in these cases. High intraocular pressure and low-grade intraocular inflammation after the surgery may also contribute to the development of corneal edema, and topical antiglaucoma agents and corticosteroids may be helpful in reducing the corneal swelling.

If the corneal endothelium cannot recover, persistent corneal edema including bullous keratopathy may develop (Figure 15-9). Repeated rupture of epithelial bullae

causes corneal scarring with loss of visual acuity. Possibly contributing to the development of bullous keratopathy are decompensation due to preexisting endothelial disease, chronic postoperative inflammation, and corneal contact with the iris, vitreous, or intraocular lens implant (especially anterior or iris-fixated lenses).[67,68] The inadvertent surgical stripping of Descemet's membrane may cause segmental or diffuse corneal swelling that requires viscoelastic tamponade or wound closure with large suture bites for repair.

Topical steroids may be used to reduce the inflammation that occurs with persistent postoperative corneal edema. Hypertonic drops during the day and ointment at night may help to maintain corneal transparency and prevent the formation of epithelial bullae. A bandage soft lens can promote epithelialization of ruptured bullae. When significant permanent scarring occurs, penetrating keratoplasty is often necessary to restore useful vision.

Epithelial Down-Growth

When a limbal wound site has good apposition, the incision is closed initially by a down-growth of subconjunctival tissue that normally stops at the inner margin of the incision. If the inner incisional margin closure is incomplete, fibroblastic overgrowth of the corneal or conjunctival epithelium into the anterior chamber can occur.[69,70]

Incomplete margin closure can be seen with wound malposition, wound hemorrhage, uveal or vitreous incarceration into the wound, chronic postoperative uveitis, or traumatic wound gap.[70] Other factors thought to contribute to the development of epithelial down-growth include excessive regenerative scarring of the stroma, a wide Descemet's membrane perforation, and damaged or absent endothelium at the wound margins.[71,72]

As the down-growth continues to replicate within the eye, a membrane forms and begins to envelop anterior chamber structures. A distinct demarcation line on the corneal endothelium indicates the limit of invasion onto the posterior corneal surface. The involved corneal region is usually edematous. If a significant portion of the trabecular meshwork becomes obstructed, a secondary glaucoma develops that is very resistant to medical therapy.

Epithelial down-growth must be removed surgically, and a variety of methods have been attempted, including cryopexy, stripping of the membrane, and excision of involved intraocular tissue.[70] Penetrating keratoplasty is only marginally successful, and most grafts fail because of recurrence of the down-growth.[70] Removing all the down-growth tissue is extremely difficult, and therefore regrowth of the membrane often occurs.

Dellen

A dellen is an oval-shaped lesion of the peripheral cornea that develops adjacent to an area of limbal elevation. Poor lid apposition next to the elevated area causes incomplete spreading of the precorneal tear film with subsequent desiccation of the corneal epithelium. Vascular deprivation or localized neurotrophic damage of the limbus after cataract surgery may also cause dellen formation.[73] The margins of a dellen are sharply demarcated, and the base is clear without infiltration. Pooling of vital stains in the base is typical. Patients may complain of slight irritation or photophobia, but visual acuity is usually unaffected. A dellen must be distinguished from infectious corneal ulceration, as well as corneal melting caused by severe inflammation. When lubricating ointment is applied to the involved area and the eye patched for 20 minutes, a dellen will typically rehydrate and the cornea will demonstrate near normal thickness.

Dellen are managed with topical ocular lubricants. Patching of the eye with application of antibiotic ointment is indicated in severe cases. A bandage soft contact lens may promote resolution by maintaining even wetting of the corneal surface. When possible, surgical removal of any limbal mass should be considered when chronic and recurrent dellen form.

Wound Dehiscence

Wound dehiscence that occurs within 1 day after cataract surgery is usually the result of poor surgical technique, although coughing, bending, and rubbing of the eye by the patient may disrupt the wound site. Later causes include blunt ocular trauma and chronic application of topical or subconjunctival corticosteroids, which delay wound healing.[74] Wound dehiscence may appear as an obvious gaping of the incision. If the wound site is hidden by overlying conjunctiva, shallow bleb formation may be present. Other signs of wound dehiscence include intraocular pressure lower than 5 mm Hg, a shallow anterior chamber, or Seidel's sign. Seidel's sign is characterized by the staining of leaking aqueous by sodium fluorescein (Color Plate 15-I). A fistula may develop from persistent wound leakage, with secondary complications including chronic inflammation, infection, or epithelialization of the wound track.[75] Fistulas may need to be closed with a corneal graft.

If wound leakage is minor and the anterior chamber fully formed, a wound dehiscence will usually reseal with a pressure patch. Topical antibiotics should be instilled to prevent infection. A soft bandage lens or tissue adhesive may also be used to promote closure of the wound. The incision site must be resutured when the anterior chamber is extremely shallow and iridocorneal touch is evident.

Iris prolapse is a complication of wound dehiscence that typically occurs secondary to inadequate wound closure, postoperative trauma, or a rapid increase in intraocular pressure (Figure 15-10). It must be repaired surgically. Iridocorneal touch, endophthalmitis, and chronic inflammation are complications of iris prolapse.

Persistent Foreign Body Sensation

A persistent foreign body sensation is usually secondary to an exposed suture or superficial keratitis. Epithelial disruption may be caused by inadvertent exposure to various surgical disinfecting agents, poor intraoperative irrigation of the cornea, or medications.[76] Typical epithelial defects are usually minor and quickly resolve. Ocular lubricants may be helpful, and broad-spectrum antibiotic drugs may be helpful to prevent secondary infection. If infectious keratitis is suspected, the pathogen must be identified and treated with an appropriate antimicrobial agent.

During surgery, sutures are normally trimmed, with the knots then rotated and buried. However, if a knot resurfaces, the overlying conjunctiva may erode, producing symptoms of itching, redness, and mild mucous

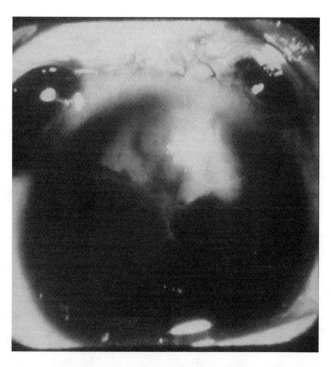

FIGURE 15-10
Iris prolapse with total hyphema from blunt trauma 4 weeks after ECCE. (Courtesy of Jack Veith, O.D.)

discharge. Sutures may spontaneously become exposed any time postoperatively. An exposed barb from a cut or broken suture may cause a focal papillary response in the superior palpebral conjunctiva.

The exposed suture must be removed when chronic erosion and irritation occur; however, the incision should be adequately healed to prevent wound dehiscence. If a suture becomes exposed shortly after surgery, lubrication drops or a soft bandage lens may promote re-epithelialization of the conjunctiva. A broad-spectrum antibiotic drop should be used to prevent secondary infection of the wound site. When wound closure is sufficient, the suture may be clipped and removed.

To remove a suture, the eye must be anesthetized with a few drops of topical proparacaine or tetracaine. If a deeper anesthesia is needed, topical xylocaine can be applied by holding a soaked cotton swab directly to the area for several minutes.[77] The patient should fixate to a point where the suture is easily accessible in the field of view of the biomicroscope. Often a suture may already be broken and jeweler's forceps may be used to easily remove the material. An intact suture must be cut, and a blade with the bevel side away from the ocular surface is an effective tool. When the suture is relatively buried, the overlying conjunctiva may have to be cut to reach the offending suture. The cut through the conjunctiva should avoid large conjunctival blood vessels. If a blood vessel is cut, a cotton swab may be applied to the bleeding site and/or a few drops of phenylephrine instilled. The suture is cut with an outward motion and removed with the forceps. The knot should not be pulled through the suture holes; rather, it may be an effective site to grasp the suture. As an alternative to suture cutting with a blade, a small tuberculin syringe needle is used. With its bevel facing the examiner, the needle is slid through the conjunctiva and under the suture. It is then rotated slightly so that the sharp edge of the bevel cuts the suture. The wound site should be inspected for gaping or leakage. Topical antibiotics to be used several times a day for a week should be prescribed.

Transient Rise in Intraocular Pressure

A transient rise in the intraocular pressure (IOP) may result from a decrease of aqueous outflow through the trabecular meshwork caused by remnant lens particles, inflammation, white blood cells, red blood cells, or residual viscoelastic materials.[78,79] Elevated IOP can be a response to topical steroid drops, and alpha-chymotrypsin, which is used for zonular lysis in intracapsular procedures, may also produce a postoperative pressure spike.

About 60% of patients will have an increase in the intraocular pressure to a level greater than or equal to 25 mm Hg within the first 24 hours after cataract surgery.[80] This rise in the postoperative intraocular pressure typically peaks between 6 and 8 hours after surgery and often returns to preoperative levels by the one-day postoperative examination.[80] If a patient has preexisting optic nerve disease, such as advanced glaucoma or ischemic optic neuropathy, a moderate elevation in IOP may cause further compromise. Because an IOP spike is difficult to predict for a particular patient, many practitioners will prescribe antiglaucoma drugs before and immediately after surgery. Topical beta blockers or oral carbonic anhydrase inhibitors are considered to be the most appropriate drugs for controlling the postoperative rise in IOP.[79] Pilocarpine is also effective in lowering the IOP postoperatively but should be avoided because of the increased risk of synechiae formation and retinal detachment. It can also increase anterior segment congestion. Epinephrine and dipivefrin are associated with the development of cystoid macular edema in aphakic and pseudophakic patients and are contraindicated. Apraclonidine is ineffective in lowering the IOP postoperatively.[79] If steroid responsiveness is the cause of elevated IOP, an alternate steroid such as fluorometic use of antiglaucoma medications.

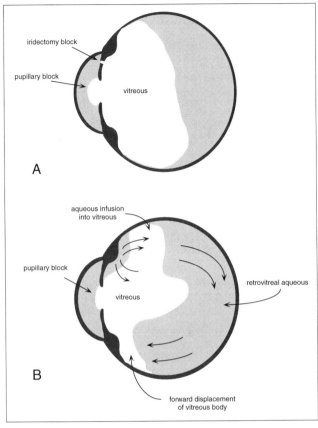

FIGURE 15-11

Schematic showing the mechanism for (A) aphakic pupillary block and (B) aphakic aqueous misdirection.

Pupillary Block Glaucoma

Pupillary block glaucoma is more prevalent in patients who have had intracapsular procedures with or without anterior chamber lens implantation and is the result of direct pupillary occlusion by the IOL optic or the anterior hyaloid face (Figure 15-11). The flow of aqueous from the posterior chamber into the anterior chamber becomes impeded and causes an increase in the posterior chamber pressure. The root of the iris then collapses forward in the anterior chamber angle and secondary angle closure occurs. The IOP rapidly rises. To prevent the development of pupillary block, a surgical iridectomy is usually performed with ICCE procedures.[81] However, an iridectomy may fail when iridovitreal adhesions develop or the iris plane shifts forward.[82] Anterior displacement of the posterior capsule may occlude the pupil in extracapsular procedures without posterior chamber lens implantation. Pupillary block glaucoma is rarely associated with the use of posterior chamber implants, since the haptics are ante-riorly angulated, thus markedly reducing the likelihood of contact between the optic and the posterior iris surface.

Although the acute rise in IOP may be medically managed, the pathway between the anterior and posterior chamber must be restored to relieve pupillary block glaucoma. Laser peripheral iridotomy (LPI) is the preferred treatment option.[81] In acute cases, LPI may be difficult to perform because of close apposition of the iris to the corneal endothelium. Additionally, corneal edema and iris congestion may interfere with laser perforation.

Aqueous misdirection, or malignant glaucoma, is a form of pupillary block glaucoma. In this disorder, the aqueous is posteriorly misdirected and collects within or behind the vitreous cavity (see Figure 15-11). The vitreous is anteriorly displaced and envelops the ciliary body and posterior iris. The anterior chamber angle is mechanically closed by the forward movement of the iris and ciliary body because of the increased pressure in the posterior segment.

Medical treatment of aqueous misdirection includes topical beta blockers or oral carbonic anhydrase inhibitors to reduce aqueous production and cycloplegics to promote the release of the entrapped aqueous. Oral hyperosmotics may help to reduce the vitreous volume. Laser capsulotomy may allow the aqueous to transverse from the posterior chamber into the anterior chamber.[82] Because the anterior vitreous face is in direct contact with the iris/ciliary body diaphragm, laser peripheral iridotomy will not relieve malignant glaucoma.

Postoperative Intraocular Inflammation

Acute postoperative intraocular inflammation is present to some degree after every type of cataract procedure and usually appears as a transient anterior uveitis. Release of inflammatory mediators after incisional injury of limbal tissue and uveal manipulation produces the mild to moderate anterior chamber reaction, which is readily treated with topical corticosteroids during the postoperative period.[83]

If the postoperative inflammatory reaction is marked in appearance, and the intraocular tissue exhibits minimal surgical disruption, endophthalmitis must be seriously considered. Endophthalmitis may result from the IOL implant, remnants of the crystalline lens, or infectious agents. Because of the aggressive intraocular behavior of some pathogens, endophthalmitis must initially be regarded as infectious until clinical evidence suggests otherwise.

The toxic lens syndrome is caused by chemical residue on the implant surface that was not removed properly after the sterilization process. A severe anterior chamber reaction with a sterile hypopyon develops within sev-

FIGURE 15-12
Postoperative bacterial endoph-thalmitis from Staphylococcus aureus. *(Courtesy of Diana Ford, O.D.)*

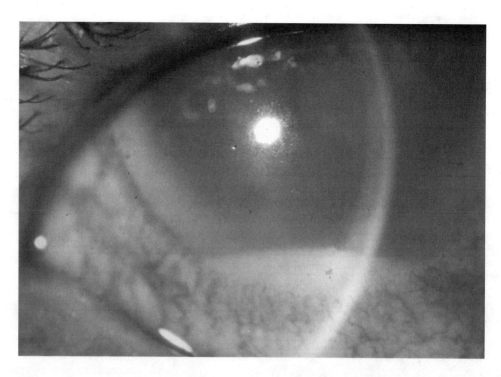

eral days of the surgery. The cornea may be mildly edematous. Aggressive management with corticosteroids, applied either topically or through subconjunctival injections, must be initiated. The IOL may have to be removed to resolve the inflammation.

Another form of postoperative uveitis is caused by remnants of the crystalline lens nucleus or cortex that were not evacuated during extracapsular cataract surgery. Lens-remnant uveitis is a granulomatous reaction occurring 1–14 days postoperatively with large mutton-fat keratic precipitates appearing on the corneal endothelium and on the surface of the implant. Lens remnants may be visualized in the anterior chamber, the pupillary space, or capsular bag. A sterile hypopyon can form. If left untreated, secondary glaucoma and cystoid macular edema may develop. Topical steroids every several hours or subconjunctival injections may reduce the inflammation; however, surgical evacuation of the lens material is usually necessary.

Although a rare complication of cataract surgery, acute infectious endophthalmitis is regarded as one of the most serious postoperative complications because of a very poor prognosis for retaining usable vision or salvaging the eye. It occurs in 0.2–0.5% of all cataract surgical procedures, with a rate of 0.072% in primary extractions and 0.3% in secondary implant procedures.[84] The infectious micro-organism is usually from a nonsterile intraocular lens or surgical field. Typically, a marked anterior chamber reaction with a rapidly developing hypopyon appears within 48 hours of the surgery (Figure 15-12). Severe ocular pain, chemosis, and corneal decompensation are other significant clinical findings of infectious endophthalmitis. Marked vitreal inflammatory cells may be present.

Most cases of acute postoperative infectious endophthalmitis are caused by highly virulent organisms, such as *Staphylococcus aureus,* various gram-negative bacteria, or fungi.[84-86] The causative pathogen must be identified by culturing the organisms from aspirated aqueous and vitreous specimens. Positive culture results are more likely to be obtained from the vitreous.

Broad-spectrum antibacterial treatment for infectious endophthalmitis should be initiated immediately after the intraocular specimens are acquired. Intravitreal antibiotics can be administered when the vitreous tap or vitrectomy is performed, and the combination of vancomycin and an aminoglycoside (amikacin or gentamicin) is a commonly used regimen for the initial treatment of presumed bacterial endophthalmitis.[84] The role of vitrectomy in the management of infectious endophthalmitis remains unclear. If the cultures produce negative results, the endophthalmitis should be treated with intraocular antibiotics. Culture-positive endophthalmitis usually requires a vitrectomy and intraocular antibiotics. Local antimicrobial ocular therapy may be supplemented with systemic antibiotics; however, most systemic antibiotics do not achieve sufficiently high intraocular concentrations.

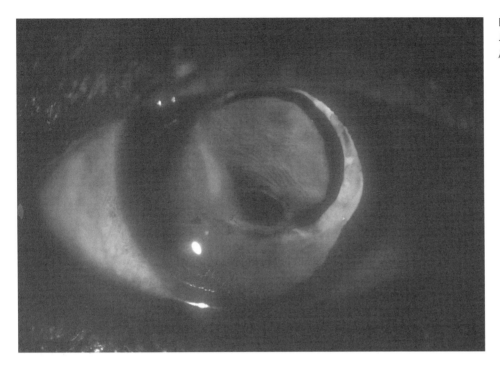

Delayed-onset or chronic postoperative infectious endophthalmitis develops weeks to months after initial cataract extraction and is characterized by a mild to moderate chronic intraocular inflammation. Organisms of low virulence, such as *Staphylococcus epidermidis* or *Propionibacterium acnes,* are usually the cause of this low-grade, smoldering infection.[86] *Propionibacterium acnes* infection often localizes to the capsular bag, where the microorganisms intermix with residual lens cortex. A white intracapsular plaque on the posterior capsule is a characteristic finding. The posterior capsule actually acts as a protective barrier, and laser capsulotomy may cause fulminant dissemination of the infection. Management includes capsular bag injection of vancomycin, a pars plana vitrectomy, and a central capsulotomy.[84,86]

Chronic postoperative intraocular inflammation may develop when the posterior capsule is torn and the anterior vitreous face is ruptured. Peripheral anterior synechiae, corneovitreal touch, and vitreous incarceration into the wound may also result in chronic inflammation. Intraocular lenses can cause persistent inflammation, particularly when they touch uveal tissue. Poorly sized, rigid, one-piece anterior chamber lenses often entrap the peripheral iris tissue or erode into the iris root or ciliary body, possibly causing recurrent hyphema, uveitis, or anterior segment ischemia.[87] These types of anterior implants often move, producing chafing of the iris and angle. Iris-fixated lenses are notorious for disruption of the iris tissue.

Posterior chamber implants may cause chafing, particularly when they are ciliary-sulcus fixated.

Opacification of the Posterior Capsule

Opacification of the posterior capsule is a common complication of extracapsular cataract surgery, with 50% of eyes demonstrating some degree of capsular changes within 5 years.[63,88,89] Opacification may develop as early as 6 months after surgery but typically occurs after 1 year. The patient will complain of a mild decrease in visual acuity or of disabling glare. Posterior capsular opacification appears as a clouding or wrinkling of the capsule caused by fibrous metaplasia of remaining anterior lens epithelium (Figure 15-13). Opacification of the posterior capsule is most likely to develop after a posterior subcapsular cataract, rather than a nuclear opacity, has been removed.[90] This tendency appears to be more related to the age group in which these types of cataracts arise. Posterior subcapsular cataracts are more common in a younger patient population, in which the anterior lens epithelium is more active. Nuclear cataracts tend to develop in older patients with relatively inactive lens epithelium.

Opacification of the posterior capsule is managed by neodymium-YAG laser capsulotomy. The restoration of vision to the previous level is almost instant. Laser capsulotomy is associated with complications, including increased intraocular pressure, posterior vitreous detach-

FIGURE 15-14
Vitreous prolapse and incarceration into the wound.

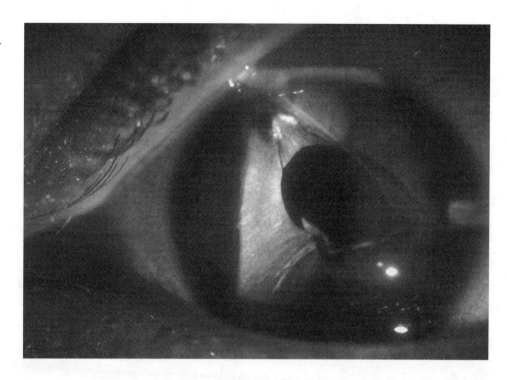

ment, and rhegmatogenous retinal detachment. Spikes in IOP after laser treatment appear to occur more frequently when the IOL is located in the ciliary sulcus rather than the capsular bag.[88] An implant placed in the capsular bag is thought to act as a physical barrier that prevents capsular debris from reaching and obstructing the trabecular meshwork. Pretreatment with 1% apraclonidine has been shown to be effective in controlling the intraocular pressure after laser capsulotomy.[78] The risk of retinal detachment after laser capsulotomy is about 1–4%, with the majority occurring within the first year after the procedure.[63,78] Male sex and axial myopia greater than 25 mm are predisposing risk factors.[78]

Postoperative Hyphema

The most common source of early postoperative hyphema is from the wound site.[91] Disruption of the newly formed blood vessels bridging the incision can occur after a Valsalva-type maneuver, with bleeding into the anterior chamber. This can be observed as a blood clot located near the inner incision border or on the adjacent iris surface. This type of hyphema is relatively minor and usually resolves without any long-term effects. The patient should be cautioned against excessive straining, and a protective shield may discourage eye rubbing. Additional topical eyedrops are generally not necessary. Hemorrhage from the ciliary body or zonular traction of the peripheral retinal vessels

may develop in the immediate postoperative period as a layered hyphema. In the late postoperative period, common sources of intraocular bleeding include iris chafing by the IOL, rubeosis irides, vitreous traction, retinal tear, and cataract wound neovascularization. If a layered hyphema has formed, topical steroid drops and cycloplegia may aid reabsorption of the blood. When the hyphema is persistent or recurs, an anterior chamber washout may be necessary to prevent the development of secondary glaucoma or permanent endothelial blood staining. Aminocaproic acid, an anti-fibrinolytic agent, has been used to treat recurrent postoperative hyphema but is associated with severe toxic side effects, particularly in elderly patients.[92]

Vitreous Incarceration

Vitreous that is incarcerated into the wound site prevents the endothelium from bridging the inner incisional margin (Figure 15-14). If the vitreous becomes externalized, infectious endophthalmitis or epithelial down-growth can develop.[93,94] When iridovitreal adhesions exist, contraction of the entrapped strand can cause distortion of the pupil, vitreoretinal traction, and retinal detachment. Chronic intraocular inflammation, corneal decompensation, and cystoid macular edema are also complications from vitreous wound incarceration. An anterior vitrectomy or laser vitreolysis may remove the adhesions from the pupillary margin and posterior corneal surface.

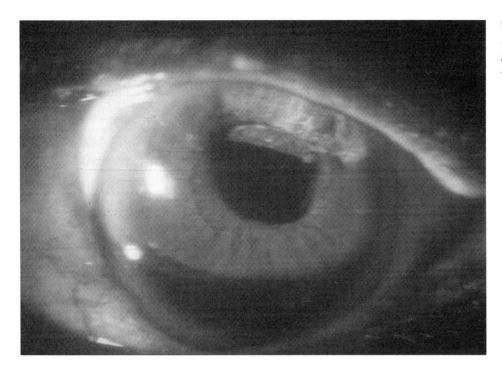

FIGURE 15-15
Pupillary capture of a uniplanar posterior chamber implant with superior iris chafing and atrophy.

Postsurgically Fixed Dilated Pupil

Although iris sphincter damage can occur from toxic, mechanical, and inflammatory causes, ischemia of the pupillary sphincter muscle is the most likely cause of an atonic pupil after cataract surgery.[78] The ciliary ganglion may also be traumatized by the retrobulbar injection; however, the pupil would demonstrate a supersensitivity constriction response to weak pilocarpine.[95] The pupil becomes fixed and dilated within 2–3 weeks after surgery, and the patient may complain of glare, photophobia, or poor cosmesis. Pupilloplasty or an opaque contact lens may reduce the symptoms.[96]

Malpositioning and Dislocation of Intraocular Lenses

The pupil can inadvertently capture the optic of a posterior chamber intraocular lens during recovery from mydriasis (Figure 15-15). "Pupillary capture" can be classified as partial when only a portion of the optic is in front of the iris plane, or total when the entire optic lies on the anterior iris surface. This has occurred most frequently with older uniplanar posterior chamber lenses. The 10- to 15-degree angulation of the haptics with newer PCIOL designs has minimized pupillary capture.[87]

Pupillary capture may cause symptoms of visual distortion or monocular diplopia, and the patient may com-

plain about the poor cosmesis of an oval pupil. Chronic contact of the implant with the iris tissue may promote pigment release, inflammation, or microhyphemas. Cystoid macular edema is a rare complication. Treatment options for pupillary capture include observation, pupillary dilation followed by miosis, manipulation of the IOL haptics with external pressure, and surgical intervention.[87,97]

If peripheral iris tissue is entrapped against the iridocorneal angle by an anterior chamber lens, distortion of the pupil parallel to the orientation of the haptic may occur; this is referred to as iris tuck. Although generally a cosmetic defect, chronic irritation and inflammation may develop. In severe cases, the anterior chamber lens implant must be removed.

A posterior chamber lens may cause peaking of the pupil because of fibroproliferation on the posterior iris surface.[98] This complication was seen more frequently with ciliary-sulcus fixated lens, but it has decreased with the advent of in-the-bag placement. If the haptics of a ciliary-sulcus fixated lens erode into the ciliary body, chronic inflammation and hyphema may result.

Inferior decentration or subluxation of a posterior chamber intraocular lens, also known as the sunset syndrome, is usually the result of inferior capsule rupture or zonular disruption that occurs either during the manual expression of the nucleus or when the IOL is being implanted into the capsular bag.[78,87,97] Other causes of implant decentration include fibrosis of the capsular bag, haptic erosion through the capsule, and misplacement of one haptic in the ciliary sulcus. These conditions may cause superior or horizontal decentration. The edge of the optic may rest in the pupillary zone, which can cause monocular diplopia, visual distortion, and separate aphakic and pseudophakic refractive zones.

Iris-fixated lenses can become decentered, subluxated, or dislocated because of excessive weight as well as movement or dilation of the pupil.[78,87,97] A dislocated iris-fixated lens can fall into the vitreous or into the anterior chamber, causing corneal endothelial touch with decompensation and development of pseudophakic bullous keratopathy. In the past, prevention of iris-fixated lens dislocation was attempted by suturing the implant to the iris.

Total dislocation of a PCIOL into the vitreous cavity may result when large posterior capsule tears are present. Capsular fibrosis may also cause excessive posterior vaulting of a hydrogel lens that may dislocate into the vitreous after laser capsulotomy.[78,87,97]

If symptoms are minimal, an opaque cosmetic contact lens may help reduce the visual disturbances caused by the optic's edge. If this is unsuccessful in relieving the symptoms associated with lens decentration, or if lens dislocation into the vitreous cavity is imminent, surgery to reposition or remove the implant is indicated. The haptic may be repositioned to an area of relative capsular stability.[78,87,97] Ciliary-sulcus fixation with and without a scleral suture, or replacement with an anterior chamber lens are other alternative treatment options. Lenses lost into the vitreous cavity are best left alone because of the technical difficulty of retrieval and an increased risk of retinal detachment during the procedure.

Windshield wiper syndrome, or pseudophakodonesis, is the movement of an intraocular lens in the posterior chamber.[78,87,97] The patient may report fluctuating vision with sudden movement or tilting of the head. Windshield wiper syndrome results when implant diameter is too small for the eye, from deformed haptics, or when an intraocular lens that was designed to be placed in the capsular bag is located in the ciliary sulcus. The intraocular lens may have to be removed if the patient is unable to tolerate the visual distortion or when severe iris chafing, inflammation, or hyphema occurs.

Cystoid Macular Edema

Cystoid macular edema (CME) is angiographically evident at 6 weeks postoperatively in 16–24% of cases; however, it only persists in 2–5% of cases for longer than 6 months.[63] Persistent CME is seen with equal frequency in extracapsular and intracapsular extractions. There are many proposed causes for the development of cystoid

macular edema, including intraocular trauma or inflammation, microscopic light toxicity, and vitreous traction on the macula.[63] Cystoid macular edema is not always apparent clinically, but the increased permeability of the perifoveal capillaries can usually be demonstrated with fluorescein angiography as a progressive hyperfluorescence during later transit phases.

Chronic CME resolves in 80% of pseudophakic patients with within 1 year, and in 95% within 2 years.[99] The resolution rate in aphakic patients without vitreous adhesions is 90% within 2 years.[99] About 90% of patients with CME will have improvement of vision to 20/40 or better within 2 years.[63] Preoperative factors indicating a poor prognosis include chronic intraocular inflammation and vascular disorders that cause macular edema, such as diabetes mellitus.[100] Cystoid macular edema is more persistent when vitreous loss or incarceration occurs. Iris-fixated and anterior chamber lenses that produce low-grade chronic inflammation are also associated with the development of CME.

Various options are available for the treatment of CME, although none has been demonstrated to be effective in the majority of cases. Corticosteroids and nonsteroidal anti-inflammatory agents are aimed at reducing the inflammatory mechanism, whereas lysis of vitreal strands by surgical or laser methods is believed to relieve mechanical factors.[100] Removal of a malpositioned intraocular lens may be helpful if excessive contact with uveal tissue is present. Acetazolamide has been shown to increase the rate of subretinal fluid absorption and promote adherence between the sensory retina and the retinal pigment epithelium.[63,78] In addition, ketorolac tromethamine 0.5% has been shown to significantly improve visual acuity in patients with cystoid macular edema.[101]

Retinal Detachment

Retinal detachment is a relatively common postoperative complication after cataract surgery and intraocular lens implantation. Between 0.5% and 2% of eyes suffer retinal detachment after uncomplicated extracapsular extraction with posterior chamber lenses.[100] Retinal detachment is more common in intracapsular than extracapsular procedures or when vitreous loss occurs. Risk factors for pseudophakic retinal detachment include age less than 70 years at the time of surgery, axial length greater than 25 mm and high myopia, retinal detachment in the other eye, and vitreoretinal precursors of retina breaks, such as lattice degeneration.[100,102] Primary or secondary capsulotomy is also a high risk factor.[103]

Retinal detachments in aphakic patients are often associated with numerous small holes that are located anterior to the equator.[103] However, in pseudophakic patients, retinal detachments tend to arise from posteriorly located, large retinal breaks. The overall success rate for anatomic reattachment is 93%.[104]

REFERENCES

1. Cataract Management Guideline Panel. Management of functional impairment due to cataract in adults. Ophthalmology 1993;100(Suppl):3S–4S.

2. Ajamian PC. Pre- and Postoperative Care of the Cataract Patient. Stoneham, MA: Butterworth-Heinemann, 1993.

3. Sherman J, Davis E, Schnider C, et al. Presurgical prediction of postsurgical visual acuity in patients with media opacities. J Am Optom Assoc 1988;59:481–8.

4. Hoffer KJ. Preoperative evaluation of the cataractous patient. Surv Ophthalmol 1984;29:55–69.

5. Bartley GB, Narr BJ. Preoperative medical examinations for patients undergoing ophthalmic surgery. Am J Ophthalmol 1991;112:725–7.

6. Guyton DL. Preoperative visual acuity evaluation. Int Ophthalmol Clin 1987;27:140–8.

7. Cinotti AA. The evaluation of indications for cataract surgery. Ophthalmic Surg 1979;10:25–31.

8. Green DG. Laser Devices in Measuring Visual Acuity. In TD Duane (ed), Clinical Ophthalmology (Vol. 1). Philadelphia: Harper & Row, 1984;1–7.

9. Smith TW, Remijan PW, Remijan W, et al. A new test of visual acuity using a holographic phase grating and a laser. Arch Ophthalmol 1979;97:752–4.

10. Lotmar W. Apparatus for the measurement of retinal visual acuity by moiré fringes. Invest Ophthalmol Vis Sci 1980;19:393–400.

11. Guyton DL. Instruments for measuring retinal visual acuity behind cataracts. Ophthalmology 1982;89:34–9.

12. Goldstein J, Hecht SD, James RJ, et al. Clinical comparison of the SITE IRAS hand-held interferometer and Haag-Streit Lotmar visometer. J Cataract Refract Surg 1988;14:208–11.

13. Faulkner HW. Laser interferometric prediction of postoperative visual acuity in patients with cataracts. Am J Ophthalmol 1983;95:626–36.

14. Goldmann H, Chrenkova A, Cornaro S. Retinal visual acuity in cataractous eyes. Determination with interference fringes. Arch Ophthalmol 1980;98:1778–81.

15. Halliday BL, Ross JE. Comparison of 2 interferometers for predicting visual acuity in patients with cataract. Br J Ophthalmol 1983;67:273–7.

16. Haugen JP, Stamper RL, Sorenson R, Newman N. The clinical value of interferometry and blue field entoptoscopy in assessing patients with cataract. Invest Ophthalmol Vis Sci 1985;26(suppl):212–4.

17. Severin TD, Severin SL. A clinical evaluation of the potential acuity meter in 210 cases. Ann Ophthalmol 1988;20:373–5.

18. Loebl M, Riva CE. Macular circulation and the flying corpuscles phenomenon. Ophthalmology 1978;85:911–7.

19. Sinclair SH, Loebl M, Riva CE. Blue field entoptic phenomenon in cataract patients. Arch Ophthalmol 1979;97:1092–5.

20. Murphy GE. Limitations of blue field entoptoscopy in evaluating macular function. Ophthalmic Surg 1983;14:1033–6.

21. Koch DD. The role of glare testing in managing the cataract patient. Focal Points 1988;VI, Mod 4:1–11.

22. Rosenthal B, Cohen J, Bosee JC, et al. Clinical use of a new contrast sensitivity vision test chart. Invest Ophthalmol Vis Sci 1985;26(Suppl):217–20.

23. Arden G. Measuring contrast sensitivity with gratings: A new simple technique for the early diagnosis of retinal and neurological disease. J Am Optom Assoc 1979;50:35–40.

24. Pelli DG, Robson JG, Wilkins AJ. The design of a new letter chart for measuring contrast sensitivity. Clin Vis Sci 1988;2:187–99.

25. Lasa MSM, Datiles MB, Podgor MJ, Magno BV. Contrast and glare sensitivity. Ophthalmology 1992;99:1046–9.

26. Neumann AC, McCarty GR, Locke J, Cobb B. Glare disability devices for cataractous eyes: A consumer's guide. J Cataract Refract Surg 1988;14:212–6.

27. Holladay JT, Prager TC, Trujillo J, Ruiz RS. Brightness acuity test and outdoor visual acuity in cataract patients. J Cataract Refract Surg 1987;13:67–9.

28. Faulkner W. Macular function testing through opacities. Focal Points 1986;IV, Mod 2:1–10.

29. Contestabile MT, Supressa F, Vincenti P, et al. Flash visual-evoked potentials and flash electroretinography in the preoperative visual prognosis of eyes with cataracts. Ann Ophthalmol 1991;23:416–21.

30. Odom JV, Chao GM, Weinstein GW. Preoperative prediction of postoperative visual acuity in patients with cataracts: A quantitative review. Doc Ophthalmol 1988;70:5–17.

31. Sadun AA, Bassi CJ, Lessell S. Why cataracts do not produce afferent pupillary defects. Am J Ophthalmol 1990;110:712–4.

32. Lam BL, Alward WLM, Kolder HE. Effect of cataract on automated perimetry. Ophthalmology 1991;98:1066–70.

33. Bullimore MA, Bailey IL. Considerations in the subjective assessment of cataract. Optom Vis Sci 1993;70:880–5.

34. Chylack LT, Leske MC, McCarthy D, et al. Lens opacification classification system II (LOCS II). Arch Ophthalmol 1989;107:991–7.

35. West SK, Taylor HR. The detection and grading of cataract: An epidemiologic perspective. Surv Ophthalmol 1986;31:175–84.

36. Sparrow JM, Bron AJ, Brown NAP, et al. The Oxford clinical cataract classification and grading system. Int Ophthalmol 1986;9:207–25.

37. Hirst LW. Clinical evaluation of the corneal endothelium. Focal Points 1986;IV, Mod 8:1–9.

38. Zavon B, Slater N. A surgical counseling plan for patients undergoing cataract surgery. J Ophthal Nurs Technol 1988;7:68–71.

39. Takeshita B, Wing V, Gallarini L. Corning CPF filters for the preoperative cataract patient. J Am Optom Assoc 1988;59:793–7.

40. Jaffe NS, Horwitz J. Lens and Cataract. In SM Podos, M Yanoff (eds), Textbook of Ophthalmology (Vol. 3). New York: Gower, 1992.

41. Jaffe NS, Jaffe MS, Jaffe GF. Cataract Surgery and Its Complications (5th ed). St. Louis: Mosby, 1990.

42. Tennant ER. Spectacles: A new look at an old stand-by. Rev Opt 1983;120:66–74.

43. Milder B, Rubin ML. The Fine Art of Prescribing Glasses Without Making a Spectacle of Yourself (2nd ed.). Gainesville, FL: Triad, 1991.

44. Alexander LJ. Aphakia and Pseudophakia. In JF Amos (ed.), Diagnosis and Management in Vision Care. Stoneham, MA: Butterworth, 1987;639–69.

45. Edmonds SA. Contact lenses: Selection grows as technology matures. Rev Opt 1983;120:65–6.

46. Olsen T. Theoretical, computer-assisted prediction versus SRK prediction of postoperative refraction after intraocular lens implantation. J Cataract Refract Surg 1987;13:146–50.

47. Sanders DR, Retzlaff J, Kraff MC. Comparison of the SRK II formula and other second generation formulas. J Cataract Refract Surg 1988;14:136–41.

48. Dang MS, Raj PPS. SRK II formula in the calculation of intraocular lens power. Br J Ophthalmol 1989;73:823–6.

49. Hope-Ross M, Mooney D. Intraocular lens power calculation. Eye 1988;2:367–9.

50. Butcher JM, O'Brien C. The reproducibility of biometry and keratometry measurements. Eye 1991;5:708–11.

51. Holladay JT, Rubin ML. Avoiding refractive problems in cataract surgery. Surv Ophthalmol 1988;32:357–60.

52. Murphy GE, Murphy CG. Minimizing anisometropia in bilateral pseudophakia. J Cataract Refract Surg 1992;18:95–9.

53. Murrill CA, Stanfield DL, VanBrocklin MD. Primary Care of the Cataract Patient. Norwalk, CT: Appleton & Lange, 1994.

54. Clompus R. Why you should determine implant power. Rev Opt 1987;124:55–62.

55. Davis DB, Mandel MR. Posterior peribulbar anesthesia: An alternative to retrobulbar anesthesia. J Cataract Refract Surg 1986;12:182–4.

56. Agapitos PJ. Cataract surgical techniques and adjuncts. Curr Opin Ophthalmol 1992;3:13–28.

57. Agapitos PJ. Cataract surgical techniques. Curr Opin Ophthalmol 1991;2:16–27.

58. Gimbel HV. Divide and conquer nucleofractis phacoemulsification: Development and variations. J Cataract Refract Surg 1991;17:281–91.

59. Smith SG, Lindstrom RL. Intraocular Lens Complications and Their Management. Thorofare, NJ: Slack, 1988.

60. Talamo JH, Stark WJ, Gottsch JD, et al. Natural history of corneal astigmatism after cataract surgery. J Cataract Refract Surg 1991;17:313–8.

61. Cory CC. Prevention and treatment of postimplantation astigmatism. J Cataract Refract Surg 1989;15:58–60.

62. Kronish JW, Foster RK. Control of corneal astigmatism following cataract extraction by selective suture cutting. Arch Ophthalmol 1987;105:1650–5.

63. Koch PS. Complications of cataract and intraocular lens surgery. Curr Opin Ophthalmol 1991;2:53–60.

64. Gelender H. Management of corneal astigmatism after cataract surgery. Refract Corneal Surg 1991;7:99–102.

65. Grabow HB. Early results of 500 cases of no-stitch cataract surgery. J Cataract Refract Surg 1991;17:726–30.

66. Levy JH, Pisacano AM. Endothelial cell loss in four types of intraocular lens implant procedures. Am Intraocular Implant Soc J 1985;11:465–8.

67. Faulkner GD. Endothelial cell loss after phacoemulsification and insertion of silicone lens implants. J Cataract Refract Surg 1987;13:649–52.

68. Cohen EJ, Brady SE, Leavitt K, et al. Pseudophakic bullous keratopathy. Am J Ophthalmol 1988;106:264–9.

69. Flaxel JT, Swan KC. Limbal wound healing after cataract extraction. Arch Ophthalmol 1969;81:653–9.

70. Kremer I, Zandbank J, Barash D, et al. Extensive fibrous downgrowth after traumatic corneoscleral wound dehiscence. Ann Ophthalmol 1991;23:465–8.

71. Swan KC. Fibroblastic ingrowth following cataract extraction. Arch Ophthalmol 1973;89:445–9.

72. Sherrard ES, Rycroft PV. Retrocorneal membranes II. Factors influencing their growth. Br J Ophthalmol 1967;51:387–93.

73. Gutner R. Dellen. Clin Eye Vision Care 1989;1:101–3.

74. Johns KJ, Sheils P, Parrish CM, et al. Traumatic wound dehiscence in pseudophakia. Am J Ophthalmol 1989;108:535–9.

75. Soong HK, Meyer RF, Wolter JR. Fistula excision and peripheral grafts in the treatment of persistent limbal wound leaks. Ophthalmology 1988;95:31–6.

76. Hwang DG, Smith RE. Corneal complications of cataract surgery. Refract Corneal Surg 1991;7:77–80.

77. Dornic DI. How to treat suture barbs. Rev Opt 1987;124:67–8.

78. Masket S. Complications of cataract and intraocular lens surgery. Curr Opin Ophthalmol 1992;3:52–9.

79. Fry LL. Comparison of the postoperative intraocular pressure with Betagan, Betoptic, Timoptic, Iopidine, Diamox, Pilopine Gel, and Miostat. J Cataract Refract Surg 1990;15:415–26.

80. Gross JG, Meyer DR, Robin AL, et al. Increased intraocular pressure in the immediate postoperative period after extracapsular cataract extraction. Am J Ophthalmol 1988;105:466–9.

81. Weinberger D, Lusky M, Debbi S, Ben-Sira I. Pseudophakic and aphakic pupillary block. Ann Ophthalmol 1988;20:403–5.

82. Tomey KF, Traverso CE. Neodymium-YAG laser posterior capsulotomy for the treatment of aphakic and pseudophakic pupillary block. Am J Ophthalmol 1987;104:502–7.

83. Meisler DM. Intraocular inflammation and extracapsular cataract surgery. Focal Points 1990;8:1–10.

84. Brod RD, Flynn HW. Advances in the diagnosis and treatment of infectious endophthalmitis. Curr Opin Ophthalmol 1991;2:306–14.

85. Mandelbaum S, Forster RK. Postoperative endophthalmitis. Int Ophthalmol Clin 1987;27:95–106.

86. Piest KL, Kincaid MC, Tetz MR, et al. Localized endophthalmitis: a newly described cause of the so-called toxic lens syndrome. J Cataract Refract Surg 1987;13:498–510.

87. deLuise VP. Complications of intraocular lenses. Int Ophthalmol Clin 1987;27:195–204.

88. Ohadi C, Moreira H, McDonnell PJ. Posterior capsule opacification. Curr Opin Ophthalmol 1991;2:46–52.

89. Solomon KD, Legler UFC, Kostick AMP. Capsular opacification after cataract surgery. Curr Opin Ophthalmol 1992;3:46–51.

90. Argento C, Nunez E, Wainsztein R. Incidence of postoperative posterior capsular opacification with types of senile cataracts. J Cataract Refract Surg 1992;18:586–8.

91. Bene C, Hutchins R, Kranias G. Cataract wound neovascularization. Ophthalmology 1989;96:50–3.

92. Goldfarb MS, Bulas KE, Rosenberg S, Lieberman TW. Aminocaproic acid treatment of recurrent postoperative hyphemas. Ann Ophthalmol 1984;16:690–7.

93. Fisher DH, Schmidt EE. A variance of the vitreous wick syndrome and its relationship to cystoid macular edema. South J Optom 1992;10:11–5.

94. McDonnell PJ, de la Cruz ZC, Green WR. Vitreous incarceration complicating cataract surgery. Ophthalmology 1986;93:247–53.

95. Saiz A, Angulo S, Fernandez M. Atonic pupil: An unusual complication of cataract surgery. Ophthalmic Surg 1991;22:20–2.

96. Lam S, Beck RW, Hall D, Creighton JB. Atonic pupil after cataract surgery. Ophthalmology 1989;96:589–90.

97. Obstbaum SA, To K. Posterior chamber intraocular lens dislocations and malpositions. Aust NZ J Ophthalmol 1989;17:265–71.

98. Hakin K, Batterbury M, Hawksworth N, et al. Anterior tucking of the iris caused by posterior chamber lenses with polypropylene loops. J Cataract Refract Surg 1989;15:640–3.

99. Bradford JD, Wilkinson CP, Bradford RH Jr. Cystoid macular edema following extracapsular cataract extraction and posterior chamber intraocular lens implantation. Retina 1988;8:161–4.

100. Wilkinson CP. Retinal complications following cataract surgery. Focal Points 1992;10:1–9.

101. Flach AJ, Jampol LM, Weinberg D, et al. Improvement in visual acuity in chronic aphakic and pseudophakic cystoid macular edema after treatment with topical 0.5% ketorolac tromethamine. Am J Ophthalmol 1991;112:514–9.

102. Nielsen NE, Naeser K. Epidemiology of retinal detachment following extracapsular cataract extraction: A follow-up study with an analysis of risk factors. J Cataract Refract Surg 1993;19:675–80.

103. Yoshida A, Ogasowara H, Jalkh AE, et al. Retinal detachment after cataract surgery: Predisposing factors. Ophthalmology 1992;99:453–9.

104. Yoshida A, Ogasawara H, Jalkh AE, et al. Retinal detachment after cataract surgery: Surgical results. Ophthalmology 1992;99:460–5.

16

Clinical Laboratory Testing

MICHELLE M. MARCINIAK AND SARA L. PENNER

As the role of optometrists as providers of primary health care continues to expand, the importance of diagnostic modalities such as laboratory testing increases. Laboratory testing is often an integral part of making a diagnosis. The potential advantages to both the doctor and the patient are numerous. Although a careful case history and examination may indicate likely disease processes affecting the eye, laboratory values may be needed to support or exclude specific diagnoses. Proper diagnosis facilitates prompt initiation of effective therapy and, if needed, referral to an appropriate specialist or subspecialist for management of the ocular condition or its underlying systemic cause. This timely referral will improve the cost effectiveness and quality of care for the patient by eliminating visits to several practitioners. Laboratory testing allows the optometrist to become involved in the total health care of the patient. In some instances, the optometrist may directly order specific laboratory tests, while in others, suggested work-ups may be made to the patient's internist or other physician. Laboratory testing as directed by the optometrist may facilitate prompt diagnosis, and knowledge of its use allows further communication with other health care professionals. This chapter discusses laboratory testing in the areas of blood chemistry, hematology, endocrinology, serology, and skin testing commonly used by eye care practitioners.

INTERPRETATION OF TEST RESULTS

It is important to remember that a laboratory test can only approximate true disease status and is secondary or confirmatory only. All laboratory results must be interpreted in the context of a thorough case history and examination. When deciding which test to select and interpreting the results, it is essential to consider the cost (Table 16-1), reference range, sensitivity, specificity, and predictive value in order to provide high-quality patient care.

Most laboratory tests have reference ranges that can be used as a general guide to help clinicians identify abnormal values (see Appendix to this chapter). Reference ranges are identified as the 95% distribution of test results in a population that is well defined in terms of race, sex, age, and health status. These reference ranges, however, should not be used as rigid indicators of normal and abnormal. The many factors that can affect test results should be considered, including medications, presence of concurrent diseases, diet, age, sex, race, and emotional status. Reference ranges can also vary between different laboratories because of differences in methods and instrumentation. Only reference values standardized by the laboratory performing the test should be used, and only values provided by the same laboratory should be compared.

The concepts of sensitivity and specificity also guide the clinician in the selection of appropriate tests and their proper interpretation. Sensitivity is the probability that the test will be positive when applied to a patient who has the disease (true-positive rate). A highly sensitive test should be selected when screening for a serious disease that is treatable or preventable to ensure that all individuals with the disease are detected. Unfortunately, a highly sensitive test will likely produce a significant number of false-positive results because of a lack of specificity. Specificity is the probability that the test will be negative when applied to a patient who does not have the disease (true-negative rate). Because specific tests are rarely positive in the absence of disease, they aid the clinician in confirming diagnostic impressions suggested by initial sensitive tests. Ideal laboratory tests are both highly sensitive and highly specific; unfortunately, most laboratory tests are less than ideal. The sensitivity and speci-

TABLE 16-1
Estimated Cost of Common Laboratory Tests

Laboratory Test	Price Range
Total cholesterol	$$
High-density lipoprotein cholesterol	$$
Triglycerides	$$
Complete blood count with differential	$
Sickle cell preparation	$$
Hemoglobin electrophoresis	$$$$$
Thyroid-stimulating hormone	$$$$$
T_4 radioimmunoassay	$$
T_3 radioimmunoassay	$$$$$
Rapid plasma reagin/VDRL	$$
FTA-ABS	$$$
Antinuclear antibody	$$$$
Rheumatoid factor	$$$$
Angiotensin-converting enzyme	$$$$$
Serum lysozyme	$$$$
HIV ELISA	$$$$$
HIV Western Blot	$$$$$
Glycosylated hemoglobin	$$$
Free T_4	$$$$
Erythrocyte sedimentation rate	$
Toxoplasmosis antibodies	$$$$$

$ = less than $15; $$ = $15–25; $$$ = $25–35; $$$$ = $35–45; $$$$$ = $45–60.

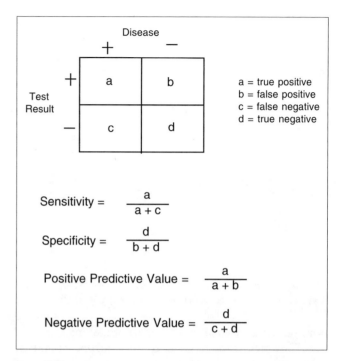

FIGURE 16-1
Calculation of sensitivity, specificity, and predictive values.

of a laboratory test are independent of the prevalence of the disease (Figure 16-1).

In contrast, while positive and negative predictive values reflect sensitivity and specificity, they are markedly affected by the disease prevalence. Positive predictive value is the probability that the disease is present when the test is positive. In a population where a disease has a low prevalence, a positive result is more likely to be false-positive, and thus, the test would have a low positive predictive value. Negative predictive value is the probability that the disease is not present when the test is negative. Thus, when the test is performed in a population with a high prevalence of a disease, a negative result is more likely to be false-negative. When interpreting and ordering laboratory tests, the clinician must consider the likelihood of the disease.

BLOOD CHEMISTRY

Glucose Determinations

Fasting Blood Glucose
Fasting blood glucose (FBG) level is reflective of the body's overall glucose metabolism. When there is an insufficient amount of insulin, an increased blood glucose level occurs,

indicating diabetes mellitus. The FBG is commonly used to screen for the presence of diabetes mellitus. It is important to obtain a fasting rather than a random serum sample because the blood glucose level is affected by dietary intake. The test requires an overnight fast of 10–16 hours. A venous plasma sample is obtained, and the glucose level is determined by various enzymatic methods (e.g., glucose oxidase, hexokinase). The National Diabetes Data Group (NDDG) has determined reference values for nonpregnant adults to be 70–115 mg/dl.[1] Values greater than 140 mg/dl are clearly abnormal, whereas values between 115 and 140 mg/dl are equivocal (Table 16-2). The FBG level may also be elevated by illness, trauma, myocardial infarction, pregnancy, endocrinopathies, certain drugs, and lack of fasting.

Oral Glucose Tolerance Test
There are some patients with impaired carbohydrate metabolism who are apparently able to compensate for the abnormality. Patients with an impaired carbohydrate metabolism demonstrate normal FBG levels.[2] These homeostatic mechanisms may be upset by a "glucose challenge," thereby unmasking the defect. The oral glucose tolerance test (OGTT or GTT) was designed for this purpose. The patient should observe a 10- to 16-hour fast the evening before, limiting fluids to water only and refraining from smoking. A baseline

TABLE 16-2
Criteria for the Diagnosis of Diabetes Mellitus

One of the four following conditions is met:
1. Classic signs or symptoms of diabetes (polydipsia, polyuria, ketonuria, and weight loss) and FBG level ≥ 140 mg/dl on one occasion only.
2. Classic signs or symptoms and nonfasting blood glucose levels > 200 mg/dl on one occasion only.
3. FBG ≥ 140 mg/dl on more than one occasion.
4. FBG < 140 mg/dl but with OGTT peak *and* 2-hour values > 200 mg/dl on more than one occasion.

FBG = fasting blood glucose; OGTT = oral glucose tolerance test.
Source: National Diabetes Data Group. Classification and diagnosis of diabetes mellitus and other categories of glucose intolerance. Diabetes 1979;28:1039–57. Copyright ® 1979 American Diabetes Association, Inc.

FBG level is obtained, followed by ingestion of a large, standardized dose of glucose. The blood glucose level is then analyzed at several time intervals (30 minutes, 1 hour, 2 hours, and 3 hours). For nonpregnant adults, a standard loading dose of 75 mg glucose or dextrose has been proposed by the NDDG. This dose is somewhat higher in pregnant women and lower in children. The glucose or dextrose may be mixed with 300 ml water and flavored with lemon juice. There are also commercial preparations available such as Glucola, a carbonated drink (Ames Co., Elkhart, IN), or Gel-a-dex, a cherry-flavored gelatin (Unitech, Sun Valley, CA).

Glucose values are expected to rise sharply after 15–60 minutes, then fall slowly, reaching the normal range within 2 hours. In patients with diabetes mellitus, glucose levels are typically greater than 200 mg/dl at the 30-minute or 1-hour peak and at 2 hours (see Table 16-2). Note that testing in pregnant women and pediatric patients requires a special testing protocol and reference ranges.

In the diagnosis of diabetes mellitus, the OGTT has high sensitivity but low specificity. Many factors can alter the outcome of the OGTT. The test should always be performed in the morning because of a diurnal variation in carbohydrate tolerance. Previous physical inactivity or limited carbohydrate intake can produce an abnormal OGTT result. A variety of other conditions can also produce abnormal OGTT values. These include various adrenal, thyroid, and pituitary abnormalities, liver or kidney disease, and alcoholism. Drugs such as steroids, thiazide diuretics, oral contraceptives, high-dose salicylates, and anticonvulsants may also produce an abnormal OGTT level. Dietary intake may likewise adversely affect the OGTT result.

The NDDG believes that there is no need to pursue OGTT testing in a patient with a sufficiently elevated FBG because the OGTT level will be abnormal in virtually all patients. However, in the presence of clinical signs and symptoms suggestive of diabetes, a normal FBG result is inconclusive and should be followed by an OGTT before diabetes mellitus is ruled out.

Glycosylated Hemoglobin

Glycosylated hemoglobin is a measure of the amount of hemoglobin A_1 ($A_{(1a)}$, $A_{(1b)}$, $A_{(1c)}$) found in the red blood cells. The degree of glycosylation parallels the concentration of blood glucose to which the erythrocyte has been exposed over its 120-day life span. The amount of hemoglobin A_1 can be measured by cationic exchange chromatography, agar gel electrophoresis, or affinity chromatography. Results are not affected by the time of day, dietary intake, exercise, administration of diabetic drugs, or emotional stress; thus, the test can be administered at any time. Normal levels are less than 8%, and levels above 12% reflect poor glycemic control. Levels may be decreased in pregnancy, hemoglobinopathies, and chronic renal failure, whereas thalassemia and iron deficiency can produce elevated levels. After glycemic control is obtained, levels will gradually return to normal. Note that glycosylated hemoglobin levels may still be elevated in patients who have only recently obtained optimal glycemic control.

Glycosylated hemoglobin provides an indicator of long-term overall glycemic control during the preceding 2–3 months, thereby providing information about the success of therapy as well as patient compliance. However, this test is not sensitive enough to be of value in establishing the diagnosis of diabetes.[3] Higher levels of hemoglobin A_1 have also been associated with the presence of diabetic retinopathy.[4]

Blood Lipid Profile

There are four major classes of lipoproteins: (1) chylomicrons, (2) very-low-density lipoproteins (VLDLs), (3) low-density lipoproteins (LDLs), and (3) high-density lipoproteins (HDLs). Each of these lipoproteins contains various amounts of cholesterol, triglycerides, phospholipids, and proteins (Table 16-3). Lipoprotein disturbances can occur as primary phenomena or secondary phenomena caused by numerous states such as renal disease, diabetes mellitus, liver disease, hypothyroidism, and chronic alcoholism. The blood lipid profile allows the hyperlipoproteinemias to be determined and classified. Certain components of the profile are also accepted as predictors of atherosclerotic risk. The greatest risk of coronary artery disease (CAD) is associated with LDLs, which carry the greatest proportion of cholesterol. The HDLs possess some capacity to remove cholesterol from tissue and con-

TABLE 16-3

The Four Major Classes of Lipoproteins and Their Relative Compositions

	Triglycerides (%)	Cholesterol (%)	Phospholipids (%)	Protein (%)
Chylomicrons	85–95	3–5	5–10	1–2
VLDL	60–70	10–15	10–15	10
LDL	5–10	45	20–30	15–25
HDL	Very little	20	30	50

VLDL = very low-density lipoprotein; LDL = low-density lipoprotein; HDL = high-density lipoprotein.
Source: Reprinted with permission from FK Widman. General Chemistry—Lipids. Clinical Interpretation of Laboratory Tests (9th ed). Philadelphia: FA Davis, 1983:257.

TABLE 16-4

Classification of the Hyperlipoproteinemias

Type	Electrophoretic Findings	Refrigerated Serum Appearance	Serum Analysis	Prevalence
1	Marked ↑ CLM ± ↓ VLDL ± ↓ LDL ± ↓ HDL	Marked cream layer – Turbidity	Mild ↑ C Marked ↑ TG	Rare
2a	– CLM Normal VLDL ↑ LDL Normal HDL	– Cream layer – Turbidity	Mild ↑ C Normal TG	Common
2b	– CLM ↑ VLDL ↑ LDL Normal HDL	– Cream layer ± Turbidity	Modest ↑ C Mild ↑ TG	Common
3	± CLM ↑ VLDL ↑ LDL Normal HDL	± Cream layer Moderate turbidity	Mild ↑ C Mild ↑ TG	Uncommon
4	– CLM ↑ VLDL Normal LDL Normal HDL	– Cream layer Moderate turbidity	± Mild ↑ C Modest ↑ TG	Very common
5	Modest ↑ CLM ↑ VLDL Normal LDL Normal HDL1	Modest cream layer Marked turbidity	Mild ↑ C Marked ↑ TG	Uncommon

CLM = chylomicrons; VLDL = very low-density lipoproteins; LDL = low-density lipoproteins; HDL = high-density lipoproteins; C = cholesterol; TG = triglycerides; ↑ = increased; ↓ = decreased; ± = present or absent.

tain protein as their main constituent, thereby exerting a protective effect against atherogenesis. The blood lipid profile includes total cholesterol, high-density lipoprotein cholesterol, low-density lipoprotein cholesterol calculation, and total triglycerides. Testing requires a fasting sample with no alcohol intake during the preceding 24–48 hours. Serum analysis is preferred to plasma analysis because anticoagulants can decrease triglyceride and cholesterol levels. Table 16-4 outlines the exact classification of the hyperlipoproteinemias. In most cases, serum cholesterol level,

triglyceride levels, and the appearance of serum when it is refrigerated are sufficient to permit accurate characterization. However, there are instances when electrophoretic studies may be necessary to make the differentiation.

Total Serum Cholesterol

Cholesterol is a steroid alcohol produced mainly in the liver and transported in the blood by the lipoproteins. It is used by the body to form steroid hormones, bile acids, and most cell membranes. The total serum cholesterol level is determined by enzymatic methods and reflects the sum total of all the cholesterol contained within the various types of lipoproteins. Age-related limits have been determined by the Expert Panel of the National Cholesterol Education Program (NCEP).[5-7] For men and women over the age of 20 years, total cholesterol values less than 200 mg/dl are acceptable. Values of 200–239 mg/dl are borderline, and values above 240 mg/dl are elevated, placing the patient in a category of high risk for coronary artery disease (Table 16-5). If an abnormal value is obtained, the test should be repeated again at the same time of day in 1–3 weeks because a 20- to 30-mg/dl physiologic variation of total cholesterol is possible.[2] Total cholesterol level may be increased in hypothyroidism, pregnancy, nephrotic syndrome, and obesity. Decreased levels are associated with hyperthyroidism, malnutrition, active infection, and liver disease. In addition, values can also be affected by use of certain drugs.

High-Density Lipoprotein Cholesterol

After precipitating out the VLDL and LDL components, measurement of the HDL fraction is obtained by centrifugation of the patient's remaining serum. The cholesterol component in this HDL fraction is then determined by enzymatic methods. The adult reference ranges are approximately 22–68 mg/dl for men and 30–80 mg/dl for women. The HDL level may be increased in patients who engage in frequent physical activity or who use moderate doses of alcohol.[8]

The ratio of total cholesterol to HDL cholesterol (HDL-C) is a useful index in estimating a patient's risk for CAD. Average risk is indicated by a ratio of 5:1, whereas 10:1 and 20:1 represent double and triple the risk, respectively.[2,9] This ratio should be interpreted in association with LDL cholesterol (LDL-C) levels, since a low ratio or increased HDL level does not entirely negate the ill effects of high LDL levels.

Low-Density Lipoprotein Cholesterol

Because direct determination is costly and only available through certain laboratories, the LDL-C fraction is most commonly calculated. This value is estimated using the Friedewald formula: LDL-C = total C – (HDL-C– 1/5 TG). The average cholesterol in VLDL is corrected for by subtracting one-fifth of the triglycerides. This formula is only accurate when triglycerides are less than 400 mg/dl. A cutoff of 130 mg/dl is advocated as the upper limit of normal by the NCEP. Borderline values range from 130 to 159 mg/dl, and values above 159 mg/dl place the patient at a risk for the development of coronary artery disease.[5,6] The cholesterol transported by the LDLs can be deposited in peripheral tissues and results in CAD and peripher-

TABLE 16-5
National Cholesterol Education Program (NCEP) Guidelines for Cholesterol Levels

Cholesterol Level (mg/dl)	Classification*
<200	Acceptable
200–239	Borderline
>240	Elevated

*For ages >20 years.
Source: The Expert Panel. Report of the National Cholesterol Education Program Expert Panel on detection, evaluation, and treatment of high blood cholesterol in adults. Arch Intern Med 1988;148:36–69, and Adult Treatment Panel II. Second report of the Expert Panel of the National Cholesterol Education Program. Detection, evaluation, and treatment of high blood cholesterol in adults. Circulation 1994;89:1329–45.

al vascular disease. Compared with LDL-C, the ratio of LDL-C to HDL-C is an even better predictor of CAD.

Triglycerides

Triglycerides are primarily contained in the chylomicrons and the VLDLs. Because chylomicrons are usually absent in fasting samples, the triglyceride determination is an accurate reflection of the VLDL level. According to the 1984 National Institutes of Health consensus conference on hypertriglyceridemia, normal serum triglyceride levels are less than or equal to 250 mg/dl. Values between 250 and 500 mg/dl are borderline, and values above 500 mg/dl are abnormal, indicating hypertriglyceridemia.[10]

The appearance of refrigerated serum provides useful clues about the triglyceride content. A turbid or lactescent quality to the sample will occur with elevated VLDL levels. Hyperchylomicronemia results in a creamy layer atop the serum.

Triglyceride levels are most beneficial in screening for and classifying hyperlipidemia. Although elevated triglycerides are frequently associated with low HDL levels, their use in determining the risk of CAD is limited. They do not directly contribute to atherosclerotic risk but are most likely markers of a high-risk lifestyle or metabolic characteristics.

Angiotensin-Converting Enzyme

In normal individuals, angiotensin-converting enzyme (ACE) is found in many cells and body fluids and functions to catalyze the cleavage of C-terminal dipeptides from a variety of peptides. The conversion of angiotensin I to the potent vasopressor angiotensin II is an illustrative example. The serum ACE level is believed to reflect the total body load of granulomatous tissue. In patients with sarcoidosis, ACE levels may be elevated because of release of this enzyme from epithelioid cells and macrophages within the sarcoid granuloma. This test alone is not specific for sarcoidosis, because elevated ACE levels may also be seen with leprosy, Gaucher's disease, primary biliary cirrhosis, histoplasmosis, hyperthyroidism, diabetes mellitus, and connective tissue diseases.

The laboratory determination of ACE levels involves a spectrophotometric determination of a biochemical reaction in which the production of one of the major reactants is dependent on the peptidase activities of ACE. The reference range for patients over 20 years of age is 6.1–21.1 U/liter. These values are somewhat higher for the under-20 age group, in which up to 42.1 U/liter may be considered normal.

In sarcoidosis, the ACE level clearly reflects the severity of the disease and may be used to monitor disease activity. Elevated ACE levels are seen in 68% of patients with stage I sarcoidosis, in 86% of patients with stage II disease, and in 92% of patients with stage III disease.[11] Topical and systemic steroids will inhibit ACE activity, potentially producing false-negative test results.

Serum Lysozyme

Lysozyme, like ACE, is released from cells within the sarcoid granuloma. Most commonly, an increase in the serum lysozyme level will parallel an increase in the ACE level, although rarely the serum lysozyme level alone will be elevated. The latter is of limited value and may be caused by numerous other conditions including leprosy, tuberculosis, pernicious anemia, Reiter's syndrome, and rheumatoid arthritis.

The ability of lysozyme to dissolve certain cell walls is the basis for laboratory testing. The organism *Micrococcus lysodieticus* is exposed to the patient's plasma. A spectrophotometer is used to determine changes in the turbidity of the solution as the enzyme attacks the organism's cell walls. The rate of clearing is proportional to the concentration of serum lysozyme. The normal reference range is 0.2–15.8 µg/ml for all ages. As with ACE level determination, false-negative results may occur if the assay is performed after institution of steroid therapy.

Baarsma et al.[12] studied 221 patients with uveitis of various causes including 12 patients with sarcoidosis. For patients with ACE levels above 50 U/liter, the test sensitivity was 84% with a 95% specificity and a predictive value of 47%. For elevated serum lysozyme levels greater than 8 µg/ml, the sensitivity dropped to 60% with a test specificity of 76% and a predictive value of only 12%. An ACE level above 40 U/liter in combination with a serum lysozyme level over 10 µg/ml results in a predictive value of 83%. In conclusion, careful interpretation of both ACE and serum lysozyme values in combination with the clinical picture is of considerable value in the diagnosis of sarcoidosis.

Metabolites

Bilirubin

Bilirubin, a by-product of hemoglobin degradation, is secreted by the liver as the major pigment in bile. Normally, only small amounts are detectable in the serum. A rise in the serum bilirubin concentration occurs with excessive destruction of red blood cells or with liver dysfunction. The reference bilirubin level for fasting adults is 0.1–1.2 mg/dl. When levels exceed 2.5 mg/dl, the abundant bilirubin stains the tissues, resulting in jaundice or scleral icterus. High levels of bilirubin are most commonly associated with liver dysfunction (e.g., hepatitis, cirrhosis, and primary or metastatic hepatic neoplasm). Certain anemias (e.g., sickle cell, hemolytic) and infectious mononucleosis may also cause increased bilirubin levels. A small chronic elevation can lead to gallstone formation. Low serum bilirubin levels are of little clinical importance.

Blood Urea Nitrogen

Urea is formed in the liver as an end-product of protein catabolism and is then excreted by the kidneys. When kidney function is compromised, urea accumulates in the blood, resulting in azotemia. Blood urea nitrogen (BUN) is a test of kidney function and can be used to determine the need for renal dialysis. For adults, reference BUN values are 10–20 mg/dl. Chronic renal failure is the most common cause of increased serum BUN. There are, however, other, nonrenal causes including gastrointestinal bleeding, excessive protein catabolism or ingestion, congestive heart failure, hypovolemia, dehydration, fever, shock, certain drugs, and burns. Levels may be slightly higher in males than females. Blood urea nitrogen values may be decreased in primary liver disease.

Creatinine

Creatinine is a nitrogenous waste product of normal protein catabolism in muscle tissue. Under normal conditions, it is filtered by the kidneys at a steady rate and excreted in the urine. Values are typically in the range of 0.7–1.5 mg/dl. Normal values are related to the overall body muscle mass and are affected by age, sex, and weight. In elderly patients, decreased muscle mass may result in decreased values. In most instances, an elevated creatinine level signals kidney dysfunction. Levels can also be altered by exercise and a diet high in proteins.

Unlike BUN, creatinine levels are not affected by dehydration or hepatic disease. Creatinine is considered a more sensitive test for kidney dysfunction than BUN; however, when used together, these two tests give the most accurate assessment of kidney function. Compared with the creatinine level, the BUN level rises more steeply in renal failure and declines more rapidly with dialysis. In severe long-term renal impairment, BUN levels will continue to increase, whereas creatinine levels will plateau because of alimentary excretion. It is important to obtain BUN and creatinine values before ordering computed tomography with contrast to be sure the patient can effectively clear the contrast dye. In patients suspected of having compromised renal function, BUN and creatine measurements should be considered when prescribing systemic drugs with renal toxicities such as acetazolamide or an aminoglycoside.

The renal system plays a vital role in maintaining the body's homeostasis. BUN and creatinine reflect renal function or, more specifically, glomerular filtration rate (GFR). Although BUN may reflect the GFR, it is also influenced by urea production and reabsorption. As previously stated, creatinine is a more direct and more sensitive assessment of the GFR. However, a normal creatinine does not necessarily indicate a normal GFR. In cases where renal compromise is suspected, additional testing is necessary if BUN and creatinine values are in the normal range.

For a healthy individual in a steady state, daily creatinine production remains fairly constant if muscle mass is not significantly changed. As part of the normal aging process, an elderly person will simultaneously have a decrease in muscle mass and loss of renal function (GFR). Thus, the kidneys are presented with decreasing amounts of creatinine and become less capable of filtering and excreting creatinine. This results in a creatinine value in the "normal" range despite abnormal renal function. BUN and creatinine measurements alone may not provide an accurate assessment of renal function. For this reason, creatinine clearance is a better index of renal function, especially in elderly persons. Creatinine clearance is an assessment of the daily quantity of urine excreted as well as the serum creatinine. It may be directly measured via 24-hour urine collection, but it is most commonly determined by calculation.

Electrolytes

Potassium
Potassium (K^+) is the major intracellular cation. It functions to maintain acid–alkaline balance, activate enzymes, process and store carbohydrates, and determine action potentials. Reference values for adults are 3.5–5.5 mEq/liter. Because the serum concentration of potassium is so small, minor changes in concentration have significant consequences. Hyperkalemia, or increased potassium level, is associated with kidney failure, massive tissue trauma (crush injury, severe burns), adrenal insufficiency, Addison's disease, potassium-sparing diuretics (e.g., spironolactone and triamterene), and hypoaldosteronism. Conditions causing hypokalemia, or decreased potassium level, include alkalosis, chronic diarrhea, potassium-depleting diuretics (acetazolamide, furosemide), vomiting, excessive ingestion of licorice, Cushing's syndrome, chronic stress, use of anti-inflammatory drugs, and hyperaldosteronism. In patients who are hypokalemic, potassium supplements should be given concomitantly with K^+-depleting diuretics.

Sodium
Sodium (Na^+) is the major cation in the extracellular space. It is responsible for maintaining fluid balance, regulating acid–alkaline equilibrium, and preserving normal muscle function. Sodium and water are physiologically closely interrelated. As the free body water level increases, sodium concentration decreases and vice versa. For adults, reference values are 136–145 mEq/liter.

Hypernatremia, or increased sodium level, normally does not occur without concurrent water retention but may be seen in association with vomiting, diarrhea, polyuria, excessive dietary intake, Cushing's syndrome, hyperaldosteronism, and excessive sweating. Symptoms of hypernatremia include dry sticky mucous membranes, flushed skin, increased body temperature, lack of tears, and thirst. Hyponatremia, or decreased sodium level, may be signaled by fatigue, weakness, apprehension, and convulsions. Conditions commonly causing hyponatremia include insufficient aldosterone, Addison's disease, congestive heart failure, renal insufficiency, and chronic diuretic use with a Na^+-restricted diet.

Chloride
Chloride (Cl^-) is the major extracellular anion. Chloride regulates the fluid pressure across cell membranes, which maintains electrical neutrality and water balance. Abnormal chloride levels rarely occur in isolation and are usually associated with changes in sodium concentration. The reference range for adults is 95–105 mEq/liter.

Excessive fluid loss (vomiting, heavy perspiration, burns, Addison's disease, and diarrhea) may produce hypochloremia or decreased chloride level. Hyperchloremia, or increased chloride level, may be found in kidney dysfunction, hyperthyroidism, anemia, heart disease, Cushing's syndrome, multiple myeloma, and dehydration.

Carbon Dioxide

Serum carbon dioxide (CO_2) level is actually a measurement of bicarbonate (HCO_3^-). It can be used to assess acid-alkaline equilibrium. Values in normal adults range from 23 to 30 mEq/liter. Increased CO_2 causes alkalosis and may be caused by vomiting, diarrhea, diuretic use, intake of excess bicarbonate, and aspirin overdose. Acidosis results from a decreased CO_2 level. Kidney and liver disease, severe dehydration, methyl alcohol poisoning, lung disease, oversedation, congestive heart failure, and head injury are all associated with decreased levels of CO_2.

Liver Function Testing

Alkaline Phosphatase

Alkaline phosphatase (ALP) is an enzyme that is responsible for mediating bone, liver, and cellular transport at alkaline pH. Levels vary with age, increasing during the first months of life, puberty, and pregnancy, reaching adult levels by age 20 years, and occasionally increasing in elderly individuals. In normal adults, values are 25–97 IU/liter. Certain drugs (e.g., penicillin, erythromycin, indomethacin, oral contraceptives, methyldopa, and antianxiety agents) can increase serum ALP levels. Pathologic increases are either caused by liver disease (intrahepatic) or bone disease (extrahepatic). Intrahepatic causes include obstructive and hepatocellular disease, jaundice, primary biliary cirrhosis, viral hepatitis, metastatic carcinoma, and space-occupying hepatic lesions. Active bone formation is associated with the extrahepatic causes. These include Paget's disease, rickets, osteomalacia, metastatic choroidal melanoma, and healing fractures. In severe orbital blowout fractures, ALP levels may rise 1 week later and will remain elevated for 6–8 weeks.

Aminotransferases

The aminotransferases (aspartate and alanine aminotransferase) catalyze the reversible transfer of an amino group between an amino acid and an alpha-keto acid. Aspartate aminotransferase (AST) was previously referred to as serum glutamic-oxaloacetic transaminase (SGOT). It is found primarily in the liver, heart, and skeletal muscle. Reference values are 7–27 U/liter. After cell injury or death, AST is released into the blood at a level directly related to the amount of damage. The level is also proportional to the time between the injury and the test. Thus, AST is used in determining the timing, initiation, and resolution of myocardial infarction. Other causes of increased serum AST levels are infectious mononucleosis, hepatitis, and metastatic or primary liver neoplasm.

Alanine aminotransferase (ALT) was previously referred to as serum glutamic-pyruvic transaminase (SGPT) and is found predominantly in the liver. Liver damage, such as in hepatitis, jaundice, or neoplasm, results in elevated ALT levels. For adults, reference values are 1–21 U/liter. Although both AST and ALT are commonly thought of as liver enzymes, ALT is found mainly in the liver, whereas AST is also present in myocardium, skeletal muscle, the brain, and the kidneys, making ALT a more sensitive and specific test for liver dysfunction. Typically these two enzyme levels rise and fall in parallel, but AST may be elevated in conjunction with a normal ALT level as occurs after myocardial infarction.

HEMATOLOGY

Complete Blood Count with Differential

The complete blood count comprises a white blood cell count, a red blood cell count, red blood cell indices, hemoglobin level, hematocrit, and platelet count. The differential yields the percentage composition of each different white blood cell type, which is useful in determining the cause of an abnormal hematologic state.

White Blood Cell Count and Differential

White blood cells (WBCs), or leukocytes, are the body's first line of defense against infection. The total WBC count is a useful tool in detecting the presence of disease. The number of WBCs per cubic millimeter of whole blood is measured by an automated cell counter. In adults, the normal reference range is $4.5–11.0 \times 10^3$ cells/μl. This range may be lower by 0.5×10^3 in blacks. The most common pathologic cause of a high WBC count, or leukocytosis, is infection, especially bacterial. However, in elderly, severely debilitated, and immunocompromised patients, the WBC count may not be elevated even in severe infection. Leukocytosis can occur in patients who are not elderly, debilitated, or immunocompromised in association with severe pain, emotional stress, pregnancy, myocardial infarction, stroke, strenuous exercise, and after epinephrine injection. An abnormally low WBC count, or leukopenia, may be secondary to certain chemical compounds, collagen vascular disease, primary hematologic disorders or bone marrow disease, exposure to ionizing radiation, viral illness, or an impaired immune system.

The percentage of each different type of leukocyte is determined by the WBC differential count. The differential count is important because while the total WBC count may be normal, abnormalities may still exist. The differ-

TABLE 16-6
White Blood Cell Count Differential, Expected Values

	Normal Values (% of Total WBCs)	Elevated	Depressed
Neutrophils	50–70	Infection Physiologic stressors Myelocytic leukemia Catecholamines Glucocorticoids Diabetic ketoacidosis Renal failure Tissue breakdown	Cancer chemotherapy Certain viral infections Aplastic anemia Immunocompromise Malnutrition
Eosinophils	0–5	Parasitic infection Allergic reaction Eczema Myelogenous leukemia Autoimmune disease Addison's disease	Elevated adrenal steroid production
Basophils	0–1	Granulocytic and basophilic leukemia Myeloid metaplasia	Hyperthyroidism Stress Prolonged steroid therapy
Lymphocytes	20–40	Viral illness Infectious mononucleosis Lymphocytic malignancy Chronic inflammation Autoimmune disease Thyrotoxicosis	HIV infection Hodgkin's disease Aplastic anemia Steroid use Renal failure Systemic lupus erythematosus Sarcoidosis
Monocytes	0–7	Viral infections Bacterial and parasitic infections Lymphoma Multiple myeloma	Not associated with specific disorders

Source: Adapted with permission from J Gawlikowski. White cells at war. Am J Nursing 1992(March):49.

ential count may be determined by automated differential counters or by manual inspection of a slide smeared with peripheral blood (i.e., blood taken from an extremity).

There are two main categories of leukocytes: granulocytes and agranulocytes. The granulocytes, or polymorphonuclear leukocytes (PMNs), are characterized by prominent cytoplasmic granules and a single multilobed nucleus. They include neutrophils, eosinophils, and basophils. The agranulocytes, which include lymphocytes and monocytes, do not contain cytoplasmic granules, have a single-lobed nucleus, and are stored in the lymph nodes, spleen, and liver. The expected values for each WBC type are outlined in Table 16-6.[13]

An increased percentage of neutrophils, or PMNs, is termed neutrophilia. Neutrophilia may be caused by bacterial infection, tissue destruction (burns, trauma, malignancy, collagen vascular disease, or infarction), toxic metabolic states (diabetic acidosis, uremia, convulsions), certain drugs (corticosteroids, lithium, epinephrine, digitalis, sulfonamides), acute hemorrhage, and hematolog-

ic disorders. Although steroid use increases the number of PMNs, it also concomitantly decreases their ability to function, and therefore the patient is more susceptible to infection. Neutrophilia is further classified as a "shift to the left" or "shift to the right." A "shift to the left" is indicative of excessive immature PMNs, or bands, in the peripheral blood. This occurs when bone marrow reserves are depleted because of severe infection or bone marrow disorders. A "shift to the right" results from an increase in the number of mature PMNs because of tissue breakdown or necrosis.

Neutropenia is characterized by a decreased number of neutrophils or PMNs in the peripheral blood. It may be secondary to aplastic anemia, hypersplenism, septicemia, chemotherapy, heredity, and vitamin B_{12}/folate deficiency. When neutropenia exists, the patient is at an increased risk for infection.

An abnormal eosinophil count is typically benign. Persistent eosinophilia is suggestive of parasitic infection, allergic disease, or some chronic dermatologic conditions.

Basophils constitute less than 1% of the total white blood cells. Although their function is poorly understood, they most likely play a role in hypersensitivity. An increased number of basophils (basophilia) is associated with chronic myelogenous leukemia and other myeloproliferative disorders. Because basophils are present in very low numbers, it is difficult to assess a decrease in their number.

Lymphocytes arise in the bone marrow and constitute 20–40% of all WBCs. Consisting of T cells and B cells, the lymphocytes mediate cellular immunity and produce antibodies. Total lymphocyte count is age-dependent. Newborns and children under 4 years old have higher counts.

Lymphocytosis is a rise in the total number of lymphocytes. Viral infection is the most common cause of lymphocytosis. This is actually a relative lymphocytosis because of the decreased granulocyte count that typically occurs following viral infection. Absolute lymphocytosis occurs in chronic lymphocytic leukemia, pertussis, infectious lymphocytosis, infectious mononucleosis, measles, mumps, toxoplasmosis, and cytomegalovirus infection. Reduction of lymphocytes is known as lymphocytopenia. Conditions associated with lymphocytopenia include systemic lupus erythematosus, burns, trauma, Hodgkin's disease, corticosteroid therapy, HIV infection, malignancy, and radiation therapy.

Monocytes are few in number but are responsible for mounting the first local defense against bacterial infection. When they enter the tissues, monocytes become macrophages that phagocytize invading antigens. Elevated levels of monocytes (monocytosis) typically occur in the recovery phase of acute viral, bacterial, or parasitic infection. Bacterial endocarditis, disseminated tuberculosis, carcinoma, and primary hematologic disorders are other potential causes of monocytosis.

Total Red Blood Cell Count

Red blood cells (RBCs), or erythrocytes, are responsible for transporting oxygen. The red blood cell count is typically determined by an automatic cell counter and is expressed as the number of RBCs per cubic millimeter. Normal adult values are 4.5–6.0×10^{12}/liter in men and 4.0–5.5×10^{12}/liter in women. Polycythemia exists when the number of circulating RBCs is above normal. Primary polycythemia is caused by hyperactive bone marrow and is a true hematologic disorder. Secondary polycythemia may be a physiologic response to high altitude or a pathologic response to hypoxia or increased levels of erythropoietin. Whether it is primary or secondary, polycythemia results in serum hyperviscosity. Conditions in which RBCs may be deficient include erythropoietin-deficient states, blood loss, systemic lupus erythematosus, leukemia, and with exposure to certain drugs (quinine, chloramphenicol) and toxic substances (lead, arsenic).

Erythrocytes may be further characterized in terms of size, shape, and structure by manual examination of a peripheral blood smear. These characteristics often provide useful information in differentiating among types of anemias and blood dyscrasias.

Hematocrit

Hematocrit is a measure of the volume of RBCs in 100 ml of blood. This measure is useful in establishing the presence and severity of anemia. The whole blood sample is centrifuged. The height of the column of packed red blood cells is then measured and compared with a column of original whole blood. The result is expressed as a percentage, and reference values are 39–49% in males and 33–43% in females. Directly related to the RBC count, the hematocrit provides information about the size, capacity, and number of RBCs. Increased hematocrit is found with severe burns, surgery, shock, dehydration, chronic obstructive pulmonary disease, and polycythemia vera. Massive blood loss, anemia, and leukemia may cause a decreased hematocrit.

Hemoglobin

Oxygen is transported through the body bound to hemoglobin in the RBCs. Hemoglobin concentration is an index of the blood's capacity to carry oxygen and carbon dioxide. Normal values may be lower in blacks than whites. The range is 12.0–15.0 g/dl in women and 13.6–17.2 g/dl in men. Values are reduced in sickle cell anemia, thalassemia, B_{12}/folate deficiency, and lead poisoning.

Red Blood Cell Indices

The RBC indices are calculated using the RBC count, hematocrit, and hemoglobin. They provide information about the size, weight, and hemoglobin concentration of RBCs. The indices include mean cell volume (MCV), mean cell hemoglobin (MCH), and mean cell hemoglobin concentration (MCHC). The MCV is an estimate of the average volume or size of a single RBC. It is calculated by dividing the hematocrit by the RBC count. Results can be classified as microcytosis, macrocytosis, or normocytosis. Normal values are 80–100 μm^3. Mean cell hemoglobin (MCH) is a measure of the average weight or amount of hemoglobin in a single RBC. It is calculated by dividing hemoglobin by the RBC count. The reference range is 26–34 pg (picogram). The MCHC is determined by dividing the hemoglobin by the hematocrit, and values should be approximately 31–37%. This is an approximation of the average concentration or the percentage of hemoglobin per cell and is helpful in identifying anemia. One should always interpret the MCH together with the MCV, since larger cells will contain larger amounts of hemoglobin. Hemoglobin content is classified as normochromic, hypochromic, or hyperchromic.

Platelet Count

Responsible for activating the blood clotting mechanism, platelets, or thrombocytes, are composed mainly of polysaccharides and phospholipids. Normal values are 150–450 $\times 10^3/mm^3$. An elevated platelet level is termed thrombocytosis. Conditions known to produce thrombocytosis include malignancy, acute bleeding, infection, splenectomy, cerebral vascular disease, and myeloproliferative syndromes. It may also result in emboli formation secondary to platelet aggregation. Thrombocytopenia, or decreased platelets, can occur in drug-induced, immunologic, and idiopathic conditions as well as after transfusion, hypersplenism, and bone marrow deficiency.

Erythrocyte Sedimentation Rate

A nonspecific hematologic test, the erythrocyte sedimentation rate (ESR) measures the rate at which RBCs settle out of anticoagulated blood in a given period of time. Normally, the downward pull of gravity is balanced by the upward current of plasma displacement, and therefore minimal settling occurs. In conditions such as injury, inflammation, malignancy, and pregnancy, there is an elevation in immunoglobulins and fibrinogen levels that leads to increased aggregation of RBCs into coin-like stacks called rouleaux. The rouleaux configuration falls faster than individual RBCs, resulting in an increased ESR. Values are also affected by age and sex.

The ESR can be determined by either the Wintrobe or the Westergren technique. In the Wintrobe technique, undiluted anticoagulated blood is allowed to settle in a long, thin, calibrated tube for 1 hour. The settled RBCs are then measured in millimeters. Reference values are in the range of 0–8 mm/hr for men and 0–15 mm/hr for women. Although it is easier to perform and more sensitive to small departures from the normal range, the Wintrobe technique is unable to reliably differentiate readings greater than 50 mm/hr. Therefore, the Westergren method is the technique of choice because it is more sensitive in the abnormal range. It is performed similar to the Wintrobe technique, but the anticoagulated blood is diluted with sodium citrate or saline. The reference ranges are typically cited as 1–10 mm/hr for men and 0–15 mm/hr for women. The ESR value is known to increase after the age of 50 years,[14] and the following formulas may be used to obtain an age-corrected value[15]:

TABLE 16-7
Signs of Temporal Arteritis

Ocular signs
    Amaurosis fugax
    Anterior ischemic optic neuropathy
    Central retinal artery occlusion
    Extraocular muscle palsies (III, IV, VI)
    Posterior segment ischemia
    Anterior segment ischemia
Nonocular signs
    Headache
    Scalp tenderness
    Jaw claudication
    Fever
    Malaise
    Weight loss
    Vertigo
    Deafness
    Myalgia

$$\text{Men: age}/2$$
$$\text{Women: (age + 10)}/2$$

Generally, the ESR is not sensitive or specific enough as a screening device for occult disease in asymptomatic patients. It may be useful in following the level of disease activity in patients with known infection or inflammation. In patients suspected of having temporal arteritis (Table 16-7), the ESR is approximately 99% sensitive and 70% specific.[16] In temporal arteritis, it is typical for the ESR to be markedly elevated to more than 50 mm/hour.[17] However, a normal ESR does not exclude the diagnosis, and further testing including temporal artery biopsy is warranted if this diagnosis is suspected. "Normal" ESR values may be found in temporal arteritis caused by prior steroid treatment, diurnal fluctuation,[18] or other systemic disease.[19]

Testing for Hemoglobinopathies

Screening for abnormal forms of hemoglobin or hemoglobinopathies may be done with the sickle cell preparation or a solubility test. Cells that contain hemoglobin S (HbS) will sickle when exposed to low oxygen tension. This principle is used in performing the sickle cell preparation. A reducing agent is added to the cell suspension and is examined 15 minutes later for sickling. If HbS is present in concentrations greater than 10%, sickling will occur, yielding a positive result. The solubility test relies on the formation of insoluble polymers when HbS is deoxygenated. This results in an increased turbidity of the solution. A test is positive if black newspaper print cannot be read through the solution because of the degree of turbidity.

These screening tests have very limited application because they only identify the presence but not the quantity of HbS and thus fail to distinguish between sickle cell trait (AS), sickle cell anemia (SS), and sickle cell C disease (SC). In addition, these tests fail to identify other hemoglobinopathies, such as thalassemia, in which HbS is not involved. False-negative results can occur if there is less than 10% HbS.

Any negative result for a screening test in a patient with clinical findings suggestive of a hemoglobinopathy and any positive screening test result should be followed with quantitative analysis by hemoglobin electrophoresis. Hemolyzed RBCs are placed on a cellulose acetate sheet and exposed to an electrical current, or electrophoresis, for 30 minutes. The charged hemoglobin molecules will move at varying rates. The cellulose acetate membrane is then stained to quantify and identify the different types of hemoglobin by their position. Hemoglobin A will migrate faster than HbS, which migrates faster than HbC. Reference values are 95–98% for HbA, 1.5–3.0% for HbA2, and 0–2% for HbF (fetal hemoglobin) in the absence of any abnormal variants (hemoglobin S, C, or E). To demonstrate other uncommon hemoglobin variants, more advanced techniques and other support media may be required.

ENDOCRINOLOGY

Thyroid Function Tests

An understanding of the various components involved in the hypothalamic-anterior pituitary-thyroid complex is essential to the discussion of the numerous assays for determining thyroid function (Figure 16-2). The hypothalamus secretes thyrotropin-releasing hormone (TRH), which influences the anterior pituitary to synthesize and secrete thyrotropin, also known as thyroid-stimulating hormone (TSH). In response to TSH, the thyroid gland synthesizes and secretes the active iodine compounds thyroxine (T_4) and triiodothyronine (T_3). Along with regulating lipid and carbohydrate metabolism, the free thyroid hormones exert a negative feedback effect on the pituitary and, to a lesser extent, the hypothalamus. Thus, increased levels of T_3 and T_4 lead to decreased levels of TSH, and decreased thyroid hormone levels initiate increased TSH secretion.

The primary assays used to evaluate thyroid function include total serum T_4 and T_3 assays, thyroid hormone-binding ratio or T_3 resin uptake, free T_4, and serum thy-

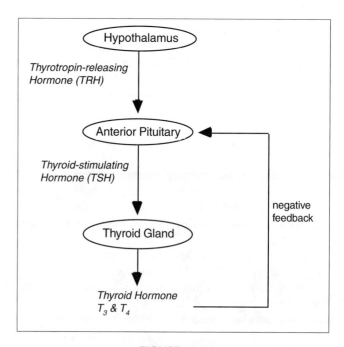

FIGURE 16-2
Hypothalamic–anterior pituitary–thyroid complex.

rotropin assay. The signs and symptoms of thyroid dysfunction are outlined in Table 16-8.

Total Serum T_4 and T_3 Assays

Almost all circulating molecules T_4 and T_3 are bound to serum proteins, the most common being thyroxine-binding globulin (TBG). Biological activity is only provided by the very small percentage of unbound thyroid hormones. Total serum thyroid hormone concentrations are a measure of all free and bound hormone. These concentrations are determined by radioimmunoassay (RIA). The RIA technique involves competitive inhibition in which a radiolabeled tracer hormone is displaced from a T_4 or T_3 antibody binding site by serum T_4 or T_3.

The normal T_4RIA reference range for adults is 4–12 μg/dl. Elevated levels are suggestive of but not diagnostic of thyrotoxicosis. Alterations in thyroid binding proteins may also produce abnormal levels. Increases in TBG, causing elevated serum T_4, may occur in a number of conditions including increased estrogen levels (e.g., pregnancy, oral contraceptive use, estrogen therapy), liver disease, certain drug use, and genetic predisposition. In contrast, nephrotic syndrome, acromegaly, androgens, glucocorticoids, malnutrition, hyperproteinemia, and genetic predisposition can produce TBG-deficient states. There are also certain drug interactions (e.g., high-dose salicylates and phenytoin) that produce a decrease in serum T_4 levels.

TABLE 16-8
Signs and Symptoms of Thyroid Dysfunction

Hyperthyroidism
　Nervousness
　Fatigue
　Weight loss despite increased appetite
　Heat intolerance
　Tachycardia
Hypothyroidism
　Lethargy
　Dry skin/hair
　Facial puffiness
　Cold intolerance
　Memory impairment
　Slowing of speech/motor abilities
　Stable/increased weight
　Bradycardia

For T_3 RIA, the nongeriatric adult range is 80–180 ng/dl. Approximately 80% of T_3 is derived from peripheral degradation of T_4, and the remaining 20% originates from direct synthesis by the thyroid gland. T_3 levels are also significantly affected by changes in the serum binding proteins. After the age of 60 years, mean serum T_3 values are known to decrease by 10–30%. Values less than 70 ng/dl do not reliably diagnose hypothyroidism because of overlapping ranges of low normal.

Generally, concomitant elevation or depression of both hormones will occur. However, some exceptions do exist (e.g., approximately 5% of adults with clinical hyperthyroidism have normal T_4 levels but elevated T_3 levels (T_3 toxicosis).[20] In Graves' disease, an increase in serum T_3 may precede an increase in T_4. Likewise, a decreased level of T_3 in the presence of normal T_4 level may be seen in conditions that impair conversion of T_4 to T_3, such as starvation, extremes of age, systemic illness, and certain drug use.

T_3 Resin Uptake Test

The T_3 resin uptake test (T_3RU) is an indirect measure of the serum thyroid binding globulin level. The test is performed by incubating radioactive T_3 with the patient's serum. Available TBG sites are bound, and the remaining radioactive T_3 is recovered on a hormone-binding resin. An elevated resin uptake indicates limited available binding sites, which may be caused by increased endogenous hormones or decreased TBG. A decreased T_3RU level is consistent with increased TBG or decreased endogenous thyroid hormones. Test results are expressed as the percentage of radioactive T_3 taken up by the resin and should be interpreted with the T_4RIA for clinical significance. Expected values are 25–35%.

Free T_4 Determination

Because only unbound thyroid hormone is metabolically active and total T_4RIA is affected by the TBG levels, it is important to obtain a measure of free T_4. Free T_4 is present in very low concentrations since 99.97% of serum T_4 is bound. Measuring this small percentage is challenging because it is difficult not to disturb the equilibrium of bound and unbound hormone. Furthermore, serum can contain other elements, such as lipoproteins, that interfere with analysis. Assessment of free T_4 can be accomplished by either direct or indirect methods.

Direct methods are mainly reserved as reference techniques, since they are technically demanding and expensive. Free T_4 is determined by separating the free hormone by equilibrium dialysis or ultrafiltration followed by quantification by radioimmunoassay or chromatography.

Indirect methods either calculate (index method) or indirectly measure (two-step and analog/one-step radioimmunoassay) the amount of free T_4. In the index methods, the amount of free T_4 is calculated by multiplying the total T_4 RIA result and T_3RU result. Expected values are between 0.7 and 2.0 ng/dl. In the presence of TBG-altering conditions, there is an inverse relationship between the T_3RU and T_4 RIA results, which may result in a normal free T_4 index in the presence of abnormal thyroid function. For example, serum T_4 is often increased in pregnancy whereas T_3RU is decreased (increased TBGs), resulting in a normal free T_4 index. High-dose salicylates or phenytoin will cause a decreased T_4 level and an elevated T_3RU (decreased TBGs), again resulting in a normal free T_4 index. In contrast, when TBG levels are not elevated and an increased amount of T_4 is produced, an elevated free index results. Therefore, a normal free T_4 index does not indicate normal thyroid function (Table 16-9).

The two-step and one-step/analog immunoassays involve indirect measurement of free T_4 with a radioactive T_4 tracer that binds the unoccupied antibody sites. The concentration of free T_4 is inversely related to the amount of antibody-bound radioactivity, and the final results are generated from a standard curve. Unlike the free T_4 index, these indirect measures are not affected by TBG-altering states.

Indirect methods are accurate in normal subjects, and a free T_4 index is usually sufficient. However, indirect methods have variable accuracy in nonthyroidal illness and extreme binding abnormalities. These tests may also be affected by serum drug, lipid, and protein levels. In these cases, results should be interpreted in the context of the clinical presentation, and if warranted, alternative testing should be ordered. Measurements of free T_4 closely reflect the hormonal states of hyper- and hypothyroidism.

TABLE 16-9
Interpretation of Thyroid Function Test Results

Pathologic State	T_3	T_4	T_3RU	FT_4	TSH	Clinical History	Thyroid Gland
↑ TBG states	↑	↑	↓	Normal	Normal	Euthyroid	No change
↓ TBG states	↓	↓	↑	Normal	Normal	Euthyroid	No change
Graves' disease	↑	↑	↑	↑	↓	Hyperthyroid	Diffuse enlargement
Toxic multinodular goiter	↑	↑	↑	↑	↓	Hyperthyroid	Nodular enlargement
Pituitary thyrotoxicosis	↑	↑	↑	↑	↑	Hyperthyroid	Diffuse enlargement
Primary myxedema	↓	↓	↓	↓	↑	Hypothyroid	Normal/small
Secondary myxedema (pituitary)	↓	↓	↓	↓	↓	Hypothyroid	Normal/small
Hashimoto's thyroiditis	↓	↓	↓	↓	↑	Hypothyroid	Enlarged

FT_4 = free thyroxine; T_3 = triiodothyronine; T_3RU = triiodothyronine resin uptake; T_4 = thyroxine; TBG = thyroxine-binding globulin; TSH = thyroid-stimulating hormone; ↑ = increased; ↓ = decreased.

Serum Thyrotropin (TSH) Assay

Determination of TSH level is accomplished by RIA techniques. An increased TSH level is 95% sensitive for primary hypothyroidism and is the single most useful test used to confirm the diagnosis.[2] Second-generation ultrasensitive assays employ a "sandwich" technique and can distinguish between hyperthyroid and low normal euthyroid conditions. The "sandwich" system involves two or more antibodies directed to different portions of the TSH molecule. One antibody is attached to a separation system and extracts the TSH from the serum. The second antibody then quantifies the bound TSH. Expected values are 0.4–6.0 mIU/liter. One should be aware that abnormal TSH values may be seen in numerous conditions other than hyperactive or hypoactive thyroid disease. Among these conditions are severe nonthyroidal disease, large doses of inorganic iodide (amiodarone), primary Addison's disease, diurnal variation, and pituitary TSH secreting tumors.

Routine thyroid function testing includes T_3 and T_4RIA, T_3RU, TSH, and free T_4 index. There may be instances in which additional investigations are warranted. For example, in euthyroid Graves' disease, other tests may include computed tomography to demonstrate enlarged extraocular muscles or alternative "thyroid function studies" to demonstrate autonomous gland function (thyroid suppression test and thyrotropin-releasing hormone). Table 16-9 outlines the general interpretation of thyroid function testing. The interpretation of thyroid function tests in patients with nonthyroidal illness is typically confusing and misleading, because alterations in thyroid function tests may not indicate thyroid dysfunction (euthyroid sick syndrome). As a general rule, the more severe the illness, the greater the degree of abnormality in thyroid function testing.

SEROLOGY

Tests for Syphilis

Infection with the spirochete *Treponema pallidum* results in the production of nonspecific antibodies (reagin) as well as specific antitreponemal antibodies, and this is the basis of the laboratory testing. The numerous serologic assays for syphilis may be divided into nontreponemal (reagin) or treponemal tests.

Reagin Tests

The basis of nontreponemal testing is the reaction between the syphilis-associated antibody known as reagin and a variety of other antigens including a mixture of cardiolipin, lecithin, and cholesterol. Nontreponemal tests include the VDRL, which is named for the Venereal Disease Research Laboratory, and the rapid plasma reagin test (RPR). The VDRL is a flocculation test in which serum is exposed to cardiolipin antigens. The presence of reagin will result in precipitation of material (flocculation) from the mixture. The results are primarily qualitative, ranging from strongly reactive to nonreactive. Quantitative information regarding the antibody titer may also be obtained, since a rising titer can indicate active disease. In primary syphilis, 4–6 weeks after the appearance of a chancre, the VDRL will be weakly positive with a titer < 1:32. As the disease progresses to secondary syphilis, the titers will rise above 1:32, and the VDRL has a sensitivity of nearly 100%.[21] The VDRL titers will then fall, and sensitivity will decrease in late stages of the disease. The VDRL will be nonreactive in approximately 39% of patients with late-stage syphilis and roughly 51% of patients with neurosyphilis.[22,23] Adequate treatment of primary or secondary syphilis often results in conversion to a nonreactive VDRL. However, treatment in late-stage disease or a history of multiple exposures may not result in seronegativity with reagin testing but should be associated with low titers. The RPR is performed and interpreted in a similar manner to the VDRL but is somewhat more sensitive yet less specific.

Because of the nonspecific nature of the VDRL and RPR tests, biologic false-positive results frequently occur in patients without syphilis who possess anticardiolipin antibodies (Table 16-10).[24] Any positive or suggestive result requires further investigation by a treponemal specific test. A patient with a reactive reagin test followed by a nonreactive treponemal antibody test is demonstrating a biologic false-positive result, and other potential causes should be considered. Although nontreponemal testing is inexpensive and simple to perform, it can only be used as a screening method because of its low specificity.

Treponemal Antibody Tests

Specific treponemal antibody tests include the fluorescent treponemal antibody absorption test (FTA-ABS) and the microhemagglutination-treponemal pallidum test (MHA-TP or TPHA). Of these, the FTA-ABS is the most frequently used. It is based on an indirect immunofluorescence technique (Figure 16-3). Test results are graded according to reactivity (1–4+). Less than 1+ is interpreted as nonreactive, whereas 1+ indicates minimally reactive (equivocal) serum and should be followed by a retest. Results of 2+ or greater are interpreted as reactive. The FTA-ABS is both highly sensitive and specific.[25] Even though false-negative results occur in approximately 10% of patients with early primary syphilis, the FTA-ABS remains the most sensitive test for *T. pallidum* infection. In the secondary stage of disease, there are virtually no false-negative results. In patients with late or tertiary syphilis, the FTA-ABS will be positive in 95–97%.[2] False-positive results may occur in less than 2% of healthy individuals (see Table 16-10). Cross-reactivity has been reported in patients with Lyme disease.

The MHA-TP is performed by exposing the patient's serum to sheep RBCs tagged with treponemal antigen. The patient's antitreponemal antibodies will combine with the tagged particles and form large insoluble aggregates that precipitate from the solution. In general, the FTA-ABS and MHA-TP are comparable; however, the MHA-TP is less expensive and somewhat more objective. In the early stages of primary syphilis, the MHA-TP is less sensitive than the FTA-ABS. Patients remain reactive to both the FTA-ABS and MHA-TP tests for years despite adequate treatment, in contrast to the VDRL and RPR tests, where patients will demonstrate falling titers or nonreactivity after successful treatment.

TABLE 16-10

Biological False-Positive Results in Treponemal and Nontreponemal Tests

Infectious causes
  Scarlet fever
  Lyme disease
  Leprosy
  HIV infection
  Viral hepatitis
  Tuberculosis
  Bacterial endocarditis
  Psittacosis
  Infectious mononucleosis
  Leptospirosis
  Lymphogranuloma venereum
  Malaria
  Measles
  Mycoplasma pneumonia
Noninfectious causes
  Chronic liver disease
  Systemic lupus erythematosus
  Connective tissue disease
  Multiple blood transfusions
  Pregnancy
  Advanced age
  Intravenous drug abuse
  Systemic malignancy

Source: Adapted with permission from CE Margo, LM Hamed. Ocular syphilis. Surv Ophthalmol 1992;37:207.

Lyme Disease

Lyme disease is caused by the spirochete *Borrelia burgdorferi*. Direct observation and culture of the organism has a very low yield. Infection is best demonstrated by the presence of IgG and IgM antibodies against the spirochete. Antibodies can be detected by either indirect fluorescent antibody (see Figure 16-3) or enzyme-linked immunosorbent assays (ELISA) (Figure 16-4), and both tests should be used when screening patients for Lyme disease.[26] Although the ELISA is generally more sensitive and specific, cases have been documented in which the ELISA failed to detect IgG and IgM antibodies but positive titers were found with the IFA.[27,28] All testing should be done in conjunction with clinical suspicion of disease, because the sensitivity and specificity of the assays are insufficient to justify screening in low prevalence populations.

The antibody response to infection with *B. burgdorferi* varies between individuals. In most cases, IgM peaks 3–6 weeks after the onset of infection and then gradually decreases in most patients. IgG antibodies develop later than IgM antibodies and will remain detectable for years. Without a doubt, seronegative Lyme disease exists. The false-negative rate may be as high as 50% in patients with

FIGURE 16-3
Immunofluorescent assay (IFA) technique. Note that if the serum does not contain antigen-specific antibodies, no fluorescence will be seen.

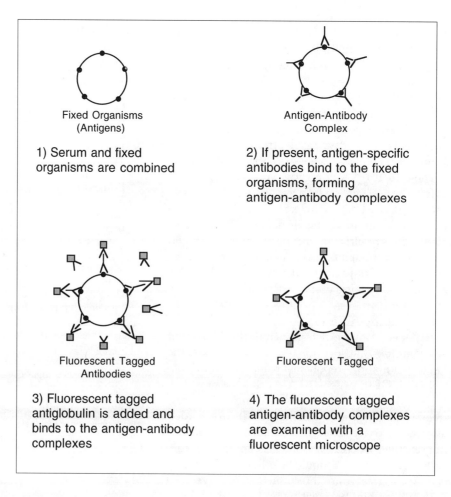

Fixed Organisms
(Antigens)

1) Serum and fixed organisms are combined

Antigen-Antibody Complex

2) If present, antigen-specific antibodies bind to the fixed organisms, forming antigen-antibody complexes

Fluorescent Tagged Antibodies

3) Fluorescent tagged antiglobulin is added and binds to the antigen-antibody complexes

Fluorescent Tagged

4) The fluorescent tagged antigen-antibody complexes are examined with a fluorescent microscope

early Lyme disease. This may be caused by early antibiotic treatment curtailing antibody production, a transient immunosuppressive effect of infection, or nonstandardization of laboratory testing. High antibody titers clinch the diagnosis, but negative results should not be used to exclude the diagnosis of clinically suggested Lyme disease. In the latter instance, the test should be repeated in 4–6 weeks if the clinical presentation suggests disease.[10]

As with FTA-ABS testing, cross-reactivity between the Lyme disease and syphilis spirochetes exists (11–22%).[29,30] In contrast, serum from patients with Lyme disease will not be reactive with RPR, VDRL, and MHA-TP testing. Smith[31] recommends the Lyme/treponemal panel, which consists of RPR with titer, FTA-ABS, Lyme IFA for IgG and IgM, and Lyme ELISA to ensure proper diagnosis.

Detection of Human Immunodeficiency Virus Infection

The acquired immune deficiency syndrome (AIDS) is caused by the human immunodeficiency virus type 1 or 2 (HIV-1 or HIV-2). Infection with the virus may be determined directly by culture or indirectly by antigenic or antibody determinations.

It is difficult, expensive, and time consuming to directly culture the virus from peripheral blood or body fluids. Although this is rarely done, the major advantage to this method is the ability to confirm infection during the first 2–3 weeks after exposure, before the development of antigenemia (antigen proliferation) or immunoglobulin production. In most cases, viral antigen may be detectable no earlier than 2 weeks after infection using radioimmunoassay, fluorescent antibody tests, or the ELISA. Antigen testing overcomes many of the problems associated with direct culture but is limited in its usefulness because the antigenemia persists for only 3–5 months.[2]

The most widely used tests are based on antibody determinations. Typically, production of immunoglobulins begins 6–10 weeks after HIV infection; although latencies of up to 5 years have been reported.[2] Routine screening is done with the ELISA for IgG and IgM (see Figure 16-4). This test is 99.5% sensitive in all populations.[32] The positive predictive value fluctuates widely depending on

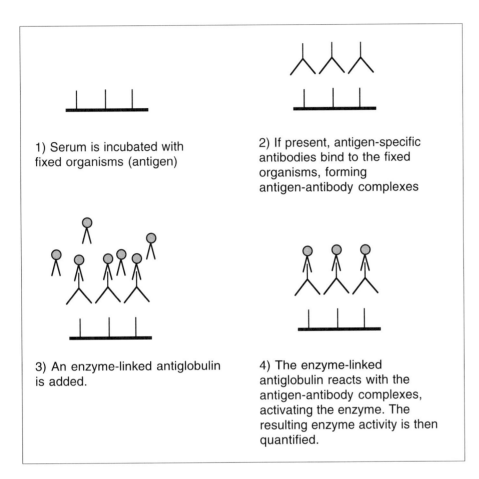

FIGURE 16-4
Enzyme-linked immunosorbent assay (ELISA). Note that if the serum does not contain any antigen-specific antibodies, no enzymatic reaction will take place.

1) Serum is incubated with fixed organisms (antigen)

2) If present, antigen-specific antibodies bind to the fixed organisms, forming antigen-antibody complexes

3) An enzyme-linked antiglobulin is added.

4) The enzyme-linked antiglobulin reacts with the antigen-antibody complexes, activating the enzyme. The resulting enzyme activity is then quantified.

the populations screened; however, in high-risk populations, specificity approaches 99.8%.[11] False-positive results occur predominantly among women and elderly patients. Because of the latency of antibody production, false-negative results have been noted when testing in early stages. Any positive result on ELISA testing on two or more occasions must be confirmed with a more specific antibody technique such as the Western blot (Figure 16-5).

The Western blot is used as a confirmatory test rather than a screening test because of its decreased sensitivity and increased specificity. The test involves electrophoretic separation of virus materials into the main protein constituents with subsequent transfer or "blotting" onto chromatography medium. The test serum is exposed to this support medium, and antibodies attach to the viral components. The antibodies are then identified by staining. False-positive results rarely occur because only few of the viral components are not specific to the HIV virus. Positive results on ELISA and Western blot have greater than 99% positive predictive value, even among low-risk populations.

In the United States, HIV-1 is the most common cause of AIDS, but HIV-2 has also been reported to cause AIDS in parts of West Africa and very rarely in the United States and Europe. Testing for HIV-2 is recommended under the following circumstances: (1) sex partner from an endemic country, (2) history of transfusion or nonsterile injection in an endemic country, (3) shared needle with a person from an endemic country or HIV-2 infected individual, or (4) suspicion of HIV disease (AIDS-associated opportunistic infection) in the absence of positive results for HIV-1 antibodies or indeterminate HIV-1 Western blot results.[33] Testing for HIV-2 is also done by ELISA for IgG and IgM and confirmed with the Western blot test. There are also combination ELISA tests that will simultaneously detect antibodies to HIV-1 and HIV-2. Sixty percent to 91% of patients infected with HIV-2 will repeatedly test positive with the HIV-1 ELISA but may demonstrate indeterminate HIV-1 Western blot results.[33] All blood has been screened for the presence of both HIV-1 and HIV-2 antibodies since 1992.

Antinuclear Antibody Test

A variety of antigenic materials in the cell nuclei of mammals exist. Numerous autoimmune conditions are asso-

FIGURE 16-5

Sequencing of HIV-1 serology. (Modified with permission from RT Davey, MB Vasudevachari, HC Lane. Serologic Tests for Human Immunodeficiency Virus Infection. In VT DeVita, S Hellman, SA Rosenberg [eds], AIDS: Etiology, Diagnosis, Treatment and Prevention. Philadelphia: Lippincott, 1992:146.)

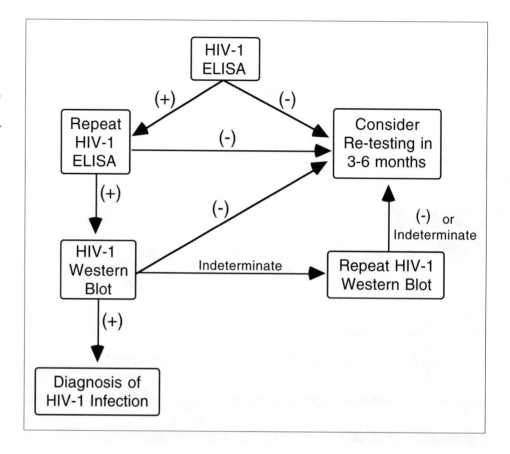

ciated with the production of autoantibodies directed against these nuclear materials. The fluorescent antinuclear antibody (FANA) test is the standard screening test for the detection of these antibodies. The antinuclear antibodies (ANA) are nonspecific and will react with any nuclei from any mammalian organ.

In the fluorescent antinuclear antibody test, an indirect immunofluorescent technique (see Appendix to this chapter) is used to detect the presence of antinuclear antibodies in sera. The antigenic substrate (mouse liver) is combined with the patient's serum, and the formation of antigen-antibody complexes is identified with a fluorescence-tagged antibody. The nuclear fluorescent pattern may be characterized as peripheral (rim), homogeneous (diffuse), nuclear, or speckled. These patterns correspond, respectively, to reactivity against DNA, histone, RNA, and extractable nuclear antigens. Because the patterns can overlap, interpretation may be challenging. However, the pattern of fluorescent staining is sometimes useful in determining the cause of a positive test result (Table 16-11). If positive, the laboratory results will include the highest dilution still giving positive results as well as the

pattern of fluorescent staining. Normal or negative results are titers less than 1:20.

The ANA will be positive, usually with a rim or diffuse pattern, in 99% of patients with systemic lupus erythematosus (SLE).[34] Researchers believe that in patients diagnosed with SLE who have a negative ANA, other nuclear antibodies exist that simply do not react with mouse liver substrate. In most of these cases, FANA testing is positive when using Hep-2 (human epithelial cell tissue culture) as the antigen substrate. Serum titers in SLE will fall during disease remission but are not affected by steroids.

Positive ANA test results can also be seen in a variety of other disorders including Sjögren's syndrome (68%), scleroderma (40%), juvenile chronic polyarthritis (22%), rheumatoid arthritis (20%), myasthenia gravis (30–50%), and drug-induced SLE.[34] Age must also be considered when interpreting test results because up to 10% of normal subjects over the age of 70 years will have a positive ANA result. False-positive results may be induced by smoking and certain drugs such as anticonvulsants, chlorpromazine, diphenylhydantoin, methyldopa, oral contraceptives, and trimethadione.

TABLE 16-11
Diseases Associated with Specific Antinuclear Antibody Fluorescent Patterns

Fluorescent Staining Pattern	Disease
Homogeneous (diffuse)	Rheumatoid arthritis
	Scleroderma
	Mixed connective tissue disease
	Systemic lupus erythematosus
Peripheral (rim)	Systemic lupus erythematosus
Speckled	Scleroderma
	Mixed connective tissue disease
	Sjögren's syndrome
Nucleolar	Sjögren's syndrome
	Scleroderma

Rheumatoid Factor

Rheumatoid factors (RFs) are thought to be autoantibodies directed against altered human IgG. RF can be found in 75–80% of adult patients diagnosed with rheumatoid arthritis (RA).[11,35] The exact biological function of RF is unknown, but it is thought to enhance the activation of complement after it interacts with the altered IgG. Detection of RF is achieved by agglutination (flocculation) of sensitized sheep RBCs or latex particles coated with altered human IgG. When combined with serum, the RF antibody combines with the altered IgG antigen, forming a large insoluble aggregate. The concentration of RF is then measured by rate nephelometry. The light scattering properties of the antigen-antibody complex are proportional to the concentration of antibody if all other variables are held constant. Rheumatoid factors occur in the forms of IgM, IgG, IgA, and IgE autoantibodies, but primarily IgM rheumatoid factors are detected. The IgG, IgA, and IgE rheumatoid factors require more sensitive and specific immunoassays for detection.

Using rate nephelometry and latex particles, expected values are expressed as titers, with 0–69 IU/ml being nonreactive. Weakly reactive results are values between 70 and 139 IU/ml, and results over 139 IU/ml are considered reactive.[11]

Because of its low sensitivity, RF is a poor screening test and negative results may be more useful than positive results. The sensitive sheep cell test is more specific for RA but is rarely used. Statistically, in patients with RA, very high titers signify severe joint disease, an increased likelihood of systemic complications, and a poor prognosis. However, in individual patients, severity of the disease cannot be predicted by the RF. Because the level of RF is relatively constant throughout the course of the disease, it cannot be used to monitor the disease activity or efficacy of treatment. RA with seronegative RF occurs in up to 25% of patients.[11] Absence of a positive RF result does not exclude the diagnosis of RA. A positive result has only a 24.4% positive predictive value for the diagnosis of RA, and a negative result has an 88.5% negative predictive value.[36]

The implications of a positive test result are not clear. RF may be a marker for severe rheumatic disease, an epiphenomenon associated with nonrheumatic illness, or a benign coincidence of age. Positive titers are found in other rheumatic diseases such as Sjögren's syndrome, systemic lupus erythematosus, systemic sclerosis, polymyositis, and mixed connective tissue disease. In these conditions, the RF has little diagnostic significance. Nonrheumatologic conditions that can cause a positive RF include bacterial endocarditis, tuberculosis, syphilis, cirrhosis of the liver, infectious or chronic hepatitis, sarcoidosis, diffuse interstitial pulmonary fibrosis, and Waldenström's macroglobulinemia. A positive titer has also been identified in 1–5% of normal subjects, and this percentage may increase with age.[35] Conditions such as osteoarthritis, ankylosing spondylitis, gout, enteropathic arthritis, Reiter's syndrome, and psoriatic arthritis are usually seronegative for RF. RF should always be interpreted in light of the clinical and physical findings.

Histocompatibility Locus Antigen

All nucleated cells have a histocompatibility locus antigen (HLA), which is expressed as glycoproteins spanning the cell surface. The HLA gene complex is located on the short arm of chromosome 6 and represents the major histocompatibility locus in humans. More than 27 antigens have been identified. Histocompatibility locus antigen typing is used to determine histocompatibility between donor and recipient for organ transplantation. The presence of specific HLAs may also be associated with an increased susceptibility to specific diseases (Table 16-12) but does not mandate the development of the disease in the patient.

The HLAs are most easily detected in lymphocytes, and because they were initially detected on human lymphocytes, these antigens have also been referred to as human leukocyte antigens (likewise abbreviated HLA). Specific antigens are identified by cytotoxic techniques. Lymphocytes are extracted and incubated with anti-HLA cytotoxic antibodies. An antigen-antibody complex will form on the cell surface, and when serum complement is added to the mixture, the lymphocyte is killed, thus identifying the antigen present.

Of these antigens, HLA-B27 has the most prognostic and diagnostic clinical relevance. The presence of

TABLE 16-12
Association Between Specific HLAs and Disease States

Associated Disease	HLAs
Ankylosing spondylitis	B27
Idiopathic anterior uveitis	B27
Multiple sclerosis	B27, Dw2, A3, and B8
Myasthenia gravis	B8
Psoriasis	A13 and B17
Reiter's syndrome	B27
Juvenile insulin-dependent diabetes mellitus	Bw15 and B8
Graves' disease	B7
Juvenile rheumatoid arthritis	B27
Behçet's disease	B51

HLA-B27 is most strongly associated with ankylosing spondylitis and Reiter's syndrome. Eighty to 90% of these patients will test positive. However, laboratory results should be interpreted with caution, because HLA-B27 has been identified in 6–8% of white and 3–4% of black normal subjects.[11]

Toxoplasmosis

Ocular toxoplasmosis is usually a presumptive diagnosis based on clinical impression with support from positive serologic testing. Tests available for the detection of serum antibodies to the parasite *Toxoplasma gondii* include the Sabin-Feldman dye test, the indirect fluorescent antibody (IFA) test, and ELISA.

The Sabin-Feldman dye test has been the gold standard for diagnosis since its development in 1948. The cell wall of *T. gondii* will normally stain with alkaline methylene blue. When the organism is exposed to test serum with toxoplasma antibodies, the cell wall is lysed, preventing dye staining. The test result will be positive early after the onset of clinical illness and remain positive for life. Although this test is associated with a relatively high sensitivity and specificity, it is very rarely used because of the difficulties and expense of maintaining live organisms.

The indirect fluorescent antibody test (IFA) detects IgG and IgM antibodies and is easier, safer, and more economical (see Appendix to this chapter). The IFA is comparable with the dye test in terms of sensitivity and specificity. After infection with toxoplasmosis, the IgG antibodies appear within 1–2 weeks, and titers peak at 6–8 weeks. Values then fall at variable rates and persist for life. The IgM antibodies can be detected as early as 5 days after infection and peak within a month. Titers will then decrease and disappear in weeks to months. In adults, IgG or IgM titers of 1:8 or greater are considered positive when testing for ocular toxoplasmosis. With acute sys-temic infection, IgG titers are often 1:1000 or greater, whereas IgM titers are typically 1:64 or greater. Because IgM cannot cross the placenta, any IgM titer in a new-born infant is highly suggestive of congenital infection. Rising titers suggest active disease or reinfection and are of greatest significance. False-negative results are rare but false-positive results may occur in patients with positive antinuclear antibodies or rheumatoid factor.

The ELISA test to detect IgG and IgM antibodies is somewhat more sensitive than the IFA (see Figures 16-3 and 16-4). It also eliminates the false-positive results caused by ANA and RF in IFA testing. A double sandwich method may be used in testing for IgM in which anti-IgM antibodies capture the serum IgM antibodies. An IgM titer of 1:256 or greater indicates acute systemic infection.

Rothova et al.[37] demonstrated positive IgG titers in 100% of patients with clinically apparent ocular toxoplasmosis; however, 58% of the controls tested positive as well. Because most adults have been previously exposed to the organism, a positive IgG titer is not discriminatory for ocular disease. A truly negative titer may actually be more diagnostically significant than a positive result when considering the possibility of ocular toxoplasmosis. A useful rule of thumb is that the patient's age in years will equal the percentage of chance of previous exposure. Because laboratories routinely test sera at low dilutions, undiluted testing must be specifically requested when ocular toxoplasmosis is suggested.

Toxocariasis

Infection with the larvae of *Toxocara canis* can be confirmed with an ELISA test (see Figure 16-4). It is important to consider the fact that 1–6% of the normal population will have titers of 1:16 or greater without evidence of *T. canis* infection.[38] As with toxoplasmosis, testing of undiluted serum must be requested when ocular toxocariasis is suggested. When a titer of 1:8 is considered to be a positive result, the ELISA is 90% sensitive and 91% specific for ocular toxocariasis.[38] Histologically proven cases of infection have been reported with titers of only 1:2.[39] Therefore, any positive titer with the appropriate clinical picture is highly suggestive of infection.

SKIN TESTING

Delayed hypersensitivity is the basis of skin testing. A soluble antigen derived from a given microorganism is injected intradermally. Significant induration and erythema at the site of injection occurs in positive tests. Erythema alone is insufficient to make a diagnosis. Failure to develop this response may be attributable to a lack of exposure to the antigen or a generalized deficiency of delayed hypersensitivity (anergy). Anergy may be induced by sarcoidosis, AIDS, and immunosuppressive therapy and is demonstrated with a panel of mumps, trichophyton, tetanus, and *Candida* skin tests. These antigens are chosen because of their high frequency of exposure.

Tuberculosis

The Mantoux method (purified protein derivative test [PPD]) is the most sensitive skin test used in making a diagnosis of *Mycobacterium tuberculosis* infection. A positive PPD, however, does not necessarily indicate active disease but is generally regarded to indicate the presence of living mycobacteria somewhere in the body. A stabilized solution of tuberculin is injected intradermally, and the results are interpreted 48–72 hours later. A skin response is evoked if the patient has systemic hypersensitivity to tuberculin antibodies. Hypersensitivity generally develops about 6 weeks after infection.

A positive or reactive PPD is defined by the resulting area of induration. In immunocompetent patients, induration of 10 mm or greater in diameter is considered positive. Induration of 5–9 mm is an equivocal response and may indicate partial anergy, recent tuberculosis infection, or atypical mycobacterium infection. Less than 5 mm induration is a negative response. In patients infected with HIV or who have certain risk factors for TB infection, test interpretation is slightly different and is outlined in Table 16-13.[40] Positive test results do not determine inactive or active disease but only suggest past exposure.

The recommended antigen is PPD tuberculin stabilized with Tween 80 in 5 tuberculin units (5 TU or 0.1 μg), which is referred to as the intermediate, standard, or critical dose. In severe infections, or if a previous history of a positive skin test is elicited, the "first strength" of PPD (0.02 μg) should be used to avoid skin necrosis. If a patient demonstrates a negative response to an intermediate strength PPD, and there is still a strong suspicion of tuberculosis, a "second-strength" PPD (5.0 μg or 250 TU) is indicated. A second-strength PPD is necessary in approximately 9–17% of patients with tuberculosis.[2] False-negative results still occur even with the use of the "second-strength" PPD. Anergy, the impaired ability to react to specific antigens, is one potential cause and may occur in very severe tuberculosis, sarcoidosis, debility, increasing age, exanthematous diseases, AIDS, or steroid therapy. With initiation of early treatment, a significant number of cases may revert to a negative PPD result. In patients over the age of 50 years, approximately 8–10% may demonstrate a "wane of activity"

TABLE 16-13
Interpretation of Purified Protein Derivative (PPD) Testing

A. Induration of ≥ 5 mm is positive in:
1. Persons with HIV infection or risk for HIV infection with unknown HIV status
2. Persons with recent close contact (household contact or unprotected occupational exposure) with persons with active TB
3. Persons with abnormal findings on chest roentgenograms consistent with old healed TB

B. Induration of ≥ 10 mm is positive in all persons who do not meet any of the above criteria but who have other risk factors for TB including:
1. High-risk groups
   a. HIV seronegative intravenous drug users
   b. Persons with other medical conditions reported to increase the risk of progressing from latent TB infection to active TB, including silicosis, gastrectomy, jejunoileal bypass surgery, body weight 10% or more below ideal, chronic renal failure, diabetes mellitus, high-dose corticosteroid and other immunosuppressive therapy, some hematologic disorders, and other malignancies
2. High-prevalence groups
   a. Foreign-born persons from high-prevalence countries in Asia, Africa, and Latin America
   b. Persons from medically underserved, low-income populations
   c. Residents of long-term care facilities (correctional facilities, nursing homes)
   d. Persons from high-risk populations in their communities, as determined by local public health authorities

C. Induration ≥ 15 mm is positive in persons who do not meet any of the above criteria

D. Recent conversion is defined on the basis of both induration and age:
1. ≥ 10-mm increase within a 2-year period in persons < 35 years of age
2. ≥ 15-mm increase within a 2-year period in persons ≥ 35 years of age
3. ≥ 5-mm increases under circumstances listed in A above

TB = tuberculosis.
Source: Adapted from Centers for Disease Control. Draft Guidelines for Preventing the Transmission of Tuberculosis in Health-Care Facilities (2nd ed). Federal Register 1993;58(195):52810–54.

many years after the infection.[2] In these cases, a booster phenomenon can occur. The initial negative PPD test will restore reactivity, and subsequent skin testing, 1–2 weeks later, will produce positive results.

Histoplasmosis

Previous exposure to the fungus *Histoplasma capsulatum* can be detected by a Mantoux skin test. Although over

80% of the patients with ocular histoplasmosis syndrome demonstrate positive histoplasmin skin tests, a fair number of patients without clinical evidence of ocular or systemic infection will test positively as well. For example, in the Mississippi and Ohio river valleys, there is a 70–90% incidence of positive skin tests among the general population.[41] In addition to this problem, administration of the skin test also carries a significant risk (18%) of reactivating ocular lesions, which can be devastating in the presence of macular lesions.[41] Skin testing is therefore not routinely recommended, and the triad of peripheral chorioretinal lesions (histo spots), peripapillary atrophy, and choroidal neovascularization is considered diagnostic.

SPECIAL CONSIDERATIONS

HIV-1/Syphilis/Tuberculosis

HIV infection affects both humoral and cell-mediated immunity. Polyclonal B-cell activation may lead to false-positive results or true-positive results at higher than expected titers with serology tests such as the RPR. In contrast, HIV infection may also cause an insufficient antibody response, leading to false-negative results or a decreased immunoreactivity causing anergy. Furthermore, coexistence of multiple diseases mandates the need for additional testing when certain conditions such as syphilis and tuberculosis are found to exist.

Because of the high prevalence of syphilis in HIV-1 patients and the possibility of more aggressive and recalcitrant disease, concomitant testing for both conditions is recommended. The majority of patients with dual infection will show typical clinical features of syphilis. However, false-positive and false-negative results must always be considered. In addition, nontreponemal titers may not decrease with adequate treatment.

A high number of individuals with HIV will also develop tuberculosis infection or reactivation.[42–45] Testing for tuberculosis infection in the presence of HIV infection is somewhat challenging, since patients frequently develop anergy and demonstrate equivocal responses with PPD testing. Because the medical management must be altered in the presence of HIV infection, HIV testing has been mandated in all persons with tuberculosis or tuberculous infection by the Advisory Committee for the Elimination of Tuberculosis (ACET).[46] Testing for HIV should be pursued in patients with tuberculosis or tuberculous infection in the context of HIV risk factors.

TABLE 16-14
Age-Related Changes in Laboratory Testing

Laboratory Test	Change with Age
Alkaline phosphatase	Gradually increases
Erythrocyte sedimentation rate	Increases
LDL cholesterol	Increases
Glycosylated hemoglobin	Increases
Oral glucose tolerance test	Increases
T_3 (triiodothyronine)	Slight decrease
Total cholesterol	Gradually increases
Triglycerides	Increase

Elderly Patients

In working with elderly patients, one is faced with a lack of age-related standards with which to compare laboratory values. There is little information regarding what constitutes a normal age-related physiologic change and what signifies a pathologic state. Abnormal laboratory findings are common in elderly patients, but few are attributable to "old age." Misinterpretation of an abnormal value as an age-related change can lead to underdiagnosis and undertreatment, whereas failure to appreciate age-related changes can lead to overdiagnosis and overtreatment. Other factors common in the management of elderly patients such as multiplicity of diseases and drug use can also make interpretation challenging. To ensure proper diagnosis and management, the clinician should be aware of the potential for age-related changes (Table 16-14).[47]

CONCLUSION

There are numerous ocular conditions that indicate the need for laboratory evaluation. Laboratory workup should be tailored, based on a carefully developed list of differential diagnoses rather than a "shotgun" approach (Table 16-15). This promotes efficiency and cost effectiveness. When used in conjunction with a thorough ophthalmic examination, laboratory testing will improve patient care, lead to more efficient diagnosis, and allow prompt medical management. Numerous tests require interpretation within the context of the entire clinical picture, and laboratory testing alone is seldom diagnostic.

TABLE 16-15

Suggested Laboratory Examinations for Selected Ocular Conditions

Ocular Findings	Laboratory Tests*	Etiologic Considerations
Anterior uveitis	CBC	Nonspecific
	ESR	Nonspecific
	ANA	Lupus
	FTA-ABS, RPR	Syphilis
	PPD/anergy panel	Tuberculosis
	ACE, serum lysozyme	Sarcoidosis
	Lyme IFA, ELISA (endemic areas only)	Lyme disease
Cotton wool spot	FBG	Diabetes
	ANA	Collagen vascular disease
	CBC	Anemia, leukemia
	HIV ELISA	AIDS
Episcleritis/scleritis	RF	Rheumatoid arthritis
	ANA	Lupus
	ESR	Nonspecific
	FTA-ABS, RPR	Syphilis
Low-tension glaucoma/optic atrophy	CBC	Hematologic disorders
	ESR	Temporal arteritis/nonspecific
	ANA	Lupus
	FTA-ABS, RPR	Syphilis
	ACE, serum lysozyme	Sarcoidosis
Periphlebitis	FTA-ABS, RPR	Syphilis
	ACE, serum lysozyme	Sarcoidosis
	Hb electrophoresis	Sickle cell disease
Posterior uveitis	Toxoplasma titers	Toxoplasmosis
	ACE, serum lysozyme	Sarcoidosis
	FTA-ABS	Syphilis
Retinal neovascularization	FBG	Diabetes
	Hb electrophoresis	Sickle cell disease
	ACE, serum lysozyme	Sarcoidosis

*Clinical diagnosis may require additional testing such as blood pressure, carotid duplex, fluorescein angiography, chest x-ray films, etc. Laboratory tests listed for each condition are not all-inclusive and should serve as a starting point in making a differential diagnosis.

REFERENCES

1. National Diabetes Data Group. Classification and diagnosis of diabetes mellitus and other categories of glucose intolerance. Diabetes 1979;28:1039–57.
2. Ravel R. Clinical Laboratory Medicine: Clinical Application of Laboratory Data (5th ed). Chicago: Year Book, 1989;214, 269, 361, 466, 489, 566.
3. Folling I. The clinical value of glycated hemoglobin and glycated plasma proteins. Scand J Clin Lab Invest 1990;50(Suppl 202):959–8.
4. Singh R, Prakash V, Shukla PK, et al. Glycosylated hemoglobin and diabetic retinopathy. Ann Ophthalmol 1991; 23:308–11.
5. The Expert Panel. Report of the National Cholesterol Education Program Expert Panel on detection, evaluation, and treatment of high blood cholesterol in adults. Arch Intern Med 1988;148:36–69.
6. Laboratory Standardization Panel, National Cholesterol Education Program. Current status of blood cholesterol measurement in clinical laboratories in the United States. Clin Chem 1988;34:193–201.
7. Adult Treatment Panel II. Second report of the Expert Panel of the National Cholesterol Education Program. Detection, evaluation, and treatment of high blood cholesterol in adults. Circulation 1994;89:1329–45.
8. Pagana KD, Pagana TJ. Mosby's Diagnostic and Laboratory Test Reference. St. Louis: Mosby-Year Book, 1992;465.
9. Fischbach F. A Manual of Laboratory and Diagnostic Tests (4th ed). Philadelphia: Lippincott, 1988;368.
10. Consensus Conference. Treatment of hypertriglyceridemia. JAMA 1984;251:1196–200.
11. Leavelle DR. Mayo Medical Laboratories: Interpretive Handbook (5th ed). Rochester, MN: Mayo Medical Laboratories, 1988;13, 79–80, 101, 133–4.
12. Baarsma GS, LaHey E, Glasius E, et al. The predictive value of serum angiotensin converting enzyme and lysozyme levels in the diagnosis of ocular sarcoidosis. Am J Ophthalmol 1987;104:211–7.
13. Gilbertsen VA. Erythrocyte sedimentation rates in older patients. Postgrad Med 1965;38:A44–A52.
14. Gawlikowski J. White cells at war. Am J Nursing 1992; March, pp 44–51.
15. Miller A, Green M, Robinson D. Simple rule for calculating normal erythrocyte sedimentation rate. Br Med J 1983;286:266.
16. Griner PF, Panzer RJ, Greenland P. Clinical Diagnosis and the Laboratory: Logical Strategies for Common Medical Problems. Chicago: Year Book, 1986;488.
17. Beri M, Klugman MR, Kohler JA, Hayreh SS. Anterior ischemic optic neuropathy: VII. Incidence of bilaterality and various influencing factors. Ophthalmology 1987;94:1020–8.
18. Jones JG, Hazleman BL. ESR in polymyalgia rheumatica and giant cell arteritis. Ann Rheum Dis 1983;42:702–44.
19. Litwin MS, Henderson DR, Kirkham B. Normal sedimentation rates and giant cell arteritis. Arch Intern Med 1992;152:209.
20. Rives KL. Endocrinologic Diagnosis. In ZA Karicioglu (ed), Laboratory Diagnosis in Ophthalmology. New York: Macmillan, 1987;243–50.
21. Pursch A. Clinical Diagnosis and Management by Laboratory Methods. Philadelphia: Saunders, 1979;1886–92.
22. Harner RE, Smith JL, Israel CW. The FTA-ABS test in late syphilis: A serologic study in 1985 cases. JAMA 1968;203:545–8.
23. Hooshmand H, Escobar MR, Kopf SW. Neurosyphilis: A study of 241 patients. JAMA 1972;219:726–9.
24. Margo CE, Hamed LM. Ocular syphilis. Surv Ophthalmol 1992;37:203–20.
25. Currie JN, Coppeto JR, Lessell S. Chronic syphilitic meningitis resulting in superior orbital fissure syndrome and posterior fossa gumma. J Clin Neuro-ophthalmol 1988;8:145–55.
26. Winward KE, Smith JL, Culbertson WW, Paris-Hamelin A. Ocular Lyme borreliosis. Am J Ophthalmol 1989;108:651–7.
27. Craft JE, Grodzicki RL, Steere AC. Antibody response in lyme disease: Evaluation of diagnostic tests. J Infect Dis 1984;149:789–95.
28. Russell H, Sampson JS, Schmid GP, et al. Enzyme-linked immunosorbent assay and indirect immunofluorescence assay for Lyme disease. J Infect Dis 1984;149:465–70.
29. Magnarelli LA, Anderson JF, Johnson RC. Cross-reactivity in serological tests for Lyme disease and other spirochetal infections. J Infect Dis 1987;156:183–8.
30. Hunter EF. Evaluation of sera from patients with Lyme disease in the FTA-ABS test for syphilis. Sex Transm Dis 1986;18:232–6.
31. Smith JL, Crumpton BC, Hummer J. The Bascom Palmer Eye Institute Lyme/Syphilis Survey. J Clin Neuro-ophthalmol 1990;10:255–60.
32. Davey RT, Vasudevachari MB, Lane HC. Serologic Tests for Human Immunodeficiency Virus Infection. In VT DeVita, S Hellman, SA Rosenberg (eds), AIDS: Etiology, Diagnosis, Treatment, and Prevention (3rd ed). Philadelphia: Lippincott, 1992;141–55.
33. O'Brien TR, George JR, Epstein JS, et al. Testing for antibodies to human immunodeficiency virus type 2 in the United States. MMWR 1992;41:1–9.
34. Sacher RA, McPherson RA, Campos JM. Widmann's Clinical Interpretation of Laboratory Tests (10th ed). Philadelphia: FA Davis, 1991;257–61.
35. Schumacher RH, Klippel JH, Robinson DR. Primer on the Rheumatic Diseases (4th ed). Atlanta: Arthritis Foundation, 1988;83–92.
36. Shmerling RH, Delbanco TL. How useful is the rheumatoid factor? An analysis of sensitivity, specificity, and predictive value. Arch Intern Med 1992;152:2417–20.
37. Rothova A, van Knapen F, Baarsma GS, et al. Serology in ocular toxoplasmosis. Br J Ophthalmol 1986;70:615–22.
38. Pollard ZF, Jarrett WH, Hagler WS, et al. ELISA for diagnosis of ocular toxocariasis. Ophthalmology 1979;86:743–9.
39. Kielar RA. Toxocara canis endophthalmitis with low ELISA titer. Ann Ophthalmol 1983;15:447–9.
40. Centers for Disease Control. Draft guidelines for preventing the transmission of tuberculosis in health-care facilities (2nd ed). Federal Register 1993;58:52810–54.

41. Parker JA, Nozik RA. Laboratory Tests in Diagnosis of Uveitis. In ZA Karicioglu (ed), Laboratory Diagnosis in Ophthalmology. New York: Macmillan, 1987;185–205.

42. Pitchenik A, Cole C, Russell BW, et al. Tuberculosis, atypical mycobacteriosis, and the acquired immunodeficiency syndrome among Haitian and non-Haitian patients in south Florida. Ann Intern Med 1984;101:641–5.

43. Sunderam G, McDonald RJ, Maniatis T, et al. Tuberculosis as a manifestation of the acquired immunodeficiency syndrome (AIDS). JAMA 1986;256:362–6.

44. Braun MM, Turman BI, Maguire B, et al. Increasing incidence of tuberculosis in a prison inmate population. JAMA 1989;261:393–7.

45. Theuer CP, Hopewell PC, Elias D, et al. Human immunodeficiency virus infection in tuberculosis patients. J Infect Dis 1990;162:8–12.

46. Centers for Disease Control. Tuberculosis and human immunodeficiency virus infection: Recommendations of the advisory committee for the elimination of tuberculosis (ACET) MMWR 1989;38:236–50.

47. Melillo KD. Interpretation of laboratory values in older adults. Nurse Prac 1993:(July);59–70.

APPENDIX

*Representative Reference Laboratory Values**

Laboratory Test	Reference Ranges
Alanine aminotransferase (ALT)	1–21 U/liter
Alkaline phosphatase (ALP)	25–97 U/liter
Angiotensin-converting enzyme (ACE)	6.1–21.1 U/liter
Antinuclear antibody (ANA)	titer <1:20
Aspartate aminotransferase (AST)	7–27 U/liter
Bilirubin	0.1–1.2 mg/dl
Blood urea nitrogen (BUN)	10–20 mg/dl
Carbon dioxide, serum (CO_2)	23–30 mEq/liter
Chloride (Cl^-)	95–105 mEq/liter
Creatinine	0.7–1.5 mg/dl
Erythrocyte sedimentation rate (ESR)	Men: age/2
	Women: (age + 10)/2
Fasting blood glucose (FBG)	Normal: 70–115 mg/dl
	Borderline: 116–140 mg/dl
	Abnormal: >140 mg/dl
Free T_4 index (FTI)	0.7–2.0 ng/dl
Glycosylated hemoglobin	Normal: <8%
	Abnormal: >12%
Hematocrit	Men: 39–49%
	Women: 33–43%
Hemoglobin electrophoresis	95–98% HbA
	1.5–3.0% HbA2
	0–2.0% HbF
High-density lipoprotein (HDL) cholesterol	Men: 22–68 mg/dl
	Women: 30–80 mg/dl
Low-density lipoprotein (LDL) cholesterol	Normal: <130 mg/dl
	Borderline: 130–159 mg/dl
	Abnormal: >159 mg/dl
Mean cell hemoglobin (MCH)	26–34 pg
Mean cell hemoglobin concentration (MCHC)	31–37%
Mean cell volume (MCV)	80–100 μm^3
Oral glucose tolerance test (OGTT)	Baseline FBG: 70–115 mg/dl
	Peak: <200 mg/dl
	2 hour: <140 mg/dl
	3 hour: 70–115 mg/dl
Platelets	150–450 × 10^3/mm^3
Potassium (K^+)	3.5–5.0 mEq/liter
Rheumatoid factor (RF) (latex/rate nephelometry)	Nonreactive: 0–69 IU/ml
	Mildly reactive: 70–139 IU/ml
	Reactive: >139 IU/ml
Serum lysozyme	0.2–15.8 μg/ml
Sodium (Na^+)	136–145 mEq/liter
Thyroxine radioimmunoassay (T_4RIA)	4–12 μg/dl
Thyroid-stimulating hormone (TSH)	0.4–6.0 milliunits/liter
Total cholesterol	Normal: < 200 mg/dl
	Borderline: 200–239 mg/dl
	Abnormal: >239 mg/dl
Total red blood cell (RBC) count	Men: 4.5–6.0 × 10^{12}/liter
	Women: 4.0–5.5 × 10^{12}/liter
Total white blood cell (WBC) count	4.5–11.0 × 10^9/liter
Triglycerides	Normal: <250 mg/dl
	Borderline: 250–500 mg/dl
	Abnormal: >500 mg/dl
Triiodothyronine radioimmunoassay (T_3RIA)	80–180 ng/dl
Triiodothyronine resin uptake (T_3RU)	25–35%

*Exact reference ranges vary for each laboratory. All values listed are for adults.

17

Ocular Microbiology and Cytology

DIANE P. YOLTON

Many inflammatory diseases of the external eye can be diagnosed on the basis of the patient's history, signs, and symptoms. Sometimes, however, the findings are rather ambiguous, and despite the best clinical workup, a diagnosis is not possible. In such cases, a few simple procedures such as microscopic examination of stained lid, conjunctival, or corneal samples will often give more clues regarding the underlying cause. Accurate identification of the majority of organisms causing ocular infections encountered in routine practice can easily be accomplished in the office. Often, simple procedures involving sample collection, preparation, and microscopic examination will quickly provide insight regarding the patient's condition. For those cases in which immediate examination is not sufficient to identify the problem, cultures can be grown using readily available media and a small incubator. Armed with knowledge provided by these techniques, the clinician can then prescribe specific therapy for the patient.

If the clinician does not wish to examine or culture specimens directly, in-office specimens can be obtained and then sent to a hospital (use of hospital laboratories may require that the optometrist have hospital privileges) or a private laboratory (private laboratories are located in most cities of significant size and will usually accept specimens from any qualified practitioner) for evaluation.

To properly obtain, examine, or send biological specimens for evaluation, knowledge of a few simple techniques is required. Furthermore, to understand the significance of what is seen in the microscope or reported by the laboratory, basic knowledge regarding the cytology and microbiology of the normal and infected human eye is needed.

DIAGNOSTIC PROCEDURES

When a patient presents with an ocular inflammation, one of the first steps is to identify the causative agent.

Obviously prognosis and treatment are quite different depending on whether the agent is a virus, fungus, allergen, or bacterium. Often, one of the best ways to make this differentiation involves collecting a specimen of the affected ocular cells (and possibly the causative agent itself) for staining or culturing.

Obtaining Ocular Specimens

Samples of conjunctival or corneal cells, along with any organisms present, can easily be obtained by using a Kimura platinum spatula or similar instrument. The blade of the spatula is initially flame heated for sterilization and then allowed to cool. If necessary, the area to be sampled can be anesthetized. Since proparacaine is less antiseptic than cocaine, tetracaine, and other topical anesthetics, it is preferred for obtaining specimens that will be cultured to assess bacterial or fungal growth.[1] The spatula is gently but firmly scraped across the area to be sampled using enough pressure to remove a superficial layer of cells. Material from the spatula is then transferred to a glass slide for staining and examination, or to a suitable medium for culturing. As an alternative, the sample may be collected using a premoistened cotton-tipped swab, as discussed in a later section.

Giemsa and Diff-Quik Staining

Studying the cytologic features of ocular scrapings can be a rapid and effective method for evaluating or diagnosing many external ocular diseases. To demonstrate the cytologic features of scrapings, Giemsa stain is typically used in laboratories.[2] For office use, however, the Diff-Quik stain (Baxter Scientific Products, McGraw Park, IL) (Figure 17-1) is often preferred. It gives results similar to traditional Giemsa staining, but it is more easily incor-

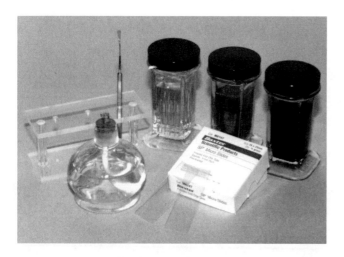

FIGURE 17-1
Materials used for a Diff-Quik stain preparation. These include the Kimura spatula and an alcohol lamp for its sterilization, glass microscope slides, and the Diff-Quik solutions.

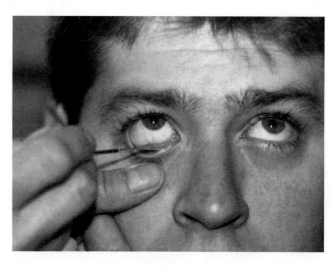

FIGURE 17-2
Obtaining a specimen from the inferior palpebra conjunctiva with a sterile Kimura platinum spatula. The conjunctival surface should blanch slightly when it is scraped.

porated into routine practice.[3] To perform Diff-Quik staining, a specimen is collected by scraping the involved conjunctiva or cornea with a sterile Kimura spatula (Figure 17-2). Alternatively, the specimen can be collected by using a cotton-tipped swab,[3] or a sterile plastic disc,[4] but the best results are usually obtained by using a spatula.[5] The specimen is then smeared onto a clean microscope slide (Figure 17-3) and allowed to air dry. Relatively small, thin smears are more easily interpreted than are large, thick ones. The dried slide is next immersed into the Diff-Quik fixative using five 1-second dips (Table 17-1). Similar immersions follow into the two Diff-Quik dye solutions (Figure 17-4). The slide is next gently rinsed, allowed to air dry, and observed under the microscope using 100× and 400× powers.

Epithelial Cells

In a conjunctival smear, epithelial cells normally are seen singly, in clusters, or in sheets. These cells are rectangular in shape with round or oval dark blue-purple nuclei and large amounts of light blue cytoplasm (Color Plate 17-I). Epithelial cell changes may be associated with a variety of disease states. For example, cytoplasmic inclusion bodies, which appear as dark, blue-purple granular clusters in the cytoplasm of epithelial cells, are usually indicative of chlamydial infection (inclusion bodies are more easily detected in samples from patients with neonatal inclusion conjunctivitis and are more difficult to observe in adult inclusion conjunctivitis and trachoma).

Keratinization of epithelial cells can be seen in patients with xerophthalmia or severe keratoconjunctivitis sicca. The earliest changes of keratinization occur in the nucleus, where the nuclear material becomes clumped and vesicular. In more advanced cases, keratin granules are seen in the cytoplasm. Strands and clusters of dark blue-purple–stained mucus and fibrin can sometimes be observed in smears. Mucus may be prominent in allergic or dry eye conditions, whereas fibrin is typical of purulent diseases such as bacterial conjunctivitis.

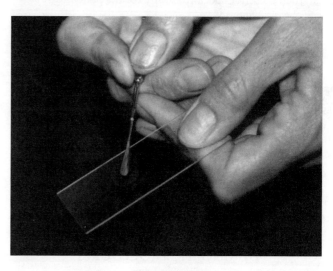

FIGURE 17-3
Preparation of a smear on a microscope slide for Diff-Quik staining.

TABLE 17-1
Procedure for the Diff-Quik Stain

1. Air dry specimen on slide for 5 minutes.
2. Immerse slide (five 1-second immersions) in solution No. 1 (triarylmethane in methyl alcohol); allow excess to drain
3. Immerse slide (five 1-second immersions) in solution No. 2 (xanthene dye); allow excess to drain
4. Immerse slide (five 1-second immersions) in solution No. 3 (thiazine dye mixture); allow excess to drain
5. Rinse slide gently with tap water.
6. Air dry and observe slide with light microscopy (100×, 400×).

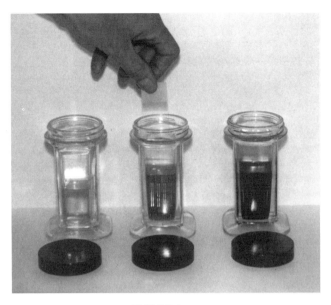

FIGURE 17-4
Staining a specimen smear with the Diff-Quik system.

Inflammatory Cells

Five basic types of inflammatory cells may be found in conjunctival samples from diseased eyes stained with the Giemsa or Diff-Quik techniques: polymorphonuclear neutrophils (PMNs), lymphocytes, monocytes, plasma cells, and eosinophils.[2,3,6,7] In comparison with the rectangular shape of the epithelial cells, inflammatory cells appear oval or round.

PMNs (or "polys") have multilobed nuclei that stain dark blue-purple, and and they exhibit fine, barely visible pink granules in the cytoplasm (see Color Plate 17-I). Classically, an abundance of PMNs indicates a bacterial infection.

Lymphocytes are cells with round, regular nuclei that stain solidly blue-purple (Figure 17-5). Because these cells vary in size, the amount of pale blue cytoplasm surrounding the nucleus ranges from a thin crescent to a medium band. Monocytes are typically larger than lymphocytes, exhibit more cytoplasm, and have kidney-bean–shaped nuclei. Both monocytes and lymphocytes are mononuclear-type cells and are the predominant cells in viral infections.

Eosinophils are identified by the red- or pink-stained granules in their cytoplasm. Their dark, blue-purple nuclei are segmented, with an average of two segments each (see Color Plate 17-I). Eosinophils are fragile cells that are frequently ruptured during preparation, so broken cells with free eosinophilic granules are commonly observed.[8] An eosinophilic response is almost pathognomonic of an allergic disease such as vernal, atopic, hay fever, or giant papillary conjunctivitis.[9,10] However, eosinophils are not always detected in patients with allergy symptoms, so the absence of these cells in a specimen does not rule out allergy as the cause of the patient's problem. Diagnosis is also complicated by the fact that a delay between the onset of allergic symptoms and the appearance of eosinophils is common. For example, in drug and cosmetic allergies, eosinophils often are not found until 10–14 days after contact. In many cases, the eosinophilia response can also vary considerably from day to day.

Plasma cells have eccentric nuclei with dark-blue cytoplasm. These cells produce antibodies and are frequently seen in chlamydial infections.

The significance of the various findings from conjunctival samples is summarized in Table 17-2. The intensity of the cellular response can be estimated by counting the number of inflammatory cells per 100 epithelial cells. Usually only one or two PMNs, lymphocytes, or monocytes are seen per 100 epithelial cells, but in acute bacterial conjunctivitis more than 100 PMNs per 100 epithelial cells are often found. In herpes simplex and adenoviral conjunctivitis, typically between 50 and 100 lymphocytes and monocytes per 100 epithelial cells can be counted.

Bacterial and fungal cells can also be observed with the Giemsa stain. Both of these cell types stain blue-purple. Their presence indicates that a smear prepared with Gram stain, as well as culturing, may be helpful with diagnosis.

Gram Stain

Gram stain allows preliminary identification of bacteria causing an infection by revealing the microscopic morphology of the bacteria as well as their specific gram reaction (coloration). Gram stain can be quickly accomplished in the office and only requires easily obtainable solutions consisting of gentian (crystal) violet, iodine, decolorizing agent, and safranin (Figure 17-6). As with the Diff-Quik stain, Gram stain involves obtaining a specimen with a spatula or swab and smearing it evenly in a thin layer on a microscopic slide. The specimen is then fixed with heat

FIGURE 17-5

Lymphocytes from a patient with adenoviral conjunctivitis (arrow). Epithelial cells are also present. Monocytes are larger than most lymphocytes and have a cytoplasm that stains light blue with a single, irregularly shaped (bean-shaped), medium-blue nucleus that often looks foamy or vacuolated. Monocytes are often observed in viral and chlamydial infections.

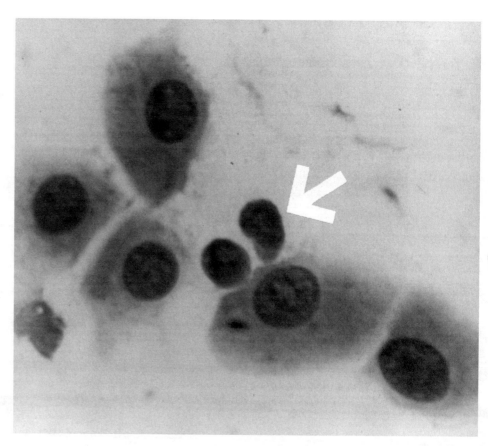

TABLE 17-2

Cytology of Giemsa-Stained Conjunctival Samples

Observation	Implication
Predominance of poly-morphonuclear neutrophils	Bacterial conjunctivitis

Predominance of lymphocytes and monocytes	Viral conjunctivitis
	  Adenovirus
	  Herpes simplex virus

Mixed response of poly-morphonuclear neutrophils, monocytes, lymphocytes	Chlamydial conjunctivitis

Presence of eosinophils	Allergic conjunctivitis
	  Vernal
	  Hay fever
	  Atopic
	  Giant papillary
	    conjunctivitis

Presence of epithelial cell changes	
Cytoplasmic inclusion bodies	Chlamydial infection
Keratinization	Keratoconjunctivitis sicca, xerophthalmia
Increased goblet cells	Keratoconjunctivitis sicca, chronic conjunctivitis

or methanol, and an alternating stain and rinse procedure is performed (Table 17-3).

Interpretation of specimens prepared with Gram stain involves observation of the slide using light microscopy (1,000×). Gram-positive bacteria retain the initial crystal violet stain and therefore appear deep violet in color. Gram-negative bacteria lose their violet color in the decolorizer and stain red or pink by the safranin counterstain. All gram-negative bacteria are consistent in their reaction (i.e., they will always appear red or pink). Gram-positive bacteria, however, may have variable staining properties according to the staining technique and the age of the bacteria. Best results are obtained with young bacteria that are not overly decolorized.

Culturing Bacteria and Fungi

To positively identify specific bacteria or fungi, it is often necessary to obtain a sample of the infectious agent for growth in a suitable culture medium. This process produces large numbers of bacteria or fungi that can be examined with staining techniques, and it allows the effects of the bacteria on a specific culture media to be assessed.

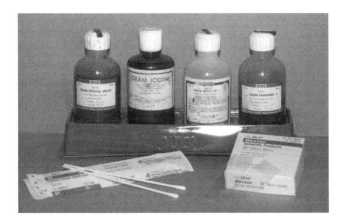

FIGURE 17-6

Materials used for Gram staining. These include sterile, cotton-tipped applicators, glass microscope slides, and the Gram stain solutions. Not pictured are an alcohol lamp and Kimura spatula, which is commonly used as an alternative for specimen collection.

TABLE 17-3

Procedure for a Gram Stain

1. Spread film of specimen on slide.
2. Allow smear to air dry.
3. Heat-fix the smear by passing the slide rapidly through a flame three times.
4. Stain with crystal violet (1 minute).
5. Rinse with tap water.
6. Stain with iodine (1 minute).
7. Rinse with tap water.
8. Rinse briefly with decolorizer.
9. Quickly rinse with tap water.
10. Stain with safranin (30 seconds).
11. Rinse with tap water.
12. Gently blot or air dry.
13. Examine slide with oil immersion microscopy (1,000×).

Culturing also provides an opportunity for evaluating the effectiveness of antibacterial or antifungal drugs.

Routine and special purpose media recommended for the growth of bacteria are listed in Table 17-4. Blood agar (5% defibrinated sheep's blood in a trypticase-soy agar base) is suitable for growing the majority of bacteria. Chocolate agar (polypeptone agar base enriched with hemoglobin and specific nutrients) is used to cultivate fastidious pathogens such as *Haemophilus* and *Neisseria*. In suspected gonococcal or meningococcal infections, specimens can be inoculated onto Thayer-Martin medium, which selectively facilitates growth of *Neisseria* in the presence of other contaminating bacteria. Blood, chocolate, and Thayer-Martin plates should be incubated in an atmosphere that contains 3–10% CO_2 (which can be obtained by using a candle jar, CO_2 incubator, or Ziploc bag with a CO_2 generator) at 37°C for a minimum of 48 hours.

A number of selective and nonselective media are available for the isolation of anaerobic bacteria (those that do not grow readily in the presence of oxygen), but fluid thioglycolate medium is generally used for culturing these bacteria (see Table 17-4).

The medium most commonly used for growing fungi from ocular infections is Sabouraud's agar containing chloramphenicol or gentamicin (but not cycloheximide) to reduce the growth of bacteria. To culture fungi with this medium, plates should be incubated at 27°C.

To simplify the growth of common ocular pathogens in the office, a convenient culturing system called the Bullseye Respiratory Culture System (Bioclinical Systems, Jacksonville, FL) can be used. This system is actually designed for growing respiratory bacteria but is usable for ocular pathogens. It consists of a single plate containing different types of media, each designed to facilitate the growth of a different type of bacteria (Figure 17-7). In the center of the

TABLE 17-4

Suggested Culture Media for Use in Ophthalmic Practice

Suspected Infection	Blood Agar	Chocolate Agar	Thayer-Martin Agar	Sabouraud's Agar	Fluid Thioglycolate Medium
Blepharitis	+	+			
Acute bacterial conjunctivitis	+	+			
Chronic conjunctivitis	+	+			
Hyperacute conjunctivitis		+	+		
Neonatal conjunctivitis	+	+	+		
Canaliculitis	+	+		+	+
Dacryocystitis	+	+		+	+
Corneal ulcer	+	+		+	+
Endophthalmitis	+	+		+	+
Orbital/preseptal cellulitis	+	+		+	+

Source: Modified from L Wilson, R Sexton. Laboratory Diagnosis in Ocular Disease. In TD Duane (ed), Clinical Ophthalmology. Hagerstown, MD: Harper & Row, 1979;4(1):3.

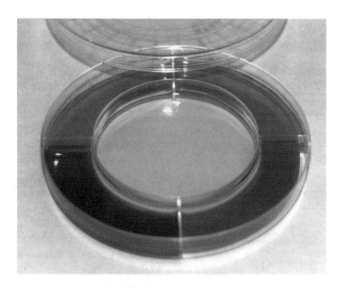

FIGURE 17-7
Culture plate from the Bullseye Respiratory Culture System showing the five sections (Bioclinical Systems, Jacksonville, FL).

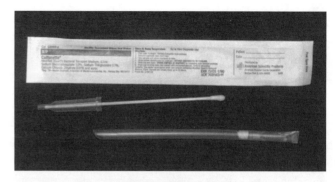

FIGURE 17-8
The Culturette device used for collecting and transporting ocular specimens (Baxter Scientific Products).

plate is a well for testing the susceptibility of bacteria to various antibiotics. This system is designed to be used in an office setting and comes complete with descriptive material to help in identifying the bacteria that are grown.

Submitting Specimens to a Laboratory

Although culturing and identifying most common pathogenic bacteria and fungi is relatively easy, some clinicians prefer to send specimens to a hospital or private laboratory for these procedures. A device used for collecting and transporting ocular specimens is the commercially available Culturette (Baxter Scientific Products, McGraw Park, IL) (Figure 17-8). The Culturette consists of a self-contained cotton-tipped swab that is used to collect the specimen. After collection, the swab is submerged into modified Stuart's transport medium (supplied in the Culturette), and the Culturette is closed. Swabs without transport medium should not be used for submitting specimens because the specimen will dry out and organism viability may be lost. If the Culturette is mailed to a laboratory, postal regulations should be consulted regarding shipment of biological specimens.

Techniques for Obtaining Specimens to Be Cultured

Lids

To obtain a lid culture, a sterile cotton swab premoistened with sterile, unpreserved saline is wiped across the anterior lid margin of both the upper and lower lids of one eye and inoculated onto blood agar by gently rolling the swab tip over the surface of the agar. The same swab can then be used to inoculate a chocolate agar plate. This procedure should be repeated for the left eye using a second swab.

Conjunctiva

To obtain a conjunctival culture, the lower lid is everted and the palpebral conjunctival surface wiped with a sterile, moistened cotton swab along the entire lower cul-de-sac. The swab is then used to inoculate the agar plates as previously described. A conjunctival culture of the upper conjunctiva can also be obtained with upper lid eversion (Figure 17-9). This procedure should be repeated with a fresh swab for the other eye.

To reduce the number of plates needed for each patient, one plate of each medium (e.g., blood and chocolate) can be used to culture the lids and conjunctiva of both eyes. This is done by streaking material from the right conjunctiva horizontally onto one quadrant of each plate, streaking material from the right lid in the form of an "R," streaking material from the left conjunctiva vertically in another quadrant, and finally streaking the material from the left lid in the form of an "L" (Figure 17-10).

Cornea

To obtain material for culturing from a central corneal ulcer, sampling must be performed in a deliberate and meticulous manner.[11] Complete workup of a corneal ulcer requires sampling of material from the lid and conjunctiva as well as from the ulcer itself. Material from the conjunctiva and lid margins of both eyes is cultured on blood, chocolate, and Sabouraud's agars. Sabouraud's agar is used to culture fungi, which rarely cause problems of

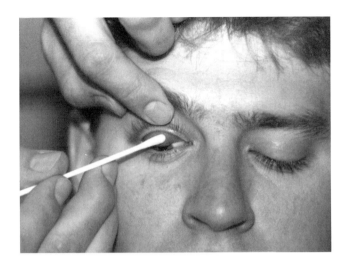

FIGURE 17-9
Obtaining a culture specimen from the superior tarsal conjunctiva with a premoistened sterile swab.

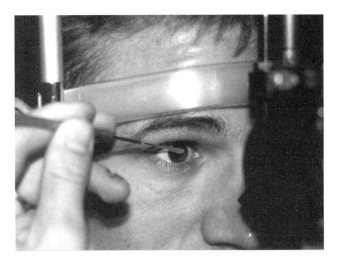

FIGURE 17-11
Obtaining a corneal specimen using a sterile platinum spatula.

the lid and conjunctiva but do cause corneal ulcers. Both eyes are cultured because results from the noninvolved eye are often useful for comparative purposes.

Corneal material for culture is best obtained by scraping areas of ulceration or suppuration with a sterile Kimura spatula (flame heated and then allowed to cool). This procedure is ideally done with the aid of a slit amp. After the instillation of one or two drops of 0.5% proparacaine (Figure 17-11), both the advancing edge and central base of the ulcer are scraped. This must be done because some organisms (e.g., *Streptococcus pneumoniae*) are found more readily at the active edge of the ulcer, whereas others (e.g., *Moraxella*) are found more readily at the base of the ulcer.[12]

To obtain adequate specimens, the ulcer must be scraped multiple times. Each scraping should consist of a series of short, moderately firm strokes made in one direction only,

with care taken not to touch the lashes or the lids. The material obtained from the scraping is placed on microscope slides for staining with Giemsa, Diff-Quik, or Gram stains, and any special stains suggested by the clinical appearance of the lesion or the results of an earlier culture. Having prepared these slides, the ulcer is scraped again and the material obtained is inoculated onto blood, chocolate, and Sabouraud's agars by lightly streaking both sides of the spatula over the surface to produce a row of separate inoculation marks (C streaks) (Figure 17-12). Each additional scraping should be plated as a new row of streaks. Care should be taken not to penetrate the surface of the agar because the recognition and isolation of bacteria and fungi in cut streaks of agar is difficult and could delay diagnosis. It must be understood that to adequately sample an ulcer, 15–20 separate scrapings should be made. Trying to spread the material obtained

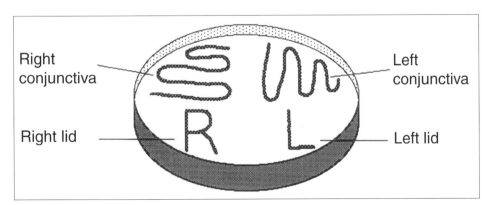

Right conjunctiva

Right lid

Left conjunctiva

Left lid

FIGURE 17-10
An example streaking convention used for conjunctival and lid cultures.

FIGURE 17-12
Inoculation of corneal scrapings onto the surface of agar medium in "C" streaks.

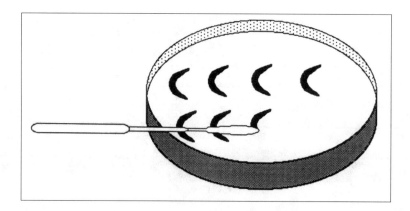

from only a few scrapings onto all of the slides and plates will usually produce unsatisfactory results.

Thioglycolate broth should also be inoculated by transferring material from the spatula onto a tryptic soy broth–saturated calcium alginate swab or by swabbing the ulcer directly with a fresh cotton-tipped swab. The swab is then pushed to the bottom of a tube containing the thioglycolate broth to ensure placement of the inoculum within the reduced oxygen zone. The shaft of the swab is next broken off against the inside edge of the tube, and the broken portion of the shaft touched by the clinician is discarded. No part of the shaft touched by the clinician should ever enter the tube.

Other Infection Sites

Specimens from other ocular tissues can also be cultured using the methods just described. For preseptal cellulitis, the source of the specimen could be drainage from the abscess if the wound is open, or material aspirated by a needle in the case of a closed lesion. For orbital cellulitis, the presence of an open wound or drainage site allows material to be obtained via aspiration with a syringe. Material from an intraorbital abscess or infected sinus can be obtained by needle aspiration. In the case of dacryoadenitis, a cotton swab can be used to collect material along the conjunctiva. With dacryocystitis or canaliculitis, conjunctival cultures should be obtained in the standard manner with additional material obtained by expressing material from the punctal opening.

Interpretation of Cultures

Interpreting the significance of growth from lid and conjunctival cultures requires familiarity with the normal, indigenous microflora of the eye (Table 17-5). Typically, surveys of normal conjunctiva and lids reveal *Staphylococcus epidermidis* as the most frequent inhabitant of the external eye.[13–15] Other bacteria, including the diph-

TABLE 17-5
Normal Flora of the External Eye

Organism	Percentage
Staphylococcus epidermidis	75–90
Diphtheroids (e.g., *Corynebacterium xerosis*)	20–33
Staphylococcus aureus	20–25
Alpha-hemolytic streptococci	2–6
Haemophilus (children under age 3 years)	3
Pneumococcus	1–3
Gram-negative rods	0–5

Source: Modified from HB Fedukowicz. External Infections of the Eye (2nd ed). New York: Appleton-Century-Crofts, 1978;260.

theroids (*Corynebacterium xerosis, Corynebacterium pseudodiphtheriticum*) and *Staphylococcus aureus,* are also found with significant frequencies in the normal population. The incidence of diphtheroids increases markedly in the 30- to 50-year age group. Pneumococci and streptococci are found occasionally in children under 5 years of age. Small numbers of certain pathogenic microorganisms such as *S. aureus, Haemophilus* sp., and *Pseudomonas* sp. can be present normally without producing disease.

Quantifying the relative number of bacteria in conjunctival samples can be of considerable value (Table 17-6). For example, in a case of suspected bacterial conjunctivitis, the cultivation of 10–15 colonies of *S. epidermidis* would usually be regarded as normal flora (Figure 17-13) and would not suggest infection, but a confluent growth of this organism would suggest that it was causing the disease.

Indigenous organisms in the preocular tear film can be cultured in infectious and noninfectious keratitis and will appear on the inoculation marks (C streaks) from the corneal specimen. Growth outside the inoculation marks should be disregarded as contamination. Recognition of

TABLE 17-6

Quantitation of Growth from Lid and Conjunctival Cultures

Finding	Grade
< 50 colonies	Count and record
> 50 isolated colonies	1+
Colonies too numerous to count, early coalescence	2+
Mass growth, coalescence	3+

Source: Modified from KR Wilhelmus, TJ Liesegang, MS Osato, DB Jones. Laboratory Diagnosis of Ocular Infections. In SC Specter (ed), Cumitech 13A. Washington, DC: American Society for Microbiology, 1994.

the indigenous flora is aided by sparse growth and the appearance of the same organisms in the culture of the ipsilateral conjunctiva. The appearance of colonies of the same organism on two or more streaks is sufficient to incriminate this isolate as the cause of an infection. Growth of the same bacterium in thioglycolate broth provides additional confirmation. Aerobic bacteria growing in thioglycolate broth, but not identified on one of the solid media plates, should be suspected as a contaminant. As a rule, in untreated, fresh bacterial corneal ulcers, the infecting organism is present in such sufficient numbers that there is little difficulty in finding it on a slide prepared with Gram stain or with culturing.

The majority of fungi causing keratitis can be detected within 5–7 days on Sabouraud's agar. However, ocular cultures should be kept for a minimum of 3 weeks to ensure that all fungi present in the culture have had a chance to develop.

Antibiotic Susceptibility Testing

Antibiotic susceptibility of bacteria can be tested using two techniques: disc diffusion or antibiotic dilution. To determine antibiotic susceptibility using disc diffusion, a uniform "lawn" of the pathogen is inoculated onto the surface of a plate, and small discs containing individual antibiotics are then placed on the plate. The plate is incubated, and zones of bacterial growth inhibition are measured (Figure 17-14). According to the diameter of the zone of inhibition, the bacteria are considered to be resistant (R), intermediately susceptible (I), or susceptible (S) to the antibiotics in the discs.

In the second type of susceptibility testing, serial dilutions of the antibacterial drug are inoculated with the test organism to determine the minimal inhibitory concentration (MIC), which is defined as the lowest concentration of antibiotic allowing no apparent growth of the bacteria (Figure 17-15). The selection of antibacterial drugs for susceptibility testing of ocular isolates is listed in Table 17-7.

OCULAR MICROBIOLOGY

A variety of microorganisms can cause ocular infections. The following sections discuss some of the more clinically important bacteria, viruses, fungi, and protozoans.

Bacteria

Bacteria are a diverse group of single-celled microorganisms that typically produce their own energy and cellular components. Structurally, bacteria have a rigid cell wall,

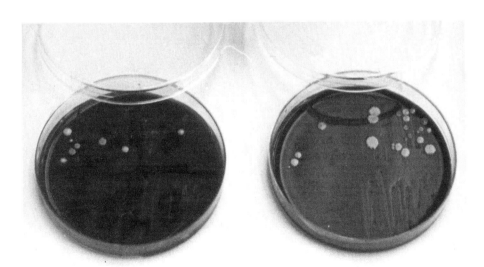

FIGURE 17-13

Blood (left) and chocolate (right) agar plates showing colonies of normal conjunctival flora (S. epidermidis). Greater numbers of colonies that become confluent would suggest pathologic infection by the organism.

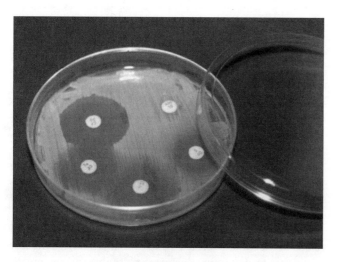

FIGURE 17-14
Disc diffusion plate for antibiotic susceptibility testing. The amount of inhibition of bacterial growth surrounding the antibiotic-laced disc indicates relative susceptibility.

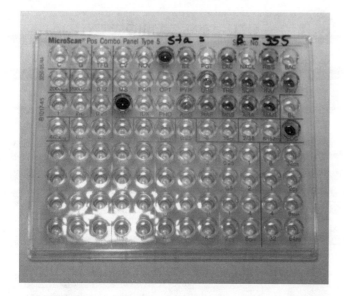

FIGURE 17-15
Microtiter plate for antibiotic minimum inhibitory concentration (MIC) testing. Bacteria are inoculated into varying concentrations of antibiotic. The MIC is the lowest concentration of antibiotic allowing no apparent bacterial growth.

a cell membrane composed of phospholipids and proteins, genetic deoxyribonucleic acid (DNA) lying free in the cytoplasm, and ribosomes that are involved in protein synthesis (Figure 17-16). The largest division of bacteria, the "true" bacteria, can be subdivided into groups on the basis of their Gram stain reaction, their cell shape,

TABLE 17-7
Recommended Anti-Infective Drugs for Use in Susceptibility Testing for Ocular Isolates

1. Neomycin
2. Polymyxin B
3. Gentamicin
4. Tobramycin
5. Tetracycline
6. Bacitracin
7. Sulfacetamide
8. Erythromycin
9. Ampicillin
10. Ciprofloxacin
11. Trimethoprim

and the arrangement patterns they form with other similar bacterial cells. Using Gram stain, bacteria stain either gram-positive (purple) or gram-negative (pink or red) depending on their cell wall components. Three different cell shapes are displayed among bacteria: spherical cells are called *cocci,* rod-shaped cells are called *bacilli,* and spiraled cells are called *spirilla.* With respect to arrangement patterns, cocci are arranged as pairs, chains, or in clusters; rods appear singly, as pairs, or in chains; and spirilla appear as individual cells, although they may tangle together.

Even though there are many species of true bacteria, only a few are pathogenic in humans. The most common pathogens and the ocular infections they cause are discussed in the following section.

Staphylococci

Staphylococci are typically gram-positive, spherical bacteria that are arranged in grape-like clusters (Figure 17-17). Young cocci stain strongly gram-positive, but many older bacteria become gram-negative. Because of this, diagnosis from direct smears can be difficult and culturing might be necessary to confirm the diagnosis of staphylococcal infection. Staphylococci can easily be cultured on routine media such as blood and chocolate agars. Colonies are typically round, discrete, smooth, raised, glistening, and 1–2 mm in diameter.

The genus *Staphylococcus* has at least 20 species.[15-17] *S. aureus* and *S. epidermidis* are among the most frequently encountered members of the normal skin flora. *S. epidermidis* has been cultured from up to 82% of normal eyelids and 83% of normal conjunctivas and *S. aureus* from up to 45% of normal eyelids and conjunctivas.[13,14,18]

For many years *S. aureus* was considered pathogenic, whereas *S. epidermidis* was considered to be part of the normal flora and not a potential cause of infection. *S. aureus* is still a major pathogen for humans, but *S. epi-*

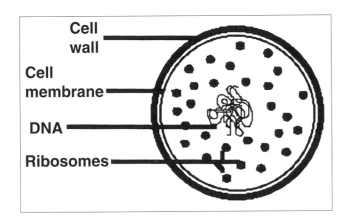

FIGURE 17-16
Schematic of a sphere-shaped bacterium showing cell wall, cell membrane, ribosomes, and nuclear material. Bacteria do not have a nuclear membrane surrounding the DNA.

dermidis and other species are now being isolated from infections.[19,20] For example, *S. epidermidis* can cause blepharoconjunctivitis in patients using eye cosmetics contaminated with the organism.[21]

To distinguish *S. aureus* from *S. epidermidis* and the other staphylococcal species, a simple laboratory test known as the coagulase test is used.[22] The test is based on the fact that *S. aureus* liberates the enzyme coagulase, which has the ability to clot human plasma, whereas *S. epidermidis* and the other species of staphylococci do not. *S. aureus* can also be differentiated from *S. epidermidis* by growth on mannitol salt agar because *S. aureus* ferments the mannitol, causing a color change in the medium, whereas *S. epidermidis* does not. In culture on blood agar, *S. aureus* often produces a hemolysis that causes destruction of red blood cells in the agar, creating a clear area around the colonies. In contrast, *S. epidermidis* does

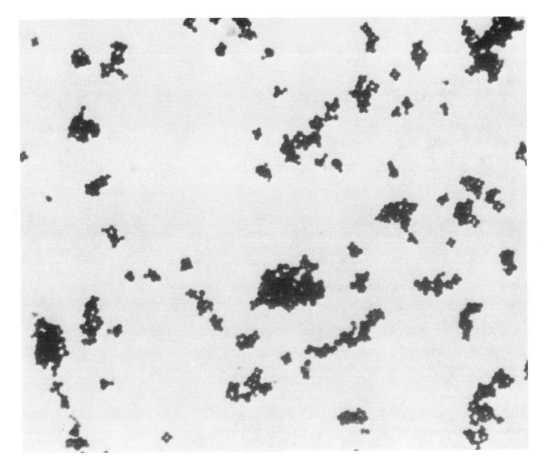

FIGURE 17-17
Staphylococcus aureus. *Note the spherical-shaped organisms arranged in clusters. (Gram stain; original magnification 250×.) (Reprinted with permission from JD Bartlett. Clinical Ocular Microbiology and Cytology. In JE Terry [ed], Ocular Disease: Detection, Diagnosis and Treatment. Springfield, IL: Thomas, 1984;402–35.)*

not produce such a clear area, which forms another basis for differentiation of the two species. In addition to these tests, new and rapid methods for differentiating and speciating *S. aureus* and the coagulase-negative staphylococci have been developed.[20,23,24]

Blepharitis   Diseases produced by staphylococci cover a wide spectrum, from the simplest localized infection of the skin, to focal infections of deep tissues and potentially fatal septicemia and disseminated disease. The source of invading staphylococci is often the patient's own endogenous, resident staphylococci but may be transferred from other infected individuals.

Staphylococci are the most common cause of simple infections of the eyelid, but they can also cause more severe diseases such as corneal ulcers. In staphylococcal blepharitis, the bacteria usually infect the lash follicles, causing lid and lash crusts and collarettes along with ulcers on the lid margins. Sixty to 80% of patients with a clinical diagnosis of staphylococcal blepharitis have *S. aureus* culturable from their lids or conjunctiva, and the majority of these patients also have coagulase-negative strains.[25,26] A characteristic shared by *S. aureus* and some strains of coagulase-negative staphylococci, and one that might be involved in the pathogenesis of blepharitis, is their ability to produce lipolytic enzymes that can modify eyelid gland lipids and result in outflow stasis.[25,27]

Complications of staphylococcal blepharitis include tylosis (callus formation) and madarosis caused by inflammation of the lash follicles. Other complications, including secondary conjunctivitis, superficial punctate keratopathy (most marked on the lower cornea), phlyctenules, and marginal corneal infiltrates, seem to be either allergic or toxic reactions to staphylococcal by-products.[28,29]

Conjunctivitis   Both *S. aureus* and *S. epidermidis* can cause acute mucopurulent and chronic conjunctivitis in children or adults.[30-34] Staphylococcal conjunctivitis typically involves the lower palpebral conjunctiva and has an associated mucopurulent discharge. Marginal corneal infiltrates are not uncommon. If untreated, the infection can become chronic.

Corneal Ulcers   Both *S. aureus* and *S. epidermidis* produce corneal ulcerations that have a similar appearance; however, those caused by *S. aureus* are generally more severe and associated with more complications.[12,35] A staphylococcal ulcer is usually yellowish-white and round to oval in shape with distinct borders, but the tissue surrounding the ulcer margin is often blurred by stromal infiltrate and edema. The infection may initially be superficial, but, if inadequately treated, can progress to a stromal abscess that may lead to perforation.

Other Ocular Problems   Staphylococci are associated with many ocular conditions besides blepharitis, conjunctivitis,

and corneal ulcers. Staphylococci are the most common bacteria to cause external hordeola by infecting individual Zeis and Moll glands, and internal hordeola by infecting meibomian glands. They can also cause dacryocystitis,[36] preseptal and orbital cellulitis,[37] endophthalmitis,[38] and secondary infections in patients with trachoma, pemphigus, and keratomalacia. In addition, superimposed staphylococcal infections can cause serious complications in measles, influenza, and adenoviral infections.

Streptococci

Streptococci are gram-positive, spherical bacteria that are typically arranged in chains, although at least one species occurs in pairs (Figure 17-18). Streptococci are distinguished from staphylococci (which are also gram-positive cocci) by the use of the catalase test. Streptococci are catalase-negative whereas staphylococci are catalase-positive.

The most common classification of the streptococci is based on their action on blood agar. *Beta hemolysis* produced by streptococci results in a complete lysis of red blood cells in the medium. *Alpha hemolysis* produced by other streptococci results in an incomplete hemolysis with a brownish or greenish discoloration to the medium. There are also some streptococci that do not produce hemolysis and thus do not change the red blood cells in the medium.

To culture streptococci, an enriched medium is required. Blood agar plates are routinely used for primary isolation and determining the type of hemolysis. Increased CO_2, obtained by the use of a CO_2 incubator, candle jar, or Ziploc bag with CO_2-generating ampules, produces the best growth of the bacteria and full development of the hemolysis.

Several species of streptococci are important causes of ocular disease. *Streptococcus pyogenes* occurs in chains. On blood agar, colonies are pinpoint, grayish, and slightly opalescent with a 2- to 4-mm zone of beta hemolysis (clear agar) surrounding the colonies. In contrast to other beta-hemolytic streptococci, *S. pyogenes* is sensitive to bacitracin, and a disc containing this antibiotic will inhibit its growth on blood agar. Further characterization of the beta-hemolytic streptococci is done by Lancefield serologic typing, with the majority of the pathogenic beta-hemolytic streptococci (*S. pyogenes*) falling into group A.[39]

While *S. pyogenes* causes many systemic diseases such as erysipelas, pharyngitis, scarlet fever, rheumatic fever, and acute glomerulonephritis, it is an infrequent cause of eye infections. Conjunctivitis caused by *S. pyogenes* is rare, but when it occurs it is frequently severe with pseudomembrane or true membrane formation.[40] Preseptal cellulitis of the lid, orbital cellulitis,[37] dacryocystitis,[36] and endophthalmitis[38] can also be caused by *S. pyogenes*.

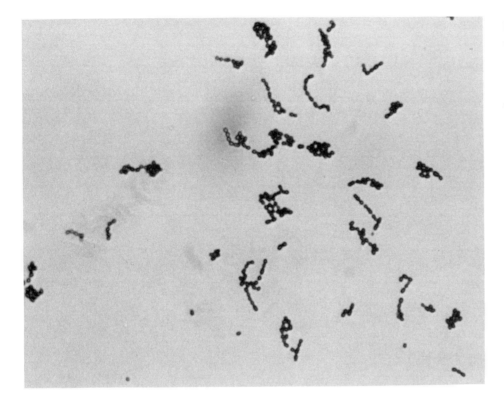

FIGURE 17-18
Streptococcus organisms are typically spherical and arranged in chains (Gram stain; original magnification 250×.) (Reprinted with permission from JD Bartlett. Clinical Ocular Microbiology and Cytology. In JE Terry [ed], Ocular Disease: Detection, Diagnosis and Treatment. Springfield, IL: Thomas, 1984;402–35.)

The viridans group of streptococci are gram-positive cocci that most commonly occur in chains. On blood agar they produce alpha hemolysis with a greening of the agar. They are distinguished from *S. pneumoniae* on the basis of the optochin test. The compound optochin does not inhibit the growth of viridans streptococci, but it does inhibit the growth of *S. pneumoniae*. Viridans streptococci (e.g., *S. mutans, S. mitis, S. sanguis*) are part of the normal respiratory system flora, but they can produce systemic diseases such as subacute endocarditis. Viridans streptococci are not common ocular pathogens, but they have been isolated from patients with conjunctivitis,[30] corneal ulcers,[12] dacryocystitis,[36] and postoperative endophthalmitis.[38]

Streptococcus pneumoniae, or pneumococcus (formerly called *Diplococcus*), is a common bacterium frequently inhabiting the upper respiratory tract of humans. Up to 70% of normal, asymptomatic individuals harbor pneumococci in their throats. The highest carrier rates are found among grammar school– or preschool-aged children and their parents.

Pneumococcus is a gram-positive coccus, usually occurring in pairs or a short chain of pairs, although it may be found singly. Characteristically these organisms are bullet-shaped with the bases of the bullets adjacent to one another. Many strains of this organism produce a polysaccharide capsule, which makes the organisms more virulent by preventing or delaying their destruction. *Streptococcus pneumoniae* causes alpha hemolysis on blood agar with a typical greenish discoloration of the blood around each colony. Differentiation from other alpha-hemolytic streptococci, such as the viridans streptococci, can be made on the basis of growth inhibition by optochin and cell solubilization by bile.

Conjunctivitis Pneumococci are occasionally found in the conjunctiva as transient members of the normal flora[13,14]; however, they are more often found as the cause of a variety of ocular diseases. *S. pneumoniae* is one of the most common causes of acute bacterial conjunctivitis in adults and children.[30,32] This infection occurs most frequently in northern climates during the winter and is often associated with a common cold. In pneumococcal conjunctivitis, as in most types of bacterial conjunctivitis, a mucopurulent discharge is usually produced, and many PMNs are found in a conjunctival scraping. Petechial hemorrhages of the bulbar conjunctival vessels are frequently seen, and chemosis, lid swelling, and enlarged preauricular lymph nodes may occur. As in many other types of conjunctivitis, superficial punctate keratopathy can occur.

Corneal Ulcers *Streptococcus pneumoniae* is a common cause of central corneal ulcers characterized as serpiginous or creeping, spreading most often toward the center of the cornea.[12,35] The ulcer usually progresses rapidly, extends

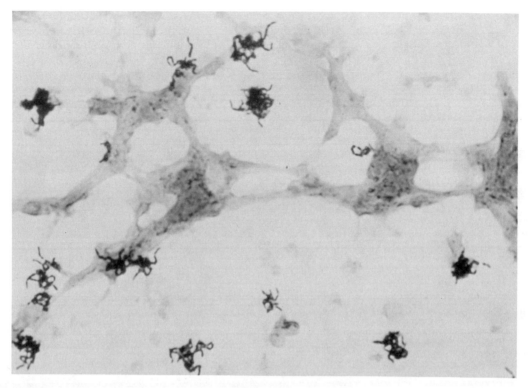

FIGURE 17-19

Corynebacteria. Note the slender, club-shaped pleomorphic rods. (Gram stain; original magnification 250×.) (Reprinted with permission from JD Bartlett. Clinical Ocular Microbiology and Cytology. In JE Terry [ed], Ocular Disease: Detection, Diagnosis and Treatment. Springfield, IL: Thomas, 1984;402–35.)

into the deep stroma, and often leads to corneal perforation. Extensive corneal tissue damage, as well as sterile hypopyon formation, which characterizes a pneumococcal corneal infection, is caused by the rapid production of bacterial exotoxins.[41] Pneumococcus, like most bacteria, is unable to penetrate intact corneal epithelium; thus ulcer development usually occurs after a corneal abrasion.

Corynebacteria

Corynebacterium species have striking morphologic features that differentiate them from other bacteria. These organisms are characteristically gram-positive, large, slender, pleomorphic rods that are straight or slightly curved (Figure 17-19). These bacilli arrange themselves at various angles to each other and are frequently considered to make patterns resembling Chinese characters. They often stain irregularly because of the presence of metachromatic granules in their cytoplasm.

Corynebacteria are nonfastidious bacteria that grow readily on many bacteriologic media. On blood agar, colonies are usually small, grayish, and granular. Beta hemolysis may be slight or absent. Species differentiation between the corynebacteria can be made on the basis of differential sugar fermentation.

Corynebacteria that are part of the normal flora of the body are often referred to as *diphtheroids.* This is because when they are stained with Gram stain, they resemble *C. diphtheriae,* the bacterium causing diphtheria. The diphtheroids, *C. xerosis* and *C. pseudodiphtheriticum,* are considered to be normal human flora. They are characteristically associated with epithelial cells and can be found in up to 33% of normal conjunctivae.[13,14]

Although diphtheria is now rare, *C. diphtheriae* can be a cause of conjunctivitis after pharyngeal diphtheria in children aged 2–8 years. Two primary clinical types of corynebacterial conjunctivitis are recognized: pseudomembranous and true membranous.[36] The pseudomembrane can be removed without resultant bleeding, whereas removal of a true membrane results in significant bleeding.

Neisseria

Neisseria are gram-negative bacteria appearing as kidney-shaped cells arranged in pairs (diplococci) (Color Plate 17-II). A number of species including *N. sicca* and *N.*

flavescens are commonly found among the normal flora of the upper respiratory tract. Two *Neisseria* species are pathogenic for humans: *N. gonorrhoeae* (also known as gonococcus) and *N. meningitidis* (also known as meningococcus). In a smear prepared with Gram stain, these two species are characteristically found within PMNs, which is a feature that is important for their identification. In general, any gram-negative diplococci found within PMNs are presumed to be one of the pathogenic *Neisseria* species.

Since the pathogenic *Neisseria* are both fragile and fastidious organisms, their isolation and identification is best accomplished by direct culture on Thayer-Martin or chocolate agar in a 2–10% CO_2 environment at 37°C. On chocolate agar, the colonies are unpigmented, glistening, large, mucoid, semitranslucent, and odorless.

Classically, the *Neisseria* have been differentiated on the basis of their capabilities to ferment various sugars, but coagglutination and enzyme immunoassay tests have been introduced to rapidly identify the different species of *Neisseria*.[42]

Conjunctivitis   Although ocular infections by *N. gonorrhoeae* and *N. meningitidis* are uncommon, their rapid progression and concomitant tissue destruction make them important organisms. In the eye, *N. gonorrhoeae* causes purulent conjunctivitis. Infection during the neonatal period can be caused by inoculation of the eyes during birth. Infection during adolescence and adulthood is usually caused by self-inoculation from infected genitalia. Gonococcal conjunctivitis of the newborn (gonococcal ophthalmia neonatorum) is characterized by an incubation period of 1–3 days with involvement usually being bilateral. The conjunctivitis is associated with a copious purulent discharge and with markedly swollen lids that are difficult to open. In adults, gonococcal conjunctivitis is similar in appearance but is usually unilateral, with the right eye most frequently involved in right-handed patients.

Keratitis   *N. gonorrhoeae* can infect intact nonkeratinized epithelial cells, and thus, peripheral or central corneal ulcers may occur as an extension of conjunctivitis. Neonatal gonococcal conjunctivitis is commonly complicated by a purulent keratitis; this can be particularly severe in untreated cases. The keratitis begins as a yellowish infiltrate and progresses to ulceration very rapidly. In some cases this can lead to perforation and panophthalmitis. Adult gonococcal conjunctivitis can also lead to similar corneal complications.

The meningococcus, which can be found in the oropharynx of healthy persons, causes meningitis. This organism is an infrequent but serious cause of bacterial conjunctivitis and keratitis similar to that caused by *N. gonorrhoeae*.

Prophylaxis   Gonococcal ophthalmia neonatorum is prevented by topical application of erythromycin or tetracycline ointment to the conjunctiva of newborns. Although instillation of silver nitrate solution is also effective and is the classic method for preventing this infection, silver nitrate causes conjunctival irritation. Therefore, the use of silver nitrate has been largely replaced by use of antibiotic ointment.

Moraxella

Moraxella are small gram-negative bacilli, coccobacilli, or cocci. They are nonfermentative and oxidase-positive. Moraxella are members of the normal flora of the upper respiratory tract and occasionally cause infection.

Blepharoconjunctivitis   *M. lacunata* is described in the older literature as a common cause of angular blepharoconjunctivitis, but now *S. aureus* is a more commonly implicated.[43,44] *Moraxella* species are relatively infrequent sources of conjunctival infection, but when they do cause infection, it usually is in the form of a chronic follicular conjunctivitis.

Corneal Ulcers   *Moraxella* corneal ulcers are rare but most commonly found in alcoholic or immune-suppressed patients.[45] Clinically, the ulcer often starts centrally, or inferiorly in areas of exposure. An anterior stromal abscess forms, which may then spread deeply into the cornea. These ulcers are often painless but almost invariably cause a large hypopyon if allowed to progress.[46] Although *Moraxella* is sensitive to most antibiotics, its ulcerative lesions are very slow to heal.

Haemophilus

Haemophilus aegyptius is of great historic interest because it was one of the first pathogens isolated from the eye. However, it is the closely related (or possibly identical) species, *H. influenzae*, that is most often encountered in the United States.[36] *H. influenzae* usually appears as a tiny, gram-negative coccobacillus, but long filamentous forms can sometimes develop in culture. This organism has a tendency to resist staining and is easily missed on microscopic examination. Because these gram-negative rods are difficult to distinguish from other important gram-negative rods, culturing may be required for identification.

Chocolate agar is an excellent culture medium for *H. influenzae*, and an environment of increased CO_2 favors growth. The colonies are tiny, glistening, translucent, pinpoint structures, with a dew-drop appearance. They have a pronounced, sweet odor.

Sometimes several colonies of *Haemophilus* can be isolated from a healthy eye but always in numbers significantly less than would be the case if an infection caused by this organism was present. *H. influenzae* is a frequent isolate from the upper respiratory tract of healthy carriers, especially children. Usually these respiratory isolates have a type b polysaccharide capsule (the capsule is a coating the bacteria places outside of its cell wall to protect it from phagocytosis). The type b capsule is significant because *Haemophilus* with such a capsule can cause serious infections. Fortunately, a vaccine against *H. influenzae* with the type b capsule has been developed.

Although conjunctivitis can often be caused by strains with type b capsules, it is equally caused by *Haemophilus* strains that are noncapsulated.[47] In contrast, periorbital cellulitis is more frequently caused by *H. influenzae* strains with type b capsules.[48]

Conjunctivitis   Clinically, *H. influenzae* is one of the most common causes of acute mucopurulent conjunctivitis.[30,32] This type of conjunctivitis is especially prevalent in younger children during warm weather in southern climates. Enlarged, tender preauricular glands can occur along with patchy conjunctival hemorrhages and corneal limbal infiltrates.[30] This infection is highly contagious and can become epidemic.

Other Infections   *H. influenzae* is occasionally found in the pus from lacrimal sac infections,[49] and cases of periorbital cellulitis associated with *Haemophilus* have been reported.

Enterics

Members of the very large family of enteric bacteria are widely distributed in the environment, particularly where fecal contamination is present. Although bacilli in the enteric group are part of the normal human flora, they can sometimes be pathogenic. Enterics of ocular significance include *Escherichia, Shigella, Klebsiella, Serratia, Proteus,* and *Enterobacter.*

The organisms in this group are all gram-negative rods of moderate size. They are morphologically indistinguishable from each other, and their genus identification from a smear is impossible. Identification of different members of this group is usually accomplished through biochemical and fermentation tests. Enterics are easily cultured on many bacteriologic media and grow rapidly. Colonies are semitranslucent and mucoid, with a tendency to become confluent. All members of this family are oxidase-negative, and this is therefore a useful differential feature for distinguishing this group from nonenteric, gram-negative rods, which are oxidase-positive (e.g., *Pseudomonas*).

Conjunctivitis   Enterics are not the leading cause of any specific ocular diseases but are isolated from most types of eye infections. Bacterial conjunctivitis caused by members of this family occurs more commonly among older adults, tends to be chronic, is often associated with a blepharitis, and is not infrequently seen in those with a pre-existing outer eye disorder.[33,50] Although there is no single, predominant organism responsible for such infections, most of those isolated represent enteric flora and were probably self-inoculated as the result of poor hygienic practice.

Corneal Ulcers   The enterics such as *Escherichia, Shigella, Klebsiella, Proteus,* and *Enterobacter* are isolated from corneal ulcers.[35] Until recently *Serratia marcescens* was considered to be a benign saprophyte found in water, soil, and food. However, it is now being isolated more frequently from central corneal ulcers in extended-wear contact lens patients.[51,52]

Other Infections   The enteric organisms are occasionally isolated from lacrimal system infections, preseptal and orbital cellulitis,[37] and endophthalmitis.[38] An extremely sensitive and rapid test for the diagnosis of endophthalmitis caused by gram-negative bacteria is the *Limulus* lysate assay for the bacterial endotoxin produced by these organisms.[53]

Pseudomonas aeruginosa

Pseudomonas aeruginosa is a well-known gram-negative rod indistinguishable in a Gram stain preparation from gram-negative enteric and other nonenteric bacilli. Therefore, differential diagnosis requires culturing and biochemical testing.

One of the most distinctive characteristics of *P. aeruginosa* is its production of two soluble pigments: a deep-blue pyocyanin and a yellowish-green, fluorescent pigment. Together, these pigments color the medium, but not the colonies, a bluish-green. The culture possesses a strong, sweet, hay-like odor. In many cases, these unique cultural characteristics enable an early preliminary diagnosis to be made. In some instances, early diagnosis also can be made in situ by using an ultraviolet lamp to demonstrate fluorescence of the cornea if there has been a sufficient amount of pigment production.

Pseudomonas aeruginosa is a common cause of bacterial keratitis in humans.[12] *Pseudomonas* is not a member of the normal flora of the external eye but is a transient opportunist rarely found in a healthy eye.[13,14] The organism is unable to infect the intact cornea, so infection typically follows some impairment of the corneal tissue. Contact lens patients with culture-positive ulcers are most often infected with gram-negative bacilli, and *P. aeruginosa* is the most often cultured bacterium.[54] These bacteria can enter the eye from contaminated products such as contact lens solutions or containers[55] or from the hands during contact lens manipulation.[56]

Infection with *P. aeruginosa* is of serious concern because ulcers caused by this organism can progress rapidly and perforate within 48 hours.[57] During the infection, a collagenase is produced, so that even if the bacteria are killed by antibiotics, corneal destruction can still continue.[58]

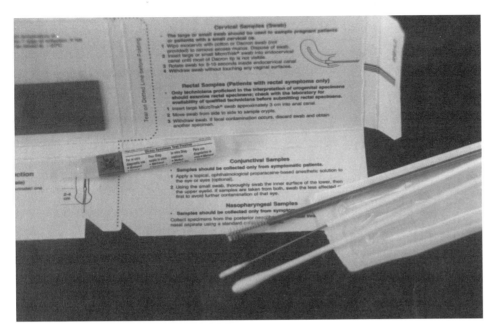

FIGURE 17-20
Opened contents of Syva's Micro-Trak chlamydial direct specimen collection kit. An ocular specimen from the palpebral conjunctiva is smeared onto a glass microscopic slide and then fixed with acetone contained in the vial. The specimen is then forwarded to a laboratory for analysis. Individual chlamydial elementary bodies can be identified with this method.

Chlamydia trachomatis

In contrast to the true bacteria discussed previously, *Chlamydia* are special microorganisms: They are obligate, intracellular organisms that cannot reproduce outside of a host cell. The ocular pathogen *C. trachomatis* is divided into several serotypes (serotypes are antigenically different versions of the same bacterial species). Serotypes A, B, Ba, and C are usually associated with classic endemic trachoma, and serotypes D through K are associated with acute conjunctivitis and sexually transmitted infections.

Chlamydia have two distinct forms: the initial body and the elementary body. The initial body is the replicative form found within the cytoplasmic inclusion bodies of host cells, and the elementary body is the extracellular form that transmits the infection between cells.

To identify ocular infections with *C. trachomatis,* several techniques are available: (1) morphologic identification of chlamydial cytoplasmic inclusion bodies by Giemsa or Diff-Quik staining of smears, (2) use of fluorescein-labeled monoclonal antibodies (FAB) to the chlamydial antigen, (3) isolation of the organism in cell cultures, (4) identification of chlamydial antigen by enzyme-linked immunoassay (EIA), (5) use of a DNA probe for chlamydial DNA, and (6) detection of antibodies to *C. trachomatis* in serum, tears, or other secretions.

Diff-Quik Stain   In Diff-Quik–stained smears, chlamydial initial bodies are seen as clusters of distinct, blue-purple clumps, known as inclusion bodies, within the cytoplasm of infected conjunctival epithelial cells.[13,59–60]

The inclusion bodies present as multiple, discrete, round granules typically aggregating in the form of a cap over the cell nucleus, or, less commonly, scattered in the cytoplasm. The cytoplasmic inclusion bodies are typically easy to observe in inclusion conjunctivitis of newborns but may be difficult to demonstrate in inclusion conjunctivitis of adults.[60] In trachoma, inclusions are usually found only when PMNs are present. The prevalence of chlamydial inclusions increases progressively with the presence of other inflammatory cells.

Direct Fluorescent Antibody (DFA) Smear   Commercially available fluorescein-labeled antibody to *C. trachomatis* is now widely available for the detection of chlamydial organisms in smears.[61] With prepared smears, individual elementary bodies are identified as brightly fluorescing extracellular particles, but the intracellular inclusions are not as easily identified.[61] At least ten elementary bodies must be identified for a positive test result. The technique requires a fluorescent microscope and an experienced microscopist. However, it is widely available, and the collection of an ocular specimen for a DFA test is easily performed (Chlamydia MicroTrak, Syva, Inc., Palo Alto, CA; Pathfinder, Kallstad Diagnostics, Chasta, MN) (Figure 17-20).[62]

For conjunctivitis patients, a local anesthetic is instilled, and the smallest Dacron swab from the kit is used to vigorously swab the most affected area of the conjunctiva. Even though the instructions in the kit recommend use of the Dacron swab, better results have been reported by using a spatula to obtain the sample.[63] The specimen is then transferred onto the MicroTrak slide supplied in the collection kit, fixed with acetone (which comes in a vial in each kit), and allowed to completely air dry. The kit is then closed and labeled for delivery to the laboratory. This test has good sensitivity for all forms of chlamydial infections: trachoma and inclusion conjunctivitis in adults and newborns.[63,64]

Cell Culture   Although isolation of *C. trachomatis* in cell culture is clearly the definitive way to identify this agent,[60] facilities for *Chlamydia* culturing are not widely available, the procedure takes 3–6 days, and it is relatively expensive. However, cell culture is the standard against which all new techniques are measured.

Enzyme Immunoassay   EIA techniques have been developed to detect chlamydial antigens in clinical specimens. (Examples of EIA kits for *Chlamydia* include Chlamydiazyme, Abbott Laboratories, North Chicago, IL; MicroTrak Chlamydia EIA, Syva, Inc., Palo Alto, CA.) For enzyme immunoassays, chlamydial antibody is coated onto a solid phase such as polyvinyl or polystyrene microtiter cups. The test specimen is then added, and any *Chlamydia* present are bound to the "capture" antibodies. After washing, the bound *Chlamydia* are detected through the addition of enzyme-labeled chlamydial antibody followed by a substrate on which the enzyme acts to produce a colored product. The advantages of EIAs are that they do not require expensive equipment or highly trained personnel, and that they are useful for testing a small or large number of samples. This technique appears to be both sensitive and specific for the detection of *C. trachomatis* in conjunctival specimens.[65]

DNA Probe   Another diagnostic procedure for *Chlamydia* involves using a DNA hybridization reaction to detect chlamydial DNA in clinical specimens.[66,67] A DNA probe is a piece of DNA that can recognize and specifically hybridize to complementary DNA sequences, even in the midst of other totally unrelated DNA. DNA probes labeled with radioisotopes have been used to identify and characterize regions of chromosomal DNA that are unique to *Chlamydia*. The label is used to monitor or quantitate the ability of a DNA probe to hybridize to its complementary (target) DNA sequences. Tests that use radioactive markers have limited usefulness in the office, but several DNA probes that use enzymes for quantification are being developed.[68]

Detection of Antibodies   Detection of antibodies in serum or tears is typically not useful for the diagnosis of ocular chlamydial infections in individual patients because the infections are chronic (as in trachoma) and endemic in most populations. The most common tests used to detect antibodies to *Chlamydia* are complement fixation, enzyme immunoassay, and microimmunofluorescence.

Chlamydial Infections   The clinical syndromes associated with *C. trachomatis* infections occur in two distinct epidemiologic patterns. One pattern is the classic, blinding endemic trachoma seen in developing countries. This is spread by eye-to-eye transmission. The second pattern is associated with sexually transmitted strains of *C. trachomatis*. These strains produce urethritis and epididymitis in men and cervicitis and salpingitis in women. When self-inoculated into an adult eye, they cause *inclusion conjunctivitis,* which is a follicular conjunctivitis that may be difficult to distinguish from the early inflammatory phases of endemic trachoma. These strains can also be transmitted from infected mothers to the eyes and lungs of newborns, causing neonatal conjunctivitis and pneumonia. *C. trachomatis* is the leading cause of ophthalmia neonatorum in the United States.[69]

Whereas sexually transmitted chlamydial infections of the eye rarely cause permanent visual loss, the involvement of other sites (e.g., respiratory and genital tracts) produces significant morbidity in both adults and neonates.

Actinomycetes

The actinomycetes are filamentous bacteria with fungus-like characteristics insofar as morphology and disease mechanisms are concerned. Gram stain reveals grampositive branching filaments, pleomorphic diphtheroid-like rods, or both. Growth is best on brain-heart infusion or blood agar under anaerobic conditions. Usually there is no growth on Sabouraud's agar. Isolation can also be achieved using thioglycolate broth.

Actinomyces israelii is a frequent cause of chronic canaliculitis.[70,71] The infected canaliculus becomes red, swollen, and tender. Pressure over the swelling will sometimes expel pus and "sulfur granules" from the puncta. The "sulfur granules" obtained from the canaliculus can be crushed on a microscopic slide, mixed with saline, and stained with Gram or Giemsa stain to reveal the organism.

Viruses

Viruses are the smallest entities recognized as microorganisms. A virus contains only a single species of nucleic acid, which may be either DNA or RNA. A virus lacks constituents fundamental for growth and multiplication; therefore its duplication strictly depends on host cells. In a complete virus particle (virion), viral nucleic acid is surrounded by a protective protein coat (capsid) that consists of many identical subunits. The proteins on the capsid have a specific affinity for complementary receptors on the surfaces of susceptible cells. They also contain antigenic determinants that are responsible for the production of protective antibodies by the infected animal.

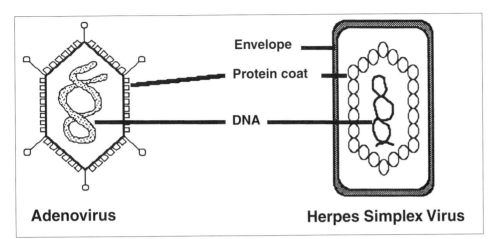

FIGURE 17-21
Schematic of an adenovirus (left) and a herpes simplex virus (right). Note both viral particles contain DNA and a protein coat, but the herpes virion has an additional outer envelope enclosing the nucleocapsid.

The capsid has icosahedral symmetry if the capsid is isometric, or helical symmetry if it is tubular. The combined nucleic acid and capsid is called the nucleocapsid. For some viruses, the nucleocapsid is surrounded by an envelope composed of the nuclear or cell membrane of a previously infected cell (Figure 17-21).

Viruses depend on host cells for multiplication. For a virus to replicate, it must invade (infect) a host cell and control metabolic processes. After new viral nucleic acid and protein are produced, new viruses are released from the host cell to infect other host cells. This type of infection produces an acute disease that is usually limited by the response of the patient's immune system. Alternatively, a few viruses are able to invade cells and then become latent. In these cases, the viral DNA becomes incorporated into the host cell's DNA and becomes protected from the host's immune system. At future times, this viral DNA can be stimulated to produce new virions, which cause recurrent disease states.

Some of the more important human viruses, their characterization, and the diseases they cause are outlined in Table 17-8. The following discussion considers the two major groups of viruses that are most important to the ophthalmic practitioner: herpesvirus and adenovirus.

Herpesvirus Group

The herpesvirus group includes four distinct members: herpes simplex virus (HSV), varicella-zoster virus (VZV), Epstein-Barr virus (EBV), and cytomegalovirus (CMV).
Herpes Simplex Virus   There are two types of HSV: type 1 (HSV-1), which is associated with infections involving the eyes, mouth, and skin above the waist; and type 2 (HSV-2), which usually affects the skin including and surrounding the genitalia. A primary systemic infection with HSV-1 occurs in most children; but in 85–99% of cases, the infection is subclinical with only mild, flu-like respiratory symptoms.[72] If ocular manifestations occur during primary infection, a follicular conjunctivitis is usually a presenting feature. Clusters of vesicles on periorbital and eyelid skin, diffuse epithelial keratitis, and microdendrites may also occur. In the United States, 60% of the population has been infected with HSV-1 by 5 years of age, and 90% has been infected by the age of 15 years.[72] Generally, the primary infection is controlled by the host's immune system, but often the virus becomes latent in the trigeminal ganglion, allowing for later recurrences. During these episodes, the virions produced in the trigeminal ganglion move through the sensory nerves to the cornea and infect the epithelial cells, producing a characteristic superficial dendritic lesion. In some instances, the virus can also cause stromal keratitis characterized by infiltration and necrosis, or it can cause disciform keratitis characterized by stromal edema. Stromal involvement is frequently accompanied by uveitis. In addition to affecting the eye, HSV-1 can also cause recurrent herpes labialis, characterized by "cold sores" or "fever blisters" on the skin around the mouth.

HSV-2 is a sexually transmitted disease that usually causes genital infection. As with a HSV-1 infection, the primary HSV-2 infection allows the virus to become latent, and the disease may become recurrent.
Varicella-Zoster Virus   In a nonimmunized host, the primary infection with VZV produces "chickenpox." The virus is thought to enter the body through the respiratory tract, and, after a 2-week incubation period, the classic vesicular rash of chickenpox breaks out on the skin. Immunity to reinfection with varicella from another person is lifelong, with second attacks of chickenpox being virtually unknown.

Once the primary infection has occurred, the virus remains latent in sensory ganglia (e.g., the trigeminal ganglion) for the patient's life. When triggered by stress,

TABLE 17-8

Classification of Some Important Human Viruses

Virus Family	Nucleic Acid	Capsid Symmetry	Envelope	Systemic Diseases	Ocular Diseases
Hepadnavirus	DNA	Icosahedral	+	Hepatitis B	
Papovavirus	DNA	Icosahedral	–	Warts	

Adenovirus	DNA	Icosahedral	–	Respiratory infections	Follicular conjunctivitis
					  Pharyngoconjunctival fever
					  Epidemic keratoconjunctivitis

Herpesvirus	DNA	Icosahedral	+	Chickenpox Shingles Cold sores Genital herpes Mononucleosis	Herpes zoster ophthalmicus Herpes simplex keratitis Cytomegalovirus retinitis
Poxvirus	DNA	Complex	Complex coat	Smallpox vaccinia	Molluscum contagiosum
Picornavirus	RNA	Icosahedral	–	Polio Intestinal infections Colds	
Reovirus	RNA	Icosahedral	–	Respiratory and intestinal infections	
Togavirus	RNA	Icosahedral	+	Encephalitis Yellow fever Rubella	
Orthomyxovirus	RNA	Helical	+	Influenza	
Paramyxovirus	RNA	Helical	+	Measles Mumps Respiratory infections	
Rhabdovirus	RNA	Helical	+	Rabies	
Retrovirus	RNA	Helical	+	AIDS	
Arenavirus	RNA	Helical	+	Encephalitis Meningitis	
Coronavirus	RNA	Helical	+	Colds Respiratory infections	

Source: Modified from JO Oh. Definition, Structure, and Classification of Viruses. In W Tasman, EA Jaeger (eds), Duane's Clinical Ophthalmology (2nd ed). Philadelphia: Lippincott, 1989;4(2):2.

reduced immunity, or other factors, the virus can reactivate, producing the syndrome of *zoster (shingles)*. During a zoster episode, the virus replicates in the sensory ganglion and migrates along the sensory nerves to the skin or eye. Signs and symptoms include neuralgic pain and vesicular eruption in the areas supplied the sensory nerves from the affected ganglion.

Herpes zoster ophthalmicus usually first manifests as a unilateral neuralgia in the region innervated by the ophthalmic division of the trigeminal nerve. The virus then produces vesicles on the skin corresponding to the distribution of the nerve. Hutchinson's sign (vesicles on the side of the tip of the nose) signals nasociliary nerve involvement and is associated with a 50–85% incidence of ocular involvement. Complications include conjunctivitis, scleritis, iridocyclitis, and glaucoma. A number of corneal lesions can also occur, such as coarse punctate keratitis, mucous plaques, dendrites, subepithelial infiltrates, stromal infiltrates, disciform kerati-

tis, deep interstitial keratitis, ring abscess, and central, paracentral, and peripheral ulceration.[73]

Epstein-Barr Virus   In early childhood, Epstein-Barr virus (EBV) infection is usually subclinical; however, in adolescence and early adulthood, it is the principal cause of infectious mononucleosis.[74] EBV infection is common throughout the world, with 90% of adults having antibodies to the virus. Conjunctivitis is the most common ocular manifestation of EBV infection. Unilateral or bilateral conjunctival hyperemia may be accompanied by an extensive follicular reaction, membrane formation, or subconjunctival hemorrhage. Other reported features include epithelial or stromal keratitis, palpebral edema, uveitis, dacryoadenitis, dacryocystitis, chorioretinitis, and optic neuritis. Since the disease is usually limited by the immune system, treatment is primarily symptomatic.

Cytomegalovirus   About 1% of infants born in the United States are infected with cytomegalovirus. The majority have subclinical but chronic infections; 10% have cytomegalic inclusion disease.[75] Adults frequently show serologic evidence of previous CMV infections, but clinical illness is rarely recognized in healthy individuals. Cytomegalovirus can cause clinical disease, however, in immunocompromised adults. Cytomegalovirus retinitis is a necrotizing infection leading to full-thickness destruction of the retina that can result in total loss of vision. This infection is common in patients with AIDS, with up to 32% of AIDS patients developing CMV retinitis.[76,77]

Adenovirus

Adenoviral infection is worldwide, mainly causing acute respiratory diseases, as well as pharyngoconjunctival fever (PCF) and epidemic keratoconjunctivitis (EKC). The serologic characteristics of the adenoviruses have been studied intensively, and at least 31 different types have been identified (serotyping is based on the fact that viruses of the same type can have different coat proteins). Serotype 4 viruses are found in acute respiratory diseases of adults, while types 1 and 2 are found in children with these conditions. Type 3 is a common finding in follicular conjunctivitis and PCF,[78,79] whereas type 8 is the most common isolate from EKC.[80] Acquired immunity to adenovirus infection is long lasting, and recurrent episodes of infection by the same serotype are extremely rare.

Pharyngoconjunctival Fever Pharyngoconjunctival fever is commonly caused by a serotype 3 adenovirus, but other serotypes can also cause this disease.[81] Pharyngoconjunctival fever is typically characterized by pharyngitis, fever, and a nonpurulent follicular conjunctivitis. Adenopathy (usually submaxillary) and high fever are commonly present. The conjunctivitis, which lasts about 3 weeks, is often unilateral and typically involves the lower fornix. Epidemics of PCF usually occur during the summer, infecting children 4–9 years old. Swimming pools may be a source of infection.[81]

Adenovirus can also cause follicular conjunctivitis without the systemic symptoms or sore throat. This condition usually occurs in winter, either sporadically or in small epidemics. The preauricular nodes, but not the maxillary nodes, are enlarged and tender. Without isolation of the virus, these cases pose a diagnostic problem, since they can be easily confused with other forms of follicular conjunctivitis.

Epidemic Keratoconjunctivitis Epidemic keratoconjunctivitis is usually caused by a serotype 8 adenovirus, but other serotypes have also been implicated.[78] Epidemic keratoconjunctivitis typically presents as an acute follicular conjunctivitis that is not accompanied by respiratory symptoms and only rarely by a low grade fever. Epidemic keratoconjunctivitis is usually unilateral at onset and accompanied by preauricular lymphadenopathy. The conjunctivitis typically runs a 7–10-day course.

Corneal involvement usually sets EKC apart from the other forms of adenoviral disease. On about the seventh day of the infection, central, focal epithelial lesions develop that stain with fluorescein. During the second week, subepithelial infiltrates form under some of these lesions. The subepithelial infiltrates may cause considerable photophobia and discomfort, and although they typically resolve within several days, they may persist for months in some individuals. Central infiltrates are the distinctive feature of EKC and cause the transient visual loss associated with this condition.

Laboratory Identification of Viruses

There are three basic approaches to the detection and identification of viruses causing ocular disease: (1) direct examination of clinical specimens for the virus or viral antigens using fluorescein-tagged antibodies, (2) examination of clinical specimens for viral antigen using EIA, (3) cultivation and identification of the virus from clinical specimens, and (4) serologic evaluation based on the demonstration of a significant increase in viral antibody during the patient's illness.

Although collection of viral specimens can easily be done in the office, actual culturing and identification techniques require special procedures that are currently best done in a laboratory. In the future, however, kits will probably become available to allow the identification of viruses right in the office environment.

Direct Fluorescent Antibody (DFA) Smear Direct examination of clinical specimens permits the most rapid identification of viral agents. Detection of herpes simplex, varicella-zoster virus, adenovirus, and cytomegalovirus can be achieved with the use of antibodies tagged with fluorescein.[82,83]

In viral conjunctivitis, collection of an adequate sample for direct observation can be achieved by everting the lower eyelid and swabbing or scraping the conjunctiva carefully but thoroughly. Eye discharge is not a useful specimen and should be gently removed before proceeding. The specimen is then transferred to a microscope slide and the smear fixed with acetone. Fluorescein-labeled antibodies against a specific virus are next added to the smear and incubated. After washing, the slide is read using a fluorescence microscope. For the diagnosis of adenoviral conjunctivitis and EKC, a positive specimen would show intense fluorescence in the cytoplasm or nucleus of epithelial cells.[84] This same technique can be used with corneal scrapings to detect HSV infection.[85]

Enzyme Immunoassay For enzyme immunoassays, specific viral antibody is coated onto a solid phase such as polyvinyl or polystyrene microtiter cups.[86] The test specimen is then added, and any viruses or viral antigens present are bound to the "capture" antibodies. After washing, the bound viruses or viral antigens are detected through the addition of enzyme-labeled viral antibody followed by a substrate on which the enzyme acts to produce a colored product.

Enzyme immunoassay methods have been used to diagnose ocular adenoviral conjunctivitis[87] and herpes simplex keratitis.[86] The enzyme methods are thought to be more sensitive than immunofluorescence staining because the enzyme produces a continuous action on the substrate, thereby amplifying the reaction.

Each of the immunologic tests should be conducted with proper controls, because these methods have a potential for nonspecific reactivity that can lead to false-positive results.

Cultivation   Viral cultivation requires specialized materials and technology, but in recent years new approaches have been developed that permit more rapid and efficient laboratory identification of viral isolates. The first step in the successful isolation is to collect a specimen during the early, acute phase of illness, before the immune system has had a chance to reduce the population of the virus.

To obtain a conjunctival sample for virus isolation, a dry cotton swab should be rubbed over the upper and lower tarsal conjunctiva and fornix of the involved eye, and then agitated in and squeezed into a viral transport medium, such as Hanks', Stuart's, or Leibovitz-Emory. To minimize the potential inhibitory effect of the swab materials, the tip of the swab should not be broken into the medium. The transport medium should always be kept cold but not frozen for maximum preservation of the virus.

Because viruses grow only within living cells, the collected material must be inoculated onto a susceptible tissue culture. The cells used for cultivation are usually from monkey kidney, human embryonic kidney, or chicken or mouse embryos. It is important that the suspected virus be matched with an appropriate tissue. Cultures are observed at intervals of 1–2 days for signs of cytopathic effect (CPE), which occurs as virions infect and kill the tissue cells. Most CPEs can be readily observed even in unfixed, unstained cell cultures.

The most rapid and efficient way to definitively identify viruses is to use fluoroscein-labeled antibodies to stain infected cultures.[82] This procedure can give results within hours of the recognition of any CPE. Newer quick culture techniques allow HSV[88] and adenovirus[88,89] growth, isolation, and identification within 48 hours.

Serologic Diagnosis   Serologic diagnosis is based on the demonstration of a significant increase (fourfold or more) in serum antibodies to a given virus over the course of an illness. This requires comparing the antibody levels in an acute-phase serum specimen to the levels in a pre-illness–phase or convalescence-phase specimen. Since pre-illness–phase specimens are seldom available, and it is necessary to wait for the disease to run its course to obtain a convalescence-phase specimen, assessment of acute viral infections with serologic assessment techniques can be difficult.

Serodiagnosis of ocular adenoviral infections can sometimes be made by the detection of rising antibody titers to adenovirus in patients during acute conjunctivitis.[90] However, serum antibody titers are not diagnostic in ocular HSV infections because most individuals already have high circulating titers, and when recurrent infection occurs, the level of serum antibody changes only slightly and is unrelated to the timing of the recurrence.[72] In addition, cross-reacting antibodies have been found for HSV and VZV.[91] Therefore, in many cases serodiagnosis is not a useful tool for identification of ocular viral infections.

Fungi

The fungi (molds and yeasts) are an extremely large and diverse group of microorganisms ranging in size and complexity from simple unicellular yeasts (Figure 17-22) to multicellular molds and mushrooms. The main structural component of a multicellular fungus is a filamentous tube containing cytoplasm with nuclei spaced at irregular intervals. In some fungi, these tubes are interrupted at numerous points by septations or cross-walls. An individual filament is called a hypha, and an entire mat of hyphae is referred to as a mycelium. Some hyphae can differentiate into structures that produce reproductive cells called spores. The differentiation of the filamentous fungi into genera and species is based on the morphologic arrangement of the reproductive structures and spores.

Yeast fungi, such as *Candida albicans,* are unicellular. They appear as small, ovoid, or cylindrical cells (four or five times as large as staphylococci) with pseudohyphae (atypical chains or filaments resembling hyphae). Budding yeast forms can sometimes be seen within clinical specimens (see Figure 17-22).

Fungal Keratitis

Fungal corneal infection is rare, with an estimated 300 cases occurring in the United States each year.[92] Fungal keratitis occurs most often after injury or surgery or when host resistance is decreased. The increased incidence of fungal corneal ulcers observed in recent years has been attributed to the widespread use of corticosteroids (which depress the immune system), and possibly to broad-spectrum antibiotic use (which reduces the population of bacteria that would normally compete with the fungi).

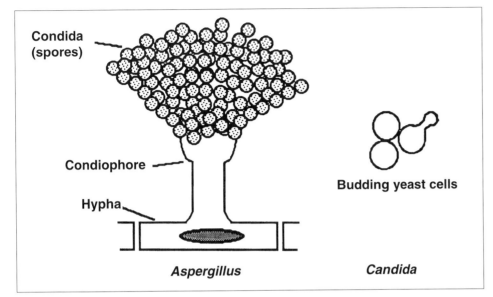

FIGURE 17-22
Schematic of Aspergillus, *a filamentous fungus (left), and* Candida, *a yeast fungus (right).*

The incidence of fungal corneal infections has a geographic distribution, with these ulcers being more common in tropical countries and in the southeastern United States, chiefly Florida. Although at least 35 genera of fungi have been cultured from mycotic corneal ulcers, the most frequent causes of fungal ulcers in the United States are the filamentous species *Aspergillus, Fusarium solani,* and *Acremonium* (formerly *Cephalosporium*), and the yeast *Candida albicans.*[92,93]

There are several features of corneal ulcers that suggest a filamentous fungal cause. The surface of the ulcer is often gray or dirty white with a dry, rough texture. The margins are delicately irregular and contain feather-like extensions into the adjacent stroma beneath the intact epithelium. Under high slit-lamp magnification, there is an impression that these areas contain branching and infiltrating hyphae. There may be focal areas of infiltration or "satellite lesions" separated from the primary lesion. Although these specific features may be diagnostic, the different fungal genera can create a biomicroscopic picture as diverse as that produced by any other group of microbial pathogens.

The most important step in early diagnosis of fungal keratitis is prompt and meticulous laboratory investigation. It is unlikely that each sample obtained by scraping the cornea with a Kimura spatula will contain hyphal fragments, so it is essential to inoculate each medium with multiple scrapings and prepare two or more slides for each stain.

Jones[94] has reported that identification of fungi in corneal scrapings can be obtained in approximately 50% of cases by using Giemsa or Gram stains. Fungi also can be visualized without staining by using 20% potassium hydroxide to remove the debris in the scrapings, thus revealing any fungi present. However, Giemsa and Gram stains have proven to be more reliable than potassium hydroxide for the identification of fungal organisms in corneal specimens.[95]

In addition to stained slides, corneal samples should be cultured for fungi. The medium most commonly used in cultivating fungi from ocular infections is Sabouraud's agar. Alternative fungal isolation media are glucose-peptone yeast extract broth with chloramphenicol, brainheart infusion broth with antibiotic, and fresh blood agar.[95,96] The culture material must be immediately inoculated onto the agar plates with "C" inoculation streaks, and the agar plates should be incubated at 27°C. On Sabouraud's medium, the fungal growth rate is slow, usually requiring more than 1 week before enough fungi are available for examination and identification.

The filamentous colonies formed by fungi are usually powdery, prickly, cottony, or leathery in consistency. Yeast colonies are soft and bacteria-like, consisting only of budding cells. Once fungal growth has been noted, it should be subcultured onto a sporulation medium such as potato-dextrose agar, cornmeal agar, or Czapek agar. Traditional and newer methods allow for further identification of specific fungi from the cultures.[97,98]

Seborrheic Blepharitis

Some uncertainty exists regarding the role played by *Pityrosporum ovale* in the etiology of seborrhea.[99] The typical yeast-like budding bodies of this fungus are gram-positive and vary in form, being either spherical or ovoid as

TABLE 17-9
Interpretation of Gram Stain

Gram Stain Reaction and Microscopic Morphology	Most Probable Causative Organism	
	Conjunctivitis	Corneal Ulcer
Gram-positive		
Cocci in clusters	*Staphylococcus* sp.	*Staphylococcus* sp.
Cocci in chains	*Streptococcus* sp. but not *S. pneumoniae*	*Streptococcus* sp. but not *S. pneumoniae*
Bullet-shaped diplococci	*S. pneumoniae*	*S. pneumoniae*
Rods	Diphtheroids	*Corynebacterium* sp., *Bacillus* sp.
Filaments	Actinomycetes	Fungus
Gram-negative		
Diplococci	*Neisseria* sp.	*Neisseria* sp.
Diplobacilli	*Moraxella* sp.	*Moraxella* sp.
Rods	*Haemophilus influenzae*	*Pseudomonas aeruginosa*, enterics

Source: Modified from L Wilson, R Sexton. Laboratory Diagnosis in Ocular Disease. In TD Duane (ed), Clinical Ophthalmology. Hagerstown, MD: Harper & Row, 1979;4(1):13.

collected from lid margin scrapings. These budding yeasts are plentiful in scrapings from seborrheic blepharitis,[100] and, in some patients, if ketoconazole cream is applied to the affected areas, the organisms are significantly reduced in number with improvement in the condition.[101] This suggests that these fungi are involved in seborrheic blepharitis. However, because these fungi do not seem to be involved in other infections, and because a mechanism for the infection has not been found, *P. ovale* may be present secondary to the blepharitis, rather than the primary cause.

Protozoans

Protozoans are unicellular organisms with a well-organized nucleus enclosed in a nuclear membrane. *Acanthamoeba* is a genus of free-living, freshwater ameba found in soil, water, hot tubs, swimming pools, and the human throat. This protozoan exists in two forms: the multiplying trophozoite and the resistant cyst.

Acanthamoeba has been reported to be the pathogen responsible for a severe keratitis found in soft-contact lens wearers who use homemade saline solutions.[102,103] The keratitis is characterized by stromal infiltration (often ring-shaped) and vascularization accompanied by persistent epithelial defects and severe pain. This infection is commonly confused with HSV stromal keratitis or fungal keratitis.

Several methods can be used to diagnose *Acanthamoeba* keratitis. In Giemsa-stained corneal specimens, clear, refractive, circular bodies, which are *Acanthamoeba* cysts, are noted.[104] In corneal scrapings stained with lactophenol cotton blue, *Acanthamoeba* cysts are seen as double-walled structures that stain a darker blue than the

surrounding tissues.[105] *Acanthamoeba* can also be identified in corneal specimens using calcofluor white.[106]

Acanthamoeba can be isolated from corneal scrapings by plating onto a nonnutrient agar that has been coated with *Escherichia coli*,[107] but the most rapid, accurate diagnostic technique is DFA staining of a corneal scraping or biopsy sample. Using this procedure, the cysts and trophozoites fluoresce very brightly.[108]

USE OF CYTOLOGIC AND MICROBIOLOGIC PROCEDURES IN THE MANAGEMENT OF OCULAR DISEASE

In routine practice, the management of anterior segment disease is often straightforward and based on characteristic signs and symptoms. However, when diagnosis is difficult, staining or culturing specimens can prove quite valuable. Cytologic testing using the Diff-Quik system can usually determine if a condition is bacterial, viral, or allergic, and subsequent testing with Gram stain can help identify any bacteria present. If a bacterial infection is present, knowledge of what tissue is involved and relative frequencies with which various bacteria infect the particular tissue can aid in identifying the specific bacterial pathogen (Table 17-9). For example, frequency of occurrence would suggest that *Haemophilus influenzae* should be the presumptive diagnosis if gram-negative rods were seen in association with a conjunctivitis, and *Pseudomonas aeruginosa* would be the presumptive diagnosis if gram-negative rods were found in a scraping from a corneal ulcer.

Outlined in Table 17-10 are examples of conditions, including neonatal conjunctivitis, follicular conjunctivi-

TABLE 17-10

Conditions in Which Laboratory Studies are Helpful or Mandatory

Helpful
    Allergic conjunctivitis
        Vernal
        Atopic
    Chronic conjunctivitis
    Follicular conjunctivitis
    Canaliculitis
    Dacryocystitis
    Persistent blepharitis
    Infectious eczematous conjunctivitis
Mandatory
    Neonatal conjunctivitis
    Hyperacute conjunctivitis
    Membranous conjunctivitis
    Central corneal ulcers (not herpetic)
    Postoperative infections
    Endophthalmitis
    Severe chronic conjunctivitis
    Parinaud's oculoglandular syndrome
    Periocular abscess

Source: Modified from JH Brinser, A Weiss. Laboratory Diagnosis in Ocular Disease. In W Tasman, EA Jaeger (eds), Duane's Clinical Ophthalmology. Philadelphia: Lippincott, 1992;4(1):2.

tis, bacterial corneal ulcers, and fungal ulcers, for which cultures and stained slides would be especially useful in making a proper diagnosis. The table also presents several ocular conditions for which cytologic and microbiologic studies would be considered clinically and medicolegally mandatory.

Because neonatal conjunctivitis has a variety of causes, its laboratory investigation should include stain preparations using Giemsa and Gram stains, as well as genera-tion of bacterial cultures using Thayer-Martin and chocolate media (Table 17-11).[109] Since *Neisseria gonorrhoeae, Haemophilus influenzae,* and *Chlamydia trachomatis* can all produce a significant, hyperacute purulent conjunctivitis, conjunctival sampling with a spatula (rather than a swab) is important to reveal inclusion bodies caused by chlamydial infection. Since most causes of neonatal conjunctivitis involve a sexually transmitted disease (i.e., passed from mother to newborn), the parents should also be examined and treated appropriately.

Since most cases of follicular conjunctivitis are viral, a preponderance of lymphocytes or monocytes is usually demonstrated with the Diff-Quik stain.[110] Other causes of follicular conjunctivitis include inclusion conjunctivitis caused by *Chlamydia,* drug-induced toxic reactions, and bacterial causes produced by species such as *Moraxella.* The appropriate laboratory investigation of follicular conjunctivitis is presented in Table 17-12.

The laboratory investigation of corneal ulcers has been given considerable attention in the literature.[12,35,92-96] Because Gram staining has a 65% accuracy rate for correctly identifying the responsible organism, it is the single best guide for the initial treatment of corneal ulcers.[92] Results from Gram stain preparations can be obtained rapidly and offer a valuable guide to the selection of an initial antibiotic at a time when culture material is still being processed (Table 17-13).

In addition to the widely accepted methods used to identify bacteria and fungi, various commercial kits, strips, and other detection and identification devices for office use are becoming available in increasing numbers. General references,[111] local laboratories, and the literature supplied by kit manufacturers should be consulted for more information about new procedures.

TABLE 17-11

Laboratory Investigation of Neonatal Conjunctivitis

Cause	Cytology	Gram Stain	Culture
Neisseria	PMNs	Gram-negative intracellular diplococci	Growth on chocolate agar, Thayer-Martin agar ($\uparrow CO_2$)

Other bacteria
  Staphylococcus
  Haemophilus
  Enterics
	PMNs	Gram-positive or gram-negative organisms	Growth on blood agar, chocolate agar ($\uparrow CO_2$)

Chlamydia	Equal numbers of PMNs and lymphocytes; cytoplasmic inclusion bodies	No organisms	Negative or normal flora
Chemical (silver nitrate)	Epithelial cells	No organisms	Negative or normal flora
Herpes simplex virus	Lymphocytes	No organisms	Negative or normal flora

PMNs = polymorphonuclear neutrophils.

TABLE 17-12
Laboratory Investigation of Follicular Conjunctivitis

Disease	Cytology	Gram Stain	Culture
PCF/EKC	Lymphocytes	No organisms	Negative or normal flora
Herpes simplex	Lymphocytes	No organisms	Negative or normal flora
Newcastle disease	Lymphocytes	No organisms	Negative or normal flora
Adult chlamydial conjunctivitis	Lymphocytes, PMNs; infrequent cytoplasmic inclusion bodies	No organisms	Negative or normal flora
Chronic trachoma	Lymphocytes, PMNs; infrequent cytoplasmic inclusion bodies	No organisms	Negative or normal flora
Chronic drug toxicity	Not known	No organisms	Negative or normal flora
Chronic molluscum toxicity	Not known	No organisms	Negative or normal flora
Moraxella blepharoconjunctivitis	Few, if any, PMNs	Gram-negative diplobacilli	Growth on blood agar

PCF = pharyngoconjunctival fever; EKC = epidemic keratoconjunctivitis; PMNs = polymorphonuclear leukocytes.
Source: Modified from CR Dawson, JD Sheppard. Follicular Conjunctivitis. In W Tasman, EA Jaeger (eds), Duane's Clinical Ophthalmology. Philadelphia: Lippincott, 1992;4(7):45, 11.

TABLE 17-13
Selection of Initial Antibiotic Therapy for Bacterial or Fungal Keratitis Based on the Gram Stain Results

Gram Stain Reaction and Microscopic Morphology	Initial Antibiotic Therapy	
	Topical	Subconjunctival
Gram-positive cocci	Cephaloridine or cefazolin or ciprofloxacin	Cephaloridine or cefazolin
Gram-positive bacilli	Gentamicin or tobramycin	Gentamicin or tobramycin
Gram-negative cocci	Penicillin G or bacitracin	Penicillin G
Gram-negative bacilli	Gentamicin or tobramycin (and carbenicillin)	Gentamicin or tobramycin (and carbenicillin)
Hyphae, yeasts, or pseudohyphae	Natamycin	None
Two or more bacteria or no organisms	Cephaloridine or cefazolin and gentamicin or tobramycin or ciprofloxacin	Cephaloridine or cefazolin and gentamicin or tobramycin

Source: Modified from RL Abbot, MA Abrams. Bacterial Corneal Ulcers. In W Tasman, EA Jaeger (eds), Duane's Clinical Ophthalmology (2nd ed). Philadelphia: Lippincott, 1989;4(18):20; and D Jones. Decision-making in the management of microbial keratitis. Ophthalmology 1981; 88:814–20; and HM Leibowitz. Clincal evaluation of ciprofloxacin 0.3% ophthalmic solution for treatment of bacterial keratitis. Am J Ophthalmol 1991;112:345–75.

REFERENCES

1. Kleinfeld J, Ellis PP. Effects of topical anesthetics on growth of microorganisms. Arch Ophthalmol 1966;76:712–5.
2. Kimura SJ, Thygeson P. The cytology of external ocular disease. Am J Ophthalmol 1955;39:137–44.
3. Babenko P, Sherman J. A rapid ocular smear technique for optometrists: A preliminary report. J Am Optom Assoc 1979;50:67–70.
4. Hershenfeld S, Kazdan JJ, Mancer K, et al. Impression cytology in conjunctivitis. Can J Ophthalmol 1981;16:76–8.
5. Hyndidiuk RA, Seideman S. Clinical and Laboratory Techniques in External Ocular Disease and Endophthalmitis. In HB Fedukowicz. External Infections of the Eye (2nd ed). New York: Appleton-Century-Crofts, 1978;266.
6. Thelmo W, Csordas J, Davis P, et al. The cytology of acute bacterial and follicular conjunctivitis. Acta Cytol 1972;16:172–7.
7. Hanser SA, Moor WA, Stickle AW. Cytology of allergic conjunctivitis. Arch Ophthalmol 1952;47:728–33.
8. Abelson MB, Madiwale N, Weston JH. Conjunctival eosinophils in allergic ocular disease. Arch Ophthalmol 1983;101:555–6.
9. Jennings B. Mechanisms, diagnosis, and management of common ocular allergies. J Am Optom Assoc 1990;(Suppl)61:S32–41.
10. Allansmith MR. Giant papillary conjunctivitis. J Am Optom Assoc 1990;(Suppl)61:S42–6.
11. Jones DB. Decision-making in the management of microbial keratitis. Am Acad Ophthalmol 1981;88:814–20.
12. Abbot RL, Abrams MA. Bacterial Corneal Ulcers. In W Tasman, EA Jaeger (eds), Duane's Clinical Ophthalmology (2nd ed). Philadelphia: Lippincott, 1989;Vol 4(18):1–34.
13. Locatcher-Khorazo D, Seegal BC (eds). Microbiology of the Eye. St. Louis: Mosby, 1972;13–23, 41–62.

14. Yolton DP, Meier RF. Normal bacteria of the healthy conjunctiva. Rev Optom 1978;115(a):85–7.

15. Kloos WE. Natural populations of the genus Staphylococcus. Annu Rev Microbiol 1980;34:559–92.

16. Giger O, Charilaous CC, Cundy KR. Comparison of the API Staph-Ident and DMS Staph-Trac systems with conventional methods used for the identification of coagulase-negative staphylococci. J Clin Microbiol 1984;19:68–72.

17. Kloos WE, Wolfshohl JF. Identification of Staphylococcus species with the API Staph-Ident system. J Clin Microbiol 1983;16:509–16.

18. Soudakoff PS. Bacteriologic examination of the conjunctiva. Am J Ophthalmol 1954;38:374–6.

19. Grasmick AE, Naito N, Bruckner DA. Clinical comparison of the AutoMicrobic system gram-positive identification card, API Staph-Ident, and conventional methods in the identificaion of coagulase-negative Staphylococcus spp. J Clin Microbiol 1983;18:1323–8.

20. John JF, Gramling PK, O'Dell NM. Species identification of coagulase-negative staphylococci from urinary tract isolates. J Clin Microbiol 1978;8:435–7.

21. Wilson LA, Julian AJ, Ahearn DG. The survival and growth of microorganisms in mascara during use. Am J Ophthalmol 1975;79:596–601.

22. Fedukowicz HB (ed). External Infections of the Eye (2nd ed). New York: Appleton-Century-Crofts, 1978;114.

23. Woolfrey BF, Lally RT, Ederer MN. An evaluation of three rapid coagglutination tests: Sero-Stat, Accu-Staph, and Staphyloslide for differentiating Staphylococcus aureus from other species of staphylococci. Am J Clin Pathol 1985;81:345–7.

24. Aldridge KE, Kogos C, Sanders CV, et al. Comparison of rapid identification assays for Staphylococcus aureus. J Clin Microbiol 1984;19:703–4.

25. McCulley JP, Dougherty JM, Deneau DG. Classification of chronic blepharitis. Am Acad Ophthalomol 1982; 89:1173–80.

26. Dougherty JM, McCulley JP. Comparative bacteriology of chronic blepharitis. Br J Ophthalmol 1984;68:524–8.

27. Osgood JK, Dougherty JM, McCulley JP. The role of wax and sterol esters of meibomian secretions in chronic blepharitis. Invest Ophthalmol Vis Sci 1989;30:1958–61.

28. Thygeson P. Bacterial factors in chronic catarrhal conjunctivitis—role of toxin-forming staphylococci. Arch Ophthalmol 1937;18:373–87.

29. Theodore FH. Allergy in Relation to Ophthalmology. In D Locatcher-Khorazo, BC Seegal (eds), Microbiology of the Eye. St. Louis: Mosby, 1972;160–1.

30. Stenson S, Newman R, Fedukowicz H. Laboratory studies in acute conjunctivitis. Arch Ophthalmol 1982;100:1275–7.

31. McGill JI. Bacterial conjunctivitis. Trans Ophthalmol Soc UK 1986;105:37–40.

32. Brook I. Anaerobic and aerobic bacterial flora of acute conjunctivitis in children. Arch Ophthalmol 1980;98:833–5.

33. Thygeson P, Kimura SJ. Chronic conjunctivitis. Trans Am Acad Ophthalmol Otolaryngol 1963;67:494–517.

34. Stenson S, Fedukowicz H, Newman R. Laboratory studies in chronic conjunctivitis. Ann Ophthalmol 1983; 15:1160–4.

35. Liesegang TJ, Forster RK. Spectrum of microbial keratitis in south Florida. Am J Ophthalmol 1980;90:38–47.

36. Locatcher-Khorazo D, Seegal BC (eds). Microbiology of the Eye. St. Louis: Mosby, 1972;63–85.

37. Weiss A, Friendly D, Eglin K, et al. Bacterial periorbital and orbital cellulitis in childhood. Ophthalmology 1983;90:195–203.

38. Forster RK, Abbott RL, Gelender H. Management of infectious endophthalmitis. Ophthalmology 1980;87:313–9.

39. Facklam RR, Carey RB. Streptococci and Aerococci. In EH Lennette, A Balows, WJ Housler Jr, HJ Shadomy (eds), Manual of Clinical Microbiology (4th ed). Washington, DC: American Society for Microbiology 1985; 4:154–75.

40. Fedukowicz HB, Stenson S. External Infections of the Eye (3rd ed). Norwalk, CT: Appleton-Century-Crofts, 1985;25.

41. Johnson MK, Allen JH. Ocular toxin of the pneumococcus. Am J Ophthalmol 1971;72:175–80.

42. Morello JA, Janda WM, Bohnhoff M. Neisseria and Branhamella. In EH Lennette, A Balows, WJ Housler Jr, HJ Shadomy (eds), Manual of Clinical Microbiology (4th ed). Washington, DC: American Society for Microbiology, 1985;4:184.

43. Thygeson P. Etiology and treatment of blepharitis—a study in military personnel. Arch Ophthalmol 1946;36:445–77.

44. Mitsui Y, Hinokuma S, Tanaka C. Etiology of angular conjunctivitis. Am J Ophthalmol 1951;34:1579–86.

45. Baum J, Fedukowicz HB, Jordan A. A survey of Moraxella corneal ulcers in a derelict population. Am J Ophthalmol 1980;90:476–80.

46. Fedukowicz H, Horwich H. The gram-negative diplobacillus in hypopyon keratitis. Arch Ophthalmol 1953; 49:202–11.

47. Davis DJ, Pittman M. Acute conjunctivitis caused by Haemophilus. Am J Dis Child 1950;79:211–22.

48. Powell KR, Kaplan SB, Hall CB, et al. Periorbital cellulitis—clinical and laboratory findings in 146 episodes, including tear countercurrent immunoelectrophoresis in 89 episodes. Am J Dis Child 1988;142:853–7.

49. McCord CD: The Lacrimal Drainage System. In W Tasman, EA Jaeger (eds), Duane's Clinical Ophthalmology (2nd ed). Philadelphia: Lippincott, 1989;4(13):1–25.

50. Wilson LA. Bacterial Conjunctivitis. In W Tasman, EA Jaeger (eds), Duane's Clinical Ophthalmology (2nd ed). Philadelphia: Lippincott, 1989;4(5):1–16.

51. Templeton WC III, Eiferman RA, Synder JW, et al. Serratia keratitis transmitted by contaminated eyedroppers. Am J Ophthalmol 1982;93:723–6.

52. Lass JH, Haaf J, Foster CS, Belcher C. Visual outcome in eight cases of Serratia marcescens keratitis. Am J Ophthalmol 1982;92:384–90.

53. McBeath J, Forster RK, Rebell G. Diagnostic limulus lysate assay for endophthalmitis and keratitis. Arch Ophthalmol 1978;96:1265–7.

54. Weissman BA, Mondino BJ, Pettit TH, Hofbauer JD. Corneal ulcers associated with extended-wear soft contact lenses. Am J Ophthalmol 1984;97:476–81.

55. Cooper RL, Constable IJ. Infective keratitis in soft contact lens wearers. Br J Ophthalmol 1977;61:250–4.

56. Adams CP, Cohen EJ, Laibson PR, et al. Corneal ulcers in patients with cosmetic extended-wear contact lenses. Am J Ophthalmol 1983;96:705–9.

57. Krachmer JH, Purcell JJ. Bacterial corneal ulcers in cosmetic soft contact lens wearers. Arch Ophthalmol 1978; 96:57–61.

58. Kessler E, Mondino FJ, Brown SI. The corneal response to Pseudomonas aeruginosa mouse corneal infections. Infect Immun 1982;35:461–4.

59. Naib ZM. Cytology of ocular lesions. Acta Cytol 1972; 16:178–85.

60. Clyde WA Jr, Kenny GE, Schachter J. Laboratory Diagnosis of Chlamydial and Mycoplasmal Infections. In WL Drew (ed), Cumitech 19. Washington, DC: American Society for Microbiology, 1984.

61. Tam MR, Stamm WE, Handsfield HH, et al. Culture-independent diagnosis of Chlamydia trachomatis using monoclonal antibodies. N Engl J Med 1984;310:1146–50.

62. Reed K. Rapid, inexpensive confirmation of chlamydial infection. J Am Optom Assoc 1988;59:46–8.

63. Taylor PB, Burd EM, Tabbara KF. Monoclonal antibodies in the laboratory diagnosis of trachoma. Int Ophthalmol 1988;12:81–6.

64. Taylor HR, Fitch CP, Murillo-Lopez F, Rapoza P. The diagnosis and treatment of chlamydial conjunctivitis. Int Ophthalmol 1988;12:95–9.

65. Hammerschlag MR, Roblin PM, Cummings C, et al. Comparison of enzyme immunoassay and culture for diagnosis of chlamydial conjunctivitis and respiratory infections in infants. J Clin Microbiol 1987;25:2306–8.

66. Enns RK. DNA Probes: An overview and comparison with current methods. Lab Med 1988;19:295–300.

67. Kohne DE. Application of DNA probe tests to the diagnosis of infectious disease. Am Clin Prod Rev 1986;5:20–9.

68. Goltz S, Todd J, Kline S, et al. DNA probes for diagnosis of sexually transmitted diseases. Am Clin Prod Rev 1986;5:30–5.

69. Ostler HB. Oculogenital disease. Surv Ophthalmol 1976;20:233–46.

70. Pine L, Hardin H, Turner L, Roberts SS. Actinomycotic lacrimal canaliculitis—a report of two cases with a review of the characteristics which indentify the causal organism, Actinomyces israelii. Am J Ophthalmol 1960;49:1278–88.

71. Hagedoorn A. Concretions in a lacrimal canaliculus caused by actinomyces. Arch Ophthalmol 1940;23:689–92.

72. Binder PS. Herpes simplex keratitis. Surv Ophthalmol 1977;21:313–31.

73. Mondino BJ, Brown SI, Mondzelewski JP. Peripheral corneal ulcers with herpes zoster ophthalmicus. Am J Ophthalmol 1978;86:611–4.

74. Andiman Warren A. The Epstein-Barr virus and EB virus infections in childhood. J Pediatr 1979;2:171–82.

75. Onorato IM, Morens DM, Martone WJ, et al. Epidemiology of cytomegaloviral infections: Recommendations for prevention and control. Rev Infect Dis 1985;7:479–97.

76. Schuman JS, Orellana J, Friedman AH, Teich SA. Acquired immunodeficiency syndrome (AIDS). Surv Ophthalmol 1987;31:384–410

77. Holland GN, Pepose JS, Pettit TH, et al. Acquired immune deficiency syndrome ocular manifestations. Am Acad Ophthalmol 1983;90:859–72.

78. Dawson CR. Follicular Conjunctivitis. In W Tasman, EA Jaeger (eds), Duane's Clinical Ophthalmology (2nd ed). Philadelphia: Lippincott, 1989;4(7):2, 4–7.

79. Darougar S, Walpita P, Thaker U, et al. Adenovirus serotypes isolated from ocular infections in London. Br J Ophthalmol 1983;67:111–4.

80. Dawson CR, Hanna L, Wood TR, Despain R. Adenovirus type 8 keratoconjunctivitis in the United States: III. Epidemiologic, clinical and microbiologic features. Am J Ophthalmol 1970;69:473–80.

81. Turner M, Istre G, Beauchamp H, et al. Community outbreak of adenovirus type 7a infections associated with a swimming pool. South Med J 1987;6:712–5.

82. Minnich LL, Smith TF, Ray CG. Rapid Detection of Viruses by Immunofluorescence. In S Specter (ed), Cumitech 24. Washington, DC: American Society for Microbiology, 1988.

83. Cepko CI, Whetstone CA, Sharp PA. Adenovirus hexon monoclonal antibody that is a group specific and potentially useful as a diagnostic reagent. J Clin Microbiol 1983;17:360–4.

84. Vastine DW, Schwartz HS, Yamashiroya HM, et al. Cytologic diagnosis of adenoviral epidemic keratoconjunctivitis by direct immunofluorescence. Invest Ophthalmol Vis Sci 1977;16:195–200.

85. Lee SF, Storch GA, Reed CA, et al. Comparative laboratory diagnosis of experimental herpes simplex keratitis. Am J Ophthalmol 1990;109:8–12.

86. Schmidt NJ. Symposium on medical virology—rapid viral diagnosis. Med Clin North Am 1983;67:953–72.

87. Wiley L, Springer D, Kowalski RP, et al. Rapid diagnostic test for ocular adenovirus. Ophthalmology 1988; 95:431–3, 442.

88. Walpita P, Darougar S. Double-label immunofluorescence method for simultaneous detection of adenovirus and herpes simplex virus from the eye. J Clin Microbiol 1989; 27:1623–5.

89. Darougar S, Walpita P, Thaker U, et al. Rapid culture test for adenovirus isolation. Br J Ophthalmol 1984;68:405–8.

90. Koc JS, Wigand R, Weil M. The efficiency of various laboratory methods for the diagnosis of adenovirus conjunctivitis. Zentralbl Bakteriol Mikrobiol Hyg 1987;263:607–15.

91. Schmidt NJ. Further evidence for common antigens in herpes simplex and varicella-zoster viruses. J Med Virol 1982;9:27–36.

92. Jones DB. Fungal Keratitis. In W Tasman, EA Jaeger (eds). Duane's Clinical Ophthalmology (2nd ed). Philadelphia: Lippincott, 1989;4(21):1–13.

93. Kolodner H. Fungal corneal ulcers. Int Ophthtlamol Clin 1984;24:17–24.
94. Jones BR. Principles in the management of oculomycosis. Am J Ophthalmol 1975;79:719–51.
95. Wilson LA, Sexton RR. Laboratory diagnosis in fungal keratitis. Am J Ophthalmol 1968;66:646–53.
96. O'Day DM, Akrabawi PL, Head WS, Ratner HB. Laboratory isolation techniques in human and experimental fungal infections. Am J Ophthalmol 1979;87:688–93.
97. Holmberg K. New diagnostic methods in medical mycology. Scand J Infect Dis 1982; Suppl 36:121–6.
98. Pincus DH, Salkin IR, McGinnis MR. Rapid methods in medical mycology. Lab Med 1988;19:315–20.
99. Parunovic A, Halde C. Pityrosporum orbiculare—its possible role in seborrheic blepharitis. Am J Ophthalmol 1967;63:815–20.
100. Thygeson P, Vaughan, DG. Seborrhiec blepharitis. Trans Am Ophthalmol Soc 1955;52:173–203.
101. Ostler HB. Blepharitis. In W Tasman, EA Jaeger (eds), Duane's Clinical Ophthalmology (2nd ed). Philadelphia: Lippincott, 1989;4(22):1–7.
102. Moore MB, McCully JP, Luckenback M, et al. Acanthamoeba keratitis associated with soft contact lenses. Am J Ophthalmol 1985;100:396–403.
103. Stehr-Green JK, Bailey TM, Brandt FH, et al. Acanthamoeba keratitis in soft contact lens wearers. JAMA 1987;258:57–60.
104. Moore MB, McCulley JP, Newton C, et al. Acanthamoeba keratitis: A growing problem in soft and hard contact lens wearers. Ophthalmology 1987;94:1654–61.
105. Thomas PA, Kuriakose T. Rapid detection of Acanthamoeba cysts in corneal scrapings by lactophenol cotton blue staining [letter.] Arch Ophthalmol 1990; 108:168.
106. Silvany RE, Luckenbach MW, Moore MB. The rapid detection of Acanthamoeba in paraffin-embedded sections of corneal tissue with calcofluor white. Arch Ophthalmol 1987;105:1366–7.
107. Larkin DFP, Kilvington S, Easty DL. Contamination of contact lens storage cases by Acanthamoeba and bacteria. Br J Opthalamol 1990;74:133–5.
108. Epstein RJ, Wilson LA, Visvesvara GS, Plourde EG. Rapid diagnosis of Acanthamoeba keratitis from corneal scrapings using indirect fluorescent antibody staining. Arch Ophthalmol 1986;104:1318–21.
109. Rotkis WM, Chandler JW. Neonatal Conjunctivitis. In W Tasman, EA Jaeger (eds), Duane's Clinical Ophthalmology (2nd ed). Philadelphia: Lippincott, 1989;4(6):1–7.
110. Dawson CR. Follicular conjunctivitis. In W Tasman, EA Jaeger (eds), Duane's Clinical Ophthalmology (2nd ed). Philadelphia: Lippincott, 1989;4(7):1–19.
111. Lennette EH, Balows A, Hausler WJ Jr, Shadomy HJ (eds). Manual of Clinical Microbiology (4th ed). Washington, DC: American Society for Microbiology, 1985.

18

Ophthalmic Radiology

CHRIS J. CAKANAC AND JACK E. TERRY

The technology of imaging techniques has changed vastly since Wilhelm Röntgen discovered x-rays in the 1890s. Plain roentgenography, computed tomography (CT), and magnetic resonance imaging (MRI) are radiologic techniques that have become instrumental in the diagnosis and management of ophthalmic disorders.

Although clinicians in almost every medical specialty order radiologic studies, the interpretation of those studies requires advanced training and is the primary duty of the radiologist. An ophthalmic clinician cannot readily expect to possess the skills and expertise of the radiologist; however, the ophthalmic clinician must realize his or her responsibility in diagnosing a patient's condition and work in conjunction with the radiologist to achieve this goal. To facilitate communications, the ophthalmic clinician should strive to attain a level of competence in dealing with radiologic data.[1]

PLAIN FILM X-RAYS

Basic Principles of X-Rays

An x-ray is a form of electromagnetic radiation of extremely short wavelength. This gives x-rays special penetrating properties. X-rays used for roentgenography have a wavelength of approximately 0.1240 angstroms.[2]

The essential characteristic of x-rays that gives them their diagnostic value is that they do not penetrate all tissues to the same degree. The roentgenographic properties of anatomic tissues range from radiolucent (x-rays pass through the tissue without being absorbed) to radiopaque (x-rays are heavily absorbed). X-rays that penetrate tissue are able to sensitize a photographic film placed adjacent to the structures being evaluated, and the subsequent image yields information about anatomic configuration and composition.

X-rays were originally produced in a tube resembling the vacuum tubes used in electronics. The tube has a filament that, when electronically heated, causes a stream of high-energy electrons to flow from a negative electrode (cathode) to a positive electrode (anode). When the electrons hit the anode, a portion of their energy is emitted at the x-ray portion of the electromagnetic spectrum. In this process, most of the electron energy is actually transformed to heat, with less than 1% of the energy becoming x-rays.[3]

The x-rays are directed out of the tube toward the anatomic structures of interest. Photographic film is positioned along the body opposite the side from which the x-rays are produced. As the x-rays exit the body, they sensitize the film according to the level of electromagnetic radiation that passes through the structures it traverses.

Harmful Effects of X-Rays

X-rays have proved to be of benefit in both the diagnosis and treatment of disease. However, it is important that those who use x-rays be aware of their hazards. Alpha rays, beta rays, gamma rays, neutron rays, and x-rays are all forms of ionizing radiation that can produce biological effects. This radiation can remove electrons from atoms, causing them to become ions, hence the term ionization. Several terms are used to define quantities of ionizing radiation and its effects. The "roentgen" is the international unit for the quantity of ionizing radiation. It is defined as the amount of radiation needed to produce 2.083×10^9 ion pairs in 1 cc of air at normal temperature and pressure (NTP) of $0°C$ and 760 mm Hg.

"Rad" is an acronym for "radiation absorbed dose" and is the dose of an ionizing radiation accompanied by the absorption of 100 ergs of energy per gram of absorbing material. The rad is a more useful unit for quantifying ionizing radiation because it is the absorbed radiation that will ultimately cause any biological effects.

Superficial injuries, hematopoietic changes, induction of tumors, reduction of life span, cataracts, sterility, and genetic variations are considered potential hazards of exposure to x-rays. However, the doses used in x-ray examinations are so low that these effects are not observed, assuming that the appropriate precautions are employed. Although the use of x-rays in medicine has grown, technical refinements have decreased the overall exposure. Providing that there is a proper indication for the use of x-rays on a patient and that the radiation is used with precision and precaution to the patient and examiner, the use of x-rays under most circumstances is unlikely to be harmful.[3]

Orbital X-Ray Techniques

For most bones of the skeleton, isolated images can be projected onto x-ray film without interference from other structures. However, it is somewhat more difficult to obtain isolated images of the bones of the orbit. There are 22 relatively small bones that compose the skull, and the proximity of these bones makes it impossible to isolate a single bone by means of x-ray technique. Interpretation of the x-ray film is complicated by the superimposed shadows of nearby bones as well as by movement of the head during exposure, which often causes image blurring.

It is a general rule in radiology that two views of an anatomic part be obtained 90 degrees from one another.[4] A routine series of films for the orbit usually consists of one or two films in a posteroanterior projection and one film in a lateral projection of the affected side. Occasionally additional films in the oblique or submentovertical projections may aid in diagnosis.[5]

Posteroanterior Views

With a posteroanterior (PA) view the x-ray beam strikes the posterior aspect of the body, passes through the body, and then sensitizes a film plate after exiting the anterior side. This is the opposite of an anteroposterior view, in which the film plate is placed along the posterior aspect of the patient with the beam striking the anterior aspect of the patient first.

In the straight posteroanterior view, the x-ray beam is aimed directly at the back of the skull at the nasion. One drawback with this view is that the petrous ridges of the skull project directly into the orbits, which can obscure meaningful details of the orbital contents. To avoid this, a Caldwell and a Waters PA view is most frequently used for visualizing the orbits.

Caldwell View The Caldwell view is a PA projection of the orbit taken while the patient is lying with the face

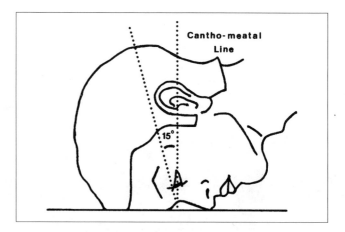

FIGURE 18-1
To obtain a Caldwell PA view for examination of the orbits, the patient's forehead and nose rest on the plane of the x-ray table. X-rays are aimed 15 degrees cephalad relative to the cantho-meatal line toward the glabellar region located between the eyebrows. (Reprinted with permission from GM Gombos. Handbook of Ophthalmic Emergencies [2nd ed]. Garden City, NY: Medical Examination, 1977.)

downward. The head is positioned so that the forehead and nose are resting on the plane of the x-ray table (Figure 18-1). With the head in this position, the cantho-meatal line (an imaginary line connecting the temporal canthus and the opening of the external auditory canal) is perpendicular to the film. The x-ray tube is then angled 15 degrees cephalad relative to the cantho-meatal line and aimed at the glabella (the region between the eyebrows).[6]

Advantages of the Caldwell view are that the orbital rims and the roofs of the orbit are easily visualized because the petrous ridges are projected downward. In addition, the lateral orbital wall (the greater wing of the sphenoid) is seen plainly, and a portion of the orbital surface of the lesser wing is seen near the medial wall. The superior orbital fissure and foramen rotundum also can be visualized (Figure 18-2).

Waters View The Waters view is another common PA view used to visualize the orbital and periorbital structures. Again, the patient lies prone with the face directed toward the table on which he or she is positioned. The head is then angled back so that the chin rests on the table and is positioned above the lower third of the film (Figure 18-3). With the head in this position, the nose is 1.5 inches off the table, and a view is rendered of the maxillary antra separated from the superimposed petrous bones.[6] Care must be taken not to angle the head too far back or distortion of this area will result; however, if the head is not angled back enough, the petrous bones will block the

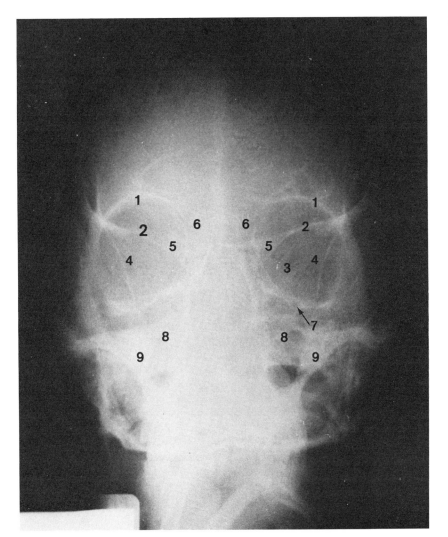

FIGURE 18-2

The normal posteroanterior appearance of the skull and orbits (Caldwell view). The orbital rim (1) is bilaterally shown as a somewhat circular radiopaque band. The sphenoid ridge (2) is shown arching across the film. A radiolucent superior orbital fissure (3) is shown medial to the greater wing of the sphenoid (4), forming the lateral orbital wall. The lesser wing forms the superomedial wall (5), which is located next to the ethmoidal sinuses (6). The small hole (7) on the inferior orbital rim is the infraorbital foramen. The maxillary antrum (8) is located below the inferior orbital rim with the petrous bone (9) covering the lower third of the sinus.

antra. To avoid these problems, the ideal head position is the cantho-meatal line at an angle of 37 degrees to the film plane with the x-ray beam centered at the root of the nose perpendicular to the center of the film. This will allow remnant x-rays to exit the head just below the nose.

Advantages of the Waters view are that the petrous ridges are projected downward and the antral contours are shown fully without distortion. In addition, there is a clear view of the maxillary antrum, the inferior orbital rim, the lateral wall, and the frontal and ethmoidal sinuses (Figure 18-4).

Rhese View

The optic canal is best seen with the head in the Rhese position, and x-ray films of this position are usually taken from both sides for the sake of comparison. For this view, the patient lies down with the head positioned so that the chin, zygoma, and nose rest on the table. When in this position, the sagittal plane of the skull should form a 53-degree angle with the film plane. This view clearly shows the optic canal, the ethmoid cells, the lesser wing of the sphenoid, and the superior orbital fissure.

Lateral View

Lateral views (Figure 18-5) are usually obtained to locate foreign bodies. The patient should lie on his or her side with the outer canthus placed on the table. The x-ray tube is aimed vertically through the canthus.

If the previous views do not provide an adequate view of the orbital floor, the examiner can use the method of Fueger and Milauskas. These investigators found that the anterolateral orbital floor is flat, whereas the posterior aspect of the floor bulges. In this method, the head is positioned as in the Caldwell view, but the x-ray beam is at a 30-degree angle caudal to the cantho-meatal line instead of 15 degrees cephalad. This allows a better view of the

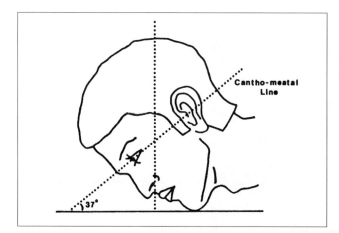

FIGURE 18-3
To obtain a Waters PA view, the patient's chin rests on the x-ray table and his or her head is angled backward so that the cantho-meatal line is at an angle of 37 degrees to the film plane. The x-ray beam is directed toward the root of the nose and perpendicular to the film plane. (Reprinted with permission from GM Gombos. Handbook of Ophthalmic Emergencies [2nd ed]. Garden City, NY: Medical Examination, 1977.)

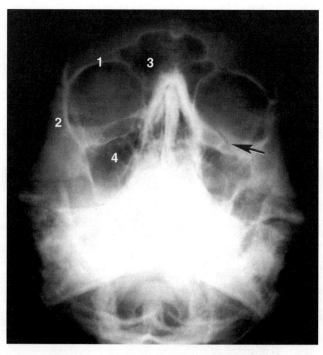

FIGURE 18-4
Plain film, Waters view. A blowout fracture is exhibited along the inferior aspect of the left orbit (arrow). Some of the structures that are highly visible include the superior orbital rim (1), the zygomatic arch (2), and the frontal (3) and maxillary (4) sinuses. (Reprinted and modified with permission from CJ Cakanac. Diagnostic Imaging Techniques. In B Blaustein [ed], Ocular Manifestations of Systemic Disease. New York: Churchill Livingstone, 1994.)

posterior orbital floor. For the anterolateral part of the orbital floor, the head is rotated about 20 degrees toward the affected side. In this position, the glabello-meatal line is perpendicular to the film, and the x-ray tube is at an angle of 35 degrees with respect to this line. These two projections are beneficial in the detection of orbital blowout fractures.

Submentovertical View

The submentovertical projection is used to examine primarily the zygomatic arches. Fractures of the zygomatic arch can be difficult to find without this view. With the submentovertical view, the film is placed against the top of the patient's head and the x-ray beam is aimed under the patient's chin.[6] Figure 18-6 demonstrates a submentovertical view showing displacement of the zygomatic arch.

Indications and Contraindications for X-Ray Studies

In the past, the plain x-ray film was the only means available for evaluating orbital fractures, tumors, and foreign bodies, but the presence of foreign bodies is now usually investigated with ultrasonography and CT scanning, since these modalities give more information for effective removal. Plain films are, however, sometimes used to grossly rule out the presence of foreign bodies. Plain films

are commonly used when a suspected foreign body is metallic in nature, because metallic objects are highly visible in contrast to soft-tissue structures. However, x-ray films are not as beneficial as CT scanning and MRI in the evaluation of soft-tissue lesions such as most tumors or demyelination.

The plain film today has its primary use in ruling out orbital fractures. CT scans are very accurate in evaluating complex fractures, but plain films remain popular because of their low cost, universal availability, and ability to detect the overwhelming majority of orbital fractures.

The contraindication for x-ray studies is pregnancy. As previously mentioned, x-rays are ionizing radiation, which is harmful to the fetus.

X-Ray Diagnosis

A prerequisite for the interpretation of x-ray films is a clear understanding of the anatomy involved because the examiner must be able to relate the two-dimensional films

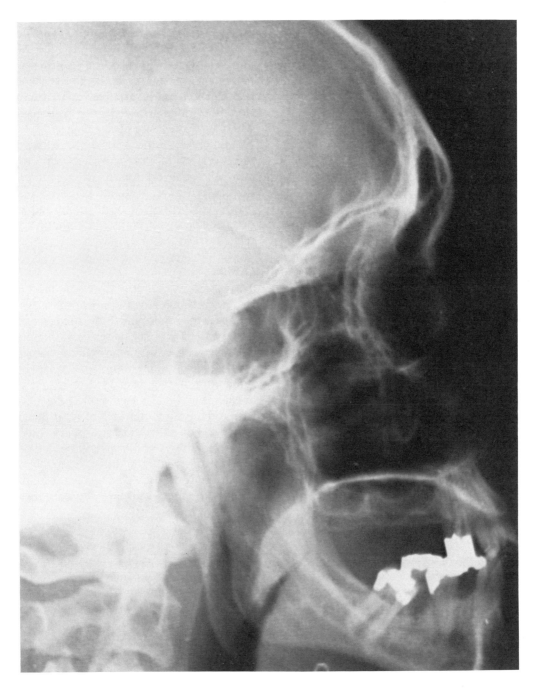

FIGURE 18-5
A normal plain film, lateral view. The lateral view is especially helpful for evaluation of the posterior orbital floor.

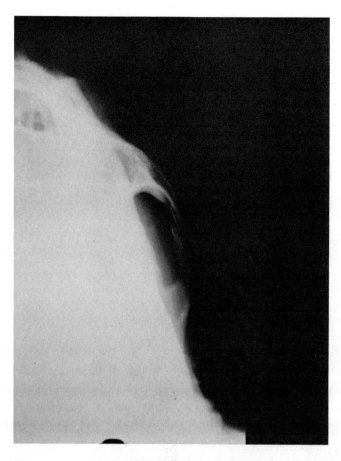

FIGURE 18-6
Submentovertical view of the zygomatic and maxillary bone demonstrating displacement of the zygomatic arch.

to an actual three-dimensional structure. The film should include sufficient structural anatomy to allow the interpreter to realize the area of the body that is represented. When reading films, it is difficult to determine the front-to-back position of structures. Magnification can give a clue to location, since structures that are located closest to the film will have the least magnification and greatest detail. The original film-to-target distance controls the amount of magnification that results. An x-ray film is labeled relative to right and left, which is obviously helpful in gaining orientation while reading the film.

To achieve a three-dimensional perspective, a structure should be radiographed from at least two sides. Usually an anteroposterior or posteroanterior view and a lateral view are taken. Oblique views can also provide important information. This method of using multiple views allows overlapping structures to be separated.[3]

During interpretation of an ophthalmic study, the symmetry of the orbital margins, the orbital walls, the sphe-

noid ridges, the anterior clinoid process, the superior orbital fissures, and the temporal lines (along temporal bones) should be noted for any normal variations and pathologic changes. Some examples include bone indentations and fossa formations, dehiscences (splits), erosions and invasions, hyperostosis (bone hypertrophy), and increased density of soft tissues.

An increase in the volume of soft tissue and signs of increased orbital pressure (demonstrated by the presence of a larger orbit with changes in the contours and density of the walls) should be noted. In addition, it is helpful to observe the optic canals and adjacent structures, the paranasal sinuses, and the sella turcica and its related structures.

Orbital Fractures

The existence of an orbital fracture must be proven and the fracture managed appropriately so that in some instances the binocular vision and cosmetic appearance of the patient will not be seriously compromised. Various types of orbital fractures have characteristic associated signs and symptoms based on the involvement of the soft intraorbital contents. With these signs and symptoms as clues, the clinician can estimate the nature of the fracture and have a better idea of what imaging technique would be best suited for confirmation of the fracture.

The radiologic techniques used in managing orbital fractures are different than those required for other skeletal parts because the orbital bones are broad, thin, and joined at various angles. Multiple views are required for their visualization.

Superior Fractures   Fractures to the frontal portion of the orbital roof are uncommon because of the thickness of the bone. As a result of superior fractures, however, cerebrospinal fluid can drain from the cranial vault through the fracture site into the orbit. Possible clinical signs of superior fractures include ptosis, exophthalmos, and superior ecchymosis. If this area is fractured laterally, levator muscle function can be affected. Central fractures may damage the supraorbital nerve, and medial fractures may involve the frontal sinus and trochlea.

A cephalocaudad force (downward force from above) usually splinters the superior orbital rim and pushes fragments downward. In contrast, a force along the long axis of the orbit may fracture the rim and extend posteriorly to the anterior cranial fossa. It is unusual for the fracture to extend all the way to the optic canal.[3]

Lateral Fractures   The lateral portion of the orbital rim is strongest, which is beneficial because it is the most exposed portion and therefore the most likely to be injured.[7] The zygomatic frontal suture is the weakest part of the lateral wall.[4] The direction of the force causing a fracture can be estimated by the degree of depression of the zygomatic bone, the anterior or posterior displacement of the zygomatic arch, and malar protrusion. Commonly, the traumatic force is so great that the floor of the orbit and lateral wall of the maxillary sinus are concurrently involved, resulting in a floating malar bone; this is referred to as a tripod fracture.[7] This must be treated quickly because the inferior and lateral support of the eye are reduced as a result of the movement of the zygomatic bone.[4]

Fractures in the lateral wall can involve the lacrimal gland and can cause restriction of the mandible and pain upon opening the mouth and chewing if the damaged zygomatic arch contacts the coronoid process of the mandible. Distortion of the outer canthus may also occur because the lateral canthal ligament inserts here on the zygoma. Anesthesia of the lateral aspect of the cheek may be present if the zygomatic nerve is damaged. A zygomatic fracture is illustrated in Figure 18-6.

Medial Fractures Many fractures of the thin medial wall remain undetected. The medial wall forms the limit of the interorbital space, with the roof of this space being the cribriform plate. The contents of this space include the ethmoid sinuses, the turbinate bones, and the nasal septum. If the nasal bones are damaged, the underlying septa will collapse. Damage to the medial wall may occur with fractures of the frontal bone and the maxilla. As a result of its thinness, the medial wall can be fractured if the hydraulic intraorbital pressure is rapidly increased, similar to the manner in which blowout fractures occur to the orbital floor.

The lacrimal sac and the medial canthal ligament are located adjacent to the medial wall; therefore, medial wall fractures can involve these structures.[7] A fracture that extends through the lamina papyracea to the cribriform plate can lead to cerebrospinal fluid rhinorrhea.[4] Orbital emphysema and crepitus commonly occur from the direct communication created by medial wall fractures between the orbit and sinus cavity. An abduction deficit can also manifest if tissue entrapment occurs within a medial wall fracture site.

Inferior Fractures When a blunt object hits the eye, the force is transmitted by way of the closed hydraulic system of the eyeball. This causes a rapid elevation of intraorbital pressure, which is released by the expulsion of the orbital soft tissues through the thin orbital floor or medial wall.[4] In this type of fracture, bone fragments are pushed downward, and the orbital contents can herniate through the fractured area (see Figure 18-4). The most common clinical sign of the blowout fracture is restriction of upward gaze because of the involvement of the inferior oblique and/or inferior rectus muscles. Vertical diplopia is a common symptom. Enophthalmos may also

be present if orbital fat is pushed through the rupture, and inferior ecchymosis is common.

Foreign Body Localization

Radiologic techniques are critical to the ophthalmic practitioner in the localization of both intraocular and intraorbital foreign bodies. As in all diagnostic procedures, the history can give clues to the nature of the foreign body. As stated previously, plain films can be useful for detecting a foreign body, although CT provides more localizing information if surgical removal is anticipated.

COMPUTED TOMOGRAPHY

Despite the ease and economy of plain films, CT is the imaging technique of choice for many ocular conditions because it provides greater information than plain films. Extraocular muscles, the optic nerve, and major blood vessels can be distinguished in conjunction with bone. Visual field defects, oculomotor anomalies, proptosis, and traumatic injury can be effectively evaluated with CT scanning. The orbit images well with CT scanning because of the large differences in density between important orbital structures and the surrounding orbital fat.

Basic Principles

CT scanning uses an x-ray tube and collimators to produce a narrow x-ray beam aimed at a very thin slice of tissue. This differs from the broad x-ray beam aimed at a large area used in plain film evaluations. The instrumentation for receiving the x-rays as they leave the body also differs. CT uses a series of x-ray detectors instead of film. As opposed to one image from one projection, a CT scanner analyzes many pictures from many different angles as the x-ray tube and detectors rotate through an arc around the object of interest. The picture information from the entire arc is analyzed by computer, which creates a cross-sectional image.[8] The process is then repeated for additional slices of variable thicknesses through the area of interest.

Images can be obtained in three different orientations: the sagittal, axial, or coronal anatomic planes (Figure 18-7).[9] The most commonly used orientation for viewing the head is the axial orientation.[10] This consists of horizontal sections taken from the top to the bottom of the head. This is also the most common plane for evaluating the orbit; however, thinner slices must be used to carefully view the detailed orbital anatomy. A typical head scan will consist of 5-mm axial slices.[11] Thinner slices of 1.5 mm are generally recommended for the orbit.[10]

p.t. gland

- blow out
- Graves
- on twmon

FIGURE 18-7

Illustration of the sagittal, axial, and coronal planes for imaging. (Modified with permission from RA Zimmerman, LT Bilaniuk, M Yanoff, et al. Orbital magnetic resonance imaging. American Journal of Ophthalmology. 1985;100:312–7. Published with permission from The American Journal of Ophthalmology. Copyright © The Ophthalmic Publishing Company.)

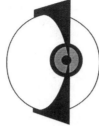
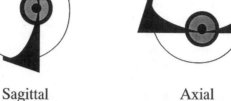
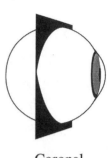

Sagittal   Axial   Coronal

Coronal sections are vertical slices taken from the front of the face to the back of the head. This is the next most common orientation for orbital evaluation. It allows the diameter of the extraocular muscles and optic nerve to be evaluated, thus making it effective for diagnosing Graves' disease and optic nerve tumors. It also has value in localizing foreign bodies when used in conjunction with axial sections.[10]

Sagittal sections are the least used orientation for orbital evaluation. These are vertical sections taken laterally from left to right. Sagittal scans are most helpful for evaluating changes in the floor or roof of the orbit.[10] They are also quite useful in evaluating the sella turcica and pituitary gland.

Sagittal and coronal tissue scans are obtained in two different ways: They may be obtained by directly scanning the body, or they may be recreated via computerized analysis of axial scans. Each method has certain advantages depending on the situation. Reformatting axial scans exposes the patient to less radiation, shortens scan times, and provides less patient repositioning. The disadvantage of reformatting is that some resolution of detail is lost. Direct scanning continues to provide the best evaluation of minute tissue details.[12]

Contrast-enhancing agents may be used concurrently with CT scanning at the clinician's or radiologist's discretion. These are iodine-based dyes given intravenously to increase the visualization of highly vascular tissues. With contrast enhancement, lesions such as tumors or aneurysms may appear brighter on imaging. The orbit possesses a natural contrast background of orbital fat, thus allowing excellent visualization without the injection of contrast agents. Thus, contrast administration is not usually required to distinguish intraorbital pathologic conditions.[13] Contrast enhancement should be used when evaluating areas around the orbit, such as the sella turcica, visual pathways, or brain. Contrast enhancement is of no value in the evaluation of foreign bodies or fractures.

As with most intravenous dyes, risks exist in the use of contrast-enhancing agents. Allergic reactions are well documented with the use of the various contrast media.[10] This can be as mild as itching or hives or as severe as anaphylaxis. In addition, toxic conditions have occurred in patients with impaired kidney function.[5] This results from the inability of the kidneys to remove the contrast agent from the body. Before contrast enhancement is ordered for a patient, allergy to iodine must be ruled out. If kidney disease is documented or suspected, determinations of blood urea nitrogen (BUN) and creatinine levels may be necessary to assess renal clearance before a contrast medium is used.[10]

Indications and Contraindications to Computed Tomographic Scanning

CT is indicated for complicated fractures, localizing foreign bodies for removal, and many types of soft-tissue pathologic conditions. Orbital fractures that need obvious repair, that carry a high possibility for muscle entrapment, or that involve many bones are better evaluated with CT scanning than plain films (Figure 18-8). Although plain films are very effective at detecting foreign bodies, a foreign body for which surgical removal is imminent is better evaluated with a CT scan. Metal particles as small as 0.05 mm can be detected with CT scanning.[14] Materials that are less radiopaque, such as wood or glass, may need to be somewhat larger to be visualized on CT scans. A common recommendation for evaluating intraorbital or intraocular foreign bodies is axial and coronal sections at 1- to 2-mm intervals.[15]

Orbital tumors can be visualized very well with CT scanning because the orbit has thin bones and an excellent contrast background of fat. Tumors of the posterior fossa are better left to MRI because the thicker surrounding bones obscure detail during CT scanning. Orbital tumors that contain calcium image especially well with CT.[16]

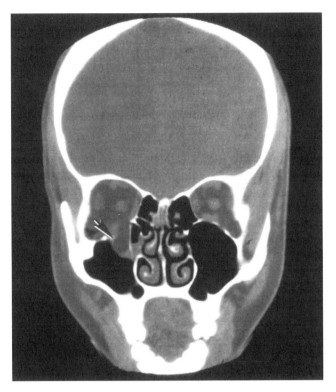

FIGURE 18-8
Coronal CT scan exhibiting a right blowout fracture with entrapped herniated tissue in the maxillary sinus (arrow). (Reprinted with permission from CJ Cakanac. Diagnostic Imaging Techniques. In B Blaustein [ed], Ocular Manifestations of Systemic Disease. New York: Churchill Livingstone, 1994.)

Thus, conditions such as optic nerve head drusen, meningiomas, and retinoblastomas may image as well or better with CT scanning than with MRI.[17] CT remains the imaging technique of first choice for many of these conditions.

Like plain films, CT scanning uses ionizing radiation. It is therefore contraindicated in the care of pregnant women or women suspected of being pregnant.

Computed Tomography Diagnosis

Mass Lesions

CT is an excellent means of evaluating the size, shape, and interaction of mass lesions with other tissues and bones. These characteristics help determine the cause of the lesion. The most common tumor of the globe is the retinoblastoma.[18] This tumor usually occurs in children before 3 years of age and often has an autosomal dominant inheritance pattern. Retinoblastoma is most often unilateral, but it is known to occur bilaterally. The common clinical presentation is an infant with leukocoria

(white pupil) and strabismus. The tumor itself is composed of malignant retinal cells and exhibits a whitish appearance due to the calcium content of the lesion. On CT scanning, retinoblastoma appears as a bright, high-density mass with obvious calcification within the globe.[19] If not treated, the tumor can extend beyond the globe, which greatly affects the prognosis. The cure rate for lesions confined to the globe is approximately 90%[19]; this decreases to about 20% when the lesion extends beyond the globe.

Another calcium-containing tumor that is readily diagnosed with CT scanning is a meningioma. This is a tumor of the leptomeninges, which are composed of the pia mater and arachnoid. The leptomeninges provide a covering over the surface of the brain. Tumors of this type account for 15% of all brain tumors, and due to its meningeal covering, optic nerve involvement can occur. Demographically, meningiomas are most common during middle age and more frequently affect women.[16] With CT scanning, the tumor appears as a bright, high-intensity mass enveloping a darker, lower intensity optic nerve (Figure 18-9). A pathognomonic radiologic finding for meningioma is the tram track sign. This is a cross-hatched appearance along the optic nerve. It indicates the optic nerve is separate from the tumor, and helps differentiate meningioma from other lesions.[18]

Tumors of the chiasm and posterior fossa are imaged better with MRI. These are discussed further in the section on MRI diagnosis.

Infiltrative Lesions

Proptosis may often require CT scanning to establish a definitive diagnosis. The most common cause of proptosis in adults is Graves' ophthalmopathy.[16] In addition to proptosis, eyelid retraction, lagophthalmos, and exposure keratitis may be observed. Gaze limitations and optic neuropathy are additional complications. The proptosis is usually bilateral, which helps to differentiate it from other causes. The pathophysiology for Graves' disease is characterized by an infiltration of lymphocytes, plasma cells, and mucopolysaccharides into the extraocular muscles, which causes them to enlarge. Most commonly involved are the medial and inferior rectus muscles.[18]

CT is of great value in differentiating Graves' ophthalmopathy from other conditions. With this disease, the belly of the extraocular muscle is expanded, but the area where its tendon inserts on the globe is spared.[20] Conditions of orbital pseudotumor and lymphoma may be ruled out. Orbital pseudotumor is an inflammation of the extraocular muscles, sclera, and orbital fat. Most frequently, the disorder occurs in young adults. Clinical findings include a painful proptosis (usually unilateral), motility limita-

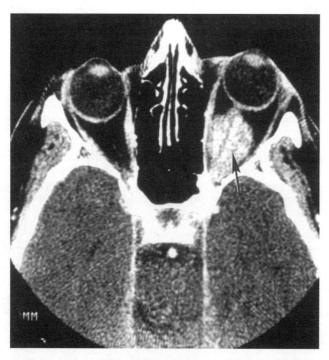

FIGURE 18-9

Axial CT scan with contrast enhancement showing a meningioma of the left optic nerve (arrow). Proptosis of the globe is evident. (Reprinted with permission from CJ Cakanac. Diagnostic Imaging Techniques. In B Blaustein [ed], Ocular Manifestations of Systemic Disease. New York: Churchill Livingstone, 1994.)

tions, and possibly vision loss.[16] A CT scan will exhibit expansion and inflammation of the entire extraocular muscle, including its scleral insertion.[18]

Pseudotumor, cellulitis, and neoplastic disease may all cause the orbital contents to have a diffuse inflammation. These pathologic entities can appear similar on CT scans, which makes diagnosis by appearance alone very difficult. Tissue biopsies may be indicated to ascertain the exact cause if the clinical presentation is unclear.[21]

Stroke

Occlusion of blood vessels within the brain can result in stroke. A leading cause of stroke is atherosclerosis, in which plaques can embolize from the carotid, vertebral, or basilar arteries. Heart disease such as endocarditis, prosthetic valve placement, or mitral disease can also cause emboli. Infarction of cerebral tissue occurs when emboli occlude smaller vessels and obstruct blood flow. Most commonly, the middle cerebral arteries are involved in the brain. In addition to the obstructed blood flow in the brain, emboli can reach the vascular system of the

eye, causing events such as retinal artery occlusion and ischemic optic neuropathy.

MRI or CT scanning can be used to evaluate infarction. Despite the sensitivity of MRI, CT scanning is currently used more often to evaluate acute stroke because of its wider availability and because it is possible to distinguish between pathologic states that can mimic infarction, such as subdural hematoma and tumor.

Brain infarction can be detected with CT scanning 6–12 hours after the occlusive event. The initial appearance of an infarcted region is characterized by a loss of density in the gray matter with a subsequent loss of the usual differentiation between white and gray matter.[18] After 48 hours, a low-density edema may be observed as the blood-brain barrier breaks down. Cystic changes in the affected area are a later finding on CT scans. Contrast enhancement enables tissue changes to be observed for up to 3 months. Many experts recommend that patients with stroke symptoms for less than 48 hours undergo a CT scan without contrast to avoid obscuring the early but more subtle findings. Those patients with stroke symptoms of longer duration are best evaluated with contrast enhancement.

Infarction can be detected with T_2-weighted MRI scans as early as 1 hour after the occlusive signal (see next section). Gadolinium contrast is quite helpful in confirming this diagnosis.

MAGNETIC RESONANCE IMAGING

MRI became available in the 1980s and began a new era in diagnostic imaging. Unlike CT scanning and plain films, which rely on ionizing radiation, MRI uses radio and magnetic waves. The images produced by MRI are the result of the actual chemical and physical properties of the tissues instead of their capacity to absorb x-rays. This makes MRI extremely sensitive to the subtle biochemical changes of degeneration or demyelination or other pathologic tissue processes.[16]

Basic Principles

Much of the basic theory of MRI is based on the properties of the hydrogen atom. Hydrogen is found almost everywhere in the body, most often in the form of water. A hydrogen atom has an odd number of protons, which gives it a small magnetic field as it spins. These magnetic fields have a specific direction and a certain amount of force. In the normal state in the body, these magnetic fields are randomly oriented and their forces tend to cancel each other. However, if the body is put within a very strong magnetic field, these small magnetic fields of the hydrogen atoms align themselves with the direction of the stronger external magnetic field. The characteristics of these small magnetic forces can then be measured and used to generate images.

In clinical use, a patient's body is placed within the tubular bore of a large magnet. The magnetic fields of the hydrogen atoms then align. Next, radio waves of a specific frequency are momentarily directed perpendicular to the alignment of the magnetic field. This disrupts the alignment and spin of the hydrogen atoms. After the radio waves are turned off, the fields of the hydrogen atoms again realign themselves with the external magnetic field. An antenna surrounding the body measures various aspects of these small fields as they return to alignment with the external magnet. Computer-assisted analysis is then used to create images from the signals detected.

Two of the variables measured are referred to as T_1 and T_2. T_1 is the time it takes for the hydrogen atom fields to realign with the external magnetic field after being disrupted by the pulse of radio waves. This time is determined by the chemical state of the tissue. T_1 is also called the spin-lattice function.[16] Generally, T_1 best illustrates normal anatomy. T_2 occupies a much shorter time period than T_1. When the external magnet is applied, the magnetic forces of the hydrogen atoms align with it but continue to "spin" or "precess" independently about their axes. With application of the radio pulse, the spinning becomes exactly the same for a brief moment. This is called *phase coherence.* When the radio pulse is removed, this phase coherence gradually returns to random spinning. The time it takes for this decay of phase coherence is called T_2. It is also called the spin-spin function. T_2 images are based mostly on the physical state of the tissue and are usually thought to highlight areas of pathologic involvement.

Because cortical bone has little hydrogen content, it does not image well with MRI. This is an advantage when areas of tissue surrounded by bone are being studied but a disadvantage if the bone itself needs to be evaluated. The differing water content between white and gray matter of the brain allows these tissue types to be clearly distinguished with MRI.[16]

For the eye and orbit, orbital fat appears as a bright (hyperintense) background with the vitreous, optic nerves, and extraocular muscles being dark or hypointense on a T_1-weighted image (Figure 18-10A). The brightnesses of these structures tend to reverse with T_2 weighting (Figure 18-10B). The T_1 and T_2 weighting variables can be changed by the technician performing the scan to achieve the most desirable images of the area of interest.

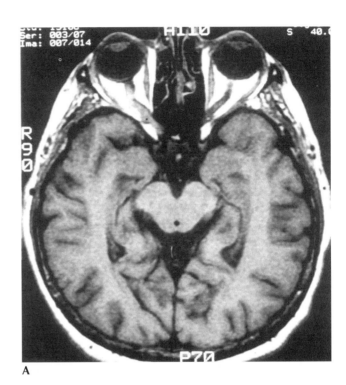

A

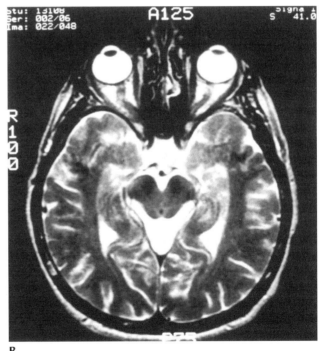

B

FIGURE 18-10

A. A normal axial MRI scan, which is T_1 weighted. The vitreous, optic nerves, and extraocular muscles are dark, with a bright background of orbital fat. B. Note the reversal of images with T_2 weighting. (Reprinted with permission from CJ Cakanac. Diagnostic Imaging Techniques. In B Blaustein [ed], Ocular Manifestations of Systemic Disease. New York: Churchill Livingstone, 1994.)

Indications and Contraindications for Magnetic Resonance Imaging

For studying most pathologic states of soft tissue, MRI has become the preferred imaging technique. As mentioned previously, bone does not image with MRI. This makes MRI superior for scanning areas surrounded by dense bone, allowing tissues to be imaged without the artifacts from bone that are often seen with CT scanning. This makes MRI the test of choice for scanning the posterior fossa, where many CT artifacts are caused by the surrounding thick petrous bones. Thus, indications for MRI include many pathologic entities found in this area such as cranial neuropathies, gaze palsies, nystagmus, and papilledema.[17]

MRI is also more sensitive than CT scanning for detecting demyelination. Therefore, it has become a standard test to support the often elusive diagnosis of multiple sclerosis.

Compared with CT scans and plain films, radiation exposure is not a factor of concern because x-rays are not used in MRI. Despite this, many experts suggest avoiding the use of MRI during the first trimester of pregnancy as a precaution, since the effects, if any, of strong magnetic waves on the developing fetus are not known.[10] Due to the strong magnetic field encountered with MRI, the presence of a metallic foreign body is a contraindication for its use. A history of a previous or a possible orbital or ocular foreign body requires thorough investigation to rule out its presence before proceeding with MRI. Metallic surgical clips from previous intracranial surgery are also a contraindication. Although metallic dental fillings are not a contraindication, they do produce artifacts that can blur the images obtained. The metallic components found in some life support systems can prevent patients dependent on them from being placed within an MRI unit.[10] Pacemakers can also be a contraindication to MRI because it may interfere with their electronics and cause them to malfunction.[16]

Other problems encountered with performing MRI result from the narrow confines of the instrumentation. Patients who have claustrophobic tendencies may need to be sedated before scanning. Certain MRI scanners may not accommodate very obese patients.

Magnetic Resonance Imaging Diagnosis

Mass Lesions

Gliomas are common malignant brain tumors. These tumors arise from neuroectoderm. In children, gliomas are most commonly located in the posterior fossa, whereas in adults they are usually supratentorial. Gliomas may involve the optic nerve, occurring most commonly in chil-

dren 2–6 years of age. One-fourth of these cases are associated with neurofibromatosis.[16] Ocular signs and symptoms of an optic nerve glioma include painless proptosis, visual loss, optic atrophy, and strabismus. On T_1 and T_2 MRI images, the tumor appears as a fusiform or bulbous expansion of the optic nerve. Involvement of the chiasm, geniculate body, or optic radiations can also occur.

An astrocytoma is a type of malignant glioma involving the central nervous system that occurs in both adults and children. This tumor consists of abnormal astrocytes mixed with normal tissue and often involves the ventricles, cerebrum, cerebellum, or brain stem.[18] MRI reveals a high-intensity mass representing tumor and edema. The tumor can also be imaged with CT scanning, which will show a low-density mass with varying amounts of calcification.[16]

Pituitary adenomas are tumors arising from the pituitary gland. Pituitary adenomas classically cause chiasmal compression, which leads to a bitemporal visual field defect. These tumors have been classified according to cell type (eosinophilic, basophilic, or chromophobic) as well as according to hormonal secretion characteristics. Most commonly, pituitary adenomas occur in young women and secrete prolactin, causing galactorrhea and amenorrhea. Tumors that secrete adrenocorticotropic hormone cause Cushing's syndrome, and those secreting growth hormone result in acromegaly and gigantism. Some pituitary adenomas are nonsecreting and will not produce symptoms until their size increases to the point where it compresses the chiasm and other structures.[18] Those tumors less than 1 cm in diameter are referred to as microadenomas and those larger than 1 cm are referred to as macroadenomas.[16] As mentioned, the classic ocular finding with a pituitary adenoma is a bitemporal visual field defect that is denser above the midline than below. A bitemporal loss occurs because nasal fibers decussate at the chiasm. The defects are denser superiorly because the tumor directly compresses the inferior aspect of the chiasm, which receives axons from the inferior retina.

Pituitary adenomas are routinely imaged with MRI. Because the bones of the sella turcica can interfere with CT images, MRI has become the preferred modality for imaging this region.[17] Secreting adenomas appear as round, low-intensity lesions within the pituitary gland. The gland itself can appear to have an upward convexity.[18] Sagittal and coronal scans are extremely helpful in visualizing the chiasm (Figure 18-11). With the use of MRI enhancing agents, the tumor appears less prominent than the gland itself.[22]

Ocular Motility Defects

Deficits in ocular motility can occur from neoplasm, trauma, aneurysm, ischemia, and demyelination.[23] MRI is the

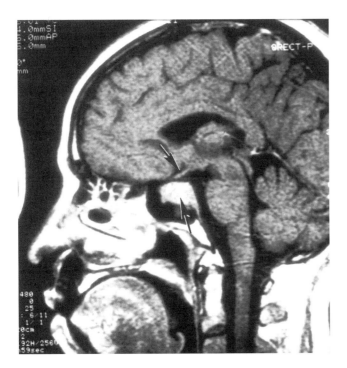

FIGURE 18-11
A sagittal MRI demonstrating a pituitary adenoma. The position of the optic chiasm (upper arrow) is noted above the tumor (lower arrow).

preferred method for imaging in these conditions. Virtually the entire intracranial course of the third, fourth, and sixth cranial nerves can be imaged with MRI, which will rarely miss a mass or aneurysm large enough to cause a gaze palsy. However, defects caused by small ischemic lesions can be difficult to document with any imaging modality, including MRI.[22]

MRI has an inherent advantage over CT scanning in the diagnosis of nystagmus, because nystagmus is often caused by posterior fossa lesions. Other supranuclear motor defects such as Parinaud's syndrome can be evaluated quite well with MRI. In addition, MRI can detect small brain stem lesions, such as those in the medial longitudinal fascicles responsible for an internuclear ophthalmoplegia.[22]

Visual Field Defects
MRI is commonly used in the evaluation of unexplained visual field defects. Disorders of the chiasm most often cause a bitemporal hemianopia.[24] The classic cause is a pituitary adenoma, but a similar presentation can occur from meningiomas, craniopharyngiomas, or gliomas.[23]

Optic tract lesions produce incongruous hemianopias. They are rare and usually also have pupillary involve-

ment.[25] Pathologic conditions causing optic tract lesions are generally the same as those resulting in chiasmal dysfunction.

Temporal lobe lesions can disturb the radiations passing around this area, thus causing hemianopias denser above the midline.[25] Additional symptoms can include visual hallucinations and psychomotor seizures.[23] Lesions of this region in older patients are usually vascular in nature. In children, they are often compressive in nature.

Parietal lobe lesions tend to produce hemianopias denser below the midline.[25] Parietal lesions also produce asymmetric optokinetic nystagmus. Other symptoms include alexia and agraphia.[24] Parietal lobe lesions are usually vascular in nature or the result of various tumors (e.g., astrocytomas, gliomas, metastases).[24]

Occipital lobe disorders produce very congruous hemianopias.[25] Bilateral lesions can cause cortical blindness. Vascular lesions of the posterior cerebral arteries of the vertebrobasilar system most commonly cause occipital defects.[24]

Because of the greater ability of MRI to differentiate soft tissues, it is superior to CT scanning for detecting and evaluating optic tract and visual radiation lesions. An exception, however, may be a visual field defect related to acute trauma, in which case it can take longer than 12 hours to obtain useful images with MRI if hemorrhage is present.

Demyelination
MRI can demonstrate demyelinating plaques in the optic nerve and brain that were previously impossible to diagnose with CT scans. Periventricular demyelinating plaques are more easily demonstrated and are suggestive of multiple sclerosis in a patient with an appropriate history (optic neuritis, internuclear ophthalmoplegia, paresthesias, etc.). It should be noted that unidentified bright objects (UBOs) found on MRI studies can be mistaken for demyelinating plaques. Unidentified bright objects have no clinical consequences and are seen in normal individuals, especially with increasing age.

Future Developments
Enhanced MRI images are being obtained with fat suppression techniques, contrast agents, and surface coils. The latter involves placing the antenna or coil in closer proximity to the tissue being scanned to increase the signal-to-noise ratio. A surface coil can be placed on the skin surrounding the orbit to yield an enhanced image.

Contrast agents have become available for MRI. They contain gadolinium rather than iodine as with CT. These agents are used only with T_1 images and particularly enhance those lesions that manifest an abnormal blood-brain-barrier or increased vascularity. They are especially useful for identifying meningiomas, lymphomas, and occult disease missed with other techniques.[22] Gadolinium appears to exhibit minimal side effects other than transient headaches. Its effects during pregnancy are not well known.[22]

Fat suppression techniques help to suppress the bright signal from orbital fat on T_1 images.[26] This aids in the visualization of lesions that might otherwise be obscured by the fat signal. The technique is particularly useful with optic nerve meningiomas, which were previously poorly imaged with MRI. The combination of surface coils, gadolinium contrast, and fat suppression is helping to eliminate any advantage CT scanning has had for studying the orbit.

Currently under development are positron emission tomography (PET) and single-photon emission computed tomography (SPECT). These involve labeling photon molecules with radioisotopes, which provide a great deal of physiologic and anatomic information about the brain. Future areas of study will most likely investigate blood flow in ischemic situations and injury sites from Alzheimer's disease and multiple sclerosis.[18]

REFERENCES

1. Pfeffer RL. Roentgenography of exophthalmos with notes on the roentgen ray in ophthalmology. Am J Ophthalmol 1943;26:724–41.
2. Semat H, Baumel P. Fundamentals of Physics. New York: Holt, Rinehart, and Winston, 1974;4–24.
3. Meschan I. An Atlas of Anatomy Basic to Radiology. Philadelphia: Saunders 1975:186–94.
4. Gombos GM. Handbook of Ophthalmologic Emergencies (2nd ed). New York: Medical Examination, 1977:109–20.
5. Lombardi G. Orbital pathology and contrast media. Radiol Clin North Am 1972;1:115–28.
6. Meschan I. Radiographic Positioning and Related Anatomy (2nd ed). Philadelphia: Saunders, 1967;230–40.
7. Vinik M, Garjone F. Orbital fractures. AJR 1966;97:607–13.
8. Lee SH, Rao K. Cranial Computed Tomography and MRI (2nd ed). New York: McGraw-Hill, 1983;1–21.
9. Meschan I, Farrer-Meschan R. Orbital Roentgen Signs in Diagnostic Imaging. Philadelphia: Saunders 1985;454–72.
10. Tower H, Oshinskie L. An introduction to computed tomography and magnetic resonance imaging of the head and visual pathways. J Am Optom Assoc 1989;60:619–27.
11. Carter B. CT of the Head and Neck. New York: Churchill Livingstone, 1985:20–38.
12. Peyster R, Hoover E. Computed Tomography in Orbital Disease and Neuro-ophthalmology. Chicago: Year Book, 1984:1–9.
13. Hammerschlag S, Hesselink J, Weber A. Computed Tomography of the Eye and Orbit. Norwalk, CT: Appleton-Century-Croft, 1983:23–8.
14. Haik B. Advanced imaging techniques in ophthalmology. Int Ophthalmol Clin 1986;26:79–99.
15. Deutsch T, Feller D. Management of Ocular Injuries. Philadelphia: Saunders, 1985:109–19.
16. Elster A. Cranial Magnetic Resonance Imaging. New York: Churchill Livingstone, 1988:1–15, 337–73.
17. Slamovits TL, Gardner TA. Neuroimaging in neuro–ophthalmology. Ophthalmology 1989;96:555–68.
18. Stimac GK. Introduction to Diagnostic Imaging. Philadelphia: Saunders, 1992:455–531.
19. Pomeranz S. Craniospinal Magnetic Resonance Imaging. Philadelphia: Saunders, 1989;231–79.
20. Newton TH, Bilaniuk LT. Radiology of the Eye and Orbit. New York: Raven, 1990;9.2–9.31.
21. Vaughan D, Asbury T. General Ophthalmology. Los Altos: Lange, 1980;163–78.
22. Kaufman DI, Pernicone JR. Advances in MRI and their impact on neuro-ophthalmology. Semin Ophthalmol 1992;7:2–22.
23. Dornic DI. Ophthalmic Pocket Companion. Oklahoma City: Vision Educational Foundation, 1990;18–29.
24. Newman N. Neuro–ophthalmology: A Practical Text. Norwalk, CT: Appleton & Lange, 1992;3–51.
25. Bajandas F, Kline L. Neuro-ophthalmology Review Manual Thorofare, NJ: Slack, 1988;3–43.
26. Levin LA, Rubin P. Advances in orbital imaging. Int Ophthalmol Clin 1992;32:1–22.

19

Neurologic Testing

DANIEL K. ROBERTS AND DENNIS E. MATHEWS

The optometrist must, on occasion, decide if a particular clinical case requires neurologic consultation. In other cases, an understanding of the initial deficits can be helpful in the overall management of patient with a neuro-ophthalmic dysfunction. In either of these situations, a thorough knowledge of basic neurologic testing techniques and principles can be indispensable. This chapter provides an overview of methods for evaluating patients with suspected neurologic deficits. Figure 19-1 shows instrumentation and materials that are useful for basic neurologic screening techniques.

Among ophthalmic clinical signs and symptoms that might indicate need for a basic neurologic workup are visual field deficits indicative of central nervous system (CNS) lesions, exophthalmos, motility disturbances (ophthalmoplegia, nystagmus), pupillary disorders (Horner's syndrome, Adie's syndrome, light-near dissociation), and transient visual loss. Other general symptoms that may indicate neurologic disease are unexplained headaches, vertigo, aphasia, paresis, paresthesias, confusion, tinnitus, and ataxia.

The basic neurologic examination can be designed to evaluate four major systems: (1) cognition, or higher cortical function; (2) cranial nerve function; (3) sensorial function; and (4) motor function.

NEUROLOGIC HISTORY

In addition to questions pertinent to the routine optometric examination, there is obviously a significant amount of information that can be helpful when dealing with a patient suspected of having neurologic disease. Table 19-1 outlines a number of items helpful in the general neurologic review. As with any symptoms that may be encountered during routine eye examination, positive findings may be followed up with inquiries about their severity, frequency, duration, onset, alleviating or aggra-

vating factors, and other circumstances surrounding their presentation. The benefits of a thorough general medical history (past and present, patient and family) including the use of medications are straightforward and will not be reviewed further within this discussion.

As shown in Table 19-1, information pertaining to the patient's mental status is primarily obtained within the neurologic history. Because of its complexity, evaluation of the mental status is discussed separately.

MENTAL STATUS EVALUATION

Observation of a patient's mental state is a routine component of the overall neurologic evaluation. Usually, only a relatively brief investigation is performed. However, if there is a suspected abnormality, a more extensive examination may be required. Attention to the patient's mental state should begin immediately on greeting the patient, and it should proceed throughout the taking of the history and the actual physical examination. Before a more detailed evaluation of mental state that requires specific questions about orientation, memory, and so forth, a general rapport should be established with the patient.

There are a number of different methods for classifying the mental status evaluation. This discussion, however, will not attempt to provide a complex organizational scheme. Rather, it will simply review some of the more basic components of mental state that are relevant to general neurologic screening. A summary of these components is provided in Table 19-2.

Physical Appearance

A patient's level of hygiene, appropriateness of dress, and posture can all yield useful information regarding his or

FIGURE 19-1

Items and materials useful for basic neurologic screening examinations. These include a 500- to 1000-Hz tuning fork; vials of aromatic substances such as coffee, cinnamon, or peppermint; vials of substances to evaluate taste (should include bitter, salty, sour, and sweet substances); a 3 × 5-inch card labeled with the words "bitter," "salt," "sour," and "sweet"; a drinking cup; cotton balls; a reflex hammer; cotton-tipped applicators; empty test tubes; tongue depressors; and a safety pin.

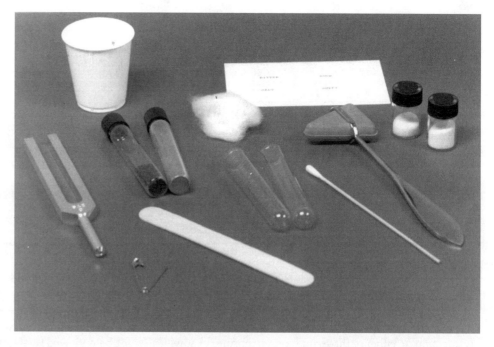

her mental state. If these appear to be inconsistent with the patient's background, position in society, or previous habits, an indication of mental deterioration may be evident. Whereas unusual characteristics may be nonspecific for a particular disorder, they may nonetheless be fairly good indicators of general abnormalities such as an organic brain disease or psychiatric dysfunction. Poor posture, refusal to make eye contact, and lack of facial expression may indicate depression.

Psychiatric diseases and organic mental illness may also be associated with a number of easily observable physiologic changes. Therefore, the examiner should observe the patient for signs such as tremors, sweating, or wide palpebral fissures. The patient may also be specifically asked about the presence of anorexia, weight loss, nausea, vomiting, diarrhea, palpitations, fatigue, and sleep dysfunction.

General Behavior

Physical appearance obviously reflects a patient's behavior, but there are other considerations as well. For example, it is important to detect signs of emotional instability that may be manifested by excessive irritability, euphoria, or unresponsiveness. Unexpected reactions by a patient to a particular topic or event may be noteworthy and can indicate marked mood swings or instability. A catastrophic reaction consisting of crying or a refusal to continue may be a nonspecific sign of diffuse brain disease. Often, a fair-

ly accurate analysis of the patient's mood can be determined through routine questioning and observation during the examination. Occasionally, it may be necessary to specifically question the patient regarding his or her general mood over the past weeks or months.

Speech patterns are an important component of behavior and should be noted. Speaking that is slow, fragmented, or too rapid may be noteworthy. Close attention to word selection and pronunciation is also important. Aphasia is a general term describing the inability of persons to express themselves properly through speech. It may also describe a loss of verbal comprehension. Various forms of aphasia may indicate specific etiologic factors. For example, motor aphasia describes the condition in which a patient knows precisely what he or she wants to say but is unable to do so because of lack of motor control stemming from a lesion in Broca's area in the cerebral cortex. Amnesiac aphasia refers to the loss of memory for words, and auditory aphasia refers to the incomprehension of spoken words. Lesions involving several locations within the CNS can result in various forms of aphasia. Abnormal volume or pitch of speech can indicate an innervational problem to the laryngeal musculature.

Other behavioral characteristics that should be noted during the neurologic screening include the development of personality characteristics such as introversion, obsessiveness, delusional changes, distractibility, loss of former interests, paranoia, hypochondriasis, aggressiveness, or other neurotic tendencies.

TABLE 19-1
The Neurologic History

Mental status
  Emotional instability—depression, anxiety, aggressiveness
  Memory loss
  Difficulty concentrating
  Confusion
  Psychiatric disorders
Sensory system
  Loss of smell or taste
  Visual changes—amaurosis, visual acuity reduction, diplopia
  Numbness
  Unusual pain
  Presence of paresthesias
  Loss of hearing, presence of tinnitus, vertigo
Motor system
  Weakness
  Transient paralysis
  Difficulty walking
  Falling
  Dropping things
  Difficulty swallowing
  Difficulty speaking
General
  Handedness
  Headache
  Seizures
  Fainting
  Constitutional symptoms—fever, nausea, vomiting, diarrhea, fatigue, anorexia, weight loss
  Exposure to environmental hazards
  Drug or alcohol abuse
  Impotence
  Difficulty urinating

TABLE 19-2
Mental Status Evaluation

Physical appearance
  Note level of hygiene, appropriateness of dress, posture
  Note physiologic changes such as tremors, sweating, widened palpebral fissures
General behavior
  Note emotional instability such as excessive irritability, euphoria, unresponsiveness, catastrophic reactions
  Speech patterns
  Introversion
  Obsessiveness
  Delusional changes
  Distractibility
  Loss of former interests
  Paranoia
  Hypochondriasis
General knowledge and orientation
  Knowledge of persons, place, time
  Knowledge of presidents, cities
Memory
  Immediate: Digit span test—repeat series of numbers 1, 8, 3, 6, 9
  Recent: Yesterday's meals, dress
  Remote: Birthday, birthplace, wedding date
Higher intellectual function
  Basic arithmetic calculations
    4×7?
    $10 - 5$?
    $60 - 3 = 57 - 3 = 54 = ?$
  Word similarities: dog–cat, etc.
  Judgment: What would you do if you found someone's lost wallet?

General Knowledge and Orientation

General knowledge can usually be evaluated during casual interaction with the patient. As the history proceeds, the patient should exhibit reasonable knowledge about such facts as his or her phone number, address, location of employment, names of children, and so forth. Obviously, however, general knowledge can vary considerably depending on such factors as a person's educational status or occupation, and these variables should be considered. Specific questions may be asked if necessary, such as the names of presidents or cities. Most persons should be oriented to the current year, month, day, and time of day. Recollection of their present location (country, state, city, address) and who they are (name, occupation) should also be demonstrated.

Memory

Memory is a complicated process requiring several components of brain function. Disturbance of any of these components can lead to defective memory. Therefore, memory dysfunction is a common symptom of organic brain disease. In addition to basic recollection of facts, memory can be tested with a few specific techniques. Memory can be categorized into three types: immediate, recent, and remote.[1] For memory to be evaluated properly, the patient should be able to adequately concentrate on a task given. Therefore, a judgment regarding the presence of an appropriate attention level should first be made.

A simple method to evaluate immediate memory is the digit span test.[1] Here, the patient repeats a series of numbers relayed by the examiner. Normally, a person should be able to immediately repeat approximately seven numbers in the same order in which they were presented.

Recent memory refers to the recollection of information pertaining to a somewhat ill-defined time period consisting of the past several minutes or hours, or the last one to two days. It is tested by asking the patient to recall information such as what he or she had for breakfast or lunch, what he or she wore the day before, or what he or she did a few hours before the examination.

Remote memory refers to information that should be known to the patient for years such as his or her birth date, wedding date, or birthplace.

Higher Intellectual Function

Higher intellectual function refers to the ability to reason or solve problems. Once again, because of the complexity of these processes and the brain centers involved in them, abnormality is often exhibited with organic brain disease. Simple tests include providing the patient with basic arithmetic calculations. For example, "What is 4×7?" or "What is $24 - 8$?" Tasks may also be given such as having the patient subtract 3 from 60, and 3 more from that number, and so on. Verbal reasoning and abstract thought can be tested by asking the patient to indicate how each of the following words is alike[1]:

dog – cat
bird – airplane
blue – yellow
hot – cold
tree – flower

Judgment also requires higher intellectual processing and may be impaired with many mental disorders. This is tested by asking the patient what he or she would do in various hypothetical situations. For example: What would you do if you found a wallet that someone had lost? What would you do if a tornado was reportedly on its way?

CRANIAL NERVE EVALUATION

An understanding of the 12 cranial nerves serves as a substantial basis for many components of the neurologic examination. There are a number of very simple tests that can be applied within the general optometric setting to evaluate the function of the cranial nerves. Table 19-3 provides a listing of the cranial nerves, their basic functions, and respective methods of evaluation.

Olfactory Nerve (Cranial Nerve I)

Asking the patient whether he or she ever perceives smells that are not actually present is important in evaluating the olfactory system (olfactory hallucination). In addition, loss of smell (anosmia), perversion of smell (parosmia), and loss of smell discrimination should also be investigated. Symmetry of olfaction can be tested by covering one of the patient's nostrils and having the patient smell with the other. Such substances as cinnamon, peppermint, wintergreen,

lemon oil, or coffee may be used for this test. Decreased smell on one side relative to the other is especially noteworthy, since unilateral loss can indicate acute neurologic dysfunction of the olfactory system. Smell normally decreases gradually with age, but acute loss can indicate such diseases as temporal lobe disease, frontal lobe lesions, meningioma of the sphenoid ridge, and parasellar lesions.[2]

Optic Nerve (Cranial Nerve II)

Visual acuities and visual fields are important in the evaluation of the optic nerve. Most important in the visual field evaluation for patients suspected of having neurologic disease are deficits that include junctional scotomata, bitemporal or binasal field defects, and homonymous field loss. Homonymous field defects indicate postchiasmal disease. Often, neurologic field changes are large and dense, which may make them easy to evaluate with gross testing. Consequently, confrontational field testing is often helpful in examination. Further evaluation with such instruments as the tangent screen or the automated perimeter can be more specific and sensitive in qualifying field loss and should be used when possible. Careful attention should be given to the vertical meridian during visual field testing of patients with suspected neurologic disease. Defects frequently respect this plane because of the anatomic distribution of the visual pathways. Visual field testing is discussed in Chapter 8.

Of obvious importance in the evaluation of optic nerve function is pupillary testing. Not only can relative conduction deficits of the optic nerve be detected via the swinging flashlight test, but additional anomalies of neurologic importance can also be identified with pupillary testing. Pupillary defects and their relationship to optic nerve function and other neurologic abnormalities are discussed in detail in Chapter 9.

Color vision testing should always be performed when optic nerve function is being evaluated. Although there are a number of different methods for assessing color vision, convenient tests such as the pseudoisochromatic plates or the Farnsworth Panel D–15 test are commonly used (see Chapter 7). As a general rule, optic nerve disease tends to cause color vision loss that is most pronounced in the red-green color spectrum.[3] The relative importance of color vision evaluation in optic nerve function stems from the fact that it is a very sensitive indicator of conduction deficits of the optic nerve, often demonstrating dysfunction well before conventional testing techniques such as Snellen acuity measurements. The entire visual field can even be plotted with color targets, searching for relative defects between quadrants of a single eye or for relative loss between eyes. Formal plotting of the visual field can be performed with instrumentation equipped with colored targets as well as

TABLE 19-3
Cranial Nerve Function and Evaluation

Cranial Nerve	Function	Screening Methods
I. Olfactory	Sensory: Smell	Presentation of aromatic odors (coffee, cinnamon, peppermint, etc.) one nostril at a time
II. Optic	Sensory: Sight	Visual acuity, color vision, visual field testing, pupillary testing, observe for nerve head atrophy
III. Oculomotor	Motor: Levator palpebrae, superior rectus, medial rectus, inferior rectus, inferior oblique Parasympathetic: Pupil, ciliary body	Motility testing, pupils, accommodation
IV. Trochlear	Motor: Superior oblique	Motility testing
V. Trigeminal	Sensory (all three branches): forehead, face, cornea, conjunctiva, iris, lacrimal gland, sinus and mouth mucosa, teeth, ears	Evaluation of forehead, cheek, and chin for sharp, dull, and light touch sensation. Evaluate blink reflex after corneal stimulation
	Motor: Mandibular division—muscles of mastication	Observe for signs of muscular atrophy. Palpate muscles for tone during forceful jaw closure
VI. Abducens	Motor: Lateral rectus	Motility testing
VII. Facial	Sensory: Soft palate, taste to anterior two-thirds of tongue	Evaluate taste with salt, sugar solutions
	Motor: Facial muscles, buccinator, scalp, auricle, stapedius, platysma, digastric Parasympathetic: Lacrimal and parotid glands	Evaluate ability to wrinkle brow, raise eyebrows, puff out cheeks, purse lips, smile, forcefully close eyes
VIII. Acoustic	Sensory: Cochlear division—hearing	Repetition of examiner's spoken words, identification of unknown sound, acknowledgment of sound, Weber and Rinne tests
	Vestibular division—equilibrium	Doll's head maneuver, caloric testing
IX. Glossopharyngeal	Sensory: Nasopharynx, soft palate, posterior one-third of tongue, carotid reflex	Evaluate gag reflex. Evaluate taste with bitter, sour solutions
	Motor: Pharyngeal muscles	Evaluate gag reflex, swallowing, movement of palate, uvular deviation, observation of speech
	Parasympathetic: Salivary glands	
X. Vagus	Sensory: Larynx, pharynx, abdominal and thoracic viscera, posterior aspect of external auditory meatus	Evaluate gag reflex
	Motor: Muscles of base of tongue, larynx, pharynx, abdominal and thoracic organs Parasympathetic: Abdominal and thoracic organs	Evaluate gag reflex, swallowing, movement of soft palate, uvular deviation, observation of speech
XI. Spinal accessory	Motor: Cranial division—some pharyngeal muscles	
	Spinal division—trapezius and sternocleidomastoid muscles	Rotation of head to right and left, shrug shoulders
XII. Hypoglossal	Motor: Muscles of tongue and strap muscles of neck	Observe for atrophy or fasciculations or deviations of tongue. Observe mobility and strength

white targets. In some instances, a simple method using red ocular pharmaceutical bottle caps can be performed for screening purposes. With this technique the examiner simply asks the patient to fixate on a red cap (or other object) with one eye at a time and then to compare the relative brightness between the eyes. Conduction defects of the optic nerve typically cause the cap to appear "less red" or "washed out" relative to a normal eye. The visual field of a single eye can be evaluated by slowly moving a single cap through the field, noting any sudden change in its brightness, particularly along the vertical meridian. In addition, two caps can be held simultaneously within

different quadrants of the visual field and the patient asked to compare their relative brightness simultaneously. This latter method can be helpful in evaluating for the presence of the extinction phenomenon that may occur with neurologic field defects.

Cranial Nerves III, IV, VI: Ocular Motility Testing

When evaluating a patient with a motility deficit, three areas should be considered in the differential diagnosis. These include neurogenic deficits (nerve palsies), restrictive or myogenic deficits (such as Graves' ophthalmopathy and Duane's retraction syndrome), and neuromuscular junction disease (such as myasthenia gravis). To separate motility deficits in these three areas, motility testing should be performed. Cover testing for determination of the objective angle of deviation in different fields of gaze should be performed. The subjective angle of deviation by such tests as the Maddox rod or red lens test may be used as the objective angle in acute diplopia cases, since these patients all have normal correspondency and central fixation unless there is underlying long-standing strabismus unrelated to the acute problem. Subtle deviations, such as small vertical deviations, may be more easily quantitated by subjective means of evaluation than by objective tests.

Versions and ductions should be performed on all patients with ocular motility deficits to disrupt the fusional system and expose movement characteristics related to consensual innervation between the two eyes. This testing can help to differentiate between neurogenic and myogenic abnormalities.

Forced duction testing should always be performed when necessary on patients with ocular motility deficits to rule out mechanical restriction of movement of the globe. This test may be performed by anesthetizing the eye with a topical anesthetic and having the patient attempt to move the eye in the direction of palsy while the examiner pushes the eye with a cotton-tipped applicator. If this is not adequate to evaluate eye movement, tissue forceps may be used to grab and tug the conjunctiva and extraocular muscle at its insertion into the globe on the side opposite the desired direction of movement. Free movement indicates lack of mechanical restriction, and further tests will determine if the cause of the weakened muscle is neurogenic, myogenic, or neuromuscular junction in nature. Further information on motility testing is provided in Chapter 10.

Oculomotor Nerve (Cranial Nerve III)

The oculomotor nerve provides motor innervation to the superior rectus, inferior rectus, medial rectus, inferior oblique, and levator muscles. Chapter 10 provides a detailed discussion on motility testing for the function of cranial nerve III. In addition to motor innervation to these muscles, the oculomotor nerve also supplies parasympathetic innervation to the eye for accommodation and efferent pupillary responses (pupillary constriction). Thus, pupillary evaluation is also a very important step in cranial nerve screening. Pupillary testing is discussed in detail in Chapter 9.

In a complete third nerve palsy, the eye will be tropic and turned down and outward. There is also ptosis and a dilated pupil on the involved side. Often the pupil may be unaffected in a third nerve palsy. This has etiologic significance because classically, pupillary sparing indicates an ischemic vascular cause such as diabetes mellitus, and pupillary involvement indicates a compressive cause such as may be seen with an aneurysm of the posterior communicating artery.[4] As discussed in Chapter 9, neurologic pupillary dysfunction may occur in isolation of third nerve extraocular muscle involvement. Lesions involving the sympathetic or parasympathetic innervation to the pupil can result in abnormalities of major neurologic significance such as Horner's syndrome, the dorsal midbrain syndrome, Argyll Robertson pupil, or a tonic pupil (Adie's pupil).

Trochlear Nerve (Cranial Nerve IV)

The only function of the trochlear nerve is to provide innervation to the superior oblique muscle. The fascicular portion of this nerve leaves its midbrain nucleus and decussates in the anterior medullary velum over the cerebral aqueduct before exiting the dorsal aspect of the brain stem. Therefore, axons from each brain stem nucleus provide innervation to the contralateral superior oblique muscle. The primary action of this muscle is infraduction, with secondary and tertiary actions of intorsion and abduction. Paresis of the fourth nerve results in a hyperdeviation of the involved eye and is best identified with the Parks three-step procedure described in detail in Chapter 10. The hyperdeviation caused by a trochlear nerve palsy is classically greater with gaze to the opposite of the side of the affected muscle and also greater with the head tilted toward the affected side. Diplopia is often noticeably worse when gaze is at near with the eyes directed downward and inward.

Abducens Nerve (Cranial Nerve VI)

The sixth cranial nerve supplies motor innervation to the lateral rectus muscle, which abducts the eye. Classically, a paresis of the abducens nerve presents as an inward turned eye with a greater deviation at far than near and that is greater with gaze toward the affected side. Differentiating a sixth nerve paresis from other causes of abductional deficit is discussed in more detail in Chapter 10.

Trigeminal Nerve (Cranial Nerve V)

The trigeminal nerve provides sensory innervation to a number of structures including the skin of the forehead and face, the cornea, conjunctiva, iris, lacrimal gland, sinus, mouth mucosa, teeth, and ears. Two of its branches, the ophthalmic and maxillary, provide sensory innervation only; the mandibular branch supplies sensory input as well as motor innervation to the muscles of mastication.

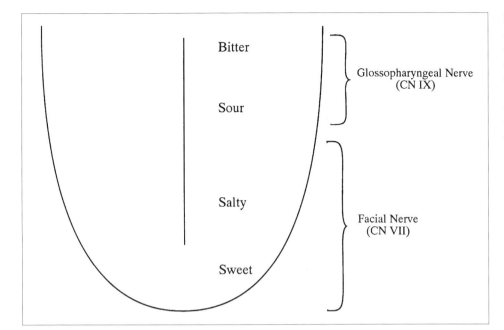

FIGURE 19-2
Schematic of the tongue illustrating sensory taste zones. The facial nerve provides sensory innervation to the anterior two-thirds (salty, sweet) and the glossopharyngeal nerve provides sensory innervation to the posterior one-third (bitter, sour).

Sensory innervation of the fifth nerve is tested by evaluating all three areas of the face (forehead, cheek, chin) for sharp, dull, and light touch sensation. Temperature sensation may also be evaluated, but this is not usually necessary if the other sensation responses are normal. With the patient's eyes closed, testing is performed by randomly applying the sharp or dull tips of a device such as a safety pin to both sides of the three facial divisions. The patient is asked to identify whether he or she perceives a sharp or dull sensation. Light touch can be tested by gently stroking the various facial sections with a cotton wisp or a twisted section of tissue paper. Here, the patient simply identifies when any sensation is felt. Temperature discrimination can be tested with the application of test tubes filled with hot or cold water to the same six facial regions (i.e., three regions on both the right and left sides of the face).

Facial Nerve (Cranial Nerve VII)

The facial nerve is a complex nerve having motor, sensory, and autonomic function. Its motor component supplies innervation to the facial muscles, the buccinator (cheek muscle), the scalp, the auricle of the ear, the stapedius muscle of the middle ear, the platysma (depresses the jaw), and the posterior belly of the digastric. Sensory innervation is provided to the soft palate, and taste sensation is also supplied to the anterior two-thirds of the tongue (salty and sweet tastes). Parasympathetic innervation is provided via branches of the facial nerve to the lacrimal and parotid glands.

The seventh nerve is responsible for the glabellar reflex, which is a manifestation of a trigeminal–facial nerve reflex system. Tapping of the glabellar region between the eyebrows will cause exaggerated eyelid closures and openings in cases of basal ganglia disease such as parkinsonism. Normally, relative suppression of this reflex can be maintained. The corneal reflex loop is also part of a trigeminal–facial nerve reflex. Here, touching the cornea causes reflex closure of the eyes. The seventh cranial nerve is also involved in the Bell's phenomenon reflex, whereby upward deviation of the eyes occurs in response to forced closure of the eyelids. Intactness of the reflex (which is not present in approximately 15% of normal subjects) indicates that absence of voluntary upward gaze is a result of a supranuclear lesion and that nuclear and infranuclear mechanisms are functioning properly.[2]

Motor function of the facial nerve is evaluated by having the patient perform a series of facial expressions. These include wrinkling the brow, raising the eyebrows, puffing out the cheeks, pursing the lips, smiling, and forcefully closing the eyes. Sensory function is generally tested by evaluating the patient's sense of taste. This is done by applying various substances to appropriate regions of the patient's tongue and asking the patient to identify the substance. The anterior portions of the tongue provide the tastes of saltiness and sweetness (Figure 19-2); therefore, substances such as salt and sugar are used. Vials of various substances should by stored in the office for this purpose. To apply a given material, an applicator stick is used to place it on one side of the tongue at a time and in the appropriate taste location (i.e., sweet substances more anterior than salty substances). The patient keeps the tongue protruded until he or she points to the name of the material on a card listing various possibilities (see Figure 19-1). Both sides of the tongue are tested, although separately, and the patient should be allowed to rinse the mouth with water between each trial.

The seventh nerve leaves its nucleus in the ventral part of the pons, then travels through the dorsal pontine region in the floor of the fourth ventricle and loops over the sixth nerve nucleus before exiting in the intermediate aspect of the pons. Because of the location of the facial nerve in its fascicular pathway through the pons, seventh nerve dysfunction is usually exhibited in the presence of sixth nerve nuclear disease.

Because it innervates the stapedius muscle of the middle ear, facial nerve palsy can yield hyperacusis on the affected side. In addition, because the seventh nerve provides sensory innervation to a small region including the external auditory canal and tympanic membrane, herpes zoster of the geniculate ganglion can result in vesicular eruptions involving the external auditory canal, neuralgia, and facial nerve palsy (Ramsay Hunt syndrome).

As with other cranial nerves, facial nerve palsies may result from many different types of CNS lesions, too numerous to list here. Of significant notoriety is the condition referred to as Bell's palsy, whereby an isolated, partial, or complete seventh nerve paresis occurs idiopathically. This relatively common neurologic disorder is seen not infrequently by optometrists because the initial symptoms are often related to corneal exposure from incomplete lid closure.

Acoustic Nerve (Cranial Nerve VIII)

The eighth cranial nerve has two main branches, the cochlear division and the vestibular division. The cochlear branch provides sensory information via end organs of the inner ear (cochlea). The vestibular division functions to control equilibrium. In addition to the structures of the inner ear (the vestibular labyrinth consisting of the semicircular canals, utricle, and saccule) and the vestibular nerve, the vestibular system as a whole consists of the four vestibular nuclei located within the medulla, the cerebellum, neck proprioception innervation through the reticular system, the coordination system of the medial longitudinal fasciculus, and some input from the basal ganglia (i.e., caudate nucleus, lentiform nucleus, amygdaloid body, and claustrum) and possibly, the substantia nigra.

Evaluation of the auditory component of the eighth cranial nerve actually begins immediately on conversing with the patient. Any particular difficulty the patient has hear-

ing the examiner's questions should be noted. However, there are a number of easily administered screening methods for this purpose as well. Commonly, the examiner covers one of the patient's ears and then whispers toward the other from a distance of 1–2 feet. The patient is asked to repeat the words he or she hears. Other methods include the use of a ticking watch or lightly rubbing the fingers together to produce subtle yet audible sounds. Obviously, more sophisticated methods for evaluating the level of hearing are available but are not practical for the routine optometric setting.

If a deficit is noted, differentiation between sensorineural (eighth nerve disease) and conductive (middle ear disease) hearing loss can be made with the Weber and Rinne tests. These tests use a 500- to 1000-Hz tuning fork to compare hearing via bone conduction with that by air conduction. The Weber test is performed by tapping the tines of the tuning fork and then holding its base in contact with the vertex of the skull along the midline (Figure 19-3A). Sound should normally be heard equally between the two ears. If middle ear disease is present (conductive hearing loss), then the sound will seem louder to the deaf ear. If eighth nerve disease is present (sensorineural hearing loss), the vibratory sound will seem louder to the normal ear.[5]

The Rinne test is performed by tapping the tines of the tuning fork and placing its base against the mastoid bone (Figure 19-3B). The examiner then times the interval until sound is no longer perceived by the patient. As soon as the sound disappears, the tines are placed 1–2 cm away from the auditory canal (Figure 19-3C) and the interval until sound is no longer heard is again measured. Normally, air-conducted sound should be heard for a time period twice as long as bone-conducted sound. If a conductive hearing loss is present, bone-conducted sound will be heard longer than or for a period equal to that for air-conducted sound. In the presence of neural hearing loss, air-conducted sound will be heard longer than but not twice as long as bone-conducted sound.[6]

Although vestibular function is not normally checked with routine cranial nerve screening, the vestibular end-organ system in the inner ear can be evaluated with simple tests. The "doll's head maneuver" checks the function of the utricles and saccules, which assist in the perception of the position in space of the head at rest and give one a sensation of being upright. The doll's head maneuver can be done on a comatose patient. If the head is moved quickly up or down, the eyes should remain fixed toward their original direction of gaze despite rotation of the head. In the presence of abnormal input from the vestibular system, instability of eye position may result during this test.

Caloric testing is a simple procedure that can be used to evaluate the intactness of the vestibular end organ,

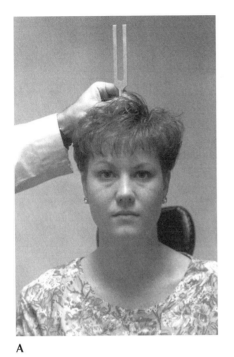
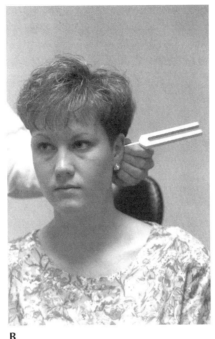
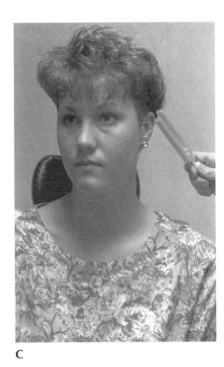

A   B   C

FIGURE 19-3

The Weber and Rinne tests to differentiate between sensorineural (eighth nerve disease) and conductive (middle ear disease) hearing loss. A. The Weber test is performed by placing the base of a vibrating tuning fork in contact with the skull at the midline. If the sound seems louder to the deaf ear, then middle ear disease is present; if the sound seems louder to the normal ear, then eighth nerve disease is present. B. The Rinne test is performed by initially placing the base of a vibrating tuning fork against the mastoid bone and timing the interval until sound is no longer perceived. C. Immediately upon disappearance of the sound, the tines are placed 1–2 cm away from the auditory canal. If middle ear disease is present, bone-conducted sound will be heard longer than or for a period equal to that for air-conducted sound. If eighth nerve disease is present, air-conducted sound will be heard longer than but not twice as long as bone-conducted sound.

vestibular nerve, and the pathways between the vestibular nuclei and the nuclei of the nerves supplying innervation to the extraocular muscles. During this test, caloric stimulation of the semicircular canals is performed by irrigating the external auditory canal with either cold or warm water. The resulting convection in the endolymph fluid affects the innervational impulses of the vestibular nerve, which then cause a conjugate lateral deviation of the eyes to one side or the other depending on the temperature of the water used. In a normal, alert patient a correctional conjugate saccade occurs back toward primary gaze position in an attempt to prevent constant deviation of the eyes to one side. In a comatose patient, however, the eyes remain deviated. Within a few minutes the eyes will gradually return to the midline. A useful mnemonic with which to remember the expected directional eye movement is COWS: Cold–Opposite; Warm–Same. Here, the directional indicators (opposite, same) refer to direction of the fast phase of the nystagmus. Therefore, when an alert

patient has his or her right ear irrigated with cold water, a nystagmus results with its fast phase toward the left side. A comatose individual will exhibit a tonic deviation of the eyes that remains to the right side (Table 19-4).

In an alert or comatose patient who has disease affecting cerebral cortical function without disease involving the oculovestibular reflex arc, expected responses should occur during caloric testing. Absent or diminished responses would occur when a lesion involves portions of the brain stem important in the oculovestibular reflex arc. Abnormal responses may also occur in situations of vestibular end organ or vestibular nerve disease, and with paresis of the nerves innervating the extraocular muscles.

To perform caloric testing, the patient is placed supine with the head elevated 30 degrees. The orientation is ideal because it places the horizontal semicircular canals in a vertical position. The alert patient should maintain the eyes in primary gaze. Before testing begins, the examiner should examine the external auditory canals for any

TABLE 19-4
Caloric Testing: COWS: Cold–Opposite; Warm–Same

Irrigation of external auditory canal with **cold** water causes:
1. Normal, alert patient: Jerk nystagmus with fast phase away from irrigated side.
2. Comatose patient with normal brain stem function: Sustained deviation of eyes toward irrigated side.
3. Comatose patient with unilateral brain stem disease: No deviation of the eyes when lesion side is irrigated. Sustained deviation of eyes toward the irrigated side when it is contralateral to the brain stem lesion.

blockage and the eardrums for evidence of perforation. Approximately 10 ml of ice-cold water is typically injected into the external auditory canal with a soft, plastic tube attached to a syringe. The tube should be inserted so that it remains a few millimeters from the eardrum. A kidney-shaped basin may be placed beneath the ear to catch the water that drains out. The eye movement response should occur within several seconds. Once the response has disappeared, the opposite ear is tested in a similar manner.

Vestibular disease often is associated with vertigo, oscillopsia, and nystagmus. If oscillopsia is present, then nystagmus will most probably be present as well. The presence of nystagmus should be noted in these cases, and it is important to include the notation of the direction of the fast phase, the amplitude of the nystagmus, any change in amplitude or fast phase with fields of gaze, and any change with cover of one eye or the other when the nystagmus is measured. Dampening of nystagmus on convergence should also be noted. End-organ disease usually yields pure horizontal or vertical nystagmus. Nystagmus with a rotatory or cyclotorsional component most probably has a CNS cause.

Evaluation of the vestibulocochlear system and particularly the vestibular system can be very important in evaluating the possibility of such diseases as Ménière's disease, vestibulobasilar disease, acoustic neuroma, and Cogan's interstitial keratitis. In all of these cases, vertigo with or without nystagmus may be present.

Glossopharyngeal Nerve (Cranial Nerve IX)

The ninth cranial nerve has multiple functions, providing motor innervation to the voluntary muscles of the pharyngeal region used for swallowing and phonation, sensory innervation to the nasopharynx and the posterior one-third of the tongue (bitter and sour tastes), and parasympathetic input to the salivary glands. It also provides the afferent loop of the gag reflex (the vagus nerve supplies the efferent loop) and sensory innervation to the soft palate. The carotid reflex also relies on partial innervation from the glossopharyngeal

nerve. The vagus nerve also has a contributory role. The carotid reflex is characterized by increased blood pressure and heart rate on external compression over the bifurcation of the common carotid artery. It is here that branches of the glossopharyngeal and vagus nerves form the carotid sinus plexuses.

The sensory function of taste innervated by the glossopharyngeal nerve can be evaluated at the same time that taste sensation is evaluated for the facial nerve. Bitter and sour substances are used, however, and their placement is within the posterior one-third of the tongue (see Figure 19-2). Because of the close relationship of the glossopharyngeal and vagus nerves in the innervational control of some structures, neuronal deficit of either of these nerves will result in similar dysfunction. Therefore, a few screening tests will simultaneously evaluate both nerves. For example, loss of the gag reflex may be found with lesions of the ninth or tenth cranial nerves. This is evaluated by lightly touching the back of the throat with a cotton-tipped applicator. During precipitation of the gag reflex, upward movement of the soft palate should occur as well as contraction of the pharyngeal muscles.

Lesions of either the glossopharyngeal or vagus nerves may affect movement of the soft palate. To evaluate this, the patient opens his or her mouth widely and says "Ah." The right and left sides of the soft palate should rise and fall symmetrically without resultant deviation of the uvula. In the presence of unequal innervation to both sides of the pharyngeal musculature, the uvula will point toward the stronger side (greater elevation of the soft palate on the right side results in deviation of the uvula to the right).

Motor function can also be evaluated by testing the patient's ability to swallow. As the patient sips from a glass of water, any particular difficulty should be noted. No retrograde flow of fluid should occur through the nose. Because the muscles of the pharynx are involved with speaking and other throat sounds, the examiner should also observe the patient for hoarseness or irregular speech. Lesions involving the ninth or tenth cranial nerves can result in difficult swallowing or speaking.

Vagus Nerve (Cranial Nerve X)

The vagus nerve is a very complex structure, providing innervation to many different structures of the body. Among those receiving sensory innervation are the larynx, pharynx, internal organs of the abdomen and thorax, posterior aspect of the auricle of the ear, and the posterior aspect of the external auditory meatus. Motor innervation from the vagus nerve goes to voluntary muscles of the larynx, pharynx, and the base of the tongue. Therefore, as discussed in the section on the glossopharyngeal nerve, the vagus nerve plays a role in speaking and swallowing. The vagus also supplies autonomic parasympathetic innervation to abdominal and thoracic organs. It is therefore critical for a number of involuntary functions of the digestive system (secretion of digestive enzymes, peristalsis), heart, bronchi, and lungs. As discussed in the preceding section, the vagus nerve also participates in the gag and carotid reflexes. Screening methods for the tenth cranial nerve were also reviewed in the section on the glossopharyngeal nerve because of the difficulty in separating out some of the ninth and tenth cranial nerve functions. Similar evaluation includes testing the gag reflex, observation of the soft palate and uvular deviation, and noticing any difficulty with swallowing or speaking (hoarseness, nasal quality).

Spinal Accessory Nerve (Cranial Nerve XI)

The eleventh cranial nerve provides motor innervation only. The nerve is divided into two parts, a cranial portion and a spinal portion. The cranial segment originates from four or five rootlets arising from the medulla, and the spinal segment comes from anterior gray column nuclei situated as low as the fifth cervical segment. In addition to the glossopharyngeal and vagus nerves, the cranial portion of the spinal accessory nerve also provides some motor input to muscles necessary for speech and swallowing. The spinal portion of the eleventh cranial nerve sends motor axonal fibers to the trapezius and sternocleidomastoid muscles.

Isolated screening of the spinal accessory nerve is typically done through evaluation of trapezoidal and sternocleidomastoidal muscular function. To test their strength, the examiner provides resistance as the patient attempts to shrug the shoulders, and then as the patient rotates the head to the right or left as if to look to either side (Figure 19-4).

Hypoglossal Nerve (Cranial Nerve XII)

The hypoglossal nerve provides purely motor function to muscles of the tongue and to strap muscles of the neck. Screening methods normally concentrate on the appearance and function of the tongue. To begin, the patient protrudes the tongue straight outward. Deviation can indicate relative weakness of the muscles on one side. Stronger muscles will push the tongue away from their direction; therefore, the tongue will point toward the affected side in instances of hypoglossal nerve palsies. Other actions used to evaluate muscular function include actively pointing the tongue from one side to the other and curling it upward and downward. Strength can be evaluated by externally palpating the resistance encountered as the patient force-

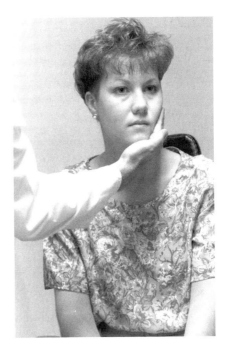

FIGURE 19-4

One method to screen for spinal accessory nerve (cranial nerve XI) function is to evaluate sternocleidomastoid muscular strength. The examiner provides resistance as the patient attempts to rotate the head to either side.

fully presses the tongue against either inside cheek wall. Careful attention to tongue-induced speech abnormalities should also be given by listening for difficulty in pronouncing lingual sounds needed for words containing the letters l, t, d, or n. Simple examination for gross changes in the tongue's appearance such as atrophy or fasciculation can also help identify paretic situations.

BRAIN STEM CONSIDERATIONS

When evaluating subcortical CNS lesions of the oculomotor system, it is important to remember the general association of the cranial nerves with the area of the brain stem.[7] The rule of fours may be used, meaning there are three groups, each having four groups of cranial nerves associated with the major parts of the brain stem. Beginning with the medulla are cranial nerves IX, X, XI, and XII, and their nuclei, which are placed within this area. Cranial nerves V, VI, VII, and VIII have their nuclei within the pontine area. Cranial nerves III and IV have their nuclei within the mid-brain area, cranial nerve I is associated with the limbic system directly, and cranial nerve II is associated with the thalamus through the lateral geniculate body.

With subcortical lesions of the CNS, a potpourri of clinical signs are seen, usually with alternating neurologic deficits (both sides of the body may be involved in varying ways).

Medulla Lesions

Large lesions of the basal part of the medulla produce cranial nerve palsies on the ipsilateral side with contralateral hemiplegia. This occurs because of involvement of the predecussated pyramids of the medulla, which carry cortical spinal fibers to the body. The ipsilateral cranial nerve nuclei of IX, X, XI, and XII may be directly involved; therefore, ipsilateral palsies of the cranial nerves are noted.

Middle involvement of the medulla not only may cause cranial nerve palsies and contralateral hemiplegia but may also involve the lateral spinal thalamic tract and nucleus ambiguus. The lateral spinal thalamic tract is postdecussated; therefore, contralateral hemiparesis may occur. The nucleus ambiguus is involved in motor innervation of cranial nerves IX and X, and disease may cause difficulty in swallowing and phonation.

Upper medulla lesions, which may result from occlusion of the posterior inferior cerebellar artery, cause involvement of the solitary nucleus, the inferior cerebral peduncle, and the vestibular nuclei (which may result in nystagmus). Alternating analgesia (or hemiparesis) can be associated with involvement of the medial lemniscus, which contains the decussated fibers of the dorsal white column after synapse at the nucleus gracilis and nucleus cuneatus. The inferior cerebellar peduncle may also be involved, which may be associated with nystagmus as well as nonpyramidal motor insufficiency.

To summarize, disease of the medulla typically causes cranial nerve palsies of the nuclear type involving nerves IX, X, XI, and XII, possible contralateral hemiparesis, reduced taste sensation due to solitary nucleus involvement, nystagmus, and nonpyramidal motor deficit.

Pontine Lesions

Inferior pontine compression or infarction can cause alternating abducens palsy where esotropia associated with abducens palsy on the ipsilateral side is associated with contralateral hemiplegia and with involvement of corticospinal fibers. Further compression of the inferior pons within this area can cause nucleus involvement of cranial nerve VII, causing complete facial nerve palsy that is referred to as Millard-Gubler's syndrome. Continued compression within the area more medially under the fourth ventricle can yield involvement of the medial longitudinal fasciculus, which then presents with internuclear ophthalmoplegia on the contralateral side, causing the syndrome of Foville.

Lesions within the cerebellopontine angle can cause involvement of cranial nerves V, VII, and VIII, resulting in sensory dysfunction, tinnitus, vertigo, hearing loss, and facial palsy on the ipsilateral side. Acoustic neuromas are frequent lesions within this area.

Involvement of the middle pontine area causes alternating trigeminal palsy as a result of involvement of the ipsilateral spinal nucleus of the trigeminal nerve, yielding ipsilateral somatosensory deficit of the face and possible motor deficit of the muscles of mastication on the ipsilateral side if the motor nucleus of the trigeminal nerve is involved. Contralateral palsy of the body and the lower cranial nerves are noted because of involvement of the corticobulbar and corticospinal fibers before decussation.

To summarize, involvement of the pontine area yields palsies of cranial nerves V, VI, and VII with contralateral body and lower brain stem paresis. External lesions of the cerebellopontine angle yield palsies of cranial nerves V, VII, and VIII.

Midbrain Lesions

Large lesions involving the basal membrane can produce a combination of third nerve palsy with pupillary involvement and contralateral hemiplegia. Contralateral inferior brain stem involvement may also be noted in those cranial nerves that have motor function. This is called Weber's syndrome.

Involvement of the tegmentum of the midbrain produces Benedikt's syndrome. Here, the medial lemniscus is involved as well as cranial nerve III and the superior cerebellar peduncle. The result is a complete third nerve palsy with a contralateral loss of proprioception and vertigo.

Involvement of the dorsal area of the midbrain in the superior colliculus area causes light-near dissociation of the pupil and superior gaze palsy (Parinaud's syndrome). The superior gaze palsy is most likely associated with involvement of the rostral medial longitudinal fasciculus and associated vertical eye movement centers within the midbrain.

To summarize, midbrain lesions cause third nerve palsies with pupillary involvement, contralateral hemiplegia, contralateral proprioceptive disorders, and vertigo. The very dorsal part of the midbrain can cause light-near dissociation with superior gaze palsies.

SENSORY EVALUATION

The sensory system is quite extensive and includes many more nerves than those contributed by the cranial nerves.

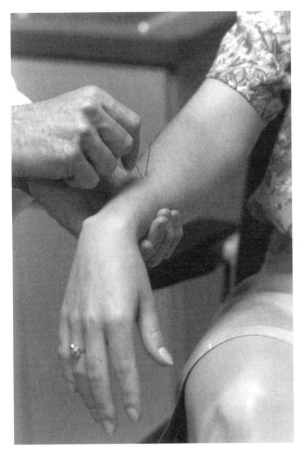 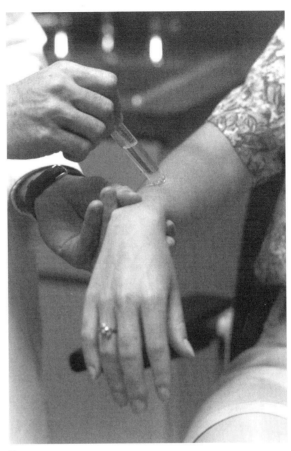

A   B

FIGURE 19-5

Methods for evaluating sensory dysfunction include testing for pain and temperature sensation. A. Pain sensation can be evaluated by alternately touching areas of the body with the sharp and dull ends of a safety pin. With the eyes closed, the patient should correctly identify the "sharp" or "dull" stimulus. B. Temperature sensation can be tested by alternately touching the body with test tubes filled with hot and cold water.

In addition to those discussed with cranial nerve evaluation, there are other simple screening methods that can help identify neurologic disease. Sensory dysfunction can result from almost any lesion involving the cerebrum, brain stem, or spinal column.

In addition to facial sensation, which is evaluated during cranial nerve testing, additional areas that may be evaluated include the lower arms, hands, abdomen, lower legs, and feet. Included among the sensory functions that can be tested are temperature, light touch, pain, deep pressure, and vibration. Sensory functions that require greater levels of interpretation include two-point discrimination, point location, the extinction phenomenon, stereognosis (the ability to identify objects by feel), and graphesthesia (the ability to identify figures drawn on the skin by feel). Dysfunction with these latter functions may indicate

abnormality within the sensory cortex or posterior columns of the spinal cord. When testing sensory function, it is helpful to compare symmetric locations on both sides of the body. The patient's eyes are closed during each of these tests.

In a manner similar to that for sensory screening described for cranial nerve V, temperature sensation can be evaluated by alternately touching the skin with test tubes filled with hot or cold water, pain sensation can be evaluated with alternate application of the sharp and dull parts of a safety pin, and light touch sensation can be tested with a cotton wisp or twisted piece of tissue paper (Figure 19-5). Deep pressure sensation may be evaluated by firmly squeezing the calf, biceps, and trapezius muscles. Mild discomfort should be acknowledged. Temperature and deep pressure are usually not tested unless superficial pain sensation appears defective, as demonstrated with the sharp point of the safety pin. Vibration sense is tested by placing the base of a tuning fork on bony prominences at several locations throughout the body (e.g., elbow, ankle, finger joints).

Two-point discrimination is tested by lightly placing the tips of two safety pins or similar objects at various locations on the skin. The distance between the instruments is gradually closed until two points can no longer be discriminated. Occasionally, only one point can be used to mix the responses. Distances will vary from one part of the body to another but should be symmetric between the two sides.

Point location is performed by simply touching the skin at various spots and asking the patient to identify the particular site. The extinction phenomenon is performed by simultaneously touching corresponding sensory locations on each side of the body with a sharp instrument. The patient identifies the number and location of the areas touched. Both should be felt. This technique, whereby variations are also applied to the testing of special sensory systems of vision and hearing, may enhance relative sensory loss on one side of the body.

Graphesthesia is tested by drawing a letter or number on various potions of the body with a blunt instrument. The patient should identify the character (Figure 19-6). Stereognosis is evaluated by placing a familiar object such as a coin in the patient's hand and asking the patient to identify it.

MOTOR FUNCTION

The motor system is highly complex, combining input from many different parts of the peripheral and central nervous systems. Contributing to the final common pathway of efferent impulses extending from the spinal cord to the neuromuscular junction are various neuronal systems within the brain. The pyramidal system consists of motor impulses originating from nuclei located within the cerebral cortex; the extrapyramidal system is composed of nuclei located within the basal ganglia, which function in a number of complex processes such as proprioception; and the cerebellar system aids in the coordination of muscular movements. As with other components of the neurologic examination, a thorough examination of the motor system is not practical from an optometric standpoint; nevertheless, there are some basic screening tests that may aid in the identification of nervous system disease. As with other screening techniques, absence of a recognizable abnormality does not absolutely exclude serious disease.

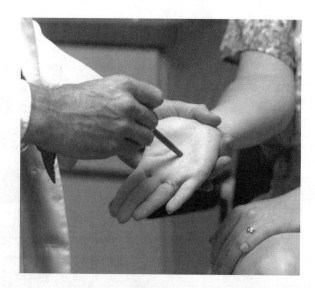

FIGURE 19-6
Graphesthesia is tested by drawing a character such as a letter or number on the palm of a patient's hand and then asking the patient to identify the character.

Evaluation of the motor system may actually begin immediately on interaction with the patient. The patient should be observed for gait abnormalities, unusual posture, or evidence of abnormal movements. Any sign of muscular wasting, fasciculations, or hypertrophy also should be noted. Lower motor neuron lesions (brain stem to neuromuscular junction) are generally manifested by muscle flaccidity and atrophy.[5] In addition, hyporeflexia or areflexia and fasciculations may be present. CNS lesions resulting in lower motor neuron disease usually occur ipsilateral to the side exhibiting muscular weakness and dysfunction; however, upper motor neuron disease (cerebral cortex to brain stem) is generally manifested by contralateral muscular dysfunction, muscular spasticity, and hyperreflexia.[5] Muscular atrophy is usually minimal.

To screen for motor weakness, it is not practical to provide a detailed examination of all muscular groups. Rather, a few basic screening tests can be performed. It should be kept in mind that a loss of strength or power may be manifested by either weakness of a movement (upper motor neuron disease) or by weakness of one or more muscles (lower motor neuron disease). Depending on early examination results, concentration could be directed toward one or the other, with detailed analysis as necessary. When quantifying muscular strength, a common grading scale is as follows[1]:

5: Normal strength
4: Full movement, but contraction can be overcome by examiner

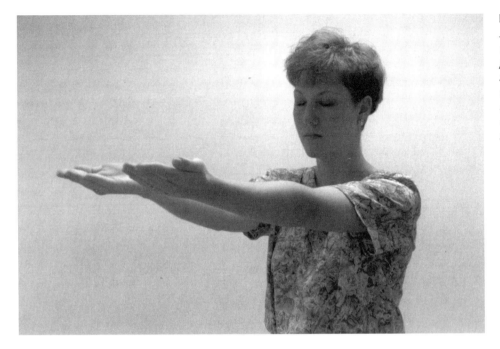

FIGURE 19-7
A method of screening for motor weakness consists of having the patient hold the arms outstretched and parallel to the ground with the palms facing upward (with the eyes closed). The patient is observed for any tendency of an arm to droop or rotate.

3: Full movement against gravity, but not against added resistance
2: Movement only without gravity in opposition
1: Only slight movement possible
0: No movement

There are several basic screening techniques. Have the patient hold the arms outstretched and parallel to the ground with the palms facing upward for 30 seconds (Figure 19-7). The eyes should be closed. Look for any tendency of an arm to droop or rotate. By having the patient lower the arms and then raise them again simultaneously, unilateral weakness may be exhibited by asymmetry of motion. Difficulty with these actions can be indicative of variable abnormality including hemiparesis of central origin, cerebellar disease, or weakness of peripheral origin. To screen for leg weakness, the patient lies supine and then lifts both legs simultaneously. Any asymmetry is noted. These postural tests may show abnormal results, despite normal findings with direct strength testing.

Direct strength testing is done by having the patient perform a number of isolated movements with the examiner providing an opposite resistance. Arm and shoulder, hand and wrist, and lower-extremity strength can be evaluated via a number of different techniques.

Coordination and Fine Motor Control

Smooth and accurate movements require input from several components of the motor system. Incoordina-tion is relatively easy to detect and can be very helpful in the identification of neurologic disease. Poor performance with the following tests can be indicative of cerebellar disease.

Rapid Alternating Movements

Have the seated patient rapidly pat the superior aspect of the thighs with the palm and back of the hands alternatively (Figure 19-8A). Both hands should be relatively symmetric in their movements, although the nondominant side is often a little slower and less controlled. Another technique is to have the patient rapidly touch each finger in succession to the thumb (Figure 19-8B). Each hand is tested separately. The speed should be gradually increased with both of these testing methods. Various lesions of the nervous system can result in slow, awkward movements.

Finger-to-Nose Test

In the finger-to-nose test, the patient alternately touches the index fingers to the nose and then to the examiner's finger, which is held about 2 feet in front of the patient. The technique is performed one arm at a time. Another method is to have the patient alternately touch the nose with the index fingers of the right and left hands. The patient's eyes are closed, and each arm is outstretched to either side after the nose is touched (Figure 19-8C). Irregular, jerky movements, as well as an overshooting (past-pointing) commonly occur with cerebellar disease.

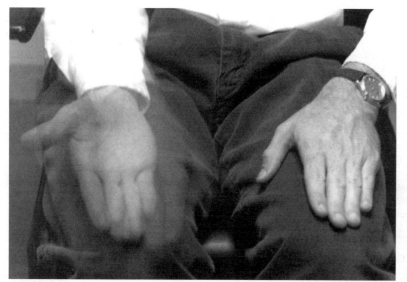
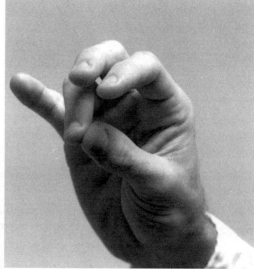

A   B

FIGURE 19-8
Screening coordination and fine motor control. Poor performance may be indicative of cerebellar disease. A, B. Performance of rapid alternating movements. C. Finger-to-nose test.

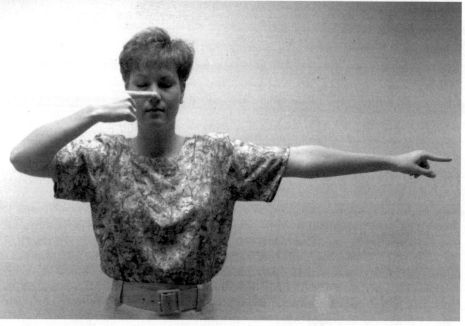

C

Observation of Gait

Have the patient walk across the examining room barefooted, and watch for any abnormality of gait and balance. Normally the gait will be smooth and regular. Notice any swaying, shuffling, asymmetry of step between each leg, or other anomalous movement. The arms should swing rhythmically as well. To increase difficulty, have the patient walk around a chair or similar object. Heel-to-toe walking can also be helpful to enhance an abnormality.

Romberg Test

The Romberg test is performed with the patient standing erect with the feet together and arms to the side. The patient is then asked to close his or her eyes. The examiner observes the patient carefully for loss of balance. The examiner should be prepared to catch the patient in case he or she begins to fall. The Romberg test is positive when the patient can maintain balance with the eyes open, but not with them closed. A positive test result is indicative of proprioceptive dysfunction.[8] Although well known,

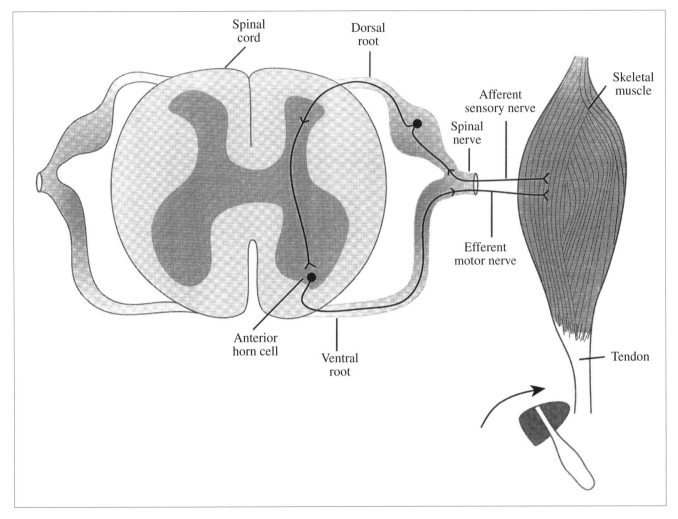

FIGURE 19-9

Schematic representation of the reflex arc. On tapping of the muscle tendon, muscle stretch receptors send an impulse through sensory fibers of the peripheral nerve to the spinal nerve, through the dorsal root nerve, and then on to synapse with motor neurons located within the anterior horns of the spinal column or on motor nuclei of the lower brain stem. Efferent impulses travel through the ventral root and spinal nerve to the motor neuron, which illicits contracture of the associated muscle.

the test is not extremely sensitive.[1] Vestibular or cerebellar disease may cause unsteady posture even with the eyes open, whereas visual input is better able to suppress a proprioceptive deficit.[1]

Reflexes

The sudden stretching of a muscle results in a reflexive contraction because of a simple reflex arc existing between the muscle and the CNS. The reflex is involuntary and therefore lends itself to pure objective evaluation. The afferent pathway of the arc extends from the muscle to cell bodies located within the dorsal root ganglia (Figure 19-9). Fibers from these cells then extend to synapse on motor neurons located within the anterior horns of the spinal column or on lower brain stem motor nuclei. The efferent aspect of the arc consists of the motor neuron extending to innervate skeletal muscle. The presence of the stretch reflex depends on the integrity of this pathway, and characteristics of the reflex response may yield important information relative to neurologic disease.

Clinically, the reflex response is elicited via the tapping of various muscle tendons of the body with a reflex hammer. Sudden stretching of the tendon produces a corresponding stretch to its muscle, and thus elicits the reflex response. The amplitudes of responses can vary consid-

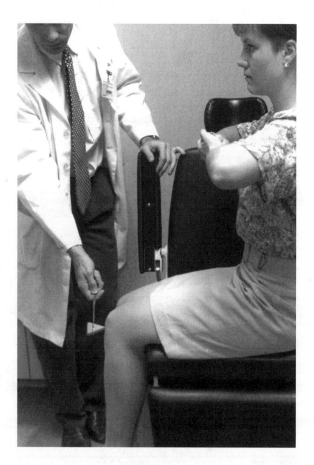

FIGURE 19-10

Isometric muscular contraction in one part of the body can enhance conduction within the reflex arc elsewhere in the body. Jendrassik's maneuver consists of interlocking the hands and pulling in opposite directions while the reflexes of the lower extremities (e.g., the patellar reflex) are tested.

erably from person to person, and their interpretation requires some experience by the examiner. Whereas the precipitation of the reflex response indicates the integrity of the reflex arc, its absence does not necessarily indicate an interrupted arc. There are a number of factors, normal and abnormal, that may suppress the reflex response. When evaluating the reflex response the following grading system is commonly used[1,2,5]:

4+: Very brisk, hyperactive response. Evidence of disease and associated with clonus.

3+: Brisk response, slightly greater than normal. Possibly indicative of disease.

2+: Normal, expected response.

1+: Reduced response, barely present.

  0: No response, possibly indicative of disease.

TABLE 19-5

Superficial and Deep Tendon Reflexes [1,5,8]

	*Spinal Level**	*Normal Response*
Superficial reflexes		
Abdominal	T-7 through T-12	Umbilicus moves toward area of stimulation
Cremasteric	L-1	Scrotum elevates on side of stimulation
Plantar	S-1, S-2	Big toe moves downward (abnormal response: big toe moves upward—Babinski's sign)
Deep tendon reflexes		
Biceps	C-5, C-6	Flexion of the elbow
Brachioradialis	C-5, C-6	Pronation of the forearm and flexion of the elbow
Triceps	C-6, C-7, C-8	Extension of the elbow
Patellar	L-2, L-3, L-4	Extension of the knee
Achilles	S-1	Flexion of the foot

*Sometimes variable depending on source.

Source: Data from RL Rodnitzky. Van Allen's Pictorial Manual of Neurologic Tests (3rd ed). Chicago: Year Book, 1988; HM Seidel, JW Ball, JE Dains, GW Benedict. Mosby's Guide to Physical Examination. St. Louis: Mosby, 1987; WEM Pryse-Phillips, TJ Murray. Essential Neurology (4th ed). New York: Medical Examination, 1991.

If no response is obtained during reflex testing, response reinforcement can be elicited with Jendrassik's maneuver. This consists of the patient interlocking the fingers of each hand and then pulling in opposite directions while reflexes of the lower extremities are tested (Figure 19-10). It is best to strike the tendon as soon as the isometric muscle contraction is applied. If no reflex is present even during this maneuver, then disease is likely.

As shown by the reflex grading scheme, increased responses (hyperreflexia) are potentially significant for disease, as is a diminished response (hyporeflexia or areflexia). Hyporeflexia or areflexia typically indicate lower motor neuron disease, and hyperreflexia usually denotes upper motor neuron lesions.

Reflexes are categorized as two types: superficial and deep tendon (Table 19-5). Superficial reflexes are mediated through a spinal arc, as are deep tendon reflexes; however, their precipitation also depends on the higher located corticospinal tract. They are based on cutaneous stimulation rather than muscle stretch. Superficial reflexes include the abdominal, cremasteric, plantar, and gluteal reflexes. Well known is the application of the plantar reflex for the evaluation of disease of the pyramidal tract. Testing this reflex is performed by stroking the lateral aspect of the foot all the way from the heel to the ball, then curv-

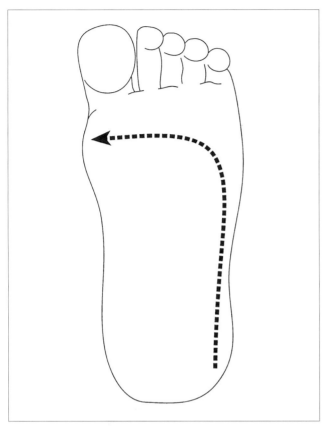

FIGURE 19-11
The plantar reflex is elicited by stroking the bottom of the foot as shown. Plantar flexion should normally occur. Babinski's sign, evidence of pyramidal tract disease, is present when dorsiflexion of the big toe occurs.

ing medially to also stroke the entire side-to-side dimension of the ball of the foot (Figure 19-11). Normally, plantar flexion should occur. Babinski's sign, which is evidence of pyramidal tract disease, is considered present when dorsiflexion of the big toe occurs. Babinski's sign is considered normal, however, when it is present in children younger than 2 years of age. Deep tendon reflexes are typically used for routine screening within the optometric setting. Those typically tested include the biceps, brachioradialis, triceps, patellar (knee), and Achilles (ankle) reflexes (Figure 19-12).

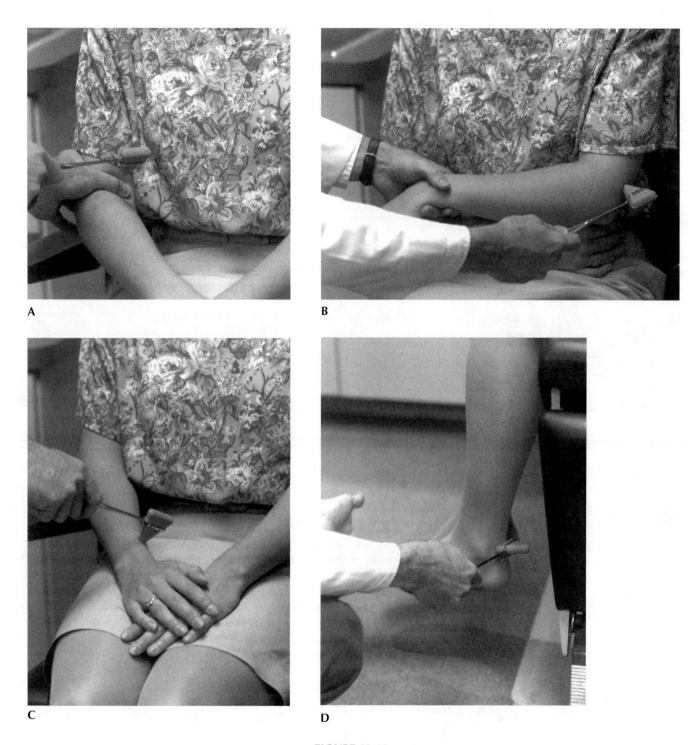

A

B

C

D

FIGURE 19-12
Deep tendon reflex testing. A. Biceps. B. Triceps. C. Brachioradialis. D. Achilles.

REFERENCES

1. Rodnitzky RL. Van Allen's Pictorial Manual of Neurologic Tests (3rd ed). Chicago: Year Book, 1988.
2. Adams, RD, Victor M. Principles of Neurology (5th ed). New York: McGraw-Hill, 1993.
3. Walsh TJ. Neuro-ophthalmology: Clinical Signs and Symptoms (3rd ed). Philadelphia: Lea & Febiger, 1992.
4. Miller NR. Walsh and Hoyt's Clinical Neuro-Ophthalmology (4th ed, Vol II). Baltimore: Williams & Wilkins, 1985.
5. Seidel HM, Ball JW, Dains JE, Benedict GW. Mosby's Guide to Physical Examination. St. Louis: Mosby, 1987.
6. Bates B, Hoekelman RA. A Guide to Physical Examination (2nd ed). Philadelphia: Lippincott, 1979.
7. Manter JT. Essentials of Clinical Neuroanatomy and Neurophysiology. Philadelphia: FA Davis, 1961.
8. Pryse-Phillips WEM, Murray TJ. Essential Neurology (4th ed). New York: Medical Examination, 1991.

20

Sphygmomanometry

T. MICHAEL GOEN AND JACK E. TERRY

The measurement of systemic blood pressure is an extremely useful procedure in the detection of disease. For eye care practitioners, it is not only helpful in the evaluation of pathologic processes affecting the eye, but routine measurement also provides an avenue to evaluate a significant segment of the population who might not otherwise be examined in this regard. Hypertension affects at least 58 million Americans,[1] many of whom are unaware of their condition. If hypertension is diagnosed early, the benefits of treatment in the reduction of attendant morbidity and mortality are clearly evident.[2,3]

Sphygmomanometry is an established and accepted procedure used to measure blood pressure. It is an inexpensive test, yielding efficient and diagnostically productive results.[4] In light of the prevalence of systemic hypertension and the relative ease and accuracy of identifying this disorder, an optometrist who performs sphygmomanometry on a routine basis is in a position to detect systemic hypertension at a relatively early stage.

BLOOD PRESSURE

Systemic arterial blood pressure (BP) represents a force against the wall of blood vessels resulting from cardiac output and total peripheral (vascular) resistance. *Cardiac output* is calculated as the *pulse rate* multiplied by the *stroke volume* (blood pumped by each ventricle per beat). The resulting product yields the blood volume pumped per minute, or blood flow.[5,6]

Figure 20-1 illustrates the forces influencing BP. The force driving blood through a vessel is represented by a piston acting as the heart. With each stroke of the piston, a new supply of blood (an increased volume) is thrust into the vessel. The lengths of the horizontal arrows denote the relative quantities of blood flowing into and out of

the artery; the incoming flow (left arrow) is larger than the outgoing flow (right arrow) during systole. This produces a higher pressure within the vessel, represented by the larger vertical arrows at point *S* (systole). An expansion of the elastic artery occurs because of the increased volume. With the vessel distended and the piston between strokes, the artery recoils. In doing so, the pressure is maintained at a relatively high level between strokes of the pump, represented at point *D* (diastole) with the smaller arrows. Noninvasive manometers measure the pressure in the arteries at stages *D* and *S*. If one could look farther along the arterial tree, the vessels would become narrowed until eventually the arterioles would be producing approximately 50% of the total peripheral resistance because of their smaller (and variable) diameters.

Systole is the BP in the arteries at the height of pulsation from the contraction of the heart as blood is forced out through the vessels. It is normally about 120 mm Hg in a young adult. Diastole is the pressure in the arteries during cardiac relaxation after the blood has been pushed out of the heart and is maintained by the elastic recoil of the large arteries. It is about 80 mm Hg in a young adult. The two measurements of BP are always reported together, the systolic pressure first, then the diastolic pressure. For example, a normal BP would be recorded as 120/80. The difference between the systolic and the diastolic pressure is called the *pulse pressure.*

MEASUREMENT OF BLOOD PRESSURE

Sphygmomanometer

Clinically, BP is routinely determined indirectly by means of a sphygmomanometer. Mercury and aneroid sphygmomanometers involve the use of a rubber compression

FIGURE 20-1

Schematic representation of the forces influencing blood pressure. The piston represents the heart, which forces blood through an artery. During systole, more blood is forced into the artery (large horizontal arrow) than is forced out (smaller horizontal arrow). This produces a higher pressure in the artery (S = systole), which causes an expansion of the vessel (longer vertical and oblique arrows). Between strokes the distended artery recoils, thus maintaining a relatively high arterial pressure (D = diastole). (Reprinted with permission from JE Terry. The measurement of systemic arterial blood pressure. J Am Optom Assoc 1976;47:571–7.)

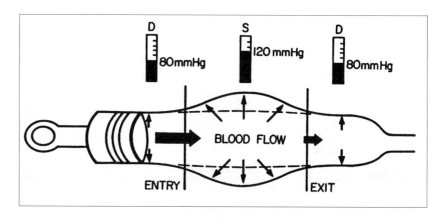

bag (bladder) in an unyielding cuff, which is wrapped around the upper arm and can be inflated (and deflated) in controlled steps sufficient to shut off blood flow to the limb. Other necessary items are an inflating bulb, a manometer gauge for measuring the pressure in the cuff, and a controlling exhaust valve. This system does not permit continuous measurement of BP, but the maximum (systolic) and minimum (diastolic) values can be obtained over the testing interval.

Indirect sphygmomanometry has been found to be most accurate when the cuff width is approximately 40% of the limb circumference,[7] or 12–14 cm in normal-sized adults.[8-10] When a standard-size cuff is used on a very large muscular or obese arm, measurements may be erroneously high because the air pressure applied within the cuff must be higher to overcome a greater tissue resistance and to impede blood flow sufficiently in the artery. Conversely, measurements may be underestimated if the standard-size cuff is used on children or adults with unusually thin arms. According to a survey conducted in 1989, only 20% of optometrists who have BP measuring equipment have more than one cuff size.[7]

Burch and Shewey[9] showed (Figure 20-2) that, as cuff width is increased, mean systolic and diastolic pressures decrease until a width of about 12 cm is reached. No marked effect of the bladder length on BP levels was found. Standard arm cuffs used clinically contain a rubber bladder 23 cm long and 12.0–12.5 cm wide and afford accurate indirect BP determinations in the adult population.

A stethoscope is required for listening to the BP sounds unless an electronic sphygmomanometer is used. Most stethoscopes consist of two heads: a larger, flat diaphragm, which is more effective in magnifying high-pitched sounds; and a smaller, concave bell, which is more effective in detecting low-pitched sounds. The Amer-

ican Heart Association[11] has recommended auscultation with the bell surface; however, the flat diaphragm is still used extensively in clinical practice. Use of the bell, as opposed to the diaphragm, results in a higher systolic measurement.[11,12]

Three types of manometers (i.e., the automatic, mercury, and aneroid) are commonly used for the noninvasive measurement of BP (Figure 20-3). The aneroid sphygmomanometer makes use of a metal bellows, which elongates with the application of pressure. A gear sector transmits this motion to the indicator needle.

Automatic sphygmomanometers use the same basic measuring principles as the aneroid and mercury manometers; however, they also contain a small-diameter microphone mounted inside the cuff. The function of the microphone is, of course, to register the systolic and diastolic pulsations in place of the examiner's stethoscope. Most devices provide a digital read-out of the BP after measurement.

An advantage of the automatic sphygmomanometer is that observer error and bias are reduced. The mercury and aneroid methods require a simultaneous coupling of hearing and sight to obtain the BP measurement. Because the microphone is mounted in the cuff, superior acoustical coupling is achieved.[13] Little skill is necessary when using an automatic sphygmomanometer and therefore an automatic sphygmomanometer offers the advantage of self-administration.

Several studies yielding varied results have been conducted to determine the reliability of automatic sphygmomanometers.[14-20] Some automatic devices have been found to be very reliable, whereas others over- or underestimate systolic and diastolic readings. Other disadvantages of the automatic sphygmomanometer are higher cost and the potential need for maintenance or frequent calibration.

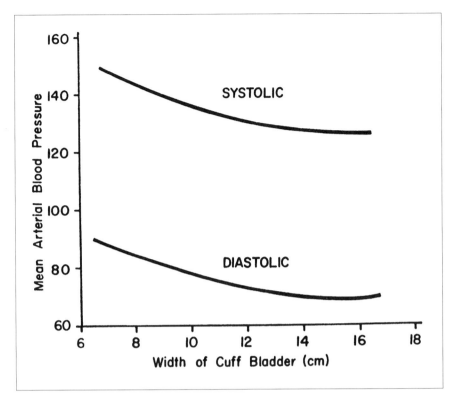

FIGURE 20-2
The relationship of the width of the cuff bladder to mean blood pressure. As the width of the cuff bladder is increased, measured blood pressure will be lower. (Modified from GE Burch, L Shewey. Sphygmomanometric cuff size and blood pressure recordings. JAMA 1973;225:1215–8.)

Technique

The most common site for measuring BP is over the brachial artery, which can be palpated in the antecubital fossa. The left arm is preferred because its arteries are located anatomically closer to the aorta as it leaves the heart. To find the pulse, the examiner's middle three fingers are placed on the patient's antecubital fossa and light pressure is applied until the rhythmic expansion of the artery can be felt. The approximate position of the brachial artery is shown in Figure 20-4.

The approximate center of the inflatable bladder is aligned with the brachial artery so that the lower margin is about 2.5 cm above the elbow. Next, the cuff is wrapped smoothly and firmly around the upper arm of the patient. The exhaust valve on the manometer must be closed so the bag can be inflated.

The patient's arm and its muscles should be relaxed and supported at the level of the heart on a firm surface. Once again, the brachial artery is located, and the stethoscope positioned over it. If an automatic device is being used, it is necessary to align the microphone with the artery. At this point, with an automatic sphygmomanometer, the examiner should simply follow the directions on how to measure the BP for that particular device. For the mercury and aneroid sphygmomanometers, the stethoscope must not touch clothing or the pressure cuff. Its bell should

be applied snugly with no space between skin and stethoscope, but not too firmly, because heavy pressure will distort the artery and produce extraneous sounds.

The manometer gauge is held in a position that allows the examiner to see it directly. The cuff is then rapidly inflated by pumping the rubber bulb until no sounds can be heard through the stethoscope, or about 30 mm Hg above the point at which the brachial pulse disappears. At this point the inflated cuff acts as a tourniquet, thereby collapsing the brachial artery and blocking its blood flow (Figure 20-5A).

The air from the cuff is gradually released (2–3 mm Hg/second) by opening the exhaust valve screw with the forefinger and thumb, observing at the same time the gauge on the manometer. The examiner should note the exact point on the gauge at which the first regular, soft thumping sounds begin. This reading is the systolic pressure. Blood begins to flow at a very high velocity at this point because of the small vessel opening and large pressure gradient. As the cuff pressure is lowered further, the duration of blood flow through the artery per cycle of heart contraction becomes longer (Figure 20-5B and C). The tapping sounds become louder as the cuff pressure is lowered still further. While the cuff continues to deflate, the sounds continue to change. They will gradually reduce in intensity, and the loud, regular thumping

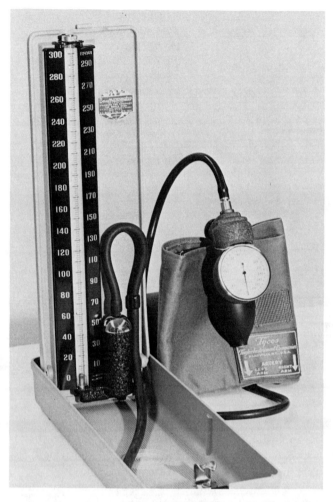

FIGURE 20-3

The mercury manometer (left) and the aneroid manometer (right) are both commonly used to measure systemic blood pressure. (Reprinted with permission from JE Terry. The measurement of systemic arterial blood pressure. J Am Optom Assoc 1976; 47:571–7.)

TABLE 20-1

Auditory Phases of Sphygmomanometry

Phase I	Systolic: First appearance of soft regular tapping sounds.
Phase II	Murmur of swishing quality is heard.
Phase III	Sounds are crisper and increasing in intensity.
Phase IV	Distinct, abrupt *muffling* of sounds so that a soft, blowing quality is heard.
Phase V	Diastolic: Sounds disappear completely.

Source: Reprinted with permission from JE Terry. The measurement of systemic arterial blood pressure. J Am Optom Assoc 1976;47:571–7.

ment procedures as a sequence of five phases, with phase I representing the systolic pressure, phase IV representing muffling, and phase V representing the complete disappearance of all sounds or the diastolic pressure.[22]

There are several methods available to enhance Korotkoff's sounds, allowing for a more accurate BP reading. Korotkoff's sounds will be longer and louder as the pressure differential between the blood under the cuff and that in the distal vessels below the cuff is increased. As the cuff is being inflated, the venous return is impeded long before the arterial input. Hence, if inflation is slow, blood is trapped in the forearm with each cardiac contraction and the pressure differential is lessened. Rapid inflation is necessary to decrease the amount of blood in the forearm and therefore obtain louder sounds.

Another means of augmenting sounds is to have the patient raise the arm for several seconds to enhance the drainage of venous blood before inflating the cuff. The cuff is inflated while the arm is elevated. The arm is then returned to the normal heart-level position for measurement of BP.

In a third procedure, vasodilation of the vessels in the forearm and hand can be obtained by instructing the patient to open and close the fist rapidly eight to ten times after the cuff is inflated above the systolic level. This produces an increase in the blood-holding capacity of the forearm. Any one or all three of these procedures may be used with benefit in individual cases.

In some patients, Korotkoff's sounds over the brachial artery may disappear as cuff pressure is decreased and then reappear at a lower level. This early disappearance of sounds (second phase) is called an *auscultatory gap* and can lead to confusion during measurement. For example, the sounds may be heard first at 195 mm Hg, disappear at 175 mm Hg, and reappear at 135 mm Hg. If the examiner inflates the cuff only to 150 mm Hg before deflating, it may then be assumed that 135 rather than 195 mm Hg is the systolic pressure. An auscultatory gap should be suspected if no phase II murmur is heard and the pulse pressure (difference between systolic and diastolic pressures) is low. A gap is more likely to occur if inflation of the cuff is too slow.

will finally change to soft, dull sounds (Figure 20-5D). The initial point at which all sounds disappear is recorded as the diastolic pressure. With the cuff pressure at this level or lower, blood flow is unrestricted and nonturbulent (Figure 20-5E). After the diastolic pressure has been noted, the remaining air in the cuff is released by opening the exhaust valve. If it is necessary to pump air into the cuff to repeat a measurement, a minute should be allowed to lapse for free blood flow in the brachial artery.

The sounds heard during the auscultatory determination of BP are produced by the blood turbulence and vibration. These auditory cues are known as Korotkoff's sounds.[21] Table 20-1 summarizes the changes noted in BP measure-

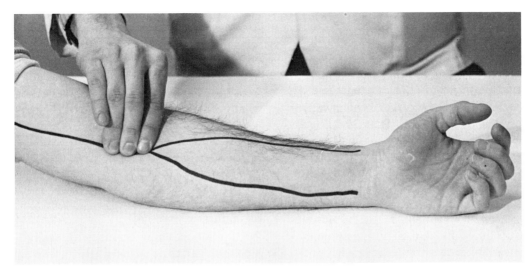

FIGURE 20-4

The left arm's brachial artery, its position outlined, is being palpated with the middle three fingers before its bifurcation into the ulnar and radial arteries. (Reprinted with permission from JE Terry. The measurement of systemic arterial blood pressure. J Am Optom Assoc 1976;47:571–7.)

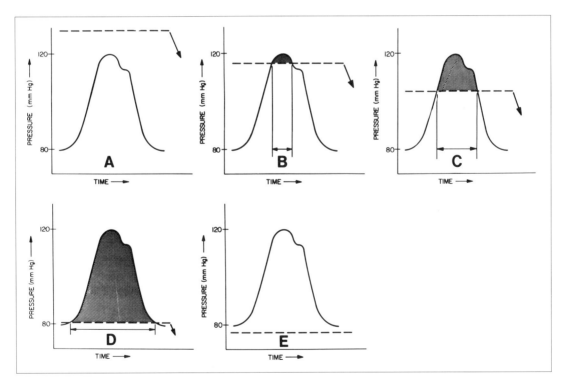

FIGURE 20-5

Graphs of the various stages of blood pressure measurement. Dashed lines represent cuff pressure; solid bell-shaped curve represents arterial blood pressure; shaded zones indicate relative amounts of turbulent blood flow through artery. A. Cuff pressure higher than systolic pressure—no blood flow and no sounds. B. Cuff pressure just lower than systolic pressure—some blood flow occurs during systole, creating audible sounds. C. Cuff pressure well below systolic pressure—blood flow increases, causing higher intensity sounds. D. Cuff pressure only slightly higher than diastolic pressure—vascular resistance is low, resulting in high blood flow and very muffled sounds. E. Cuff pressure below diastolic pressure—blood flow unrestricted with no audible sounds. (Reprinted with permission from JE Terry. The measurement of systemic arterial blood pressure. J Am Optom Assoc 1976;47:571–7.)

SYSTEMIC HYPERTENSION

As mentioned previously, an average, normal BP for a young adult is approximately 120/80 mm Hg. Normal BP, however, is difficult to define on an individual basis and actually represents a range that may be shifted upward or downward depending on the person. Table 20-2 lists the current classification of blood pressure for adults age 18 years and under.

Because the average BP that will cause pathologic alterations in any given individual is not known, other factors can be helpful in the diagnosis of hypertension and in determining the need for treatment. Through epidemiologic evidence, certain high-risk variables governing the development of cardiovascular complications have been identified. These include the magnitude of the BP, the persistence of pressure elevation, age, sex, race, family history of hypertension, diabetes, and the degree of target organ damage (e.g., the ocular fundus).

Persistence of Elevation

It is well known that BP can vary considerably within a normal and hypertensive person over a single 24-hour period and from day to day. Armitage et al.[23,24] noted a large intrasubject variability (25–30 mm Hg) when a series of 40 BP measurements were performed on 20 different occasions. Consequently, a single recording of BP can be quite misleading.

Prognostically, it is important to note that the risk of complications is three or more times higher in patients with persistent hypertension than in those whose diastolic pressures moderately fluctuate above and below 90 mm Hg.[25,26] Cardiovascular complications and end-organ damage are therefore more related to average BP than to occasional transient elevations. Multiple measurements are consequently much better at establishing the extent and persistency of pressure elevations.

Age

A rule of thumb for approximating the average normal BP for a given patient based on age is as follows[27]:

$$\text{Systolic} = (106 \text{ mm Hg}) + (0.6 \times \text{patient age})$$
$$\text{Diastolic} = (74 \text{ mm Hg}) + (0.15 \times \text{patient age})$$

Thus, a 60-year-old patient would have an estimated BP of 142/83 mm Hg.

Numerical data listing the male and female mean systolic and diastolic pressures for different age groups are illustrated in Table 20-3. Evident from these data is that systolic pressures typically increase at a higher rate than diastolic pressures with advancing age.

The younger a patient at the onset of hypertension, regardless of the pressure magnitude, the greater is the reduction in life expectancy. Insurance data have shown that even a modest elevation of BP is associated with greater morbidity when it appears at a relatively early age.[28] Diastolic essential hypertension normally appears in the 30- to 50-year age range and rarely begins in either the young or old.

Sex

Men of all ages have about twice as high a morbidity and mortality rate as compared with women,[29,30] who appear to better tolerate elevated BP. For example, with a BP of 150/100 mm Hg at age 45 years, life expectancy reduction in men is four years greater than in women.[31] Contributing factors in this relationship such as occupation, stress, and physical activity remain controversial.

Race

Blacks have, on average, higher systolic and diastolic BPs than whites.[32–34] In addition, hypertension is twice as prevalent in blacks of all ages, and it tends to be more severe.[35] The devastating mortality levels for black hypertensives are particularly apparent when subdivided by age. The reported death rates from hypertension and hypertensive heart disease are about six to seven times higher in blacks than in whites for the group under age 50 years. In the over-50 category, the death rates are approximately 2.5 times higher in blacks, which largely reflects the higher prevalence of hypertension alone. Hence, hypertension in a black person at a relatively young age carries an extremely high risk.

Family History

Schweitzer et al.[36] summarized the long-recognized impression that essential hypertension tends to be familial. A family history is important for two reasons: It suggests essential rather than secondary hypertension, and it may have negative prognostic implications.[37] Platt[38] reported that a middle-aged sibling of a patient with severe essential hypertension had about eight times the chance of having a diastolic pressure of 100 mm Hg or greater than a randomly selected patient. Hence, a history of relatively early death in a parent or sibling with hypertensive complications (e.g., stroke, renal failure, or congestive heart failure) makes the patient with borderline or mild hypertension more likely to progress to a more severe stage.

130/85.

Table 20-2
Classification of Blood Pressure for Adults Aged 18 Years and Older[a]

Category	Systolic (mm Hg)	Diastolic (mm Hg)
Normal[b]	<130	<85
High normal	130–139	85–89
Hypertension[c]		
Stage 1 (mild)	140–159	90–99
Stage 2 (moderate)	160–179	100–109
Stage 3 (severe)	180–209	110–119
Stage 4 (very severe)	≥210	≥120

[a]Not taking antihypertensive drugs and not acutely ill. When systolic and diastolic pressures fall into different categories, the higher category should be selected to classify the individual's blood pressure status. For instance, 160/92 mm Hg should be classified as stage 2, and 180/120 mm Hg should be classified as stage 4. Isolated systolic hypertension is defined as a systolic blood pressure of 140 mm Hg or more and a diastolic blood pressure of less than 90 mm Hg and staged appropriately (e.g., 170/85 mm Hg is defined as stage 2 isolated systolic hypertension).

In addition to classifying stages of hypertension on the basis of average blood pressure levels, the clinician should specify presence or absence of target-organ disease and additional risk factors. For example, a patient with diabetes and a blood pressure of 142/94 mm Hg, plus left ventricular hypertrophy, should be classified as having "stage 1 hypertension with target-organ disease (left ventricular hypertrophy) and with another major risk factor (diabetes)." This specificity is important for risk classification and management.
[b]Optimal blood pressure with respect to cardiovascular risk is less than 120 mm Hg systolic and less than 80 mm Hg diastolic. However, unusually low readings should be evaluated for clinical significance.
[c]Based on the average of two or more readings taken at each of two or more visits after an initial screening.
Source: Reprinted with permission from the Fifth Report of the Joint National Committee on Detection, Evaluation, and Treatment of High Blood Pressure (JNCV). Arch Intern Med 1993;153:154–83.

TABLE 20-3
Age, Sex, and Blood Pressure

Age (years)	Systolic (mm Hg)	Diastolic (mm Hg)	Age (years)	Systolic (mm Hg)	Diastolic (mm Hg)
0–4 M F	94	61	50–54 M	135	83
			F	137	84
5–9 M F	102	56	55–59 M	138	84
			F	139	84
10–14 M F	113	59	60–64 M	142	85
			F	144	85
15–19 M	121	69	65–69 M	143	83
F	118	67	F	154	85
20–24 M	123	76	70–74 M	145	82
F	116	72	F	159	85
25–29 M	125	78	75–79 M	146	81
F	117	74	F	158	84
30–34 M	126	79	80–84 M	145	82
F	120	75	F	157	83
35–39 M	127	80	85–89 M	145	79
F	124	78	F	154	82
40–44 M	129	81	90–94 M	145	78
F	127	80	F	150	79
45–49 M	130	82	95–106 M	146	78
F	131	82	F	149	81

Source: Reprinted with permission from JE Terry. The interpretation of systemic arterial blood pressure. Part II: Headaches and systemic hypertension. J Am Optom Assoc 1976;47(No. 10):1293–1302.

Diabetes Mellitus

Both diabetes mellitus and hypertension are important, although independent, risk factors for cardiovascular, vascular, and renal disease. A positive correlation has been observed between increased blood serum glucose levels and hypertension.[39] The prevalence of hypertension in diabetics is more than twice that in the nondiabetic population.[35,40,41] Hypertension in a diabetic heightens the risk and accelerates the course of nephropathy, atherosclerosis, retinopathy, stroke, and cardiovascular disease.[42,43]

The underlying mechanisms that initiate and sustain hypertension in the diabetic population are poorly understood. However, some have suggested that diabetes can

TABLE 20-4

Recommendations for Follow-Up Based on Initial Set of Blood Pressure Measurements for Adults

Initial Screening Blood Pressure (mm Hg)[a]		
Systolic	*Diastolic*	*Follow-Up Recommended*[b]
< 130	< 85	Recheck in 2 yrs
130–139	85–89	Recheck in 1 yr[c]
140–159	90–99	Confirm within 2 mos
160–179	100–109	Evaluate or refer to source of care within 1 mo
180–209	110–119	Evaluate or refer to source of care within 1 wk
≥ 210	≥ 120	Evaluate or refer to source of care immediately

[a]If the systolic and diastolic categories are different, follow the recommendation for the shorter time follow-up (e.g., 160/85 mm Hg should be evaluated or referred to source of care within 1 month).
[b]The scheduling of follow-up should be modified by reliable information about past blood pressure measurments, other cardiovascular risk factors, or target-organ disease.
[c]Consider providing advice about life-style modifications.
Source: The Fifth Report of the Joint National Committee on Detection, Evaluation, and Treatment of High Blood Pressure (JNC V). Arch Intern Med 1993;153:154–83.

be considered a model of premature aging, since many of the disturbances in BP regulation seen in diabetics are similar to those seen in elderly patients.[39] Because the incidence of hypertension increases with age, a diabetic with advanced age-related changes would have a greater likelihood of having hypertension.

Target Organ Damage

The most important aspect of the optometric eye examination with regard to hypertension is observation of the fundus. The presence of arteriolar narrowing, hemorrhages, exudates, nicking, tortuosity, and optic disc edema are prognostically unfavorable[8] and will be discussed at length with regard to hypertensive retinopathy in another section. Daubs[44] concluded that fundus evaluation was not a reliable screening test for hypertension unless performed by a highly skilled examiner. A plausible explanation of this view is that patients must be chronically hypertensive for a period of years before observable retinal damage and characteristic changes are observed. After this period of prolonged pressure, the effects of treatment may be much less beneficial than if started years earlier.

Criteria for Referral

The criteria used when considering referral of a hypertensive patient should include the following considerations: magnitude of all BP readings, persistence of elevation, age, sex, race, family history, and damage to a target organ such as the ocular fundus. Guidelines for follow-up based on an initial set of blood pressure measurements are shown in Table 20-4. These guidelines provide that adults who have

systolic pressure higher than 210 mm Hg or a diastolic pressure greater than 120 mm Hg should be referred immediately. Someone with a blood pressure of 160/85 mm Hg should be referred to receive additional follow-up and care within 1 month. The purpose of the BP recheck, of course, is to define those patients whose pressure has returned to normal from those with a sustained increase in BP, which warrants treatment or further evaluation.

SECONDARY HYPERTENSION

The hypertension in more than 90% of all hypertensive patients is of the previously discussed essential idiopathic variety. In these patients, elevated BP develops without an identifiable cause. This is in contrast to secondary hypertension, in which an identifiable systemic disorder is responsible for the elevation of BP.

Several epidemiologic studies suggest that salt intake has a significant role in the development of hypertension.[45–47] The primary link relating salt to hypertension is its ability to increase the extracellular volume in the tissues through plasma volume. Normally, excess salt in the diet can be handled by the normal kidney without expanding extracellular fluid volume. However, in the presence of renal dysfunction, a moderate sodium intake expands this volume, thereby contributing to hypertension. Todian[48] suggested that if not predisposed, an individual is unlikely to develop high BP while maintaining a reasonable daily salt intake. However, someone susceptible to hypertension may only be able to avoid the disease throughout life by remaining on a low-salt diet. It has been suggested, though, that only the most restrictive of low-sodium diets has any effect on BP.[49]

Toxemia of pregnancy is an acute, vasospastic, sodium-retaining disease that is characterized by moderate to severe hypertension and associated edema. In the United States, toxemia develops in 7% of women during their first pregnancy; in economically depressed areas the incidence may reach 30%.[37] It occurs more often during first pregnancies, in those over 35 years of age, and in those carrying more than one fetus.[50]

Although toxemia commonly begins after the twenty-fourth week (last trimester) of gestation and frequently only a few days before delivery, it may begin earlier. Its onset may be insidious or abrupt. Hypertension is usually an early sign. Headaches and visual disturbances are frequent but not universal. Ophthalmoscopy may reveal narrowing and spasm of the retinal arterioles, and the fundus may appear glistening or wet. Exudates and hemorrhages tend to be late occurrences in severe cases. Clearly, the optometrist's examination of pregnant patients should include sphygmomanometry and a careful fundus evaluation.

Oral contraceptives have been implicated in aggravating preexisting hypertension or precipitating its onset.[51,52] It also has been found that BP increases slowly and may take several months or years after oral contraceptives are administered to become significantly elevated.[53,54] Fortunately, systemic hypertension improves gradually when the medication is withheld.[53,55,56]

Although all of the causes of secondary hypertension are too numerous to discuss in detail, Table 20-5 lists many others. During the evaluation of a patient with suspected hypertension, all of these should be kept in mind as potential underlying etiologic factors. By far the most common cause of secondary hypertension is renal parenchymal or vascular disease (occlusion of a renal artery). Because the kidneys play an important role in the maintenance of normal BP, this is not surprising. Relative to the etiologic contribution of kidney disease to the development of hypertension, there are two main categories: (1) renovascular hypertension associated with excessive renin secretion, and (2) chronic renal insufficiency associated with volume excess.

MALIGNANT ARTERIAL HYPERTENSION

Malignant (accelerated or fulminating) arterial hypertension is a serious state that occurs in approximately 5% of the population with diagnosed essential hypertension.[57] Whereas essential hypertension is defined as a systolic pressure reading of 140 mm Hg or higher or a diastolic reading of 90 mm Hg or higher (based on an average of two pressure readings made on two separate occasions),[1]

TABLE 20-5
Causes of Secondary Hypertension

Renal disease
    Occlusion of renal artery
    Glomerulonephritis
    Pyelonephritis
    Obstructive uropathy
    Polycystic renal disease
    Collagen disease of the kidney
Pheochromocytoma
Hyperthyroidism
Primary aldosteronism
Cushing's syndrome
Coarctation of the aorta
Myxedema
Oral contraceptives

malignant hypertension is generally defined as severe hypertension with evidence of acute target-organ damage.[58] Such damage may include effects on the eye, cardiac damage such as left ventricular failure, renal disease, or signs of neurologic compromise stemming from hypertensive encephalopathy.[59] Systolic BP is generally 200 mm Hg or higher and diastolic BP 120 mm Hg or higher.[58]

Usually, malignant arterial hypertension develops rapidly in patients already diagnosed with essential arterial hypertension. Only rarely does it occur in previously normotensive individuals or children. Patients with malignant hypertension have been found to have high levels of angiotensin II and aldosterone.[57] Angiotensin II is an extremely potent peripheral vasoconstrictive agent that results in increased peripheral resistance. Aldosterone works to increase sodium resorption, resulting in increased water resorption in the kidneys, which in turn increases total blood volume. The combined increase in peripheral resistance and blood volume produces a rapid and severe rise in BP throughout the body.[58]

Malignant arterial hypertension may, on occasion, arise secondary to several systemic conditions. Such conditions include acute renal failure (nephrosis, glomerulonephritis, unilateral atrophic kidney), adrenal tumors (Cushing's syndrome, pheochromocytomas), connective tissue disorders (periarteritis nodosa, lupus erythematosus, progressive systemic sclerosis), toxemia of pregnancy, catecholamine excess, previous vascular surgery, congestive heart failure, eclampsia, cerebral vascular accidents, and central nervous system tumors.[57,58,60]

Often patients suffering from malignant hypertension will have visual symptoms of blurred vision. In addition, patients may report scotomas and spots before the eyes.

Although the essential feature of malignant arterial hypertension is often considered by practitioners to be the appearance of optic disc edema (Figure 20-6), disc swelling

FIGURE 20-6
Optic disc edema secondary to malignant arterial hypertension. The margins of the disc are blurred and there are associated hemorrhages in the superficial nerve fiber layer. Note that in this example there are relatively few other fundus changes except for small flame-shaped hemorrhages and arteriolar narrowing.

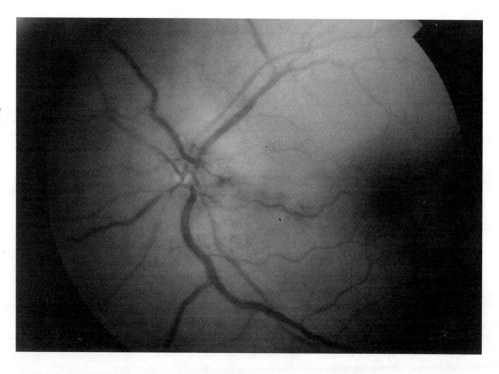

is not always associated with malignant hypertension and should not be considered necessary for diagnosis of the disease.[61,62] As a note regarding proper use of terminology, "papilledema" is not currently considered an appropriate term to describe disc edema secondary to hypertension; rather, the use of the term is reserved for disc swelling secondary to increased cerebrospinal fluid pressure.

GENERAL COMMENTS

Low BPs of 95/55 to 100/60 mm Hg, unless accompanied by significant patient symptoms (lethargy, weakness, dizziness, faintness), are typically not of clinical significance.[8] In fact, these patients may actually have a greater life expectancy than those with higher pressures.[50] Some patients have become unduly alarmed concerning the presence of insignificant low BP. Of course, hypotension is occasionally a symptom of a serious underlying condition. Some of the most significant causes of hypotension include Addison's disease, acute myocardial infarction, hemorrhage, and shock.

Patients with elevations of systemic arterial blood pressure are usually asymptomatic. Hence, hypertension has been appropriately referred to as "the silent disease."[63] When symptoms are present, however, headaches are the most consistent symptom related to the increased blood pressure, and other complaints may include dizziness, palpitations, and easy fatigability.[50]

Systolic hypertension is the condition in which the systolic BP is elevated while the diastolic is at a normal or reduced level, thus resulting in a widened pulse pressure value. It is most commonly seen in elderly patients in whom the wall of the aorta has become less pliable because of arteriosclerosis.

The effects of hypertension will often follow an asymptomatic latent period. The damage occurring to the cardiac, renal, and central nervous system (including the retina) is a manifestation of the accelerated vascular changes resulting from high BP, which, if unaltered because of nontreatment, may ultimately result in symptomatic illness and death.[64]

Left ventricular hypertrophy is the initial means of cardiac compensation for the excessive work load imposed by increased blood pressure. Eventually, the chamber's contractibility deteriorates, and heart failure results. Angina pectoris may occur concomitantly, since accelerated coronary arterial disease or increased myocardial oxygen requirements may exceed the blood flow capacity of the coronary circulation.[64]

The neurologic effects of long-standing hypertension may be divided into retinal and central nervous system changes. The retinal manifestations will be reviewed in another section, as will headaches. Dizziness, light-headedness, vertigo, and visual impairment may be observed. With severe and prolonged hypertension, patients may develop focal or widespread vascular infarction or hemorrhage, resulting in damage to the brain. The small focal

TABLE 20-6
Grades of Vascular Retinopathies

Degree	*A. Hypertension*[a] General A/V[b] Narrowing	Hemorrhages	Exudates	Papilledema[c]	*B. Arteriolar Sclerosis* Light Reflex	Arteriovenous Crossing Defects
Normal	3/4–3/5	0	0	0	Fine, yellow line, red blood column	0
Grade I	1/2	0	0	0	Earliest increase in light reflex	Mild compression of the venules
Grade II	1/3	0	0	0	More marked	Compression or elevation of the venules
Grade III	1/4	+	+ (macular star)	0	Copper wire	Right angle deviation, nicking
Grade IV	Fine cords	+	+	+	Silver wire	Distal congestion

[a]Based on the Keith-Wagener-Barker method classification of hypertensive retinopathy.[65]
[b]Ratio of arteriolar/venule diameter; 0 = absent; + = present.
[c]Regarding current usage, "papilledema" should actually be reserved for disc edema secondary to increased intracranial pressure.

changes may be manifested as personality changes, whereas the larger lesions may produce major strokes.

Briefly stated, general measures the physician may initially employ on a mildly hypertensive patient are relief of stress, control of diet, and regular exercise.[29] Since hypertension is a chronic disease, a therapeutic program must be maintained for the duration of a patient's life. The optometrist should encourage patients who are under hypertensive treatment to maintain a consistent therapeutic regimen, since medical noncompliance is undoubtedly one of the greatest problems in the successful management of hypertension.

HYPERTENSIVE FUNDUS CHANGES

Ophthalmoscopy provides an exceptional opportunity to observe and study the changes in the retinal vessels caused by hypertensive vascular disease. Historically, many of the classifications used to evaluate severity of hypertensive fundus changes were based on ophthalmoscopic interpretation of retinal arteriolar changes. With the advent of fundus fluorescein angiography and a better understanding of the pathophysiology of the various fundus lesions, additional insights into the classification of hypertensive retinopathy have been obtained.

Hypertensive Retinopathy Classification

Some practitioners still use a classification of hypertensive retinopathy based on the Keith-Wagener-Barker method,[65] which ranks fundus changes from grades I–IV. A summary of this can be found in Table 20-6, part A. Although this method has the advantage of avoiding ter-

minology semantics, it has some limitations because of potential examiner bias.

Arteriolar Attenuation

Much emphasis is placed on the ophthalmoscopic evaluation of arteriolar attenuation in spite of the proven subjective nature of the finding. A study by the World Health Organization[66] found a 33% ± 12% intraobserver disagreement and a 42% ± 17% interobserver disagreement among experts evaluating narrowing of the retinal arterioles in hypertensive patients. In a different study, Cogan[67] determined that "Over-interpreting arterial narrowing in the fundus is a common failing. When one knows the patient has hypertension, one tends to attach undue significance to questionable changes." The unreliability of assessing arteriolar narrowing has also been stressed by Stokoe and Turner[68] and Evelyn et al.[69]

A more accurate assessment of arteriolar attenuation can be achieved with fundus angiography. This is because fluorescein mixes in the plasma traveling adjacent to the vessel wall, thus revealing the entire width of the blood column. Ophthalmoscopy and color fundus photography show only the width of the central column of red blood cells.[70] By using fluorescein angiography in rhesus monkeys who suffered from malignant arterial hypertension, Hayreh et al.[70] demonstrated that ophthalmoscopically identified arteriolar attenuation is often an artifact secondary to retinal edema masking part of the arteriole, and that arteriolar attenuation is not as predominant in malignant hypertension as once believed.

Hemorrhages

It is well documented that retinal hemorrhages often develop in hypertensive patients. Hemorrhages can occur in the nerve fiber layer or in deeper layers of the retina. They often present initially in the radial peripapillary retinal capillaries.[71,72] Later on, in the course of hypertensive retinopathy, the location of hemorrhages becomes more variable.[71] Hemorrhages result when capillary blood flow is so impaired that nutritional damage to the vessel walls and retinal tissue occurs.[73] Retinal hemorrhages are generally of no great significance in the course of hypertensive retinopathy; however, it has been noted that an increase in the frequency of hemorrhaging generally precedes a more serious arterial hypertensive state.[74]

Cotton Wool Spots

Historically, the term *exudate* has been used to describe a variety of fundus lesions that are white, yellow, or gray and that occur in definite patches varying from barely visible dots to abnormalities occupying a large portion of the fundus. Falling into this category have been "hard exudates" and "cotton wool spots," which both occur in hypertensive retinopathy. Cotton wool spots (CWSs) are sometimes referred to as "soft exudates"; however, this term is confusing relative to their actual pathophysiology and may imply a relationship to hard exudates. In reality, hard exudates and cotton wool spots are unrelated with regard to the precise mechanism of their development. Hence, it is preferable not to use the term exudate with reference to cotton wool spots.

Cotton wool spots appear as white or gray fluffy opacities having indistinct, edematous edges and surfaces. These spots result from focally obstructed terminal retinal arterioles caused by swelling and disruption of the vessel walls. Fluorescein angiography reveals focal retinal capillary nonperfusion distal to the site of the occlusion.[75-77] The whitish coloration of these lesions is produced by swelling of the nerve fiber layer within the ischemic zone. As the focal swelling resolves, the cotton wool area may gradually disappear (in 3–6 weeks) ophthalmoscopically. However, permanent obliteration of the retinal capillaries may be demonstrated by fluorescein angiography.

The presence of cotton wool spots is significant in the development of hypertensive retinopathy. It is believed that CWSs develop earlier and with higher incidence in cases where the arterial hypertension is more accelerated.[78]

In the past, CWSs and focal intraretinal periarteriolar transudates (FIPTs) have been mistakenly considered as one entity, with FIPTs being a precursor of CWSs. Whereas CWSs are acute focal retinal ischemic lesions located mainly in the nerve fiber layer of the retina, FIPTs are exudative retinal lesions of the deeper retinal layers (therefore explaining their round or oval shape), caused by a breakdown of the blood-retinal barrier in precapillary retinal arterioles.[78]

During fluorescein angiography, FIPTs show dilation of the precapillary terminal retinal arterioles rather than capillary nonperfusion, as is seen with CWSs. In addition, FIPTs last only 2–3 weeks and resolve completely without leaving any permanent ophthalmoscopic, microvascular, or fluorescein angiographic abnormality.[78]

Exudates

Exudates are more yellow and exhibit a more discrete border and smoother surface than CWSs. The contents of these outer plexiform layer exudative foci consists largely of albumin, fibrin, or mixed substances. Red blood cells may also be present.[79] After their initial formation, exudates undergo a process of ingestion by phagocytes, which are fat-laden cells, giving them a more intensely white or creamy color. Generally, they are seen irregularly scattered across the retina. Because of the anatomic peculiarity of the outer plexiform layer within the macular region (Henle's fiber layer), deposition of exudates in this portion of the retina frequently becomes radially arranged and forms a star-like pattern, referred to as a "macular star" (Figures 20-7 and 4-22).

Optic Disc Edema

Optic disc edema occurs in the most severe hypertensive states (see Figure 20-6). Patients frequently have a BP above 200/140 mm Hg.[50] Electron microscopy has shown that edema results from swelling and leakage from injured arterioles derived from the circle of Haller.[80,81] The ultrastructural changes that occur in hypertensive disc edema are similar to the changes that develop in the retina proper.[82] That is, throughout the neural tunic, a severe rise in BP causes an increase in the tissue blood flow resulting from a failure of the local autoregulation system. Normally, autoregulation is effective over a wide range of systemic arterial pressures but fails at the extremes. At the upper limit, failure seems to be related to muscle necrosis, when the tension in the vessel wall becomes too great for the smooth muscle to sustain contraction.[75,77] The arterioles then dilate, and the tension in the wall increases. As the vessel distends, the increased diameter allows the pressure to be transmitted to the most distal segments of the arteriolar bed and proximal capillaries. The resulting increased mean capillary pressure allows more fluid to flow out of the vessel than returns into the distal capillary. As a result, fluid accumulates in the extracellular spaces and edema results. The exact mechanism by which this fluid in the interstitial spaces swells the nerve fiber axons is not entirely known, but it may result from a cellular osmotic pressure gradient.

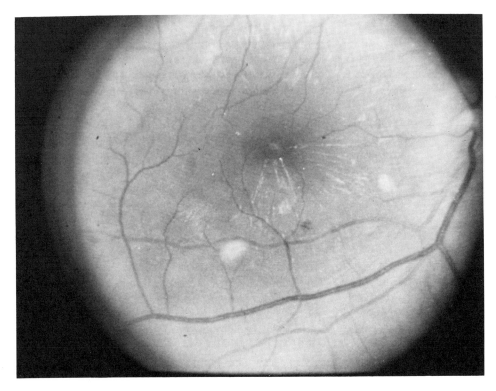

FIGURE 20-7
Exudative "macular star" found in hypertensive retinopathy. A few small flame-shaped hemorrhages and cotton wool spots are also present.

Occasionally optic disc edema occurs in hypertension without (or before) the development of additional retinopathy changes.[64] Such cases are difficult to distinguish from intracranial tumors, since varying degrees of arteriolar attenuation may be the only distinguishing sign. If the diastolic pressure is much below 140 mm Hg in these patients, cerebral tumors should be strongly suspected.[79]

Arteriosclerotic Retinopathy

Arteriosclerosis is a general term that includes several types of degenerative arterial disease.[83] Some types of arteriosclerosis occur only in large arteries, some in arterioles, and some throughout the arterial system. It should be remembered that the retinal arterial tree is primarily arteriolar in nature except for the central retinal artery and its first branches.

The normal progression of aging is associated with sclerotic changes, but these changes may be prematurely accelerated through sustained high BP. Therefore, arteriosclerotic changes are frequently seen in hypertensive patients, but the two are not exclusively linked to each other. Involutional or senile sclerosis is the term given to the normal straightening and narrowing of the retinal arterioles seen with aging.

There are six forms of arteriosclerosis in Bell's[75] classification, two of which produce changes in the retinal arter-ial system that are visible ophthalmoscopically. These are intimal atherosclerosis and diffuse arteriolar sclerosis. Each is a distinct disease entity, and each causes a characteristic retinal picture. The following sections discuss these two entities as well as involutional (senile) sclerosis.

Involutional Arteriosclerosis

Involutional arteriosclerosis is a progressive replacement fibrosis involving the media of arteries and arterioles. It is associated with aging and is seen almost universally after the age of 60 years.[79,83]

The retinal vessels in geriatric patients are uniformly narrower, paler, and less brilliant, since the light reflex from the convex arteriolar surface is of diminished intensity and less distinct than normal. Diffuse narrowing of the vessel lumen associated with thickening of the wall and a reduction in the translucency account for the paler color and duller arteriolar reflex. Vessels are diffusely straighter in their course and branch more acutely than the arterioles seen in younger individuals. This occurs because there is a lessening of the vessel wall elasticity and contraction along the length of the arteriole, which results in a straightening of the course of the vessel.

Intimal Atherosclerosis

Intimal atherosclerosis is a patchy, nodular, lipid infiltration of the intima (the inner coat) of large arteries.[84]

Because the central retinal artery and its first branches are true arteries with an internal elastic lamina and a complete tunica muscularis, atherosclerotic changes in the eye will only be seen at or around the disc. Atherosclerosis is responsible for most myocardial infarctions, cerebrovascular accidents, and other arterial occlusions.[84] If the central retinal artery is occluded, a characteristic cherry-red spot develops in the macula, surrounded by pale ischemic retina and a severely attenuated arterial tree.[85]

The central retinal artery within the optic nerve, particularly at the level of the lamina cribrosa, is the main ocular site of involvement in atherosclerosis. Friedenwald[86] pointed out the difficulty in making an ophthalmic diagnosis of atherosclerosis, since it generally only affects the artery within the substance of the optic nerve. However, atherosclerotic vessel wall plaques may extend out to the main branches as far as the first or second bifurcation from the optic disc and are considered to be outposts of a larger lesion upstream. Vessel wall changes may reach sufficient thickness to be observed ophthalmoscopically as a localized, irregular, whitish sheath surrounding an arterial blood column caused by atheromatous projection into a vessel lumen.

Since the atherosclerotic lesion in the retinal artery usually produces minimal if any ophthalmoscopic change, its presence is usually based on inference. Fibrosis of the atheroma in its central branch may, by contraction, shorten the artery and displace the retinal arteries toward the disc. Arterioles will then become straighter, and bifurcations will occur at more acute angles. A marked reduction in blood flow may result, causing attenuation of vessels within the retinal arterial tree.

Transient diminution of vision because of temporary occlusion of the retinal vessels by atheromatous emboli has been reported. Atherosclerosis is also more commonly seen systemically in men over the age of 30 years but may occur independent of age, sex, or elevated BP.[87]

Diffuse Arteriolar Sclerosis

Physiologic hypertonus is the initial arteriolar response associated with elevated BP. This vasoconstriction is ultimately followed by hyperplasia of the muscular media of the vessel wall and a lessening of the arterial wall elasticity. These changes are most marked when sustained hypertension of moderate to severe degree acts on young cellular arterioles.[88] A stage of reactive sclerosis is eventually reached in which the vessel wall is relatively fibrotic and acellular. This diffuse arteriosclerotic thickening of the small arteries and arterioles (rather than the spotty plaque-like lesions of intimal atherosclerosis) results from subendothelial deposition of hyalin and lipids. Ultimately, arteriolar sclerosis results in thickening of the walls and narrowing of the lumen of arterioles as a response to vascular hypertension.

Light Reflex   The normal arterial light reflex seen during ophthalmoscopy originates on the surface of the blood column. If circulation is momentarily interrupted by digital pressure on the globe, the reflex will disappear. Pathologic changes in the reflex caused by sclerotic loss of transparency originate on the vessel wall itself and remain visible after cessation of the circulation from digital pressure.[89] This differentiation is critical, because the intensity of the arteriolar reflex varies a great deal among normal individuals. As such, less attention is currently directed toward changes in the light reflex in systemic disease.[90] Even with this, widening of the light reflex is considered an early sign of arteriolar sclerosis.[50,82]

The first change in arteriolar sclerosis is widening of the arteriolar light reflex because of an increase in vessel wall thickness and an associated increase in its refractive index. Initially, the widening of the light reflex occurs nonuniformly. As the light streak increases in width, it eventually becomes so wide that it occupies most of the vessel surface. A subtle color change also becomes more observable. The light reflex becomes gradually more yellowish-orange, then coppery (hence the term "copper wire"). Finally, in the end-stage form of arteriolar sclerosis, the vessel wall is so thickened and opaque by replacement fibrosis that the underlying blood column is completely concealed. It then appears as a white, silver-wire chord, even though blood is still circulating through it.

Crossing Defects   Some of the most revealing areas for evaluation of arteriolar sclerosis within the retina are the arteriovenous crossing points. Arterioles usually cross over the venules while sharing a common adventitial coat of fibrous tissue that binds them together in a figure eight configuration. Thus, as an arteriole thickens, displacement or compression of a contiguous venule results. The "nicking sign" then may be observed. Nicking is a characteristic finding in arteriolar sclerosis. Nicking is a tapering of a venule on either side of a crossing (Figures 20-8A and 20-9), whereby its blood column is partially hidden by a common adventitial coat.[91]

The diagnostic significance of the nicking sign is that it occurs almost regularly in arteriolar sclerosis. Involutional sclerosis may occasionally have focal arteriovenous crossing changes associated with it but these are not as generalized as with arteriolar sclerosis. This difference serves to differentiate the two conditions. Furthermore, nicking is an early change that is occasionally well developed at a time when few other ophthalmoscopic changes are observed.

Initially, when there is only minimal venous impediment from arteriolar compression, minor indentation

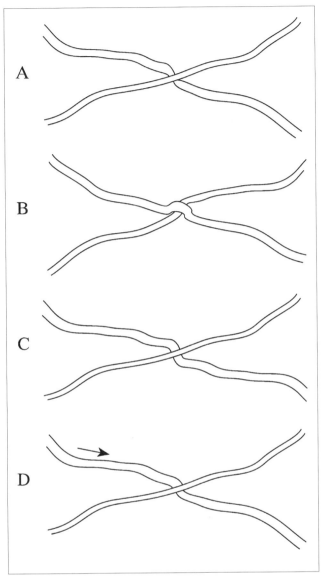

FIGURE 20-8

Arteriovenous crossing changes in arteriolar sclerosis. A. Apparent tapering (nicking) of a venule as it crosses below an arteriole. B. Displacement of a venule into more superficial retinal layers (venule crossing over an arteriole). C. Abrupt deviation in the lateral course of a venule. D. Dilatation (banking) of a venous segment distal to the location at which it crosses under an arteriole (arrow denotes direction of blood flow within the venule). (Courtesy of Daniel K. Roberts, O.D.)

of the venule may occur without congestion or attenuation. In more advanced cases, there is greater interference with circulation. A displacement of the vein into the depth of the retina ("compression") or an elevation ("humping") of the vein over the arteriole (Figure 20-8B) can re-establish free circulation. The deeper into the

retina the vein is displaced, the more indistinct and thinner it will appear. Due to the common adventitial sheath, venules may exhibit an abrupt turn (S-shaped bend or right-angle deviation) at its crossing with an arteriole, which is apparently due to a straightening of the arteriole (Figures 20-8C and 20-9). Severe sclerosis, with compression or constriction, impedes venous flow to such an extent that dilation and swelling ("banking") of the distal venous segment results (Figures 20-8D and 20-9).

Occasionally, a series of punctate hemorrhages and possibly a circumscribed slate-colored, superficial area of retinal edema can be found surrounding an arteriovenous crossing site, which may reflect significant venous congestion.[89] Eventually, the venous branch may become completely occluded at the arteriovenous crossing, resulting in pronounced hemorrhaging in the involved retinal region. Nicking of a venule, a change in its course, or an apparent interruption by a crossing arteriole provide evidence that the vessel wall is involved. A summary of the classification of arteriolar sclerosis is given in Table 20-6, part B.

Arteriolar sclerotic changes are usually classified into two types. The first, replacement fibrosis, may develop in slowly progressing, moderately severe hypertension, which is associated with a systolic BP in the range of 170–200 mm Hg and a diastolic pressure usually less than 100 mm Hg. Increased collagen and elastic tissue along with a loss of cellular detail in all vessel layers are the common histologic changes. The second type of changes, hyperplastic thickening and fibrinoid necrosis, occur as acute responses to a sudden marked elevation of the BP that exceeds 200/120 mm Hg. Vessels that have been the site of involutional necrosis are generally not involved, since these changes appear to protect the arterioles from the effects of severe hypertension. If ophthalmoscopic examination of a patient with known vascular hypertension reveals no arteriolar sclerosis, then the hypertension is probably not severe or is of recent onset. If the changes of replacement fibrosis are present, the disease is likely to be long-standing, affecting arterioles throughout the body, with the amount of sclerosis serving as an index to the duration of the hypertension. If the changes are hyperplastic thickening and fibrinoid necrosis, the hypertension is severe and probably of recent onset.

Prognostically, because arteriolar sclerosis affects arterioles uniformly throughout the systemic circulation, funduscopic changes reflect changes elsewhere (e.g., the brain, kidneys, and heart). In contrast, intimal atherosclerosis occurs in a localized, spotty fashion so that the eye may be extensively involved, whereas little or no change has occurred elsewhere in the body.

FIGURE 20-9

Advanced fundus changes associated with malignant arterial hypertension. The arrow pointing left denotes "nicking" of a venule as well as deviation of its course. The arrow pointing up denotes dilatation of a venous segment distal to an arteriovenous crossing (banking). The arterioles are markedly attenuated, and extensive hemorrhaging and exudative changes are present. (Courtesy of Daniel K. Roberts, O.D.)

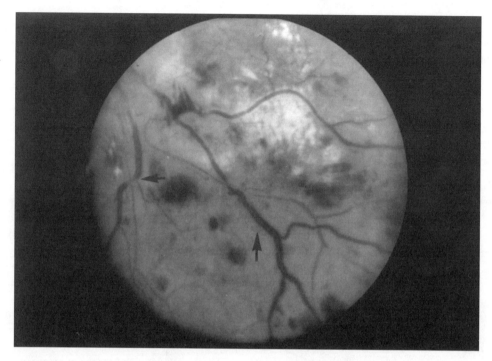

OTHER CONSIDERATIONS RELEVANT TO SYSTEMIC HYPERTENSION

Increased BP may indicate systemic disease, have ocular manifestations, or be related to psychosocial factors such as anger, denial, repression, or interpersonal anxiety.[92] This section will encompass the related topics of intraocular pressure, glaucoma, related pharmacologic relevance, and headaches.

Intraocular Pressure and Glaucoma

Systemic arterial BP has long been known to influence intraocular pressure.[93–95] This alteration may result from BP fluctuations associated with pulse, respiration, asphyxia, vagal nerve stimulation, coughing, postural changes, and neck compression.[94] However, these changes in intraocular pressure are short-lived. If BP is artificially elevated, intraocular pressure will likewise increase, but it will quickly return to its original level within a matter of a few seconds to minutes. These rapid ocular pressure fluctuations associated with the cardiac cycle and respiration are manifested as small second-to-second variations in tonometric readings, which are especially visible when an applanation tonometer is used. Fluctuation may be as much as 2–3 mm Hg.[86]

The relationship between chronic systemic hypertension and glaucoma has always been thought-provoking.

Throughout the years, investigators have come to varying conclusions about the correlation. Several studies have reported a relationship between elevated systemic BP and elevated intraocular pressure but have failed to find an association between elevated systemic BP and glaucomatous field loss.[96–101]

A study at the Wilmer Institute[102] matched 94 individuals with well-documented glaucomatous visual field loss with 94 controls and found that the greatest association between glaucoma and arterial BP was found in patients with an elevated diastolic pressure (90 mm Hg or higher). This same association has been reported by other investigators.[103,104] No association was found between elevated systolic pressure and glaucoma. In fact, although statistically insignificant, elevated systolic pressure seems to afford some protection against glaucoma.[100,102]

The effect of treatment of systemic hypertension adds further confusion to the study of its association with glaucoma. Successfully treated systemic hypertension will decrease the perfusion of blood to the optic nerve when compared with untreated systemic hypertension. Since glaucoma is not defined by ocular pressure level alone but is related to the vascular supply (or lack thereof) to the optic nerve,[105] a decreased perfusion may increase the susceptibility of the optic nerve to ischemic damage, even in the presence of normal levels of intraocular pressure. This can result in glaucomatous field loss and provides an etiologic basis for low-tension glaucoma. In fact, low systemic BP, hemodynamic crises, and rigorous antihypertensive therapy have all been postulated as risk factors in patients with low-tension glaucoma.

Leighton and Phillips[106] found that in patients who were suffering from low-tension glaucoma, the systemic arterial BP was significantly less than that of closely matched patients with open-angle glaucoma. Morgan and Drance[107] reported a marked difference in blood transfusion histories of glaucoma patients compared with their normal controls, suggesting that acute hypotensive episodes sufficient to require transfusion may lead to visual field and disc changes. These conditions included severe shock, hemorrhage, or hypotension occurring during or after surgery, and myocardial infarction. Schwartz[108] suggested that these hypotensive episodes may operate in the same fashion as a persistently low vascular pressure in the presence of normal levels of ocular pressure.

Several reports have stressed the development of glaucomatous damage associated with the inducement of a severe reduction in BP during therapy of systemic hypertension.[109-113] Feldman et al.[111] closely examined the vascular status of 58 chronic simple glaucoma patients who had large-vessel disease (carotid or vertebrobasilar) and who also had BP lower than that of similarly aged normal individuals. A combination of low systemic BP with a relative obstruction in the large vessels was found to cause a reduced supply of blood to the eyes and greater susceptibility to damage. Other conclusions were that greater optic ischemia occurs (1) in patients with high intraocular pressure, (2) in those who had a major hemodynamic crisis during which tissue perfusion was impaired, and (3) in those who have low systemic BP, ranging from 100/60 to 120/70 mm Hg in conjunction with clinically normal vasculature. Francois and Neetens[110] concluded that patients having increased ocular pressure with low BP have the worst prognosis and develop the most rapid deterioration in the visual field and disc excavation. These phenomena were more pronounced if vascular sclerosis was present, resulting in a reduced lumen diameter and a marked increase in resistance, corresponding to reduction in tissue perfusion of the optic nerve head in the prelaminar region.

Drance[109] compared various systemic abnormalities in low-tension glaucoma patients and found that in the vast majority, hemodynamic crises (e.g., gastrointestinal hemodynamic crises, uterine hemorrhages, cardiac arrest, and severe hypotension during anesthesia) and low BP levels occurred statistically more frequently than in ocular hypertensive or normotensive individuals matched for age and sex. This again suggests an ischemic process to the optic nerve with a decrease in tissue perfusion.

Although Demailly et al.[114] did not find an association between patients with low-tension glaucoma and conditions associated with low systemic BP, they did report a statistically significant difference in BP between standing and lying positions in the low-tension glaucoma group (systolic BP: –6.9 mm Hg) when compared with the open-angle glaucoma control group (systolic BP: –1.5 mm Hg). Their study suggests that postural hypotension could play a role in the pathogenesis of low-tension glaucoma.

Pharmacologic Considerations

Phenylephrine hydrochloride is a commonly used adrenergic agent in the practice of optometry. Its primary action is as a direct alpha-receptor agonist that is effective for pupillary dilation without an appreciable cycloplegic effect. It is also a powerful vasoconstrictor and may cause a rapid rise in systemic BP by increasing the total peripheral resistance if enough is absorbed systemically after cul-de-sac instillation through either the conjunctival vessels or the nasal and oral mucosa.[90,115] If total peripheral resistance increases significantly, the diastolic pressure will rise more rapidly than the systolic pressure, resulting in a decrease in pulse pressure (difference between diastolic and systolic pressure). Compared with rises elicited by epinephrine, the phenylephrine response occurs more slowly and persists longer. When this drug is used prudently, however, in the concentration of 2.5% phenylephrine (single instillation) on noninflamed eyes, systemic complications are rare.[116]

Heath and Geiter[117] reviewed the clinical experiences and observations reported with the use of 2.5% phenylephrine. Their investigation into the effect of 2.5% phenylephrine on the elevation of BP was performed using a variety of subjects, both normal individuals and patients with eye disease. They found that the BP was not increased in 98% of the cases and only slightly increased (5 mm Hg) in 2%.

McReynolds et al.[118] reported the case of a 35-year-old man who developed posterior synechiae after an iritis. A cotton wick soaked with 10% phenylephrine was placed in the lower cul-de-sac. The patient quickly complained of a severe throbbing occipital headache. His BP was found to be 230/130, although it had previously been 118/68. To substantiate the findings of Heath and Geiter, McReynolds et al.[118] then studied the effects of 2.5% phenylephrine on 100 hypertensive patients. No elevation was found in 94% of the cases, while only 6% showed an increase in diastolic pressure of 10 mm Hg or less. They summarized that phenylephrine may cause minor toxic effects that include anxiety, tremor, palpitation, and headache, all of which are transient and nondangerous with a wide margin of safety.

Lansche[63] reported an incident in which a patient whose eyes had been previously anesthetized, resulting in marked conjunctival hyperemia and some disruption of the corneal epithelium, developed a systemic reaction after the instillation of 10% phenylephrine. The effect was characterized by an occipital headache, palpitation, hypertension (230 mm Hg systolic), paleness, tachycardia, trembling, and excessive perspiration.

Wilensky and Woodward[119] also reported a case of acute systemic hypertension after the topical ocular use of 10% phenylephrine. A 76-year-old man with chronic open-angle glaucoma whose BP averaged 150/110 mm Hg was given one drop of proparacaine followed by three drops of phenylephrine to each eye over a 12-minute period. Fifteen minutes later, his BP was 270/170 mm Hg. However, they concluded that it was not possible to determine whether the rise in BP represented a drug overdose or an individual idiosyncrasy unrelated to dosage.

In a controlled study of ten healthy students, the responses to several circulation variables were followed after the application of three drops of 10% phenylephrine (same as previous report). The results showed no significant changes of circulation variables without observable side effects.[120]

The conclusions seem to support the contention that while phenylephrine hydrochloride has an important use in optometric practice, some precaution should be taken. Increased systemic absorption may occur in rare instances such as a highly hyperemic and inflamed eye or when there is a disruption in the integrity of the cornea. Also, possible idiosyncrasies may occur in highly hypertensive patients.

Headaches

Headaches are a common initial symptom in ophthalmic practice,[121] since many patients associate discomfort and pain emanating anywhere in the cranial vault with an eye problem. Among the various causes, headache from hypertension should not be disregarded or overlooked, since it has been shown that at least 33% of all persons with mild hypertension have headaches. Since hypertension is frequent in the general population, it is usually difficult to prove that it is the sole cause of recurrent headaches. However, headache is the most consistent symptom directly associated with hypertension, especially with diastolic BPs of over 100 mm Hg. These headaches are commonly localized to the occipital region, present on awakening in the morning, and subside spontaneously after several hours.[50]

Nick and Tenon[122] examined 72 patients suffering from hypertensive headaches. They found that discomfort was characterized by an early morning onset (second half of the night or dawn) and a regression in intensity by early afternoon. The pain was typically occipital but could be localized elsewhere. The investigators also found that hypertensive headaches occurred mainly in women during the fifth decade of life, some of whom also had migraine. Emotion was thought to be an important precipitating factor.

The widespread belief that headaches are a reliable symptom in milder degrees of hypertension is not entirely supported.[29,123,124] Classical hypertensive headaches do tend to be associated with the presence of retinopathy.[30,125] This holds special significance to the optometrist who may closely correlate symptoms with retinal damage. Weiss[126] examined 6,672 subjects and correlated the level of diastolic pressure and headache symptoms with the presence of hypertensive retinopathy. The author chose grade II, III, and IV retinopathies (Keith-Wagener-Barker classification), consisting of marked arteriolar narrowing, arteriovenous compression, increased arteriolar light reflexes, retinal hemorrhages (type and size not specified), hard exudates, and cotton wool spots, to classify the presence or absence of ocular damage. It was found that 40% of the individuals with at least grade II retinopathy had a diastolic pressure greater than 90 mm Hg, whereas only 9% of those without retinal changes had a pressure exceeding this level. Thus, headaches may be a significant presenting symptom, especially among patients with diastolic pressures of 100 to 130 mm Hg or greater[116] who also are found to manifest significant hypertensive retinopathy (grade II or greater).

REFERENCES

1. The Fifth Report of the Joint National Committee on Detection, Evaluation, and Treatment of High Blood Pressure (JNC V). Arch Intern Med 1993;153:154–83.
2. Veterans Administration Cooperative Study Group on Antihypertensive Agents. Effects of treatment on morbidity in hypertension. Results in patients with diastolic blood pressures averaging 115 through 127 mm Hg. JAMA 1967;202:1028–34.
3. Veterans Administration Cooperative Study Group on Antihypertensive Agents. Effects of treatment on morbidity in hypertension. II: Results in patients with diastolic blood pressure averaging 90 through 114 mm Hg. JAMA 1970;213:1143–52.
4. Daubs J. Cost-efficiency of optometric screening. Opt J Rev Optom 1974;111:9–18.
5. Vander AJ, Serman JH, Luciana DS. Human Physiology: The Mechanisms of Body Function. New York: McGraw-Hill, 1970.
6. Guyton AC. Textbook of Medical Physiology (4th ed). Philadelphia: Saunders, 1971.

7. Good GW, Augsburger AR. Role of optometrists in combatting high blood pressure. J Am Optom Assoc 1989;60: 352–5.

8. Prior JA, Silberstein JS. Physical Diagnosis: The History and Examination of the Patient (4th ed). St. Louis: Mosby, 1973.

9. Burch GE, Shewey L. Sphygmomanometric cuff size and blood pressure recordings. JAMA 1973;225:1215–8.

10. Kirkendall WM, Burton AC, Epstein FH, Freis ED. Recommendations for human blood pressure determination by sphygmomanometers. Circulation 1967;36:980–8.

11. Kirkendall WM, Feinleib M, Freis ED, et al. Recommendations for human blood pressure determination by sphygmomanometers. Subcommittee of the AHA post graduate education committee. Circulation 1980;62:1145A–55A.

12. Mauro AM. Effects of bell versus diaphragm on indirect blood pressure measurement. Heart Lung 1988;17:489–94.

13. Saba JM. Indirect blood pressure measurement. Medical Electronics and Data 1971;(Sept/Oct).

14. McCaughan D. Comparison of an electronic blood pressure apparatus with a mercury manometer. J Advancement Med Inst 1966;(Nov/Dec).

15. Rebenson-Piano M, Holm K, Foreman MD, et al. An evaluation of two indirect methods of blood pressure measurement in ill patients. Nurs Res 1989;38:42–5.

16. Borow KM, Newburger JW. Noninvasive estimation of central aortic pressure using the oscillometric method for analyzing systemic artery pulsatile blood flow: Comparative study of indirect systolic, diastolic, and mean brachial artery pressure with simultaneous direct ascending aortic pressure measurements. Am Heart J 1982; 103:879–86.

17. Venus B, Mathru M, Smith RA, et al. Direct versus indirect blood pressure measurements in critically ill patients. Heart Lung 1985;14:228–31.

18. Fortmann SP, Marcuson R, Bitter PH, et al. A comparison of the sphygmetrics SR-2 automatic blood pressure recorder to the mercury sphygmomanometer in population studies. Am J Epidemiol 1981;114:836–44.

19. LaBarthe DR, Hawkins MC, Remington RD. Evaluation of performance of selected devices for measuring blood pressure. Am J Cardiol 1973;32:546–53.

20. Polk BF, Rosner B, Feudo R, et al. An evaluation of the Vitastat automatic blood pressure measuring device. Hypertension 1980;2:221–7.

21. Dorland's Medical Dictionary (25th ed). Philadelphia: Saunders, 1974.

22. Central Committee for Medical and Community Program. Recommendations for human blood pressure determination by sphygmomanometers. New York: American Heart Association, May 1967.

23. Armitage P, Rose GA. The variability of measurements of casual blood pressure. I: A laboratory study. Clin Sci 1966;30:325–35.

24. Armitage P, Fox W, Rose GA, Tinker CM. The variability of measurements of casual blood pressure. II: Survey experience. Clin Sci 1966;30:337–44.

25. Lew EA. Blood Pressure and Mortality, Life Insurance Experience. In J Stamler (ed), The Epidemiology of Hypertension. New York: Grune & Stratton, 1967.

26. Sokolow M, Werdegar D, Kain HK, Hinman AT. Relationship between level of blood pressure measured casually and by portable recorders and severity of complications in essential hypertension. Circulation 1966;34:279–98.

27. Terry JE. The interpretation of systemic arterial blood pressure. Part I. Glaucoma, papilledema and pharmacology. J Am Optom Assoc 1976;47:1119–27.

28. Society of Actuaries. Build and Blood Pressure Study (Vols 1 and 2). Chicago: Society of Actuaries, 1959.

29. Pincherle G, Robinson D. Mean blood pressure and its relation to other factors determined at a routine executive health examination. J Chron Dis 1974;27:245–60.

30. Badran RH, Weir RJ, McGuiness JB. Hypertension and headache. Scott Med J 1970;15:48–51.

31. Fries ED. Age, race, sex and other indices of risk in hypertension. Am J Med 1973;55:275–80.

32. Gordon T, Devine B. Hypertension and hypertensive heart disease in adults, US 1960–62. Vital and Health Statistics, Series 11, No. 13. Washington DC: US Department of Health, Education, and Welfare, 1966.

33. Borhani NO, Barkman TX. The Alameda County Blood Pressure Study. Berkeley, CA: State of California Department of Public Health, 1968.

34. Dustan HP. Racial differences in hypertension. VA Practitioner 1989;3:4–12.

35. Freis ED. The clinical spectrum of essential hypertension. Arch Intern Med 1974;133:982–7.

36. Schweitzer MD, Clark EG, Gearing FR. Genetic factors in primary hypertension and coronary disease. J Chron Dis 1963;45:1093–108.

37. Laragh JH. Hypertension Manual. New York: Yorke Medical Books, 1974.

38. Platt R. Heredity in hypertension. Lancet 1963;1:899–904.

39. Sowers JR. Hypertension associated with diabetes. VA Practitioner 1989;3:30–6.

40. Sowers JR, Tuck ML. Hypertension associated with diabetes mellitus, hypercalcemic disorders, acromegaly and thyroid disease. Clin Endocrinol Metab 1981;10:631–56.

41. A multicenter study, United Kingdom Prospective Diabetes Study III. Prevalence of hypertension and hypotensive therapy in patients with newly diagnosed diabetes. Hypertension 1985;7:2:II-8–II-13.

42. Asplund K, Hagg E, Lithner F, et al. The natural history of stroke in diabetic patients. Acta Med Scand 1980;207:417–24.

43. Chanal P, Inglesby DV, Slightholm M, et al. Blood pressure and the progression of mild background diabetic retinopathy. Hypertension 1985;7:11–79.

44. Daubs J. Funduscopy in the assessment of cardiovascular risk. Opt J Rev Optom 1972;109:29–31.

45. Schechter, PJ, Horwitz D, Henkin RI. Salt preference in patients with untreated and treated essential hypertension. Am J Med Sci 1974;267:320–6.

46. Sazaki N. The relationship of salt intake to hypertension in the Japanese. Geriatrics 1964;19:735.

47. Dahl LK. Salt and hypertension. Am J Clin Nutr 1972;25: 231–44.

48. Todian L. Na/Hypertension revisited. USV Q J Med Mandates 1975;97:FM:10.

49. Freis ED. The Modern Management of Hypertension. Washington DC: Veterans Administration, 1973.

50. Wintrobe MM, et al. Harrison's Principles of Internal Medicine (7th ed). New York: McGraw-Hill, 1974.

51. Woods JW. Oral contraceptives and hypertension. Lancet 1967;2:653–4.

52. Tapia HR, Johnson CE, Strong CG. Effect of oral contraceptive therapy on the renin-angiotensin system in normotensive and hypertensive women. Obstet Gynecol 1973;41:643–9.

53. Weinberger MH, Collins RD, Dowdy AJ, et al. Hypertension induced by oral contraceptives containing estrogen and gestagen. Effects on plasma renin activity and aldosterone excretion. Ann Intern Med 1969;71: 891–902.

54. Dunn FG, Jones JV, Fibe R. Malignant hypertension associated with use of oral contraceptives. Br Heart J 1975; 37:336–8.

55. Laragh JH, Sealey JE, Ledingham JG, Newton MA. Oral contraceptives. Renin, aldosterone, and high blood pressure. JAMA 1967;201:918–22.

56. Lund JO. Oral contraceptives and hypertension. Clin Sci Mol Med 1973;45(Suppl 1):317S–20.

57. Robbins SL, Cotran RS, Kumar V. Pathological Basis of Disease (3rd ed). Philadelphia: Saunders, 1984;1041–7.

58. Williams HW. The eye in malignant hypertension. Clin Eye Vision Care 1990;4:172–85.

59. Reuler JB, Magarian GJ. Hypertensive emergencies and urgencies: Definition, recognition and management. J Gen Intern Med 1988;3:64–74.

60. McRae RP, Liebson PR. Hypertensive crisis. Med Clin North Am 1986;70:749–67.

61. Kincaid-Smit P, McMicael J, Murphy EA. The clinical course and pathology of hypertension with papilledema (malignant hypertension). Q J Med 1958;27:117–52.

62. Sevitt LH, Evans DJ, Wrong OM. Acute oliguric renal failure due to accelerated (malignant hypertension). Q J Med 1971;40:1217–44.

63. Lansche RK. Systemic reactions to topical epinephrine and phenylephrine. Am J Ophthalmol 1966;61:95–8.

64. Platt R. Hypertensive retinopathy and its medical treatment. Qtrly J Med 1954;23:441–9.

65. Keith NM, Wagener HP, Barker NW. Some different types of essential hypertension: Their course and prognosis. Am J Med Sci 1939;197:332–43.

66. Michaelson IC, Eliakim M, Avashalom A, et al. An approach to the investigation of the vascular changes in the fundus of the eye in hypertension and arteriolosclerosis. In E Weigelin (ed), Acta XX Cone Ophthalm Germania, Part I. Amsterdam: Excerpta Medica, 1967; 207–19.

67. Cogan DG. Ophthalmic Manifestations of Systemic Vascular Disease. Philadelphia: Saunders, 1974;74–8.

68. Stokoe NL, Turner RWD. Normal retinal vascular patterns. Arterio-venous ratio as measure of arterial calibre. Br J Ophthalmol 1966;50:21–40.

69. Evelyn KA, Nicholis JVV, Turnbull W. A method of grading and recording. The retinal changes in essential hypertension. Am J Ophthalmol 1958;45:165–79.

70. Hayreh SS, Servais GE, Virdi PS. Retinal arteriolar changes in malignant arterial hypertension. Ophthalmologica 1989;198:178–96.

71. Hayreh SS, Servais GE. Retinal hemorrhages in malignant arterial hypertension. Int Ophthalmol 1988;12:137–45.

72. Dollery CT, Henkind P, Paterson JE, et al. Ophthalmoscopic and circulatory changes in focal retinal ischaema. Br J Ophthalmol 1966;50:285–324.

73. Scheie HG. Evaluation of ophthalmoscopic changes of hypertension and arteriolar sclerosis. Arch Ophthalmol 1953;49:117–38.

74. Becker RA. Hypertension and Arteriolosclerosis. In EA Jaeger, WE Benson (eds), Clinical Ophthalmology. Philadelphia: Harper & Row, 1981;11:1–21.

75. Gass JD. A fluorescein angiographic study of macular dysfunction secondary to retinal vascular disease. III. Hypertensive retinopathy. Arch Ophthalmol 1968;80:569–82.

76. Haining WM. The Optic Papillary and Peripapillary Microcirculation in Disease. The Wm. Mackenzie Centenary Symposium on the Ocular Circulation in Health and Disease. St. Louis: Mosby, 1969.

77. Duke-Elder SS. System of Ophthalmology (Vol 10). St. Louis: Mosby, 1967.

78. Hayreh SS, Servais GE, Virdi PS. Cotton-wool spots (inner retinal ischemic spots) in malignant arterial hypertension. Ophthalmologica 1989;198:197–215.

79. Ballantyne AJ, Michaelson IC. Textbook of the Fundus of the Eye (2nd ed). Baltimore: Williams & Wilkins, 1970.

80. Ashton N. The eye in malignant hypertension. Trans Am Acad Ophthalmol Otolaryngol 1972;76:17–22.

81. Saunders MD. Ocular Disorders Associated with Systemic Diseases. In TD Vaughan, T Asbury (eds), General Ophthalmology (11th ed). Norwalk, CT: Appleton-Century-Crofts, 1986.

82. Trevor-Roper PD. The Eye and Its Disorders. Boston: Little, Brown, 1974.

83. Leishman R. The eye in general vascular disease, hypertension and arteriosclerosis. Br J Ophthalmol 1957;41: 642–9.

84. Jampol LM. Ocular manifestations of selected systemic diseases. In: Part 7 – Medical Ophthalmology. 1633–40.

85. Hogan MJ, Zimmerman LE. Ophthalmic Pathology: An Atlas and Textbook (2nd ed). Philadelphia: Saunders, 1962.

86. Friedenwald JS. Retinal and Choroidal Arteriosclerosis. In F Riley, A Sorsby (eds), Modern Trends in Ophthalmology. New York: Paul B. Noeter, 1940.

87. Scheie H. Adler's Textbook of Ophthalmology (8th ed). Philadelphia: Saunders, 1969.

88. Sorsby A. Modern Ophthalmology (Vol. 2), Systemic Aspects. Washington, DC: Butterworths, 1963.

89. Salus R. A contribution to the diagnosis of arteriosclerosis and hypertension. Am J Ophthalmol 1958;45:81–92.

90. Newell FW, Ernest JT. Ophthalmology Principles and Concepts (3rd ed). St. Louis: Mosby, 1974.

91. Elwyn H. The changes in the fundus of the eye in arterial hypertension. Arch Ophthalmol 1960;49:365–70.

92. Sommers-Flanagan J, Greenberg RP. Psychosocial variables and hypertension: A new look at an old controversy. J Nerv Ment Dis 1989;177:15–24.

93. Fink H. Blood pressure, blood flow and intraocular pressure. Ophthalmol Res 1974;6:338–45.

94. Moses RA (ed). Adler's Physiology of the Eye (5th ed). St. Louis: Mosby, 1970.

95. Duke-Elder SS. System of Ophthalmology, IV: Physiology of the Eye and of Vision. St. Louis: Mosby, 1968.

96. Cullen AP, Sharp HR, Moore SV, McCoy DE. Systemic blood pressure as a diagnostic tool in glaucoma. Am J Optom Physiol Opt 1974;51:414–8.

97. Kahn HA, Leibowitz HM, Ganley JP, et al. The Framingham study. II. Association of ophthalmic pathology with single variables previously measured in the Framingham heart study. Am J Epidemiol 1977;106:33–41.

98. Kahn HA, Milton RC. Alternative definitions of open-angle glaucoma. Effect on prevalence and associations in the Framingham eye study. Arch Ophthalmol 1980;98:2172–7.

99. Leske MC, Podgor MJ. Intraocular pressure, cardiovascular risk variables and visual field defects. Am J Epidemiol 1983;118:280–7.

100. Bulpitt CJ, Hodes C, Everitt MG. Intraocular pressure and systemic blood pressure in the elderly. Br J Ophthalmol 1975;59:717–20.

101. Klein BE, Klein R. Intraocular pressure and cardiovascular risk factors. Arch Ophthalmol 1981;99:837–9.

102. Katz J, Sommer A. Risk factors for primary open angle glaucoma. Am J Prev Med 1988;March/April 4:104:110–4.

103. Wilson R, Walker AM, Dueker DK, Crick RP. Risk factors for rate of progression of glaucomatous visual field loss. A computer-based analysis. Arch Ophthalmol 1982;100:737–41.

104. Wilson MR, Herztmark E, Walker AM, et al. A case-control study of risk factors in open angle glaucoma. Arch Ophthalmol 1987;105:1066–71.

105. Hayreh SS. Optic disc changes in glaucoma. Br J Ophthalmol 1972;56:175–85.

106. Leighton DA, Phillips CI. Systemic blood pressure in open-angle glaucoma, low tension glaucoma, and the normal eye. Br J Ophthalmol 1972;56:447–53.

107. Morgan RW, Drance SM. Chronic open-angle glaucoma and ocular hypertension. An epidemiological study. Br J Ophthalmol 1975;59:211–5.

108. Schwartz B. Shock and low-tension glaucoma. N Engl J Med 1973;288:417–8.

109. Drance SM, Sweeney VP, Morgan RW, Feldman F. Studies of factors involved in the production of low tension glaucoma. Arch Ophthalmol 1963;89:457–65.

110. Francois J, Neetens A. The deterioration of the visual field in glaucoma and the blood pressure. Docum Ophthalmol 1970;28:70–132.

111. Feldman F, Sweeney VP, Drance SM. Cerebro-vascular studies in chronic simple glaucoma. Can J Ophthalmol 1969;4:358–64.

112. Kenney AH. Ocular Examination: Basis and Technique. St. Louis: Mosby, 1970.

113. Kolker AE, Hetherington J. Becker-Shaffer's Diagnosis and Therapy of the Glaucomas (3rd ed). St. Louis: Mosby, 1970.

114. Demailly P, Cambien F, Plouin PF, et al. Do patients with low tension glaucoma have particular cardiovascular characteristics? Ophthalmologica 1984;188:65–75.

115. Hamilton WF (ed). American Physiological Society: Handbook of Physiology. Section 2: Circulation. Baltimore: Williams & Wilkins, 1965.

116. Garston MJ. A closer look at diagnostic drugs for optometric use. J Am Optom Assoc 1975;46:39–43.

117. Heath P, Geiter CW. Use of phenylephrine hydrochloride in ophthalmology. Arch Ophthalmol 1949;41:172–7.

118. McReynolds WU, Havener WH, Henderson JW. Hazards of the use of sympathomimetic drugs in ophthalmology. Arch Ophthalmol 1956;56:176–9.

119. Wilensky JT, Woodward HJ. Acute systemic hypertension after conjunctival instillation of phenylephrine hydrochloride. Am J Ophthalmol 1973;76:156–7.

120. Haltmann HW, Meyer W. Problems of the side effects of Neo-Synephrine. A Von Graefes Arch Klin Exp Ophthalmol 1972; 185:221.

121. Leslie WJ, Greenberg DA. Headache: Discussion, classification and differential diagnosis for the optometrist, Part I. J Am Optom Assoc 1974;45:827–32.

122. Nick J, Tenon H. Hypertensive headache, a critical study. Coeur Med Interne 1970;9:495–9.

123. Smith AT. Symptoms in hypertension. Br Med J 1973;5851:443–52.

124. D'Alessandro R, Benassi G, Lenzi PL, et al. Epidemiology of headache in the Republic of San Marino. J Neurol Neurosurg Psychiatry 1988;51:21–7.

125. Stewart IM. Headache and hypertension. Lancet 1953;1:1261–5.

126. Weiss NW. Relation of high blood pressure to headache, epistaxis and selected other symptoms. N Engl J Med 1972;287:631–3.

II

Treatment and Management of Common Ocular Disorders

21

Diseases of the Lids and Lashes

DEBRA J. BEZAN

Disorders affecting the lids and lashes are among the most frequent problems encountered by eye care practitioners. Associated pathologic states are quite numerous and can result in a wide variety of conditions. Because of the intricate relationship of the lids with the anterior surface of the globe, conditions affecting the lids may not only result in localized disturbances but also often lead to significant problems involving the cornea and conjunctiva.

REVIEW OF EYELID ANATOMY

Although the eyelids may be structurally divided in different ways, their basic components include (1) the skin and subcutaneous fascia, (2) the orbicularis oculi muscle and its submuscular fascia, (3) the orbital septum, (4) retractor muscles, (5) the tarsi, and (6) the conjunctiva[1-3] (Figure 21-1).

The skin of the lids is among the thinnest in the body. It is very loose and elastic, allowing for marked stretching and rapid opening and closure. The orbicularis muscle, a circular muscle that lies just below the subcutaneous fascia, is innervated by the seventh cranial nerve and serves to close the eyelids. The orbicularis muscle can actually be divided into two basic zones—i.e., the palpebral zone (which is further subdivided into the pretarsal and preseptal zones), and the orbital zone.

The orbital septum is a layer of fascia that lies posterior to the orbicularis muscle and its submuscular fascia. It serves as a barrier between the orbital contents and lid.

The main retractor of the upper lid is the levator palpebrae superioris, which is innervated by the third cranial nerve. Tendinous extensions from this muscle course through the lid with insertions into the skin and subcutaneous tissue as well as the anterior surface of the tarsal plate. Serving to provide secondary elevation of the upper

lid is Müller's muscle, which consists of sympathetically innervated smooth muscle fibers that arise from the inferior surface of the levator palpebrae. Retraction of the lower lid is supplied by the inferior palpebral muscle of Müller, which originates from extensions of the inferior rectus. Müller's muscle fibers of the lower lid insert within the conjunctiva of the lower fornix as well as the inferior tarsal plate.

The tarsal plate is composed of dense connective tissue. Within the upper and lower tarsi are parallel rows of meibomian glands extending from the lid margins. On lid eversion, these glands are visible through the overlying translucent tissue as long, slender, vertically oriented, yellowish streaks. There are about 30–40 of these sebaceous glands in the upper lid and about 20–30 in the lower lid. Oily secretions from these glands, draining from the meibomian orifices located posterior to the lash line along the lid margin, contribute to the most superficial layer of the tear film.

Other eyelid glands include the accessory lacrimal glands of Krause and Wolfring, which contribute to the middle, or aqueous, layer of the tear film. The glands of Krause are located predominantly within the subconjunctival tissue of the upper fornix, with some in the lower fornix as well. The glands of Wolfring are located mainly within the supratarsal conjunctiva of the upper lid; a few are also present in the lower lid.

Located near the lid margins are the glands of Zeis and Moll. The glands of Zeis communicate directly with lash follicles and produce sebaceous secretions. The glands of Moll, found near the roots of the lashes, are modified sweat glands.

The conjunctiva is very closely adherent to the tarsi, and it is the innermost structure of the eyelid. The mucocutaneous junction formed at the lid margin between terminations of the skin and the conjunctiva is referred to as

FIGURE 21-1
*Schematic section of the upper
and lower eyelid. (Courtesy of
Daniel K. Roberts, O.D.)*

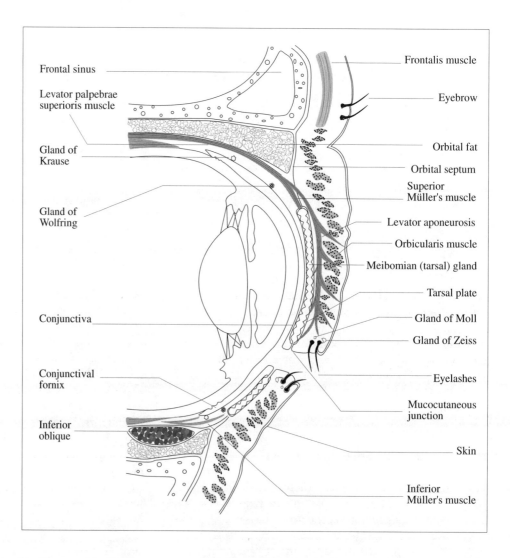

the gray line. An incision along this line would split the tarsal plate and conjunctiva from more anterior structures including the orbicularis muscle, lash follicles, and skin. Goblet cells are contained within the conjunctiva, which are the main source of mucin within the tear layer.

INFLAMMATORY CONDITIONS
OF THE LIDS

Angular Blepharitis

Angular blepharitis is usually caused by gram-positive *Staphylococcus* or gram-negative *Moraxella* species, although other gram-negative bacteria and some fungi such as *Candida* are occasional causative organisms. It is characterized by edema and hyperemia of the lids, particularly near the lateral canthus. The skin in this area may appear macerated (softened), excoriated (cracked),

or ulcerated, and is often tender. Angular blepharitis may also have an associated conjunctivitis.[4,5]

Maceration of the skin at the canthus that is caused by proteases produced by *Moraxella* species usually responds well to zinc sulfate ointment applied topically three times a day. The treatment of choice for gram-positive staphylococcal angular blepharitis is topical bacitracin or erythromycin ointment. Most staphylococcal species are also sensitive to chloramphenicol, aminoglycosides (neomycin, gentamicin, tobramycin), fluoroquinolones (ciprofloxacin, norfloxacin), and trimethoprim, although these are not considered to be the drugs of first choice.[6-9]

Staphylococcal Marginal Blepharitis

As the name implies, staphylococcal marginal blepharitis primarily involves the lid margins. The primary pathogen is *S. aureus*; however, *S. epidermidis*, which is usually considered to be normal flora, is often found in cultures of patients with this condition. Staphylococcal marginal blepharitis is more common in women than men and tends to become a chronic condition with exacerbations and remissions.[6,10]

Characteristic signs include red, inflamed eyelids, crusting with collarette formation on the cilia, and focal areas of lid ulceration. In chronic cases, madarosis (loss of lashes) or tylosis (thickening of the lid margins) may be noted. Internal or external hordeola may also occur (Figure 21-2). Staphylococcal marginal blepharitis is often associated with a mild conjunctivitis, dry eye, and epithelial disruption of the lower one-third of the cornea secondary to the release of staphylococcal exotoxins. Occasionally, marginal corneal infiltration, ulceration, or phlyctenule formation may occur.[6,10,11]

Good lid hygiene is the mainstay of the management of most types of blepharitis. This involves loosening crusts with warm compresses followed by cleaning the lid margins with a commercial lid scrub or nonirritating baby shampoo at least twice a day for several weeks. Applying bacitracin or erythromycin ointment to the lid margin after lid scrubs is effective against most staphylococcal species that cause marginal blepharitis.[6,10,11]

Seborrheic Blepharitis

Seborrheic blepharitis can be found alone or in combination with staphylococcal blepharitis or meibomianitis. Primary seborrheic blepharitis tends to be a chronic condition, and affected patients are typically older than those who develop staphylococcal blepharitis. Primary seborrheic blepharitis is characterized by minimal erythema and inflammation compared with staphylococcal or mixed staphylococcal/seborrheic blepharitis. The lids and lashes exhibit a greasy scale or scurf. This condition is often associated with seborrheic dermatitis affecting other areas such as the scalp, brows, nasolabial folds, and behind the ears.[6,10-12]

Management is similar to that of any chronic blepharitis, with warm compresses and lid hygiene being the primary mode of therapy. Topical antibiotic ointments may be applied if there is an associated bacterial component.[6,11,12] Associated seborrheic dermatitis of the scalp may be treated with a selenium sulfide–based shampoo.[13]

Mixed Staphylococcal and Seborrheic Blepharitis

Mixed staphylococcal/seborrheic blepharitis has features common to both conditions. Patients typically have both collarettes and greasy scurf on the lashes. The lids tend to be more inflamed than in primary sebor-

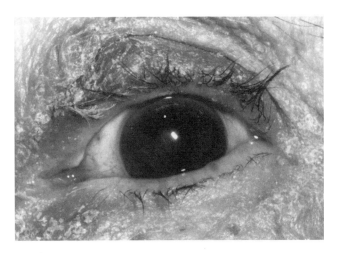

FIGURE 21-2
Staphylococcal marginal blepharitis. An internal hordeolum is also present.

rheic blepharitis, although to a lesser extent than in staphylococcal blepharitis. The combined conditions are often associated with seborrheic dermatitis and keratoconjunctivitis sicca.[6,10-12]

Mixed staphylococcal/seborrheic blepharitis is chronic with frequent exacerbations that can be controlled with diligent lid hygiene and the application of topical bacitracin or erythromycin ointment two to four times a day. Artificial tear solutions may be added to treat associated dry eyes.[11]

Seborrheic Blepharitis with Meibomian Dysfunction

Seborrheic blepharitis with meibomian dysfunction can be subdivided into two categories: seborrheic blepharitis with meibomian seborrhea and seborrheic blepharitis with secondary meibomianitis. In the former condition patients tend to exhibit the mild signs of seborrheic blepharitis combined with excessive meibomian secretion and foaming of the tear film. These patients often complain of a burning sensation, especially in the morning.[6,12] Seborrheic blepharitis with secondary meibomianitis has similar signs except that there are patchy areas of inflammation and blockage of the meibomian glands. During periods of exacerbation these patients tend to be more symptomatic than those with meibomian seborrhea. Both subgroups frequently have associated keratoconjunctivitis sicca. This is presumably attributable to the change in tear film stability associated with meibomian gland dysfunction.[6,12]

The mainstay of treatment for these types of chronic blepharitis is proper lid hygiene. Warm compresses are used to help drain oils in blocked glands and remove debris from the lids. Meibomian massage performed by gently pressing the lid against the globe with a finger to express the contents of the glands to the lid margin may help to treat areas of blockage. Management of associated seborrheic dermatitis and dry eye may also be indicated.[6,12]

Primary Meibomianitis

Primary meibomianitis is characterized by generalized blockage of the meibomian glands and inspissation or "pouting" of the orifices along the lid margins. The lids tend to be thickened and inflamed with minimal crusting or scurf on the lashes (Figure 21-3). These patients often have a punctate keratopathy caused by secondary dry eye or acne rosacea. The term *secondary meibomianitis* is often used to describe the situation where only a few glands are involved secondary to such conditions as seborrheic blepharitis.

Lid hygiene, including warm compresses, meibomian gland expression, and lid scrubs, is the first line of treatment for primary meibomianitis. Topical therapy with antibiotic ointments has also been shown to be helpful. Oral therapy with tetracycline, 250 mg four times a day, may be needed to control inflammation. Tetracycline is thought to inhibit bacterial lipases and decrease free fatty acid production. This, in turn, helps re-establish tear film stability. Oral tetracycline therapy is typically continued for a minimum of 6 weeks, and some patients, especially those with rosacea, may need a long-term dosage of 250 mg per day to maintain control of the condition. When tetracycline is contraindicated, such as in pregnant or lactating women, erythromycin should be substituted.[6,12]

Hordeolum

Hordeola are localized, acute staphylococcal infections of the sebaceous glands of the lids. Other terms for hordeola are styes and acute chalazia. Internal hordeola involve the meibomian glands, whereas external hordeola involve the glands of Zeis and Moll. These lesions often occur in association with chronic staphylococcal blepharitis and are also common in diabetics and immunocompromised patients (see Figure 21-2). Hordeola present as focal, tender, erythematous nodules on the lid. As inflammation progresses, these lesions may spontaneously drain purulent material.[14,15]

Most hordeola respond well to warm compresses applied to the affected area three or four times a day. If the lesion is starting to "point," epilating adjacent lashes or opening the area with a stab incision may help it drain. Treating a draining hordeolum with a topical antibiotic ointment such

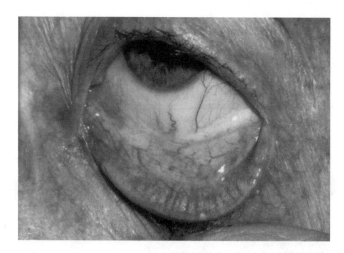

FIGURE 21-3
Easy visualization of swollen meibomian glands associated with primary meibomianitis.

as bacitracin or one of the aminoglycosides may help prevent recurrence by reducing the bacteria in the purulent discharge. Hordeola that are recurrent or associated with other staphylococcal infections may be treated with oral tetracycline, erythromycin, dicloxacillin, or cloxacillin, 250 mg four times a day for 2 weeks.[14,15]

Chalazion

A chalazion is a focal granuloma of a meibomian gland that is often a sequela of staphylococcal or seborrheic blepharitis or meibomitis. In contrast to a hordeolum, it appears as a relatively nontender, nonerythematous lump on the lid.[16]

Small chalazia often respond to conservative treatment with warm saline compresses applied three or four times a day for several weeks. Chalazia up to 6 mm in size that do not resolve with hot pack therapy may respond to intralesional injection with 0.5–2.0 ml of 5%, 10%, or 20% triamcinolone. A second treatment in a week may be needed. Larger or more recalcitrant lesions, especially those present for more than 6 months, may require surgical incision and curettage. Recurrent lesions should be biopsied because basal cell and sebaceous gland carcinomas can masquerade as chalazia.[16,17]

Preseptal Cellulitis

Preseptal cellulitis is a generalized inflammation of the lid anterior to the orbital septum. It is usually caused by *S. aureus* in adults, although it is occasionally associated with streptococcal or anaerobic species. In young children

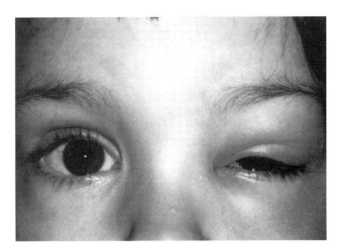

FIGURE 21-4
Swollen lid and periorbital tissue associated with preseptal cellulitis.

Haemophilus influenzae should be ruled out, as this organism can cause life-threatening bacteremia or meningitis. The routes of entry of these microbes include traumatic injuries such as puncture wounds, penetrating foreign bodies, and lacerations, or spreading from other sites of infection such as hordeola, dacryocystitis, and sinusitis. Preseptal cellulitis presents as an edematous, tender, erythematous lid that is warm to the touch (Figure 21-4). It has no associated proptosis or extraocular motility restriction, and there is minimal pain on eye movement. The lack of these signs and symptoms is helpful in differentiating it from orbital cellulitis.[18]

Systemic antibiotic therapy is often indicated in treating preseptal cellulitis. If staphylococcal or streptococcal species are suspected, agents that can be used include amoxicillin, ampicillin, cefaclor, trimethoprim/sulfamethoxazole, erythromycin, or tetracycline. If cultures or the clinical picture indicate *Haemophilus influenzae*, intravenous nafcillin or oxacillin combined with ceftazidime followed by oral therapy with comparable drugs is an effective regimen.[18] Oral ampicillin may also be used with success.[19]

PARASITIC INFESTATIONS

Demodicosis

Demodicosis is a condition caused by an overabundance of the mite species *Demodex folliculorum* or *Demodex brevis* that normally inhabit the eyelids. This condition is more common in older adults and diabetics. It is characterized by chronic itching and burning of the eyelids. Although the signs of demodicosis are minimal, the clin-

ician may note mild crusting and a cuffing or "tenting" of dead epithelial cells surrounding the base of the cilia. Madarosis and bacterial infections are occasionally present. Mites may also be observed clinging to epilated lashes when viewed under a clinical microscope.[20-22]

Although demodicosis is a chronic condition, symptoms can be controlled with lid scrubs and heavy application of an ophthalmic ointment such as bacitracin/polymyxin B, petrolatum, or mercuric oxide to the lid margins on a nightly basis. Ointments are believed to inhibit the nocturnal migration of the parasites. Pilocarpine gel 4% has also been shown to be effective but is more likely to cause undesirable ocular side effects than the other ointments.[20,22]

Phthiriasis

Phthiriasis is infestation of the cilia by the pubic louse, *Phthirus pubis* (Figure 21-5A). The lashes are less frequently infested by the head louse, *Pediculus humanus capitis,* a condition termed *pediculosis.* These infestations are often associated with poor hygiene, and phthiriasis is usually transmitted through sexual contact. Both conditions are characterized by chronic itching and mild inflammation of the lids. Clinically the adult lice may be seen clinging to the cilia, and egg cases or "nits" attached to the lashes can be present as well (Figure 21-5B). Brownish crusts are often noted at the base of the lashes.[23,24]

The initial therapy consists of removal of the adult lice and nits with forceps or freezing them with a cryoprobe. Topical ointments, such as white petrolatum or yellow mercuric oxide, applied twice a day for 7–10 days are somewhat effective in smothering the parasites. Other agents such as physostigmine ointment, A-200 pyrinate solution, or gamma benzene hexachloride shampoo are effective but can be toxic to the cornea or cause central nervous system side effects. Laundering clothing and bedding in very hot water is also helpful in preventing reinfestation.[23]

VIRAL INFECTIONS

Verrucae

Verrucae (warts) are a type of papillomatous lesion caused by papillomavirus. They are most frequently found in children and young adults. They may be multilobular or attached to the lid via a pedunculated stalk (verruca vulgaris), or they may be more rounded and flattened with a cauliflower-like surface (verruca plana). Lesions located on the lid margin can cause a chronic keratoconjunctivitis by shedding viral particles and toxins into the eye.[25]

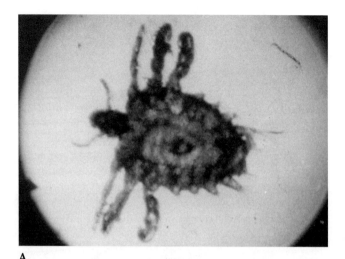

A

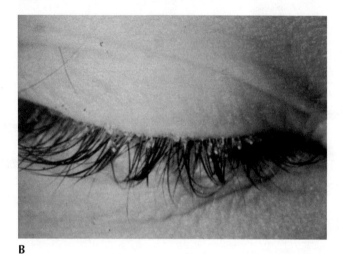

B

FIGURE 21-5
A. Phthirus pubis. *B. Clinical infestation of the eyelid cilia. Adult lice as well as egg cases or "nits" cling to the lashes.*

Verrucae often resolve spontaneously, although they frequently recur. Removal of verrucae is indicated if they cause chronic keratoconjunctivitis or if they are undesirable cosmetically. Topical application of dichloroacetic acid is usually effective in removing verrucae. The acid causes the lesion to whiten immediately and fall off a few days later. Occasionally a second application is needed. Surgical excision, electrocautery, and cryoablation have also been used successfully to remove verrucae.[25]

Molluscum Contagiosum

Molluscum contagiosum, a dermal condition caused by a pox virus, is only mildly contagious. It may be spread by venereal contact or by sharing contaminated cosmetics. Characteristic lesions are dome-shaped, skin-colored papules with an umbilicated center. Lesions on the lid margins can shed toxins into the cul-de-sac, producing a follicular keratoconjunctivitis.[26]

Molluscum contagiosum tends to be self-limiting, although it may be progressive in patients with AIDS or who are otherwise immunosuppressed.[27] If desired, molluscum lesions may be removed via simple excision or incision and curettage. Cryosurgery and chemical cauterization are also effective but can produce excessive scarring.[26]

Herpes Simplex

Herpes simplex virus (HSV) is a very common organism infecting approximately 90% of the population in the United States by the age of 15 years. Primary herpes simplex is usually spread by direct contact with an infected individual. Most primary cases are subclinical, but those who have overt ocular signs typically show vesicular lesions on the lids and a follicular conjunctivitis (Figure 21-6). These signs may be accompanied by fever, gingivostomatitis, and lymphadenopathy. Although dendritic keratitis is the hallmark of recurrent ocular HSV infections, only one-third to two-thirds of patients with primary ocular infections will also have corneal involvement.[28,29]

The vesicular lid lesions of primary HSV infections are usually self-limiting. Topical antivirals such as vidarabine ointment have been used to treat these lesions, but because of the potential for toxic pharmaceutical reactions, it has been recommended that antivirals only be used when the cornea is also involved.[29]

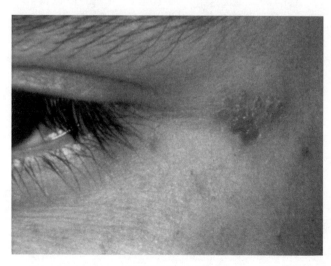

FIGURE 21-6
Early vesicle formation secondary to herpes simplex.

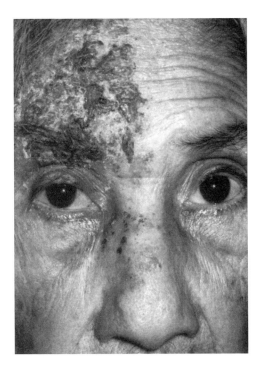

FIGURE 21-7
Marked cutaneous eruptions respecting the facial midline in a patient with herpes zoster.

Varicella-Zoster

The varicella virus causes two systemic conditions with ocular manifestations: chicken pox and herpes zoster. The primary infection, chicken pox, is a highly contagious disease typically found in children. It is characterized by fever, malaise, and pruritic lesions of the skin including the eyelids. These lesions progress from macules to papules, vesicles, pustules, and finally to crusts.[30]

After the primary infection, the varicella virus resides latent in the dorsal root ganglia. If there is a decrease in the effectiveness of the patient's immune system, the virus will reactivate and cause herpes zoster. This is a disease primarily affecting older adults, although it may affect immunocompromised individuals of any age, such as young adults with AIDS.[31] Herpes zoster is characterized by vesicular skin lesions that form a pattern honoring the midline of the body (Figure 21-7) This represents the sensory dermatome innervated by the involved dorsal root ganglion. The ophthalmic branch of the trigeminal ganglion is commonly involved, and when the nasociliary branch is affected, lesions are usually seen on the tip of the nose (Hutchinson's sign). This sign is usually associated with ocular involvement. In addition to vesicular eruptions and occasional scarring of the lids, herpes zoster can cause keratitis, conjunctivitis, scleritis, iridocyclitis,

chorioretinitis, optic neuritis, extraocular muscle paresis, cataracts, and secondary glaucoma.[32]

The lid lesions of both chicken pox and herpes zoster usually resolve spontaneously. However, topical antibiotic ointments such as bacitracin, tetracycline, erythromycin, or gentamicin may be applied as a prophylactic treatment against secondary bacterial infection. Antibiotic/corticosteroid combination ointments may be used to manage particularly inflamed lid lesions of herpes zoster.[30,32] Oral acyclovir has been shown to be helpful in lessening the duration and severity of the symptoms of herpes zoster in doses of 600–800 mg administered five times a day for a week. This is most effective if the therapy is initiated within 48–72 hours of the appearance of the skin lesions. Intravenous acyclovir may be indicated in severe cases.[33,34] Oral corticosteroids, analgesics, sedatives, and antidepressants are frequently used to treat postherpetic neuralgia and accompanying depression. Cimetidine helps reduce the gastrointestinal upset caused by oral corticosteroid therapy and may also aid in relieving the pain and itching of the skin lesions. Topical capsaicin cream is also helpful in treating specific areas of neuralgia.[34]

ALLERGIC REACTIONS

Type I Hypersensitivity Reactions

Type I hypersensitivity reactions (anaphylactic, immediate, IgE-mediated) affecting the lids include hay fever blepharoconjunctivitis and angioneurotic edema. Pollens or molds are usually the sensitizing agent in hay fever blepharoconjunctivitis, whereas reactions to foods, drugs, or insect stings cause angioneurotic edema. In type I reactions, after a previous sensitizing exposure, subsequent contact with the antigen will cause mast cells to release histamine and other chemical mediators. Signs include lid and conjunctival edema and excessive tearing, often accompanied by allergic rhinitis. The hallmark symptom is itching.[35,36]

The best way to manage allergic blepharitis is to avoid contact with the antigen. If this is not possible, oral antihistamines such as chlorpheniramine maleate, diphenhydramine hydrochloride, or terfenidine may provide symptomatic relief. Topical mast cell stabilizers can be helpful in preventing subsequent histamine release, and cool compresses can be used as supportive therapy. Topical corticosteroids may be used if the above therapies are not effective.[35,36]

Type IV Hypersensitivity Reactions

Allergic contact blepharitis is a type IV (delayed, cell-mediated) hypersensitivity reaction. It requires a previous exposure to the allergen, and subsequent exposures

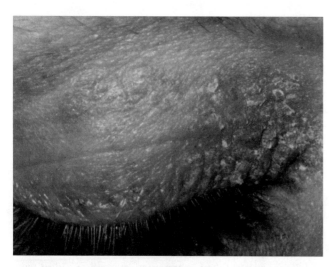

FIGURE 21-8
Primary irritant blepharitis resulting from eye shadow make-up.

result in papular or vesicular eruptions that appear on the lid 24–72 hours after contact. Itching is the typical symptom. Common allergens causing allergic contact blepharitis include poison ivy or oak, nail polish, nickel, dyes, preservatives (e.g., benzalkonium chloride, thimerosal, EDTA), and drugs (e.g., aminoglycosides, antivirals, and beta-blockers).[35–37]

Another type of contact blepharitis is the primary irritant form. It is not a true hypersensitivity response and does not require a previous sensitizing exposure. In this reaction, mild erythema and a scaly eruption of the lids occurs within minutes to hours of contact with the offending agent (Figure 21-8). Common irritants include cosmetics, soaps, contact lens solutions, and medications. Unlike true allergic reactions, the chief symptom in primary irritant blepharitis is typically burning rather than itching.[35,36]

The best management of contact blepharitis is to avoid contact with the offending agent. If this is not possible, cool compresses with water or Burrow's solution applied three or four times a day may provide symptomatic relief. Calamine lotion can be helpful in drying exudative vesicles such as those seen in reactions to poison ivy. Topical corticosteroid creams or ointments may also be used to manage the symptoms; however, only mild corticosteroids such as 1% hydrocortisone should be used, and the dosage should be kept to a minimum to avoid side effects (e.g., atrophy of the lid tissue and elevated intraocular pressure). In severe cases of contact blepharitis, oral corticosteroid therapy may be necessary to control the symptoms.[35,36]

Mixed Hypersensitivity Reactions

Vernal and atopic keratoconjunctivitis have characteristics of both type I and type IV hypersensitivity reactions. Vernal keratoconjunctivitis is more common in children and has seasonal exacerbations, whereas atopic is more common in adults and is not seasonal. With either condition, a personal or family history of allergies is common. In both conditions lid edema may accompany papillary conjunctivitis and keratopathy. In chronic cases the lid has a scaly, corrugated appearance (lichenification). Moderate to severe itching is the classic symptom.[36,38]

Management of both of these conditions is essentially a combination of the treatment strategies for type I and type IV reactions. This includes cool compresses, topical and oral antihistamines, mast cell stabilizers, corticosteroids, and, if possible, avoidance of allergens.[36,38]

BENIGN LID TUMORS

Squamous Papilloma

Squamous papilloma is a benign epithelial tumor that is commonly found on the lids of older adults. It is a cauliflower-like, multilobed lesion, with each lobe having a central vascular core (Figure 21-9). It is similar in appearance to a verruca but is not of viral origin.[39,40]

If cosmetically undesireable, squamous papillomas may be removed by surgical excision, cryoablation, or chemical cauterization with dichloroacetic acid.[39,40]

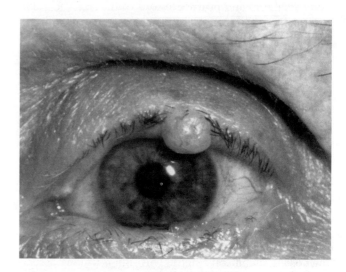

FIGURE 21-9
Squamous papilloma, a benign epithelial tumor, is characterized by a cauliflower-like, multilobed lesion.

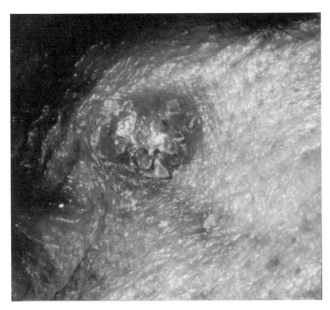

FIGURE 21-10
Keratoacanthoma. Note the central crater filled with keratin debris.

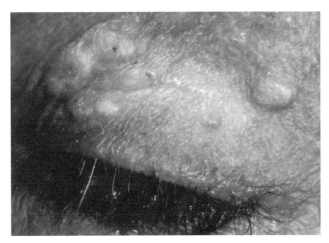

FIGURE 21-11
Sebaceous inclusion cysts.

Nevi

Nevi (moles) are common benign melanocytic tumors. They are located in the dermis or at the dermoepithelial junction. They vary widely in color and shape (i.e., flat, domed, or pedunculated) and can occur in any age group.[41]

Most nevi remain benign and only need to be surgically excised for cosmetic considerations. Some acquired dysplastic nevi, however, can develop into malignant melanoma. It is therefore important to carefully monitor large, irregularly shaped, or pigmented nevi for change. These lesions should be biopsied if changes are noted.[41,42]

Keratoacanthoma

Keratoacanthoma is a skin lesion that is found most commonly in middle-aged and older adults. It is usually a firm, elevated, reddish lesion exhibiting a central crater filled with keratin debris (Figure 21-10). Although benign, keratoacanthomas grow rapidly and are often mistaken for malignant lesions such as basal cell and squamous cell carcinomas.[39,43,44]

Conservative management of keratoacanthomas involves careful monitoring, as many of these lesions resolve spontaneously without treatment. Large or recalcitrant lesions, and particularly those involving the lid margin or lashes, can be removed with surgical excision, curettage, or electrocautery.[43,44]

Inclusion Cysts

The most common types of inclusion cysts found on the lids are congenital epidermoid, acquired epidermal, and sebaceous cysts (Figure 21-11). Epidermoid and epidermal cysts are formed when squamous epithelial cells are trapped under the cutaneous surface. Hyperplastic sebaceous glands form sebaceous cysts, which appear as yellowish, doughnut-shaped lesions that may have associated comedones (blackheads). These are most commonly found in sun-exposed areas of the skin in older adults.

For cosmetic purposes, inclusion cysts may be surgically excised. It is important to completely remove the inner wall of the cyst to prevent recurrence.[39,40,43]

Xanthelasma

Xanthelasma (xanthoma) is a yellow, plaquelike lesion that is typically found on the lids near the nasal canthus (Figure 21-12). It is composed of cells containing cholesterol and other lipids. These lesions are more commonly found in adults with hyperlipidemia or diabetes.

Xanthelasmas may be removed surgically or with dichloroacetic acid if they are cosmetically unacceptable. A serum lipid panel should also be ordered to rule out hyperlipidemia in these patients.[43,44]

Keratoses

There are two basic types of keratoses that involve the lids: seborrheic and actinic. Seborrheic keratoses are benign brownish lesions that are most commonly seen in older patients (Figure 21-13A). They have a waxy or slightly

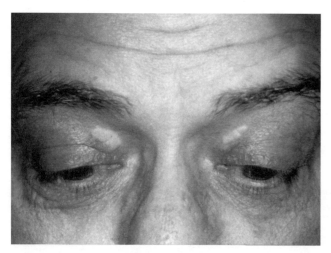

FIGURE 21-12
Xanthelasma lesions are typically yellow, plaquelike lesions occurring on the lids near the nasal canthus.

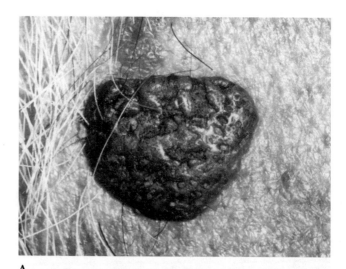

A

B

FIGURE 21-13
A. Seborrheic keratosis. The borders are well-defined and the surface is waxy and slightly scaly. B. Actinic keratosis. These lesions are yellowish and have a very scaly, rough appearance.

scaly surface, well-defined borders, and a characteristic "stuck on" appearance.

Actinic keratoses, although benign, are precursors to squamous cell carcinomas in 25% of cases. They are most commonly found in older adults on areas of the skin that have been chronically exposed to the sun. Actinic keratoses are yellowish, rough, crusty lesions that bleed easily (Figure 21-13B). They occasionally form cutaneous horns.[39,40]

Keratoses should be monitored carefully and can be removed with cryotherapy, electrocautery, or surgical excision. Judicious application of sunscreens can prevent the occurrence of actinic keratoses.[39,40,45]

MALIGNANT LID TUMORS

Basal Cell Carcinoma

Basal cell carcinomas are the most common type of skin cancer in the United States and account for approximately 90% of all malignant eyelid tumors. They usually occur in fair-skinned older adults in areas of the skin that have received chronic sun exposure. A basal cell carcinoma typically presents as a nodular lesion with pearly borders that may have telangiectatic vessels coursing over them. The center of the lesion is often umbilicated and may erode, resulting in a "rodent ulcer" appearance (Figure 21-14).[45,46]

Basal cell carcinomas rarely metastasize but can be locally invasive and destructive to tissues if left untreated. Those lesions in the nasal canthus region, in particular, can be lethal if they invade beyond the orbit. Basal cell carcinomas are treated by surgical excision, cryosurgery, electro-

surgery, irradiation, or combinations of these modalities. They may also be prevented through the conscientious use of sunscreens and by avoiding excessive sun exposure.[45,46]

Squamous Cell Carcinoma

Squamous cell carcinomas are the second most common type of skin cancer occurring in the United States and are typically found in fair-skinned older adults. Although uncommon on the lids, the lesions occasionally present there as elevated, scaly red plaques. They bleed easily and often have a central ulceration that is covered by a serosanguinous crust.[45,46]

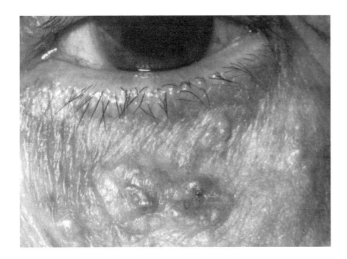

FIGURE 21-14
Basal cell carcinomas typically present as a nodular lesion with an umbilicated or eroded center.

Squamous cell carcinoma, unlike basal cell, is likely to metastasize to regional lymphatics. Therefore, aggressive surgical removal of these lesions is the treatment of choice.[45,46]

Malignant Melanoma

Malignant melanomas, although uncommon, account for approximately 65% of skin cancer–related deaths. They are derived from melanocytes and may develop from a dysplastic nevus or a lentigo maligna (Hutchinson's freckle), or they may appear spontaneously. A simple mnemonic, "ABCD," can help the practitioner remember the main clinical features of melanoma: "A" refers to *Asymmetry* of the lesion, either horizontal or vertical; "B" refers to *Border* irregularity; "C" refers to *Color* variation within a single lesion, ranging from black to blue, red, or white; and "D" refers to the *Diameter* of the lesion, which is typically greater than 6 mm.[42,47]

Any pigmented lesion exhibiting the features mentioned or that has changed in size or shape suggests a malignant melanoma, and the patient should be referred immediately for biopsy and possible treatment. Tumors that are surgically excised before they reach a depth of 0.75 mm usually have not yet metastasized; deeper tumors have a poorer prognosis and a higher associated mortality rate.[45,47]

Kaposi's Sarcoma

In the United States, Kaposi's sarcoma is usually associated with AIDS and is found in at least one-third of AIDS patients. It is also seen in patients on immunosuppressive

therapy, such as those receiving renal transplants. The nodular or plaquelike skin lesions of Kaposi's sarcoma range in color from pink to dark purple and may become ulcerated. They are most commonly found on the extremities but occasionally occur on the lids.[48,49]

Kaposi's sarcoma lesions on the lids are usually slowly progressive and are managed conservatively. The treatment of choice is radiation therapy. Other treatments include surgical excision, electrosurgery, topical immunotherapy, and systemic chemotherapy.[50]

LID POSITION AND FUNCTION ANOMALIES

Ptosis

Ptosis, a condition in which the upper lid droops in the position of primary gaze, can be classified as either congenital or acquired. Congenital ptosis can further be subdivided into three groups: myogenic (abnormality in the levator muscle), neurogenic (abnormality in the innervation to the muscles of elevation), and aponeurotic (abnormality in the levator aponeurosis.)

Most forms of acquired ptosis can also be classified as myogenic, neurogenic, and aponeurotic. Conditions that can cause acquired ptosis include muscular dystrophy, myasthenia gravis, third nerve palsies, Horner's syndrome, surgical trauma, dermatochalasis, and blepharochalasis.[51]

Treatment of ptosis is based on the underlying pathophysiologic cause. Correction of severe congenital ptosis should be done as early as possible to prevent amblyopia. It is corrected with a variety of surgical procedures including aponeurosis tightening, external levator resection, Müller's muscle shortening, and frontalis suspension. Acquired ptosis is occasionally managed with a spectacle-mounted ptosis crutch; however, surgical procedures similar to those used in congenital ptosis are usually preferred. Dermatochalasis, sometimes classified as pseudoptosis rather than true ptosis, is treated with blepharoplasty.[51-53]

Blepharospasm

Blepharospasm is an intermittent or constant, involuntary, forced closure of the eyelids. It may be secondary to dry eye, other types of keratitis, or neurologic conditions such as Parkinson's disease. Benign essential blepharospasm has no known cause. It is more common among older people and frequently involves the lower face and oropharynx in addition to the eyelids. This condition may be aggravated by bright light, fatigue, stress, and certain activities, such as driving.[54]

The management of secondary blepharospasm is aimed at treating the underlying cause. For example, ocular lubricant therapy is used to treat blepharospasm secondary to dry eye. Benign essential blepharospasm is often resistant to therapy, although various medications have been used with some success. These drugs include oral anticholinergics, dopamine agonists, benzodiazepines, and antidepressants. Injections of botulinum A toxin at several sites on the lid often provide relief for several months. Those cases that do not respond well to medical therapy can often be managed surgically.[55,56]

Myokymia

Lid myokymia is an intermittent tremor of the orbicularis muscle. These tremors are often not apparent to an observer but can be quite annoying to the patient. They are sometimes precipitated by stress, fatigue, anxiety, anemia, bright light, corneal or conjunctival lesions, or the use of certain drugs including alcohol and tobacco.[57,58]

Often the patient with lid myokymia simply needs reassurance that it will probably resolve spontaneously. If the condition persists, topical antihistamine drops such as antazoline or pheniramine administered four times a day can be effective. In severe or recalcitrant cases, oral promethazine, tripelennamine, or quinine may be needed to provide relief.[57,58]

Lid Retraction

Lid retraction is characterized by the presence of visible sclera between the limbus and lid margin while the eyes are directed in primary gaze. Retraction of the upper lids is usually secondary to Graves' disease (thyroid ophthalmopathy), but is occasionally caused by tumors, surgical overcorrection of ptosis, or Marcus Gunn's jaw-winking syndrome. Retraction of the lower lids is usually iatrogenic, although it can also be associated with ectropion or Graves' disease. Lid lag is a sign often accompanying lid retraction in Graves' disease. Excessive retraction of the lids can lead to exposure keratitis.[59]

Management of the dry eye symptoms associated with lid retraction usually involves the frequent use of ocular lubricants. Cosmetic repair of lid retraction can be done with several different surgical procedures. In the case of Graves' disease, surgical repair should not be initiated until the condition is stable.[59,60]

Ectropion

Ectropion is a partial or complete outward turning of the lower eyelid margin. It is classified as congenital, aton-

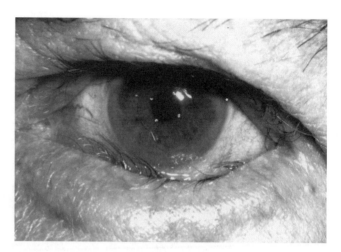

FIGURE 21-15
Entropion of the lower lid with trichiasis.

ic, cicatricial, or inflammatory (allergic). Atonic ectropion can be further classified as involutional, which is caused by age-related tissue relaxation, or paralytic, which is usually caused by seventh nerve palsy or paresis. Chronic ectropion can cause epiphora, exposure keratitis, and conjunctival keratinization.[61]

The use of topical lubricants, moisture chambers, or taping the temporal portion of the lower lid can provide temporary relief from the symptoms associated with ectropion. These therapies are particularly helpful in ectropion secondary to conditions that tend to resolve, such as Bell's palsy. Thermal cautery, lateral tarsorrhaphy, and other surgical techniques are more effective for managing long-standing ectropion such as the involutional type.[61]

Entropion

Entropion is an inward turning of the upper or lower lids that usually causes the cilia to come in contact with the cornea or conjunctiva (trichiasis) (Figure 21-15). This should not be confused with distichiasis, a condition in which there is an extra row of cilia growing near the meibomian orifices. Entropion can be either unilateral or bilateral and can be classified as congenital, involutional, spastic, or cicatricial. Involutional entropion usually involves the lower lid and is caused by age-related changes to the lid muscles and adnexal tissues. Spastic entropion is associated with ocular inflammation, irritation, or surgical trauma. It can occur in any age group but is most common among the elderly.[62]

Applying tape to evert the lid margin is an inexpensive temporary therapy for entropion. Lid suturing techniques can also provide short-term relief. Epilating, freezing cilia with a cryoprobe, or laser ablation can alleviate corneal irritation from associated trichiasis. Various surgical procedures, including horizontal lid tightening and retractor repair, provide a more permanent solution to entropion.[62,63]

Floppy Eyelid Syndrome

Floppy eyelid syndrome is a condition in which the tarsus is pliable and rubbery, allowing the lid to be very easily everted. It is associated with chronic papillary conjunctivitis and punctate epithelial keratitis, presumably caused by pillow contact when the lids evert during sleep. The patient usually complains of irritation, foreign body sensation, and excessive mucous discharge that is worse on awakening.[64]

Lid patching or shielding at night can be used to prevent lid eversion in patients with floppy eyelid syndrome. Surgical techniques aimed at lid shortening or tightening have also been shown to be effective.[65]

LID TRAUMA

Blunt Trauma

Blunt trauma to the lids typically causes ecchymosis (bruising) and edema. Patients with these signs and a history of trauma should be further evaluated for other manifestations of ocular injury such as orbital fracture, hyphema, iridocyclitis, angle recession, cataract, lens subluxation, commotio retinae, retinal tears, choroidal ruptures, or optic nerve avulsion.[66]

Lid edema secondary to trauma tends to resolve over a few days without treatment; however, cool compresses can provide some immediate symptomatic relief and help to reduce swelling. Ecchymosis also tends to resolve spontaneously over a period of days to weeks.[66]

Lacerations

Lid lacerations can range from mild to severe. The presence of any type of lid laceration warrants further investigation to rule out penetrating injuries to the globe and intraocular foreign bodies.[66,67]

In most cases, surgical repair of lid lacerations should be done as soon as possible to prevent undesirable sequelae such as cicatricial entropion, ectropion, or lid notching. Complex cases may involve repair of the globe or lacrimal drainage system in addition to repair of the lids. After repair, a topical antibiotic ointment such as bacitracin is applied to the wound site, and

an oral antibiotic such as dicloxacillin or cephalexin is administered if wound contamination is suspected. In all laceration cases, the patient's tetanus prophylaxis history should be reviewed, and immunization updated, if necessary.[67]

Thermal Burns

A number of agents can cause thermal burns to the lids, including open flames, gunpowder, cigarette ashes, molten metals, and scalding liquids. The eyelid often bears the brunt of these types of injuries in a reflexive effort to spare the cornea and conjunctiva. Manifestations of thermal burns include erythema and edema in superficial burns, blistering and exudation in partial-thickness burns, and necrosis and loss of sensation in full-thickness burns. Charring or loss of lashes may also be noted.[66,68]

Cool compresses can be applied immediately after a burn to reduce lid edema, and antibiotic ointments such as erythromycin or tetracycline can be applied topically as a prophylaxis against secondary infection. More severe burns can be protected with medical silicone rubber (Silastic) foam. Mild to moderate burns tend to resolve without complications, whereas severe burns may result in cicatricial lid deformities that require surgical repair.[66,68]

Chemical Injuries

Numerous chemicals can cause injuries to the lids ranging from mild to severe. In general, alkaline chemicals cause more penetrating and severe injuries to ocular tissue than acids. Chemical burns can cause lid edema, crusting, and sloughing.[69]

Another relatively common type of chemical injury is termed "super glue tarsorrhaphy," or inadvertent adhesion of the upper and lower cilia with cyanoacrylate adhesive. This renders the patient temporarily unable to open the eye.[70]

Chemical burns to the lid should be irrigated immediately with water or saline for several minutes. Other ocular tissues should also be carefully examined for signs of contact with the chemical. After irrigation, the affected lid tissues should be topically treated with an antibiotic ointment such as erythromycin to prevent secondary infection. Severe chemical injuries to the lids may require surgical repair.[69]

Cyanoacrylate adhesions can be quickly managed by cutting off the adherent cilia. Another treatment consists of patching the eye overnight with an eye pad soaked in water or saline. This usually allows the lids to be separated with minimal discomfort the following day.[70]

REFERENCES

1. Jones LT. The Orbital Adnexa. In LT Jones, MJ Roch, JD Wirtschaffer (eds), Ophthalmic Anatomy. Rochester, MN: American Academy of Ophthalmology and Otolaryngology 1970;39–56.
2. Moses RA. The Eyelids. In RA Moses (ed), Adler's Physiology of the Eye: Clinical Application (7th ed). St. Louis: Mosby, 1981;1–15.
3. Warwick R. Eugene Wolff's Anatomy of the Eye and Orbit (7th ed). Philadelphia: Saunders, 1976;181–237.
4. Glasser DB. Angular blepharitis caused by gram-negative bacillus DF-2. Am J Ophthalmol 1986;102:119–20.
5. Baum J. Moraxella. In FT Fraunfelder, FH Roy (eds), Current Ocular Therapy (3rd ed). Philadelphia: Saunders, 1990;29–30.
6. Bowman RW, Dougherty JM, McCulley JP. Chronic blepharitis and dry eyes. Int Ophthalmol Clin 1987;27:27–35.
7. Cokington CD, Hyndiuk RA. Insights from experimental data on ciprofloxacin in the treatment of bacterial keratitis and ocular infections. Am J Ophthalmol 1991;112:25–8.
8. Nozik RA, Smolin G, Knowlton G, Austin R. Trimethoprim-polymyxin B ophthalmic solution in treatment of surface ocular bacterial infections. Ann Ophthalmol 1985;17:746–8.
9. Steinert RF. Current therapy for bacterial keratitis and bacterial conjunctivitis. Am J Ophthalmol 1991;112:10–4.
10. McCulley JP, Dougherty JM, Deneau DG. Classification of chronic blepharitis. Ophthalmology 1982;89:1173–80.
11. Brown DD, McCulley JP. Staphylococcal and Mixed Staphylococcal/Seborrheic Blepharoconjunctivitis. In FT Fraunfelder, FH Roy (eds), Current Ocular Therapy (3rd ed). Philadelphia: Saunders, 1990;525–7.
12. Holsted M, McCulley JP. Seborrheic Blepharitis. In FT Fraunfelder, FH Roy (eds), Current Ocular Therapy (3rd ed). Philadelphia: Saunders, 1990;522–4.
13. Bartlett JD. Diseases of the Eyelids. In JD Bartlett, SD Jaanus (eds), Clinical Ocular Pharmacology (2nd ed). Stoneham, MA: Butterworth, 1989;463–5.
14. Diegel JT. Eyelid problems. Blepharitis, hordeola, and chalazia. Postgrad Med 1986;80:271–2.
15. Fraunfelder FT. Hordeolum. In FT Fraunfelder, FH Roy (eds), Current Ocular Therapy (3rd ed). Philadelphia: Saunders, 1990;510–1.
16. Perry HD, Serniuk RA. Conservative treatment of chalazia. Ophthalmology 1980;87:218–21.
17. Vidaurri LJ, Jacob P. Intralesional corticosteroid treatment of chalazia. Ann Ophthalmol 1986;18:339–40.
18. Friedberg MA, Rapuano CJ. Preseptal Cellulitis. In Wills Eye Hospital Office and Emergency Room Diagnosis and Treatment of Eye Disease. Philadelphia: Lippincott, 1990;137–40.
19. Bartlett JD. Diseases of the Eyelids. In JD Bartlett, SD Jaanus (eds), Clinical Ocular Pharmacology (2nd ed). Stoneham, MA: Butterworth, 1989;466–7.
20. Fulk GW, Clifford C. A case report of demodicosis. J Am Optom Assoc 1990;61:637–9.
21. Clifford CW, Fulk GW. Association of diabetes, lash loss, and Staphylococcus aureus with infestations of eyelids by Demodex folliculorum. J Med Entomol 1990;27:467–70.
22. English FP. Demodicosis. In FT Fraunfelder, FH Roy (eds), Current Ocular Therapy (3rd ed). Philadelphia: Saunders, 1990;106–8.
23. Kincaid MC. Pediculosis and Phthiriasis. In FT Fraunfelder, FH Roy (eds), Current Ocular Therapy (3rd ed). Philadelphia: Saunders, 1990;115–7.
24. Kairys DJ, Webster HJ, Terry JE. Pediatric ocular phthiriasis infestation. J Am Optom Assoc 1988;59:128–30.
25. Melore GG. Verrucae and their treatment. South J Optom 1985;3:20–5.
26. Groden LR, Arentsen JJ. Molluscum Contagiosum. In FT Fraunfelder, FH Roy (eds), Current Ocular Therapy (3rd ed). Philadelphia: Saunders, 1990;87–8.
27. Kohn SR. Molluscum contagiosum in patients with acquired immunodeficiency syndrome [letter]. Arch Ophthalmol 1987;105:458.
28. Darouger S, Wishart MS, Viswalingam ND. Epidemiological and clinical features of primary herpes simplex virus ocular infection. Br J Ophthalmol 1985;69:2–6.
29. Simon JW, Longo F, Smith RS. Spontaneous resolution of herpes simplex blepharoconjunctivitis in children. Am J Ophthalmol 1986;102:598–600.
30. Pavan-Langston D. Varicella-zoster ophthalmicus. Int Ophthalmol Clin 1975;15:171–88.
31. Sandor EV, Millman A, Croxson TS, Midvan D. Herpes zoster ophthalmicus in patients at risk for the acquired immune deficiency syndrome (AIDS). Am J Ophthalmol 1986;101:153–5.
32. Marsh RJ. Herpes Zoster. In FT Fraunfelder, FH Roy (eds), Current Ocular Therapy (3rd ed). Philadelphia: Saunders, 1990;82–4.
33. Cobo LM, Foulks GN, Liesegang T, et al. Oral acyclovir in the therapy of acute herpes zoster ophthalmicus. Ophthalmology 1985;92:1574–83.
34. Friedberg MA, Rapuano CJ. Herpes Zoster Virus. In Wills Eye Hospital Office and Emergency Room Diagnosis and Treatment of Eye Disease. Philadelphia: Lippincott, 1990;76–9.
35. Hogan JD. Pruritis. In FT Fraunfelder, FH Roy (eds). Current Ocular Therapy (3rd ed). Philadelphia: Saunders, 1990;188–91.
36. Abelson MB, Allansmith MR. Ocular Allergies. In G Smolin, RA Thoft (eds), The Cornea (2nd ed). Boston: Little, Brown, 1987;307–21.
37. Jennings BJ. Allergic contact dermatitis. J Am Optom Assoc 1985;56:474–8.
38. Rich LF, Hamifin JM. Ocular complications of atopic dermatitis and other eczemas. Int Ophthalmol Clin 1985;25:61–76.
39. Findley HM. Eyelid tumors. South J Optom 1986;4:60–4.
40. Rodriquez-Sains RS. The aging face: commonly encountered tumors and cutaneous changes. Adv Ophthal Plast Reconstr Surg 1983;2:9–18.
41. Lazarus GS, Goldsmith A. Diagnosis of Skin Disease. Philadelphia: FA Davis, 1981;4–13.
42. Freidman RJ, Rigel DS, Kopf AW. Early detection of malignant melanoma: the role of the physician examination and self examination of the skin. CA 1985;35:4–25.

43. Smith ME. The Eyelids. In ME Smith (ed), External Disease and Cornea. Basic and Clinical Science Course. San Francisco: American Academy of Ophthalmology, 1988;143–206.

44. Friedberg MA, Rapuano CJ. Malignant Tumors of the Eyelid. In Wills Eye Hospital Office and Emergency Room Diagnosis and Treatment of Eye Disease. Philadelphia: Lippincott, 1990;140–3.

45. Kaminester LH. Skin cancer—diagnosis and treatment. Hosp Med 1990;26:99–115.

46. Stegman SJ. Basal cell carcinoma and squamous cell carcinoma: recognition and treatment. Med Clin North Am 1986;70:95–107.

47. Chanda JJ. The clinical recognition and prognostic factors of primary cutaneous malignant melanoma. Med Clin North Am 1986;70:39–55.

48. Bezan D. An overview of dermatology for primary care providers. J Am Optom Assoc 1991;62:138–45.

49. Muggin FM, Lonberg M. Kaposi's sarcoma and AIDS. Med Clin North Am 1986;70:139–54.

50. Safai B. Kaposi's Sarcoma. In FT Fraunfelder, FH Roy (eds), Current Ocular Therapy (3rd ed). Philadelphia: Saunders, 1990;294–6.

51. Beard C, Sullivan JH. Ptosis—current concepts. Int Ophthalmol Clin 1978;18:53–73.

52. Anderson RL, Dixon RS. Aponeurotic ptosis surgery. Arch Ophthalmol 1979;97:1123–8.

53. Cohen MB. Case history: use of a bilateral ptosis crutch. N Engl J Optom 1987;40:26–7.

54. Jankovic J, Ford J. Blepharospasm and orofacial-cervical dystonia. Clinical and pharmacological findings in 100 patients. Ann Neurol 1983;13:402–11.

55. Engstrom PF, Arnoult JB, Mazow ML, et al. Effectiveness of botulinum toxin therapy for essential blepharospasm. Ophthalmology 1987;94:971–5.

56. Gillum WN, Anderson RL. Blepharospasm surgery: an anatomical approach. Arch Ophthalmol 1981;99:1056–62.

57. Jaffe NS, Shults WT. Lid Myokymia. In FT Fraunfelder, FH Roy (eds), Current Ocular Therapy (3rd ed). Philadelphia: Saunders, 1990;513.

58. Bartlett JD. Diseases of the Eyelids. In JD Bartlett, SD Jaanus (eds), Clinical Ocular Pharmacology (2nd ed). Boston: Butterworth, 1989;477.

59. Heffernam JT, Tentel RR. Lid Retraction. In FT Fraunfelder, FH Roy (eds), Current Ocular Therapy (3rd ed). Philadelphia: Saunders, 1990;514–5.

60. Cooper WC. The surgical management of the lid changes in Graves' disease. Ophthalmology 1979;86:2071–80.

61. Frueh BR, Schoengarth LD. Evaluation and treatment of the patient with ectropion. Ophthalmology 1982;89:1049–54.

62. Dailey RA. Entropion. In FT Fraunfelder, FH Roy (eds), Current Ocular Therapy (3rd ed). Philadelphia: Saunders, 1990;502–5.

63. Wesley RE, Collins JW. Combined procedure for senile entropion. Ophthalmic Surg 1983;14:401–5.

64. Culbertson WW, Ostler HB. The floppy eyelid syndrome. Am J Ophthalmol 1981;92:568–75.

65. Moore MB, Harrington J, McCulley JP, et al. Floppy eyelid syndrome management including surgery. Ophthalmology 1986;93:184–8.

66. Eagling EM, Roper-Hall MJ. Eye Injuries: An Illustrated Guide. Philadelphia: Lippincott, 1986;4.2–5.4.

67. Friedberg MA, Rapuano CJ. Eyelid Laceration. In Wills Eye Hospital Office and Emergency Room Diagnosis and Treatment of Eye Disease. Philadelphia: Lippincott, 1990;25–9.

68. Burns CL, Chylack LT. Thermal burns: the management of thermal burns of the lids and globe. Ann Ophthalmol 1979;11:1358–68.

69. Pfister RR. Chemical injuries of the eye. Ophthalmology 1983;90:1246–53.

70. Raynor LA. Treatment for inadvertent cyanoacrylate tarsorrhaphy. Arch Ophthalmol 1988;106:1033.

22

Diseases of the Conjunctiva, Cornea, and Sclera

GARY E. OLIVER

Diseases of the conjunctiva, cornea, and sclera are encountered worldwide and affect patients of any age, race, sex, or socioeconomic level.[1] Conjunctivitis and keratitis may originate from both infectious and inflammatory causes. Potential causes include allergy, bacteria, dermatologic conditions of the eyelids, mechanical irritation, toxins, trauma, viruses, and systemic diseases. Conjunctivitis is often related to epidemic outbreaks of infectious disease in endemic environments. Keratitis is often directly related to contact lens wear. Episcleritis and scleritis are frequently related to systemic inflammatory diseases and require appropriate laboratory testing to accurately assess associated causes. In many cases, primary conjunctivitis is self-limiting and resolves without intervention. However, keratitis usually requires intervention with pharmaceutical agents. Although episcleritis is frequently self-limiting, topical steroid therapy usually improves patient comfort and lessens the duration and severity of the disease. Management of scleritis must be aggressive. Treatment with topical and systemic steroids is necessary to avoid sight-threatening consequences.

As with any ocular disease process, the clinician's ability to properly manage these conditions depends on his or her ability to recognize and properly diagnose the numerous clinical presentations of a particular entity. Timely therapy with the appropriate medication can lessen the severity and reduce both the duration and morbidity of the disease. This chapter discusses the most frequently encountered diseases of the conjunctiva, cornea, and sclera, with emphasis on both diagnosis and treatment of each condition.

REVIEW OF ANATOMY

Conjunctiva

The conjunctiva is a mucous membrane that, anatomically and clinically, may be divided into three sections: palpebral or tarsal conjunctiva, fornix conjunctiva, and bulbar conjunctiva.[2] The conjunctiva covers the inner portions of the eyelids and is reflected onto the globe over the anterior episclera and sclera. Developing from surface ectoderm, the membrane consists of nonkeratinized epithelium overlying a substantia propria or stroma containing connective tissue and a rich vascular network. The palpebral conjunctiva begins at the posterior lid margin and extends posteriorly toward the fornix. The keratinized epithelium of the eyelids gradually transforms into the moist stratified epithelium forming the mucous membrane of the conjunctiva.

Mucin-secreting goblet cells, the main source of mucin within the tear layer, are found in the conjunctival fornix tissue.[3] Loss of goblet cell density may result in complications ranging from mild dry eye to severe cicatricial changes. Most of the immune system cellular components are found in the substantia propria. Accumulations of lymphocytes, lymphoid follicles, neutrophils, plasma cells, and mast cells are located within the stroma and proliferate extensively in conjunctival inflammatory disease. This proliferation leads to the formation of papillae and follicles.[4-7]

The conjunctival fornix encircles the anterior portion of the globe, beginning and ending at the medially located plica semilunaris and caruncle.[6] The fornix is loosely adherent to the underlying stroma with a fold of tissue that permits free motion during eye movements. An abundance of lymphoid follicles and inflammatory cells are found in the lower fornix. The accessory lacrimal glands of Krause are predominantly located in the substantia propria of the superior conjunctival fornix, with a few glands situated in the lower fornix as well.

The conjunctiva is reflected onto the globe from the fornix to form the bulbar conjunctiva, which overlies Tenon's capsule and merges with the limbal cornea.[2]

Many sensitive unmyelinated nerve fibers and free nerve endings are found in the limbal conjunctival substantia propria along with a complex network of perilimbal vessels and vascular arcades. Medially, the bulbar conjunctiva is bordered by the caruncle, which forms a mucocutaneous junction between the bulbar conjunctiva and the epidermis of the skin. Accessory lacrimal glands may occasionally be located in the caruncle.[2]

Cornea

The cornea consists of five distinct layers that form a transparent, refracting surface for the eye. This avascular, acellular tissue must be properly hydrated to maintain its transparency. The five layers anterior to posterior include the epithelium, Bowman's membrane, the stroma, Descemet's membrane, and the endothelial cell layer (Figure 22-1).[7]

The epithelial layer is composed of multiple layers of nonkeratinized squamous epithelium overlying a basal layer of cuboidal cells that secrete a basement membrane. The epithelial cells are joined by tight junctions and attached to Bowman's membrane by hemidesmosomes. The quality of the hemidesmosomal junctions plays an important role in recurrent corneal erosion and some corneal dystrophies.

Bowman's layer is a hyalinized layer of stroma that covers the entire cornea except for the most peripheral 1 mm of tissue adjacent to the limbus. Bowman's layer does not regenerate if damaged.

The stroma, which constitutes 90% of the corneal thickness, consists of layers of collagen lamellae, which run parallel to the corneal surface. Keratocytes within the stroma produce the collagen material. Although many ciliary vessels are present at the limbus, the stroma is avascular. It does contain numerous unmyelinated nerves that also traverse through the epithelium.

Descemet's membrane is a true membrane that can regenerate following insult. Schwalbe's line forms the peripheral termination of Descemet's membrane as well as the anterior boundary of the trabecular meshwork. The innermost or most posterior corneal layer is the endothelium, a single layer of cuboidal cells rich in mitochondria. These cells regulate corneal hydration through an active transport mechanism.[2,7] Nourishment to the cornea is provided by the aqueous humor, limbal vasculature, and tear film. The mechanical flushing effect of the tear film along with its circulating immunoglobulins and enzymes provide a natural defense against infection for the cornea.[8]

Sclera

The scleral layer of the globe provides the eye with most of its rigidity and shape. The thickness of the sclera ranges from 0.3 mm at the extraocular muscle insertion sites to 1 mm elsewhere. Anteriorly the sclera joins with the cornea and posteriorly it joins with the dural covering of the optic nerve. The sclera is composed of closely packed, interlacing layers of collagen; there are scattered dendritic melanocytes along its inner side forming the lamina fusca adjacent to the choroid. Emissary channels within the sclera permit penetration by the ciliary vessels, nerves, and vortex veins.[2,7] The optic nerve penetrates the back of the eye through the modified scleral structure known as the lamina cribrosa. Here, scleral collagen fibers actually interdigitate between bundles of nerve axons. Occasionally, a bending of the long anterior ciliary nerves toward the scleral outer surface produces Axenfeld's anomaly, a benign pigmented spot that is usually located posterior to the limbus overlying the ciliary body.[9] The outer surface of the sclera consists of the episclera, a highly vascularized, fine elastic layer that blends superficially with Tenon's capsule, which is a relatively loose, avascular connective tissue layer that surrounds the globe. Anteriorly, near the limbus, Tenon's capsule diminishes in thickness as it blends with the episcleral tissue as well as the overlying conjunctiva (Figure 22-2).[7] The blood vessels of the episclera contribute to the nourishment of the sclera.

CLINICAL SIGNS OF INFLAMMATION

Conjunctiva

The clinical signs exhibited by the conjunctival inflammatory response usually depend on the nature of the causative agent. Acute or chronic conjunctivitis may exhibit any of the five clinical manifestations of conjunctival inflammation, including chemosis, hyperemia, discharge or exudate, papillae, and follicles (Table 22-1). Increased vascular permeability resulting from the ocular response to antigens, infectious agents, toxins, or other environmental stimuli, such as smoke or wind, often results in hyperemia, chemosis, or exudative discharge. Exudative conjunctival discharge may be serous, mucoid, purulent, fibrinous, or hemorrhagic.[10,11] Fibrinous cellular debris may cause the formation of membranes or pseudomembranes, which is a sign of severe inflammation requiring aggressive management. "True" conjunctival membranes are firmly attached to the underlying epithelium and when removed cause bleeding because of a denuding of the epithelial surface. "Pseudomembranes" are more loosely attached to the conjunctival epithelium and are more easily removed, causing little or no bleeding.[11]

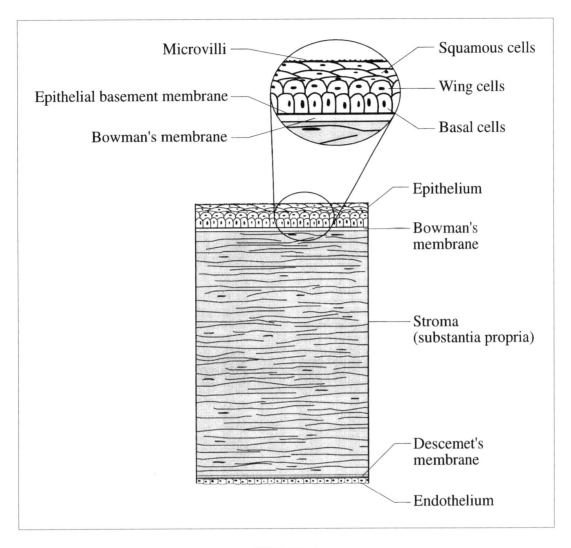

FIGURE 22-1

Anatomy of the cornea. The five basic layers of the cornea include the epithelium, Bowman's membrane, the stroma, Descemet's membrane, and the endothelial cell layer. The epithelium consists of five to six layers of cells that become thinner in shape the more superficial their location. The most superficial squamous epithelial cells exhibit tiny microvilli, which are covered by the mucin layer of the tear film. The deepest epithelial cells are the basal cells, which are columnar in shape and have rounded tops. Bowman's membrane is relatively invisible clinically and is acellular. It blends with the underlying stroma, which accounts for about 90% of the corneal thickness. Descemet's membrane is the basement membrane for the single layer of flattened endothelial cells along the posterior corneal surface. (Courtesy of Daniel K. Roberts, O.D.)

Papillary conjunctival hypertrophy represents a nonspecific inflammatory response occurring commonly with allergic or bacterial conjunctivitis (Figure 22-3). Individual papillae are characterized by usually small but variably sized conjunctival elevations that contain a tiny central vascular tuft. The central vessel is the source of cellular infiltration of the substantia propria by inflammatory cellular material such as eosinophils, lymphocytes, mast cells, and polymorphonuclear leukocytes.[2,10,11] Diffusely distributed, small papillae give the conjunctiva a velvety appearance.

Follicles result from focal lymphoid hyperplasia commonly in response to chlamydial, viral, or toxic causes. Their clinical appearance consists of elevated, rounded lesions that

FIGURE 22-2

Anatomy of the sclera. The three layers of the sclera include the episclera, the stroma, and the innermost layer, the lamina fusca. The episclera, which blends with the scleral stroma, is composed of loose connective tissue and is highly vascularized compared with the relatively avascular stromal layer. The episclera blends superficially with Tenon's capsule, an even looser connective tissue layer that is relatively avascular. Clinically, the episclera can be identified by its immobile and deeper vasculature compared with the conjunctival blood vessels, which are more superficial and may shift slightly during blinking. The lamina fusca is exaggerated in the drawing and is actually characterized by modified inner scleral lamellae, which blend with the suprachoroidal and supraciliary lamellae. (Courtesy of Daniel K. Roberts, O.D.)

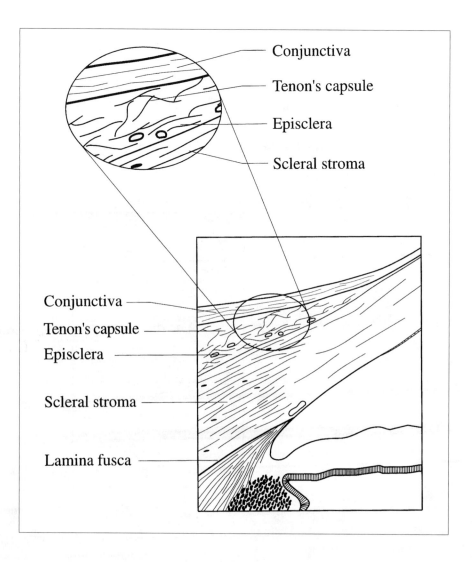

are translucent to whitish-gray in color (Figure 22-4). Small vessels may course along their surface, but there is no central vascular tuft. Germinal cells (immature lymphocytes) and macrophages are found in the central portion of the lesions with mature cells occurring peripherally. Follicles are routinely observed near the fornices of the normal eye and in this instance do indicate specific disease. In pathologic conditions they may be more pronounced than usual near the fornices and commonly occur more centrally along the lower palpebral conjunctival surface. In some situations follicles may be fairly pronounced along the superior palpebral surface, and they may occur near the limbus as well.[2,10,11] Limbal follicles are often secondary to chlamydial disease.

Cornea

Corneal insult may be characterized by edema, neovascularization, superficial punctate keratopathy, infiltra-tion, ulceration, or combinations of these.[12,13] Limbal injection, either segmental or circumlimbal, is the most easily recognizable and frequently encountered clinical response to corneal irritation and may be caused by any condition affecting the cornea such as abrasion, infectious ulceration, toxic irritation, immune responses, drying, or contact lens-related hypoxia.[12,14]

Leukocytic infiltration of the cornea occurs in many infectious and inflammatory conditions and its location, delineation, density, and color as well as the characteristics of the overlying epithelium are often important in determining the cause of conditions affecting the cornea[13] (Table 22-2). The precise cellular composition of corneal infiltrates depends on the nature of the immunologic response. For example, acute infectious disease typically causes greater infiltration of polymorphonuclear leukocytes or monocytes, whereas chronic infection results in mononuclear cell infiltration.[2]

TABLE 22-1

Clinical Manifestations of Conjunctival Inflammation

Clinical Entity	Physical Appearance	Pathophysiologic/Histologic Findings
Chemosis	Edematous, swollen tissue	Increased vascular permeability
Hyperemia	Pale to bright red engorged vessels	Increased vascular permeability
Exudates		
Serous	Clear, watery discharge	Increased vascular permeability
Mucoid	Clear to yellowish tinged, translucent, sticky or stringy discharge	Increased mucus from goblet cell irritation
Mucopurulent	Yellowish white, less translucent, sticky discharge	Increased mucus combined with inflammatory cells, such as eosinophils and macrophages
Purulent	Yellowish white to yellowish green tinged, opaque, thick discharge	High concentration of inflammatory cells, such as polymorphonuclear leukocytes and macrophages
Fibrinous	White, opaque, flat appearing discharge that follows contour of conjunctiva and may be attached to the underlying tissue	High degree of fibrin mixed with inflammatory cells, such as polymorphonuclear leukocytes and macrophages
Hemorrhagic	Red streaked discharge that may also have any of the above characteristics	Red blood cells in discharge from increased vascular permeability or trauma
Papillae	Elevations of conjunctival epithelium and stroma with a delineating margin and small central vascular tuft; when papillae are small, conjunctiva has velvety appearance	Cellular infiltration of the substantia propria by inflammatory cellular material such as eosinophils, lymphocytes, mast cells, and polymorphonuclear leukocytes
Follicles	Elevated, avascular, rounded lesions, translucent to whitish gray, commonly located in fornices; small vessels may course along surface; no central vascular tuft is present	Germinal cells (immature lymphocytes) and macrophages constitute central portion with mature cells forming the periphery

Source: Reprinted and modified with permission from GE Oliver, CJ Quinn, JJ Thimons. Diseases of the Conjunctiva. In JD Bartlett, SD Jaanus (eds), Clinical Ocular Pharmacology (3rd ed). Boston: Butterworth-Heinemann, 1995;633.

Ulceration of the cornea occurs in the presence of high concentrations of inflammatory cells, offending microbial organisms (especially those that secrete collagenolytic or proteolytic enzymes), bacterial toxins, or toxic chemicals. Persistent mechanical irritation of the cornea may provide the initial insult to the corneal epithelium leading to the accumulation of inflammatory cells. Mucopurulent or purulent exudate in the presence of an epithelial defect is always an indication to rule out bacterial ulcerative keratitis and should be managed as such until proven otherwise.[2,12,13]

Episclera and Sclera

Inflammation of the episclera and sclera typically causes increased vascular permeability and hyperemia. Conjunctival injection can be relatively easily differentiated from superficial and deep episcleral injection with careful stereoscopic slit lamp examination because of a relatively superficial location and slight movement exhibited during blinking or on digital pressure through the lid margin. Under gross observation, conjunctival injection is more bright red in color, whereas episcleral injection may exhibit a relative violaceous hue that is most pronounced when the deepest episcleral vessels are engorged.

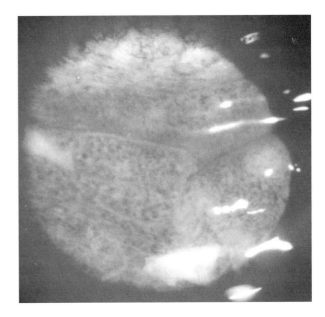

FIGURE 22-3

Papillary hypertrophy of the lower palpebral conjunctiva. Clinically, papillae are small, closely packed elevations with reddish tips that are caused by a centrally located dilated vessel tuft. (Courtesy of Sara L. Penner, O.D.)

FIGURE 22-4
Follicular hypertrophy of the lower palpebral conjunctiva. Follicles are rounded, dome-shaped, translucent elevations. They are much larger than most papillae and are found routinely near the fornices. They may occur normally or they may also result from chlamydial, viral, and toxic causes. (Courtesy of Sara L. Penner, O.D.)

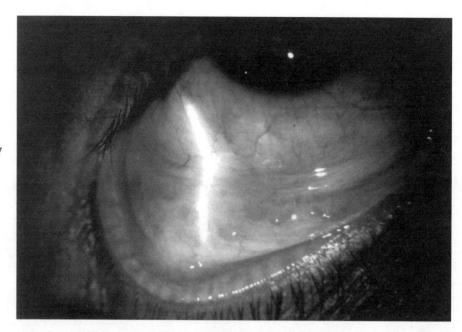

TABLE 22-2
Clinical Differentiation of Corneal Infiltrates

Characteristic	Noninfectious	Infectious
Location	Peripheral	Central
Margins	Distinct	Hazy or not well defined
Depth	Isolated to single layer of cornea	Involves multiple layers of cornea
Overlying epithelium	Intact, although mild overlying stippling stain is possible	Distinct epithelial break or defect
Color	White or grayish white	Dark gray or yellowish or green tinge
Size	No correlation	No correlation
Anterior chamber reaction	No correlation	No correlation

Differentiating between superficial injection within the parietal episcleral layer and injection of the deeper visceral episcleral layer can be more challenging. Injection within both of these layers occurs with episcleritis and scleritis, but the pronounced deep injection may be indicative of scleritis, a more serious disease than episcleritis.[15,16] Scleritis will always produce a concurrent episcleritis, but scleral inflammation will not always be present when there is episcleral inflammation. Infiltration and nodule formation may occur with either condition and may be helpful in differentiation. Episcleral nodules are more superficial and are moveable with pressure from the lid, but scleral nodules are fixed and distort the contour of the translucent or opaque scleral tissue, which can be visualized with a thin slit beam.

BACTERIAL DISEASES

Acute Bacterial Conjunctivitis

Acute bacterial conjunctivitis typically causes a red eye characterized with a mucopurulent or purulent discharge. Hyperemia is usually diffuse in nature and tends to be more intense within the palpebral and fornix conjunctiva compared with the limbal region. This may result, in part, from a higher concentration of bacterial toxins becoming trapped and accumulating in the fornix regions.

Patients often report pronounced foreign body sensation as well as other relatively nonspecific complaints such as photophobia, burning, general discomfort, and aching. Although common with other conditions affecting the eye such as the viral infection epidemic keratoconjunctivitis, adhesion of the eyelids upon waking is usually more typical of a prominent mucopurulent discharge associated with bacterial infections of the eye. In many cases of acute bacterial conjunctivitis, the fellow eye becomes involved 2–3 days later.

Acute bacterial conjunctivitis is most often caused by *Staphylococcus aureus*, *Streptococcus pneumoniae*, or *Haemophilus influenzae*.[17] The latter two organisms may sometimes cause an associated infectious otitis media in pediatric patients.[18,19] Although acute bacterial conjunctivitis is often diagnosed based on clinical presentation, conjunctival scrapings and smears may help confirm the diagnosis. Cytologic examination with a Giemsa-type stain or Diff-Quik (Baxter Scientific Products, McGraw Park, IL) staining usually shows increased numbers of polymorphonuclear leukocytes.

Since most acute bacterial conjunctivitides are self-limiting, therapy is designed to minimize patient symptomatology, lessen the duration of disease, and prevent recurrence or spread to the fellow eye. Topical broad-spectrum antibiotic solutions are effective for treating mild to moderate acute bacterial conjunctivitis. Gentamicin, tobramycin, or trimethoprim/polymyxin B solutions applied four times a day for 7–10 days is an appropriate initial dosage.[20,21] In more severe cases, ciprofloxacin, norfloxacin, or ofloxacin may be indicated.[22–25] An antibiotic ointment such as bacitracin/polymyxin B or gentamicin may be easier to administer in pediatric cases. All patients with severe purulent conjunctivitis and those who do not respond to initial therapy should undergo cytologic examination and culturing of specimens. Identification of a particular bacterial cause should then be managed with more specific therapy based on antibiotic sensitivity testing.

Chronic Bacterial Conjunctivitis

Chronic bacterial conjunctivitis often presents bilaterally with nonspecific symptoms; these may include general discomfort, foreign body sensation, burning, tearing, and sticky eyelids. The conjunctiva may exhibit mild diffuse hyperemia, a mucoid or mucopurulent discharge, and a papillary or mixed reaction. The condition is often associated with blepharitis. In long-standing cases, there may be secondary corneal involvement consisting of epithelial edema, limbal injection, superficial neovascularization, and peripheral infiltrates.

Staphylococcus aureus and *Moraxella lacunata* are very common offending microbial organisms, and *Staphylococcus epidermidis* may be implicated as well. Overgrowth of normal bacterial flora occurs often, especially in the presence of chronically altered tear film composition, which is frequently associated with chronic blepharitis, either primary or secondary to conditions such as acne rosacea. Environmental factors such as air pollution, allergies, and contact lens wear may influence the nature of the host's immunologic response to the offending organism. Studying the cytologic features of conjunctival scrapings as well as culturing of specimens are often useful in evaluating chronic bacterial conjunctivitis. Scrapings usually demonstrate an increased number of polymorphonuclear leukocytes.[17,26,27]

Proper lid hygiene is critical in the management of chronic bacterial conjunctivitis. Lid therapy consisting of warm compresses, lid massage, and lid scrubs is often necessary for satisfactory resolution. Concurrent application of a bacitracin/polymyxin B or erythromycin ointment three times a day for 10 days along with the lid hygiene regimen may be helpful to eradicate the lid bacterial component. Trimethoprim/polymyxin B or gentamicin solution four times a day for 10 days can be effective in managing the conjunctivitis.

Hyperacute Bacterial Conjunctivitis

Hyperacute bacterial conjunctivitis is characterized by a sudden, rapid onset of purulent conjunctivitis with a copious discharge, chemosis, and severe hyperemia. The rapidly forming purulent discharge reaccumulates quickly if it is wiped away (Figure 22-5). There is often associated pain and tenderness of the globe, periorbital discomfort, and lid swelling. Concurrent preauricular lymphadenopathy and preseptal cellulitis with associated fever occur in many cases. If not managed properly, hyperacute conjunctivitis can lead to conjunctival membrane or symblepharon formation as well as to bacterial keratitis that could possibly cause ulceration and perforation.

Neisseria gonorrhoeae is the most common cause of hyperacute conjunctivitis afflicting primarily neonates and sexually active adolescents or young adults.[17] A less frequent cause is *Neisseria meningitidis*.[28] Several other pathogens can also cause hyperacute conjunctivitis, including *Staphylococcus aureus*, *Streptococcus* species, *Haemophilus influenzae*, *Escherichia coli*, and *Pseudomonas aeruginosa*.[17] Laboratory assessment consisting of both conjunctival scrapings/smears and cultures with antibiotic sensitivity testing is mandatory in the treatment of hyperacute conjunctivitis (Table 22-3).

Treatment must be aggressive, since potentially blinding complications may result. After the collection of smear and culture specimens, appropriate topical antibiotic therapy should be immediately instituted. A fluoroquinolone antibiotic or a fortified antibiotic solution is often indicated for the therapy of hyperacute conjunctivitis.[22–25,29] As examples, topical ciprofloxacin, norfloxacin, or

FIGURE 22-5
Copious purulent discharge associated with hyperacute bacterial conjunctivitis. (Reprinted with permission from GE Oliver, CJ Quinn, JJ Thimons. Diseases of the Conjunctiva. In JD Bartlett, SD Jaanus [eds], Clinical Ocular Pharmacology [3rd ed]. Boston: Butterworth-Heinemann, 1995;641.)

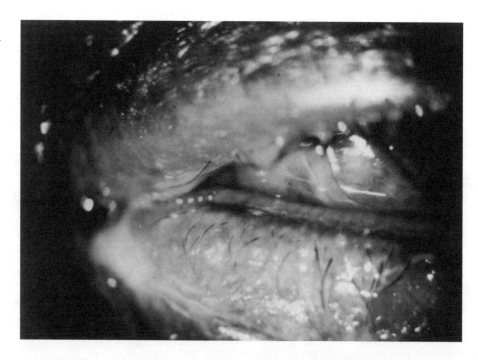

TABLE 22-3
Standard Microbiologic Analysis for Routine Assessment of External Ocular Disease

Culture techniques
Inoculate all of the following media
   1. Blood agar
   2. Chocolate agar
   3. Thioglycolate broth
   4. Sabouraud's agar

Smear techniques
Stain microscope slide smear as follows
   1. Bacterial analysis—Gram stain
   2. Inflammatory cell analysis—Giemsa stain

Special tests
Commercial detection kits are available for herpes simplex, *Chlamydia trachomatis*, and general viruses (i.e., adenovirus)

ofloxacin should be administered initially every hour. After laboratory results of the conjunctival scrapings or cultures are known, fortified bacitracin, gentamicin, tobramycin, cefazolin, or carbenicillin solutions can be substituted for the initial therapy if indicated. Dosages are tapered as the condition responds.

If *Neisseria gonorrhoeae* is confirmed, 1 g ceftriaxone intramuscularly with 1 g probenecid orally should be given daily for up to 5 days.[27,30] If *Staphylococcus aureus, Streptococcus* species, *Haemophilus influenzae, Escherichia coli,* or *Pseudomonas aeruginosa* are identified or suspected, adjunct systemic therapy with an appropriate penicillin or cephalosporin should be added to the topi-

cal regimen. Depending on the coverage desired, therapy may include 500 mg amoxicillin three times a day orally for 10 days or cephalexin 250 mg four times a day orally for 10 days for an average adult. Frequent irrigation of the conjunctival fornices with normal saline will help remove the purulent exudate, thus permitting better antibiotic contact with the affected tissues.

Phlyctenular Keratoconjunctivitis

Phlyctenular keratoconjunctivitis is characterized by an irritated or painful red eye characterized with inflammatory conjunctival or corneal nodules that form as a result of a delayed, or cell-mediated, hypersensitivity response to foreign antigenic material. The nodules most often form near the limbus but may occasionally occur away from this location in isolation within the conjunctiva or cornea. Limbal phlyctenules appear as white, elevated mounds of tissue with surrounding haziness and infiltration. Sectoral conjunctival injection may be very marked adjacent to the lesions.

Limbal phlyctenules may remain in the same location, undergoing spontaneous resolution after necrosis and flattening of the elevated mound. They may also migrate toward the central cornea, causing a track of scarring and vascularization (Figure 22-6). Multiple attacks of corneal phlyctenulosis may lead to severe visual loss, a more common occurrence in underdeveloped countries where therapy is often inadequate.

Historically, the offending antigen has been noted to be *Mycobacterium tuberculosis*, but most cases in the Unit-

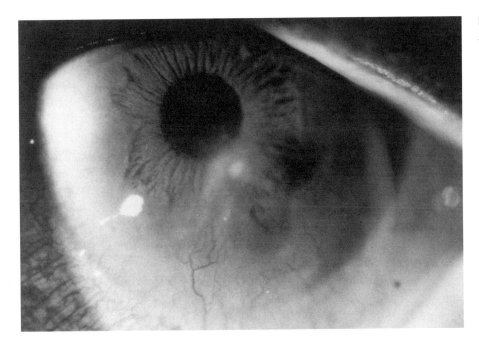

FIGURE 22-6
A corneal phlyctenule that has migrated toward the central cornea, creating a trail of thinning and vascularization. Treatment with topical corticosteroids resulted in clearing of the infiltrate and involution of the associated neovascularization. (Courtesy of Vasvi Amin-Babu, O.D., and Daniel K. Roberts, O.D.)

ed States are caused by *Staphylococcus aureus*.[31] *Chlamydia trachomatis* should be considered as a possible cause in children.[32] Other possible etiologic agents include *Candida albicans*, coccidioidomycosis, gonococci, and intestinal parasitic infection. Phlyctenular keratoconjunctivitis is sometimes associated with infectious eczematoid blepharitis and contact lens wear. Unless related to contact lens wear, phlyctenular keratoconjunctivitis tends to be more common in children or women. Phlyctenular nodules are usually composed of polymorphonuclear leukocytes, macrophages, and T-lymphocytes.[33]

Topical steroids such as 1.0% prednisolone acetate or 0.1% dexamethasone administered every 2–4 hours usually provide effective resolution when there is no evidence of associated infection. Topical antibiotic/steroid solutions, such as gentamicin/prednisolone acetate or tobramycin/dexamethasone, are sometimes used when there is doubt regarding active bacterial infection. If an active staphylococcal infection is demonstrated through culturing, appropriate therapy should be provided according to sensitivity testing if not responsive to initial therapy or if recurrence is a problem. Oral antimicrocial treatment may be indicated for some infections (e.g., chlamydial).

Tuberculosis should be ruled out with appropriate laboratory investigation in all cases of phlyctenulosis, especially because of the resurgence of the disease in the United States. Tuberculosis-induced phlyctenulosis may initially respond to topical corticosteroidal therapy, but recurrence would be expected. Treatment of the underlying tuberculitic infection is effective in eliminating the related ocular con-

dition. When *Chlamydia* is suspected in pediatric cases, oral tetracycline or erythromycin, depending on the age of the child, may be necessary.[32]

Angular Conjunctivitis

Angular conjunctivitis causes a sectoral inflammation that is usually located at the lateral canthus but may also involve the nasal canthus. The conjunctiva is hyperemic and may exhibit a papillary or follicular response depending on the specific cause. A mucoid-type discharge with complaints of sticky eyelids in the mornings are common. Angular conjunctivitis is usually secondary to angular blepharitis, which manifests with desquamated and ulcerated skin caused either by *Moraxella lacunata* or *Staphylococcus aureus*. The clinical manifestations of the condition may appear consistent with nonspecific chronic bacterial conjunctivitis.[34]

When caused by *M. lacunata*, satisfactory resolution can be achieved with topical 0.25% zinc sulfate solution four times a day, 0.5% erythromycin ointment three times a day, or 1% tetracycline ointment three times a day. Staphylococcus-related angular conjunctivitis can be managed with trimethoprim/polymyxin B solution four times a day or bacitracin ointment three times a day.[34]

Ophthalmia Neonatorum

Ophthalmia neonatorum, conjunctivitis in the neonate, requires special consideration and prompt management because of its increased potential for complications. The

FIGURE 22-7
Multiple corneal infiltrates associated with nonulcerative bacterial keratitis. Serratia marcescens, *a gram-negative rod, was cultured from the palpebral conjunctiva and the contact lens case of this soft contact lens wearer.*

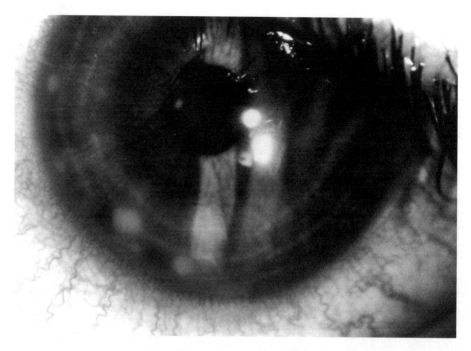

entity occurs in up to 12% of all newborns.[35] Etiologic diagnosis may be difficult since most clinical signs are nonspecific. The condition is characterized by acute onset of hyperemia, chemosis, lid edema, and mucopurulent or purulent exudate beginning 5–21 days postpartum.

Although the offending organism cannot be determined in many cases of ophthalmia neonatorum, a laboratory investigation consisting of both conjunctival scrapings/smears and cultures with antibiotic sensitivity testing is mandatory. The leading cause of ophthalmia neonatorum is *Chlamydia trachomatis,* occurring in approximately 2–6% of all newborns.[36] The high incidence of this infection is because up to 13% of women shed *Chlamydia* from the urogenital tract during the third trimester of pregnancy.[36] The high incidence of infection may also be related to the ineffectiveness of silver nitrate in preventing chlamydial infections. Other common causes of ophthalmia neonatorum are *Neisseria gonorrhoeae,* and *Pseudomonas aeruginosa, Staphylococcus aureus,* and herpes simplex virus.

Passage through an infected birth canal carries an increased risk of neonatal infection leading to ophthalmia neonatorum. Premature membrane rupture and prolonged delivery can also increase exposure to pathogens. Determination of the offending organism causing ophthalmia neonatorum is imperative, since serious complications can result such as corneal scarring or perforation, endophthalmitis, pneumonia, septicemia, encephalitis, and death.[37] Although infections that cause ophthalmia neonatorum may occur in utero or during delivery, they may also occur after birth. Herpes simplex infection is a rela-

tively unusual but important neonatal infection implicated in 5–10% of cases with conjunctivitis.[38]

Culturing of specimens and sensitivity testing should be done on all infants with conjunctivitis so that specific therapy can be instituted if the condition does not respond to an initial therapy. When a bacterial cause exists, treatment of the acute conjunctivitis is similar to that for any other hyperacute conjunctivitis. Broad-spectrum topical antibiotics with low toxicity, such as trimethoprim/polymyxin B or 0.3% gentamicin solution four times a day to every 2 hours or topical 0.5% erythromycin or 1% tetracycline ointments four to six times daily. In addition, systemic treatment with intramuscular cefotaxime (50 mg/kg) may be effective.[30,39] Although the optimal treatment for chlamydial infection has not been determined, systemic erythromycin (40–50 mg/kg/day in four divided doses for 14 days) may be used for *C. trachomatis* infections. Treatment of herpes simplex neonatal conjunctivitis may include topical 1% trifluridine every 2 hours. Systemic therapy with acyclovir may be indicated in the presence of viremia and disseminated disease.[40]

Bacterial Keratitis

Bacterial keratitis can be categorized as nonulcerative or ulcerative. Nonulcerative keratitis may be caused by primary bacterial infection but more likely is secondary to (1) exotoxins liberated in the presence of infectious blepharitis or conjunctivitis (Figure 22-7), (2) mechanical irritation, or (3) trauma. Most instances of ulcerative bacterial ker-

TABLE 22-4
Antibiotic Susceptibility of Selected Bacterial Pathogens

Organism	Topical Pharmaceutical Agent
Actinomyces sp.	Bacitracin, gramicidin, tetracycline
Cornyebacterium sp.	Bacitracin, ciprofloxacin, erythromycin, gramicidin
Escherichia coli	Ciprofloxacin, gentamicin, neomycin, norfloxacin, ofloxacin, polymyxin B, tobramycin, trimethoprim
Haemophilus sp.	Ciprofloxacin, gentamicin, norfloxacin, ofloxacin, polymyxin B, sulfonamides, tobramycin, trimethoprim
Moraxella sp.	Ciprofloxacin, erythromycin, neomycin, norfloxacin, ofloxacin, polymyxin B, trimethoprim
Neisseria sp.	Bacitracin, ciprofloxacin, erythromycin, neomycin, norfloxacin, ofloxacin, tetracycline
Proteus sp.	Ciprofloxacin, gentamicin, neomycin, norfloxacin, ofloxacin, tobramycin, trimethoprim
Pseudomonas sp.	Ciprofloxacin, gentamicin, norfloxacin, ofloxacin, polymyxin B, tobramycin
Serratia sp.	Ciprofloxacin, gentamicin, neomycin, norfloxacin, ofloxacin, tobramycin, trimethoprim
Staphylococcus sp.	Bacitracin, ciprofloxacin, erythromycin, gentamicin, gramicidin, norfloxacin, ofloxacin, tobramycin, trimethoprim
Streptococcus sp.	Bacitracin, ciprofloxacin, erythromycin, gentamicin, gramicidin, norfloxacin, ofloxacin, trimethoprim

Note: Additional antibiotics may be effective as demonstrated by antibiotic sensitivity testing.
Source: Data from G Smolin, RA Thoft. The Cornea (3rd ed). Boston: Little, Brown, 1994;5:135.

atitis occur in eyes with predisposing risk factors.[41,42] Only four pathogens can invade an intact, healthy cornea. These organisms are *Neisseria gonorrhoeae, Corynebacterium diphtheriae, Listeria* species, and *Acanthamoeba* species. All other microbial pathogens require an entry port in the form of an epithelial defect to establish an active infection.[17] The wearing of contact lenses, use of contaminated cosmetics or medications, or the presence of other corneal disease, such as herpes simplex, also increase the risk of keratitis because of the potential for corneal abrasion and possible alterations in the normal bacterial flora.[43,44]

The most common causes of bacterial keratitis are *Staphylococcus aureus, Streptococcus pneumoniae, Pseudomonas aeruginosa, Staphylococcus epidermidis,* and other *Streptococcus* species.[17] *Streptococcus pneumoniae* and *Pseudomonas aeruginosa* are more common in corneas with no underlying pathologic condition, whereas infections of *Staphylococcus aureus, Staphylococcus epidermidis,* and other *Streptococcus* species usually are secondary to compromised corneas.

Clinically, patient symptomatology includes varying degrees of pain, photophobia, redness, and reduced visual acuity. Superficial keratitis is typically characterized by punctate staining with or without associated infiltration. Early ulceration of the epithelium may exhibit smooth, rolled margins, and frequently there is underlying infiltrate. All ulcerations or infiltrates with overlying epithelial defects potentially have an infectious cause. A tissue specimen for laboratory analysis must be obtained in these cases by scraping the cornea before instilling a therapeutic pharmaceutical agent. Specimens should be taken for both culture and smear (see Table 22-3). A smear prepared with Gram stain can provide the clinician with valuable insight for initial empirical therapy.

Although the clinical appearance of the three most common corneal ulcers can sometimes be distinctive, laboratory workup is still mandatory. *Staphylococcus aureus* ulcers appear as a localized, grayish-white infiltrated site that may exhibit microabscesses. *Streptococcus pneumoniae* usually has a history of rapid onset, 24–48 hours after an abrasion of the cornea. This grayish, circumscribed lesion often spreads erratically toward the central cornea and has rough-appearing undermined edges. *Pseudomonas aeruginosa* infection often develops in patients with recent exposure to warm, moist environments, such as whirlpools, bath water, and swimming pools, or who use old eye cosmetics or wear contact lenses. The most virulent strains of *Pseudomonas* produce rapidly developing ulcers that are highly necrotic because of destruction of the corneal collagen by the enzyme protease. These ulcers, if not properly managed, can lead to rapid descemetocele formation with corneal melting within 24 hours. Endophthalmitis, orbital cellulitis, and septicemia may subsequently ensue. Patients frequently have ocular pain 1–3 days after trauma or contact lens wear. Infiltrates with ulceration, necrosis, and a greenish mucopurulent discharge constitute the clinical findings.[17,45]

Superficial or nonulcerative keratitis should be initially treated with a topical aminoglycoside or fluoroquinolone antibiotic[27,45] (Table 22-4). Gentamicin, tobramycin, ciprofloxacin, or ofloxacin is commonly used. In the presence of significant risk factors, such as the wearing of extended-wear soft contact lenses, tobramycin or ciprofloxacin are more appropriate.

If ulcerative keratitis is present, the initial therapy after the collection of culture and smear specimens may consist of the following regimens[27,45–47]: (1) two drops of ciprofloxacin every 15 minutes for the first 6 hours fol-

TABLE 22-5
Topical Concentrations of Fortified Antibiotics for Ocular Therapy

Pharmaceutical Agent	Concentration
Amikacin sulfate	10–50 mg/ml
Bacitracin	5,000–10,000 units/ml
Carbenicillin	4 mg/ml
Cefamandole	50 mg/ml
Cefazolin	50 mg/ml
Erythromycin	50 mg/ml or 5 mg/g ointment
Gentamicin	8–15 mg/ml
Methicillin sodium	50 mg/ml
Penicillin G	100,000 units/ml
Polymyxin B	1–2 mg/ml
Tobramycin	8–15 mg/ml
Vancomycin	50 mg/ml

Sources: Data from Physician's Desk Reference for Ophthalmology (23rd ed). Oradell, NJ: Medical Economics, 1995; and G Smolin, RA Thoft. The Cornea (3rd ed). Boston: Little, Brown, 1994;5:136.

TABLE 22-6
Viral Causes of Ocular Disease

Adenoviruses
Herpes simplex (HSV1 and HSV2)
Varicella-zoster
Epstein-Barr
Coxsackie A24
Enterovirus 70
Molluscum contagiosum
Papilloma virus
Mumps
Rubeola
Rubella
Newcastle
Vaccinia

lowed by two drops every 30 minutes for the remainder of the first day, or (2) a regimen consisting of a fortified aminoglycoside and cephalosporin, one drop of each applied every 30 minutes. The aminoglycoside may be either gentamicin or tobramycin combined with cefazolin (Table 22-5). If the Gram stain results indicate gram-positive organisms, gentamicin is preferred; if gram-negative, tobramycin combined with carbenicillin is often preferred. Patients should be instructed to continue therapy during sleep hours, or topical bacitracin or tobramycin ointment to be used at bedtime may sometimes be prescribed. The initial follow-up visit should be in 24 hours. Clinical findings at follow-up and results of the laboratory analysis determine the remaining course of therapy.

VIRAL DISEASES

General Viral

Although many different viruses are implicated in ophthalmic disease, most general viral conjunctivitides are caused by an adenovirus (Table 22-6). Forty-seven immunologically distinct serotypes of adenoviruses have been identified as potential causes of viral conjunctivitis.[48] Most adenoviral infections initially involve the upper respiratory tract, nasal mucosa, or sinuses. Epidemic outbreaks of adenoviral conjunctivitis have been recognized as distinct clinical entities including epidemic keratoconjunctivitis (EKC) and pharyngoconjunctival fever (PCF). Although many different adenoviral serotypes have been identified as the causative agents of both EKC and PCF,

most studies indicate serotypes 8, 19, 29, and 37 as the etiologic agents of EKC, and serotype 3 and occasionally serotypes 4 or 7 as causes of PCF. Epidemic outbreaks of adenoviral disease occur via direct contact with infected patients, contact with contaminated ophthalmic instruments or solutions, and contact with shared environmental settings, such as swimming pools.

Ophthalmic viral disease is usually a clinical diagnosis, and laboratory studies are rarely necessary. General viral disease usually presents as an acute conjunctivitis with diffuse hyperemia, chemosis, foreign body sensation, tearing, and mild lid edema. Corneal involvement is variable, often including a punctate keratitis, subepithelial infiltration, or both. Infection usually begins unilaterally and becomes bilateral after 2–3 days. Preauricular node involvement is variable. Often there is a history of recent cold or influenza.

Viral conjunctivitis is usually self-limiting, with most cases resolving spontaneously over approximately 10–21 days. Supportive therapy is usually indicated for acute symptoms, including cold compresses, topical vasoconstrictors, and artificial tears. Patients with viral conjunctivitis also should be counseled regarding proper hygiene and infection control in their home, work, and social environments. They should be advised to wash their hands frequently and avoid sharing bed linens, towels, and so forth. Adenoviral infections may be particularly contagious, and infected individuals will continue to shed viral particles in tears and from the nasopharynx for 2 weeks.[49]

Infection control is important in the clinician's office to prevent the spread of viral disease. Tonometer probes and other ophthalmic equipment should be appropriately disinfected. Barrier protection (disposable latex gloves) is indicated when examining patients with viral conjunctivitis. Careful handwashing before and after patient examination is mandatory.

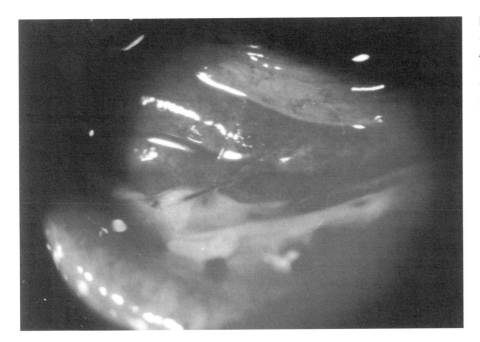

FIGURE 22-8
Pseudomembrane of the lower palpebral conjunctiva secondary to epidemic keratoconjunctivitis. An eyelash is caught in the inflammatory debris. (Courtesy of Sara L. Penner, O.D.)

Epidemic Keratoconjunctivitis

Epidemic keratoconjunctivitis (EKC) initially presents similar to a nonspecific viral conjunctivitis except that frequently the signs and symptoms are more severe. Often there is a dull, achy pain in the involved eye, as well as moderate foreign body sensation, photophobia, and significant periorbital lid edema. Tender preauricular and submandibular lymphadenopathy on the side of involvement is common.

Marked conjunctival hyperemia and chemosis is often present, and there may be a mixed papillary/follicular reaction. Pseudomembranes commonly form, which represent the accumulation of mucus and inflammatory debris and indicate severe inflammation (Figure 22-8).[50,51] They must be aggressively managed to avoid subsequent conjunctival scarring and symblepharon formation (Figure 22-9). Petechial hemorrhages are common and diffuse subconjunctival hemorrhage may occasionally develop. A superficial punctate keratitis may develop with subsequent formation of characteristic subepithelial infiltrates (SEIs) within the central cornea approximately 1–2 weeks after the initial onset. The SEIs help distinguish EKC from other viral conjunctivitides. The development of SEIs in patients with EKC causes increased pain and photophobia and may result in reduced visual acuity. Frequently, infiltrates will persist for many weeks or months, and anterior stromal scarring may occur (Figure 22-10).[50]

Treatment of EKC usually is supportive. Many cases can be successfully managed with cold compresses, topical vasoconstrictors, and artificial tears. Although the role of top-ical steroids remains controversial, they may be indicated in the presence of pseudomembranes and when patient symptoms are debilitating, usually when SEIs are pronounced in the visual axis. Steroid therapy will lessen the severity of the immune response and improve visual acuity. However, suppressing the immune response may interfere with elimination of the viral antigen and ultimately prolong the course of the disease. Patients treated with topical steroidal therapy require close monitoring for several weeks with gradual tapering of the steroid medication. Occasionally, patients may develop a steroid dependence, making withdrawal more difficult. Subsequent discontinuation of steroids or withdrawal that is too quick may result in recurrence or worsening of subepithelial infiltration.[52]

The existence of an EKC-like variant of herpes simplex keratoconjunctivitis requires the clinician to be absolutely certain of the diagnosis before prescribing topical steroids.[53] Steroids should be prescribed with caution, and patients should be advised regarding the potential risks and benefits before treatment is instituted.

Topical antibiotics are usually not indicated in the management of EKC. Although the viral conjunctivitis can be severe, the risk of secondary bacterial infection is low. Use of antiviral medication for the management of adenoviral conjunctivitis has not been proved effective.[54]

Pharyngoconjunctival Fever

Pharyngoconjunctival fever (PCF) is usually a contagious childhood disease characterized by a unilateral or bilater-

FIGURE 22-9
Permanent, asymptomatic symblepharon formation after epidemic keratoconjunctivitis. (Courtesy of Daniel K. Roberts, O.D.)

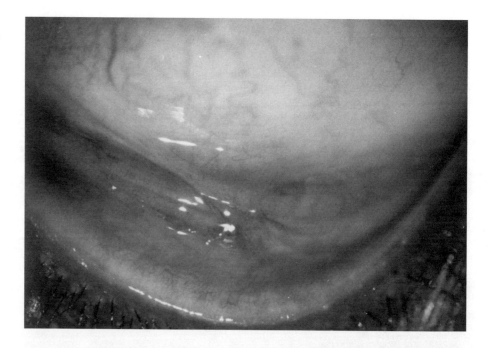

FIGURE 22-10
Anterior stromal scarring secondary to central subepithelial infiltrates associated with epidemic keratoconjunctivitis.

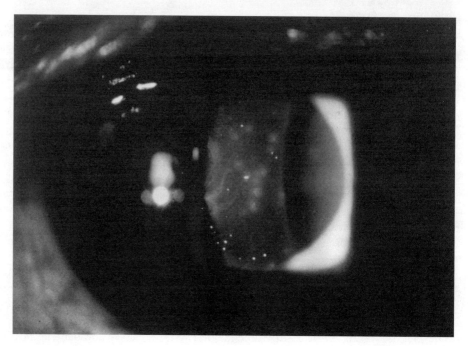

al follicular conjunctivitis, fever, and pharyngitis. The associated fever often ranges from 101–104°F (38.3–40°C).[55] In many cases only one or two findings of the clinical triad are present. The most prominent sign is tearing. Clinical findings usually include hyperemia, prominent follicles, and nontender preauricular lymphadenopathy. In more severe clinical presentations, there may be a superficial punctate epithelial keratitis with subepithelial opacities.

Supportive therapy consisting of cold compresses and topical vasoconstrictors usually lessen symptoms in most cases of PCF. Topical steroids are rarely necessary.

Herpes Simplex

Approximately 70% of the United States population exhibits immunologic evidence of prior infection with herpes simplex virus (HSV) by the age of 15–20 years. This percentage increases to 97% by age 60 years.[56] Herpes simplex virus is an encapsulated DNA virus that has two serotypes, type 1 (nonvenereal) and type 2 (venereal). Primary HSV infection is subclinical 85–90% of the time.[57] Although the ocular involvement of the two types is clinically indistinguishable, type 1 is demonstrated in approximately 85% of clinically active adult cases.[58] Herpetic eye disease is the leading cause of infectious blindness in the United States, with approximately 0.5–1.5 cases/1,000 persons.[59]

Primary HSV ocular infections typically present as a blepharoconjunctivitis in children between the ages of 6 months and 5 years. Although the nonvenereal, type 1–related infection predominates in children, the venereal, type 2 HSV infection may occur in both newborns and adults. In newborns, a type 2 ocular infection presumably results from contact with the virus in the infected birth canal, while in adults it occurs by auto-inoculation after sexual contact with an infected partner.

Type 1 and type 2 HSV infections are commonly characterized by recurrent episodes of disease months or years after initial infection. Potentially up to 50% of patients with HSV ocular involvement will experience a second episode within 2 years of their initial disease presentation.[60]

Herpes simplex blepharoconjunctivitis is typically characterized by follicular conjunctivitis as well as cutaneous vesicular lesions located on or near the lid margin. Lid lesions, when present, exhibit an erythematous base and may ulcerate and have a honey-yellow crusty border. The bulbar and palpebral conjunctiva is usually diffusely hyperemic, and patients may complain of an acute onset of tearing, burning, foreign body sensation, and photophobia. Whereas most cases are unilateral, the fellow eye may show involvement 3–7 days after the initial symptoms in the first eye.

Because herpes simplex and adenoviral conjunctivitis are often indistinguishable in the absence of corneal or lid involvement, unilaterality is an important clinical sign, with EKC more commonly becoming bilateral. Although not typical of most cases, pseudomembranes may form in HSV ocular infection, which is another potential similarity to EKC.[38] Nontender or tender preauricular lymphadenopathy also commonly occurs in HSV infection.

Herpes simplex keratitis (HSK) has several presentations. A diffuse punctate epitheliopathy and subepithelial infiltrates may be seen in concert with blepharoconjunctivitis. Occasionally, corneal filaments are noted. The classic dendritic or geographic corneal ulcer usually occurs during later reactivation of the disease. The epithelial dendritic ulcers of HSK are characterized by the presence of terminal end bulbs, which help distinguish these lesions

from those caused by the Epstein-Barr or varicella-zoster viruses. The corneal dendritic ulcers of HSK demonstrate diffuse staining with sodium fluorescein, and rose bengal dye characteristically stains the border tissue of dendrites. Rose bengal staining may be helpful in differentiating between noninfectious persistent epithelial defects and geographic herpetic lesions, the latter of which stain with rose bengal dye.

The most serious presentation of HSK is the sight-threatening stromal, or disciform, keratitis that typically occurs in patients who have had repeated attacks of epithelial keratitis. Herpetic stromal keratitis is characterized by a relatively large zone of stromal edema and infiltration. Posterior corneal folds may be evident, and keratic precipitates may be present underlying the area of inflammation. An anterior chamber reaction may be present, and intraocular pressure can be significantly elevated. A variable epithelial defect often overlies the stromal disease, and in many instances an epithelial dendrite progresses into stromal disease, especially when inadvertently managed with topical steroids without concurrent antiviral therapy.

Herpes simplex blepharoconjunctivitis is usually benign and self-limited.[61,62] Topical vasoconstrictors, such as naphazoline, or other supportive treatment may be recommended. Occasionally prophylactic therapy with antiviral agents to prevent corneal involvement is used but is typically not necessary. When used, however, the primary therapeutic agent is 1% trifluridine solution applied every 2–4 hours with an additional dose at bedtime. Dosage should not exceed 9 drops per day and may be tapered after there is evidence of clinical improvement. Therapy should be continued for an additional 3–5 days after the conjunctivitis resolves. Instead of trifluridine solution, 3% vidarabine ointment applied every 3 hours (5 times daily) may be effective. Although vidarabine ointment may be applied directly to the lid lesions, it may not significantly affect their resolution. Idoxuridine 0.1% solution is more irritating than either trifluridine or vidarabine and may not be as effective because of resistant strains of herpes simplex. Also, its usage often results in hypersensitivity or toxic reactions. Conjunctival scarring has been reported with chronic topical applications of idoxuridine.[63]

Steroids are contraindicated for the treatment of herpes simplex conjunctivitis, since their use will increase virus replication. Topical antibiotics are not indicated for management of herpes simplex blepharoconjunctivitis unless there is suspected secondary bacterial infection.

Herpes simplex dendritic epithelial keratitis is usually treated with 1% trifluridine solution initially applied every 2 hours with a dose at bedtime to achieve 9 drops per day. The dosage may be tapered to four times a day after the epithelial dendrite resolves. Therapy should be continued for 5–7 days after resolution of the dendritic ulcer to inhibit any active virus remaining within epithelial cells before they are normally shed. If trifluridine solution is not well tolerated or ineffective, 3% vidarabine ointment applied five times per day may be substituted.

Whereas topical steroids are specifically contraindicated in dendritic keratitis, they may be useful in severe cases for reducing stromal inflammation that causes tissue destruction and scarring. If needed in this situation, topical steroids, such as 1% prednisolone acetate, may be used judiciously with concurrent antiviral therapy. The antiviral therapy must be continued while the steroid is tapered. Antiviral therapy should then be continued on a daily basis for 2–3 weeks after the steroid is discontinued to ensure elimination of any residual viral particles. Referral to a corneal specialist may be necessary for disciform keratitis.

Herpes Zoster Ophthalmicus

The most common ocular manifestation caused by the herpes varicella-zoster virus is an acute conjunctivitis characterized by hyperemia, chemosis, and occasionally follicular hyperplasia. Other ocular manifestations may include the development of keratitis (punctate, dendritic, or disciform), uveitis, and increased intraocular pressure. Cranial nerve palsies, optic neuritis, and retinitis have also been described.[64] These ophthalmic manifestations usually follow the development of vesicular skin lesions within the sensory dermatome innervated by the ophthalmic division (first division) of the trigeminal nerve (cranial nerve V). The involved dermatome obeys the vertical midline and its overall extent depends on which branches of the ophthalmic division are affected. If only the frontal nerve is involved, then the forehead, the upper lid, and possibly a portion of the conjunctiva will show inflammatory signs. More pronounced ocular involvement typically occurs if the nasociliary nerve is affected. Classically, significant ocular involvement is more likely to occur if the sides or tip of the nose exhibit the vesicular cutaneous lesions (Hutchinson's sign).

Herpes zoster (HZ), which actually affects other dermatomes of the body more often than the face, results from reactivation of the dormant varicella-zoster virus. This is the same virus typically acquired during childhood and manifested as chicken pox. The incidence and severity of herpes zoster infection increases with age.[65] An increased incidence of herpes zoster is also associated with immune compromise. Peak incidence occurs between 50 and 75 years of age. In young patients with no history of malignancy or immunosuppression, HZ infection may be the presenting sign of AIDS-related complex (ARC) or

AIDS.[66] Ocular lesions occur in approximately 50–71% of patients who develop active herpes zoster infection involving the ophthalmic division of the trigeminal nerve.[67]

Although patient symptoms associated with mild to moderate acute conjunctivitis or episcleritis may be helped with topical vasoconstrictors such as naphazoline solution four times a day, the management of herpes zoster–related ocular disease usually requires topical steroids. Prednisolone sodium phosphate 1% or fluorometholone alcohol 0.1% applied four times a day will usually achieve satisfactory resolution. Careful monitoring for the development of keratitis, anterior uveitis, and increased intraocular pressure is necessary. If keratitis or anterior uveitis occurs, topical steroids are often used more aggressively than in the presence of conjunctivitis or episcleritis alone. Concurrent antiglaucoma therapy, including beta-blockers, oral carbonic anhydrase inhibitors, or both, may be indicated in instances of increased intraocular pressure.

It should be remembered that the anterior uveitis in herpes zoster ophthalmicus (HZO) may be related to ischemic necrosis of the iris and may have a very severe and protracted course that is relatively unresponsive to steroidal therapy. Cataracts and steroid-induced glaucoma are relatively common complications in some HZO patients because of the protracted course of therapy sometimes required. Recurrence of ocular inflammation may develop up to years after the initial cutaneous eruption and can be a source of diagnostic confusion when mild external signs went unnoticed or were forgotten. Vigilance should be maintained during the withdrawal of steroidal therapy, because tapering too quickly can precipitate a rebounding of inflammation.

Oral acyclovir, 800 mg five times per day, has been shown to lessen the severity and hasten the recovery of acute HZO, especially if treatment is initiated within 72 hours of the skin eruption.[68] Postherpetic neuralgia syndrome, which occurs in approximately 20% of these patients, may also be reduced by oral acyclovir therapy.[69–71] Some dermatologists advocate oral prednisone as well to prevent postherpetic neuralgia from the skin dermatome involvement.

CHLAMYDIAL DISEASES

Chlamydial infections are a common cause of venereal disease, with 3–5 million new cases per year in the United States.[72] The disease is relatively asymptomatic in terms of urogenital symptoms, although nonspecific urethritis and chronic vaginal discharge are not uncommon. Ocular infection commonly occurs from autoinoculation by an infected individual.

Chlamydial infections represent the most common cause of chronic conjunctivitis.[34] Inclusion conjunctivitis is caused by *Chlamydia trachomatis*, serotypes D–K and occasionally serotype B. Trachoma is usually caused by serotypes A, B, Ba, and C. Although *Chlamydia trachomatis* is the common etiologic agent for trachoma and adult inclusion conjunctivitis, the two diseases are distinctly different in their clinical and epidemiologic characteristics.

Trachoma and its complications represent a serious world health problem and today remain a major cause of preventable blindness. The incidence of trachoma is highest in the unhealthy, dirty, crowded conditions typically associated with a low socioeconomic environment. Approximately one-seventh of the world's population is affected by trachoma, although in the United States the disease is mostly limited to native American populations living in the southwest.[38] In addition to trachoma and inclusion conjunctivitis, *Chlamydia trachomatis* is also responsible for lymphogranuloma venereum and other venereal diseases.

Adult Inclusion Conjunctivitis

Inclusion conjunctivitis is usually seen in sexually active teens or adults. Patient complaints include red eyes and foreign body sensation associated with a watery or mucopurulent discharge. The onset may be acute or chronic with unilateral or bilateral involvement. Clinically, conjunctival hyperemia is noted, often with follicular hyperplasia. Commonly, instead of primarily a follicular hyperplasia, a mixed papillary and follicular hypertrophy of the lower palpebral conjunctiva is found. Corneal involvement may include punctate keratopathy, micropannus, and central or peripheral subepithelial infiltrates. Preauricular lymphadenopathy very frequently occurs on the affected side and can be a very helpful diagnostic sign.

As in other cases of chronic conjunctivitis, conjunctival cultures and cytology scrapings can be helpful in diagnosis. Several laboratory tests have been used to establish a diagnosis of inclusion conjunctivitis.[73,74] Classically, Giemsa staining reveals numerous epithelial intracytoplasmic inclusion bodies. However, these are not found very often clinically in adult patients.

Treatment of inclusion conjunctivitis must include oral therapy, since topical medications alone are not sufficient for chlamydial disease. The usual adult regimen is 250 mg tetracycline four times a day for 21 days. An alternative treatment consists of 100 mg doxycycline two times a day for 7 days followed by 50 mg two times a day for 14 days.[75] Adjunct therapy with 1% tetracycline solution or ointment four times a day may lessen the patient's symptoms. Doxycycline has a less frequent dosing schedule and has

TABLE 22-7
World Health Organization Criteria for the Diagnosis of Trachoma

The diagnosis of trachoma should be made when at least two or more of the following clinical signs are present:
  Superior palpebral conjunctival follicles
  Limbal follicles
  Herbert's pits
  Conjunctival scarring
  Limbal corneal vascularization or pannus

Source: CR Dawson, BR Jones, ML Tarizzo. Guide to Trachoma Control. In Programmes for the Prevention of Blindness. Geneva: World Health Organization, 1981;12–20.

better intestinal absorption that is less affected by dietary consumption, particularly dairy products. For lactating women, children under 8 years of age, or patients sensitive to tetracycline, erythromycin is an effective alternative, with the dosage being 250 mg four times a day for 14 days for adults and 40–50 mg/kg/day for 14 days for children. A careful medical history must be obtained in these cases so that the urogenital infection is adequately treated, as well as any sexual partners. Azithromycin 1 g/day has also been shown to be effective.[76]

Trachoma

Trachoma, in its early stages, presents as a chronic follicular conjunctivitis that has a predilection for the superior tarsal and bulbar conjunctiva (Table 22-7). As time passes, the conjunctival reaction becomes papillary in nature and the follicular character of the infection can be obscured. Symptomatic patients may complain of photophobia, tearing and mucoid or mucopurulent discharge. Limbal edema and superior bulbar conjunctival hyperemia may be apparent, and conjunctival follicles that form at the limbus are characteristically found, especially in severe disease.

Primary corneal involvement often includes superior epithelial keratitis and superficial superior pannus formation. A wide variety of corneal infiltrates (superior, diffuse, limbal) may occur, and marginal ulcerations are not uncommon. As the disease progresses, conjunctival subepithelial scarring begins to replace the acute inflammatory signs. This scarring can result in entropion and trichiasis, which may cause corneal ulceration and scarring, the major blinding complications of trachoma.

The involution of limbal follicles results in sharply demarcated limbal depressions known as Herbert's pits, which are considered pathognomonic for trachoma. Patients with severe conjunctival scarring can develop a host of other secondary complications including severe dry eye syndrome and punctal stenosis. The course of trachoma is usually staged according to the MacCallen classification system, which is based solely on the conjunctival findings.[77,78]

In areas endemic for trachoma, the presence of two of the typical signs (i.e., upper tarsal follicles, corneal pannus, or limbal follicles) is sufficient for diagnosis of trachoma. Laboratory studies may be quite useful in mild cases, either by isolation of chlamydial organisms in tissue culture or detection of chlamydial antibodies in serum or tears by immunofluorescent assay. In nonendemic populations, trachoma must be differentiated from other causes of chronic follicular conjunctivitis such as *Moraxella*, adenoviral infection, herpetic infection, molluscum contagiosum, and chemical conjunctivitis. A history should be carefully obtained to determine whether the patient has traveled to an area where trachoma is endemic. The predilection of trachoma to affect the upper palpable conjunctiva as well as the superior cornea is of great diagnostic value.

Trachoma usually responds to a 3-week course of oral tetracycline 250 mg four times a day or oral erythromycin 250 mg four times a day. The clinical response itself is relatively slow and may not be significant for 3–4 months after therapy is started. Reinfection rates are high, especially in endemic areas. In pregnant patients and children under the age of 8 years, tetracycline is contraindicated because it can discolor the teeth and depress bone marrow in premature infants. Once again, topical treatment alone is generally considered ineffective for a complete cure; however, topical tetracycline or erythromycin may be applied as adjunctive therapy. In patients with severe conjunctival cicatrization, surgical intervention may be required to correct trichiasis and entropion and to prevent the possibility of corneal scarring. In those patients with significant corneal scarring and decreased vision, penetrating keratoplasty can be considered once the disease has been controlled.[79,80]

FUNGAL DISEASES

Fungal causes of conjunctivitis and keratitis are not common but are seen in patients who have diabetes mellitus, suffer penetrating trauma involving organic matter, or are immunocompromised. Fungal corneal ulcers may be precipitated by the overuse of topical ocular steroids. Patients who poorly maintain their soft contact lenses and lens cases may also be at risk, since fungal organisms have been cultured from these items. *Candida*, *Fusarium*, and *Aspergillus* species are the more commonly identified

opportunistic pathogens. Microsporidial keratoconjunctivitis has been identified as a potential ocular complication in immunocompromised patients.[81,82]

The *Candida* species conjunctivitis is characterized by scattered, raised, white patchy areas similar to thrush lesions. Fungal corneal ulcers tend to have grayish stromal infiltrates with irregular, epithelial ulceration and associated hypopyon. With time, stromal infiltration progresses posteriorly and there may be formation of an endothelial plaque at the ulcer site. The borders of the infiltrate may not be well delineated, and there may be featherlike projections extending outward from the primary area of infiltration. The presence of satellite lesions adjacent to or completely separated from the primary lesion is characteristic of fungal infections.

Prompt laboratory investigation is essential in the diagnosis of fungal keratitis. Specimens for culture and smear analysis should be taken from all ulcers.[81,83] Conjunctival scrapings often reveal the increased presence of polymorphonuclear leukocytes. Preparations of corneal specimens with Giemsa and Gram stains may demonstrate hyphae formations. Since an individual scraping may not show hyphal fragments, it is important to collect multiple specimens, inoculating each medium several times. Specimens collected from the base of a fungal corneal ulcer are more likely to yield hyphal fragments than specimens collected elsewhere.

Agents effective in treating fungal infections include nystatin, amphotericin B, and natamycin. Ketoconazole and miconazole have also been shown to be effective. High dosages are often used initially and then tapered as the condition responds to therapy.[84] On initial confirmation of a fungal infection, 5% natamycin instilled every hour is often the regimen of choice; this is effective against most types of fungal keratitis. If the condition is unresponsive and depending on the results of culture and sensitivity testing, other agents are used. Topical cycloplegia is typically administered in the presence of fungal keratitis, and antiglaucoma medications may also be necessary depending on the degree of anterior chamber inflammation.

PARASITIC DISEASE

Acanthamoeba

Acanthamoeba keratitis is characterized by a red eye with moderate to intense pain that is more severe than expected by the clinical findings. The organisms, *Acanthamoeba polyphaga* or *Acanthamoeba castellani*, and their spores become embedded in the corneal stroma, forming an ulceration surrounded by an immune ring. Stromal edema, subepithelial perineural opacities, and anterior uveitis often accompany the infection. Hypopyon is rarely present. The use of contact lens saline made from salt tablets and swimming while wearing contact lenses in improperly chlorinated hot tubs and pools have been implicated as causative factors for the infection. The ulcer may have a dendritic appearance, leading to a misdiagnosis of herpes simplex keratitis. The *Acanthamoeba* organism is difficult to visualize in corneal scrapings but may be cultured on nutrient agar. The cysts may be detected on calcifluor white–stained, paraffin-embedded sections.[85]

Topical 0.1% propamidine solution or 0.15% ointment applied every 30 minutes initially and fortified neomycin 20 mg/ml have been shown to be effective in many cases. However, the prognosis is always guarded with *Acanthamoeba* keratitis, and additional oral therapy with miconazole or ketoconazole may be necessary. Topical clotrimazole continues to be studied for its effectiveness against *Acanthamoeba* keratitis and may be beneficial. The use of topical steroids is controversial. Unfortunately, despite medical therapy, many patients require penetrating keratoplasty because of severe corneal scarring.[86]

ALLERGIC DISORDERS

Seasonal Allergic Conjunctivitis

Complaints of constant or intermittent itchy, red, watery eyes with or without a clear to whitish, sticky mucoid discharge are typical of seasonal allergic conjunctivitis. The condition tends to be bilateral, although there may be some degree of asymmetry. Fluctuating visual acuity may occur if there is a mucoid discharge because of the mucus spreading across the cornea. Clinical findings include edema and erythema of the eyelids with mild to moderate conjunctival hyperemia and chemosis. Rubbing of the eyes to relieve itching intensifies the chemosis. Small papillae may be present on the tarsal conjunctiva. The cornea is usually unaffected but may show fine stippling staining with sodium fluorescein in prolonged or recurrent episodes.

Many patients will associate their ocular symptoms with systemic conditions such as asthma, hay fever, rhinitis, or seasonal sinusitis.[87] A medical history of systemic allergies with complaints of perennial or seasonal exacerbation is common.[87-89] Younger patients, 15–40 years of age, who live in warmer climates seem to be most susceptible. A familial predisposition for the development of allergic conjunctivitis is common.[88,90,91] Conjunctival scrapings stained with Giemsa may demonstrate an eosinophilic response.

TABLE 22-8
Systemic Antihistamines for Adjunct Treatment of Allergic Ocular Diseases

Chlorpheniramine maleate	2–4 mg q4–6h
Clemastine fumarate	1.34–2.68 mg q4–6h
Diphenhydramine HCl	25–50 mg q4–6h
Terfenadine	60 mg q12h
Astemizole	10 mg qd
Promethazine HCl	25 mg qhs
Loratadine	10 mg qd

Source: Data from Physician's Desk Reference (49th ed). Oradell, NJ: Medical Economics, 1995.

Seasonal allergic conjunctivitis is a type I immediate IgE immunoglobulin hypersensitivity reaction in which the conjunctival tissue becomes infiltrated with eosinophils and mast cells that degranulate, releasing histamine and other inflammatory mediators. Other mediators include precursors of prostaglandins, thromboxanes, and leukotrienes.[92,93] The reaction often takes less than 30 minutes. Pharmacologic management of seasonal allergic conjunctivitis includes topical vasoconstrictor/antihistamines, mast cell stabilizers, and nonsteroidal anti-inflammatory solutions. Naphazoline 0.02% or 0.05% solution may reduce conjunctival congestion; however, the addition of a topical antihistamine such as 0.05% levocabastine, 0.05% antazoline, or 0.3% pheniramine will improve results because the histamine response is also decreased. The mast cell stabilizers, 4% cromolyn sodium and 0.1% lodoxamide, and a nonsteroidal anti-inflammatory agent, 0.5% ketorolac tromethamine, applied four times a day have all been shown to be effective agents for reducing patient symptoms.[94-96] These agents may also be used for prophylactic therapy to prevent additional seasonal episodes. Systemic antihistamines, particularly at bedtime, are useful for reducing lid edema (Table 22-8). Cold compresses will also help alleviate the lid edema and chemosis. Topical steroids are rarely needed for seasonal allergic conjunctivitis except in severe exacerbations of the disease.

Contact Allergies

Contact ocular allergies are usually type IV, cell-mediated or delayed, hypersensitivity responses that take hours or days to develop. Type IV reactions are mononuclear cell responses in which T-lymphocytes rather than antibodies interact with the antigen. Although type I and type IV reactions cause some of the same clinical findings, type IV cases tend to be more severe with more papillary hypertrophy.[90]

Unilateral cases typically result from a contact cause such as reactions to cosmetics, perfumes, soaps, detergents, insect foreign bodies, and topical drugs such as neomycin, sulfacetamide, atropine, and timolol.[97-99] Contact lens solution preservatives such as thimerosal and benzalkonium chloride have also been implicated. Contact lens solution–related reactions tend to be less severe that those that occur secondary to topical drugs.[100,101]

In addition to removal of the offending allergen, contact allergies typically require topical steroids for satisfactory resolution. Topical steroidal ointments such as 0.5% or 1% hydrocortisone or 0.025% or 0.1% triamcinolone may be applied to the affected skin region until the condition resolves.[102] Prednisolone sodium phosphate 1% or fluorometholone alcohol 0.1% may be applied directly to the ocular surface for relief of symptoms if necessary. Systemic antihistamines may be required in some cases to achieve symptomatic relief. Examples include chlorpheniramine, diphenhydramine, terfenadine, astemizole, and loratadine (see Table 22-8). Cold compresses may also be helpful to reduce symptoms.

Chronic Allergic Conjunctivitis

Chronic allergic conjunctivitis is characterized by complaints of itching, burning, dryness, foreign body sensation, and photophobia. The eyelids are often erythematous and eczematous with crusting. Careful examination is needed to rule out a secondary staphylococcal infection. Follicles may be present in chemical or drug hypersensitivity reactions.[103] A clear, watery, or whitish mucoid discharge that has a stringy texture may accumulate in the conjunctival fornices.

The cornea may demonstrate punctate staining with sodium fluorescein and there may be extensive papillary hypertrophy. The presence of peripheral corneal subepithelial infiltrates can indicate chronic *Staphylococcus aureus* involvement. Grayish subepithelial infiltrates are common in chemical preservative hypersensitivity reactions.[97]

Conjunctival smears are useful in evaluating chronic allergic conjunctivitis. Scrapings stained with Giemsa stain demonstrate a higher number of eosinophils with some scattered basophils and mast cells.[87,104]

Management of chronic allergic conjunctivitis is similar to that for simple allergic conjunctivitis. An exception is that chronic disease usually requires treatment of the underlying lid disease or other offending agents. In addition, more prolonged use of medications is often necessary, sometimes requiring weeks or months of therapy.

Giant Papillary Conjunctivitis

Giant papillary conjunctivitis (GPC) refers to a papillary conjunctivitis that is most often associated with contact lens wear. Similar clinical findings are also encountered in patients wearing an ocular prosthesis or in those with an exposed suture barb after cataract surgery. Complaints of itchy, burning eyes with mucoid discharge during or after contact lens wear are common. Intense itching on lens removal is a common complaint. Fluctuating vision may be reported and patients may frequently remove their lenses to clean them. Clinically, the upper palpebral conjunctiva demonstrates hyperemia and giant papillae, sometimes 1 mm or greater in size (Figure 22-11). Mild diffuse bulbar injection may be present. Conjunctival scrapings reveal primarily basophils and mast cells with some eosinophils.[105]

The pathogenesis of GPC is not totally understood. Protein deposits on contact lenses may initiate a combination type I and type IV immune reaction, or mechanical irritation of the conjunctival surface may play a role. Possibly, both processes may be involved concurrently, or there may be situations where one factor or the other is primarily involved.

Refitting and modification of contact lenses, incorporating new lens materials and parameters is often the treatment of choice. Temporary discontinuance of contact lens wear may be necessary for satisfactory resolution. More frequent enzymatic cleaning, hydrogen peroxide disinfection, and the use of disposable or frequent replacement lenses may also be beneficial. Topical 4% cromolyn sodium or 0.1% lodoxamide solution four times a day for 7–14 days before restarting contact lens wear may be helpful in milder cases. Discontinuance of contact lenses may be necessary in severe cases.

Vernal Keratoconjunctivitis

Most patients with vernal keratoconjunctivitis (VKC) complain of intense itching with a thick, ropy, white-to-yellowish discharge that requires removal from the eyes several times per day. Other symptoms include burning, foreign body sensation, general discomfort, photophobia, blepharospasm, tearing, and blurred vision from mucus in the tear film. The discharge tends to accumulate at the inner canthus in the mornings. Vernal keratoconjunctivitis is a bilateral disease but may be asymmetric. Clinical findings include giant cobblestone papillae on the superior palpebral conjunctiva, pseudoptosis, Horner-Trantas' dots, and thick, ropy, white-to-yellowish discharge. The excessive cellular infiltration creating the marked papillary hypertrophy causes the pseudoptosis. The multiple, polygonal, cobblestone-shaped papillae are 1 mm or larger.[105] The papillary surfaces are less rounded than those papillae seen in giant papillary conjunctivitis; this fact may be helpful in the differential

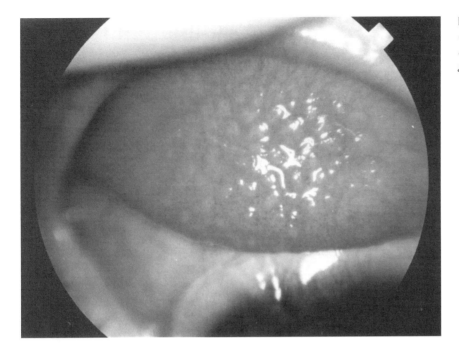

FIGURE 22-11
Giant papillae of the upper palpebral conjunctiva associated with giant papillary conjunctivitis.

diagnosis. The inferior palpebral conjunctiva is involved to a lesser degree.

Focal or confluent gelatinous limbal lesions with or without papillary hypertrophy create a second presentation of the disease. On regression of these limbal lesions, residual eosinophilic cell accumulations form the characteristic Horner-Trantas' dots. Vernal keratoconjunctivitis is a recurrent, seasonal condition with exacerbations typically during warmer months, and it is more prevalent in warm, dry climates. Most patients are males between 4 and 20 years old and have the disease for a period of 4–10 years.[106-108] Asthma, hay fever, perennial allergic rhinitis, or other atopic conditions are often reported in the patient's or family medical history.[107]

A diffuse superficial punctate keratitis with focal epithelial erosions and micropannus is commonly seen involving the superior cornea. A shallow oval, immune ulcer may form on the superior cornea and may contain accumulations of mucus, inflammatory cells, or other necrotic debris. The ulcer may last for weeks and eventually may form a ring scar.[109]

Conjunctival scrapings stained with Giemsa will have a mixed triad of eosinophils, basophils, and mast cells.[105] A tremendous influx of mast cells into the conjunctival epithelium and substantia propia occurs in VKC. The conjunctival epithelium in VKC has mast cell levels approaching $15,000/mm^3$ when normally few or no cells are present.[110-112] On degranulation the high numbers of mast cells lead to increased tear levels of histamine and other inflammatory mediators, such as prostaglandin and leukotriene precursors.[110,113,114] These increased tear levels of inflammatory mediators have a toxic effect on conjunctival cells, resulting in conjunctival inflammation, ptosis, and corneal epithelial lesions.[115] The development of VKC surrounds a complex immunologic reaction involving both IgE- and IgG-mediated responses. Elevated levels of locally produced IgE, IgG, and IgM have been isolated from the tears of these patients.[116] The IgG antibodies often lead to an elevation of complement factors.

Cold compresses, topical antihistamines-vasoconstrictors, mast cell stabilizers, and steroids may all be necessary to manage VKC. Adjunct systemic antihistamines and steroids may be needed for exacerbations. Avoidance of the offending allergen(s) is the ultimate cure. Topically applied 0.05% naphazoline/0.5% antazoline, 4% cromolyn sodium, 0.1% lodoxamide, or 0.5% ketorolac tromethamine solutions four times a day may provide relief from symptoms for prolonged periods.[99-101]

Moderate to severe exacerbations of the disease after sufficient allergen exposure are best managed with topical steroids, such as 1% prednisolone acetate or 0.1% fluorometholone alcohol. The steroids may be best prescribed in a pulse fashion, one drop every 2 hours for 48–72 hours, then tapering in an appropriate manner. Systemic antihistamines provide effective adjunct therapy for vernal conjunctivitis patients, especially when given at bedtime (see Table 22-8). In severe cases with multiple exacerbations, a 1-week pulse of oral prednisone given several times per year may help alleviate the patient's symptoms.[117] Aspirin, an inhibitor of cyclo-oxygenase, also has been shown to be effective in reducing conjunctival inflammation, limbal cellular infiltration, and superficial punctate keratitis in patients who did not respond well to cromolyn sodium.[111,118] The recommended dosage is 0.5–1.5 g/day, depending on age.

TOXIC DISEASES

Toxic conjunctivitis and keratitis may result from overuse of topical medications, chronic exposure to foreign chemicals (such as contaminated eye cosmetics), and molluscum contagiosum.[119] Chronic or overuse of many topical medications including antibiotics, miotics, vasoconstrictors, or other ocular medications with chemical preservatives, such as thimerosal, can lead to a toxic conjunctivitis or keratitis. Eye cosmetics often become contaminated with bacteria, particularly *Pseudomonas aeruginosa*, which elaborate toxins. Diagnosis of toxic keratoconjunctivitis is aided by a careful history with particular attention to the patient's past medication history. The patient should be questioned directly about the use of over-the-counter (OTC) eye preparations and contact lens solutions.

Most ocular toxic reactions involve the conjunctiva and present with variable injection and a chronic follicular hyperplasia. There may be a mild-to-moderate mucoid discharge. In some cases, epithelial keratinization may be seen. Corneal signs can include epithelial edema, limbal injection, superficial neovascularization, and peripheral infiltrates.

The primary treatment is to remove the offending agent. Patients with chronic conjunctivitis who have been treated with a number of ophthalmic preparations without success should discontinue use of all topical medications for several days. Old eye cosmetics should be discarded. Unpreserved artificial tears will lubricate the globe and hasten resolution of the irritation. Judicious use of topical steroids such as 0.12% prednisolone acetate or 0.1% fluorometholone may be needed in severe cases. In instances where molluscum contagiosum is the cause of chronic follicular conjunctivitis, simple excision of the lesions is generally the preferred treatment. Molluscum lesions, which are caused by a poxvirus, are small, umbilicated papular lesions that may occur along the lid margin and rarely on the conjunctiva or cornea. The keratoconjunctivitis that results from molluscum lesions is caused by a toxic reaction to viral particles shed into the eye rather than a direct infectious process.

OCULAR SURFACE DISEASES

Tear Film Abnormalities

Symptoms caused by tear film abnormalities can be very mild or consist of severe pain and photophobia. Most patients report dry, burning, scratchy sensations often associated with a mild mucoid discharge. Occasionally, the patient may have increased tearing because of the irritation. Tear film abnormalities can involve all three layers of the tear film and may be either primary or secondary disorders. Aqueous deficiency of the tear film has multiple causes such as age-related changes in the lacrimal gland, medication use (e.g., antihistamines or beta-adrenergic blockers), or it may be related to systemic conditions such as Sjögren's syndrome.

Primary Sjögren's syndrome is characterized by keratoconjunctivitis sicca and dryness of other mucous membranes of the body such as the mouth, nasopharynx, and vagina. Aqueous deficiency in Sjögren's syndrome is related to inflammatory activity within the lacrimal gland, which becomes infiltrated with lymphocytes. Sjögren's syndrome is more common in women at or near menopause, although it can occur in men and younger women. When associated with connective tissue disease such as rheumatoid arthritis, the constellation of findings is referred to as secondary Sjögren's syndrome.

Definitive diagnosis of Sjögren's syndrome is accomplished via biopsy of the accessory lacrimal glands or labial tissue. Sodium fluorescein dye will stain damaged corneal epithelium in the aqueous-deficient patient and help define the volume of the tear meniscus. Rose bengal dye will stain desiccated, devitalized cells, outline any corneal filament formations, and provide a more sensitive test of conjunctival/corneal integrity than fluorescein dye, however.[120] Additional testing for aqueous tear deficiency is outlined in Chapter 11.

Tear lipid abnormalities are commonly overlooked in evaluating dry eye patients and are usually associated with lid margin aberrations, blepharitis, and meibomianitis. Contact lens wear also can significantly alter the quality and composition of both the lipid and mucin components of the tear film, thereby leading to dry eye problems. Tear mucin deficiencies are related to goblet cell dysfunction, which may be secondary to chemical burns, chronic conjunctivitis, ocular pemphigoid, hypovitaminosis A, and Stevens-Johnson syndrome.

The conjunctiva in ocular pemphigoid, hypovitaminosis A, and Stevens-Johnson syndrome often develops squamous metaplasia, which leads to goblet cell destruction, keratinization, and conjunctival scarring. Symblepharon formation is common, and patients with Stevens-Johnson syndrome may also have loss of accessory lacrimal glands and stenosed duct orifices.

Measurement of the tear break-up time (TBUT) can be helpful in the diagnosis of mucin deficiency. The mucin layer is necessary for the even spreading of the more superficially located aqueous and lipid tear layers. Although the diagnostic importance of this test can be somewhat variable, a TBUT of longer than 15 seconds is traditionally considered normal, 10–15 seconds is considered borderline, and less than 10 seconds is considered abnormal.

Most tear film abnormalities can be managed with frequent instillation of artificial tear solutions during waking hours. The dosage may range from several times per hour to only a few times daily depending on severity of symptoms. Ocular lubricating ointments at bedtime help prevent desiccation during sleep.[120] Punctal occlusion by silicone plugs or with electric or laser cautery can help prolong existing tears in the eye.[121]

Lid Abnormalities Affecting the Tear Film

Lagophthalmos, ectropion, unresolved Bell's palsy, and other lid closure problems cause the tear film to be poorly spread over the conjunctival and corneal surfaces leading to exposure keratoconjunctivitis. The symptoms and clinical findings are similar to those described with tear film deficiencies including burning, tearing, foreign body sensation, mucous discharge, tear film debris, and punctate keratopathy. The inferior cornea is typically the site of most pronounced epithelial disruption with lid closure problems.

To help prevent exposure and drying during sleep, the use of lubricating ointments or lid taping can be helpful. During the day, artificial tears and ointments are generally the mainstay of treatment. The frequency of instillation is adjusted according to individual need in these cases. Surgical intervention may be necessary to correct lid position in instances where lubricating therapy is not sufficient.

Dellen

Corneal dellen may cause an acute red eye and complaints of pain and photophobia. A mild mucoid discharge may be present. Clinically, dellen appear as round to oval corneal excavations usually located peripherally. With mild dellen the excavations only involve the epithelium, but stromal thinning may occur in more severe cases. The most common sites of involvement are at 3 and 9 o'clock adjacent to elevated conjunctival tissue such as caused by a pinguecula or pterygium. Elevated filtering blebs, pronounced chemosis, and other types of conjunctival and corneal masses may also cause the localized nonwetting that results in

TABLE 22-9
Clinical Characteristics of Corneal Dystrophies and Degenerations

Dystrophies	Degenerations
Bilateral	Unilateral or bilateral
Symmetric	Asymmetric
Central location	Peripheral or midperipheral location
Avascular	Often vascularized
Hereditary	
Slowly progressive	
Usually early onset	

dellen lesions. Diffuse epithelial edema, superficial neovascularization, and scarring may form in chronic cases. Dellen must be differentiated from persistent epithelial defects that can be caused by herpes simplex virus.[122,123]

Dellen, which are associated with localized drying, are treated with bland lubricating ointments and artificial tears. Ointments are generally more effective than tears alone because of a more prolonged contact time. Occasionally, the eye may need patching therapy to achieve a satisfactory resolution. Although artificial tears are helpful in the resolution of dellen, elimination of the cause of the localized drying is the ultimate treatment. Consequently, conjunctival tumors or other lesions may require surgical excision in some cases to prevent recurrence of the lesion. With lubricating therapy, most dellen lesions resolve in 24–48 hours.

CORNEAL DYSTROPHIES

In general, corneal dystrophies are usually inherited, not associated with any other primary corneal or systemic disease, initially involve one layer of the cornea, and are most often bilateral, although asymmetry may exist between the eyes.

The age of onset and degree of severity vary among the different corneal dystrophies. The corneal dystrophies are usually classified according to the affected layer of the cornea (Table 22-9).

Epithelial Basement Membrane Dystrophy

Epithelial basement membrane dystrophy (EBMD) is a dominantly inherited condition that is also known as Cogan's dystrophy or map, dot, or fingerprint dystrophy.[124] It may occur at any age. Epithelial basement membrane dystrophy is characterized by bilateral, although occasionally unilateral, grayish-white dots or lines that form in the region of the epithelial basement membrane.

FIGURE 22-12
Grayish-white, "putty-like" deposits, or dots, occurring in epithelial basement membrane dystrophy. (Courtesy of Leonard V. Messner, O.D.)

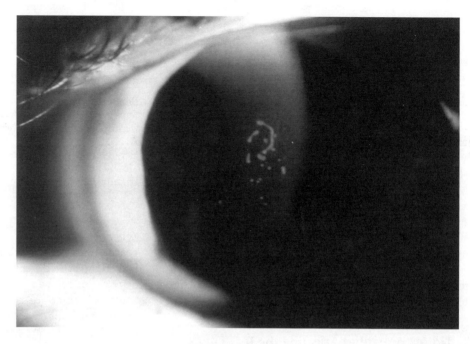

The dots represent clear-to-white microcysts that contain cellular debris. These microcysts form when basal epithelial cells become trapped by an abnormal basement membrane. They may have a putty-like appearance, and they may be variable in shape and size, occurring up to a few millimeters in length or width (Figure 22-12). Maplike lines consist of irregularly shaped, thin lines at the level of the epithelial basement membrane, which may form geographic or fingerprint-like patterns. The different types of lesions may occur alone or in combination with one another. These clinical findings result from abnormal synthesis of the basement membrane, which leads to thickening and extension of the basement membrane into the epithelium, causing abnormal misoriented basal epithelial cells, intraepithelial microcysts, intercellular edema, fibrillar material between the basement membrane and Bowman's layer, and reduction of hemidesmosomes.[125]

Recurrent corneal erosions can result from breaks in the loosely attached epithelium surrounding the basement membrane lesions. Although most patients with EBMD are asymptomatic, complaints of foreign body sensation, irritation, photophobia, and blurred vision are common when recurrent erosions are present.[125,126] Recurrent erosions classically develop upon opening the eyes after sleeping due to friction from the upper lids causing a shearing away of the inadequately attached epithelium. Recurrent corneal erosions account for the primary clinical significance of this disorder.

Epithelial basement membrane dystrophy may be dominantly inherited, thereby accounting for its classification as a corneal dystrophy. Occasionally, trauma to the epithelial layer, surgical or otherwise, can result in changes similar to classic EBMD.

Epithelial basement membrane dystrophy is generally treated with artificial tears and hypertonic solutions or ointments such as 2% or 5% sodium chloride. Corneal erosions caused by EBMD often require pressure patching with concomitant use of topical cycloplegics and antibiotic ointments. After epithelial healing, the frequency of recurrent erosion may possibly be reduced by continuing a hypertonic ointment at bedtime for several weeks even though no symptoms persist. In some cases, a bandage soft contact lens may be useful to protect the fragile epithelium until it firmly reattaches to the basement membrane. Debridement of loose epithelium from recurrent erosion sites is frequently necessary to prevent additional microcystic formations and promote re-epithelialization. Stromal puncture has been shown to be an effective procedure in some cases of persistent recurrent erosion.[127]

Meesmann's Juvenile Epithelial Dystrophy

Meesmann's juvenile epithelial dystrophy is an autosomal dominant disorder that begins in the first year of life. It is characterized by tiny, round, grayish-white cysts that are diffusely scattered or form a whorl-like pattern occurring predominantly in the interpalpebral zone of the cornea. Over time, the cysts, which contain glycogen and other cellular material, migrate toward the epithelial surface. The cysts appear relatively transparent in retro-illumination. The corneal epithelium and basement membrane are thickened and there is a diffuse grayish subepithelial appearance. Frequently, there is decreased corneal sensitivity. Meesmann's dystrophy is gradually progressive with few symptoms in early life, although mild irritation, photophobia, and blurred vision may occur during later years.[125,128] The exact pathophysiologic process causing this disorder is unknown.

Most patients do not require any treatment since visual acuity usually remains unaffected. A lamellar keratoplasty may be required in severe cases.

Reis-Buckler's Dystrophy

Reis-Buckler's dystrophy is an autosomal dominant condition that appears in the first decade of life. It is characterized by irregular, semitransparent lesions at Bowman's layer that develop into a grayish-white fishnet or honeycomb pattern in the central cornea with fine granulations in the anterior stroma in advanced cases. The midperipheral cornea often becomes involved, and increased corneal thickness and decreased corneal sensitivity are typical findings. Because of the abnormal Bowman's membrane and disruption of the overlying epithelial basement membrane, the corneal epithelium often becomes irregular and recurrent erosions are prone to occur. Bowman's layer is characterized by irregular collagen fibrils and fibroblast activity. It eventually disintegrates in later stages of the dystrophy with subsequent scar formation.[125,129,130] Generally, visual acuity does not become affected until the second or third decade of life.

Small corneal erosions associated with Reis-Buckler's dystrophy may be managed with artificial tears, lubricants, and hypertonic solutions or ointments. Larger abrasions may require pressure patching along with topical cycloplegia and antibiotic therapy. Soft bandage contact lenses may also be useful in some situations. As the dystrophy worsens, superficial keratectomy becomes necessary.

Granular Dystrophy

Granular dystrophy is an autosomal dominant, bilateral, and relatively symmetric stromal condition. It is characterized by discrete, central grayish-white opacities in the anterior stroma that appear in the first decade of life. The 0.2- to 0.4-mm round or oval lesions often have frayed irregular borders and appear randomly distributed with clear stroma between them. The peripheral stroma is unaffected. Occasionally, the dots coalesce to form linear or arcuate chains. As the clear anterior stroma opacifies and the lesions extend into the central stromal tissue, visual acuity gradually decreases to 20/200 or worse.[125] The granular lesions consist of a noncollagenous hyaline material that may push through Bowman's layer, indenting the basal epithelial cells. Although the exact cause is unknown, there is no correlation to collagen degeneration or excess keratocyte synthesis.[131] The surface corneal epithelium usually remains intact.

Granular dystrophy does not typically cause visual symptoms until later in life, and many patients may never develop loss of vision. Therefore, often no treatment is required. If treatment is required because of decreased visual acuity, lamellar or penetrating keratoplasty may be indicated. Although these surgical measures are effective, the condition may recur within the graft tissue.[132,133] Rarely, recurrent corneal erosions may complicate the later stages of the disease. They are managed with standard patching therapy, artificial tears, hypertonic agents, and possibly soft bandage contact lenses.

Macular Dystrophy

Macular dystrophy is an autosomal recessive, bilateral, symmetric dystrophy appearing in the first decade of life. It tends to be more severe than the autosomal dominant dystrophies. It is characterized by a diffuse stromal haze, focal grayish-white stromal opacities, and an irregular Descemet's membrane with corneal guttata. Unlike granular dystrophy, the peripheral stroma becomes cloudy in macular dystrophy. As the dystrophy progresses during the second and third decades, the lesions extend posteriorly to the endothelium, leading to dense stromal cloudiness and a graying of Descemet's membrane with subsequent reduced visual acuity. The surface epithelium usually remains smooth until later stages, when opacities break through Bowman's membrane and cause an irregular refractive surface and recurrent erosion.

The stromal opacities are composed of excess glycosaminoglycan concentrations, an acid mucopolysaccharide, which can also be found between the stromal collagen fibrils. The extracellular glycosaminoglycan causes the stromal hazing and clustering of the stromal fibrils, which results in decreased corneal thickness.[125,134,135] Macular dystrophy is distinguished from systemic mucopolysaccharidoses by the absence of systemic or other ocular clinical signs.[136]

Penetrating keratoplasty is the treatment of choice for macular dystrophy. Although the condition can recur in the graft, keratoplasty using a large graft, leaving a minimum of host tissue, may have a more favorable long-term prognosis.[137,138]

Lattice Dystrophy

Lattice dystrophy is an autosomal dominant, bilateral, symmetric condition that usually appears in the first decade of life. Asymmetric and unilateral cases with later onsets have been reported, often exhibiting fewer symptoms and good visual acuity.[139,140] The clinical appearance of lattice dystrophy includes translucent refractile lines; discrete, round, subepithelial white dots or dashes; anterior stromal dots; and a diffuse central stromal haze. The filamentary lines may develop into a dense network radiating throughout the cornea. Recurrent corneal erosions may develop over the lines or dots.

The refractile lines and corneal deposits are composed of amyloid, which results either from collagen degeneration due to lysosomal enzymes released from the abnormal keratocytes or from synthesis of amyloid from the abnormal keratocytes.[125] This process is not associated with any primary or secondary amyloidosis of the cornea but may appear in patients with systemic amyloid.[141,142]

Corneal erosions associated with lattice dystrophy may require pressure patching along with other appropriate therapy including topical cycloplegia and antibiotic therapy to prevent secondary bacterial infection and ulceration. For severe and recurrent erosions, bandage soft contact lenses or stromal puncture therapy may be effective.[127] Lamellar or penetrating keratoplasty is often required in advanced cases, but like some other dystrophies, lattice opacifications can recur in graft tissue.[143]

Fuchs' Endothelial Dystrophy

Fuchs' dystrophy is a bilateral, asymmetric condition that usually appears in middle age. It occurs more often in women, particularly those who are postmenopausal.[144,145] The clinical manifestations of Fuchs' dystrophy may be divided into three clinical stages that progressively develop over a period of 10–20 years. The first stage is characterized by asymptomatic, central, irregular, sometimes pigmented corneal guttata posterior to Descemet's membrane. The guttata are composed of collagen and may initially present around 30 years of age. Occasionally, associated pigmentation occurs in a well-delineated geographic zone within the central cornea (Figure 22-13). Descemet's membrane becomes thickened during the later part of this first stage.

The second stage is typified by blurred visual acuity caused by developing stromal and epithelial edema. Folds in Descemet's membrane caused by the pronounced edema are often evident. As the second stage of the condition advances, pronounced epithelial edema may produce painful bullae and recurrent corneal erosions. The corneal edema associated with Fuchs' dystrophy tends to worsen during sleep because of limited tear evaporation under the closed eyelid, and therefore patients usually complain of worse visual acuity on awakening.

Subepithelial connective tissue forms in the third stage of Fuchs' dystrophy, with less corneal edema being present but with greater loss of visual acuity.[145,146] Potential complications include infectious keratitis, corneal neovascularization, and glaucoma.[145,147]

The corneal edema in Fuchs' endothelial dystrophy is best managed with hypertonic solutions and ointments. Five percent sodium chloride ointment is most commonly used at bedtime; a 2% or 5% solution is helpful during the day to avoid the deleterious blur caused by ointments. To help alleviate the early morning blur, patients may direct a hair dryer toward their corneas to facilitate evaporation and reduce the epithelial edema. It may be helpful to use antiglaucoma medication to reduce intraocular pressure, thereby lessening the force of aqueous flow into the stroma. This may be especially helpful if intraocular pressure is abnormally high initially. Epithelial erosions caused by ruptured bullae may require bandage contact lenses, and stromal puncture may also be beneficial.[127] Penetrating keratoplasty is usually successful in severe cases.[145]

Posterior Polymorphous Dystrophy

Posterior polymorphous dystrophy (PPD) is a stable or slowly progressive unilateral or bilateral endothelial dystrophy that is probably present at birth. Most patients are asymptomatic with no reduction of visual acuity. The inheritance pattern is usually autosomal dominant, but it can also be autosomal recessive. Clinical findings include small, grouped vesicles, larger geographic blister-like lesions, broad bands, and gray sheets that protrude posteriorly and appear as thickenings of Descemet's membrane. As Descemet's membrane becomes irregular, it develops a peau d'orange appearance in retroillumination.[145,148] The 0.2- to 0.4-mm blister-like lesions, seen best in retroillumination, are surrounded by a diffuse gray halo. They can be found anywhere on the posterior cornea and do not affect visual acuity. The broad bands associated with PPD are formed by translucent, elevated ridges that are approximately parallel.[149] The band-shaped lesions can be about 1 mm in width and extend across the entire corneal diameter (Figure 22-14). Corneal edema and peripheral iridocorneal adhesions may form with progression of the dystrophy. Elevated intraocular pressure and glaucoma occur in 15% of cases.[145,148,149]

Histologically, PPD is characterized by multilaminar collagen layers posterior to Descemet's membrane and a multilayered epithelial-like morphology of the endothelium.[145,150] The presence of broad iris adhesions to a prominent Schwalbe's line or higher, as well as other anomalies

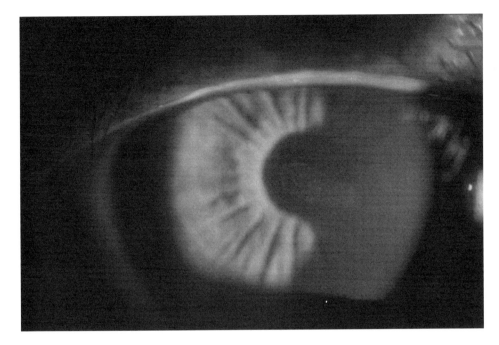

FIGURE 22-13
Geographic zone of endothelial pigmentation associated with Fuchs' endothelial dystrophy. The irregular quality of the posterior cornea causing a shagreen-like appearance can be appreciated as it is retroilluminated against the pupillary border. (Courtesy of Michelle L. Cornick, O.D., and Daniel K. Roberts, O.D.)

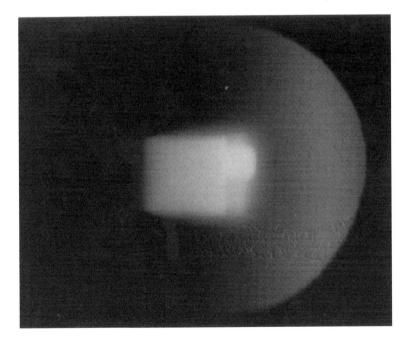

FIGURE 22-14
Posterior polymorphous dystrophy may occasionally cause prominent posterior corneal band-shaped lesions, which may extend across the entire cornea. (Courtesy of Daniel K. Roberts, O.D.)

of the iris and iridocorneal angle structures, suggest the condition could be related to other conditions resulting from ocular mesenchymal dysgenesis.[148,151]

Corneal edema associated with PPD may be managed with standard hypertonic therapy, including the use of sodium chloride solution and ointment, although the effects from this therapy may be minimal. Severe cases with pronounced edema and corneal opacification require penetrating keratoplasty. The prognosis of penetrating keratoplasty is less favorable when iridocorneal adhesions are present.[145,148] Associated glaucoma is managed with standard measures.

CORNEAL DEGENERATIONS

Arcus

Corneal arcus is a common, bilateral benign degeneration most often noted in patients 50 years of age or older. The clinical appearance is a 1- to 2-mm wide, grayish-white ring located in the peripheral cornea and separated from the limbus by a clear zone. The ring is composed of lipid material within the stroma. Arcus in younger patients may be associated with hypercholesterolemia.[152]

Corneal arcus does not require treatment. However, laboratory investigation for hyperlipidemia is indicated for younger patients.

Band Keratopathy

Band keratopathy is typified by calcium deposits in the anterior corneal stroma, epithelial basement membrane, and Bowman's layers. The deposits form a white horizontal band within the interpalpebral zone. Other clinical features include clear holes within the band, a clear margin or lucid zone at the limbus, and slight corneal edema. The peripheral cornea is most affected early on; however, with progression the central cornea becomes prominently involved as well. Symptoms include irritation, redness, tearing, photophobia, and blurred vision. Band keratopathy is usually associated with chronic ocular inflammatory conditions, or it may occur in association with systemic diseases involving disturbances of calcium metabolism such as juvenile rheumatoid arthritis, hyperparathyroidism, vitamin D toxicity, and uremia.[153]

If significant irritation and blurred vision exist, removal of the calcium deposit may be attempted by chelation with ethylenediamine tetra-acetic acid (EDTA). In this procedure, the epithelium is first mechanically debrided and then an EDTA-soaked sponge is applied to the opacified region for a period of time, followed by repeated rubbing of the affected area. Lamellar keratoplasty may be considered if EDTA chelation is unsuccessful.[153,154]

Keratoconus

Keratoconus is a noninflammatory, usually bilateral and progressive, thinning and ectasia of the central cornea frequently resulting in anterior stromal scarring and reduced visual acuity. It typically causes symptoms in the second and third decades of life. The condition demonstrates increased visibility of the corneal nerves, inferior corneal steepening, and posterior stromal vertical striae (Vogt's striae). Classically, on inferior gaze, the ectatic cornea causes an outward distortion of the lower lid, a well-

TABLE 22-10
Corneal Iron Lines

Entity	Description
Hudson-Stähli line	Horizontal line in inferior cornea
Fleischer ring	Base of cone in keratoconus
Stocker-Busacca line	Leading edge of inactive pterygium
Ferry line	Edge of filtering bleb
Superficial corneal scar	Breakdown of corneal epithelium after traumatic injury
Metallic foreign body scar	Deposition of iron from oxidation of metallic foreign body
Congenital spherocytosis	Brownish-yellow deposits

known phenomenon referred to as Munson's sign. The base of the ectatic area, or "cone," portion of the cornea is identified by a partial or complete Fleischer ring, a brownish arcuate line or oval ring characterized by iron deposition. Various types of iron deposition affecting the cornea are contrasted in Table 22-10.

Initially, keratoconus presents with progressively increasing myopia and high degrees of irregular astigmatism. With advancing disease, progressive thinning and ectasia occur, and visual acuity becomes less satisfactory as irregular astigmatism progresses. In more advanced disease, ruptures may occur in Descemet's membrane, creating marked corneal edema, a situation referred to as acute hydrops. Acute hydrops typically resolves but is recurrent, eventually causing pronounced scarring. Although the etiology is uncertain, keratoconus may be associated with hay fever, asthma, allergies, eczema, eye rubbing, Down's syndrome, connective tissue disorders, and contact lens wear.[155]

Various contact lens fitting modalities may be successful in the early stages of keratoconus by eliminating the effects of the irregular astigmatism. As the disease progresses, a penetrating keratoplasty frequently becomes necessary because of contact lens intolerance, hydrops formation, or corneal scarring. Occasionally, 5% sodium chloride solution may provide temporary symptomatic relief for acute hydrops.[156,157]

Mooren's Ulcer

Mooren's ulcer is a painful, chronically progressive ulceration that begins in the peripheral cornea and moves circumferentially and toward the central cornea. The ulceration characteristically exhibits a central, elevated, and undermined leading edge. The progression eventually involves the central cornea with occasional perforation. In the wake of the ulcer's active leading edge is a thinned vascularized stroma. Symptoms include intense pain, photophobia, redness, and decreased visual acuity. A concurrent anterior uveitis may exist.

Mooren's ulcers can be divided into two categories. Unilateral ulcers comprise 75% of the cases and tend to occur in older age groups. These ulcers are typically milder. The remaining ulcers usually occur in men 20–30 years of age and which tend to be more progressive. They are bilateral in 60–80% of cases.

Mooren's ulcers are thought to have an autoimmune etiology. They may develop after surgical procedures, trauma, foreign bodies, and chemical burns.[158,159] One report indicates a possible relationship of Mooren's ulcer with hepatitis C infections.[160]

Topical 1% prednisolone acetate every 30 minutes is required day and night until the progression is halted, followed by a slow tapering of the drug over 2 months until final resolution is achieved. Systemic immunosuppressive agents are indicated if pain or progression continues with topical therapy. Cycloplegia with topical 1% atropine is typically necessary to decrease ciliary spasm and improve comfort, and prophylactic topical antibiotics may be prescribed to help prevent secondary infection. Topical cyclosporin A may be effective in some cases of Mooren's ulcer. Penetrating keratoplasty may be successful for some endstage cases.[161-164]

Pellucid Marginal Degeneration

Pellucid marginal degeneration is characterized by a 1- to 2-mm wide bilateral thinning of the inferior cornea, causing a corresponding ectasia and high degrees of irregular astigmatism. Although Descemet's folds may form, there is no associated infiltration, scarring, or vascularization. Similar to keratoconus, acute hydrops can occur because of rupture of Descemet's membrane. Pellucid degeneration is found equally in both sexes, is possibly hereditary, and usually occurs between the ages of 20 and 40 years. The etiology may be similar to that for keratoconus.[155,158]

The typical photokeratoscopic image associated with pellucid marginal degeneration is an egg-shaped mire pattern. This is created by a vertical flattening of the cornea centrally and a steepening inferiorly (Figure 22-15). Computerized topographic analysis of pellucid degeneration shows the corneal distortion similarly as there being irregular against-the-rule astigmatism centrally and with-the-rule astigmatism inferiorly (Color Plate 22-I).

Contact lenses are initially fitted in the management of pellucid marginal degeneration in an attempt to eliminate the effects of the irregular astigmatism. If unsuccessful, surgical measures including penetrating keratoplasty may be required.[155,158]

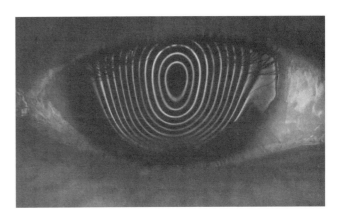

FIGURE 22-15
Photokeratoscopic image of pellucid marginal degeneration. A classic egg-shaped mire pattern is exhibited. There is vertical flattening of the cornea centrally and steeping inferiorly. (Courtesy of Daniel K. Roberts, O.D., and Pamela J. Boyce, O.D.)

Pterygium

Pterygia are triangle-shaped, vascularized elevations of connective tissue on the bulbar conjunctiva that also encroach onto the cornea, frequently threatening the visual axis (Figure 22-16). Usually located nasally, pterygia intertwine with the corneal epithelium and Bowman's layer. Histopathologically, there is a degeneration of the subepithelial bulbar conjunctival stroma and subepithelial collagen. During active growth, the leading edge of a pterygium can exhibit a slightly translucent zone with associated corneal edema. A faint, brown, iron deposition line, referred to as a Stocker-Busacca line, is commonly observed anterior to the leading corneal edge during inactive phases (see Table 22-10). Chronic environmental irritation from exposure to ultraviolet light, air pollution, dust, and wind may contribute to pterygium formation.[165,166]

Most pterygia only require annual monitoring. When tear film wetting problems or corneal dellen develop, artificial tears are usually beneficial. Inflamed pterygia may require topical corticosteroids for several days. When encroachment of a pterygium threatens the visual axis, surgical excision is indicated and should be performed before the leading edge involves the visual axis.[167-170] Recurrence of pterygia may follow their excision. Refractive error may be influenced by larger pterygia causing with-the-rule astimatism due to corneal flattening created in the horizontal meridian. Occasionally, irregular astigmatism may develop and cause visual blur that is not correctable with spectacles.

FIGURE 22-16
Pterygia are vascularized, triangle-shaped lesions that typically extend onto the cornea nasally at the epithelial and Bowman's membrane layers. Larger lesions may cause corneal distortion or even directly involve the visual axis.

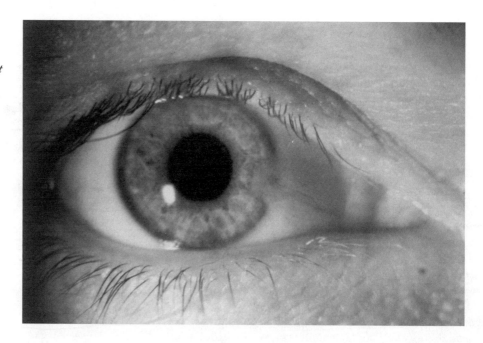

Salzmann's Nodular Degeneration

Salzmann's nodular degeneration is typified by elevated, grayish-white or bluish-gray nodules in the peripheral cornea with alternating thickening and thinning of the epithelium. The nodules have semitransparent margins with adjacent clear cornea and no neovascularization. The nodules are variable in size and are composed of recently formed collagen involving Bowman's layer and the anterior stroma. The condition is usually asymptomatic. Salzmann's degeneration is most common in elderly women and frequently develops after injuries or keratitis.[171]

Terrien's Marginal Degeneration

Terrien's degeneration is characterized by a very slowly progressive marginal corneal thinning that often begins at the superior limbus with injection, lipid deposition, and furrowing, which eventually forms a peripheral corneal gutter. The gutter steadily deepens with vascularized scar formation. The corneal epithelium remains intact while nonulcerative destruction of Bowman's layer and the stromal lamellae ensues. Pseudopterygia are typical of Terrien's marginal degeneration and are characterized by vascularized extensions that cross areas of thinning from the conjunctiva obliquely in meridians usually other than at 3 and 9 o'clock (Figure 22-17). Spontaneous perforation can occur. The degeneration is usually bilateral and often occurs in 20- to 40-year-old men. Visual acuity may be reduced because of irregular astigmatism formation.[155,158]

Conservative management is indicated for most cases of Terrien's marginal degeneration; only the induced astigmatism warrants correction. Some cases are characterized by recurrent episodes of inflammation, and in these instances, topical steroids can be used on a short-term basis to quiet the eye. For advanced cases with severe corneal thinning and irregular astigmatism, various surgical procedures have been attempted including excision of opacified tissue with suturing of the gutter walls and penetrating keratoplasty. Scleral contact lenses have been used in some patients. Because of the high risk of perforation or rupture of the thinned cornea in advanced cases, the eyes should be protected from trauma.[172]

CORNEAL AND CONJUNCTIVAL TRAUMA

Injuries to the conjunctiva and cornea result from many household, school, sport, or workplace activities. Children and young adults are particularly at risk. One study[173] found that 40% of eye injuries were caused by foreign bodies involving the conjunctiva or cornea, but clinical findings may also include chemical or thermal burns and abrasions, lacerations, or contusions from blunt trauma.

Abrasions, Contusions, and Lacerations

Direct trauma is the most frequent cause of abrasions, contusions, and lacerations to the conjunctiva or cornea. The nature of the contact instrument usually determines

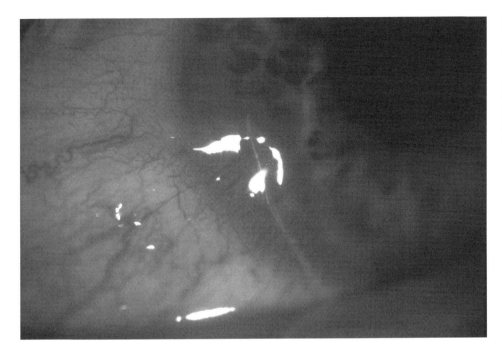

FIGURE 22-17
Pseudopterygium located infero-temporally that is associated with Terrien's marginal degeneration. These vascularized extensions typically cross areas of peripheral corneal thinning in areas other than 3 and 9 o'clock. (Courtesy of Daniel K. Roberts, O.D.)

the type of wound. For example, a large, blunt object may only cause a contusion, whereas a sharp pencil point is more likely to lacerate.

Abrasions of the conjunctiva and cornea are highlighted with sodium fluorescein dye. Corneal abrasions are delineated by relatively sharp margins and usually only involve the epithelial layers. Lacerations may involve all corneal layers and result in perforation of the globe. Whenever a corneal laceration is present, Seidel's test (see Color Plate 15-I) should be performed to rule out perforation with aqueous or vitreous leakage.

Conjunctival lacerations frequently result in loose conjunctival tissue flaps. The white sclera may be visible, flanked by clumping of conjunctival tissue, chemosis, and hemorrhage. The sclera must be carefully evaluated to rule out any perforation of this tissue. Most conjunctival contusions result in subconjunctival hemorrhages.[174] Occult perforation and the presence of an intraocular foreign body should always be considered when ocular injury occurs in the setting of possible projectile objects.

Conjunctival and corneal abrasions should be irrigated with sterile normal saline to remove any foreign material. Loose corneal epithelial tissue should be debrided, particularly if the eye is to be patched. Abrasions may be prophylactically treated with topical broad-spectrum antibiotics until wound healing occurs. Conjunctival and small corneal abrasions usually do not require patching, but patching is usually required for large corneal abrasions or in patients with considerable pain.

– Aculor tid
– Tobrex / Polysporin

Conjunctival lacerations may also be managed with topical broad-spectrum antibiotics. Frequently, conjunctival lacerations will require patching along with other appropriate measures including topical cycloplegia and the instillation of a topical broad-spectrum antibiotic ointment. Sutures are not needed for uncomplicated conjunctival lacerations.[175] Small corneal lacerations may self-seal immediately after the injury, but more extensive corneal lacerations usually require sealing with cyanoacrylate glue or sutures.

No specific therapy is required for conjunctival contusions since most only involve subconjunctival hemorrhages, which are self-limiting. Artificial tears may improve patient comfort.[174] In all instances of corneal and conjunctival trauma, other parts of the eye should be explored for trauma-related conditions and these should be managed appropriately if found.

Burns

Chemical burns of the conjunctiva usually result from inadvertent splashes of chemicals into the face or from hydrogen peroxide contact lens solutions. Occasionally patients may directly insert a chemical irritant into the eye. The latter injuries are often more severe. Thermal burns frequently are caused by cigarettes, curling irons, or overexposure to ultraviolet light. It is absolutely crucial with chemical burns to determine whether the offending chemical is acid or alkaline in nature. If the clinician is unfamiliar with the chemical, assistance is available by contacting the local poison control center for information.

After a thermal or chemical burn, the conjunctiva and cornea must be carefully assessed for the depth of the injury. Most acid burns will cause superficial epithelial damage as indicated with sodium fluorescein. Blanching of the conjunctival blood vessels is possible in severe cases. Alkaline burns from chemicals such as lye or lime usually blanch the conjunctival vessels and cause more severe injury because of their collagenolytic capabilities. Melting of the conjunctival, corneal, or scleral tissue can ensue from alkaline burns. Thermal burns may cause either superficial or severe injury depending on the contact time of the offending agent.[174,176]

Chemical burns require copious irrigation of the conjunctiva and cornea with normal saline. The saline lavage should be continued for approximately 30 minutes for acid and alkali burns (or until a neutral pH is obtained for alkali burns). Prophylactic topical broad-spectrum antibiotics should be used during the post-traumatic period to prevent secondary infection. Careful monitoring for signs of fibroblast activity and scar formation is necessary for several days after acid burns and for weeks after alkali burns. Topical steroids may be indicated to reduce cicatricial changes and the possibility of symblepharon formation. Acetylcysteine 20% may help reduce collagenase activity.

Since secondary glaucoma can result if there is significant corneal involvement, intraocular pressure should be closely monitored in alkali burn patients. Most conjunctival and corneal thermal burns are treated similar to acid burns. Frequent instillation of nonpreserved artificial tears is also important for keeping the tissue well lubricated in burn injuries.[12,174,176]

Foreign Bodies

Environmental foreign material consisting of dirt, dust, glass, or metal may contact and adhere to the conjunctiva or cornea. The workplace is a frequent source of ocular foreign body material, particularly when protective eyewear is not worn. After a thorough case history is obtained from the patient reporting an ocular foreign body, the eye must be carefully assessed. When uncertain regarding the nature or location of a foreign body, lid eversion is often required to complete a thorough search for the object or objects. Occasionally a double lid eversion may be required. Topical anesthesia may be necessary to evaluate the eye in some patients exhibiting marked discomfort and photophobia.

Fluorescein dye may be used to identify foreign body tracking along the corneal surface or other signs of epithelial disruption. Seidel's test is helpful in ruling out global

perforation and especially should be performed when there has been the possibility of projectile objects entering the eye, such as may occur when hammering metal on metal.

Most ocular foreign bodies are superficial and are usually found on the superior palpebral conjunctival or temporal corneal regions. When foreign bodies are embedded in the conjunctiva, a subconjunctival hemorrhage or conjunctival granuloma may envelop the impact site, and there may be surrounding hyperemia. Corneal wound sites may exhibit associated abrasion, edema, and infiltration. A rust ring may form around a metallic corneal foreign body.

Copious lavage with normal saline will loosen and remove many superficial foreign bodies. Swabbing the affected conjunctival area with a moistened cotton-tipped applicator can be effective with some foreign bodies, especially when they are larger and not embedded. Care must be taken, however, not to force a foreign object further into the corneal or conjunctival tissue. Cotton-tipped applicators may not be desirable instruments for removing corneal foreign bodies because of the amount of epithelial disruption that they may cause. When foreign material is difficult to visualize, as with fiberglass particles, swabbing the fornices can be effective. Any swabbing should be followed by a saline lavage.

Embedded objects in either the conjunctiva or cornea may be removed with a needle or foreign body spud. Corneal rust rings are commonly removed with an Alger brush burr. A broad-spectrum topical antibiotic coverage, such as gentamicin or bacitracin/polymyxin B ointment, should be applied to the eye after removal of a foreign body to prevent secondary infection. The antibiotic should be continued until the wound site has healed. Pressure patching with cycloplegia and instillation of a topical broad-spectrum antibiotic ointment may be indicated with larger wound sites or when a foreign body has been relatively deeply embedded.[174]

MISCELLANEOUS DISORDERS

Superior Limbic Keratoconjunctivitis

Superior limbic keratoconjunctivitis (SLK) is a chronic or acute inflammatory condition involving the superior bulbar and palpebral conjunctiva.[177] It is characterized by thickening of the bulbar conjunctiva, injection (Figure 22-18), punctate staining involving the cornea and conjunctiva along the superior limbal region, papillary hypertrophy, and sometimes filamentary keratitis (Table 22-11). Superior punctate keratoconjunctivitis stains with rose bengal as well as fluorescein, a sign that is often very helpful in the

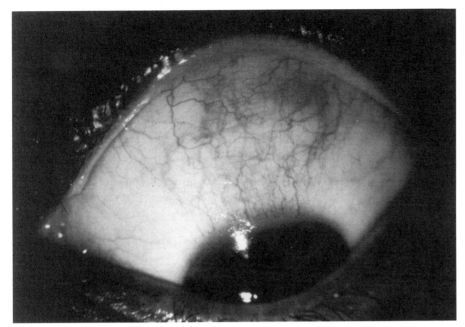

FIGURE 22-18
Superior limbic keratoconjunctivitis is typified by sectoral superior bulbar injection. The superior limbal region classically exhibits punctate staining with rose bengal. Superior corneal pannus, chemosis, and papillary hypertrophy of the upper tarsus are common. (Courtesy of Scott Robison, O.D.)

TABLE 22-11
Common Causes of Corneal Filaments

Diabetes mellitus
Epithelial basement membrane dystrophy
Herpes simplex keratitis
Keratoconjunctivitis sicca
Extended patching of the eye
Recurrent erosion
Superior limbic keratoconjunctivitis

diagnosis of this disorder. Superior limbic keratoconjunctivitis is usually bilateral but may occur unilaterally and can affect individuals of all ages. The condition can last years and typically has a chronic remitting and relapsing course. There is an increased incidence of thyroid dysfunction in patients with SLK.

Patients with SLK typically experience dry eye–type symptoms and exhibit some keratinization of the bulbar conjunctival epithelial cells. Symptoms may include burning, foreign body sensation, tearing, blepharospasm, photophobia, and blurred vision. Symptoms are markedly worse when filaments are present.

Treatment is supportive in mild cases of SLK, consisting of artificial tears and topical vasoconstrictors. Topical mast cell stabilizers and nonsteroidal anti-inflammatory agents may be beneficial. More severe cases may require 0.5% silver nitrate applied to the superior bulbar conjunctival region. Bandage contact lenses may be helpful in the management of filamentary keratitis and

topical acetylcysteine may relieve mucus accumulation related to filament formation. Following improvement, there may be recurrence of symptoms, and surgical resection of the superior bulbar conjunctiva is sometimes used in severe cases to provide temporary relief.[12,178,179]

An SLK-like presentation has been reported to occur in soft contact lens wearers using thimerosal-preserved solutions.[180] Temporary discontinuance of contact lens wear and switching to preservative-free saline and other solutions typically eliminates the condition.

Pinguecula

Pingueculae are small, yellowish-white elevations on the nasal or temporal bulbar conjunctiva and exhibit a degenerative process similar to pterygia. While there is no encroachment onto the cornea, pingueculae can become inflamed, resulting in a pingueculitis. This frequently occurs in conjunction with dry eye syndrome or keratoconjunctivitis sicca. Large pingueculae may occasionally cause corneal dellen formation.

Artificial tears are appropriate if a pinguecula becomes irritated from dry eye syndrome. Topical 0.12% prednisolone phosphate solution or another similar steroid for several days is usually effective for pingueculitis.

Subconjunctival Hemorrhage

Hemorrhages from small transient breaks in the conjunctival vessels can accumulate in the subconjunctival space, creating a bright red appearance to the affected area. The approximate site of the original leakage may sometimes be identified by an area of denser hemorrhage accumulation. Although the majority of subconjunctival hemorrhages result from Valsalva type stress, they can also ensue from infectious conjunctivitis, systemic hypertension, or trauma. Other disorders may also be implicated.

Subconjunctival hemorrhages do not require treatment. However, associated systemic disease should be ruled out, especially if recurrent. Subconjunctival hemorrhages spontaneously reabsorb into the conjunctival lymph or vascular networks within 10–14 days.

Thygeson's Superficial Punctate Keratitis

Thygeson's superficial punctate keratitis is a bilateral, chronic condition typically seen in patients under 40 years of age. It is characterized by coarse, discrete, elevated interepithelial, whitish-gray dot-like or oval opacities in the central cornea. The lesions frequently stain with sodium fluorescein, and there is no underlying stromal inflammation. The condition will resolve without therapy within days or weeks, but recurrences are common. Individuals may be afflicted with these recurrent inflammatory episodes for months or even years. Occasionally, there may be residual subepithelial opacities on resolution of the epithelial disease. Typical symptoms include foreign body sensation, photophobia, tearing, and blurred vision. The etiology of Thygeson's disease is unknown.[181]

Topical steroids such as 1% prednisolone sodium phosphate or 0.1% fluorometholone solution four times a day provide symptomatic relief within several days but are not curative. Artificial tears may help reduce foreign body sensation, and therapeutic soft contact lenses have been shown to be beneficial in some cases.[182]

Episcleritis

Diffuse Episcleritis
Episcleritis is an acute, nonspecific inflammation of the loose episcleral connective tissue overlying the sclera. It is a benign, self-limited inflammatory condition that is usually unilateral but may occur bilaterally. Symptoms include tearing, foreign body sensation, mild pain, tenderness, and photophobia. The clinical presentation is typically a localized, nonelevated, sectoral redness within the interpalpebral area that lasts for 2–4 weeks. Occasionally, there is an associated mild anterior chamber reaction. Diffuse episcleritis is more common in women and may recur. The etiology is unknown, but its occurrence may be related to herpes simplex and polyarteritis nodosa. A laboratory workup is usually not performed for initial presentations.[12,15]

The treatment of mild diffuse episcleritis may be supportive; however, topical steroids are commonly used to hasten its resolution. On response to therapy, topical steroids should be tapered to prevent rebounding of the inflammation.

Nodular Episcleritis
Nodular episcleritis comprises about 20% of all cases of episcleritis. The symptoms and clinical findings are similar to those of diffuse episcleritis with the exception of nodule formation and a longer duration of the disease. Frequently, nodular episcleritis last 4–6 weeks. Episcleritis nodules, which are composed of large mononuclear cells, are raised and may be 2–3 mm in diameter. Helpful in the differentiation of nodular scleritis, the episcleritis nodules move freely over the sclera on palpation. Mild iritis is a common associated finding, and the condition may be associated with conditions such as rheumatoid arthritis, herpes simplex infection, herpes zoster ophthalmicus, Epstein-Barr virus, polyarteritis nodosa, syphilis, and tuberculosis. Laboratory workups are often productive in nodular episcleritis.[12,15]

Topical steroids are generally used to treat nodular episcleritis. Slow tapering over several weeks is often necessary to prevent a recurrence of the inflammation.

Scleritis

Scleritis is a more serious inflammation of the sclera that may involve the anterior or posterior segment. A commonly used classification system is shown in Table 22-12. Anterior scleritis is far more common than posterior scleritis and the condition may be bilateral or unilateral. Anterior scleritis can be subclassified into diffuse, nodular, and necrotizing scleritis. Posterior scleritis usually presents with choroiditis or chorioretinitis but may also have associated nonrhegmatogenous retinal detachment, macular edema, and venous occlusion. Appropriate diagnosis and management are critical for successful resolution of scleritis.

Anterior scleritis is characterized by deep and superficial vascular injection and congestion that has a violaceous hue over the inflamed tissue. The deep injection does not blanch with topical 2.5% phenylephrine solution. Unlike simple episcleritis, the contour of the deep scleral tissue may appear altered or elevated when a thin slit beam is passed over the involved regions. This observation can occasionally be helpful in differentiating between the two conditions. Symptoms include tenderness, tearing, photophobia, and severe pain that often radiates to surrounding facial structures. There is a variable amount of overlying episcleral inflammation, and the conjunctiva usually demonstrates moderate chemo-

TABLE 22-12
Classification of Scleritis

I. Anterior scleritis
   A. Diffuse
   B. Nodular
   C. Necrotizing
      1. With inflammation
      2. Without inflammation (scleromalacia perforans)
II. Posterior scleritis

Source: PG Watson, SS Hayreh. Scleritis and episcleritis. Br J Ophthalmol 1976;60:163–91.

sis and hyperemia. Although the peripheral cornea may become infiltrated or vascularized in anterior scleritis, marginal corneal ulceration is only an occasional complication. Anterior scleritis may be idiopathic or related to systemic disease such as rheumatoid arthritis, herpes zoster ophthalmicus, Epstein-Barr virus, gout, and systemic lupus erythematosus.[12,15]

The clinical appearance of nodular anterior scleritis is similar to that of diffuse anterior scleritis with the exception of tender, fixed nodules, which usually form on the superior sclera. The nodules do not necrotize. Most cases are associated with systemic disease.[12,15]

Necrotizing scleritis with inflammation is distinguished by an initial inflammatory reaction that leads to thinning of the sclera accompanied by intense, progressively worsening pain. The necrotic sclera has a bluish appearance because of visibility of the underlying uveal tissue and has surrounding areas of inflammation. Marginal corneal ulceration can occur. Necrotizing scleritis is often associated with rheumatoid arthritis or herpes zoster ophthalmicus.[12,15]

Although necrotizing scleritis without inflammation (i.e., scleromalacia perforans) is not accompanied by intense inflammation or pain, nodules and staphyloma may form. Most cases occur in women over 40 years of age with rheumatoid arthritis. Other associated systemic diseases include polyarteritis nodosa, rheumatoid arthritis, and systemic lupus erythematosus.[12,183]

Posterior scleritis is often accompanied by anterior scleritis, but when it is not, its diagnosis is less straightforward. Associated signs and symptoms may include extreme pain and global tenderness, proptosis, limited mobility, exudative retinal detachment, and disc edema. After resolution, the overlying retina may be pale and exhibit pigmentary changes corresponding to the region of scleral inflammation. Pigmentation may give the appearance of a "high water" mark at the posterior border of involvement.

Scleritis is primarily treated with oral therapy, which usually initially consists of nonsteroidal anti-inflammatory agents such as indomethacin or flurbiprofen. Since some patients respond to one nonsteroidal drug but not another, different agents may be tried. If nonsteroidal therapy is ineffective, then oral corticosteroids are usually tried. In patients resistant to these therapies, especially those with severe necrotizing scleritis, immunosuppressive therapy may be instituted. Cyclophosphamide is typically used. Intravenous pulse therapy with methylprednisolone is indicated in those patients who have vasculitis-associated destructive disease. Early identification and treatment of scleromalacia perforans is necessary, otherwise the tissue damage related to underlying arteriolar obstruction will not be halted.

Scleritis may require long-term therapy, so some patients do poorly because they are intolerant to the drugs used. Although topical corticosteroidal therapy is insufficient to control the inflammation caused by scleritis, it may improve subjective patient comfort and therefore may be useful in the management of these cases. Topical therapy may be beneficial for the maintenance of those patients already brought under control with systemic medications.

REFERENCES

1. National Center for Health Statistics, JP Ganley, J Roberts. Eye Conditions and Related Need for Medical Care Among Persons 1–74 Years of Age—United States 1971–1972. Vital and Health Statistics. Series 11, No. 228. DHHS Pub (PHS)83–1678. Public Health Service. Washington, DC: US Government Printing Office, March 1983.
2. Apple DJ, Rabb MF. Ocular Pathology. Clinical Applications and Self Assessment. St. Louis: Mosby-Year Book, 1991;58–111, 456–93.
3. Greiner JV, Henriquez AS, Covington MS, et al. Goblet cells of the human conjunctiva. Arch Ophthalmol 1981; 99:2190–7.
4. Sachs EH, Wieczorek R, Jakobiec FA, Knowles DM. Lymphocytic subpopulations in the normal human conjunctiva: a monoclonal antibody study. Ophthalmology 1986;93: 1276–83.
5. Spinak M. Cytological changes of the conjunctiva in immunoglobulin-producing dyscrasias. Ophthalmology 1981;88:1207–11.
6. Allansmith MR, Greiner JV, Baird BS. Number of inflammatory cells in the normal conjunctiva. Am J Ophthalmol 1978;86:250–9.
7. Warwick R (ed). Eugene Wolff's Anatomy of the Eye and Orbit (7th ed). Philadelphia: Saunders, 1976;48–51, 206.
8. Tiffany JM, Bron AJ. Role of tears in maintaining corneal integrity. Trans Ophthalmol Soc UK 1978;98:335–8.

9. Crandall A, Yanoff M, Schaffer D. Intrascleral nerve loop mistakenly identified as a foreign body. Arch Ophthalmol 1977;95:497–8.

10. Friedlaender MH. Allergy and Immunology of the Eye. New York: Raven, 1993;55.

11. Yanoff M, Fine BS. Ocular Pathology. Philadelphia: Lippincott, 1989;216–9.

12. Ostler HB. Diseases of the External Eye and Adnexa. Baltimore: Williams & Wilkins, 1993;137–9, 194, 253–6, 261–8, 782–4.

13. Kenyon KR, Chaves HV. Morphology and Pathologic Response of Corneal and Conjunctival Disease. In G Smolin, RA Thoft (eds), The Cornea. Scientific Foundations and Clinical Practice. Boston: Little, Brown, 1994;85–9.

14. Mannis MJ. Therapeutic Contact Lenses. In G Smolin, RA Thoft (eds), The Cornea. Scientific Foundations and Clinical Practice. Boston: Little, Brown, 1994;724.

15. Watson PG, Hayreh SS. Scleritis and episcleritis. Br J Ophthalmol 1976;60:163–91.

16. Watson PG. The diagnosis and management of scleritis. Ophthalmology 1980;87:716–20.

17. Limberg MB. A review of bacterial keratitis and bacterial conjunctivitis. Am J Ophthalmol 1991;112:2S–9S.

18. Giglotti F, Williams WT, Hayden FG et al. Etiology of acute conjunctivitis in children. J Pediatr 1981;98:531–6.

19. Weiss A, Brinser JH, Nazar-Stewart V. Acute conjunctivitis in childhood. J Pediatr 1993;122:10–4.

20. Baum J. Therapy for ocular bacterial infection. Trans Ophthalmol Soc UK 1986;105:69–77.

21. Nozik RA, Smolin G, Knowlton G, Austin R. Trimethoprim-polymyxin B ophthalmic solution in treatment of surface ocular bacterial infections. Ann Ophthalmol 1985;17:746–8.

22. Leibowitz HM. Antibacterial effectiveness of ciprofloxacin 0.3% ophthalmic solution in the treatment of bacterial conjunctivitis. Am J Ophthalmol 1991;112:29S–33S.

23. Huber-Spitzy V, Arocker-Mettinger E, Baumgartner I. Efficacy of norfloxacin in bacterial conjunctivitis. Eur J Ophthalmol 1991;1:69–72.

24. Gwon A. Topical ofloxacin compared with gentamicin in the treatment of external ocular infection. Ofloxacin Study Group. Br J Ophthalmol 1992;76:714–8.

25. Gwon A. Ofloxacin vs. tobramycin for the treatment of external ocular infection. Ofloxacin Study Group II. Arch Ophthalmol 1992;110:1234–7.

26. Mannis MJ. Bacterial Conjunctivitis. In TD Duane, EA Jaeger (eds), Clinical Ophthalmology (Vol 4). Hagerstown, MD: Harper & Row, 1990;5–6.

27. Foulks GN. Bacterial Infections of the Conjunctiva and Cornea. In DM Albert, FA Jakobiec (eds), Principles and Practice of Ophthalmology (Vol 1). Philadelphia: Saunders, 1994;164–70.

28. Moraga FA, Domingo P, Barquet N, et al. Invasive meningococcal conjunctivitis. JAMA 1990;264:333–4.

29. Donnenfeld ED, Schrier A, Perry HD, et al. Penetration of topically applied ciprofloxacin, norfloxacin, and ofloxacin into the aqueous humor. Ophthalmology 1994;101:902–5.

30. Haimovici R, Roussel TJ. Treatment of gonococcal conjunctivitis with single-dose intramuscular ceftriaxone. Am J Ophthalmol 1989;107:511–4.

31. Thygeson P. The etiology and treatment of phlyctenular keratoconjunctivitis. Am J Ophthalmol 1951;34:1217–36.

32. Culbertson WW, Huang AJ, Mandelbaum SH, et al. Effective treatment of phlyctenular keratoconjunctivitis with oral tetracycline. Ophthalmology 1993;100:1358–66.

33. Jakobiec FA, Lefkowitch J, Knowles DM. B- and T-lymphocytes in ocular disease. Ophthalmology 1984;91:635–54.

34. Rapoza PA, Quinn TC, Terry AC, et al. A systematic approach to the diagnosis and treatment of chronic conjunctivitis. Am J Ophthalmol 1990;109:138–42.

35. Sandstorm KI, Bell TA, Chandler JW, et al. Microbial causes of neonatal conjunctivitis. J Pediatr 1984;105:706–11.

36. Chandler JW, Alexander, ER, Pheiffer TA, et al. Ophthalmia neonatorum associated with maternal chlamydia infections. Trans Am Acad Ophthalmol Otolaryngol 1977;83:302–8.

37. Burns RP, Rhodes DH. Pseudomonas eye infection as a cause of death in premature infants. Arch Opthalmol 1961;65:517–25.

38. Arffa RC. Grayson's Diseases of the Cornea. St. Louis: Mosby-Year Book, 1991;118, 151, 242.

39. Lepae P, Bogaerts J, Kestelyn P, Meheus A. Single-dose cefotaxime intramuscularly cures gonococcal ophthalmia neonatorum. Br J Ophthalmol 1988;72:518–20.

40. Chandler JW, Rotkis WM. Ophthalmia neonatorum. In TD Duane, EA Jaeger (eds), Clinical Ophthalmology (Vol 4). Philadelphia: Harper & Row, 1984;6–7.

41. Gudmundsson OG, Ormerod LD, Kenyon KR. Factors influencing predilection and outcome in bacterial keratitis. Cornea 1989;8:115–21.

42. Hyndiuk RA. Experimental *Pseudomonas* keratitis. Trans Am Ophthalmol Soc 1981;79:540–624.

43. Schein OD, Glynn RJ, Poggio EC, et al. The relative risk of ulcerative keratitis among users of daily-wear and extended-wear soft contact lenses. A case-control study. N Engl J Med 1989;321:773–8.

44. Schein OD, Wasson PJ, Boruchoff SA, Kenyon KR. Microbial keratitis associated with contaminated ocular medications. Am J Ophthalmol 1988;105:361–5.

45. Ogawa GSH, Hyndiuk RA. Bacterial Keratitis and Conjunctivitis: Clinical Disease. In G Smolin, RA Thoft (eds), The Cornea. Scientific Foundations and Clinical Practice. Boston: Little, Brown, 1994;126–8, 133–42.

46. Baum JL. Initial therapy of suspected microbial corneal ulcers: I. Broad antibiotic therapy based on the prevalence of organisms. Surv Ophthalmol 1979;24:97–105.

47. Leibowitz HM. Clinical evaluation of ciprofloxacin 0.3% ophthalmic solution for treatment of bacterial keratitis. Am J Ophthalmol 1991;112:34S–48S.

48. Hierholzer JC, Wigand R, Anderson LJ, et al. Adenoviruses from patients with AIDS: a plethora of serotypes and a description of five new serotypes of subgenus D (types 43–47). J Infect Dis 1988;158:804–13.

49. Dawson C, Hanna L, Wood TR, Despain R. Adenovirus type 8 keratoconjunctivitis in the United States. Epidemic, clinical and microbiologic features. Am J Ophthalmol 1970;69:473–80.

50. O'Day DM, Guyer B. Clinical and laboratory evaluation of epidemic keratoconjunctivitis due to adenovirus types 8 and 19. Am J Ophthalmol 1976;81:207–15.

51. Kivela T, Tervo K, Ravila E, et al. Pseudomembranous and membranous conjunctivitis: immunohistochemical features. Acta Ophthalmol 1992;70:534–42.

52. Laibson PR, Dhiri S, Onconer J. Corneal infiltrates in epidemic keratoconjunctivitis. Arch Ophthalmol 1970;84:36–40.

53. Darougar S, Hunter PA, Viwalingam M, et al. Acute follicular conjunctivitis and keratoconjuctivitis due to herpes simplex virus in London. Br J Ophthalmol 1978;62:843–9.

54. Ward JB, Siojo LG, Waller SG. A prospective, masked clinical trial of trifluridine, dexamethasone, and artificial tears in the treatment of epidemic keratoconjunctivitis. Cornea 1993;12:216–21.

55. D'Angelo LJ, Hierholzer JC, Keenlyside RA, et al. Pharyngoconjunctival fever caused by adenovirus type 4: report of a swimming pool-related outbreak with recovery of virus from pool water. J Infect Dis 1979;140:42–7.

56. Smith IW, Peutherer JF, MacCallum FO, et al. Incidence of *Herpesvirus hominis* antibody in the population. J Hyg 1967;65:395–408.

57. Darrell RW. Ocular Infections Caused by the Herpes Virus Group. In D Locatcher-Khorato, BC Seegal (eds), Microbiology of the Eye. St. Louis: Mosby-Year Book, 1972;302–12.

58. Hanna L, Ostler HB, Keshishyan BA. Observed relationship between herpetic lesions and antigenic type of *Herpesvirus hominis*. Surv Ophthalmol 1976;21:110–4.

59. Liesengang TJ, Melton J, Daly PJ, Ilstrup DM. Epidemiology of ocular herpes simplex: incidence in Rochester, Minn., 1950 through 1982. Arch Ophthalmol 1989;107:1155–9.

60. Nahias AJ, Starr SE. Infections Caused by Herpes Simplex Viruses. In PD Hoperich (ed), Infectious Diseases. Hagerstown, MD: Harper and Row, 1977;272.

61. Simon JW, Longo F, Smith RS. Spontaneous resolution of herpes simplex blepharoconjunctivitis in children. Am J Ophthalmol 1986;102:598–600.

62. Ostler MB. The management of ocular herpesvirus infections. Surv Ophthalmol 1976;21:136–40.

63. Lass JH, Thoft RA, Dohlman CH. Idoxuridine-induced conjunctival cicatrization. Arch Ophthalmol 1983;101:747–50.

64. Marsh RJ, Dudley B, Kelly V. External ocular motor palsies in ophthalmic zoster: a review. Br J Ophthalmol 1977;61:677–82.

65. Rogers RS, Tindal JP. Geriatric herpes zoster. J Am Geriatr Soc 1971;19:495–504.

66. Sandor EV, Millman A, Croxson TS, Mildvan D. Herpes zoster ophthalmicus in patients at risk for the aquired immune deficiency syndrome (AIDS). Am J Ophthalmol 1986;101:153–5.

67. Strommen GL, Pucino F, Tight RR, et al. Human infection with herpes zoster: etiology, pathophysiology, diagnosis, clinical course, and treatment. Pharmacotherapy 1988;8:52–68.

68. Schwab IR. Oral aycyclovir in the management of herpes simplex ocular infections. Ophthalmology 1988;95:423–30.

69. Hoang-Xuang T, Buchi ER, Herbort CP, et al. Oral acyclovir for herpes zoster ophthalmicus. Ophthalmology 1992;99:1062–71.

70. Bowsher D. Acute herpes zoster and post-herpetic neuralgia: effects of acyclovir and outcome of treatment with amitriptyline. Br J Gen Prac 1992;42:244–6.

71. Harding SP, Lipton JR, Wells JCD. Natural history of herpes zoster ophthalmicus: predictors of postherpetic neuralgia and ocular involvement. Br J Ophthalmol 1987;71:353–8.

72. Judson FN. Assessing the number of genital chlamydial infections in the United States. J Reprod Med 1985;30:269–72.

73. Sheppard JD, Kowalski RP, Meyer MP, et al. Immunodiagnosis of adult chlamydia conjunctivitis. Ophthalmology 1988;95:434–42.

74. Darougar S, Treharne JD, Minassian D, et al. Rapid serologic test for the diagnosis of *Chlamydia* ocular infections. Br J Ophthalmol 1978;62:503–8.

75. Viswalingam ND, Daroughar S, Yearsley P. Oral doxycyline in the treatment of adult chlamydial ophthalmia. Br J Ophthalmol 1986;70:301–4.

76. Stamm WE. Azithromycin in the treatment of uncomplicated genital chlamydial infections. Am J Med 1991;91:19S–22S.

77. McCallan A. The epidemiology of trachoma. Br J Ophthalmol 1931;15:369.

78. Al-Rifai KM. Trachoma through history. Int Ophthalmol 1988;12:9–14.

79. Darougar S, Viswalingam N, El-Sheikh H, et al. A double-blind comparison of topical therapy of chlamydial ocular infection (TRIC infection) with rifampicin or chlortetracycline. Br J Ophthalmol 1981;65:549–52.

80. Tabbara KF, Cooper H. Minocycline levels in tears of patients with active trachoma. Arch Ophthalmol 1989;107:93–5.

81. Jones BR, Clayton YM, Oji EO. Recognition and therapy of oculomycosis. Postgrad Med J 1979;55:625–8.

82. Rosberger DF, Serdarevic ON, Erlandson RA, et al. Successful treatment of microsporidial keratoconjunctivitis with topical fumagillin in a patient with AIDS. Cornea 1993;12:261–5.

83. Parrish CM, O'Day DM, Hoyle TC. Spontaneous fungal corneal ulcer as an ocular manifestation of AIDS. Am J Ophthalmol 1987;104:302–3.

84. Foster CS. Candidiasis. In FT Fraunfelder, FH Roy (eds), Current Ocular Therapy 3. Philadelphia: Saunders, 1989;56–9.

85. Stehr-Green JK, Bailey TM, Visvesvara GS. The epidemiology of *Acanthamoeba* keratitis in the United States. Am J Ophthalmol 1989;107:331–6.

86. Cohen EJ, Parlatto CJ, Arentsen JJ, et al. Medical and surgical treatment of *Acanthamoeba* keratitis. Am J Ophthalmol 1987;103:615–25.

87. Friedlander MH, Okumoto M, Kelley J. Diagnosis of allergic conjunctivitis. Arch Ophthalmol 1984;102:1198–9.

88. Bloch-Michel E. Chronic allergic conjunctivitis. Int Ophthalmol Clin 1988;28:321–3.

89. Dart JKG, Buckley RJ, Monnickenda M, Prasad J. Perennial allergic conjunctivitis: definition, clinical characteristics and prevalence. A comparison with seasonal allergic conjunctivitis. Trans Ophthalmol Soc UK 1986; 105: 513–20.

90. Roitt I. Essential Immunology. Oxford: Blackwell, 1974; 132–5, 148–55.

91. Jay JL. Clinical features and diagnosis of adult atopic keratoconjunctivitis and the effect of treatment with sodium cromoglycate. Br J Ophthalmol 1981;65:335–40.

92. Abelson MB, Soter NA, Simon MA, et al. Histamine in human tears. Am J Ophthalmol 1977;83:417–8.

93. Bisgaard H, Ford-Hutchinson AW, Charleston S, Taudorf E. Production of leukotrienes in human skin and conjunctival mucosa after specific allergen challenge. Allergy 1985;40:417–23.

94. Abelson MB, Schaefer K. Conjunctivitis of allergic origin: immunologic mechanisms and current approaches to therapy. Surv Ophthalmol 1993;38:S115–S132.

95. Caldwell DR, Verin P, Hartwich-Young R, et al. Efficacy and safety of lodoxamide 0.1% vs. cromolyn sodium 4% in patients with vernal keratoconjunctivitis. Am J Ophthalmol 1992;113:632–7.

96. Ballas Z, Blumenthal M, Tinkelman DG, et al. Clinical evaluation of ketorolac tromethamine 0.5% ophthalmic solution for the treatment of seasonal allergic conjunctivitis. Surv Ophthalmol 1993;38:S141–S148.

97. Fisher AA. Cosmetic dermatitis of the eyelids. Cutis 1984;34:216.

98. Fernandez-Vozmediano JM, Blasi NA, Romero-Cabrera MA, Carrascosa-Cerguero A. Allergic contact dermatitis to timolol. Contact Dermatitis 1986;14:252.

99. Hatinen A, Terasvirta M, Fraki JE. Contact allergy to components in topical ophthalmologic preparations. Acta Ophthalmol (Copenh) 1985;63:424–6.

100. Sendele DP. Chemical hypersensitivity reactions. Int Ophthalmol Clin 1982;26:25–34.

101. Fisher AA. Allergic reactions to contact lens solutions. Cutis 1985;36:209–11.

102. Friedlander MH. Contact allergy and toxicity in the eye. Int Ophthalmol Clin 1988;28:317–20.

103. Hogan MJ, Zimmerman LE. Ophthalmic Pathology. Philadelphia: Saunders, 1962;232.

104. Abelson MD, Madiwale N, Weston JH. Conjunctival eosinophils in allergic ocular disease. Arch Ophthalmol 1983;101:555–6.

105. Allansmith MR, Baird RS, Greiner JV. Vernal conjunctivitis and contact lens-associated giant papillary conjunctivitis compared and contrasted. Am J Ophthalmol 1979;87:544–55.

106. Neumann E, Gutmann MJ, Blumenkrantz N, Michaelson IC. A review of four hundred cases of vernal conjunctivitis. Am J Ophthalmol 1959;47:166–72.

107. Allansmith MR, Frick OL. Antibodies to grass in vernal conjunctivitis. J Allergy Clin Immunol 1963;34: 535–43.

108. Foster CS, Duncan J. Randomized clinical trial of topically administered cromolyn sodium for vernal keratoconjunctivitis. Am J Ophthalmol 1980;90:175–81.

109. Buckley RJ. Vernal keratopathy and its management. Trans Ophthalmol Soc UK 1981;101:234–8.

110. Allansmith MR, Ross RN. Ocular allergy and mast cell stabilizers. Surv Ophthalmol 1986;30:229–44.

111. Abelson MD, Butrus SI, Weston JH. Aspirin therapy in vernal conjunctivitis. Am J Ophthalmol 1983;95:502–5.

112. Henriquez AS, Kenyon KR, Allansmith MR. Mast cell ultrastructure: comparison in contact lens associated giant papillary conjunctivitis and vernal conjunctivitis. Arch Ophthalmol 1981;99:1266–72.

113. Allansmith MR, Baird RS. Percentage of degranulated mast cells in vernal conjunctivitis and giant papillary conjunctivitis associated with contact lens wear. Am J Ophthalmol 1981;91:71–5.

114. Abelson MB, Baird RS, Allansmith MR. Tear histamine levels in vernal conjunctivitis and other ocular inflammation. Ophthalmology 1980;87:812–4.

115. Woodward DF, Ledgard SE, Nieves AL. Conjunctival immediate hypersensitivity: re-evaluation of histamine involvement in the vasopermeability response. Invest Ophthalmol Vis Sci 1986;27:57–69.

116. Ballow M, Mendelson L. Specific immunoglobin E antibodies in tear secretion of patients with vernal conjunctivitis. J Allergy Clin Immunol 1980;66:112–8.

117. Allansmith MR. Vernal Conjunctivitis. In TD Duane (ed), Clinical Ophthalmology (Vol. 4). Philadelphia: Lippincott, 1988;7.

118. Meyer E, Kraus E, Zonis S. Efficacy of antiprostaglandin therapy in vernal conjunctivitis. Br J Ophthalmol 1987; 71:497–9.

119. Lee OS Jr. Keratitis occurring with *Molluscum contagiosum*. Arch Ophthalmol 1944;31:64–7.

120. Holly FJ. Diagnostic methods and treatment modalities of dry eye conditions. Int Ophthalmol 1993;17:113–25.

121. Dohlman CH. Punctal occlusion in keratoconjunctivitis sicca. Ophthalmology 1978;85:1277–81.

122. Baum JL, Mishima S, Boruchoff SA. On the nature of dellen. Arch Ophthalmol 1968;79:657–62.

123. Tragakis MP, Brown SI. The tear film alteration associated with dellen. Ann Ophthalmol 1974;6:757–61.

124. Laibson PR, Krachmer JH. Familial occurrence of dot (microcystic), map, fingerprint dystrophy of the cornea. Invest Ophthalmol 1975;14:397–9.

125. Waring GO, Rodrigues MM, Laibson PR. Corneal dystrophies. I. Dystrophies of the epithelium, Bowman's layer and stroma. Surv Ophthalmol 1978;23:71–122.

126. Trobe JD, Laibson PR. Dystrophic changes in the anterior cornea. Arch Ophthalmol 1972;87:378–82.

127. McLean EN, MacRae SM, Rich LF. Recurrent erosion. Treatment by anterior stromal puncture. Ophthalmology 1986;93:784–8.
128. Nakanishi I, Brown SI. Ultrastructure of epithelial dystrophy of Meesmann. Arch Ophthalmol 1975;93:259–63.
129. Rice NSC, Ashton N, Jay B, Blach RK. Reis-Buckler's dystrophy: a clinicopathological study. Br J Ophthalmol 1968;52:577–603.
130. Hogan MJ, Wood I. Reis-Buckler's corneal dystrophy. Trans Ophthalmol Soc UK 1971;91:41–57.
131. Garner A. Histochemistry of corneal granular dystrophy. Br J Ophthalmol 1969;53:799–807.
132. Miller HU. Granular corneal dystrophy Groenouw type I. Clinical aspects and treatment. Acta Ophthalmol 1990; 68:384–9.
133. Stuart JC, Mund ML, Iwamuto T, et al. Recurrent corneal granular dystrophy. Am J Ophthalmol 1975;79:18–24.
134. Klintworth GK, Smith CF. Macular corneal dystrophy: studies of sulfated glycosaminoglycans in corneal explant and confluent stromal cell cultures. Am J Pathol 1977; 89:167–82.
135. Quantock AJ, Meek KM, Ridway AE, et al. Macular corneal dystrophy: reduction in both corneal thickness and collagen interfibrillar spacing. Curr Eye Res 1990; 9:393–8.
136. Klintworth GK, Vogel FS. Macular corneal dystrophy—an inherited acid mucopolysaccharide storage disease of the corneal fibroblast. Am J Pathol 1964;45:565–86.
137. Akova YA, Kirkness CM, McCartney AC, et al. Recurrent macular corneal dystrophy following penetrating keratoplasty. Eye 1990;4:698–705.
138. Newsome DA, Hassell JR, Rodrigues MM, et al. Biochemical and histological analysis of "recurrent" macular corneal dystrophy. Arch Ophthalmol 1982;100: 1125–31.
139. Rabb MF, Blodi F, Boniuk M. Unilateral lattice dystrophy of the cornea. Trans Am Acad Ophthalmol Otolaryngol 1974;78:440–4.
140. Harding RB, Lalle PA, Kasik K. Unilateral lattice dystrophy of the cornea. J Am Optom Assoc 1982;53:477–9.
141. Francois J, Hanssens M, Teuchy H. Ultrastructural changes in lattice dystrophy of the cornea. Ophthalmic Res 1975;7:321–44.
142. Klintworth GK. Current concepts on the ultrastructural pathogenesis of macular and lattice corneal dystrophies. Birth Defects 1971;7:27–31.
143. Meisler D, Fine M. Recurrence of the clinical signs of lattice corneal dystrophy (type I) in corneal transplants. Am J Ophthalmol 1984;97:210–4.
144. Cross HE, Maumenee AE, Cantolino SJ. Inheritance of Fuchs' endothelial dystrophy. Arch Ophthalmol 1971; 85:268–72.
145. Waring GO, Rodriques MM, Laibson PR. Corneal dystrophies. II. Endothelial dystrophies. Surv Ophthalmol 1978;23:147–68.
146. Stocker FW. The Endothelium of the Cornea and Its Clinical Implications. Springfield, IL: Thomas, 1971;79–109.

147. Buxton JN, Preston RW, Riechers R, Guilbault N. Tonography in corneal guttata. A preliminary report. Arch Ophthalmol 1967;77:602–3.
148. Cibis GW, Krachmer JA, Phelps CD, Weingeist TA. The clinical spectrum of posterior polymorphous dystrophy. Arch Ophthalmol 1977;95:1529–37.
149. Rubenstein RA, Silverman JJ. Hereditary deep dystrophy of the cornea associated with glaucoma and ruptures in Descemet's membrane. Arch Ophthalmol 1968;79: 123–6.
150. Rodrigues MM, Waring GO, Laibson PR, Weinreb S. Endothelial alterations in congenital corneal dystrophies. Am J Ophthalmol 1975;80:678–89.
151. Grayson M. The nature of hereditary deep polymorphous dystrophy of the cornea. Its association with iris and anterior chamber dysgenesis. Trans Am Ophthalmol Soc 1974;72:516–59.
152. Winder AF. Factors influencing the variable expression of xanthelasmata and corneal arcus in familial hypercholesterolemia. Birth Defects 1982;18:449–62.
153. Lembach RG, Keates RH. Band keratopathy: its significance and treatment. Perspect Ophthalmol 1977;1:13–6.
154. Bokosky JE, Meyer RF, Sugar A. Surgical treatment of calcific band keratopathy. Ophthalmic Surg 1985;16:645–7.
155. Krachmer JH, Feder RS, Belin MW. Keratoconus and related noninflammatory corneal thinning disorders. Surv Ophthalmol 1984;28:293–322.
156. Smiddy WE, Hamburg TR, Kracher GP, Stark WJ. Keratoconus: contact lens or keratoplasty? Ophthalmology 1988;95:487–92.
157. Belin MW, Fowler WC, Chambers WA. Keratoconus: evaluation of recent trends in the surgical and nonsurgical correction of keratoconus. Ophthalmology 1988;95: 335–9.
158. Robin JB, Schanzlin DJ, Verity SM. Peripheral corneal disorders. Surv Ophthalmol 1986;31:1–36.
159. Murray PI, Rahi AHS. Pathogenesis of Mooren's ulcer: some new concepts. Br J Ophthalmol 1984;68:182–7.
160. Wilson SE, Lee WM, Murakami C, et al. Mooren-type hepatitis C virus-associated corneal ulceration. Ophthalmology 1994;101:736–45.
161. Martin NF, Stark WJ, Maumenee AE. Treatment of Mooren's and Mooren's-like ulcer by lamellar keratectomy: report of six eyes and literature review. Ophthalmic Surg 1987;18:564–9.
162. Hill JC, Potter P. Treatment of Mooren's ulcer with cyclosporin A: report of three cases. Br J Ophthalmol 1987;71:11–5.
163. Foster CS. Systemic immunosuppressive therapy for progressive bilateral Mooren's ulcer. Ophthalmology 1985; 92:1436–9.
164. Brown SI, Mondino BJ. Penetrating keratoplasty in Mooren's ulcer. Am J Ophthalmol 1980;89:255–8.
165. Detels R, Dhir SP. Pterygium: a geographic study. Arch Ophthalmol 1967;78:485–91.
166. Elliott R. The surgery of pterygium. Trans Ophthalmol Soc NZ 1961;13:27–34.

167. Bahrassa F, Datta R. Postoperative beta radiation treatment of pterygium. Int J Radiat Oncol Biol Phys 1983; 9:679–84.

168. Kleis W, Pico G. Thio-tepa therapy to prevent postoperative pterygium occurrence and neovascularization. Am J Ophthalmol 1973;76:371–3.

169. McCoombes JA, Hirst LW, Isbell GP. Sliding conjunctival flap for the treatment of primary pterygium. Ophthalmology 1994;101:169–73.

170. Rosenthal G, Shoham A, Lifshitz T, et al. The use of mitomycin in pterygium surgery. Ann Ophthalmol 1993;25:427–8.

171. Muir EB. Case of Salzmann's nodular corneal dystrophy. Arch Ophthalmol 1940;23:138–44.

172. Caldwell DR, Insler MS, Boutros G, Hawk T. Primary surgical repair of severe peripheral marginal ectasia in Terrien's marginal degeneration. Am J Ophthalmol 1984; 97:332–6.

173. Monestam E, Bjornstig U. Eye injuries in northern Sweden. Acta Ophthalmol 1991;69:1–5.

174. Kenyon KR, Wagoner MD. Conjunctival and Corneal Injuries. In BJ Shingleton, PS Hersh, KR Kenyon (eds), Eye Trauma. St. Louis: Mosby-Year Book, 1991;63–8, 77.

175. Casser-Locke L. Conjunctival abrasions and lacerations. J Am Optom Assoc 1987;58:488–93.

176. Wagoner MD, Kenyon KR. Chemical Injuries. In BJ Shingleton, PS Hersh, KR Kenyon (eds), Eye Trauma. St. Louis: Mosby-Year Book, 1991;79–92.

177. Theodore FH, Ferry AP. Superior limbic keratoconjunctivitis. Clinical and pathological correlations. Arch Ophthalmol 1970;84:481–4.

178. Confino J, Brown SI. Treatment of superior limbic keratoconjunctivitis with topical cromolyn sodium. Ann Ophthalmol 1987;19:129–31.

179. Passons GA, Wood TO. Conjunctival resection for superior limbic keratoconjunctivitis. Ophthalmology 1984; 91:966–8.

180. Sendele DD, Kenyon KR, Mobilia EF, et al. Superior limbic keratoconjunctivitis in contact lens wearers. Ophthalmology 1983;90:616–22.

181. Jones BR. Thygeson's superficial punctate keratitis. Trans Ophthalmol Soc UK 1963;83:245–53.

182. Goldberg DB, Schanzlin DJ, Brown SI. Management of Thygeson's superficial punctate keratitis. Am J Ophthalmol 1980;89:22–4.

183. Watson PG. The nature and treatment of scleral inflammation. Trans Ophthalmol Soc UK 1982;102:257–81.

23

Uveitis

GREGORY S. ABEL

With its varied etiologies, presentation, and course, uveitis provides an interesting challenge to diagnosis and management. The goal of the practitioner is to use the patient's history, clinical examination findings, and auxiliary test results to arrive at a correct diagnosis. Anatomically localizing the uveitis as anterior, intermediate, or posterior aids in the choice of management regimen. It is important to be aware that often the inflammation is secondary to a systemic disorder, and treatment may extend beyond topical ocular agents.

SIGNS AND SYMPTOMS OF UVEITIS

Signs

Ciliary Injection

Although diffuse bulbar injection is common with uveitis involving the anterior segment, circumlimbal vessels are typically more prominently dilated (Color Plate 23-I). This injection pattern may be more easily appreciated if the lids are spread widely apart. With eversion of the lower lid, injection of the bulbar tissue is typically more pronounced than the palpebral tissue. While prominent bulbar injection is usually present with anterior uveal inflammation, it is important to note that some forms of uveitis, especially those that are insidious in onset and chronic in nature, may present with a relatively white and quiet-appearing eye.

Pupillary Miosis

A common response of the pupils to anterior uveitis is that of pupil constriction. The miosis is caused by a release of prostaglandins, which are in response to iris irritation.[1] A spasm of the sphincter muscle then constricts the pupil. In the presence of conjunctivitis, the pupil size remains normal, whereas during an acute angle-closure attack it typically becomes fixed in a mid-dilated state.

Keratic Precipitates

Adhering to the endothelium, keratic precipitates (KPs) are most often visible on the inferior one-half of the cornea (Figure 23-1). Keratic precipitates consist of clusters of white blood cells (e.g., lymphocytes and plasma cells), which initially are released into the aqueous humor via the iris vasculature. The warmth of the vascularized iris and the cooler avascular cornea cause an aqeuous convection current that brings some of the inflammatory cells in contact with the posterior cornea. The precipitates often adhere to the inferior cornea in either a vertical line (Turk's line) or a base-down triangular shape (Arlt's triangle, Figure 23-2). In some cases they appear in a relatively diffuse distribution over the corneal endothelial surface.

Keratic precipitates may vary in size and appear as white or pale-colored round deposits. Traditionally, they may be classified as fine, medium, large, "mutton-fat" or greasy, or hyalinized. Mutton-fat KPs are typically large and exhibit an oily appearance along with the intervening posterior corneal surface. The importance of classifying the KP presentation is that the type of precipitate and its distribution may have etiological implications. As an example, mutton-fat KPs typically indicate a granulomatous-type inflammation that tends to be caused by certain types of systemic disorders such as sarcoidosis. Also, fine KPs that are diffusely distributed over the posterior corneal surface are more consistent with Fuchs' heterochromic iridocyclitis.

Cells in the Anterior Chamber

Normally the aqueous has no cells present within it. However, active inflammation in the iris or ciliary body results in the release of inflammatory cells (e.g., lymphocytes and monocytes) into the aqueous. Clinical diagnosis

FIGURE 23-1
Slit lamp photograph of large, mutton-fat keratic precipitates (KPs) along the posterior corneal surface.

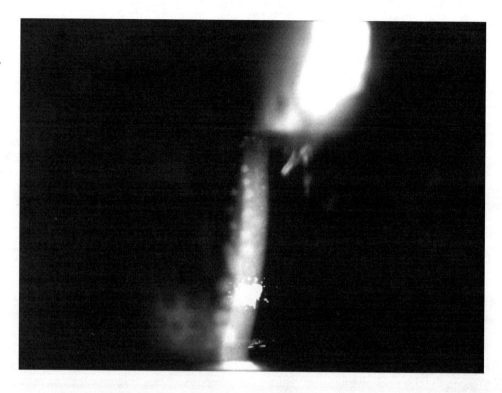

requires skill in evaluating the anterior chamber for a cellular response to the inflammation. Evaluating the anterior chamber for the presence of cells is best done with the slit lamp biomicroscope using a narrow beam of light at maximum intensity. The best visualization of any inflammatory reaction is accomplished if the room illumination is very dim and the examiner is relatively dark-adapted. The light source is directed toward the cornea from an angle of approximately 45–50 degrees. Using high magnification to focus on the cornea, the beam is slowly advanced forward so that the focus of the instrument is in the anterior chamber. With the slit lamp system properly aligned, the slit beam can be seen passing through the cornea, through the aqueous humor of the anterior chamber, and into the lens. To visualize cells and other debris, the slit beam is viewed against the backdrop of the dark pupillary aperture (see Figure 2-6). Normally the aqueous will appear essentially optically empty; however, when cells are present, they will appear as white dots moving within the beam of light via the aqueous convection currents. Flare, discussed in the next section, will be seen simultaneously as a generalized haze within the beam.

The number of cells is graded on a scale of 0 to 4+. It is important to assess and record cellular grade so that treatment efficacy can be gauged at a later time. If no cells are noted, a value of 0 is assigned to the response. As the number of cells increases, a correspondingly higher grade is assigned (Table 23-1).[2]

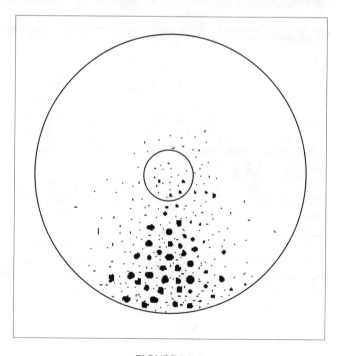

FIGURE 23-2
Common distribution of keratic precipitates (KPs) in the shape of a base-down triangle (Arlt's triangle) along the inferior aspect of the posterior corneal surface. (Courtesy of Daniel K. Roberts, O.D.)

TABLE 23-1
Grading Anterior Chamber Cells and Flare

Grade	Cells Per Field*	Flare
0	None	None
1+	5–10	Slight detection
2+	10–20	Present with iris and lens viewed clearly
3+	20–50	Present with iris and lens haze
4+	50+	Intense amount

*Cells per field as detected with a "wide beam, narrow slit."
Source: Modified with permission from MH Hogan, SJ Kimura, P Thygeson. Signs and symptoms of uveitis. I. Anterior uveitis. Am J Ophthalmol 1959;47:162–3.

Flare

Most instances of anterior chamber inflammation cause an early appearance of flare. Normal aqueous contains a low amount of protein, which may increase significantly during a uveitic attack. As a component to the inflammatory response, vascular permeability increases, allowing protein to escape.

Evaluating for both flare and cells is done simultaneously. Flare is observed as a haze within the biomicroscope light beam. It appears similar to evenly distributed smoke rising through a projector beam that traverses a dark room (Tyndall effect). Grading of flare also is done with a scale of 0 to 4+ (see Table 23-1).[2] Severe or chronic intraocu-lar inflammation may damage the walls of blood vessels, allowing flare to persist even during quiescent periods.

Iris Nodules and Granulomas

Iris nodules represent a clumping of inflammatory cells along the iris surface. Often they are overlooked during an examination because of their small size or surface dusting with pigment. Iris nodules are likely to form in the presence of a granulomatous-type inflammation but may also be found with severe nongranulomatous uveitis.

Koeppe nodules are the most common form of iris nodules. Round or oval in shape, they appear as a mass at the pupillary margin (Figure 23-3). Posterior synechiae may develop at the site of Koeppe nodule formation. Initially Koeppe nodules are translucent or whitish, but as mentioned, they may become pigmented, which may cause them to blend in with the background of the iris structure.

Busacca nodules are less often observed than Koeppe nodules, possibly in part because of their positioning away from the pupillary border. The nodules are cream-colored or white and are usually larger than Koeppe nodules. Whereas both Koeppe and Busacca nodules uncommonly occur with nongranulomatous uveitis, Koeppe nodules are more likely to do so than Busacca nodules.

Iris granulomas, which represent foci of inflammation, occur less frequently than Koeppe or Busacca nodules and may be located on the iris surface, the pupillary border, or in the anterior chamber angle. These lesions are pink,

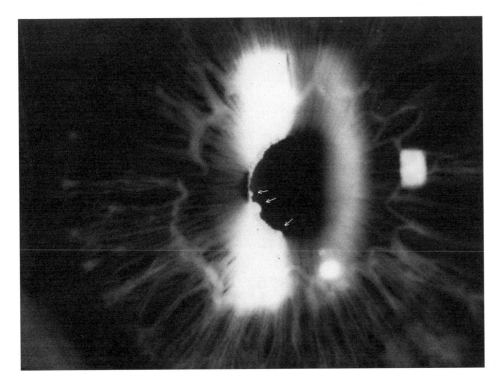

FIGURE 23-3
Koeppe nodules along the pupillary margin (arrows) in a granulomatous anterior uveitis.

FIGURE 23-4
Posterior synechia secondary to anterior uveitis.

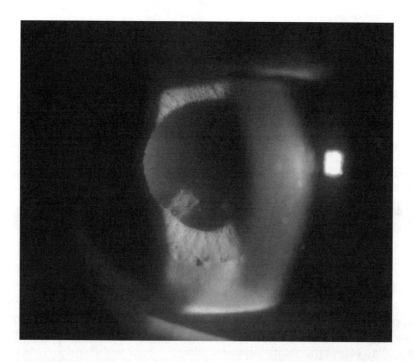

vascularized, and opaque. Usually a single, often large, granuloma is observed. Pathognomonic of granulomatous disease, this iris lesion is found with sarcoidosis, tuberculosis, and syphilis.

Synechiae

Posterior synechiae represent adhesion of the posterior iris surface onto the anterior crystalline lens surface (Figure 23-4) and are a common complication encountered as a result of anterior uveal inflammation. A major goal in the treatment of anterior uveitis is to prevent or break these attachments. If not broken soon after development, posterior synechiae can become permanent, thereby interfering with pupillary dilation. In addition, if posterior synechiae become extensive, involving 360 degrees of the pupil circumference, iris bombé results, which blocks the flow of aqueous from the posterior chamber into the anterior chamber and thus creates secondary angle closure glaucoma. Some types of anterior uveal inflammations are more likely to result in posterior synechiae than others, such as sarcoidosis. In locations where posterior synechiae have existed, fibrous tissue and pigment remnants of the attachments may remain.

Peripheral anterior synechiae (PAS) are also a complication of anterior uveal inflammation and represent a need for aggressive therapy when they occur. PAS are an adhesion between the peripheral iris and the inner wall of the eye in the region of the anterior chamber angle. In some instances, PAS may be relatively small and only extend as far anteriorly as the ciliary body or scleral spur;

in others, they may be more broad-based and they may cover the trabecular meshwork. When extensive, an obvious complication is secondary angle closure glaucoma, which is related to mechanical blockage of the flow of aqueous through the trabecular meshwork. Pupil block is not a factor here.

Intraocular Pressure

A decrease in the intraocular pressure may occur during the initial stages of an acute anterior uveitis. Here, inflammation within the ciliary body apparently causes a decrease in aqueous humor production. Later, a gradual rise in intraocular pressure may occur secondary to synechial angle closure or other mechanisms including (1) pupil block resulting from posterior synechiae or a swollen ciliary body, (2) swelling of tissue within the trabecular meshwork, or (3) obscuration of the trabecular outflow channels by inflammatory cell and debris.[3]

All patients receiving steroid therapy, either topically or orally, should routinely be examined for secondary elevation of intraocular pressure. The practitioner should be aware that so-called steroid responders who do not initially develop intraocular pressure elevation may do so months to years later.[4]

Vitreous Opacities

Inflammatory cells may occur individually within the vitreous or in "clumps." Their locus of concentration within the vitreous cavity depends on the primary location of inflammation and the underlying cause. For example,

TABLE 23-2
Grading Posterior Chamber Opacities

Grade	Opacities	Fundus Appearance
0	None	Clear
1+	Few	Clear
2+	Scattered	Mild haze
3+	Many	Blurred
4+	Dense	Unable to view

Source: Modified with permission from SJ Kimura, P Thygeson, MJ Hogan. Signs and symptoms of uveitis. II. Classification of the posterior manifestations of uveitis. Am J Ophthalmol 1959;47:172.

if an intermediate uveitis is present, the greatest number of cells occurs in the anterior vitreous. However, with a posterior uveitis, cells may be densest in the posterior vitreous or may be distributed fairly evenly throughout. A classic finding, especially associated with intermediate uveitis, is the accumulation of white cell aggregates (vitreous "puffball" or "snowball" opacities) within the anterior-inferior vitreous. Gravitational forces contribute to this presentation.

Visualizing vitreal opacities can be accomplished with a biomicroscopic lens (60 D, 78 D, 90 D lenses or the noncontact or contact Hruby lenses) or a direct or indirect ophthalmoscope. A scale of 0 to 4+ is typically used for grading the number of vitreal cells (Table 23-2).[5]

Symptoms

Pain
Spasm of the ciliary body creates a significant amount of discomfort for patients suffering from anterior uveitis. The ciliary body radiates pain via branches of the trigeminal nerve, causing discomfort within and around the globe. Pharmacologic blockade of ciliary muscle contracture helps alleviate this symptom. Topical cycloplegics, which are used for this purpose, provide the added therapeutic effect of pupillary dilation, which serves to prevent posterior synechiae formation.

Photophobia
Excessive sensitivity to light (i.e., photophobia) is well noted with anterior uveitis. Ciliary spasm due to inflammatory irritation of sensory branches of the trigeminal nerve that innervates intraocular structures including the iris and ciliary body is the cause.[6] Patients with anterior uveitis may complain of significant photophobia or pain upon accommodation. A test that can be helpful in the diagnosis of subclinical inflammation in one eye is to shine a light in the contralateral eye. If pain is felt in the eye suspected of having inflammation, then a mild or incipient

anterior uveitis may indeed exist. Overt cells and flare may not always be present, at least initially, in cases such as these. Another test is to cover the suspect eye and then have the patient focus on a near object with the other eye. Pain experienced by the occluded eye may also be evidence of early or mild anterior uveal inflammation.

Lacrimation
Excessive tearing is a common complaint of patients with an anterior uveitis. Similar to photophobia, it is attributable to irritation of sensory branches of the trigeminal nerve.[7]

Blurred Vision
Hazy or blurred vision frequently occurs with all forms of uveitis. Floating strands or spots are also a common complaint. It should be noted that from the examiner's perspective, the relative density of vitreal cells does not correlate with the level of visual impairment experienced by the patient. Although media changes may appear significant, visual acuity often remains better than expected. Aside from inflammatory debris, acuity loss may result from a number of different mechanisms, including corneal edema and opacification, cataract, and macular edema.[7]

CLASSIFICATION OF UVEITIS

Uveitis encompasses many different forms of ocular inflammation, and its classification can be accomplished with a variety of categorization schemes. Of these schemes, "naming and meshing"[8] is commonly used. Rather than using a single descriptive characteristic such as the location or clinical course of the uveitis, a combination of descriptive terms is used to provide an overall naming classification (Table 23-3). This profile is then compared with known uveitic types (meshing). Patient history, auxiliary test results, and other factors narrow the differential diagnoses.

Anatomic Position

Anterior
Anterior uveitis accounts for approximately 75% of all uveitic presentations.[9] In anterior uveitis, the iris (iritis), ciliary body (cyclitis), or a combination of the two uveal structures (iridocyclitis) may be the focus of inflammation. Whereas the locus of inflammation is not always readily evident, the distribution of cells in the anterior segment can be helpful in determining the primary site of involvement. For example, inflammatory cells will be found predominantly in the anterior chamber when an

TABLE 23-3
Classifying Uveitis

Anatomic Position	Lesion Pattern	Clinical Course	Pathology	Laterality
Anterior	Diffuse	Acute	Granulomatous	Unilateral
Iritis	Distinct	Subacute	Nongranulomatous	Bilateral
Iridocyclitis	Focal	Recurrent		
Cyclitis	Multifocal	Chronic		
Intermediate	Disseminated			
Pars planitis				
Posterior				
Choroiditis				
Chorioretinitis				
Retinochoroiditis				
Retinitis				
Panuveitis				

iritis is present. Fewer cells will be detected in the retrolental region and anterior vitreous. However, if a cyclitis primarily exists, more cells will be detected in the retrolental region and anterior vitreous. When an iridocyclitis (iris > ciliary body) or a cycloiriditis (ciliary body > iris) occurs, a less pronounced difference in inflammatory response exists between the two segments of the eye.

Intermediate

Debate has arisen over the actual anatomic boundaries of an intermediate inflammatory reaction. The International Uveitis Study Group (IUSG) first used the term "intermediate"[10] to describe this category of inflammation that involves the middle portion of the eye. In an intermediate uveitis, an inflammatory process occurs with involvement of the peripheral retina and anterior vitreous. Cellular reaction is primarily concentrated within the retrolental space and anterior vitreous, with inflammatory debris spilling over into the anterior chamber and posterior vitreous.

In most cases of intermediate uveitis, no signs of pain or injection are typically noted, and vision may remain clear unless there are pronounced floaters and dense inflammatory debris, or if other complications develop such as posterior subcapsular cataract and cystoid macular edema. There is some confusion surrounding the use of the term *intermediate uveitis* because it has been used interchangeably with the term *pars planitis*, which actually describes a specific uveitic entity that presents as an intermediate uveitis. Table 23-4 lists several conditions that may result in an intermediate uveitis. With any patient presenting with an intermediate-type inflammation, it should be remembered that there are multiple causes in addition to the idiopathic disorder known as pars planitis.

Posterior

Posterior uveitis is characterized by inflammation of the posterior uvea, the choroidal layer. Although inflammation limited to the choroid is referred to as a choroiditis, adjacent retinal structures are typically affected, hence the term *chorioretinitis*. Technically the term chorioretinitis is used to describe those inflammations that affect the choroid primarily and the retina secondarily (e.g., presumed ocular histoplasmosis syndrome). Retinochoroiditis is used to describe those inflammations that initially affect the retina and then the choroid secondarily (toxoplasmosis). Because of the close proximity of the retina and choroid, it is unlikely for significant inflammatory lesions to involve one of the layers and not the other.

Inflammatory lesions of the posterior uvea may take focal or diffuse patterns. Focal lesions (e.g., focal choroiditis, focal chorioretinitis) are fairly well demarcated and may be variable in size. The term *multifocal* (e.g., multifocal chorioretinitis) is applied when more than one lesion exists, and the term *disseminated* (e.g., disseminated chorioretinitis) is used to describe numerous lesions scattered throughout the fundus or a large portion of the fundus (Figure 23-5). Unlike focal lesions, diffuse lesions (diffuse choroiditis) may be characterized by poorly defined regions of inflammation in which the margins between affected and unaffected regions are difficult to discern, especially with magnification that is too high.

A classic sign of posterior uveitis is the presence of vitreal cells. Vitreous cellular response may be mild or marked depending on the severity and cause of the inflammation. Likewise, the concentration and distribution of cells within the vitreous may vary as well. More peripheral uveal inflammations may concentrate cells within the anterior vitreous, whereas lesions closer to the posterior pole may cause vitreal cells to cluster more posteriorly

TABLE 23-4

Major Conditions That May Produce the Clinical Picture of Intermediate Uveitis

Birdshot retinochoroidopathy
Fuchs' heterochromic iridocyclitis
Idiopathic vitritis of the elderly
Lyme disease
Multiple sclerosis
Pars planitis
Sarcoidosis
Syphilis
Toxocariasis
Toxoplasmosis
Tuberculosis

Source: CE Pavesio, RA Nozik. Anterior and intermediate uveitis. Int Ophthalmol Clin 1990;30:244–51.

in the vitreal cavity. Vitreal cells may be very densely concentrated over focal fundus lesions in some instances (e.g., the focal retinochoroiditis secondary to toxoplasmosis).

Newly formed fundus lesions associated with posterior uveal inflammations generally appear as lesions of the choroid and retina with fairly indistinct borders, even when the inflammation is focal in nature. These are typically variably elevated and may be associated with retinal vessel dilation, hemorrhage, or vascular sheathing.[11] As posterior uveal inflammatory lesions resolve, they flatten, typically leaving chorioretinal scars that often have pigmented margins.

Patients with active posterior uveitis may have few or no complaints depending on the severity, location, and

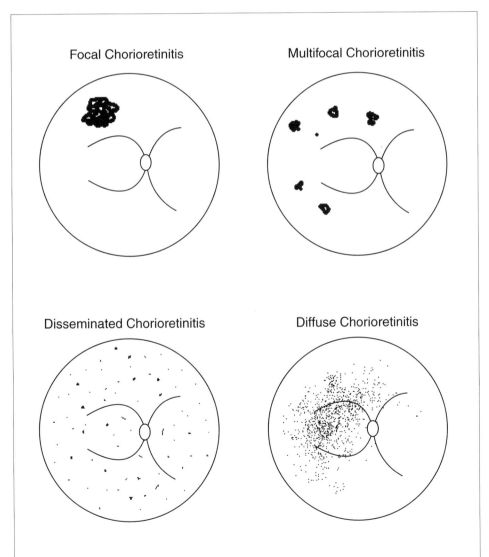

Focal Chorioretinitis

Multifocal Chorioretinitis

Disseminated Chorioretinitis

Diffuse Chorioretinitis

FIGURE 23-5

Diagram illustrating the use of the descriptive terms "focal," "multifocal," "disseminated," and "diffuse" as they apply to the classification of posterior uveitis. (Courtesy of Daniel K. Roberts, O.D.)

cause of the inflammation. Visual complaints are typically blurry or hazy vision caused by vitreal cells, macular involvement, or other secondary complications.

Panuveitis

Inflammation involving all divisions of the uvea (i.e., the iris, ciliary body, and choroid) is termed *panuveitis*. The synonym "diffuse uveitis" is occasionally used to denote this type of inflammation. Care must be taken, however, to avoid confusing this with the term as it is applied to such entities as diffuse choroiditis and diffuse chorioretinitis.

Clinical Course

Acute

Inflammation that is rapid in onset (hours to a few days) and short in duration (days to weeks) typifies an acute uveitis. An acute uveitis also typically involves the anterior segment (acute anterior uveitis) and is characterized by marked symptoms. Commonly there is pronounced circumlimbal injection, photophobia, and blurred vision.

Subacute

A subacute uveitic attack involves a speed of onset and a duration somewhere between those of acute uveitis and chronic uveitis. Onset is neither sudden nor insidious, and duration is typically weeks to months.

Chronic

Chronic uveitis denotes uveal inflammation that persists months to years. The typical chronic uveitis develops insidiously without initial patient awareness. Chronic uveal inflammations often wax and wane in their severity without total resolution ever occurring. Even though patient symptoms, if any, may disappear, signs of continued inflammation may persist. Anterior uveal inflammation tends to be more acute in nature, and posterior uveal inflammations tend to be more chronic. Any severe inflammation that is acute, recurrent, or both may eventually become chronic. Chronic, severe inflammation may damage the walls of blood vessels, causing persistent inflammatory flare and cell in the anterior chamber even when a uveitic condition is quiescent. This can cause difficulty in assessing the level of disease activity, often resulting in overtreatment.

Recurrent

Many forms of uveitis may resolve over a period of time and then recur. Intervals between inflammatory episodes are variable, being anywhere from weeks to months to years. Patient symptoms at each recurrence depend on the type and severity of inflammation that is present.

TABLE 23-5
Classic Characteristics of Granulomatous- and Nongranulomatous-Type Uveitis

Granulomatous
    Acute onset
    Marked pain
    Marked injection
    Small to medium, nongreasy, keratic precipitates (KPs)
    Short course
    No iris nodules
    Fundus involvement uncommon
Nongranulomatous
    Insidious onset
    Minimal pain
    Minimal injection
    Long (chronic) course
    Large "mutton-fat" KPs
    Iris nodules common
    Fundus involvement common

Note: There may be some overlap of these presentations, with some conditions occasionally exhibiting characteristics of both.
Source: Reprinted with permission from AC Woods. Endogenous Inflammations of the Uveal Tract. Baltimore: Williams & Wilkins, 1961;45.

Acute or chronic uveitis can be recurrent in nature, and as previously mentioned, an acute uveitis that is recurrent can eventually become chronic.

Pathology

Granulomatous and *nongranulomatous* are terms commonly used in the clinical description and classification of uveitis. They describe the type of pathologic responses found within the eye, and although it was originally intended that these different presentations would consistently indicate certain causes,[12] their correlations are not always accurate. Nevertheless, *granulomatous* and *nongranulomatous* are useful clinical terms, and various causes of uveitis do tend to yield characteristic ocular responses that can be categorized under one heading or the other. Table 23-5 lists the classical characteristics of granulomatous and nongranulomatous types of inflammations, and Table 23-6 lists the presentation of various uveitic conditions according to this descriptive classification.

Granulomatous

The formation of medium to large, greasy keratic precipitates ("mutton-fat" KPs) as well as iris nodules (Koeppe or Busacca) or granulomas is a classic response associated with granulomatous uveitis.[12] Koeppe nodules form along the pupil border, and Busacca nodules form away from the pupil border along the stromal surface of the iris. Granulomatous uveitis tends to develop insidiously and

TABLE 23-6
Typical Clinical Presentation* of Various Forms of Uveitis

Uveitis Form	Nongranulomatous	Granulomatous
Idiopathic anterior uveitis	+	—
Traumatic uveitis	+	—
Ankylosing spondylitis	+	—
Reiter's syndrome	+	—
Inflammatory bowel syndrome	+	+
Juvenile rheumatoid arthritis	+	—
Fuchs' heterochromic iridocyclitis	+	—
Herpes simplex uveitis	+	—
Herpes zoster uveitis	+ +	+
Syphilis	+	+ +
Tuberculosis	+	+ +
Glaucomatocyclitic crisis	+	—
Pars planitis	+	—
Toxoplasmosis	+	+ +
Toxocariasis	+	+ +
Behçet's syndrome	+	+
Lens-induced uveitis	+	+
Sarcoidosis	+	+ +
Lyme disease	+	+
Vogt-Koyanagi-Harada syndrome	+	+ +
Sympathetic ophthalmia	+	+ +

*i.e., nongranulomatous versus granulomatous.
+ + = occurs with greater frequency than +.

has a chronic course. Likewise, patients usually experience minimal or no pain, and their eyes may not exhibit any significant circumlimbal injection. Posterior segment involvement is more common with granulomatous uveitis than with nongranulomatous uveitis; therefore, choroidal, retinal, and vitreal involvement is more likely.

Nongranulomatous

Unlike granulomatous uveitis, nongranulomatous uveitis does not present with large mutton-fat KPs. Instead, the associated KPs tend to be small to medium and are non-greasy. Iris nodules do not typically form, and posterior segment involvement is less common. Patients with a nongranulomatous uveitis more commonly have an acute onset inflammation, and they tend to be more symptomatic, complaining of pain, photophobia, blurred vision, and prominent injection.

EVALUATION OF UVEITIS

Arriving at a diagnosis among all the possible uveitis types may prove difficult for any examiner. A thorough history must be obtained and a complete patient examination performed. Laboratory testing may also be warranted to differentiate between causes.

History

A complete patient history is invaluable in the evaluation of uveitis. Key elements may be discovered if the examiner asks the correct questions. Too often the history is performed by an office assistant or technician. Although time consuming, the practitioner must usually expand on the original history to receive adequate information.

History of Illness

Each patient should be allowed to completely describe his or her illness. Symptoms and time of onset are recorded. Does the patient note any changes or does he or she remember a similar previous occurrence? Were any medications used (request information from a previous examiner, if possible)?

Previous Ocular History

Not only should the patient's history be evaluated, but a family ocular history must also be obtained. Does the patient report any trauma, surgery, or infections? Is there a history of family eye disease?

Geographic History

Geography plays a role in the incidence of a number of types of uveitis. Some disorders may be isolated within areas of the United States or other regions of the world.

Demographic History

Age, sex, and race are details that are commonly acquired during a health evaluation. Various forms of uveitis often have a predilection for certain age groups, occur more frequently in males or females, and may be more prevalent within certain races.

Medical History

Questioning patients about their general medical history is extremely important because of the association of some forms of uveitis with systemic disease. For example, tuberculosis, syphilis, and sarcoidosis are all associated with anterior and posterior uveitis. A patient's complete personal medical history should therefore be obtained. Obviously, because patients commonly have undiagnosed disease, questioning should address the presence or absence of specific symptoms consistent with possible systemic disease. For example, the examiner may inquire specifically about fever, weight loss, arthralgias, cough, and skin lesions in attempt to rule out sarcoidosis. A complete medical history should include investigation of allergies and current medications.

Personal History

The personal component of the history may encompass a variety of areas that may be of etiologic significance in a uveitis patient. Examples include place of residence, occupation, recreational activity, sexual history, and pet ownership.

Family History

Although most causes of uveitis are not familial in nature, it is important that a family ocular and medical history be obtained, since this information can sometimes be important. For example, with a patient suspected of having uveitis associated with congenital syphilis, it is important to attempt to delineate whether the patient's mother has had syphilis. Additionally, a person with tuberculitic uveitis may also have family members with active tuberculosis.

Workup

Each time a patient is examined for a possible uveitis, there are several procedures that must be completed. A systematic examination enables the practitioner to gather data without neglecting any portion of the evaluation.

External Examination

It is important to evaluate the patient's overall features. Are there any abnormalities, ocular or otherwise, that may provide clues about the patient's health? Are there any notable superficial anomalies?

Visual Acuities

A dense grade of cells and flare in the aqueous, cells in the vitreous, cataracts, and choroidal/retinal involvement are signs or complications of uveitis that could possibly contribute to decreased acuities.

Pupils

The presence of an anterior uveitis may cause slight pupillary constriction or a sluggish response to light. Posterior synechiae may cause abnormally shaped pupils and poor reactivity.

Biomicroscopic Examination

In any patient with a uveitis, the slit lamp biomicroscope examination should be more detailed than usual. Specific attention should be given to determining the grade of inflammatory response in the anterior and posterior segments. Keratic precipitates should be specifically assessed to determine their distribution and type. The iris should be carefully examined for Koeppe and/or Busacca nodules. Any color change or atrophy of the anterior stromal layer should be noted, such as may occur in Fuchs' heterochromic iridocyclitis. The presence of rubeosis should be examined for, as well as synechiae between the posterior iris surface and crystalline lens. Gonioscopy may also be indicated to rule out the presence of peripheral anterior synechiae. With the aid of ancillary lenses, the vitreous should be carefully examined to determine the grade and distribution of inflammatory cell, if present. Retinal examination may also include use of the slit lamp biomicroscope in conjunction with ancillary lenses, especially to evaluate carefully the macula for edema.

Intraocular Pressure

As previously mentioned, intraocular pressure may be significantly affected by the presence of uveal inflammation. Intraocular pressure may be decreased in anterior uveitis as a result of slowing of aqueous production by the ciliary body, or it may be increased because of various mechanisms such as secondary angle closure and decreased outflow resulting from the presence of inflammatory debris. In instances of increased intraocular pressure, gonioscopy should always be performed in an attempt to determine the underlying mechanism.

Retinal Examination

If possible, retinal examination should be performed through a dilated pupil. The entire retina should be evaluated with the binocular indirect ophthalmoscope and the posterior pole with a slit lamp biomicroscopic indirect fundus lens and/or a direct ophthalmoscope. A fundus contact lens should be used for retinal examination when a very detailed examination with high magnification is needed for macular or peripheral retinal exam. Scleral indentation accompanying the binocular indirect examination may be required. Examination of the posterior segment should be performed on all patients with uveitis in an attempt to determine the extent of involvement, to reveal clues concerning the cause, and to rule out masquerade causes of uveitis such as retinal detachment or malignancy.

Laboratory Testing

Extensive numbers of laboratory tests are available to aid the practitioner in differentiating the causes of uveitis. Some practitioners use an extensive battery of tests in the workup of uveitis patients, but most follow a guide of targeted testing in relation to clinical findings.[13,14] Table 23-7 lists a variety of uveitic conditions and corresponding laboratory tests that may be useful in diagnosis. Usually certain etiologies or associated conditions should already be suspected before laboratory investigation, and its use should be as a confirmatory tool. The history and physical examination cannot be overemphasized in the workup of uveitis. Of course, there are certain conditions in which laboratory diagnosis is essential due to the possible lack of other overt evidence of the disease (e.g., syphilis).

PRINCIPLES OF MANAGEMENT

When therapy is initiated, there are several factors that help determine an initial regimen. These include the site(s) of inflammation (i.e., anterior, intermediate, and/or posterior segment involvement), degree of inflammation, presence or absence of secondary complications such as synechiae, elevated intraocular pressure, or macula edema, and the presence or absence of contraindications to specific medical therapy. Treatment may also depend on the specific underlying disease processes when they are identified.

Nonspecific Treatment Modalities

The general therapeutic treatment of uveitis should usually begin immediately. Anterior uveitis is typically managed successfully with topical medications, whereas posterior and intermediate uveitis often require periocular injections or systemic forms of treatment.

Mydriatics and Cycloplegics

There are two primary reasons for administration of mydriatic/cycloplegic agents: prevention of synechiae and improving the patient's comfort. The prevention of

TABLE 23-7
Laboratory Tests That May Be Helpful in the Diagnosis of Various Uveitic Entities

Uveitis Entity	Laboratory Test
Idiopathic anterior uveitis	HLA-B27
Ankylosing spondylitis	SI joint x-ray films; ESR; HLA-B27
Reiter's syndrome	HLA-B27; x-ray films of hands, knees, ankles, feet, and SI joint; ESR; body temperature; WBC; culture of urethral discharge
Inflammatory bowel disease	Gastrointestinal analysis (upper and lower GI series, etc.); HLA-B27
Juvenile rheumatoid arthritis	ANA; ESR; joint x-ray films (especially of the knee); Rh factor (negative in children with uveitis)
Syphilis	FTA-ABS or MHA-TP; VDRL or RPR
Tuberculosis	PPD skin test; chest x-ray films; ESR
Toxoplasmosis	IFA; ELISA; hemagglutination test; Sabin-Feldman dye test (*Toxoplasma* dye test)
Toxocariasis	ELISA
Histoplasmosis	Histoplasmin skin test; chest x-ray films; HLA-B7
Behçet's syndrome	Behçet's skin puncture test; HLA-B5; fluorescein angiography
Sarcoidosis	ACE; serum lysozyme; ESR; chest x-ray films; gallium scan of head, neck, thorax; biopsy of suspected granulomas
Lyme disease	IFA; ELISA
Vogt-Koyanagi-Harada syndrome	Lumbar puncture; fluorescein angiography

ACE = angiotensin-converting enzyme; ANA = antinuclear antibody; ELISA = enzyme-linked immunosorbent assay; ESR = erythrocyte sedimentation rate; FTA-ABS = fluorescent treponemal antibody absorption; GI = gastrointestinal; HLA = human leukocyte antigen; IFA = indirect fluorescent antibody; MHA-TP = microhemagglutination-treponemal pallidum; PPD = purified protein derivative; RPR = rapid plasma reagin; Rh = rheumatoid; SI = sacroiliac; VDRL = Venereal Disease Research Laboratory; WBC = white blood cell count.

posterior synechiae may be accomplished with the use of topical mydriatic solutions. Because the fully dilated pupil may also adhere to the anterior surface of the lens, a mydriatic drug that allows some gradual movement of the pupil is best. This pupillary cycling limits the amount of time the pupillary margin remains in contact with a given area of the lens. Good mobility of the iris may generally be achieved with the use of tropicamide, cyclopentolate, or homatropine. Most often, either cyclopentolate or homatropine is the drug of choice, depending on the length of response desired. Dosage may range from 1 drop every 2–3 hours to 1 drop two times per day. Duration is approximately 3–6 hours for tropicamide, 18–30 hours for cyclopentolate, and 18–36 hours for homatropine.[15]

Ciliary spasm results in complaints of pain and discomfort. Good cycloplegia is helpful in reducing patient symptoms. Once again, the strength of the cycloplegic depends on the level of inflammation. For most cases of anterior uveitis, homatropine 2% or 5% is used. The 2% solution is typically used for eyes with light-colored irises and the 5% solution for eyes with dark-colored irises.

Corticosteroids

Steroid therapy is the mainstay of ocular anti-inflammatory therapy. A variety of topical steroids are available, ranging in both strength and ocular penetration.

Steroid therapy coincides with use of a mydriatic/cycloplegic agent. Delivery may be in the form of a topical solution or suspension, periocular injection, or an oral medication. Intermediate and posterior forms of uveitis generally react poorly to topical therapy. For anterior uveitis, prednisolone acetate is commonly used because of its effective penetration of the intact corneal epithelium.[16] Dosage initially ranges from approximately every hour to four times per day, dependent on the severity of the uveitis. Tapering of topical steroidal therapy, especially after longer periods of use, is necessary to help prevent rebound inflammation.[17] A common tapering regimen for a mild, acute anterior uveitis, for example, might include an initial therapy of four times per day usage; this is then tapered to three times a day for 3 days, two times a day for 3 days, once a day for 3 days, and then discontinued. Of course, the exact tapering regimen may vary greatly depending on individual characteristics such as length and severity of inflammation. Tapering may be necessary over a period of weeks or months in some protracted cases.

Patients using any form of steroid therapy must be regularly examined for side effects. For example, "steroid responders" may develop elevated intraocular pressure after a period of weeks to months secondary to steroid use. Chronic steroid use may also lead to the formation of posterior subcapsular cataracts.

Although not used for routine cases, immunosuppressives are increasingly being used for the treatment of certain uveitic presentations, particularly in severe cases and in those patients who have not responded to other measures. For some disorders, such as Behçet's disease, immunosuppressive therapy may be indicated as a first line of treatment.[18] Immunosuppressives include drugs such as cyclosporine, azathioprine, chlorambucil, and cyclophosphamide. These agents are most commonly used in tertiary care settings.

Nonsteroidal anti-inflammatory agents are being investigated in the treatment of uveitis in hopes of suppressing inflammation without the same side effects as steroids.[19] Thus far, they have met with limited success.

Ocular Complications of Uveitis

Chronic inflammation may promote the deposition of calcium within the cornea, resulting in band keratopathy. Younger patients with juvenile rheumatoid arthritis and iridocyclitis are at a higher risk for this complication. The opacification associated with band keratopathy begins nasally and temporally near the limbus, with gradual advancement centrally across the interpalpebral area of the cornea. When visual acuity becomes diminished, removal of the calcium with chelating agents may be indicated.

Lenticular opacification may be caused by several forms of uveitis.[20] Focal anterior capsular opacities can occur due to posterior synechiae formation. Anterior subcapsular opacification may occasionally result from severe uveitis, but more common are posterior subcapsular cataracts. Their development may be hastened by the prolonged use of the corticosteroids used to treat the inflammation. Juvenile rheumatoid arthritis,[21] intermediate uveitis, and Fuchs' heterochromic iridocyclitis[22] are often associated with cataract formation.

Glaucoma associated with uveitis is caused by various inflammatory effects. Trabecular meshwork inflammation (trabeculitis) may cause congestion of outflow channels. Also, inflammatory cells and debris may mechanically block aqueous outflow, as can peripheral anterior synechiae. Posterior synechiae formation may lead to iris bombé (360-degree pupillary block), which prevents the flow of aqueous from the posterior to the anterior chamber and subsequently causes shallowing of the anterior chamber and secondary angle-closure glaucoma. Ciliary body inflammation may cause swelling and forward rotation of the lens and iris, which produces similar angle-closure results. Neovascularization of the iris may also lead to secondary angle-closure glaucoma.

The treatment of glaucoma secondary to uveitis depends on individual mechanisms. In addition to aggressive treatment to suppress intraocular inflammation, when simple mechanical blockage of the trabecular meshwork occurs by inflammatory cells and debris, beta-blockers or carbonic anhydrase inhibitors may be prescribed to decrease aqueous production. Pilocarpine is avoided because its parasympathomimetic effects lead to increased anterior segment congestion and worsening of the inflammatory response. When iris bombé exists, efforts are made to break the posterior synechiae with strong mydriatic/cycloplegic agents. Beta-blockers, carbonic anhydrase inhibitors, and oral glycerin may also be given concurrently to reduce intraocular pressure. If posterior synechiae are not broken and pupillary block remains, then surgical measures are necessary to allow the flow of aqueous from the posterior to the anterior chamber. The management of neovascular glaucoma is generally aimed at a reduction in the formation of aqueous, calming anterior segment inflammation, and improving aqueous outflow with surgical measures if necessary.

In contrast to elevated intraocular pressure, long-standing inflammation may lead to aqueous humor hyposecretion and hypotony, with severe cases resulting in phthisis bulbi. Chronic hypotony can result in degenerative changes throughout the eye.

Macular edema may result from uveal inflammation. It can cause symptoms of blurred vision associated with uveitis and can lead to permanent visual loss through macular scarring. Attempts should be made to control intraocular inflammation and chronic macular edema before this occurs. Macular edema is a common complication of pars planitis, and its development is used as the rationale for active treatment of this condition in lieu of periodic observation.

Retinal detachment can result from intermediate or posterior uveitis. In some cases, bands of condensed vitreous strands pull on the retina, causing a tractional detachment. Exudative nonrhegmatogenous retinal detachment may also occur from the accumulation of fluid beneath the retina in some uveitic conditions.

SPECIFIC UVEITIC ENTITIES

Numerous entities may cause inflammation of the uveal tract. To be all-inclusive is too extensive for a chapter of this nature. However, it is important that the more common causes or associations of uveitis be introduced. The practitioner should become acquainted with the general signs and symptoms, specific laboratory tests, and auxiliary tests that may be required in some instances. After the initial examination, further testing or a specialized consultation may contribute invaluably toward a final diagnosis.

Idiopathic Anterior Uveitis

Slightly less than one-half of anterior uveitis cases are labeled as idiopathic.[23] Inflammation may occur as either an iritis or an iridocyclitis. Clinical characteristics are that of a nongranulomatous inflammatory response. An acute,

unilateral onset is most often noted, and the process may recur in either eye.

A careful history must be obtained to help differentiate an idiopathic uveitis from one with an identifiable, hidden systemic cause. Extensive laboratory investigation is often not performed with the initial episode in a characteristic patient, provided no other overt signs or risk factors of associated systemic disease exist. However, if the inflammation recurs or does not respond well to general treatment, laboratory testing is warranted.

Although no direct cause for acute idiopathic anterior uveitis can be found, 40–50% of patients are positive for the HLA-B27 antigen.[13,24] The reason for this association is unknown. Although it is a relatively expensive test, evaluation for the HLA-B27 antigen is occasionally performed in attempt to characterize an individual's condition further. Patients with idiopathic anterior uveitis who test positive for the HLA-B27 antigen tend to have more recurrent attacks that are more severe in nature. Young men with idiopathic acute anterior uveitis tend to be HLA-B27-antigen–positive more often than others. The HLA-B27 antigen also has a strong association with acute anterior uveitis associated with Reiter's syndrome, ankylosing spondylitis, psoriatic arthritis, and inflammatory bowel disease. Since most patients who have an anterior uveitis that is related to Reiter's syndrome or ankylosing spondylitis are also positive for the HLA-B27 antigen, these disorders should be ruled out in any individuals who have an HLA-B27–associated acute anterior uveitis, particularly if they are young and male.

Management of idiopathic anterior uveitis consists of nonspecific treatment that is tailored toward the level of inflammation. The typical regimen for an acute, idiopathic anterior uveitis consists of a topical mydriatic/cycloplegic drop such as homatropine 2% or 5% and a topical corticosteroid such as prednisolone acetate 1%. Severe, recurrent cases may require periocular and oral corticosteroidal therapy.

Traumatic Uveitis

An inflammatory response to trauma may present as an iritis, iridocyclitis, or cyclitis. More widespread inflammation can also occur in more severe cases. Lid ecchymosis may be visible with accompanying pain and photophobia. Visual acuity may be decreased. Keratic precipitates are uncommon, and variable degrees of cell and flare are present. The aqueous humor may also contain some red blood cells or a frank hyphema, depending on the type and degree of structural damage to the eye. Other signs of trauma may be present, including trabecular meshwork tears, angle recession, cyclodialysis, a ring of pigment on the anterior surface of the lens (Vossius' ring), lens dislocation, commotio retinae, and retinal breaks or retinal detachment.

Because of the possibility of other ocular findings caused by the trauma, evaluation for these complications should be performed when possible. Gonioscopy is necessary to examine the angle structures, and fundus examination is indicated in all cases of traumatic uveitis. Peripheral retinal evaluation should include scleral depression to rule out subtle retinodialysis or retinal tears. This is especially true when clues to a retinal break exist such as pigment in the anterior vitreous, vitreous hemorrhage, or persistent flashes and floater symptoms. B-scan ultrasonography or neuroimaging may be necessary if no view of the posterior segment is possible. Plain x-ray films or computed tomographic (CT) scanning may be indicated if a periorbital bone fracture (e.g., blow-out fracture) is suspected.

Aside from any management that is directed toward other ocular complications, the treatment of traumatic uveitis, like that of idiopathic anterior uveitis, is nonspecific. Therapy usually consists of a topical mydriatic/cycloplegic agent and a corticosteroid. In mild cases where the anterior chamber reaction is minimal, a mydriatic/cycloplegic agent alone may suffice.

Ankylosing Spondylitis

Ankylosing spondylitis (AKS), also known as Marie-Strümpell syndrome, is a systemic rheumatologic disorder that exhibits ocular involvement in 20% of cases.[25] The most common known systemic cause of uveitis among men, AKS predominantly affects white men between the ages of 20 and 30 years. Systemic findings consist primarily of a spondylitis that typically involves the sacroiliac (SI) joint as well as arthritis involving other larger, weight-bearing joints. Aortic insufficiency and other vascular problems also occur.

Ocular characteristics include an acute iridocyclitis that is typically nongranulomatous in nature. One eye is typically affected at a time, but uveitis may recur in either, sometimes affecting one eye more often than the other. Patients with advanced spondylitis may not have complete flexion of the spine, causing them to have difficulty placing their chin in the biomicroscope for examination (Verhoeff's test).[26]

Patients with AKS may be asymptomatic for their joint disease; therefore x-ray films of the SI joint are most important, since it is the joint most commonly affected. Because of widespread inflammatory activity, the erythrocyte sedimentation rate (ESR) is often elevated and should therefore be investigated in appropriate patients. The HLA-B27 antigen test produces positive results in 80% of patients

with AKS[27] and may therefore be of benefit. It should be kept in mind, however, that the results are also commonly positive in idiopathic anterior uveitis and therefore may be of marginal benefit in the differential diagnosis.

The management of patients with AKS includes nonspecific therapy for the presence of anterior uveitis and referral to a rheumatologist for appropriate care of the systemic findings. Aggressive ophthalmic treatment may be necessary in some instances to manage secondary complications such as posterior synechiae, secondary glaucoma, and cystoid macular edema. Early identification of AKS can be of significant benefit to affected patients because appropriate physical therapy and other treatment measures may lessen long-term complications from the disease.

Reiter's Syndrome

Reiter's syndrome is a variable disease that classically produces a triad of clinical findings consisting of polyarthritis, nonspecific urethritis, and mucopurulent conjunctivitis. Ophthalmic features may also consist of iridocyclitis (20%), episcleritis, papillitis, and superficial punctate or infiltrative keratitis.[28] Other systemic features may include mucosal lesions involving the mouth and genitalia, and cutaneous lesions mainly consisting of keratoderma blenorrhagica of the soles of the feet or on the genitalia. Chronic prostatitis may occur. There is an association with other arthritic conditions since some patients with Reiter's syndrome will also develop ankylosing spondylitis. Males are affected more than females, typically between the ages of 15 and 40 years.

The iridocyclitis of Reiter's syndrome is recurrent and is characterized by an acute onset, possibly with a marked degree of cells and flare, KPs, photophobia, and pain. Although the associated findings of Reiter's syndrome, including the anterior uveitis, may be chronic and recurrent, subsequent episodes of active disease tend to be less severe. Consequently, serious complications from the anterior uveitis do not generally occur.

Nonspecific treatment is used for the anterior uveitis associated with Reiter's syndrome, which includes topical mydriatic/cycloplegic agents and corticosteroids. Management of other components of the disease, such as a treatable urethritis (e.g., chlamydial infection), should be done through consultation with specialists such as a urologist or rheumatologist.

Since arthritic symptoms or urethritis may not initially be reported by Reiter's patients, this disease should be suspected in all young male patients with recurrent mucopurulent conjunctivitis and iridocyclitis. A careful history focusing on systemic symptoms should be obtained and appropriate laboratory tests and consultation ordered. X-rays of the hands, knees, ankles, feet, and sacroiliac joints may show asymptomatic arthritis. HLA-B27 typing may be ordered but may be of marginal value in the differential diagnosis, since other forms of idiopathic uveitis also yield positive results. White blood cell count, ESR, and body temperature may all be elevated during active disease and may be evaluated. Cultures of fecal specimens may yield evidence of dysentery, and cultures of any existing urethral discharge or of the prostatic fluid may yield evidence of chlamydial infection.

Inflammatory Bowel Disease

Various forms of inflammatory bowel disease (IBD) appear to be occasionally associated with uveitis. Among them are ulcerative colitis, granulomatous colitis (Crohn's disease), and Whipple's disease. Ulcerative colitis is an idiopathic, relapsing, chronic disease characterized by diffuse ulceration of the mucosal lining of the rectum and proximal colon. The predominant symptoms include diarrhea and other gastrointestinal (GI) symptoms. Arthritis may be an associated finding, and many patients also have ankylosing spondylitis, once again demonstrating the link between uveitis and some of the various arthritic syndromes. Episcleritis and recurrent attacks of an acute anterior uveitis can occur that are often coincident with episodes of colitis.[8]

Granulomatous colitis, or Crohn's disease, is also an idiopathic, relapsing chronic disease that may be associated with ophthalmic findings including anterior uveitis. Unlike ulcerative colitis, Crohn's disease is characterized by focal inflammation within the GI tract. The terminal ilium and rectal areas are most frequently involved, but other areas of the GI tract may also be affected. Symptoms consist mainly of diarrhea and other GI disturbances. Arthritis is also a common feature of the disease. An increased prevalence of HLA-B27 antigen exists.[29] Females are affected more frequently than males.

About 10% of patients develop ocular complications, which in addition to an acute or chronic anterior uveitis may include episcleritis, scleritis, conjunctivitis, peripheral infiltrative keratitis, lid edema, extraocular muscle palsies, and optic neuritis.[8]

Whipple's disease, another GI disorder, is likewise characterized predominantly by GI symptoms, including diarrhea. Arthritis is also an associated finding. The disease occurs most commonly in men in the fifth decade of life and may be associated with bacilliform microbes within the bowel wall. Systemic tetracycline may be an effective treatment for both the systemic and ocular manifestations.

In addition to recurrent anterior uveitis, other ocular complications may include extraocular muscle palsies, gaze palsies, and nystagmus, which results from CNS involvement. Posterior segment findings include vitritis, diffuse chorioretinitis, and vasculitis.

Because of the occasional association of uveitis with GI disease, most patients with recurrent uveitis should be questioned regarding GI symptoms. If GI disease is suspected, the patient should be referred to an internist or gastroenterologist for appropriate testing, which may include radiologic GI studies, colonoscopy, or biopsy.

Anterior uveitis associated with inflammatory bowel disease is treated nonspecifically according to the level of inflammation with mydriatic/cycloplegic agents and topical corticosteroids. More aggressive therapy, such as periocular steroid injections, may be indicated in some instances. Other ocular complications are also treated as necessary.

Juvenile Rheumatoid Arthritis

Juvenile rheumatoid arthritis (JRA) is an inflammatory condition affecting young children usually between the ages of 2 and 4 years. Three subgroups of JRA are generally described based on the characteristics of the disease during the first 3 months after onset. These include systemic onset JRA (Still's disease; approximately 20% of cases), polyarticular onset JRA (approximately 40% of cases), and pauciarticular (monoarticular or oligoarticular) onset JRA (approximately 40% of cases).[30] Iridocyclitis as well as other ocular complications occur in all three types of JRA but with variations in presentation, incidence, and severity.

Systemic onset JRA is typically characterized by fever and variable combinations of lymphadenopathy, splenomegaly, hepatomegaly, maculopapular rash, and pericarditis. Arthritis, which may not be present initially, usually involves the large joints and is rarely progressive. Uveitis develops infrequently and less commonly than in the other subgroups of JRA.

When five or more joints are initially affected, JRA may be classified within the polyarticular subgroup. Systemic symptoms associated with the initial illness are less severe than in the systemic onset group. Associated iridocyclitis is also uncommon but occurs more frequently than in the systemic onset subgroup. The approximate incidence of uveitis in this group is 15% or less.[30]

Pauciarticular onset JRA, probably the most frequent form of JRA, is characterized by involvement of less than five joints within the first 3 months of onset. The systemic manifestations may be relatively mild in the pauciarticular subtype. Two forms of ocular involvement may occur. Type 1 is accompanied by a chronic iridocyclitis that is usually asymptomatic in its early course, without significant anterior chamber reaction or synechiae.[31] Later, however, patients may develop ocular symptoms as an initial identifiable manifestation of the disease. Visual acuity may be significantly reduced at this stage from band keratopathy and secondary cataract. Dense posterior synechiae may lead to iris bombé and secondary angle-closure glaucoma. The insidious onset of the iridocyclitis in these cases allows for many ocular complications to develop in this disease, and once recognized, despite intensive therapy, many of these cases worsen further, possibly leading to blindness.

Type 2 ocular involvement associated with pauciarticular JRA resembles ankylosing spondylitis with recurrent, acute iridocyclitis. Ocular involvement is often discovered earlier in these cases. Approximately 25% of patients with the pauciarticular subgroup develop uveitis,[32] and more than 78% of uveitis cases associated with JRA are type 2 ocular involvement associated with pauciarticular onset disease.[33] Pauciarticular-associated anterior uveitis is typically bilateral and nongranulomatous.

Juvenile rheumatoid arthritis should be suspected in all children with iridocyclitis. A detailed history should be obtained on such patients and should include inquiries about the presence of a febrile illness and arthralgia or arthritis. Helpful diagnostic tests include antinuclear antibody (ANA) testing, which produces positive results in 80% of JRA patients who develop iridocyclitis (ANA testing produces negative results in JRA patients who do not develop iridocyclitis). The ESR is usually elevated in JRA patients. Rheumatoid factor (Rh factor) test results are negative in children with JRA and uveitis and therefore such testing is unnecessary. X-rays of the joints may be obtained in an attempt to identify JRA. The knee is probably the most commonly affected joint.

The management of iridocyclitis associated with JRA usually consists of nonspecific therapy including topical mydriatic/cycloplegic agents and corticosteroid preparations. Since the iridocyclitis is often severe and progressive, additional measures may occasionally be necessary, including periocular corticosteroid injections or systemic therapy. Care should be taken not to overuse steroidal therapy in these patients because the use of steroids may have little effect and may actually hasten the development of cataracts or lead to steroid-induced glaucoma. Aqueous flare is often persistent in JRA patients, despite relative quiescence of the inflammation; therefore, overly aggressive anti-inflammatory therapy should not be performed in an attempt to totally eliminate this com-

ponent. Pediatric consultation should be obtained for all patients suspected of having JRA.

Fuchs' Heterochromic Iridocyclitis

Fuchs' heterochromic iridocyclitis (FHI) is commonly an asymptomatic disorder that is typically discovered during routine examination or with the development of secondary complications including cataract formation or glaucoma. It is almost always unilateral and affects both men and women, usually between the ages of 20 and 40 years. Fuchs' heterochromic iridocyclitis is probably the most often misdiagnosed uveitic entity.[8]

Ocular findings include a white and quiet eye with very mild degrees of cells and flare. Very fine, stellate or filamentous KPs are often diffusely distributed over the posterior corneal surface. Although FHI is a nongranulomatous inflammation, iris nodules may occasionally be seen along the pupil margin or on the surface of the iris.[34] They are typically small, translucent, and easily overlooked. The involved iris in FHI exhibits an anterior stromal atrophy, which causes the heterochromia. Depending on the preexisting iris color, heterochromia may actually be very difficult to detect, especially in patients with dark irides. Some loss of the posterior iris pigment epithelium may result in transillumination defects. Close evaluation of the iris surface reveals a blunting or loss of detail of the anterior stromal tissue. Fine neovascularization of the iris stroma or of the angle may occur. Posterior synechiae do not occur, although peripheral anterior synechiae have been reported. Vitreal floaters and inactive chorioretinal scars are associated posterior segment findings.

Fuchs' heterochromic iridocyclitis is a chronic disorder, and the most significant ocular complications are secondary cataract and glaucoma. There are no known systemic associations and there are no specific laboratory tests to aid in its identification. Although the mechanism is unknown, there does appear to be an occasional association between congenital ocular toxoplasmosis and FHI. Although FHI is not directly caused by infection with *Toxoplasma gondii,* the presence of this organism may somehow trigger the onset of FHI.

At the initial examination, patients may be treated with topical corticosteroids on a trial basis. However, FHI is generally unresponsive to steroidal therapy, and prolonged administration should be avoided, as this may only hasten the development of secondary cataract and glaucoma. Mydriatics are not necessary, since posterior synechiae do not develop. Most cases of FHI are probably best managed with simple monitoring at 3- to 6-month intervals. Secondary glaucoma can be managed similar to typical chronic open-angle glaucoma. When indicated, cataract surgery can be performed and generally has a good prognosis.

Herpes Simplex Uveitis

Anterior uveitis is a frequent sequela of active herpes simplex infection. It occurs with both epithelial and stromal disease, usually as an acute, mild or moderate, nongranulomatous iridocyclitis. Keratic precipitates are often present and are commonly clustered beneath stromal lesions. Intraocular pressure may be significantly elevated, despite a relatively mild appearing anterior chamber reaction. Focal iris atrophy may occur in severe or recurrent cases. Some controversy exists regarding the exact cause of the uveitis associated with the herpes simplex virus, whether it be from direct viral involvement of the uvea, hypersensitivity phenomena, or simply a response to adjacent inflammation. In most cases, anterior uveitis follows corneal involvement by a few days, whereas in others, uveitis may apparently begin without corneal involvement.[13]

Herpes simplex associated anterior uveitis is managed initially with antivirals and mydriatic/cycloplegic agents. Topical steroids should not be given in the presence of active epithelial disease but may be indicated to control residual uveitis in some instances when the epithelial disease has resolved. Antiviral therapy should be continued, however, and observation maintained for the redevelopment of active corneal disease.

Herpes Zoster Uveitis

Herpes zoster ophthalmicus (HZO), a varicella-zoster virus infection of the trigeminal nerve's ophthalmic division, produces cutaneous facial lesions respective of the midline. The tip of the nose is affected approximately 50% of the time (Hutchinson's sign),[35] and when this sign is present, ocular involvement is much more likely. Conjunctivitis, episcleritis, keratitis, and anterior uveitis are common sequelae. Associated keratitis is variable but may be characterized by dendritic or geographic epithelial lesions, sometimes resembling those caused by herpes simplex. The anterior uveitis is typically a nongranulomatous, unilateral, acute iridocyclitis, but on occasion a chronic granulomatous uveitis is seen. Inflammation may be mild or severe and usually begins within several days after the onset of skin lesions; it can develop somewhat later, however. Because of the perivasculitis caused by the virus, ischemic necrosis can occur to the iris and ciliary body, possibly causing severe inflammation that is unresponsive to therapy. Sectoral secondary iris atrophy is common,

and secondary inflammatory glaucoma is also seen. Small to medium KPs often develop with the anterior uveitis. Posterior synechiae occur, and hypopyon formation combined with hyphema is possible in severe cases.

The early use of oral acyclovir may prevent or reduce the severity of ocular complications and should be administered where possible in cases of herpes zoster ophthalmicus.[36] Corneal involvement is managed with nonspecific therapy, including topical corticosteroids and mydriatic/cycloplegic agents. Steroids are administered according to the degree of inflammation and may be necessary over a period of several months. They may have minimal effectiveness in instances where ischemic vasculitis is particularly severe. The primary goal of mydriatics and cycloplegics is to prevent posterior synechiae and decrease ciliary spasm. Secondary glaucoma also requires nonspecific therapy.

Syphilis

Known as the "great mimicker," syphilis has various ocular presentations. This sexually transmitted disease, caused by the spirochete *Treponema pallidum,* has both congenital and acquired forms. Uveitis, although a relatively uncommon complication of syphilis and one that represents only a small percentage of all uveitis cases, results from a treatable underlying cause and is therefore of great clinical significance.

Congenital syphilis, resulting from transmission of *Treponema pallidum* from mother to fetus, may lead to a variable constellation of findings. Early congenital syphilis in an infant may be characterized by a variety of skin lesions, generalized lymphadenopathy, fissured lesions around the mouth (rhagades), enlarged liver and spleen, mental retardation, meningitis, hydrocephalus, and a failure to thrive. After resolution of this stage, many individuals remain in a latent stage throughout their lives. Others develop late congenital syphilis, which may be characterized by clinical findings such as a "saddle bridged nose," "saber shins," focal or generalized chorioretinitis, optic atrophy, and the Hutchinson's triad of interstitial keratitis (IK), maldeveloped teeth (notched incisors, Hutchinson's teeth), and eighth nerve deafness.

IK typically develops between the ages of 5 and 15 years. It is characterized by an acute, bilateral, diffuse stromal inflammation that develops deep neovascularization. The keratitis may last several weeks or months and causes a significant decrease in vision. Resolution is gradual with relative clearing of the stroma and emptying of the neovascularization, leaving behind ghost vessels. A secondary anterior uveitis commonly develops along with the IK. It is treated with mydriatic and cycloplegic drops as well as corticosteroid therapy, which is also prescribed for the corneal inflammation.

Acquired syphilis results from *T. pallidum* infection in adults. The infection is categorized into primary, secondary, latent, and tertiary stages. Primary syphilis typically occurs within several days to weeks after the initial infection and is characterized by genital chancre formation. Secondary syphilis usually develops within 6 weeks of initial infection and is recognized clinically by a variety of features such as a maculopapular rash along the palms and soles, generalized lymphadenopathy, mucous membrane lesions, meningitis, periostitis, alopecia, and constitutional symptoms.

Ocular findings may occur during secondary syphilis and include iridocyclitis, multifocal or diffuse chorioretinitis, vasculitis, and neuroretinitis, the latter including an inflammation of the retina and optic nerve. The posterior segment involvement may later result in a clinical picture consisting of a "salt and pepper" retinopathy, vessel sheathing, and optic atrophy. A ring scotoma may result from the retinal changes, mimicking retinitis pigmentosa.

The iridocyclitis of acquired secondary syphilis may be granulomatous or nongranulomatous and initially may be associated with a transient prominent engorgement of the fine superficial vasculature of the iris. This is referred to as roseola. Whereas topical corticosteroid therapy may temporarily suppress existing inflammation, the uveitis associated with syphilis is typically recurrent or not responsive to therapy. Syphilis should therefore be considered in anyone with a recurrent or progressive uveitis.

Once identified as the etiologic agent, the syphilitic infection should be treated accordingly, typically with penicillin therapy. The uveitis, as long as it is present, is managed with nonspecific therapy including mydriatic/cycloplegic agents to decrease ciliary spasm and prevent synechiae formation, and tailored corticosteroid therapy to suppress inflammation.

The laboratory investigation for syphilis consists of the fluorescent treponemal antibody absorption test (FTA-ABS), which is very sensitive and specific for syphilitic infection and remains positive throughout a person's life, even after active infection is adequately treated.[37] Comparable to the FTA-ABS test is the microhemagglutination-*Treponema* pallidum test (MHA-TP), which is also a specific treponemal test. Like the FTA-ABS test, the MHA-TP test results remain positive for years despite adequate treatment. The workup should also include a nonspecific reagin test, such as the Venereal Disease Research Laboratory (VDRL) test or the rapid plasma reagin (RPR) card test. Both of these tests often become nonreactive in the later stages of syphilis or after treatment.

A reactive VDRL or RPR is generally considered evidence of active syphilis.

High on the differential diagnosis of syphilitic iridocyclitis is uveitis associated with sarcoidosis, tuberculosis, and arthritic syndromes. Appropriate laboratory investigation of these diseases should be performed as well.

Tuberculosis

Similar to syphilis, tuberculosis (TB) can produce a variety of ocular and systemic findings. Related ocular features can include anterior and posterior uveitis, phlyctenular keratoconjunctivitis, retinitis, vasculitis, and optic neuritis. Choroidal involvement may result in a focal or multifocal choroiditis, or a single, relatively large choroidal nodule can occur. The iridocyclitis associated with TB may be unilateral or bilateral and granulomatous or nongranulomatous. Like syphilis, TB causes only a small percentage of all reported cases of uveitis.[38] Also, the associated uveitis may be slowly progressive and unresponsive to treatment. TB should therefore be suspected in any patient with a recalcitrant iridocyclitis.

Helpful laboratory tests include purified protein derivative (PPD) skin testing and chest x-ray films.[39] Other methods such as cultures and biopsy of specifically involved sites may be necessary in some cases. Once a diagnosis of active TB is made, standard systemic medical therapy should be instituted. Antituberculosis therapy commonly consists of drug combinations of isoniazid, rifampin, or ethambutol. Whereas antituberculosis therapy is the ultimate treatment for related uveitis, existing ocular inflammation is controlled with nonspecific medical therapy including mydriatic/cycloplegic agents and corticosteroids.

Glaucomatocyclitic Crisis (Posner-Schlossman Syndrome)

Unilateral attacks of markedly increased intraocular pressure (usually 40–50 mm Hg or higher) accompanied by signs of mild anterior segment inflammation characterize the Posner-Schlossman syndrome. Fine KPs may be present, although possibly not initially, and there may be mild degrees of aqueous cells and flare. Corneal edema may be present, which commonly causes complaints of haloes around lights and mildly blurred vision. Externally, the eye is often relatively white and quiet but may exhibit moderate circumlimbal injection. Discomfort is usually mild and visual symptoms may be the only initial symptom. The attacks associated with glaucomatocyclitic crisis are usually recurrent over a period of years (possibly decades) and occur with variable frequency.

Episodes may occur in both eyes, but typically only one eye at a time is affected. There can be a predilection for one side. During attacks, the involved pupil may be larger. Over time, subtle heterochromia may develop, causing the condition to be included in the differential diagnosis of Fuchs' heterochromic iridocyclitis.

Although attacks may last from one to several days, resolution generally occurs without residual sequelae. Although optic nerve damage and visual field loss do not occur in most cases,[40] recurrent attacks may lead to chronic elevation in intraocular pressure with associated cupping and visual field loss. It is postulated that although usually considered an isolated ocular disease, glaucomatocyclitic crisis may be associated with the development of primary open-angle glaucoma in both eyes, and therefore all patients with this syndrome should be carefully monitored and treated as glaucoma suspects.[41]

Acute attacks are managed with topical antiglaucoma medications such as beta-blockers and with topical corticosteroids. Although posterior synechiae formation is rare, mydriatic/cycloplegic agents may be given to protect against this as well as to decrease ciliary spasm.

Pars Planitis

Pars planitis is a relatively common idiopathic disorder characterized by chronic intraocular inflammation that usually initially affects young adults and children.[42] It is often asymptomatic and discovered during routine examination. Affected eyes usually appear white and quiet externally. The disease is mostly bilateral, although asymmetric involvement is typical. A classic characteristic is a whitish material ("snowbank") overlying the inferior pars plana and pre-oral retina.[43] The "snowbank" may extend upward to involve a portion of the nasal and temporal oral regions as well. A peripheral vasculitis involving the retinal veins is often present and accompanied by sheathing of the vessel walls. Cells are located predominantly within the anterior vitreous, and cellular aggregates ("snowballs") accumulate inferiorly. The anterior chamber may contain some spillover, with mild cell, flare, and KP being present. Posterior synechiae only occasionally form.

The significant complications occurring with this disorder include cataract, cystoid macular edema, and tractional retinal detachment. Whereas the majority (possibly 80%) of patients with pars planitis require no treatment, measures must be taken to treat these complications when they occur. Anti-inflammatory therapy is usually only prescribed when macular edema reduces visual acuity to approximately 20/40. Whereas topical corticosteroidal therapy is ineffective in halting the inflammation and progression of cystoid macular edema, periocular and oral treatment may prove beneficial. In recalcitrant cases, pars plana cryotherapy and/or immunosuppressive therapy may be indicated.

Most patients with pars planitis are asymptomatic and do not develop significant ocular complications. Even patients who are symptomatic often only develop intermittent exacerbations, which gradually clear. Overtreatment, which may hasten cataract formation or cause a steroid-induced glaucoma, should be avoided.

Pronounced visual loss, if it occurs, is usually secondary to macular disruption from the chronic macular edema or from related lamellar hole formation. Tractional retinal detachment, resulting from contraction of a vascularized membrane that forms over the inferior retinal "snowbank" and ciliary body, may cause vitreous hemorrhage and displacement of the macula.

"Intermediate uveitis" has often been used interchangeably with the term "pars planitis" to describe the same specific disorder. Intermediate uveitis, however, is best used as an anatomic classification term describing inflammation located within the middle region of the eye. Pars planitis is one specific type of intermediate uveitis; a similar inflammatory picture may occur secondary to other disorders including sarcoidosis, toxocariasis, and Lyme disease.[44]

Toxoplasmosis

Toxoplasmosis is a common clinical entity caused by infestation with the intracellular protozoan parasite *Toxoplasma gondii*. On initial entry into the body, the organism becomes disseminated and may then reside in various tissues including the neuroretina, where it becomes responsible for as many as half or more of all cases of posterior uveitis in the United States.[8]

Cats are the definitive host of *T. gondii* and shed the organism in their feces. Humans become infected by direct contact with cat feces or contaminated matter, the ingestion of uncooked meat of an animal infested with the organism, or via transplacental spread. The infection may therefore present as an acquired or a congenital disorder. The initial infestation with *T. gondii* in acquired cases may cause a febrile or influenza-like illness that generally resolves over a period of days to weeks. A small percentage of cases may develop severe complications such as meningoencephalitis, but the vast majority of cases are asymptomatic. After the acute infectious phase, the *T. gondii* parasite becomes dormant within intracellular cysts. The organism may remain dormant throughout the life of the host or (as a result of immune suppression) active parasites may be released, causing disease recurrence.

Ocular toxoplasmosis rarely occurs in the acute acquired phase of infection; rather, it is typically a manifestation of recurrent disease.

Transmission of toxoplasmosis from mother to fetus only occurs if the mother is infected during pregnancy. If the fetus does become infected, the organism may be active or inactive at the time of birth. Fetal infection can result in severe congenital abnormalities or miscarriage. Most cases of congenital toxoplasmosis are inactive at birth. Healed chorioretinal lesions are ophthalmic evidence of congenital infection. Most cases of active ocular toxoplasmosis result from congenital infection. Recurrent retinochoroiditis from this type of infection typically occurs in the second, third, or fourth decades of life.

The active lesion of ocular toxoplasmosis typically consists of an elevated whitish inflammatory lesion, which represents primarily a retinitis. Coincident inflammation of the choroid occurs because of its proximity, resulting in a retinochoroiditis. Active toxoplasmosis lesions typically occur adjacent to old healed lesions that become reactivated. During active disease, the overlying vitreous contains significant amounts of inflammatory cell, possibly resulting in a marked loss of detail of the fundus. Arteritis or periphlebitis may occur within or adjacent to the foci of inflammation.

In addition to posterior segment findings, inflammatory signs commonly are present in the anterior chamber, which often includes a granulomatous-type reaction consisting of cells and flare and mutton-fat KPs.

Confirmation of suspected toxoplasmosis infection can be aided with laboratory investigation, which can include the Sabin-Feldman dye test (*Toxoplasma* dye test), indirect fluorescent antibody (IFA) testing, hemagglutination testing, and the enzyme-linked immunosorbent assay (ELISA) for toxoplasmosis. The IFA and the ELISA are the two tests most frequently used.

Associated anterior uveitis is managed nonspecifically to suppress inflammation, prevent synechiae formation, and improve patient comfort. Topical steroids are not effective against the posterior segment inflammation.

Depending on the location and extent of active toxoplasmosis fundus lesions, only observation may be necessary, with lesions typically resolving on their own. If, however, inflammation threatens the macula or if it is particularly severe, antimicrobial therapy is indicated. This typically consists of drug combinations, possibly consisting of pyrimethamine, triple sulfa (sulfadiazine, sulfamethazine, and sulfamerazine), clindamycin, and oral corticosteroids. Corticosteroids should not be used alone without concurrent antimicrobial therapy because immunosuppressive effects may actually exacerbate activity of the toxoplasmosis organism. Periocular injection may be an effective replacement for oral steroids in some patients. Other treatment modalities that have been used include cryotherapy and photocoagulation applied directly to active lesions.[45] Vitrectomy may be needed in instances of tractional retinal detachment caused by vitreal fibrosis and contraction.

Toxocariasis

Toxocariasis is a parasitic infection caused by the organism *Toxocara canis* and *Toxocara cati,* common intestinal parasites of dogs and cats, respectively. Both organisms have been isolated in humans, but *T. canis* appears to be responsible for ophthalmic complications. Human infection occurs through the ingestion of contaminated soil or food. The organism is shed by cats and dogs in their feces.

The life cycle of *Toxocara* in dogs and cats consists of ingestion of dormant *Toxocara* ova, which travel from the intestinal tract to the lungs after they mature into a larval stage. Upon reaching the lungs and eventually the trachea, the larvae are reingested. The larvae then produce ova, which are shed in the feces. In humans, mature larvae do not form and therefore additional ova are not formed and shed in the feces. Rather, the larvae travel to various organs and tissues of the body, including the eye, where they die. There is a predilection for the central nervous system, eyes, liver, lungs, and heart. At this stage, an inflammatory reaction occurs because of disintegration of the larvae. Granulomas develop at the site of larval death.

After an incubation period of several weeks to months, systemic or ocular forms of the disease can occur. The systemic form, referred to as visceral larva migrans (VLM), usually occurs in children between 6 months and 3 years of age and is characterized by fever, pneumonia, hepatomegaly, splenomegaly, and skin rash.[46] There is a good prognosis for the disease, and gradual resolution usually occurs. However, severe cases may result in death.

Ocular toxocariasis rarely occurs in association with VLM, but rather tends to affect older patients (average age 7.5 years) without signs of VLM. The ocular involvement may be discovered only on routine examination after resolution of the disorder or after a visual decrease is noted by the patient. In the eye, *Toxocara* infection takes one of three different forms: (1) endophthalmitis, (2) solitary posterior pole granuloma, or (3) peripheral granuloma.

In cases of endophthalmitis, patients exhibit dense amounts of vitreal cells and a mild anterior chamber reaction. The severe vitreal inflammation may result in vitreoretinal membranes, which can contract and cause retinal breaks and tractional retinal detachment. An isolated peripheral granuloma may be detected or it may be obscured by inflammatory debris. Dense cyclitic membranes may form behind the lens, which can contract and cause ciliary body detachment and hypotony. Patients may have strabismus and leukokoria, and may be misdiagnosed as having retinoblastoma, pars planitis, or Coat's disease. Cases of endophthalmitis related to toxocariasis respond poorly to antihelminthic drugs but do rather well after the administration of periocular or systemic steroids. Vitrectomy to remove the *Toxocara* antigens may be necessary in unresponsive cases. Photocoagulation may be warranted to stop progression of a nematode as it encroaches on the fovea or optic nerve head.[47]

Isolated posterior pole granulomas may be very benign or cause a severe visual decrease if the macula is involved. The clinical appearance of focal granulomas is that of fairly well-delineated, round, white, elevated lesions of the inner retina. Tractional forces may cause retinal folds extending away from the lesions. Small amounts of vitreal cells may be present with active lesions.

Peripheral granulomas may also be benign in nature and go unnoticed until routine examination. Others may cause visual loss as a result of contraction of vitreoretinal bands that extend from the lesion to the posterior pole. Macular displacement may occur as well as tractional or rhegmatogenous retinal detachment. Because of the fibrotic changes and vitreoretinal membrane associated with peripheral granulomas, these presentations may be confused with retinopathy of prematurity (ROP), congenital falciform retinal folds, and pars planitis. The location of the peripheral granuloma and associated fibrotic tissue is helpful in the differential diagnosis—i.e., peripheral *Toxocara* granulomas may occur in any quadrant, but ROP occurs temporally and pars planitis occurs inferiorly. In addition, ocular toxocariasis is unilateral whereas pars planitis and ROP occur bilaterally.

Although the diagnosis of ocular toxocariasis depends largely on clinical presentation, laboratory confirmation is generally acquired via ELISA testing for *Toxocara*.

Presumed Ocular Histoplasmosis Syndrome

Histoplasmosis is an infectious systemic disease caused by *Histoplasma capsulatum*. It is contracted via inhalation of dust particles carrying the fungal spores. Endemic areas are the Ohio and Mississippi River valleys. After initial infection with the *Histoplasma* organism, individuals may remain asymptomatic, develop symptoms of a nonspecific upper respiratory tract infection, or, after hematogenous spread from the lungs, develop disseminated systemic histoplasmosis, possibly characterized by lymphadenopathy, hepatomegaly, splenomegaly, and ulcerations of the oropharynx and GI tract in addition to the respiratory symptoms. Within weeks the organisms disappear from affected organs, leaving behind focal granulomatous lesions and scars.

After hematogenous spread, the *H. capsulatum* organisms may also reach the choroid, resulting in focal lesions that cause some characteristic clinical findings. The ophthalmic picture of the presumed ocular histoplasmosis syndrome (POHS) consists of peripapillary atrophy and small, focal chorioretinal lesions, which are classically peripheral but may occur throughout the fundus. These lesions, commonly referred to as "histo spots," are often white centrally and surrounded by hyperpigmentation. Occasionally, several of the "punched out" appearing chorioretinal lesions occur contiguous with one another, causing the appearance of linear streaks.

A relatively common complication of these lesions, which also have some predilection for the macula, is the development of subretinal neovascularization, which leads to the significant visual loss attributed to this disease. Rather than occurring with the initial choroiditis, subretinal neovascular membrane (SRNVM) formation is a late complication, often occurring several years later in association with histo lesions. SRNVMs may develop at peripheral lesions, in the peripapillary region, and in the macular region.

Because of the threat of SRNVM formation, patients with atrophic scars involving the macula should be aware of this potential complication and may be encouraged to use Amsler grid monitoring on a daily basis at home. This is especially true for those patients who have already developed a SRNVM in one eye. Patients with a SRNVM secondary to POHS may benefit from laser photocoagulation.[48] Patients do not benefit from antifungal therapy because active organisms do not appear to be present at this stage. Corticosteroids have been advocated by some individuals in addition to photocoagulation for the treatment of SRNVM secondary to POHS.[8]

As a result of the typical clinical appearance of POHS, diagnosis is usually made on ophthalmic appearance alone. If uncertain, the histoplasmin skin test can be used, which produces positive results in approximately 90% of patients with POHS.[49] Patients with POHS also have a high prevalence of the HLA-B7 antigen. Fluorescein angiography is helpful in the evaluation of SRNVM formation and should be performed in all cases before photocoagulation treatment.

Behçet's Syndrome

Behçet's syndrome is a systemic disorder characterized by the classic findings of recurrent episodes of aphthous ulcerations of the mouth and genitalia and uveitis. Many other characteristics may occur including various skin lesions (papules, pustules, vesicles), arthritis involving primarily the knees, thrombophlebitis, CNS involvement, GI involvement, and cardiovascular lesions. The etiology of Behçet's syndrome is unknown. Affected individuals are typically young and of Mediterranean and Far Eastern descent (especially Japan). Men are affected more commonly than women.

The ocular presentation of Behçet's syndrome may consist of an anterior, posterior, or panuveitis. Classically, patients have a recurrent, bilateral, nongranulomatous anterior uveitis that produces a hypopyon formation. Other ophthalmic features of the disease may include conjunctivitis, episcleritis, keratitis, retinal vasculitis (primarily of the retinal veins), and retinitis. Related fundus changes may include diffuse serous, exudative, and hemorrhagic leakage throughout the fundus, optic disc edema and atrophy, and prominent vascular sheathing. In 75–80% of cases, ocular involvement follows the onset of genital or oral ulceration.[50]

The diagnosis of Behçet's syndrome is primarily made on clinical grounds. Skin puncture testing often yields blistering of the skin but is a nonspecific finding. Fluorescein angiography can be helpful in identifying the typical clinical picture. A high positivity rate for the HLA-B5 antigen is associated with the disorder.

Exacerbations and remissions characterize the disease for several years, after which it may eventually resolve. Commonly, exacerbations last 2–4 weeks.[13] The long-term systemic course is generally benign; however, serious complications and even death may occur. The ocular prognosis is typically worse than systemic complications, with severe visual loss possibly resulting from the uveitis, vasculitis, retinal edema, and optic atrophy.

Milder forms of iridocyclitis can be treated well with topical steroids and mydriatic/cycloplegic agents. More severe cases may require periocular steroidal injections. Posterior segment inflammation is much less responsive, often showing little clearing with systemic corticosteroid therapy. Because of this, immunosuppressive drugs have been tried and have become the mainstay for treatment of posterior segment disease.[51]

Lens-Induced Uveitis

Three basic subtypes of lens-induced uveitis have traditionally been described. These include (1) phacoanaphylactic endophthalmitis (phacoanaphylactic uveitis, phacoantigenic uveitis), (2) phacotoxic uveitis, and (3) phacolytic glaucoma.[8] The literature is somewhat confusing concerning the categorization of the various types

of lens-induced uveitis, and subsequent misuse of terminology commonly occurs. Adding to the confusion is the fact that precise causes for all types of lens-induced uveitis are not known, and new theories have emerged casting great doubt on earlier assumptions pertaining to disorders falling into this category of uveitis.

Traditionally, phacoanaphylactic endophthalmitis was believed to result from the leakage of lens proteins into the aqueous humor, which were then recognized as foreign, causing an autoimmune response and sterile inflammation. Disruption of the lens capsule that allowed for the leakage typically resulted from trauma or intraocular surgery or occurred spontaneously. It was generally believed that once the lens proteins leaked into the aqueous humor, they reached the bloodstream where antibodies to the lens material were made. Then, 24 hours to 3 weeks after exposure of the lens protein, an immune reaction ensued within the anterior chamber because of the presence of remaining material. Clinically, the anterior chamber reaction was described as granulomatous in nature, exhibiting large mutton-fat KPs, a marked degree of cells and flare, anterior and posterior synechiae, cyclitic membrane formation, and secondary glaucoma.

Phacotoxic uveitis has traditionally been a poorly delineated category of lens-induced uveitis, often used to describe clinical presentations without increased intraocular pressure and without the more usual signs of phacoanaphylactic endophthalmitis. Patients with phacotoxic uveitis typically have mild or severe anterior segment inflammation that generally is not granulomatous in nature. Since there was occasionally a clinical picture similar to phacoanaphylactic uveitis, it has been postulated that many cases of phacotoxic uveitis simply represent a varied presentation of phacoanaphylactic uveitis.

More recent literature has reported that lens proteins are not recognized as foreign because they have been fully sequestered within the lens; on the contrary, lens proteins are recognized as "self" because otherwise, phacoanaphylactic uveitis would be seen routinely after injury and disruption of the lens capsule.[52] Since lens protein is recognized by the immune system, it is more likely that an abnormal tolerance develops to lens proteins. The reasons for this are unknown but probably involve a complicated sequence of events.

It is also clear from more recent literature that phacoanaphylactic uveitis is difficult to accurately diagnose clinically and that histopathologic examination is necessary for confirmation.[52] Usually when this disease is diagnosed through histopathologic means, it is not suspected clinically. In addition, the disorder is often not confirmed histopathologically when it is suspected clinically. Therefore, it must be remembered that it is difficult to differentiate clinically between phacoanaphylactic uveitis and other forms of inflammation, particularly postoperative uveitis. The differential diagnosis in particular should include sympathetic ophthalmia as well as postoperative endophthalmitis. Phacoanaphylactic enophthalmitis should be considered a rare response to lens injury, and other conditions should be ruled out before making this difficult diagnosis. Treatment requires topical, periocular, or systemic corticosteroids followed by extraction of the offending lens or lens material once the eye is quieted. Mydriatics and cycloplegics are indicated to prevent posterior synechiae and improve patient comfort.

Phacolytic glaucoma is characterized by minimal anterior segment inflammation and has significance because of the development of an acute elevation in intraocular pressure. Nevertheless, because of its mechanisms and the presence of some uveitic signs, it is usually categorized as lens-induced uveitis. Patients with phacolytic glaucoma usually exhibit an advanced (mature or hypermature) cataract. Lens proteins that leak into the aqueous are engulfed by large macrophages, which block trabecular meshwork outflow either by themselves or in combination with free lens proteins. There is usually only a mild cellular and flare reaction without KP formation. Diagnosis of this condition is aided by the appearance of large white particles in the aqueous, which are individual macrophages.

The initial goal in the treatment of phacolytic glaucoma is to lower the intraocular pressure with antiglaucoma medications. Miotics should be avoided. Topical corticosteroids are beneficial to suppress the inflammatory component. Once intraocular pressure is lowered to an acceptable level and the eye is quieted, cataract surgery should be performed.

Sarcoidosis

Sarcoidosis is an idiopathic, multisystem disorder that is characterized by the development of noncaseating epithelioid granulomas within various organs and tissues of the body. Signs and symptoms of the disease depend on the size or severity of involvement. There is a predilection for the lymph nodes, lungs, liver, skin, and eyes. Bones, the spleen, skeletal muscle, the heart, and the CNS are also involved. Sarcoidosis typically affects individuals between the ages of 20 and 40 years, but it may also occasionally occur in young and elderly persons. It is more common in American blacks and northern Europeans.[53] Females are affected more often than males.

Typical symptoms of sarcoidosis include fever, weight loss, and arthralgias. Common clinical findings include mediastinal lymphadenopathy (bilateral hilar lym-

phadenopathy) and diffuse pulmonary infiltration discovered on chest x-ray films; peripheral lymphadenopathy; skin lesions, which include subcutaneous nodules and frequently erythema nodosum; and granulomatous uveitis, which occurs in 15–25% of cases. Seventy percent of patients exhibit hepatic granulomas as determined with biopsy examination. Most patients with sarcoidosis probably recover fully and spontaneously from their disease over a period of months to years, and many probably develop symptoms so mild that evaluation is not sought and a diagnosis is never established. On the other hand, serious permanent sequelae such as blindness or respiratory dysfunction may occur. Death is uncommon, occurring in a small percentage of cases.

The ophthalmic manifestations of sarcoidosis are varied, with anterior uveitis (acute, recurrent, or chronic) the most common manifestation. Both eyes are usually involved, but often asymmetrically and at different times. The inflammation is usually granulomatous in nature, with complications such as anterior and posterior synechiae, secondary glaucoma, cataract formation, and band keratopathy.

Posterior segment involvement is common, characterized by a variety of possible findings including vitritis, retinal vasculitis, venous occlusion and retinal neovascularization, choroidal and retinal granuloma, and granulomatous infiltration of the optic nerve head. A classic finding is the presence of peripheral, whitish perivenous infiltrations occurring secondary to active periphlebitis. These exudative lesions around retinal vessels are often referred to as "candle wax drippings." Resolved periphlebitis usually presents as a well-defined vascular sheathing. Common with posterior segment ocular sarcoidosis are the presence of white cell aggregates clustered just above the inferior retina, known as "vitreous puffballs" or "snowball" opacities.

Other ocular findings include sarcoid granulomas involving the conjunctiva, episclera, and lacrimal gland. Lacrimal gland infiltration results in keratoconjunctivitis sicca, commonly a pronounced feature of ocular sarcoidosis. Of patients with ocular sarcoidosis, approximately 60% develop iridocyclitis, whereas 25% develop retinal vasculitis and choroiditis.[54]

Medical consultation is obtained to assist in the diagnosis of systemic sarcoidosis. Chest x-ray films are very helpful in the workup of sarcoidosis since the vast majority of patients with ocular sarcoid show abnormal findings such as hilar adenopathy and diffuse pulmonary fibrosis. Serum lysozyme and angiotensin-converting enzyme levels may be elevated in active systemic sarcoidosis but may also be elevated in other conditions such as TB and rheumatoid arthritis. Gallium scanning of the head, neck, and thorax can show increased uptake in active sarcoidosis and may produce positive results when other test results are negative.[55] Kveim skin testing may also be performed but is uncommonly used. Biopsy of suspected granulomas, occasionally of the conjunctiva, can be used to make a definitive diagnosis of sarcoidosis.

The treatment of anterior uveitis secondary to sarcoidosis is topical mydriatic/cycloplegic agents and corticosteroids.[17] Periocular injections may be necessary as well as systemic corticosteroids, especially if posterior segment disease is present. Systemic corticosteroids and occasionally immunosuppressives may be used to control systemic manifestations of the disease.

Lyme Disease

Lyme disease is an infectious, inflammatory disorder caused by the tick-transmitted organism, *Borrelia burgdorferi*. The disease is endemic to certain geographic regions of the United States, and these regions have been expanding since the disease was first recognized in Lyme, Connecticut. Affected individuals often live or spend much time outdoors in heavily wooded areas.

Typically, within a few days to one month of initial infection a reddish macular or papular skin lesion referred to as erythema chronicum migrans (ECM) develops at the tick bite site. This lesion can be quite large and occurs in the majority of infected patients. Mild constitutional symptoms may accompany the ECM; these usually last for a few weeks. Fever, lymphadenopathy, and splenomegaly can be observed. Many patients apparently become asymptomatic and have no further sequelae after resolution of the ECM. Others, however, go on to develop a variety of related findings within weeks to months. Arthritis is most commonly observed, characterized by intermittent and chronic exacerbation for several years thereafter. Prominent swelling, especially of the knees, may appear during exacerbations. A small percentage of patients develop chronic, nonepisodic arthritis. A host of CNS abnormalities occur in a small percentage of patients within weeks to months of the ECM. These include cranial neuritis, meningitis, motor and sensory radiculitis, and others. Myocardial abnormalities also occur.

The diagnosis of Lyme infection is based on clinical suspicion in conjunction with laboratory investigation. Both a Lyme IFA for IgG and IgM antibodies and a Lyme ELISA should be performed when screening for Lyme disease. Seronegative Lyme disease does exist, and the false-negative rate may be relatively high in early disease stages.

Ocular complications may include conjunctivitis, nongranulomatous and granulomatous anterior uveitis, intermediate uveitis, optic neuritis, choroiditis, and papilledema.[44,56] Because of the relatively nonspecific presentation in the eye, Lyme disease should be considered in the differential diagnosis in idiopathic presentations of these disorders.

Whereas the treatment of anterior uveitis associated with Lyme disease is nonspecific, the definitive treatment for permanent resolution is antispirochetal therapy against the *B. burgdorferi* organism. Tetracycline, penicillin, and erythromycin are commonly used medications.

Vogt-Koyanagi-Harada Syndrome

The Vogt-Koyanagi-Harada (VKH) syndrome is a multisystem disorder with the primary characteristics of anterior or posterior uveitis, CNS manifestations, and cutaneous abnormalities. The disorder, which has an unknown etiology, is more common in darkly pigmented races, especially Asians (Japanese). Adult men and women are typically affected between the ages of 20 and 50 years.

The initial manifestations of VKH syndrome are variable but may begin with meningeal signs such as headache, nausea, vomiting, and pain and stiffness in the back of the neck. Encephalopathy can occur, causing convulsions, cranial nerve dysfunction (particularly of the eighth cranial nerve, which may cause hearing impairment), vertigo, and tinnitus. Lymphocytosis occurs in the cerebral spinal fluid during acute phases of the disease.

Ocular involvement can initially manifest itself as either anterior or posterior uveitis. The anterior uveitis typically presents bilaterally, but in one eye before the other. Inflammation may be severe with marked degrees of cells and flare, KPs, synechiae formation, and secondary glaucoma. The uveitis can be granulomatous in nature characterized by mutton-fat KPs and iris nodules.

Posterior segment changes consist initially of a bilateral diffuse or multifocal choroiditis that results in exudative retinal detachment. These serous detachments are often benign and are localized to the posterior pole. Detachments may be shallow or bullous and exhibit shifting fluid. Because of gravity, the inferior fundus may show prominent detachments in addition to the posterior pole changes. In longstanding cases, the entire retina can become involved. Disc hyperemia and edema are often present, as well as increased numbers of vitreal cells. Fluorescein angiography can be helpful in delineating the choroiditis in early or atypical cases. Characteristically, leakage of dye from the choroid into the subretinal space is noted.

The cutaneous signs of VKH syndrome are variable, consisting of alopecia, poliosis, and vitiligo. These usually but not always occur after the CNS and ocular manifestations of the disease. The cutaneous lesions can eventually disappear or remain permanent.

Without treatment the visual prognosis in VKH syndrome is poor, with complications resulting from chronic anterior and posterior uveitis and longstanding exudative retinal detachment. However, aggressive local and systemic corticosteroid therapy greatly limits the ocular and systemic complications. Exudative retinal detachment may resolve after even only a few days of therapy. After resolution of the exudative retinal detachment, the fundus may appear mottled because of proliferation and atrophy of the retinal pigment epithelium.

A diagnosis of VKH syndrome is typically made on clinical grounds alone. In confusing cases, fluorescein angiography may help delineate fundus changes. Lymphocytosis of the CSF can be demonstrated in acute phases of the disease. The VKH syndrome is associated with a higher prevalence of the HLA-B22 antigen.[57]

Sympathetic Ophthalmia

Sympathetic ophthalmia, or sympathetic uveitis, is a rare disorder occurring after a penetrating injury, either traumatic or surgical, to one eye. Usually within 2–8 weeks after penetrating injury to the "exciting" eye, a panuveitis concurrently develops in the "sympathizing" eye. Occasionally, inflammation may not occur for up to 1 year after initial injury. The inflammation developing in both eyes is granulomatous in nature, exhibiting mutton-fat KPs, iris nodules, and quick-forming posterior synechiae. The earliest sign of the developing uveal inflammation is often cells in the retrolenticular region. Prominent vitritis later develops.

Fundus changes consist of signs of a diffuse, multifocal choroiditis. Small, yellow-white lesions, referred to as Dalen-Fuchs nodules, are scattered throughout each fundus at the level of the retinal pigment epithelium. Both optic nerve head edema and subretinal edema may occur, possibly resulting in exudative retinal detachment.

Mild and atypical presentations of sympathetic ophthalmia can occur, presenting as an isolated anterior uveitis, intermediate uveitis, and focal choroiditis. Confusion with phacoanaphylactic uveitis and VKH syndrome can occur.

Sympathetic ophthalmia occasionally has a mild, self-limiting course; however, the majority of cases, if untreated, exhibit chronic inflammation leading to a variety of ophthalmic complications and subsequent visual loss.

Treatment consists of aggressive topical, periocular, and systemic corticosteroid therapy.[8] Prognosis is generally good but steroid therapy is needed for months and must be tapered very gradually after inflammation has cleared. Patients must be monitored regularly because recurrence may occur up to several years after the initial

TABLE 23-8
Masquerade Syndromes

Systemic disorders
  Leukemia
  Large cell lymphoma
  Juvenile xanthogranuloma
Ocular disorders
  Retinal detachment
  Intraocular foreign body
  Retinoblastoma
  Malignant melanoma
  Retinitis pigmentosa

inflammatory episode. Treatment of recurrent attacks should be as aggressive as treatment at the initial onset of the disease. Immunosuppressives may be of benefit in recalcitrant cases.

Early enucleation of the "exciting eye," usually before any development of sympathetic inflammation, has been used in the treatment and prevention of severe inflammation in the "sympathizing eye." With the availability of corticosteroidal therapy, however, this is only recommended in instances where the "exciting eye" has no chance of retaining useful vision.[8]

Masquerade Syndromes

There are several conditions, ocular and systemic, that may result in a secondary inflammatory response in the eye and may "masquerade" as a primary anterior or posterior uveitis (Table 23-8). It is important not to confuse these disorders with primary intraocular inflammation, as they may lead to significant morbidity or even death.

Leukemia

The leukemias, which are primary disorders of the bone marrow, are characterized by malignant neoplasia of the hematopoietic stem cells. There is replacement of bone marrow by the neoplastic cells, and spillover of large numbers of the abnormal cells into the peripheral blood and other tissues. The leukemias may be differentiated into acute and chronic forms, the acute form being characterized by a rapidly progressive fatal course if untreated and the chronic form being more indolent.

The infiltration of leukemic white cells into the eye may yield a clinical picture similar to that of a primary anterior uveitis, consisting of cells and flare in the anterior chamber and even pseudohypopyon formation. Additional ocular manifestations of leukemia may include bulbar conjunctival masses, iris heterochromia, hyphema, and increased intraocular pressure.[58] Retinal vascular changes, hemorrhages, cotton-wool spots, optic disc changes, and serous detachments may also be observed.[58] Preretinal, white, elevated masses are often found on funduscopic examination.[59]

Large Cell Lymphoma

The lymphomas are malignant disorders characterized by the proliferation and accumulation of lymphoid tissue cells such as lymphocytes and histiocytes. Large cell lymphoma (histiocytic lymphoma, reticulum cell sarcoma) is a type of lymphoma characterized by the proliferation of neoplastic cells two to three times larger than normal lymphocytes. The initial feature of this disease may be the discovery of tumor formation involving tissues throughout the body including the CNS, the visceral organs, bone, or the eye. Onset occurs at approximately 50 years of age. Nearly all cases begin unilaterally, the second eye affected weeks to months after the first.[60] Malignant cells within the vitreous are at times present without an underlying retinal involvement. These cells are often misdiagnosed as an active vitritis, leading the examiner to suspect retinal and choroidal inflammatory activity. These isolated cases of vitreous cells presenting without retinal involvement point to the presence of a large cell lymphoma.[61] Vitreal samples and either computed tomographic or magnetic resonance imaging scans confirm the presence of lymphomas.

Malignant Melanoma

Malignant choroidal melanoma, as well as tumor cell invasion of the vitreous and anterior segment, may cause signs of anterior or posterior uveitis. Occasionally the clinical picture may be confusing, as the overt signs of the intraocular tumor may not be readily apparent. Careful evaluation of the iris, iridocorneal angle, and fundus are helpful in differentiating the true cause of the secondary inflammatory signs. Any fundus elevation or discoloration should be closely scrutinized. Fluorescein angiography and ultrasonography can be extremely helpful.

Retinoblastoma

Retinoblastoma is the most common of pediatric ocular malignancies. Ocular signs may include leukokoria, strabismus, and an injected, painful eye. Cells from the retinoblastoma float in the aqueous humor, resembling inflammatory cells, and are often misdiagnosed as an iridocyclitis. They may form a pseudohypopyon in some cases.[62] Differentiation from an actual hypopyon may be made by having the patient tip the head to one side. A hypopyon will move, but a pseudohypopyon will not. Large white retinal tumors with accompanying serous retinal detachments may be discovered.

The family history should be evaluated for a previously diagnosed retinoblastoma. Ultrasonography may be help-ful in detecting the malignancy. A MRI scan also provides localization of the retinoblastoma. If in doubt, a biopsy may also be performed.

Juvenile Xanthogranuloma

Juvenile xanthogranuloma is a benign disorder occurring most often in young children that may cause poorly demarcated, yellowish, fleshly tumors of the iris. Similar appearing skin lesions may also be present and can be extremely valuable in the differential diagnosis. Signs of anterior uveitis are present, and spontaneous hyphema and elevated intraocular pressure may occur.

The ocular condition is generally treated with topical corticosteroids and antiglaucoma therapy if necessary. Spontaneous regression of the tumor may occur. Radiation therapy and surgical excision may be indicated in some cases.

Retinal Detachment

Long-standing peripheral retinal detachment may cause intraocular inflammation and may mimic an idiopathic anterior uveitis. The reaction occasionally may be severe, resulting in marked degrees of cell and flare, as well as synechiae formation. This underscores the need to perform a fundus evaluation in all patients with an apparent inflammation of the anterior segment. Without examination of the posterior segment at the time of initial presentation, one often is completely unable to anticipate significant underlying causes such as peripheral retinal detachment.

Retained Intraocular Foreign Body

A retained intraocular foreign body should be considered as a possible cause of intraocular inflammation in any patient with a history of trauma, especially if the patient reports being in an environment where projectile objects are a possibility. Techniques other than those used for routine ocular examination may be necessary for the diagnosis of a retained intraocular foreign body, including ultrasonography, plain film x-rays, and CT or MRI scanning.

Retinitis Pigmentosa

The presence of vitreal cells associated with retinitis pigmentosa (RP) can occasionally cause difficulty in differential diagnosis if one is unaware of this association or if incomplete fundus examination is performed. Usually RP can be easily differentiated from primary intermediate or posterior segment inflammation by the presence of consistent signs such as a waxy, pale nerve head, attenuation of the retinal arterioles and venules, peripheral bone spicule-like clumping of the retinal pigment epithelium, and electroretinogram findings.

REFERENCES

1. Waitzman MB, King CD. Prostaglandin influences on intraocular pressure and pupil size. Am J Physiol 1967; 212:329–34.

2. Hogan MJ, Kimura SJ, Thygeson P. Signs and symptoms of uveitis. I. Anterior Uveitis. Am J Ophthalmol 1959;47: 155–70.

3. Roth M, Simmons RJ. Glaucoma associated with precipitates on the trabecular meshwork. Ophthalmology 1979;86: 1613–8.

4. Kitazawa Y. Increased intraocular pressure induced by corticosteroids. Am J Ophthalmol 1976;82:492–5.

5. Kimura SJ, Thygeson P, Hogan MJ. Signs and symptoms of uveitis. II. Classification of the posterior manifestations of uveitis. Am J Ophthalmol 1959;47:171–6.

6. Lebensohn JE. The nature of photophobia. Arch Ophthalmol 1934;12:380–90.

7. Tessler HH. Classification and Symptoms and Signs of Uveitis. In W Tasman, E Jaeger (eds), Duane's Clinical Ophthalmology (Vol. 4). Philadelphia: Lippincott, 1987;32:1.

8. Smith RE, Nozik RA. Uveitis: A Clinical Approach to Diagnosis and Management (2nd ed). Baltimore: Williams & Wilkins, 1989;23–5, 128–32, 141–5, 158–60, 180–2, 198–200, 209–11.

9. Pavesio CE, Nosik RA. Anterior and intermediate uveitis. Int Ophthalmol Clin 1990;30:244–51.

10. Bloch-Michel E, Nussenblatt RB. International uveitis study group recommendations for the evaluation of intraocular inflammatory disease. Am J Ophthalmol 1987;103:234–5.

11. Heiden D, Nozik RA. A systematic approach to uveitis diagnosis. Ophthalmol Clin North Am 1993;6:17, 21.

12. Woods AC. Endogenous Inflammations of the Uveal Tract. Baltimore: Williams & Wilkins, 1961;45.

13. Rosenbaum JT, Wernick R. Selection and interpretation of laboratory tests for patients with uveitis. Int Ophthalmol Clin 1990;30:238–43.

14. Roberts SP. Optometric utilization of clinical laboratory tests. Problems in Optometry 1991;3:90.

15. Rao NA, Forster DJ. Nonspecific Therapy of Uveitis. In NA Rao, DJ Forster, JJ Augsburger (eds), The Uvea: Uveitis and Intraocular Neoplasms (Vol. 2). New York: Gower, 1992;3:2–5.

16. Fingeret M, Potter JW. Uveitis. In JD Bartlett, SD Jaanus (eds), Clinical Ocular Pharmacology (2nd ed). Boston: Butterworth, 1989;626–8, 632–3.

17. Melton R, Thomas R. Second annual practical guide to therapeutic drugs. Optom Management 1993;May(Suppl):9–12.

18. Nussenblatt RB, Palestine AG. Uveitis: Fundamentals and Clinical Practice. Chicago: Year Book, 1989;71–5, 165–7, 219–24, 229–32, 424–5.

19. Chiou GCY, Yao QS, Chang MS, Okawara T. Prevention and treatment of ocular inflammation with a new class of non-steroidal anti-inflammatory agents. J Ocul Pharmacol 1994;10:335–46.

20. Hooper PL, Rao NA, Smith RE. Cataract extraction in uveitis patients. Surv Ophthalmol 1990;35:120–44.

21. Wolf MD, Lichter PR, Ragsdale CG. Prognostic factors in the uveitis of juvenile rheumatoid arthritis. Ophthalmology 1987;94:1242–8.

22. Liesegang TJ. Clinical features and prognosis in Fuchs' uveitis syndrome. Arch Ophthalmol 1982;100:1622–6.

23. Wakefield D, Dunlop I, McCluskey PJ, Penny R. Uveitis: Aetiology and disease associations in an Australian population. Aust NZ J Ophthalmol 1986;14:181–7.

24. Scharf Y, Zonis S. Histocompatibility antigens (HLA) and uveitis. Surv Ophthalmol 1980;24:220–8.

25. Brewerton DA, Caffrey M, Hart FD et al. Ankylosing spondylitis and HL-A27. Lancet 1973;1:904–7.

26. Abel GA, Terry JE. Ankylosing spondylitis and recurrent anterior uveitis. J Am Optom Assoc 1991;62:844–8.

27. Beckingsale AB, Davies J, Gibson JM, Rosenthal AR. Acute anterior uveitis, ankylosing spondylitis, back pain, and HLA-B27. Br J Ophthalmol 1984;68:741–5.

28. Holland EJ. Reiter's Syndrome. In DH Gold, TA Weingeist (eds), The Eye in Systemic Disease. Philadelphia: Lippincott, 1990;56–7.

29. Mallas EG, Mackintosh P, Asquith P, Cooke WT. Histocompatibility antigens in inflammatory bowel disease; their clinical significance and their association with arthropathy with special reference to HLA-B27(W27). Gut 1976;17: 906–10.

30. Rao NA, Forster DJ, Spalton DJ. Anterior Uveitis. In RA Rao, DJ Forster, JJ Augsberger (eds), The Uvea: Uveitis and Intraocular Neoplasms (Vol. 2). New York: Gower, 1992;3:5–8.

31. Talley DK. Clinical Laboratory Testing for the Diagnosis of Systemic Disease Associated with Anterior Uveitis. In JG Classé (ed), Optometry Clinics (Vol. 2). Norwalk, CT: Appleton & Lange, 1992;112–3.

32. Shaller J, Kupfer C, Wedgwood RJ. Iridocyclitis in juvenile rheumatoid arthritis. Pediatrics 1969;44:92–100.

33. Kanski JJ, Shun-Shin GA. Systemic uveitis syndromes in childhood: An analysis of 340 cases. Ophthalmology 1984; 91:1247–52.

34. Jones NP. Fuchs' heterochromic uveitis: An update. Surv Ophthalmol 1993;37:253–72.

35. Womack LW, Liesegang T. Complications of herpes zoster ophthalmicus. Arch Ophthalmol 1983;101:42–5.

36. Cobo LM, Foulks GN, Liesegang TJ et al. Oral acyclovir in the therapy of acute herpes zoster ophthalmicus: An interim report. Ophthalmology 1985;92:1574–83.

37. Tamesis RR, Foster CS. Ocular syphilis. Ophthalmology 1990;97:1281–7.

38. Schlaegel TF. Perspectives in uveitis. Ann Ophthalmol 1981;13:799–806.

39. Abrams J, Schlaegel TF. The tuberculin skin test in the diagnosis of tuberculosis uveitis. Am J Ophthalmol 1983;96: 295–8.

40. Schlossman A. Glaucomatocyclic Crisis (Posner-Schlossman Syndrome). In FT Fraufelder, FM Roy (eds), Current Ocular Therapy (3rd ed). Philadelphia: Saunders, 1990;558.

41. Kass MA, Becker B, Kolker AE. Glaucomatocyclic crisis and primary open-angle glaucoma. Am J Ophthalmol 1973;75:668–73.

42. Smith RE. Pars Planitis. In SJ Ryan (ed), Retina (Vol. 2). St. Louis: Mosby, 1989;637–46.

43. Henderly DE, Haymond RS, Rao NA, Smith RE. The significance of the pars plana exudate in pars planitis. Am J Ophthalmol 1987;103:669–71.

44. Breevald J, Rothova A, Kaiper H. Intermediate uveitis and Lyme borreliosis. Br J Ophthalmol 1992;76:181–2.

45. Ghartey KN, Brockhurst RJ. Photocoagulation of active toxoplasmic retinochoroiditis. Am J Ophthalmol 1980;89:858–64.

46. Shields JA. Ocular toxocariasis. A review. Surv Ophthalmol 1984;28:361–81.

47. Raymond LA, Gutierrez Y, Strong LE, et al. Living retinal nematode (filarial-like) destroyed with photocoagulation. Ophthalmology 1978;85:944–9.

48. Macular Photocoagulation Study Group. Argon laser photocoagulation for ocular histoplasmosis. Results of a randomized clinical trial. Arch Ophthalmol 1983;101:1347–57.

49. Kanski JJ. Uveitis: A Color Manual of Diagnosis and Treatment. London: Butterworths, 1987.

50. Michelson JB. Diffuse uveitis. Ophthalmol Clin North Am 1993;6:55–64.

51. Nussenblatt RB, Palestine AG. Cyclosporine: Immunology, pharmacology, and therapeutic uses. Surv Ophthalmol 1986;31:159.

52. Marak GE. Phacoanaphylactic endophthalmitis. Surv Ophthalmol 1992;36:325–39.

53. Jabs DA, Johns CJ. Ocular involvement in chronic sarcoidosis. Am J Ophthalmol 1986;102:297–301.

54. Obenauf CD, Shaw HE, Sydnor CF, Klintworth GK. Sarcoidosis and its ophthalmic manifestations. Am J Ophthalmol 1978;86:648–55.

55. Weinreb RN, Tessler H. Laboratory diagnosis of ophthalmic sarcoidosis. Surv Ophthalmol 1984;28:653–64.

56. Steere AC, Bartenhagen NH, Craft JE et al. The early clinical manifestations of Lyme disease. Ann Intern Med 1983;99:76–82.

57. Shimizu K. Harada's, Behçet's, Vogt-Koyanagi syndromes. Are they clinical entities? Trans Am Acad Ophthalmol Otolaryngol 1973;77:281–90.

58. Kincaid MC, Green WR. Ocular and orbital involvement in leukemia. Surv Ophthalmol 1983;27:211–32.

59. Kuwabara T, Aiello L. Leukemic miliary nodules in the retina. Arch Ophthalmol 1964;72:494–7.

60. Vogel MH, Font RL, Zimmerman LE, Levine RA. Reticulum cell carcinoma of the retina and uvea. Am J Ophthalmol 1968;66:205–15.

61. Minckler DS, Font RL, Zimmerman LE. Uveitis and reticulum cell sarcoma of brain with bilateral neoplastic seeding of vitreous without retinal or uveal involvement. Am J Ophthalmol 1975;80:433–9.

62. Shields JA, Augsburger JJ. Current approaches to the diagnosis and management of retinoblastoma. Surv Ophthalmol 1981;25:347–72.

24

Diseases of the Retina and Vitreous

Rex Ballinger

RETINAL VASCULAR DISEASE

Diabetic Retinopathy

Diabetic retinopathy is one of the most common causes of legal blindness in the United States today.[1] Approximately one-fourth of all patients with diabetes are estimated to have some form of retinopathy. The incidence and progression of retinal manifestations depends on the duration of diabetes as well as the patient's age.[2,3] When managing patients with diabetic retinopathy, it is important for optometrists to understand the natural history of the disease in the eye and the appropriate approaches to management. In order to properly follow patients with diabetic retinopathy, results from several studies should be reviewed, including the Diabetic Retinopathy Study (DRS),[2-6] the Diabetic Retinopathy Vitrectomy Study,[7,8] and the Early Treatment Diabetic Retinopathy Study (ETDRS).[9,10] These studies not only report on the natural history of the disease but have identified the risk factors for progression and have outlined when and how treatment should be given.

Although much is known about the complications associated with diabetic retinopathy,[11,12] the underlying pathogenesis is not well understood. It is reported that chronic hyperglycemia is a major pathogenic influence in the formation of diabetic retinopathy, and tight glucose control reduces the risk of retinopathy by 76%.[13] Some researchers feel there may also be an associated genetic factor for the risk of retinopathy.[14,15] That is, specific biochemical mechanisms in some tissues and organs involving glucose are affected by genetic control. Some studies suggest an immunologic association for the development of diabetes in which the HLA antigen is involved.[16] Well-known mechanisms such as the sorbitol pathway have been examined extensively, and it is believed that by altering the enzy-matic reactions of this pathway, the complications of diabetes may be decreased or controlled. The Sorbinil Retinopathy Trial, however, has shown that sorbinil, an aldose reductase inhibitor, has no effect on the outcome of retinopathy.[17] Other mechanisms involved in retinal complications of diabetes may include the nonenzymatic glycosylation of proteins or the effect of glucose on cellular genetic material.[18] Studies also suggest increases in hemoglobin A1c, oxygen level, and microvascular and hematologic changes may contribute to the development of retinopathy.[19]

Histologically, early diabetic retinopathy consists of defects in the tight junctions between capillary endothelial cells, focal thickening of the capillary basement membrane, and hyalinization of the precapillary arterioles. Eventual vessel narrowing decreases blood flow, resulting in tissue hypoxia. Later, loss of endothelial cells and pericytes, vessel occlusion, and capillary bed nonperfusion occurs.[20,21] Hematologic changes that include increased levels of plasma proteins may affect the agglutination of red blood cells in the microcirculation. Platelet aggregation may be increased as well. These factors alone or in combination can lead to partial or complete occlusion of retinal arterioles or capillaries. A summary of these changes and others that occur within the retinal vessels include basement membrane thickening, weakening of the vessel wall resulting in microaneurysm formation, increased permeability, lumen stenosis, loss of capillary circulation, and, finally, formation of new blood vessels (neovascularization) with eventual fibrous formation and traction on the retina.

Microaneurysm formation is one of the earliest clinical findings in diabetic retinopathy. Ophthalmoscopically, microaneurysms appear similar to pinpoint intraretinal hemorrhages. They commonly occur within the posterior pole and may extend into the midperiphery. Histologically, microaneurysms develop as focal capillary out-pouchings that result from loss of vessel wall pericytes. They are commonly located near areas of capillary nonperfusion in the posterior pole but may occur anywhere throughout the retina. Microaneurysms are readily identifiable on fluorescein angiographic studies as pinpoint spots of relatively early hyperfluorescence with late leakage. This leakage, and subsequent increase in hyperfluorescence, results due to the breakdown of the capillary wall and the collection of intraretinal serous fluid around the microaneurysm.

Cotton-wool spots are focal areas of nerve fiber layer infarct caused by the occlusion of adjacent capillaries. Clinically they appear as whitish lesions on the surface of the retina. Their appearance is due to the accumulation of "cytoid" bodies and stasis of axoplasmic flow within individual nerve fibers. Cotton-wool spots appear suddenly but resolve over several weeks. They may indicate the development of significant retinal capillary nonperfusion that may soon lead to neovascular tissue formation; however, they are not as predictive as once thought for the prognosis of diabetic retinopathy.

Intraretinal fluid may accumulate as diabetic retinopathy progresses, with retinal vessel breakdown, occlusion, and leakage of plasma into the interstitial retinal tissue. The resultant edema causes retinal thickening that may be observed with stereoscopic examination. As water and electrolytes are resorbed by the adjacent vascular endothelium and retinal pigment epithelium, intraretinal lipid deposits, referred to as "hard exudates," often remain. These deposits are eventually surrounded by macrophages and resorbed as well. Ophthalmoscopically, exudates appear as whitish-yellow spots with relatively distinct borders. Individual exudative foci may accumulate in a ringlike fashion, present in clusters, or coalesce into large plaquelike lesions. Exudates usually persist for several months before being resorbed. On fluorescein angiographic studies, exudates will block underlying fluorescence thereby causing intraretinal hypofluorescent spots.

Retinal edema is best observed using the slit lamp biomicroscope with a 60-D indirect lens or a fundus contact lens. Fine stereopsis is necessary. Retinal edema may be focal or diffuse and causes the tissue to appear thickened and clear or grayish-white. It is often present surrounding microaneurysms and intraretinal microvascular abnormalities (IRMAs), or in areas of nonperfusion. Fluorescein angiography may demonstrate gradual hyperfluorescence overlying foci of leakage.

Intraretinal microvascular abnormalities develop as a result of vascular remodeling. They commonly appear adjacent to areas of capillary nonperfusion. Intraretinal microvascular abnormalities are small dilated vessels that have a marked number of endothelial cells. Their structural integrity, however, is unlike that of normal retinal vessels in that they lack effective tight junctions. Intraretinal microvascular abnormalities may be difficult to view ophthalmoscopically. They often appear as fine single vessels or as multiple branches or arcades. In some cases, IRMAs may be confused with neovascularization on ophthalmoscopic examination. The differential diagnosis may be aided with fluorescein angiography. In many cases IRMAs will show mild staining adjacent to the vessels on angiographic studies whereas neovascularization will leak profusely.

Venous beading is a retinal finding that typically occurs in patients with more severe nonproliferative diabetic retinopathy. Clinically, venous beading represents localized increases in venous caliber with adjacent constrictions, an appearance likened to sausage links or beads on a string. Similar, but different, clinical features include venous dilation and tortuosity and venous loops. The etiology of venous beading is unclear; however, it is thought to result from retinal ischemia and increased retinal blood flow. Venous beading is useful in determining the progression to proliferative disease and indicates more severe retinal ischemia.

Diabetic macular edema (DME) is the leading cause of decreased visual acuity from diabetic retinopathy. One-half of patients with diabetic macular edema may lose two or more lines of visual acuity within 2 years.[22] Diabetic macular edema is characterized by focal or diffuse retinal thickening in the macula with or without associated exudates (Figure 24-1). Macular edema results from leaking microaneurysms or from other mechanisms such as diffuse vessel leakage or poor pigment epithelial function. Macular edema is usually a chronic process; however, spontaneous resolution occasionally occurs. The Early Treatment Diabetic Retinopathy Study (ETDRS) was designed to evaluate the effects of photocoagulation in patients with persistent macular edema in nonproliferative or early proliferative diabetic retinopathy.[9,10] The ETDRS definition of clinically significant diabetic macular edema (CSDME) is given in Table 24-1. If any eyes are determined to have CSDME, they may benefit from argon laser photocoagulation. Although further visual loss may be prevented with focal photocoagulation, return of visual acuity to normal once macular edema has involved the fovea is not always expected.

The clinical presentations of diabetic retinopathy may range from mild retinal hemorrhages with no impact on visual loss to total blindness from proliferative disease. The ETDRS study has conveniently grouped diabetic retinopathy into two broad categories: nonproliferative and proliferative disease. Nonproliferative disease includes

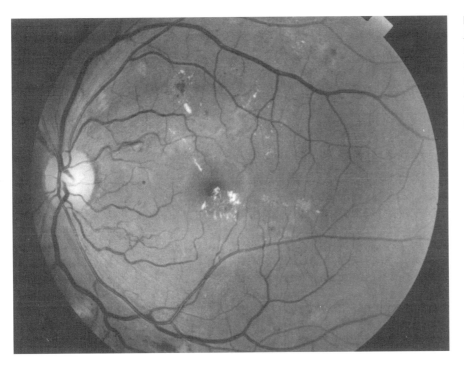

FIGURE 24-1

Nonproliferative diabetic retinopathy and clinically significant macular edema. Although retinal thickening cannot be appreciated in the photograph, hard exudates are noted close to the foveal center.

TABLE 24-1

Clinically Significant Diabetic Macular Edema

Macular edema is considered clinically significant if any of the following is present:
1. Retinal thickening at or within 500 μm (approximately one-third disc diameter) of the center of the macula
2. Hard exudates at or within 500 μm of the foveal center if associated with retinal thickening
3. An area of retinal thickening one disc diameter in size of which any part is within one disc diameter of the center of the macula

Source: Early Treatment Diabetic Retinopathy Study Research Group. Early treatment diabetic retinopathy study design and baseline patient characteristics: ETDRS Report Number 7. Ophthalmology 1991;98:741–56; and Early Treatment Diabetic Retinopathy Research Group. Fundus photographic risk factors for progression of diabetic retinopathy. ETDRS Report Number 12. Ophthalmology 1991;98:823–33.

a number of intraretinal abnormalities, whereas proliferative disease indicates new vessels forming on the surface of the retina. Nonproliferative retinopathy is further classified into stages according to severity (mild, moderate, severe, and very severe disease). This designation helps predict the risk of progression of retinopathy to more serious vision-threatening complications such as neovascularization. Nonproliferative disease includes any or all of the variety of retinal abnormalities described earlier such as intraretinal hemorrhages, IRMAs, and venous beading.

Alternatively, proliferative disease is also classified into non–high-risk and high-risk disease. Proliferative disease is marked by the formation of neovascular blood vessels and fibrous tissue formation on the optic disc, retinal surface, the posterior hyaloid face, the surface of the iris, or within the anterior chamber angle. These frail new vessels can hemorrhage, causing marked reduction in visual acuity, or the fibrous component can lead to tractional retinal detachment. Proliferative retinopathy ranges from "early" to "high-risk" to "advanced disease." Clinically there are four risk factors identified by the DRS as being associated with the increased risk of developing severe visual loss. In order of importance they are the presence of any neovascularization (NV), the presence of neovascularization on or near the optic disc (NVD), the presence of neovascularization elsewhere, and preretinal or vitreous hemorrhage (Table 24-2).

The ETDRS has shown that specific clinical findings are significant for the development of proliferative diabetic retinopathy.[23] From the least significant to the most significant, these include the amount of retinal hemorrhaging, IRMAs, and venous beading, which generally correspond to the level of retinal ischemia. Mild to moderate diabetic retinopathy may consist of one or several mild intraretinal hemorrhages, and/or cotton-wool spots, and/or hard exudates. Moderate to severe disease may consist of these changes as well as mild IRMA and/or venous beading.

TABLE 24-2

*High-Risk Characteristics of Severe Visual Loss
from Diabetic Retinopathy*

1. Retinal neovascularization
2. Neovascularization of the disc greater than one-fourth disc diameter
3. Neovascularization elsewhere if greater than one-fourth disc diameter
4. Vitreous hemorrhage associated with neovascularization

Source: Early Treatment Diabetic Retinopathy Study Research Group. Early treatment diabetic retinopathy study design and baseline patient characteristics: ETDRS Report Number 7. Ophthalmology 1991;98:741–56; and Early Treatment Diabetic Retinopathy Research Group. Fundus photographic risk factors for progression of diabetic retinopathy. ETDRS Report Number 12. Ophthalmology 1991;98:823–33.

TABLE 24-3

Grading of Severe and Very Severe Nonproliferative Diabetic Retinopathy: The ETDRS "4-2-1" Rule

Severe nonproliferative diabetic retinopathy exists if one of the following is present:	Very severe nonproliferative diabetic retinopathy exists if two or more of the following are present:
	Severe retinal hemorrhages in 4 quadrants
	Venous beading in 2 or more quadrants
	Moderately severe IRMA in 1 or more quadrants

Source: Personal communication with RP Murphy, The Retinal Institute of Maryland. Based on a modification of information given in Early Treatment Diabetic Retinopathy Research Group. Fundus photographic risk factors for progression of diabetic retinopathy. ETDRS Report Number 12. Ophthalmology 1991;98:823–33.

To facilitate grading of severe and very severe diabetic retinopathy, the ETDRS 4-2-1 rule has been adopted (Table 24-3). It is important to note the levels of risk of developing neovascularization with this classification system. Eyes with severe nonproliferative retinopathy have a 33% chance within 1 year and 27% chance within 3 years of developing neovascularization. Patients with very severe nonproliferative retinopathy have a 75% chance within 1 year and 83% chance within 3 years of developing neovascularization.

Currently it is theorized that neovascularization results from hypoxic retinal tissue that produces either an angiogenesis factor or a disruption of extracellular modulating factors.[24] As this chemical is released into the eye, proliferation of new blood vessels may occur on the surface of the retina, in the vitreous, on the surface of the iris, or in the angle. Neovascularization in the angle is particularly important as it may lead to neovascular glaucoma.

If three of the four high-risk characteristics for severe visual loss from diabetic retinopathy are noted, panretinal photocoagulation is indicated. The ETDRS has shown the rate of severe visual loss (<5/200) may be reduced by as much as 60% if timely retinal laser photocoagulation is given.[6] It is also important to realize that patients who do not meet three of the four high-risk characteristics may also be treated if there is a history of poor compliance and follow-up, or if the progression of retinopathy indicates that earlier treatment is needed. After photocoagulation, reevaluation is performed in 6–12 weeks to assess the effects of treatment. If further treatment is necessary, the same criteria are used.

Hypertensive Retinopathy

Hypertensive retinopathy is only described briefly here, as it is discussed in Chapter 20. Hypertensive retinopathy has been classified according to the changes seen in the retinal arterioles. Unfortunately, many of the classifications of hypertensive retinopathy include arteriolar-sclerotic changes that may occur in isolated older individuals and serve only to confuse the clinician. The most noted classifications are those described by Keith et al.[25] and Scheie.[26] Hypertension causes a variety of retinal changes. In the early stages, the changes range from subtle arteriolar attenuation and focal narrowing to more pronounced arteriovenous crossing changes. With long-standing cases of hypertension, sclerotic changes in the arteriolar wall are evident, resulting in a broadening of the arteriolar light reflex. In later stages there is further opacity of the vessel wall, creating a "copper wire" or "silver wire" appearance. The arteriolar wall may become completely opacified, yielding a whitened, threadlike appearance.

In the more severe forms of hypertensive retinopathy, microaneurysms, flame-shaped hemorrhages, cotton-wool spots, exudates, and disc edema may occur. These findings result from vascular wall damage and increased permeability. Microaneurysms commonly develop as well.

The clinician must understand there is wide variability of retinal findings in hypertension. Often in the older patient normal arteriosclerotic changes occur and may be mistaken as signs of hypertension. In such cases definitive evaluation is performed through routine blood pressure measurement.

Retinal Vein Occlusion

Retinal vein occlusion is the second most common retinal vascular disorder of the eye. It is a condition that primarily affects elderly persons (mean age 63 years).[27] Retinal venous occlusive disease commonly results from obstruction of venous flow at arteriovenous crossing points.[28] At these crossings both arterioles and venules share a common adventitial sheath. Thickening of the arterial wall may cause compression of the weaker walled vein, producing turbulent blood flow, endothelial cell damage with vessel degeneration, and eventual thrombus formation leading to occlusion. Although this is a viable explanation, the exact pathogenesis of venous occlusive disease is not fully understood. There appears to be an association with systemic conditions such as hypertension, diabetes, cardiovascular disease, chronic obstructive pulmonary disease, and arteriosclerosis.[15,19,29,30] Hypertension and diabetes appear to be the most significant systemic findings in venous occlusive disease.[29] Patients with venous occlusion should therefore undergo evaluation for both of these diseases. Other conditions associated with retinal vein occlusion include hyperviscosity syndromes and elevated intraocular pressure.[31]

Retinal venous occlusive disease may occur as a central retinal vein occlusion (CRVO) or branch retinal vein occlusion (BRVO). Venous occlusive disease is also classified into ischemic (nonperfused) and nonischemic (perfused) types. The ophthalmoscopic findings typically seen in venous occlusion depend on the stage of occlusion. In the earliest stage of venous occlusive disease, a small splinter hemorrhage may be seen adjacent to an area of arteriovenous nicking (Bonnet's sign).[31] As venous occlusion develops further, superficial retinal hemorrhages, retinal edema, and cotton-wool spots may be seen. Hemorrhaging may initially be minimal, later becoming more pronounced. Commonly the venules distal to the occlusion become dilated and tortuous. Collateral vascular channels may develop later in the disease with resolution of the retinal signs. In more serious forms of retinal vein occlusion, significant amounts of retinal capillary nonperfusion may occur, resulting in the development of retinal or iris neovascularization. Retinal neovascularization developing remote from the optic nerve head is commonly located at the junction of perfused and nonperfused retina. Neovascular glaucoma may result from vascular proliferation on the iris and in the anterior chamber angle.

Branch retinal vein occlusion is the most common of the venous occlusive diseases and occurs in the superotemporal quadrant in about two-thirds of all cases.[29,32] Individuals between the ages of 50 and 70 years are most frequently affected, and there is no sex predilection. Branch retinal vein occlusions are characteristically located to one side of the horizontal raphe, with occlusions nearer the optic disc producing more widespread retinal involvement. Macular edema will develop if this area of the retina is drained by the involved vein. Macular edema may be either cystoid or diffuse in nature. A reduction in visual acuity may occur, either permanent or temporary, depending on the severity and duration of fluid in this region. Reduced visual acuity may spontaneously improve with the resolution of associated intraretinal fluid and the development of collateral blood vessels.

Collateral vessels are preexisting blood vessels that become enlarged as they drain blood from the occluded area of the retina. Clinically they appear as tortuous dilated retinal vessels often seen temporal to the macular area and crossing the horizontal raphe. Collateral vessels may also form at the optic disc after branch (or central) retinal vein occlusion (Figure 24-2). These blood vessels are sometimes mistaken for retinal neovascularization.

In about one-half of all branch vein occlusions, there is significant capillary nonperfusion of the retina, and less than one-half of these will develop retinal neovascularization. Neovascularization may occur anywhere from 6 to 12 months after the occlusion, with some cases reported up to 3 years after the initial occlusion.[29] Neovascularization in venous occlusive disease is similar to that seen in diabetic retinopathy and is characterized by poorly structured blood vessels that may cause vitreous hemorrhage, vitreoretinal fibrosis, and occasionally tractional and rhegmatogenous retinal detachments. As in diabetic retinopathy, retinal neovascularization in venous occlusive disease usually develops adjacent to areas of retinal capillary nonperfusion.

The Branch Retinal Vein Occlusion Study Group[33,34] recommended that if visual acuity is reduced immediately following a BRVO, management should involve waiting for the retinal hemorrhaging to clear sufficiently so that useful fluorescein angiography can be performed. If macular edema is reducing the visual acuity to 20/40 or worse without improvement after 6 months, grid photocoagulation is recommended. If capillary nonperfusion involves the macula, then no treatment is available to improve vision.

If a large area of the retina is affected, such as in a hemicentral retinal vein occlusion (HCRVO), management involves waiting for hemorrhage to clear sufficiently so that useful fluorescein angiography can be performed. If more than five disc diameters of retinal nonperfusion are present, the patient should be followed at least every 4 months to determine if neovascularization occurs. Should neovascularization develop, sector panretinal photocoagulation is then performed in the involved area.

Central retinal vein occlusions, although less common than BRVOs, are more severe. Again, central retinal vein occlusion may occur in ischemic or nonischemic forms. The classic hallmarks of an ischemic CRVO include extensive retinal hemorrhaging in all quadrants, venous engorgement and tortuosity, severely reduced visual acuity (<20/400), large areas of retinal capillary nonperfusion,

FIGURE 24-2
Collateral vessels at the optic nerve head in a patient with previous central retinal vein occlusion.

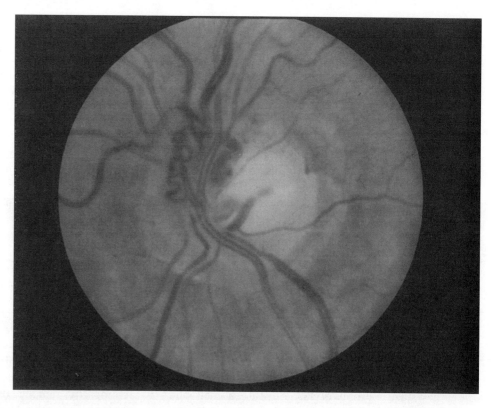

multiple cotton-wool spots, and optic disc edema. Fluorescein angiography demonstrates a prolonged retinal circulation time. The presence of an afferent pupillary defect may be indicative of ischemic disease. Reduction in visual acuity is usually secondary to macular nonperfusion.

Nonischemic retinal vein occlusions are typically characterized by mild to moderate retinal hemorrhaging, a visual acuity of 20/400 or better, and no afferent pupillary defect (Figure 24-3). Reduction in visual acuity is usually attributed to macular edema rather than capillary nonperfusion.

It is important to differentiate between ischemic and nonischemic central retinal vein occlusions. With ischemic CRVOs, 50–75% of patients will develop rubeosis and neovascular glaucoma within 3 months of the event.[29] The clinician must be aware that the onset of neovascular glaucoma can be quite rapid. In some instances it may occur within days to a few weeks after the onset of rubeosis. Patients who develop rubeosis need to be treated with panretinal photocoagulation, cryotherapy, or vitrectomy with endophotocoagulation in an attempt to prevent neovascular glaucoma from occurring or progressing.[29]

Systemic conditions associated with retinal vein occlusions include cardiovascular disease, hypertension, and diabetes. Bilateral venous occlusive disease may be associated with hyperviscosity syndromes. Intraocular pressure may also be a risk factor in the development of venous occlusive disease.

Important in the differential diagnosis of retinal vein occlusion is venous stasis retinopathy, which occurs as a manifestation of the ocular ischemic syndrome. In such cases patients exhibit a reduced central retinal artery pressure leading to retinal hypoperfusion. The underlying cause is typically atherosclerotic carotid artery occlusive disease. Classically, the retinal hemorrhaging associated with this condition is located mostly in the midperiphery, unlike a CRVO, which exhibits hemorrhage scattered throughout the fundus. Variable presentations do exist with venous stasis retinopathy, however.

Retinal Arterial Occlusion

Retinal arterial occlusions result from emboli or thrombosis of the affected vessels. Ophthalmoscopically, the retinal tissue becomes white and edematous from infarction. Onset is sudden and in some cases emboli may be seen proximally within the arterioles. There are three common types of emboli associated with arteriole occlusions. Most are typically seen lodged at the arterial bifurcations.

The most common emboli are cholesterol crystals (Hollenhorst plaques), which arise from the aortic arch or

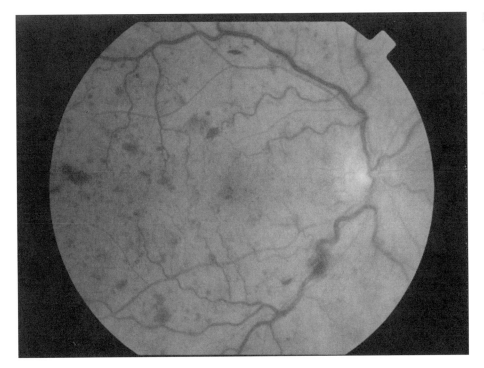

FIGURE 24-3
Central retinal vein occlusion. Note the widespread retinal hemorrhaging and tortuosity of the retinal vessels. Cotton-wool spots and disc edema are not evident in this patient.

more commonly the carotid arteries.[35] These emboli appear as bright orange to yellow and are highly refractile. Because they are very thin, they seldom occlude the blood vessels in which they are found. Cholesterol emboli may be seen for several days to weeks after an occlusive event.

Platelet-fibrin emboli arise from large vessel atherosclerosis. They are uncommon and are rarely seen within the vessels because they have the tendency to disintegrate and flow further distally within the retinal vasculature. These emboli appear dull gray to white in color and completely occlude the lumen of the blood vessel. Multiple emboli may be observed within the same arteriole. The blood column distal to the emboli appears severely attenuated or may be absent. Fragmentation of these emboli may occur, thereby allowing them to move more distally through the arteriole. Should these emboli remain lodged within the arteriole for a significant period of time, retinal infarction will occur.

Calcific emboli are small, irregular, opaque, and grayish white to yellow in color. They are less refractile than cholesterol emboli and produce high-grade retinal arteriolar occlusions. These emboli commonly arise from diseased cardiac valves or the aortic arch.

Branch retinal artery occlusions (BRAOs) may be symptomatic or asymptomatic depending on their location. The retinal tissue distal to the site of occlusion appears white and edematous. Nonfilling of the involved arterioles is apparent with fluorescein angiography (Figure 24-4). With time, however, the edema resolves and recanalization of the arterioles occurs. Permanent visual field defects develop corresponding to the area of retinal infarct. Unfortunately, specific treatment for branch retinal artery occlusion is not available except for ocular massage, which uncommonly may dislodge the emboli and cause them to move further distally. This may only be successful within the first 90 minutes of occlusion.[36]

Central retinal artery occlusions (CRAOs) are considered an ocular emergency. They produce a sudden painless loss of vision in the affected eye. The entire retina becomes pale and edematous with a central "cherry-red spot" in the macula. Similar to the occlusion site in BRAOs, the central retinal artery will eventually recanalize with resolution of the retinal edema. Several weeks after the event the retinal tissue appears normal with the exception of attenuated arterioles and optic atrophy. Arteriolar sheathing may be evident. If the patient is fortunate enough to have a cilioretinal artery supplying the fovea, visual acuity may be spared. There will, however, be severe constriction of the visual field.

Treatment for CRAO has very limited effectiveness, and if instituted, must begin within 90 minutes of the event.[36] Measures include ocular massage, reduction of intraocular pressure with topical antiglaucoma agents, oral acetazolamide, aspirin, and even anterior chamber paracentesis. The actual relative effectiveness of any one or a combination of these modalities in restoring retinal circulation is not known.

FIGURE 24-4
Fluorescein angiogram demonstrating a branch retinal artery occlusion. The superotemporal branch arteriole does not fill during the arteriovenous phase. (Courtesy of Peter A. Russo, O.D.)

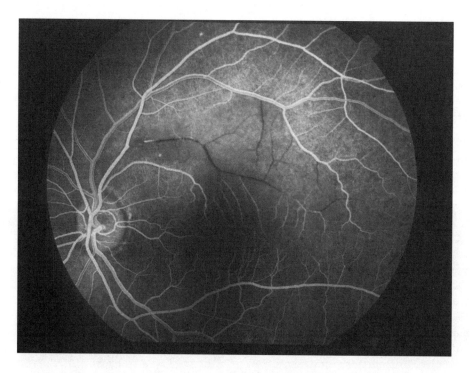

Causative conditions to be considered in arterial occlusive disease include migrainous phenomena, carotid artery disease, cardiac disease, trauma, sickle cell disease, connective tissue disorders, and infections.[37] In addition, giant cell arteritis must strongly be considered in elderly patients.

Ocular Ischemic Syndrome

Ocular ischemic syndrome (ischemic oculopathy) is typically a manifestation of atherosclerotic carotid artery disease. It usually occurs in patients 50–90 years of age (mean 65 years).[37,38] Clinically, the disease may be characterized by episcleral vascular congestion, corneal edema, uveitis, retinal hemorrhages, retinal and iris neovascularization, and cataract formation. The retinal hemorrhages typically appear as round splotchy patches in the midperipheral retina that may also extend to the posterior pole. The fundus appearance may be confused with central retinal vein occlusion. As mentioned in an earlier section, the perfusion pressure of the central retinal artery is reduced in the ocular ischemic syndrome, whereas the arterial pressure is normal in a CRVO. Ophthalmodynamometry may be useful in determining reduced central retinal artery pressure. In pronounced cases, mild digital pressure to the globe may be sufficient to demonstrate abnormal arterial pulsations that occur secondary to reduced arterial flow.

Patients with ocular ischemic syndrome may report a decrease in visual acuity, amaurosis fugax (may be light-induced), and ocular pain. The differential diagnosis includes diabetes, CRVO, polyarteritis nodosa, temporal arteritis, atherosclerosis, and hyperviscosity states.[38,39] Patients exhibiting the ocular ischemic syndrome should be evaluated for carotid occlusive disease, cardiac disease, and blood dyscrasias. Treatment includes panretinal photocoagulation, aspirin therapy, antiglaucoma therapy, and carotid endarterectomy.

Retinopathy of Prematurity

Retinopathy of prematurity (ROP), previously referred to as retrolental fibroplasia, may occur in premature (<36 weeks' gestation) and low-birth-weight infants (<2000 g) who are given supplemental oxygen.[40] With the increase in oxygen levels a vaso-occlusive effect occurs in the immature retinal vasculature. This effect leads to an ischemic retinopathy that is most pronounced in the temporal peripheral retina. The pathogenesis of the disease is not fully understood, however. Retinopathy of prematurity has also been reported in full-term infants and infants who did not receive oxygen therapy. Retinopathy of prematurity is classified according to location, extent, and severity.

Clinically, some regions of the retina may exhibit a translucent vascularized tissue that blends into a grayish nonvascularized tissue more anteriorly. Between these areas lies a well-demarcated zone that may become elevated into a ridge and develop a pinkish coloration. The more peripheral in the retina this zone is located, the better the prognosis.[41] This ridge of blood vessels may gradually involute on their own, or new blood vessels may develop that extend into the vitreous. In severe cases, vitreous hemorrhage may develop as well as rhegmatogenous, exudative, or tractional retinal detachment. Because of tractional effects within the retinal periphery, temporal dragging of the disc with situs inversus and displacement of the macula may occur. Patients with ROP commonly exhibit high myopia, strabismus, and amblyopia.

Management includes monitoring intra-arterial oxygen levels in high-risk infants. Supplemental vitamin E may be helpful during the course of oxygen therapy. High-risk infants should be evaluated between 4 and 8 weeks of age depending on their birth weight.[42] The Cryotherapy for Retinopathy of Prematurity Study (CRYO-ROP) has found that cryoablation of the residual avascular retina significantly decreases the incidence of blindness.[43]

Sickle Cell Retinopathy

Of all the forms of sickling disease, the most important with respect to ocular complications are sickle cell disease (SS), hemoglobin SC disease (SC), and sickle cell thalassemia disease (S-thal). The ocular complications are caused by the intravascular sickled cells, hemolysis, hemostasis, and thrombosis. Most clinical findings are seen in the peripheral retina. Sickle cell retinopathy may appear as nonproliferative or proliferative disease. Nonproliferative retinal findings include intraretinal refractile spots, black "sunburst" lesions consisting of retinal pigment epithelial hypertrophy and hyperplasia, and salmon patch intraretinal and subretinal hemorrhages. These findings occur at the junction of perfused and nonperfused areas of the retina. Other ocular findings include comma-shaped conjunctival capillaries, angioid streaks, branch or central retinal artery or vein occlusions, optic nerve infarction, and pseudoangiomas of the retina.

Ocular findings in proliferative sickle retinopathy have been classified according to the retinal changes that occur.[44] These include arterial occlusions (stage 1), arteriovenous anastomosis (stage 2), neovascularization or "sea fans" (stage 3, Color Plate 24-I), vitreous or preretinal hemorrhage (stage 4), and tractional retinal detachment (stage 5). Treatment includes diathermy, cryopexy, and laser photocoagulation.

Parafoveal Telangiectasis

Parafoveal telangiectasis may be congenital or acquired with an unknown etiology. Patients with the disease have mild blurring of vision caused by a leakage of fluid from juxtafoveal telangiectatic retinal capillaries that are usually present temporally. The structural abnor-

malities in this disease are similar to diabetic retinopathy.[45] Males are typically affected in congenital cases that exhibit a unilateral presentation.[46] Fluorescein angiography is useful in demonstrating the telangiectatic vessels as well as associated fluid leakage resulting in macular edema.

Idiopathic, acquired telangiectasis may be unilateral or bilateral. Patients are typically affected in the fifth or sixth decades. As in the congenital form, the telangiectatic vessels usually occur in the temporal parafoveal region. These patients may experience slow, progressive loss of vision over years due to fluid exudation from the vessels. Atrophy of the retinal pigment epithelium may occur, and in some cases a choroidal neovascular membrane may develop with an acute loss of vision. In some cases photocoagulation may be helpful in preventing further loss of visual acuity.[45]

Retinal Macroaneurysm

Retinal macroaneurysms are associated with hypertension and arteriosclerosis. Affected individuals are most commonly women in their sixth or seventh decade.[47] Retinal macroaneurysms usually occur unilaterally as a single, large, round aneurysm in a major branch retinal arteriole, usually at a bifurcation or arteriovenous crossing. They are commonly located along the temporal arcades. Approximately 50% of patients will have retinal hemorrhage surrounding the macroaneurysm.[47] There may also be a circinate pattern of intraretinal exudates and associated capillary dilatation around the lesions. Most commonly, macroaneuryms involute spontaneously without visual acuity loss; however, in some cases they may cause vitreous, preretinal, or subretinal hemorrhage, macular edema, serous retinal detachments, and vascular occlusions.[47] Macroaneurysms may require photocoagulation, especially when macular function is threatened.

Eales Disease

Eales disease is characterized by vasculitis with retinal neovascularization developing in areas of peripheral retinal vascular occlusion. Men in the third and fourth decades of life are most commonly affected. Involvement is bilateral. The etiology remains unknown. Loss of visual acuity may occur from vitreous hemorrhage or cystoid macular edema. On fluorescein angiography the appearance may be similar to that of sickle cell retinopathy. There may be an association with tuberculosis. This disease should be differentiated from collagen vascular disease, sarcoidosis, temporal arteritis, polyarteritis, systemic lupus erythematosus, Behçet's disease, acquired immunodeficiency syndrome (AIDS), toxoplasmosis, cytomegalovirus, herpes zoster, syphilis, and multiple sclerosis.[48]

MACULAR DISORDERS

Age-Related Macular Degeneration

Age-related macular degeneration (ARMD) is a common retinal disorder that is the leading cause of legal blindness in patients over age 60 years.[49] It affects the central macular area, producing a central scotoma that may severely limit a patient's ability to read or drive. The etiology of the disease remains unknown; however, several risk factors have been identified. These include age, sex, blood pressure, hyperopia, pigmentation of the iris, familial history, and ultraviolet light exposure.[50] The risk is greatest in patients over age 75 who have light irides.

Age-related macular degeneration produces a variety of clinical findings involving the choriocapillaris, Bruch's membrane, retinal pigment epithelium, and outer retinal layers of the macula. The primary lesion appears to be in the retinal pigment epithelial cell layer. Initially, retinal pigment epithelial changes include a loss of pigment granules and the accumulation of lipofuscin and residual by-products of phagocytosis. In addition, exophytic deposits accumulate between the retinal pigment epithelium and its basement membrane. Hyaline deposits (drusen) occur on Bruch's membrane. Bruch's membrane eventually thickens and becomes calcified, and breaks may develop in the layer with subsequent choroidal neovascular invasion into the sub-RPE space.

Drusen, the most common finding in ARMD, may appear clinically in several forms, including hard, diffuse, soft confluent, and calcific drusen.[51] Hard drusen are extrusions of RPE cell debris onto Bruch's membrane. They appear as small, well-demarcated, round, yellowish deposits deep within the retina. Diffuse drusen consist of basal laminar deposits and diffusely thickened Bruch's membrane. Because of its fine microscopic features, this form of drusen cannot be seen ophthalmoscopically or with fluorescein angiography. Clinically, soft drusen are much larger than hard drusen and have poorly defined borders. They may be confluent and a significant amount of pigmentary disturbance is commonly found, including RPE dropout and hypertrophy. Soft confluent drusen are associated with a higher risk of exudative macular detachments and choroidal neovascular membrane formation.[49] Calcific drusen may appear individually or in combination with other drusen types. They appear as glistening yellowish patches at or below the level of the RPE.

Visual loss in ARMD occurs from either geographic atrophy of the outer retinal layers or development of subretinal choroidal neovascularization. Geographic chorioretinal atrophy is present in about 90% of patients with ARMD; however, it accounts for only 10% of the cases with severe vision loss (20/200 or worse).[52,53] This is because extrafoveal areas are usually involved. When geographic atrophy is bilateral, symmetric, and involving the central macula, it may be confused with disorders such as Best's disease or central areolar choroidal dystrophy.

The exudative form of ARMD is seen in 10% of patients with the disease but accounts for up to 90% of cases with severe vision loss ($\leq$20/200).[51,54] In this situation, loss of visual acuity results from the development of a subretinal choroidal neovascular membrane (CNVM) either adjacent to or under the fovea. Classic CNVMs appear clinically as round to oval greenish-gray areas below the level of the RPE. There may be sub-RPE accumulation of lipids or blood with an associated pigment epithelial detachment. The clinician must always seriously consider the development of a CNVM in any patient who exhibits risk factors and reports a sudden loss, distortion, or blurring of central vision. In such cases fluorescein angiography may be indicated to evaluate for a CNVM (Figure 24-5).

Treatment for ARMD varies depending on the presentation and the visualization and location of any associated CNVM. The treatment of CNVMs is based on the results of the Macular Photocoagulation Study (MPS).[55–57] This randomized clinical trial has shown that argon laser photocoagulation is effective in treating angiographically well-defined CNVMs located at least 200 μm away from the center of the foveal avascular zone. The results of this study initially did not apply to poorly defined CNVMs, those closer than 200 μm, or those membranes beneath the fovea. However, the MPS has recently shown that subfoveal membranes or those closer than 200 μm may also benefit from argon laser photocoagulation.[58] In such cases it is understood that direct treatment to the fovea will result in immediate visual loss; however, over the course of time, better acuity will result than if the membrane were left untreated. Aside from photocoagulation, there is evidence that surgical removal of fresh subfoveal CNVMs may prove beneficial in the preservation of vision in these patients.[59,60]

The rate of recurrence of CNVMs is high in patients with ARMD, and treated patients should therefore be monitored closely for new and inadequately treated membranes. In patients with geographic atrophy, no effective treatment has been found. However, patients with this and other forms of ARMD may benefit from low vision devices. The Age Related Eye Disease Study (AREDS), a large long-term, randomized multicenter prospective study, is currently under way to evaluate whether anti-

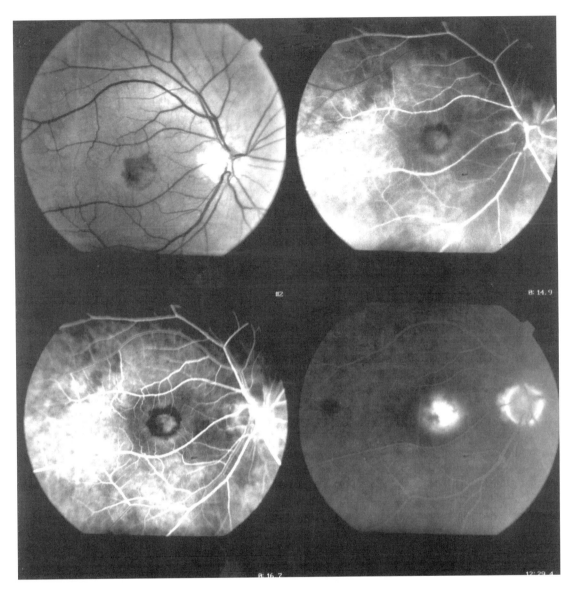

FIGURE 24-5

Subretinal choroidal neovascular membrane associated with age-related macular degeneration. Top left: Black-and-white photograph showing evidence of subretinal and intraretinal hemorrhage within the macular region. Top right and bottom left: Arteriovenous phases of a fluorescein angiogram demonstrate early hyperfluorescence of the neovascular membrane. Bottom right: Late phase of the fluorescein angiogram shows intense hyperfluorescence caused by leakage of dye from the neovascular membrane.

oxidants such as vitamins and minerals may have an effect of slowing or halting the progression of macular degeneration and cataracts.[61]

Angioid Streaks

Angioid streaks may be associated with a number of systemic conditions including pseudoxanthoma elasticum,

Paget's disease of the bone, and sickle cell anemia. Other reported conditions include hyperphosphatemia, Ehlers-Danlos syndrome, lead poisoning, trauma, pituitary disorders, and intracranial disorders.[62] The etiology of angioid streaks, however, is unknown. Histologic studies have shown calcification and thickening within Bruch's membrane, which makes it more brittle. This can lead to irregular breaks in Bruch's, degeneration of both the choriocapillaris and RPE,

FIGURE 24-6
Subtle presentation of angioid streaks. Note the small, radial, spokelike lesions emanating from the peripapillary tissue at the 3 o'clock and 5 o'clock positions (arrows). A mottling of the fundus background, referred to as a "peau d'orange" appearance, is evident.

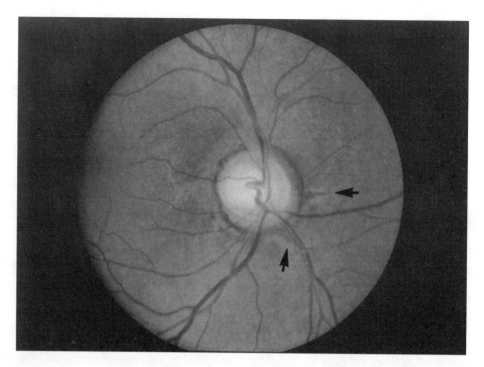

and eventual fibrovascular proliferation. Serous and hemorrhagic retinal detachments may also occur.

Clinically, angioid streaks appear as reddish-brown or gray irregular spokes radiating out from the optic nerve. In lightly pigmented individuals these streaks may be orangish or reddish in color. In some patients a mottling of the RPE in the fundus background (peau d'orange appearance) may be seen (Figure 24-6). Angioid streaks may vary in number, length, and width and are commonly seen bilaterally. On fluorescein angiography, hyperfluorescence and late staining may be found in areas of RPE thinning. Characteristic leakage and fluorescence may be demonstrated if subretinal neovascularization is present. In such cases laser photocoagulation may prevent visual loss. When angioid streaks are seen clinically, medical and dermatologic consultation can be helpful.

Choroidal Rupture

Choroidal ruptures occur from blunt trauma to the globe causing a disruption in the choriocapillaris and Bruch's membrane. In some cases a complete tear through to the sclera may be seen. Choroidal ruptures are commonly seen in the posterior pole away from the site of impact to the globe in a configuration concentric to the optic disc (Figure 24-7). Clinically, fresh choroidal ruptures appear as white to yellow-red, crescent-shaped lesions with associated retinal hemorrhage and edema. Typi-

cally, they range from one to five disc diameters in length and one-third to one-fifth of a disc diameter in width.[63] Commonly, ruptures occur singly, but up to 25% of eyes may have multiple ruptures.[64] Many choroidal ruptures are located temporal to the optic disc. Acuity loss may result from direct involvement of the macula by a rupture, causing destruction of overlying retinal tissue, or from complications associated with the development of secondary choroidal subretinal neovascularization.

Stargardt's Disease (Fundus Flavimaculatus)

Stargardt's disease and fundus flavimaculatus are described by many as variants of the same disorder.[46] It is a bilateral, symmetric, hereditary condition that most commonly occurs in the first or second decade of life (6–20 years), although some patients have been reported to be affected in midlife. The disease is characterized by a progressive loss of visual acuity caused by an excess of lipofuscin within the RPE. Initially there may be a disproportionate vision loss relative to the fundus appearance. There are autosomal dominant and recessive pedigrees, with recessive being the most common.[65] The natural history of the disease is variable, with some patients demonstrating relatively early severe visual loss, whereas others retain good vision for long periods of time.

Clinically, the disease may begin with an annular area of yellow flecks within the macular region. The flecks vary

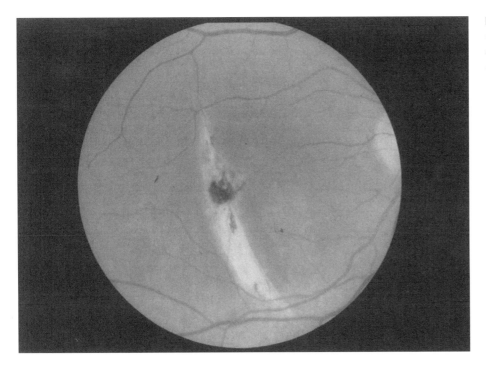

FIGURE 24-7
Crescent-shaped traumatic choroidal rupture located temporal to the macula.

in size and shape and may be confused with drusen. They may extend into the midperiphery where a more pisciform (fishtail-like) shape is exhibited. With time these lesions may fade and change in color from yellow to gray. Later the macula may take on a beaten bronze appearance or become atrophic. Visual acuity generally ranges from 20/30 to about 20/100. In the later stages of the disease, the macular appearance can be similar to that of cone-rod dystrophy.

Clinical testing should include an electro-oculogram, electroretinogram, and fluorescein angiography. The results of the electro-oculogram and electroretinogram are usually normal in the initial phases but may become subnormal as the disease progresses.[46] Both tests are helpful in distinguishing the disease from cone and rod dystrophies. Fluorescein angiography may demonstrate hypofluorescence in the macula and a lack of overall choroidal fluorescence ("dark" or "silent choroid" sign, Figure 24-8). There may also be areas of focal hypofluorescence and hyperfluorescence in the area of retinal flecks.

Currently, there is no effective medical therapy for Stargardt's disease. Management is generally limited to patient counseling and low vision therapy. In particular, genetic counseling should be provided.

Cone Dystrophies

Cone dystrophies are a group of inherited disorders primarily affecting the cones within the photoreceptor layer.

Generally these diseases are characterized by progressive bilateral loss of vision, poor color vision, and photophobia. All three inheritance patterns have been noted in the cone dystrophies with multiple genetic forms possible. Initial manifestations of cone dystrophies typically occur early in life (first or second decade) but may manifest themselves at any time from infancy to adulthood.

Clinically, there may be a relatively normal appearing fundus in the early stages of the disease, even though color vision and Snellen acuity may be reduced. Later, pronounced atrophy of the RPE with some pigmentary clumping may occur. Classically, macular lesions acquire a "beaten bronze" appearance and demonstrate a "bull's-eye" pattern. Temporal optic atrophy may be mild or pronounced. Visual acuities can vary from 20/20 early on to about 20/200 later in the disease.[46] Fluorescein angiography shows hypofluorescence in areas where the RPE is attenuated without late staining or leakage. The ERG shows a reduced or nondetectable photopic response as well as an abnormal flicker response.[65] Some patients develop an acquired nystagmus. Management of patients with cone dystrophies includes dark tinted glasses, miotics, low vision devices, and genetic counseling.

Vitelliform Dystrophy (Best's Disease)

Best's disease is an inherited autosomal dominant disease affecting the RPE within the macula. It is well known for

FIGURE 24-8
Fluorescein angiogram demonstrating the "dark choroid" sign found in Stargardt's disease. Note the lack of background choroidal fluorescence during the arteriovenous phase of the angiogram. Hyperfluorescent spots in the macula correspond to areas of RPE dropout within the macular lesion. (Courtesy of Sara L. Penner, O.D.)

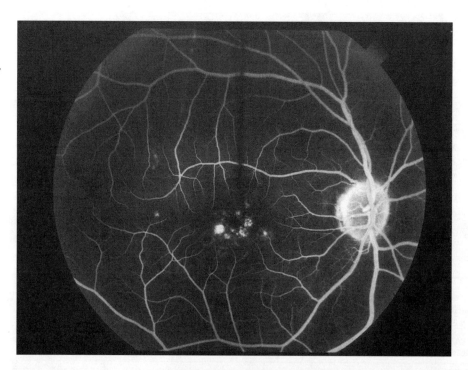

its "egg yolk" appearance early in the disease. Onset may occur in infancy or early childhood. Visual acuities in the early stages of the disease range from about 20/30 to 20/60 and are often much better than expected relative to the appearance of the fundus.[46] Progression of the disease is slow, and asymmetry between the eyes can be exhibited.

Clinically, the vitelliform lesion appears as a yellow fluid-filled cyst in the macula in the early stages of the disease. Later there is disruption of the lesion with RPE changes (Figure 24-9). Eventually the yellow material may resolve, leaving an area of atrophic RPE. In some patients there is development of subretinal fibrosis or occult choroidal neovascular membrane.[66-68] The ERG and dark adaptation are normal, whereas the EOG is markedly abnormal. Carriers of the disease may have subnormal EOGs.

Management of these patients includes evaluation for choroidal neovascular membranes with Amsler grid monitoring and angiography when indicated. Genetic counseling and low vision devices may also be helpful.

Dominant Drusen

As the name implies, dominant drusen is an autosomal dominant form of drusen that occurs at an earlier age than other usual forms of drusen. Onset is typically around the third decade but may not become pronounced until 10–20 years later.[69]

Early in the condition, drusen appear as small, round yellow dots at the level of the RPE in the posterior pole.

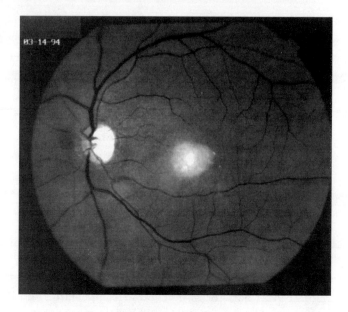

FIGURE 24-9
Late-stage atrophic macular lesion associated with vitelliform dystrophy (Best's disease).

They are usually bilaterally symmetric and can change in size and shape. Patients are generally asymptomatic in early stages. Over many years the drusen increase in number and coalesce, some eventually become calcified, and associated pigment clumping and atrophy of the RPE may occur. As the drusenoid changes progress, macular atrophy and scarring can develop with a corresponding loss of acuity.[70] Retinal edema, subretinal neovascularization, and hemorrhage may develop in some cases similar to that which occurs with age-related macular degeneration.

The EOG is usually abnormal whereas the ERG is normal or only mildly abnormal.[65] Fluorescein angiography shows transmission defects in the area of the drusen and occasional late staining. Except for cases that develop associated subretinal neovascularization, there is no treatment for the condition. Those patients with subretinal neovascular membranes may sometimes be treated with laser photocoagulation.

Myopic Degeneration

Pathologic myopia is characterized by a progressive elongation of the eye. There is general stretching and attenuation of the scleral, choroidal, and retinal layers. It is unknown whether the expansion of the eye is a result of a biomechanical response to normal intraocular pressure or is a result of some genetically determined condition.[71,72] Clinically, fundus changes may consist of peripapillary atrophy, posterior staphyloma, geographic atrophy, and disruptions in Bruch's membrane called lacquer cracks. Subretinal neovascularization is a relatively common complication causing variable visual loss depending on its location. In patients with myopic degeneration, subretinal neovascular membranes commonly exhibit a dark pigmentation overlying the lesion. This has been referred to as a Fuchs' spot (Foerster-Fuchs' spot) and is probably related to pigment epithelial hypertrophy secondary to inherent changes specific to the highly myopic fundus.

Eyes with posterior staphylomas (an outward bowing of the wall of the globe) should be examined carefully, as they may develop small retinal breaks near the fovea. These breaks may eventually lead to retinal detachment. Patients with myopic degeneration who have questionable lesions resembling choroidal neovascular membranes should be evaluated with fluorescein angiography. Eyes with extrafoveal membranes may be treated with laser photocoagulation to help prevent serious loss of vision.

Pattern Dystrophies

Pattern dystrophies are typically seen in middle-aged patients. They are characterized by various yellow, orange, or gray pigment deposits in the macular area. A bilateral, relatively symmetric presentation is typically found. An autosomal dominant inheritance mode of transmission usually occurs.[46] Visual acuity is only mildly affected until late in adult life. The findings on electroretinograms are usually normal.[73,74]

Gass[46] described four types of dystrophies: adult-onset foveomacular vitelliform dystrophy, butterfly-shaped pigment dystrophy, reticular dystrophy of the RPE, and coarse mottling of the macula. Some believe that at least some of these dystrophies are simply variations of the same disorder.

Central Areolar Choroidal Dystrophy

Central areolar choroidal dystrophy initially appears as fine mottled loss of pigmentation in the macular area. The early stages of this dystrophy usually develop in late childhood or early adulthood. Initially, patients usually have normal acuities, visual fields, ERGs, and dark adaptation. The EOG may be subnormal, however. Later, in the fourth and fifth decade, there is a slow reduction of visual acuity. This is associated with the development of round to oval areas of geographic atrophy that may be three to four disc diameters in size. Serous or hemorrhagic retinal detachments have been reported but are rare.[75-77] Late in life the visual acuity drops to about 20/200.

Early in the disease, fluorescein angiography may show mild pigment changes in the macular area with a bull's-eye configuration. Later, prominent transmission defects occur due to atrophy of the RPE. A corresponding loss of the choriocapillaris is demonstrated.

Central Serous Retinopathy

Central serous retinopathy is characterized by a serous detachment of the sensory retina, frequently involving the macula. This condition typically affects patients between 30 and 50 years of age with men being affected more often than women.[46] It is usually a self-limiting disorder, resolving spontaneously with almost complete recovery of visual acuity within 1–6 months. The condition may recur in up to 50% of all affected eyes. The etiology of the condition is not well understood. Some investigators feel stress, pregnancy, renal disease, organ transplantation, and a host of other conditions may play a role.[78]

Clinically, there is a dimness and blurring of vision with acuity reduction ranging from 20/20 to 20/200 (average 20/30). There may be a hyperopic refractive shift, metamorphopsia or micropsia on Amsler grid testing, color desaturation, and a relative central or paracentral visual field defect. On fundus examination there is typically an elevated dome of sensory retinal detachment without evidence of hemorrhage, vitritis, or iritis. Fluorescein angiography typically demonstrates a small focal hyperfluorescent leak in the RPE with percolation and accumulation of dye into the subsensory retinal space

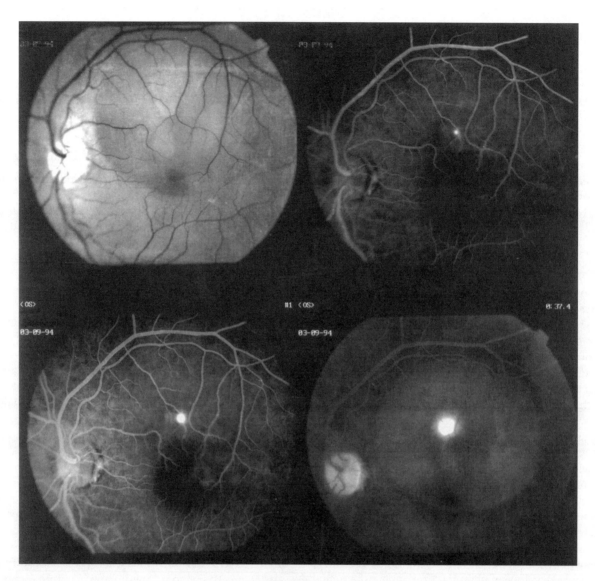

FIGURE 24-10
Central serous chorioretinopathy. Top left: Black-and-white photograph demonstrating dome-shaped eleva-
tion of the sensory retina. Top right and bottom left: Fluorescein angiograms (arteriovenous phase) showing a
hyperfluorescent spot, which denotes the location of the RPE defect that has allowed serous fluid to collect in
the subsensory retinal space. Bottom right: Late-phase fluorescein angiogram illustrating the accumulation of
dye within the subsensory retinal space corresponding to the zone of sensory retinal detachment.

corresponding to the area of detachment (Figure 24-10).
During the initial pooling of dye beneath the sensory retina, this leakage often creates a classic "smokestack"
appearance. After several minutes, the dye becomes diffusely distributed.

Many cases of central serous retinopathy are simply
monitored, as the condition is usually self-limiting. Laser
photocoagulation may be indicated for some patients, since

the procedure possibly may decrease the duration of acute
disease as well as lessen the incidence of recurrence.[79]

Macular Holes

Macular holes may occur from a variety of pathologic
processes including diabetic retinopathy, venous occlusive disease, trauma, myopic fundus degeneration, epireti-

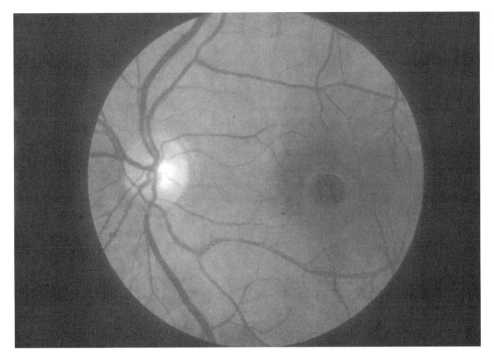

FIGURE 24-11
*Full-thickness macular hole. A
small flap of tissue is present at
the inferior border of the hole.
(Courtesy of Pamela Boyce,
O.D., and Iris Matsukado, O.D.)*

nal membrane formation, and vitreous contraction.[80-82] They most commonly occur in women in the sixth to eighth decade of life.[83] Up to 22–30% of macular holes may be bilateral.[81] Visual acuity in the affected eye usually drops to about 20/200, but some cases may remain relatively good at 20/50. Idiopathic macular holes may be caused by prefoveal vitreous cortex contraction.[84] Other holes may develop at the time of posterior vitreous detachment.

Gass[46,83,85] outlined the stages of macular hole development. He reported the earliest sign of macular hole formation as foveolar detachment (stage 1). This occurs from contraction of the prefoveal vitreous cortex without vitreoretinal separation. There may be formation of a yellow spot or ring in the center of the fovea. There is usually a decrease in visual acuity with metamorphopsia. This may resolve or progress to stage 2, which is characterized by a small, early macular hole. In this stage the yellow ring enlarges over several weeks to months with full-thickness retinal dehiscence of the foveal sensory retina. In stage 3 (3–6 months) there is a fully developed macular hole with vitreofoveal separation. Visual acuity ranges from 20/70 to 20/400 with hole formation that is approximately 500 μm in diameter. In stage 4 there is complete posterior vitreous detachment from the macula and optic nerve. There is usually a free operculum on the posterior hyaloid membrane.

Clinically, macular holes appear round and are characterized by loss of the sensory retinal tissue (Figure 24-

11). There may be a small cuff of subsensory retinal fluid surrounding the hole. Commonly, multiple, small yellowish deposits are present in the base of the hole.

High-risk characteristics for macular hole formation in the fellow eye include macular cyst with a visual acuity of 20/50 or worse, cystic retinal or pigment epithelial changes, involutional macular thinning, metamorphopsia, and low sensory detachment at the center of the macula.[86]

Rhegmatogenous retinal detachment rarely occurs secondary to macular hole formation; therefore surgical intervention such as prophylactic laser photocoagulation is rarely performed. Laser photocoagulation to limit the ring of subretinal fluid surrounding macular holes has been suggested to improve vision, but this is also rarely done.[87] Vitrectomy is occasionally carried out to help prevent complete hole formation in the fellow eyes of some patients with a unilateral macular hole who are likely to develop bilateral disease. Success in resealing holes combining vitrectomy and the use of transforming growth factor-beta (TGF-β) has been reported.[88]

Epiretinal Membrane

Epiretinal membranes are translucent fibrocellular tissue layers that develop on the inner surface of the retina. These membranes develop as a result of a variety of pathologic conditions or they may develop spontaneously. They can be associated with venous occlusive disease, diabetic retinopathy, uveitis, trauma, and intraocular surgery.[89] They also commonly occur after posterior vitreous detachments.

Histologically, epiretinal membranes are composed primarily of glial cells but may also contain myofibroblasts, fibrocytes, or RPE cells.[90] These cells proliferate on the surface of the retina and may subsequently contract, producing retinal surface wrinkling and distortion of vision.

Idiopathic epiretinal membranes typically occur in adults over 50 years of age. They are bilateral in approximately 20% of patients. Visual acuity may be affected but usually is not worse than 20/40.[83] Occasionally vision may drop to 20/100 or worse. In such cases a vitrectomy with membrane peeling can be helpful in restoring vision.

Ophthalmoscopically, epiretinal membranes appear as a glistening reflective sheet of tissue on the surface of the retina. Retinal blood vessels may appear dragged or distorted in many instances, corresponding to membrane contraction. Fine retinal folds are commonly present, causing marked metamorphopsia and decrease in visual acuity when they involve the central macula. Cystoid macular edema, retinal hemorrhages, exudates, serous detachment of the retina, and retinal holes or breaks may develop.

Macular Edema

Macular edema occurs when there is an intraretinal accumulation of fluid. Commonly associated with the development of macular edema is diabetes, hypertension, retinal vein occlusion, surgery, infection, inflammation, photocoagulation, as well as any other condition causing a breakdown of the blood-retinal barrier. Primary, idiopathic macular edema is very uncommon. Macular edema can present as a diffuse fluid accumulation or in a cystic pattern. Clinically, edema in the macula is best observed stereoscopically with either a fundus contact lens or an indirect biomicroscope lens to detect subtle thickening or frank elevation of the sensory retina. Fluorescein angiography, by demonstrating gradual hyperfluorescence corresponding to the pooling of dye in involved areas, is much more helpful in clearly delineating fluid accumulation. Cystoid macular edema exhibits a classic petaloid pattern on angiography secondary to dye accumulation within individual cystic spaces in the perifoveal tissue.

INFECTIOUS DISEASES

Toxoplasmosis

Toxoplasmosis is caused by the protozoan *Toxoplasma gondii,* a parasite in which the cat is the definitive host.[91]

The organisms, which are shed in cat feces, may remain viable as sporocysts in soil for months or years. After ingestion by humans or through transplacental transmission, the *Toxoplasma* organisms multiply intracellularly, then become encysted by the host's immune system. Encysted organisms may be found in the brain, heart, and skeletal muscle. Once encysted, the organism may remain viable throughout the life of the host. Should the immune system become depressed, there may be reactivation and dissemination of the parasites. Clinical manifestations range from asymptomatic presentation to a fulminant infection that may become fatal. Toxoplasmosis is the most common cause of necrotizing retinitis and posterior uveitis in humans.[92] The disease has also been reported as an initial manifestation of AIDS.[93] In AIDS patients toxoplasmosis is the most common cause of encephalitis.[94]

Most cases of toxoplasmosis are transmitted in utero from an infected mother, or less commonly, from ingestion of the organism. *Toxoplasma gondii* has an affinity for tissue of the central nervous system (CNS) or retina. In the CNS the organism may produce encephalitis, paralysis, cerebral calcification, convulsions, and fever. Retinochoroiditis can occur from either an initial infection or a latent reactivation from an extraocular site. The macula is often involved, but lesions may also occur elsewhere. Most lesions develop posterior to the equator. If lesions occur near the nerve head, there may be loss of the nerve fiber layer and an associated visual field defect. In AIDS patients, when *Toxoplasma* infection is found in the retina, up to 50% of patients may also have concurrent *Toxoplasma* encephalitis. A CT scan of the brain should be performed to rule out the condition.[95]

When an active infection is present in the retina, there is usually a single or multifocal whitish-yellow, slightly raised area of retinochoroiditis. These lesions also present with an overlying moderate to severe vitritis. Active lesions commonly occur adjacent to an old, healed chorioretinal toxoplasmosis scar (satellite lesions). Sites of active infection may be associated with focal serous retinal detachment. Other possible ocular complications include papillitis, retinal holes, retinal vascular occlusions, and cystoid macular edema.[96] Patients with active ocular disease commonly have concurrent iridocyclitis.

The diagnosis of active toxoplasmosis is based on clinical appearance and confirmatory laboratory test results. Many patients will test positive serologically (enzyme-linked immunosorbent assay [ELISA]) and on skin tests for infection with the organism. Treatment consists of pyrimethamine and triple sulfa along with corticosteroids, especially for those patients with lesions that threaten the macula or large peripheral lesions. Recurrences have been reported in up to 49% of cases.[97]

Toxocariasis

Toxocara canis is a common intestinal parasite of dogs.[98] Infection in humans is acquired by ingestion of the ova form of the parasite by coming into contact with contaminated soil or oral contact with the fur of puppies. Children up to 4 years of age are most often affected. Once ingested, the ova mature into larvae, which disseminate to the liver, lungs, brain, and eyes via the bloodstream. Once in the eye, the organism can produce a number of ocular complications. Most ocular findings are a result of the immune response to the organism. In many cases a destructive endophthalmitis is seen.[99] A focal retinal granuloma may develop with the larvae in the center of the lesion. There may be disciform macular or peripheral retinal detachment, peripheral retinal mass, vitritis, and cataract formation. When the lesion heals there may be a gray to white disciform scar with fibrous tissue formation and contraction. The traction on the retina may cause an appearance similar to a dragged disk. The retinal lesion may look very similar to a retinoblastoma.

Laboratory evaluation includes ELISA testing. There are, however, no hematologic or liver enzyme tests that are pathognomonic for *Toxocara* infection. Definitive diagnosis is made by liver biopsy to look for the larvae. Ultrasonographic studies will show characteristic calcified lesions.

Treatment consists of topical steroids to control inflammation caused by the organism. In certain cases, when viable larvae are visualized, laser photocoagulation may be used.[99] A vitrectomy or retinal detachment repair may be necessary in some cases.

Retinal Infections Associated with AIDS

AIDS results from infection from the human immunodeficiency virus (HIV). Patients infected with the virus can have a variety of opportunistic retinal infections. Such infections occur from viruses, bacteria, and fungi, many of which are disseminated from other systemic locations. Occasionally, discovering an ocular infection may lead to an initial diagnosis of systemic opportunistic infection. However, retinal infections occur much less frequently than those found systemically.[100] When evaluating patients with AIDS, the clinician is most likely to encounter opportunistic infections when CD4 levels drop below 200/mm³.

The most common retinal infection in the patient with AIDS is cytomegalovirus (CMV) retinitis. It occurs in up to 25% of patients with the disease and may be seen bilaterally in half of these cases.[101] Patients with CMV retinitis usually are severely immunocompromised with a CD4 level of less than 50/mm³.[102] Once a diagnosis of CMV infection has been established, survival typically ranges from 7 to 10 months.[103]

The diagnosis of CMV retinitis is based on the clinical ophthalmoscopic presentation. The earliest stages of infection are often difficult to interpret accurately. Early CMV lesions may be small, fluffy, white, and granular within the retina and may appear similar to cotton-wool spots. Smaller CMV lesions gradually enlarge into a diffuse retinitis. Active CMV retinitis may be associated with retinal vasculitis, and there may be diffuse intraretinal hemorrhaging as well as areas of retinal necrosis (Color Plate 24-II). Cytomegalovirus lesions are often characterized with an advancing edge of active retinitis with hemorrhaging, trailed by retinal necrosis behind the lesion. Because of this, lesions are often described as having a "brush fire" border. After active CMV retinitis, thin necrotic retina remains that is avascular with pigment epithelial atrophy. Up to one-third of patients may develop retinal breaks in these areas.[104,105] There is often minimal to no vitritis in the early stages of the infection, but vitreal inflammatory debris may accumulate in time. The anterior segment is also relatively quiet in most patients. Direct infection of the optic nerve by CMV may occasionally occur, resulting in an optic neuritis followed later by optic atrophy.

The clinician must be aware that up to one-half of CMV retinitis lesions begin peripherally.[106] Therefore the eyes of all AIDS patients should be routinely dilated. Treatment for CMV retinitis consists of either ganciclovir or foscarnet in induction and maintenance dosages.[107-109]

Differentiated from active CMV retinitis are noninfectious retinal changes, which, although relatively benign, may occasionally lead to the initial diagnosis of HIV infection. Noninfectious retinopathy, which may occur in one-half of all patients with AIDS, consists of cotton-wool spots, retinal hemorrhages, and microvascular abnormalities. These lesions are nonprogressive and do not require treatment. Noninfectious retinopathy is primarily observed in the posterior pole, and evidence does not suggest that existing lesions are precursor sites for infectious lesions. Rather, noninfectious retinopathy appears to be a manifestation of AIDS itself.

Because of the prevalence of noninfectious retinopathy in AIDS patients, particularly cotton-wool spots, AIDS should be heavily considered in the differential diagnosis when such changes are discovered in patients without other obvious causes for the retinal findings.

Toxoplasmosis is the second most common opportunistic ocular infection seen in AIDS. It is discussed elsewhere in this chapter. Acute retinal necrosis (ARN) is also an opportunistic infection seen in AIDS patients. It consists of a triad of clinical findings.[110] There is usually an

FIGURE 24-12
Presumed ocular histoplasmosis syndrome (POHS). Classic findings include peripapillary atrophy and chorioretinal lesions, which may appear "punched out." Macular lesions sometimes occur, which can lead to choroidal neovascular membranes.

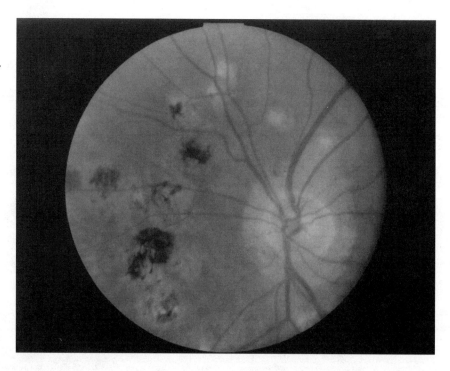

arteritis and phlebitis of the choroidal vasculature, a confluent necrotizing retinitis typically seen in the peripheral retina, and an accompanying moderate to severe vitritis. The necrotic areas enlarge and progress posteriorly and may eventually destroy the macula. Optic neuritis has also been noted. Retinal breaks and detachments are seen in up to 75% of cases.[110] Mild to moderate anterior uveitis may be present, and intraocular pressure may be elevated. Herpesvirus infection has been implicated as the etiology of the disease.[111] Syphilis, another HIV-associated infection, is discussed elsewhere in this chapter.

Fungal infections are common in AIDS patients as the immune system diminishes. Common organisms include *Cryptococcus* sp., *Candida* sp., and *Histoplasma,* all of which may produce ocular involvement.

Histoplasmosis

Histoplasmosis is a systemic disease caused by the fungal organism *Histoplasma capsulatum.* Infection is acquired through inhalation. Once inside the body a bronchopneumonia can result. During primary infection in the lungs there may be hematogenous spreading to other organs where it produces a granulomatous intracellular inflammation.[112] Ocular findings typically occur in otherwise healthy patients between 20 and 50 years of age. Most cases are found in the eastern half of the United States.[46]

In the eye, histoplasmosis classically causes a triad of clinical findings. These include peripapillary atrophy,

peripheral "punched out" foci of chorioretinal scarring, and macular lesions (Figure 24-12).[113] During active ocular infection there is a yellowish-white or gray, slightly elevated, circumscribed, focal choroidal infiltration. The chorioretinitis that develops is not commonly associated with an overlying vitritis. The choroidal lesions eventually become atrophic scars with central or eccentric pigmentation. Breaks in Bruch's membrane may develop with subsequent formation of choroidal neovascular membranes and subretinal fibrosis. This is problematic if the lesions develop near the fovea, as visual acuity may be lost from serous and hemorrhagic macular detachment and subsequent scarring.

Because the diagnosis of ocular involvement is typically made based on the funduscopic appearance alone, the term *presumed ocular histoplasmosis syndrome* (POHS) is usually used to describe the retinal picture caused by the *Histoplasma* organism. Tests are available, however, to determine if the patient has been previously exposed to *Histoplasma.* Diagnostic skin tests for histoplasmin may produce positive results in up to 90% of patients.[114] The HLA-B7 antigen has been found in association with POHS, and chest x-ray films may demonstrate calcific hilar lymph nodes typical of pulmonary histoplasmosis. Treatment for the disease includes systemic and periocular corticosteroid injections. Macular choroidal neovascular membranes may be treated with either argon or krypton laser photocoagulation.[56,57,115] Ocular histoplasmosis is usually asymptomatic and goes undetected until routine examination.

Syphilis

Syphilitic infections have been gradually increasing over the past several years in the United States.[116] Because of the associated high-risk activities of many HIV patients (e.g., intravenous drug abuse and sexual habits), there is a frequent association between syphilis and AIDS. Syphilis is caused by the spirochete *Treponema pallidum* and develops in three clinical stages: primary, secondary, and tertiary. The primary stage is characterized by chancre sores developing on mucous membranes within a few weeks after initial infection. These persist only for a few weeks. Ocular findings are rare at this stage. The secondary stage may begin a few months after the primary infection (2–12 weeks). Clinical findings occur in 60–90% of patients during this secondary stage.[117] The most common ocular manifestations include nongranulomatous anterior uveitis, diffuse chorioretinitis, and vasculitis.[118] Patients may also develop optic neuritis and perineuritis. Tertiary syphilis occurs after a latent period of time and may exhibit associated iridocyclitis, retinochoroiditis, optic atrophy, and Argyll-Robertson pupils.

In the early stages of syphilitic retinopathy, the clinical appearance includes a necrotizing chorioretinitis, which appears as a yellow-white patch, with hemorrhaging occurring infrequently. Also, gray-white patches at the level of the RPE may be seen. There may be a mild to moderate vitritis. Patients may complain of photophobia, floaters, and decreased vision.

A definitive diagnosis of syphilis is made via serologic testing. Investigation includes a nonspecific reagin test such as the Venereal Disease Research Laboratory (VDRL) test or the rapid plasma reagin (RPR) card test. A positive VDRL or RPR test indicates active syphilis, but they typically become negative in later stages or following treatment. Therefore, additional workup should include a test such as the fluorescent treponemal antibody absorption test (FTA-ABS), which is more sensitive and specific for syphilis and remains permanently positive, even after adequate treatment. The essential treatment for active syphilitic infection is antispirochetal therapy such as penicillin.

Tuberculosis

Tuberculosis is caused by *Mycobacterium tuberculosis*. Transmission occurs through airborne particles or close contact with infected persons. Active infection commonly occurs in the lungs but may involve other sites throughout the body. Ocular involvement is uncommon, occurring in only about 1–2% of patients with tuberculosis.[119] Ocular involvement can present secondary to direct infection by the bacilli or as the result of an immune-type reaction. The most common ocular presentations include chronic anterior uveitis, retinal periphlebitis, and choroiditis.[120] Choroidal infection may occur and manifests itself as a granulomatous infiltration. Vasculitis with vitreous hemorrhage can occur and is more commonly associated with primary tuberculosis.

DISORDERS OF THE PERIPHERAL RETINA

Common Anomalies

Retinal Tufts

Retinal tufts generally appear in three forms: noncystic, cystic, and zonular traction tufts. Noncystic retinal tufts appear as small, chalky white, short projections of fibroglial tissue from the surface of the retina. They are about 0.1 mm in size and appear in the peripheral retina between the equator and the ora serrata. They are seen in about 75% of all eyes, are bilateral in about half of all patients, and are commonly located inferonasally.[121-123] They usually appear in clusters and are not associated with retinal breaks.

Cystic tufts, on the other hand, are larger and appear as grayish-white elevations of retinal tissue containing microcystic spaces (Figure 24-13). They are also found between the equator and ora serrata. Cystic retinal tufts have a prevalence of 5–6%.[124] They are associated with retinal breaks such as flap tears or operculated holes, especially at the time of posterior vitreous detachment. They are found in up to 10% of all rhegmatogenous retinal detachments; however, the risk of retinal detachment is less than 1%.[124]

Zonular traction tufts are similar to cystic retinal tufts but they occur in the retinal periphery within the vitreous base. They are composed of fibroglial tissue but with projections that extend anteriorly over the surface of the retina and onto the zonules of the ciliary body. They are found in about 9% of eyes.[125] Retinal breaks may occur within the vitreous base from these lesions. Associated retinal detachment is rare, however.

Meridional Folds

Meridional folds are common developmental lesions that are elongated elevations of peripheral retinal tissue. These lesions appear whitish-gray and are somewhat translucent to opaque. Histologically, they are composed of thickened retinal tissue. Meridional folds are oriented perpendicular to the ora serrata and may align with an oral bay or dentate process. They occur in about 20% of all eyes.[126] They occasionally extend beyond the ora serrata as far posteriorly as the equator. Meridional folds are commonly bilateral, symmetric, and are frequently

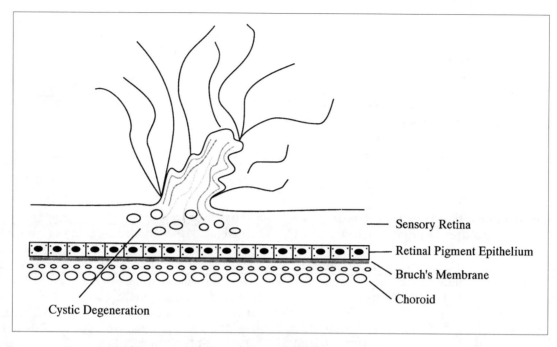

FIGURE 24-13

Schematic representation of a cystic retinal tuft. Vitreoretinal adhesion to the surface of the tuft is present, as well as cystic retinal degeneration at its base. (Courtesy of Daniel K. Roberts, O.D.)

found in the superonasal quadrant. Retinal breaks may occur at the posterior edge of these lesions.

Meridional complexes consist of larger meridional folds that align with a dentate process, extend onto the ciliary body, and merge with a ciliary process. As with meridional folds, they are frequently seen in the superonasal quadrant. They occur in about 12% of all eyes.[126] Retinal pits and breaks may occur at the posterior margin of these lesions as well.

White Without Pressure

White without pressure is characterized by a whitish retinal discoloration, typically found in the periphery. Regions of white without pressure are usually well demarcated with smooth or irregular configurations. There may be darker areas within white without pressure that can be mistaken for retinal holes. White without pressure is more commonly seen in the inferotemporal quadrant. The condition is found in about one-third of all eyes and is more common in blacks, young patients, and myopic patients.[122,127] It may vary in appearance over time and generally decreases with age. Although not fully understood histopathologically, the discoloration may be caused by irregularities of the internal limiting membrane or condensation of collagen fibrils near the surface of the retina. These interface changes may produce an atypical light

reflex from the surface of the retina. It has been suggested that areas of white without pressure coincide with abnormal vitreoretinal adherences. White without pressure is generally not associated with retinal breaks.

White with pressure occurs during scleral indentation of the peripheral retina. Its cause is not known and there is no apparent clinical significance.

Pars Plana Cysts

Pars plana cysts are translucent or transparent round cysts located anterior to the ora serrata on the pars plana. These cysts develop between the ciliary epithelial layers and may be found in up to 5–10% of individuals.[121] They increase in frequency with age. Pars plana cysts are generally not seen unless they are very large or scleral depression is used. They do not cause holes or tears in the retina and are easily differentiated from tumors. They are benign in nature but may have a striking appearance and cause concern in the clinician is not familiar with their presentation.

Retinal Degenerations

Cystoid Degeneration

Cystoid degeneration is the most common peripheral retinal degeneration of the eye. It occurs in 100% of patients

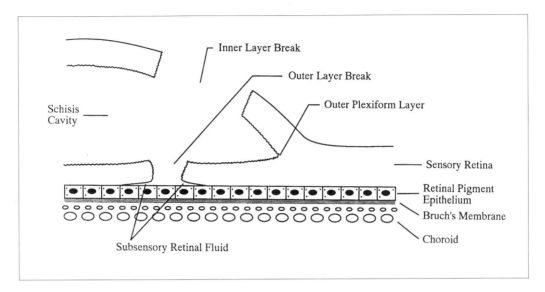

FIGURE 24-14
Schematic representation of a degenerative retinoschisis. A splitting of the sensory retina occurs at the level of the outer plexiform layer, and holes may develop within the inner or outer layers of the schisis. (Courtesy of Daniel K. Roberts, O.D.)

over the age of 8 years.[128] The condition begins at the ora serrata and extends both posteriorly and circumferentially with age. Cystoid degeneration is usually bilateral and symmetric and generally is limited to the far peripheral retina. Involved retina manifests a stippled appearance and may seem slightly elevated. Cystoid degeneration usually is benign; however, in the extreme cases it may lead to retinoschisis formation. Scleral depression may aid in its visualization.

Pavingstone Degeneration
Pavingstone degeneration is present in about 22% of the adult population.[129] It is found between the equator and ora serrata and appears as multiple discrete round areas of retinal thinning and chorioretinal depigmentation. The lesions are typically yellowish-white with pigmented margins, and larger choroidal vessels are seen clearly within these areas. Most pavingstone lesions occur in the inferior retina. Pavingstone degeneration is considered benign; however, the involved retinal tissue is thin and atrophic and may therefore easily tear should a retinal break occur adjacent to the lesion.

Retinoschisis
Retinoschisis is a splitting of the neurosensory retina in the outer plexiform layer. It occurs in about 7–10% of the population over the age of 40 years.[130,131] It is bilateral in 70–80% of cases and is commonly located in the inferotemporal quadrant. The inner layer appears smooth and

elevated, whereas the outer layer of remaining sensory retina appears irregular. Occasionally, small yellowish flecks may be seen adherent to the inner layer, which probably represents fragments of Müller's cells. Associated retinal vessels often become whitened secondary to sclerotic changes. Retinal holes may occur in either the inner or outer layers of a retinoschisis (Figure 24-14). Outer wall holes are more common and are seen in about 12% of cases.[122] Inner wall holes occur less frequently. Often, small areas of inner layer thinning appear as pseudoholes.

Of obvious importance is the differentiation of retinoschisis from retinal detachment, which is a difficult task in some cases. Table 24-4 lists characteristic features of each disorder that may be helpful in their identification.

Retinoschisis causes up to 3% of all retinal detachments.[132] Detachment may occur secondary to outer wall holes occurring alone or in the presence of outer and inner wall holes occurring simultaneously. When outer wall holes are present by themselves, associated detachments tend to occur very slowly. Secondary retinal detachments tend to occur more quickly when both outer and inner wall holes are present at the same time.[130]

Lattice Degeneration
Lattice degeneration is one of the most important vitreoretinal fundus lesions predisposing the retina to breaks and detachments. It occurs in approximately 10% of the general population.[133] Clinical appearances can vary widely; however lattice degeneration is typically characterized

TABLE 24-4
Differential Diagnosis of Retinoschisis Versus Retinal Detachment

Feature	Retinoschisis	Retinal Detachment
RPE changes	Not usually	Yes
Visual field defect	Steep margins	Sloping margins
Retinal surface	Smooth	Wrinkled
Retinal movement	Rigid	Undulates
Vitreous	Normal	Pigment dispersion

RPE = retinal pigment epithelium.

by a well-demarcated oval or band-shaped retinal lesion located between the equator and ora serrata (Figure 24-15). Lesions show a variable amount of pigmentation and sometimes exhibit crisscrossing white lines, which are sclerosed blood vessels. The retinal tissue within lattice degeneration is thinned and may develop round atrophic holes in approximately 25% of lesions.[133] Lattice lesions exhibit strong vitreoretinal attachments at their borders, which may cause retinal tears, especially at the time of posterior vitreous detachment. This more commonly accounts for retinal detachment than do atrophic holes within areas of lattice. Lattice degeneration is more commonly located in the superior and inferior periphery and occurs bilaterally up to 50% of the time.

Lattice degeneration typically develops by the second decade of life and changes little in appearance over time.[133] The pathogenesis of lattice degeneration is not well understood. Potential causes may include embryologic vascular anomalies in the retina and choroid, degeneration from vitreoretinal traction, retinal ischemia, and defects in the internal limiting membrane of the retina.[133]

Retinal Breaks and Detachment

There are three general types of retinal detachment: rhegmatogenous, exudative, and tractional. Rhegmatogenous (*rhegma*—Greek, to tear) retinal detachments occur from full-thickness retinal breaks. Causes of such retinal breaks

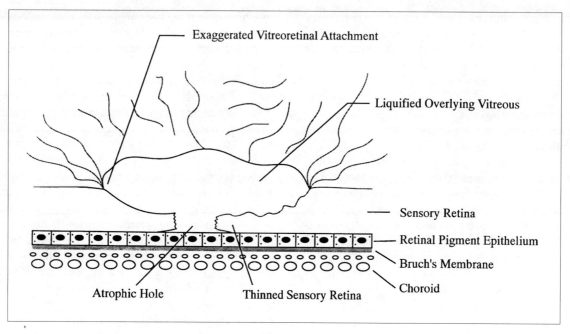

FIGURE 24-15
Schematic representation of lattice degeneration. A thinning of the sensory retina occurs and is associated with liquefaction of the overlying vitreous. Strong vitreoretinal adhesions are present at the borders of lattice degeneration, and full-thickness holes may develop within the thinned sensory retina. (Courtesy of Daniel K. Roberts, O.D.)

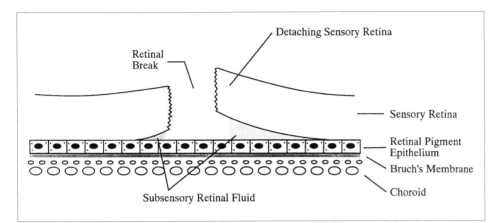

FIGURE 24-16
Retinal breaks are characterized by a splitting, or atrophic loss, of sensory retinal tissue. Accumulation of serous fluid within the subsensory retinal space may begin at the border of a retinal break. This may contribute to a progressive detachment of the sensory retina from the retinal pigment epithelium. (Courtesy of Daniel K. Roberts, O.D.)

are varied but commonly include lattice degeneration, cystic tufts, or any other focal vitreoretinal adhesions. Often these breaks occur at the time of posterior vitreous detachment. Vitreous fluid enters the subsensory retinal space through the retinal break, thereby progressively dissecting the retina from the pigment epithelium. Fresh rhegmatogenous retinal detachments typically appear as translucent retinal tissue that undulates with eye movement. The underlying choroidal vascularization is poorly visualized. If the area of detachment is large enough, or near the macula, the patient will notice associated visual field defects. Light flashes, floaters, or blurred vision are commonly observed. Retinal breaks at highest risk of progressing to detachment include flap tears or tears involving blood vessels.[122] Here tractional forces from the vitreoretinal interface continue to pull on the flap or blood vessel, causing further retinal tearing and accumulation of subretinal fluid. Tears resulting in a round, free-floating operculum are less likely to result in retinal detachment because tractional forces that may lead to further tearing are alleviated.

Risk factors for the development of retinal breaks include posterior vitreous detachment, lesions with vitreoretinal adhesions such as lattice degeneration or retinal tufts, myopia usually greater than 3 D, a familial history of retinal detachment, trauma, and retinal breaks in the fellow eye. Treatment for rhegmatogenous retinal detachments and associated breaks may include laser retinopexy, cryopexy, diathermy, or vitrectomy and scleral buckling or any combination thereof.

With most retinal breaks there is usually at least a thin margin of subsensory retinal fluid accumulation at the border of the lesion (Figure 24-16). If this "cuff" of subretinal fluid extends more than one disc diameter from the edge of the lesion it is termed a *subclinical detachment*. Scleral depression is helpful in observing this condition. As a characteristic lesion is indented, the free edge of the

sensory retina will more clearly separate from the underlying RPE; the cuff of fluid is also highlighted, becoming brighter in appearance. Subclinical detachments are usually treated even if the patient is asymptomatic.

Retinal breaks or detachments commonly exhibit pigmentation along the borders of attached and detached retina. In cases where retinal detachment has existed for some time, there is atrophy of the photoreceptors, cystoid degeneration of the outer retinal layers, and fibrous and glial proliferation. Fibroglial membranes will contract, forming fixed retinal folds. In the late stages of degeneration there is thinning of the retina that takes on a transparent appearance. The underlying RPE, Bruch's membrane, and choroid will also develop degenerative changes.

Exudative detachments result from an accumulation of fluid underneath the sensory retina without evidence of retinal breaks. These types of detachments occur from inflammatory conditions, systemic disorders, defects in the retinal pigment epithelium, subretinal neovascularization, or tumors. Characteristic detachments typically have a bullous appearance and may in extreme cases touch the back of the crystalline lens. The fluid beneath the detachment often shifts as the eye is rotated. Fluorescein angiography will show leakage and pooling in the subretinal space. Management includes treating the underlying cause of inflammation or systemic disease and possibly photocoagulation.

Tractional retinal detachments occur from vitreous traction of the retinal surface in the absence of a retinal break. Causes include inflammatory exudates, vitreous hemorrhage, trauma, proliferative retinopathy, and vitreal loss and fibrosis as a result of intraocular surgery. Diseases such as diabetic retinopathy, venous occlusive disease, sickle cell retinopathy, retinopathy of prematurity, congenital toxoplasmosis, and Eales disease may result in tractional detachment. Vitreous degenerations can also cause such detachments.

FIGURE 24-17
Schematic representation of a posterior vitreous detachment (PVD). The posterior hyaloid face detaches from the retinal surface and gradually moves forward to settle within the anterior aspect of the vitreous cavity. The hyaloid face usually remains attached at the anterior vitreal base, which straddles the ora serrata. With separation of the posterior hyaloid face, a prominent glial ring, "Weiss' ring," is commonly pulled away from the peripapillary retinal tissue. (Courtesy of Daniel K. Roberts, O.D.)

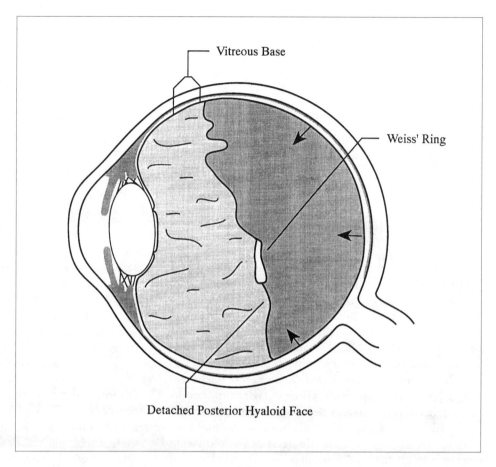

DISORDERS OF THE VITREOUS

Vitreous Detachment

The vitreous substance is composed of 99% water. The remaining 1% consists of hyaluronic acid and collagen.[123] These latter two components form a fibrillar matrix throughout the vitreous providing organization and a gel-like quality. This structure helps to support the retinal layers against the retinal pigment epithelium. The fibrillar matrix is denser in the far peripheral retina where it straddles the ora serrata and forms the vitreous base. This vitreal base extends about one disc diameter anterior and posterior to the ora serrata. Vitreoretinal adherence is very strong in this region. Other areas of strong vitreoretinal adherence occur at the optic nerve head, the macula, and along blood vessels.

As the eye ages the vitreal fibrillar matrix begins to break down (syneresis) forming lacunae of liquefied vitreous. When about 50% of the vitreous breaks down there may be disruption of the vitreous cortex, causing it to separate from the retinal surface (posterior vitreous detachment [PVD]). This event commonly occurs in the sixth and seventh decades of life. It may occur earlier in patients who are myopic, have a history of trauma, or have disease of the posterior segment. Classically, during detachment of the posterior vitreous, a ring of glial tissue is pulled from the borders of the optic nerve and remains adherent to the detached posterior hyaloid face (Figure 24-17). The glial ring, which may not be completely intact, is usually easily visualized on direct or indirect ophthalmoscopy. Symptoms associated with a PVD often include photopsias and floaters. Whereas a PVD is often a harmless and asymptomatic event, it also is a common cause of rhegmatogenous retinal detachment. Although there is no treatment for a PVD, observation is maintained after the acute PVD for the possible development of secondary retinal breaks and detachment, with management then appropriately directed toward these complications.

Asteroid Hyalosis

Asteroid hyalosis is named for the clinical appearance of floating white or yellow intravitreal opacities. These opacities are made of calcium soaps and vary in number and size between individuals. They are found in older patients and are seen monocularly in 75% of cases.[134,135] Visual acuity is rarely affected, although their presence may greatly interfere with visualization of fundus detail during ophthalmoscopic examination.

Developmental Anomalies

There may be remnants that are of developmental origin observed in the vitreous. These include Bergmeister's papilla, vascular loops, and persistent hyperplastic primary vitreous (PHPV). Bergmeister's papilla is a congenital glial remnant resulting from embryonic vasculature that extends into the vitreous from the optic nerve head. Vascular loops are retinal vessels that grow into the hyaloid canal during ocular development and persist after regression of the embryonic tissues. Persistent hyperplastic primary vitreous is mostly a unilateral condition that is associated with microphthalmia, cataract formation, shallow anterior chamber, and angle-closure glaucoma. It occurs as a persistence and proliferation of the primary vitreous and tunica vasculosa lentis. Patients may present with leukokoria and very poor vision. It is important to differentiate PHPV from retinoblastoma, as it is one of the most frequent causes of a white pupillary reflex in infants. Elongated and stretched ciliary processes extending centrally and associated with microphthalmia help to differentiate PHPV from retinoblastoma.[136]

Vitreous Hemorrhage

Vitreous hemorrhage may occur from a variety of conditions. In adults, the most common causes include diabetic retinopathy, retinal breaks, PVD, neovascularization from venous occlusive disease, and trauma. Peripheral neovascularization from causes such as sickle cell retinopathy and sarcoidosis may also lead to vitreous hemorrhage. In children the most common causes are trauma, congenital retinoschisis, and pars planitis.

Vitreous hemorrhages may vary in appearance. If the vitreous cortex (hyaloid face) is generally attached, the hemorrhage will take on the outline of the portion of the cortex detached by the hemorrhage. Sometimes it may appear boat-shaped with a flattened superior border and curved inferior border. If there is a posterior vitreous detachment the hemorrhage may be diffusely scattered in the vitreous cavity. If the posterior segment is markedly obscured by blood, diagnostic ultrasonography should be performed to determine the cause as well as to rule out the possibility of tumor or detachment.

RETINOBLASTOMA

Retinoblastoma is the most common intraocular childhood malignancy. It occurs with a frequency of 1 in 15,000.[137] It is the third most common intraocular malignancy.[28] The heritable form is transmitted in an autosomal dominant manner. The condition is seen bilaterally in 25–35% of cases.[136] Retinoblastoma may be more common in the modern world, where survival rates have been more favorable, thus increasing the gene pool. Most cases occur in children before the age of 3 years and are uncommon after the age of 7 years. A few rare cases have been reported into adolescence and adulthood.[138] Early signs of this condition include leukokoria (white pupil), visual loss, anisocoria, nystagmus, and strabismus, with strabismus being the most common initial symptom.[139] Rubeosis, hyphema, secondary glaucoma, or intraocular inflammation may also be present. Retinoblastomas typically have a white, light gray, or pink-cream coloration with blood vessels on the surface or within the tumor. The early and accurate diagnosis of retinoblastoma is important, because metastasis is common. Prognosis depends on whether "seeding" occurs within the vitreous and anterior chamber, the size of the tumor, choroidal invasion, and whether there is optic nerve or subarachnoid invasion.

Treatment for retinoblastoma has increased survival rates to 86–92% in recent years.[140] Modalities include cryotherapy, radiation, chemotherapy, and enucleation.

CHOROIDAL MELANOMA

Choroidal nevi are found in 1–6% of the population.[137] Typically they have a slate gray coloration and may be oval to round in configuration. The borders are usually well pronounced but may have a feathery appearance. They commonly range in size from 0.5 to 1.5 disc diameters, but may extend up to 5 or 6 disc diameters. Choroidal nevi are generally flat or only minimally elevated. Their location is often peripheral but they may be located anywhere within the fundus. Drusen formation may be seen on the surface of nevi.

Malignant melanomas are the most common primary intraocular malignancy. They occur equally between the sexes and may present in any age group; however, they develop more commonly in elderly persons. Patients may be asymptomatic, have visual field loss, photopsias, floaters, or ocular pain.[137] Choroidal melanomas often occur at or near the posterior pole, and may arise from preexisting nevi. Some are darkly pigmented, whereas others are light-colored or have mixed pigmentation. Small melanomas are generally well circumscribed, pigmented, and limited to the choroid, whereas larger lesions may break through Bruch's membrane, causing retinal detachment. A mushroom shape or "collar button" shape often results from extension through Bruch's membrane.

The retinal pigment epithelium overlying melanomas may appear mottled and exhibit drusenoid changes similar to that of age-related macular degeneration. Overlying some melanomas will be choroidal neovascular membranes beneath the RPE. Sometimes cystoid degeneration, pavingstone degeneration, subretinal fluid, vitreous hemorrhage and seeding, and invasion of the sclera may be seen with choroidal melanomas.[137] Treatment includes enucleation as well as irradiation followed by enucleation. The Collaborative Ocular Melanoma Study is attempting to determine the best management of this tumor.[141]

REFERENCES

1. National Society to Prevent Blindness. Vision problems in the U.S. Data Analysis. Definitions, Data Sources, Detailed Data Tables, Analysis, Interpretation. New York: National Society to Prevent Blindness, 1980;1–46.

2. Klein R, Kein BEK, Moss SE, et al. The Wisconsin epidemiologic study of diabetic retinopathy: IX. Four-year incidence and progression of diabetic retinopathy when age at diagnosis is less than 30 years. Arch Ophthalmol 1989;107:237–43.

3. Klein R, Kein BEK, Moss SE, et al. The Wisconsin epidemiologic study of diabetic retinopathy: X. Four-year incidence and progression of diabetic retinopathy when age at diagnosis is 30 years or more. Arch Ophthalmol 1989;107:244–9.

4. The Diabetic Retinopathy Study Research Group. Photocoagulation treatment of proliferative diabetic retinopathy: The second report of Diabetic Retinopathy Study findings. Ophthalmology 1978;85:82–106.

5. The Diabetic Retinopathy Study Research Group. Four risk factors for severe visual loss in diabetic retinopathy: The third report from the Diabetic Retinopathy Study. Arch Ophthalmol 1979;97:654–5.

6. The Diabetic Retinopathy Study Research Group. Preliminary report on effects of photocoagulation therapy. Am J Ophthalmol 1976;81:383–96.

7. The Diabetic Retinopathy Vitrectomy Study Research Group. Early vitrectomy for severe vitreous hemorrhage in diabetic retinopathy: Four-year results of a randomized trial: DRVS Report Number 5. Arch Ophthalmol 1990; 108:958–64.

8. The Diabetic Retinopathy Vitrectomy Study Research Group. Early vitrectomy for severe proliferative diabetic retinopathy in eyes with useful vision: Results of a randomized trial: DRVS Report Number 3. Ophthalmology 1988;95:1307–34.

9. The Early Treatment Diabetic Retinopathy Study Research Group. Photocoagulation for diabetic macular edema: ETDRS Report Number 1. Arch Ophthalmol 1985;103: 1796–1806.

10. Early Treatment Diabetic Retinopathy Study Research Group. Early treatment diabetic retinopathy study design and baseline patient characteristics: ETDRS Report Number 7. Ophthalmology 1991;98:741–56.

11. The Diabetic Retinopathy Research Group. Photocoagulation treatment of proliferative diabetic retinopathy: Clinical applications of Diabetic Retinopathy Study (DRS) findings: DRS Report Number 8. Ophthalmology 1981; 88:583–600.

12. Klein R. The epidemiology of diabetic retinopathy. Findings from the Wisconsin Epidemiologic Study of Diabetic Retinopathy. Int Ophthalmol Clin 1987;27:230–8.

13. The Diabetes Control and Complications Trial Research Group. The effect of intensive treatment of diabetes on development and progression of long term complications in insulin-dependent diabetes mellitus. N Engl J Med 1993; 329:977–86.

14. Leahy JL. Natural history of beta cell dysfunction in NIDDM. Diabetes Care 1990;13:992.

15. Darlow JM, Smith C, Duncan LPJ. A statistical and genetical study of diabetes. Empiric risks to relatives. Ann Hum Genet 1993;38:157.

16. Ziegler AG, Herskowitz RD, Jackson RA, et al. Predicting type I diabetes. Diabetes Care 1990;13:762.

17. Sorbinil Retinopathy Trial Research Group. A randomized trial of Sorbinil, an aldose reductase inhibitor, in diabetic retinopathy. Arch Ophthalmol 1990;108:1234–44.

18. Green WR, Wilson DJ. Histopathology of diabetic retinopathy. In RM Franklin (ed), Proceedings of the Symposium on Retina and Vitreous, New Orleans Academy of Ophthalmology, New Orleans, LA. March 12–15, 1992;63–81.

19. Franklin RM (ed). Retina and vitreous. Proceedings of the Symposium on Retina and vitreous of the New Orleans Academy of Ophthalmology, March 1992.

20. Bloodworth JMB, Molitor DL. Ultrastructural aspects of human and canine diabetic retinopathy. Invest Ophthalmol Vis Sci 1965;4:1037–48.

21. Speiser P, Gittelsohn AM, Patz A. Studies on diabetic retinopathy. III. Influence of diabetes on intramural pericytes. Arch Ophthalmol 1968;80:332–7.

22. Ferris FL III, Patz A. Macular edema. A complication of diabetic retinopathy. Surv Ophthalmol 1984;28:S452–61.

23. Early Treatment Diabetic Retinopathy Research Group. Fundus photographic risk factors for progression of diabetic retinopathy. ETDRS Report Number 12. Ophthalmology 1991;98:s823–33.

24. Glaser BM. Extracellular modulating factors and the control of intraocular neovascularization: An overview. Arch Ophthalmol 1988;106:603–7.

25. Keith NM, Wagener HP, Barker NW. Some different types of essential hypertension: Their course and prognosis. Am J Med Sci 1939;197:332–43.

26. Scheie HG. Evaluation of ophthalmoscopic changes of hypertension and arteriolar sclerosis. Arch Ophthalmol 1953;49:117–38.

27. Appiah AP, Trempe CL. Risk factors associated with branch vs. central retinal vein occlusion. Ann Ophthalmol 1989;21:153–7.

28. Apple DJ, Rabb MF. Ocular Pathology. Clinical Applications and Self Assessment (4th ed). St. Louis: Mosby-Year Book, 1991;293–300, 375–418.

29. Finkelstein, D, Clarkson JG. The Branch Vein Study Group. Branch and central retinal vein occlusions. In RE Smith (ed), Focal Points (Vol. V, module 12). Philadelphia: American Academy of Ophthalmology, 1987.

30. Orth DH, Patz A. Retinal branch vein occlusion. Surv Ophthalmol 1978;22:357–76.

31. Elman MJ. Systemic associations of retinal vein occlusion. Int Ophthalmol Clin 1991;31:15–23.

32. Joffe L, Goldberg RE, Magargal LE, Annesley WH. Macular branch vein occlusion. Ophthalmology 1980;87:91–8.

33. The Branch Vein Occlusion Study Group. Argon laser photocoagulation for macular edema in branch vein occlusion. Am J Ophthalmol 1984;98:271–82.

34. The Branch Retinal Vein Occlusion Study Group. Argon laser scatter photocoagulation for prevention of neovascularization and vitreous hemorrhage in branch vein occlusion: A randomized clinical trial. Arch Ophthalmol 1986;104:34–41.

35. Hollenhorst RW. Vascular status of patients who have cholesterol emboli in the retina. Am J Ophthalmol 1966;61:1159–65.

36. Hayreh SS, Kolder HE, Weingeist TA. Central retinal artery occlusion and retinal tolerance time. Ophthalmology 1980;87:75–8.

37. Brown GC. Arterial obstructive disease and the eye. Ophthalmol Clin North Am 1990;3:373–92.

38. Brown GC, Margargal LE. The ocular ischemic syndrome: Clinical, fluorescein angiographic and carotid angiographic features. Int Ophthalmol 1988;11:239–51.

39. Miller NR. Cerebral Vascular Disease. In CL Brown (ed), Walsh and Hoyt's Clinical Neuro-Ophthalmology (4th ed, Vol. 4). Baltimore, Williams & Wilkins, 1991;2210–4.

40. Ben Sira I, Nissenkorn I, Kremer I. Retinopathy of prematurity. Surv Ophthalmol 1988;33:1–16.

41. Machemer R. Description and pathogenesis of late stages of retinopathy of prematurity. Ophthalmology 1985;92:1000–4.

42. Multicenter Trial of Cryotherapy for Retinopathy of Prematurity Cooperative Group. Manual of Procedures. No. PB 88-163530. Springfield, VA: US Dept of Commerce, National Technical Information Service, 1985.

43. Cryotherapy for Retinopathy of Prematurity Cooperative Group. Multicenter trial of cryotherapy for retinopathy of prematurity: One year outcome—structure and function. Arch Ophthalmol 1990;108:1408–16.

44. The International Committee for the Classification of the Late Stages of Retinopathy of Prematurity. An international classification of retinopathy of prematurity: II. The classification of retinal detachment. Arch Ophthalmol 1987;105:906–12.

45. Green WR, Quigley HA, de la Cruz Z, Cohen B. Parafoveal retinal telangiectasis: Light and electron microscopy studies. Trans Ophthalmol Soc UK 1980;100:162–70.

46. Gass JDM. Stereoscopic Atlas of Macular Diseases: Diagnosis and Treatment (3rd ed, Vol. 1). St. Louis: Mosby, 1987;46–59, 112, 236–61, 264–6, 390–5, 686.

47. Rabb MF, Gagliano DA, Teske MP. Retinal arterial macroaneurysms. Surv Ophthalmol 1988;33:73–96.

48. Jampol LM, Isenberg SJ, Goldberg MF. Occlusive retinal arteriolitis with neovascularization. Am J Ophthalmol 1976;81:583–9.

49. Bressler NM, Bressler SB, Fine SL. Age-related macular degeneration. Surv Ophthalmol 1988;32:375–413.

50. Young RW. Pathophysiology of age-related macular degeneration. Surv Ophthalmol 1987;31:291–306.

51. Green WR, McDonnell PJ, Yeo JH. Pathologic features of senile macular degeneration. Ophthalmology 1985;92:615–27.

52. Ferris FL, Fine SL, Hyman L. Age-related macular degeneration and blindness due to neovascular maculopathy. Arch Ophthalmol 1984;102:1640–2.

53. Kini MM, Leibowitz HM, Colton T, et al. Prevalence of senile cataract, diabetic retinopathy, senile macular degeneration, and open angle glaucoma in the Framingham Eye Study. Am J Ophthalmol 1978;85:28–34.

54. Smiddy WE, Fine SL. Prognosis of patients with bilateral macular drusen. Ophthalmology 1984;91:271–7.

55. Macular Photocoagulation Study Group. Argon laser photocoagulation for senile macular degeneration: Results of a randomized clinical trial. Arch Ophthalmol 1982;100:912–8.

56. Macular Photocoagulation Study Group. Recurrent choroidal neovascularization after argon laser photocoagulation for neovascular maculopathy. Arch Ophthalmol 1986;104:503–12.

57. Macular Photocoagulation Study Group. Argon laser photocoagulation for neovascular maculopathy: Three year results from randomized clinical trials. Arch Ophthalmol 1986;104:694–701.

58. Macular Photocoagulation Study Group. Subfoveal neovascular lesions in age-related macular degeneration: Guidelines for evaluation and treatment in the macular photocoagulation study. Arch Ophthalmol 1991;109:1242–57.

59. de Juan E Jr, Machemer R. Vitreous surgery for hemorrhagic and fibrous complications of age-related macular degeneration. Am J Ophthalmol 1988;105:25–9.

60. Thomas MA, Grand G, Williams DF, et al. Surgical management of subfoveal choroidal neovascularization. Ophthalmology 1992;99:952–68.

61. Age-Related Eye Disease Study (AREDS). Bethesda, MD: National Institutes of Health, National Eye Institute (investigation in progress).

62. Clarkson JG, Altman RD. Angioid streaks. Surv Ophthalmol 1982;26:235–46.

63. Wyszynski RE, Grossniklaus HE, Frank KE. Indirect choroidal rupture secondary to blunt ocular trauma. A review of eight eyes. Retina 1988;8:237–43.

64. Godtfredson E. Re-examination of central ruptures of the choroid. Acta Ophthalmol 1942;20:337–50.

65. Cavender JC, Ai E. Heriditary Macular Dystrophies. In TD Duane, EA Jaeger (eds), Clinical Ophthalmology (Vol. 3). Philadelphia: Lippincott, 1988;1–29.

66. Weingeist TA, Kobrin JL, Watzke RC. Histopathology of Best's macular dystrophy. Arch Ophthalmol 1982;100: 1108–14.

67. Frangieh GT, Green WR, Fine SL. A histopathologic study of Best's macular dystrophy. Arch Ophthalmol 1982;100: 1115–21.

68. Deutman AF. The Hereditary Dystrophies of the Posterior Pole of the Eye. Springfield, Ill: Thomas, 1971.

69. Krill AE. Hereditary Retinal and Choroidal Diseases (Vol. 2). Hagerstown, MD: Harper & Row, 1977.

60. Deutman AF, Jansen LMAA. Dominantly inherited drusen of Bruch's membrane. Br J Ophthalmol 1970;54:373–82.

71. Hotchkiss ML, Fine SL. Pathologic myopia and choroidal neovascularization. Am J Ophthalmol 1981;91:177–83.

72. Rabb MF, Garoon I, Lafranco FP. Myopic macular degeneration. Int Ophthalmol Clin 1981;21:51–69.

73. Marmor MF, Byers B. Pattern dystrophy of the pigment epithelium. Am J Ophthalmol 1977;84:32–44.

74. Watzke RC, Folk JC, Lang RM. Pattern dystrophy of the retinal pigment epithelium. Ophthalmology 1982;89:1400–6.

75. Sorsby A, Crick RP. Central areolar choroidal sclerosis. Br J Ophthalmol 1953;37:129–39.

76. Retina and Vitreous. Basic and Clinical Science Course. Philadelphia: American Academy of Ophthalmology, 1991;137.

77. Fetkenhour CL, Gurney N, Dobbie JG, Choromokos E. Central areolar pigment epithelial dystrophy. Am J Ophthalmol 1976;81:745–53.

78. Friberg TR. Central serous chorioretinopathy. Semin Ophthalmol 1991;6:36–44.

79. Spitznas M. Central Serous Retinopathy. In SJ Ryan, AP Schachat, RB Murphy, A Patz (eds), Retina. Vol. 2. St. Louis: Mosby, 1989;217–27.

80. Frangieh GT, Green WR, Engel HM. A histopathologic study of macular cysts and holes. Retina 1981;1:311–36.

81. Smiddy WE, Michels RG, Glaser BM, deBustros S. Vitrectomy for impending idiopathic macular holes. Am J Ophthalmol 1988;105:371–6.

82. Morgan CM, Schatz H. Idiopathic macular holes. Am J Ophthalmol 1985;99:437–44.

83. Gass JDM. Idiopathic senile macular hole: Its early stages and pathogenesis. Arch Ophthalmol 1988;106:626–39.

84. Johnson RN, Gass JDM. Idiopathic macular holes: Observations, stages of formation, and implications for surgical intervention. Ophthalmology 1988;95:917–24.

85. Gass JDM, Joondeph BC. Observations concerning patients with suspected impending macular holes. Am J Ophthalmol 1990;109:638–46.

86. Morgan CM, Schatz H. Involutional macular thinning: A pre-macular hole condition. Ophthalmology 1986;93: 153–61.

87. Schocket SS, Lakhanpal V, Xiaoping M, et al. Laser treatment of macular holes. Ophthalmology 1988;95:574–82.

88. Glaser BM, Michels RG, Kuppermann BD, et al. Transforming growth factor-β2 for the treatment of full-thickness macular holes: A prospective randomized study. Ophthalmology 1992;99:1162–73.

89. Kampik A, Kenyon KR, Michels RG, et al. Epiretinal and vitreous membranes: Comparative study of 56 cases. Arch Ophthalmol 1981;99:1445–54.

90. Clarkson JG, Green WR, Massof D. A histopathologic review of 168 cases of preretinal membrane. Am J Ophthalmol 1977;84:1–17.

91. Tessler HH. Ocular Toxoplasmosis. In MF Rabb (ed), Int Ophthalmol Clin. Boston: Little, Brown, 1981;21:185–99.

92. Berrocal J. Toxoplasmosis. In DH Gold, TA Weingeist (eds), The Eye in Systemic Disease. Philadelphia: Lippincott, 1990.

93. Weiss A, Margo CE, Ledford DK, et al. Toxoplasmic retinochoroiditis as an initial manifestation of acquired immune deficiency syndrome [letter]. Am J Ophthalmol 1986;101:248.

94. Pierce EA, D'Amico DJ. Ocular toxoplasmosis: Pathogenesis, diagnosis, and management. Semin Ophthalmol 1993;8:40–52.

95. Culbertson WW. Infections of the retina in AIDS. Int Ophthalmol Clin 1989;29:108–18.

96. Tabbara KF. Ocular toxoplasmosis. Int Ophthalmol 1990;14:349–51.

97. Rothova A, Meenken C, Buitenhuis HJ, et al. Therapy for ocular toxoplasmosis. Am J Ophthalmol 1993;115:517–23.

98. Shields JA: Ocular toxocariasis. A review. Surv Ophthalmol 1984;28:361–81.

99. Fitzgerald CR, Rubin ML. Intraocular parasite destroyed by photocoagulation. Arch Ophthalmol 1974;91:162–4.

100. Pepose JS, Holland GN, Nestor MS, et al. Acquired immune deficiency syndrome: Pathogenic mechanisms of ocular disease. Ophthalmology 1985;92:472–84.

101. Ballinger R. Ocular Manifestations of AIDS. In BE Onofrey (ed), Clinical Optometric Pharmacology and Therapeutics. Philadelphia: Lippincott, 1992.

102. Holland GN. In Focal Points: An Update on AIDS-Related Cytomegalovirus Retinitis (Clinical Module, Vol. IX, Module 5). Philadelphia: American Academy of Ophthalmology, 1991.

103. Holland GN, Sison RF, Jatulis DE, et al. Survival of patients with the acquired immune deficiency syndrome after development of cytomegalovirus retinopathy. Ophthalmology 1990;97:204–11.

104. Jabs DA, Enger C, Haller J, deBustros S. Retinal detachments in patients with cytomegalovirus retinitis. Arch Ophthalmol 1991;109:794–9.

105. Sheilds W, Ai E, Fujikawa L. Cytomegalovirus retinitis: Diagnosis and management. Ophthalmol Clin North Am 1988;1:81–90.

106. Henderly DE, Freeman WR, Causey DM, Rao NA. Cytomegalovirus retinitis and response to therapy with ganciclovir. Ophthalmology 1987;94:425–32.

107. Pepose JS, Newman C, Bach MC, et al. Pathologic features of cytomegalovirus retinopathy after treatment with the antiviral agent ganciclovir. Ophthalmology 1987;94:414–24.

108. Miles J, Jacobson MA, O'Donnell JJ et al. Treatment of cytomegalovirus retinitis in patients with AIDS. Rev Infect Dis 1988;10(Suppl 3):S522.

109. Singer DRJ, Fallon TJ, Schulenberg WE, et al. Foscarnet for cytomegalovirus retinitis. (Letter). Ann Intern Med 1985;103:962.

110. Duker JS, Blumenkranz MS. Diagnosis and management of the acute retinal necrosis (ARN) syndrome. Surv Ophthalmol 1991;35:327–43.

111. Ludwig IH, Zegarra H, Zakov ZN. The acute retinal necrosis syndrome: Possible herpes simplex retinitis. Ophthalmology 1984;91:1659–64.

112. Watzke R. Histoplasmosis. In DH Gold, TA Weingeist (eds), The Eye in Systemic Disease. Philadelphia: Lippincott, 1990;200.

113. Schlaegal TF Jr. Corticosteroids in the Treatment of Ocular Histoplasmosis. In TF Schlaegal Jr (ed), Update on Ocular Histoplasmosis. Int Ophthalmol Clin. Boston: Little, Brown, 1983;23:1–49.

114. American Academy of Ophthalmology. Basic and Clinical Science Course: Retina and Vitreous. Philadelphia: American Academy of Ophthalmology, 1991–1992;66.

115. Macular Photocoagulation Study Group. Argon laser photocoagulation for ocular histoplasmosis: Results of a randomized clinical trial. Arch Ophthalmol 1983;101:1347–57.

116. Margo CE, Hamed LM. Ocular syphilis. Surv Ophthalmol 1992;37:203–20.

117. Hutchinson CM, Hook EW III. Syphilis in adults. Med Clin North Am 1990;74:1389–1416.

118. Ho AC, Guyer DR, Yannuzzi LA, Brown GC. Ocular syphilis. Classic manifestations and recent observations. Semin Ophthalmol 1993;8:53–60.

119. Donahue HC. Ophthalmologic experience in a tuberculosis sanatorium. Am J Ophthalmol 1967;64:742–8.

120. Knox DL. Syphilis and Tuberculosis. In SJ Ryan, AP Schachaat, RB Murphy, A Patz (eds), Retina (Vol. 2). St Louis: Mosby, 1989;647–54.

121. Bec P, Ravault M, Arne J-L, Trepsat C. The Fundus Periphery. Report of the French Society of Ophthalmology. New York: Masson, 1985.

122. Michels RG, Wilkinson CP, Rice TA. Retinal Detachment: Diagnosis and Management. St. Louis: Mosby, 1990.

123. Green WR. Vitreoretinal Juncture. In SJ Ryan, B Glaser, R Michels (eds), Retina (Vol. 3). St. Louis: Mosby, 1989;13–69.

124. Byer NE. Cystic retinal tufts and their relationship to retinal detachment. Arch Ophthalmol 1981;99:1788–90.

125. Foos RY. Zonular traction tufts of the peripheral retina in cadaver eyes. Arch Ophthalmol 1969;82:620–32.

126. Spencer LM, Foos RY, Straatsma BR. Meridional folds, meridional complexes, and associated abnormalities of the peripheral retina. Am J Ophthalmol 1970;70:697–714.

127. Schepens CL. Subclinical retinal detachments. Arch Ophthalmol 1952;47:593–606.

128. O'Malley PF, Allen RA. Peripheral cystoid degeneration of the retina: Incidence and distribution in 1,000 autopsy eyes. Arch Ophthalmol 1967;77;769–76.

129. O'Malley P, Allen RA, Straatsma BR, et al. Paving-stone degeneration of the retina. Arch Ophthalmol 1965;73:169–82.

130. Byer NE. Long-term natural history study of senile retinoschisis with implications for management. Ophthalmology 1986;93:1127–37.

131. Byer NE. The natural history of senile retinoschisis. Trans Am Acad Ophthalmol Otolaryngol 1976;81:OP458–OP471.

132. Hagler WS, Woldoff HS. Retinal detachment in relation to senile retinoschisis. Trans Am Acad Ophthalmol Otolaryngol 1973;77:OP99–OP113.

133. Byer NE: Lattice degeneration of the retina. Surv Ophthalmol 1979;23:213–48.

134. Bell FC, Senstrom WJ. Atlas of the Peripheral Retina. Philadelphia: Saunders, 1983.

135. Topilow HW, Kenyon KR, Takahashi M, et al. Asteroid hyalosis: Biomicroscopy, ultrastructure, and composition. Arch Ophthalmol 1982;100:964–8.

136. American Academy of Ophthalmology. Basic and Clinical Science Course. Ophthalmic Pathology and Intraocular Tumors. Philadelphia: American Academy of Ophthalmology, 1992;72.

137. Shields JA, Shields CL. Intraocular Tumors: A Text and Atlas. Philadelphia: Saunders, 1992.

138. Tamboli A, Podgor MJ, Horm JW. The incidence of retinoblastoma in the United States: 1974 through 1985. Arch Ophthalmol 1990;108:128–32.

139. Abramson DH, Fusco Marks R, Ellsworth RM, et al. The management of unilateral retinoblastoma without primary enucleation. Arch Ophthalmol 1982;100:1249–52.

140. Abramson DH, Ellsworth RM, Rozakis GW. Cryotherapy for retinoblastoma. Arch Ophthalmol 1982;100:1253–65.

141. Schachat AP. Collaborative Ocular Melanoma Study. In SJ Ryan, TE Ogden, AP Schachet (eds), Retina (Vol. 1). St. Louis: Mosby, 1989;733–6.

25

Glaucoma

Michael A. Chaglasian

A thorough understanding of the diagnosis and management of glaucoma is essential for every eye care practitioner. Glaucoma is a significant public health care problem, with over 2.25 million Americans estimated to have the disease. Since approximately one-half of these individuals have undiagnosed glaucoma, it is imperative that practitioners evaluate their patients for the disease on a regular basis.[1]

An exhaustive amount of research has been done and a large volume of literature has been published concerning glaucoma. Numerous areas have been investigated including pathophysiologic concepts underlying aqueous humor flow, axonal damage at the optic nerve head, effects on visual function, epidemiology, diagnosis, and medical and surgical management. Despite this great body of knowledge, there is still much that is not known about this complex disease.

Making a diagnosis of glaucoma requires a comprehensive ocular examination with the examiner's attention directed toward the characteristic findings that are associated with the glaucomas. All of the specific techniques and procedures used in the diagnosis and management of glaucoma are essentially routine primary care skills. Many of these techniques have already been thoroughly reviewed in this text. This chapter concentrates on those procedures that have a particular importance in the diagnosis, treatment, and management of glaucoma. Specific therapeutic strategies are outlined to guide the practitioner in a systematic and rational approach to managing patients with glaucoma.

OVERVIEW OF GLAUCOMA

Definition and Classification

There have been numerous definitions of glaucoma proposed over the past two centuries, each reflecting the current understanding of the disease at the time. It is important to establish a good definition so that there is agreement in making a diagnosis for an individual patient. A definition that encompasses our current understanding of glaucoma and also emphasizes some important characteristics is:

> Glaucoma is a family of diseases in which an optic neuropathy occurs as manifested by the death of ganglion cell axons, which results in excavation of the optic nerve head. This damage causes characteristic nerve fiber bundle defects that produce visual field loss and other abnormalities of visual function. Whereas glaucoma is more common among those persons with elevated intraocular pressure (IOP), many individuals develop the neuropathy at low or normal pressure ranges. Most glaucomas have a chronic progression that can lead to blindness.

The many different forms of glaucoma can be broadly classified into three divisions: primary, secondary, and developmental (Table 25-1). These terms refer to the presence or absence of any underlying disorder responsible for elevated IOP. Within these three divisions, subclassifications can be made based on an open-angle or closed-angle mechanism.

Primary glaucomas are believed to have a multifactorial genetic basis and no known direct contribution from other ocular or systemic disorders. There may be, however, a variety of conditions that increase the risk of developing glaucoma. The primary glaucomas are generally bilateral but often present asymmetrically. They include primary open-angle glaucoma (POAG), normal tension glaucoma, and primary angle closure.

The secondary glaucomas are unilateral or bilateral and are always associated with an ocular or systemic abnormality that interferes with the outflow of aqueous humor. They are also subdivided into open-angle and closed-angle forms.

TABLE 25-1
Classification of the Glaucomas

Primary glaucomas
    Open angle
        High tension
        Normal tension/low-tension
    Closed angle with pupillary block
        Acute angle closure
        Subacute angle closure
        Chronic angle closure
    Closed angle without pupillary block
        Plateau iris syndrome
Secondary glaucomas
    Open angle
        Pigmentary glaucoma
        Exfoliative glaucoma
        Traumatic glaucoma
        Inflammatory related
        Lens related
        Steroid induced
        Following intraocular surgery
    Closed angle
        Anterior membrane contracture
            Neovascular
            Iridocorneal endothelial syndrome
            Inflammatory related
        With pupillary block
            Lens related
            Iris bombé and posterior synechia
Developmental glaucomas
    Primary congenital glaucoma
    Associated with congenital anomalies
        Aniridia
        Axenfeld-Rieger syndrome
        Lowe's syndrome
        Marfan's syndrome
        Microcornea
        Neurofibromatosis
        Sturge-Weber syndrome

Developmental glaucomas are those associated with increased resistance to aqueous outflow because of a congenital abnormality to the anterior chamber angle. Primary congenital glaucoma is a developmental glaucoma that is not associated with some other ocular or systemic abnormality.

Understanding the classification of the glaucomas gives the practitioner information about the underlying mechanisms (or lack of mechanisms) and helps direct treatment strategies more effectively.

Epidemiology

The prevalence and distribution of open-angle glaucoma has been investigated in numerous studies. Specific numbers vary between these investigations depending on the population studied and the specific criteria for detection that were defined. Information from the Framingham Eye Study gives an incidence range of 1.2–2.1% for open-angle glaucoma.[2]

The more recent Baltimore Eye Survey used a thorough battery of screening tests including applanation tonometry, automated perimetry, and ophthalmoscopy. A positive finding during the screening prompted referral for a complete ocular examination. Among the data studied the distribution of glaucoma among blacks and whites was compared. Primary open-angle glaucoma had an overall prevalence of 1.7% for whites and 5.6% for blacks. This demonstration of a risk that is 4.7 times greater in an urban black population points out the varying distribution of the disease in the United States.[3] The Beaver Dam Eye Study of a white population in Wisconsin found a prevalence of 2.1% for POAG.[4] European population studies have regularly shown a less than 1% prevalence of open-angle glaucoma.[5–7]

The prevalence of ocular hypertension has been found to be significantly higher than primary open-angle glaucoma. Ocular hypertension, like open-angle glaucoma, is strongly correlated with age. For individuals between 30 and 39 years of age, Armaly found a 1.25% incidence of ocular hypertension, while among those 70–79 years of age, the prevalence jumped to 10.5%.[8]

The development of glaucoma in subjects with ocular hypertension is a complex question. Numerous studies have shown that the majority of ocular hypertensives will never go on to develop glaucoma. A commonly cited Swedish study found a 1.5% incidence of glaucoma in ocular hypertensives who were followed for a 5-year period.[9] Another study of 124 ocular hypertensives followed for 5–7 years revealed a 3.23% incidence.[10] It is generally assumed that ocular hypertensives will develop glaucoma at a rate of approximately 1% per year, with large differences occurring depending on age, race, and other significant risk factors.[10–13]

In attempting to identify the prevalence of low-tension glaucoma, several studies of different populations have found a range of 0.5–0.79%.[14,15] The definition of low-tension glaucoma varies among investigators and thus the results of these studies do as well. Of significance is the percentage of all glaucoma patients who have low-tension glaucoma. It is generally accepted that low-tension glaucoma is not an uncommon form of open-angle glaucoma, occurring in 20–50% of all cases of glaucoma. The general impression that low-tension glaucoma is a rare form of glaucoma probably results from an overemphasis on IOP in making a diagnosis of glaucoma.

Primary angle closure is much less common than open-angle glaucoma. Among whites the frequency of angle closure is less than 0.1%.[6] Eskimos are well known to have a higher prevalence of acute angle closure. In one study of primary angle closure, the prevalence was almost 3% of the population, and 17% were thought to have occludable angles.[16] Certain Asian populations have been found to have a higher prevalence of acute angle closure than of primary open-angle glaucoma.[17] The prevalence of chronic angle closure is much higher among blacks than acute angle closure and frequently may be misdiagnosed as open-angle glaucoma because of the absence of symptoms.[18]

Pathophysiology

Glaucomatous optic neuropathy develops from the loss and death of ganglion cell axons, most often secondary to increased IOP. Two pertinent questions come to mind. First, why and how do some individuals develop elevated IOP? Second, how does that increased pressure damage axonal fibers? To answer these two questions an overview of the trabecular meshwork and optic nerve with regard to glaucoma is presented.

Aqueous Humor Outflow

After its production in the ciliary body and circulation from the posterior to anterior chamber, the aqueous humor must ultimately exit the eye. The trabecular meshwork and Schlemm's canal provide an outflow route for approximately 85% of the aqueous.[19] The remainder exits through the uveoscleral pathway, which involves the surface of the iris, its root, and interstitial spaces of the ciliary body, ultimately reaching the suprachoroidal space. The increased IOP in glaucoma is not the result of increased aqueous production; it originates with an increased resistance to outflow, primarily at the level of the outer portion of the trabecular meshwork and the inner wall of Schlemm's canal. Histologic studies of glaucomatous eyes in comparison with normal eyes show an acceleration of normal aging changes that significantly decrease outflow.[20,21] In normal individuals these aging changes are counterbalanced by an age-related decrease in aqueous production. Glaucoma may develop in those patients with risk factors that create greater than normal physiologic changes that result in a significantly higher resistance to aqueous outflow.

Increased resistance in the trabecular meshwork has been attributed to many specific histologic changes. Important changes include the loss of endothelial cells that cover the trabecular lamellae, an increase in extracellular material (plaque) that is deposited within the meshwork, and a decrease in the number and size of giant vacuoles on the inner wall of Schlemm's canal, which are critical in the movement of aqueous into the lumen of the canal.[22,23]

Numerous other histologic changes have been reported in glaucoma patients, although there is considerable disagreement and conflicting evidence in the literature. Any resistance to outflow from inside Schlemm's canal or the aqueous drainage veins is probably minimal.[24]

Varying degrees of these and other changes ultimately lead to an elevation of IOP via decreased aqueous outflow. When the IOP rises above an individual's "critical level," damage begins to take place that ultimately destroys ganglion cell axons.

Glaucomatous Optic Neuropathy

Maintenance of axonal transport is vital to the health and integrity of ganglion cell axons. It is responsible for the transfer of nutrients and intracytoplasmic materials along the entire length of the axon.[25] The axon courses from the retinal ganglion cell through the optic nerve, chiasm, and tract to its final synapse in the lateral geniculate body. Axonal transport is an energy-dependent process requiring oxygen and glucose from a nearby blood supply. Disruption of this transport mechanism will eventually cause cell death and atrophy. Either focal hypoxia or mechanical blockage to individual axons can cause obstruction of normal transport, and within days, weeks, or months axonal swelling and ultimate cellular disintegration take place. Whether the axonal death in glaucoma is caused by a vascular or a mechanical mechanism has not yet been determined, and this point remains a source of much controversy.[26–29]

The vascular theory suggests that ischemia secondary to increased IOP decreases axonal transport. The vascular supply to the optic nerve head is derived from retinal, choroidal, and short posterior ciliary arteries. Autoregulation of blood flow in the retina can respond to varying IOP; however, this takes place to a lesser degree in the optic nerve head. Thus, a rise in IOP would cause a decrease in blood flow to the optic nerve head and an ischemic state. Evidence in support of this theory includes decreased capillarity of the optic disc in glaucoma, poor autoregulation of the short posterior ciliary arteries serving the optic nerve head, progression of cupping after decreased blood flow, and the existence of low-tension glaucoma.[27,28,30]

The mechanical theory proposes that elevated IOP produces a backward bowing of the lamina cribrosa, leading to a misalignment of the pores through which nerve fiber bundles must pass. The scleral laminar sheets then act to bend and compress bundles of axonal fibers, which leads to a stasis of axoplasmic flow and subsequent axonal death.[31,32] The mechanical theory has been supported by numerous studies but does not adequately explain optic nerve damage in low-tension glaucoma. If it is possible to have progressive glaucomatous neuropathy without increased IOP, then factors other than mechanical compression of the lamina cribrosa must be involved.[33]

At present, optic nerve damage in glaucoma is felt to be multifactorial in origin. There may be components of both vascular and mechanical mechanisms in any individual patient. Glaucoma patients with dramatically elevated IOP could have axonal damage primarily from mechanical means, whereas in patients with low-tension glaucoma, vascular ischemia may be the cause.

Diagnosis and Workup

Open-angle glaucoma is typically present without patient symptoms in the early stages; thus it is frequently diagnosed after a routine ocular examination. A complete and thorough primary care examination that includes patient history, entrance tests, refraction, slit lamp biomicroscopy, tonometry, and dilated fundus examinations with stereoscopic optic disc evaluation will detect glaucoma in a majority of patients with the disease. Additional procedures necessary in the evaluation of glaucoma patients include gonioscopy, automated threshold visual fields, and stereoscopic optic nerve head photography.

History

As with most other ocular diseases, a complete history is an essential part of the examination of a patient suspected of having glaucoma. Vital to the history is the identification of risk factors that are known to contribute to the development of glaucoma. The incidence of glaucoma is clearly age related, and there is a higher prevalence among blacks. A positive family history of glaucoma also indicates a higher risk.[34,35]

Important aspects of a patient's ocular history that should be highlighted include a history of ocular trauma, past ocular surgery, symptoms of acute pressure elevation, symptoms of uveitis, and past long-term use of topical or oral steroids. Systemic medical history must also be thoroughly reviewed. Areas of particular relevance to glaucoma include the presence of diabetes mellitus, systemic hypertension, cardiovascular disease, thyroid disease, an episode of shock or significant blood loss, cerebrovascular disease, and any respiratory disease. Each of these is associated with a higher risk for the development of glaucoma or may lead to potential complications with future medical therapy. Drug allergies, current systemic medications, and past nonocular surgery should also be clearly documented.

Entrance Tests

Pupillary testing, color vision, and confrontation fields are routine entrance tests that can provide important diagnostic information in a glaucoma suspect. Pupillary testing that reveals an afferent (Marcus Gunn) pupillary defect may signify asymmetric glaucomatous optic nerve head damage. When present, an afferent pupillary defect should also be correlated with IOP levels and visual field status. Often IOP will be higher and visual field changes will be worse ipsilateral to the afferent pupillary defect.[36]

Since automated threshold perimetry has become the standard method in assessing the status of a patient's visual field, confrontation field testing only has the role of detecting gross glaucomatous visual field loss. Color vision testing with standard clinical techniques is not sensitive enough to detect early glaucomatous changes. Several research studies have demonstrated blue-yellow dyschromatopsia in both ocular hypertension and glaucoma; however, further longitudinal studies are needed to determine the actual significance of this.[37]

Slit Lamp Examination

The slit lamp examination is directed at the identification of structural abnormalities that would be an indication of a secondary glaucoma. These secondary changes, which may contribute to increased IOP, must be identified since they may dictate the particular course of therapy. The glaucoma suspect should be screened for secondary changes or abnormalities including a narrow peripheral chamber depth (a narrow van Herrick grade depth), signs of ocular trauma (corneal scars, iridodialysis, cataract), corneal endothelial pigmentation (Krukenberg's spindle), iris transillumination, rubeosis iridis, and signs of inflammation (keratic precipitates, cells and flare). Additional findings that may be noted include exfoliative material, glaukomflecken, posterior synechiae, and lens subluxation. Clinically, the anterior segment and crystalline lens appear normal in primary open-angle glaucoma.

Tonometry

Goldmann applanation tonometry is considered the standard for IOP measurement and is the preferred technique for assessing glaucoma patients.[38] In the workup and evaluation of glaucoma suspects, it is important to establish a baseline of multiple tonometry readings. Readings should be taken at different times throughout the day in an attempt to gauge diurnal fluctuations. The diurnal variation in IOP can be as much as 30 mm Hg in a glaucoma patient; thus any single reading is unlikely to be helpful in making a definitive diagnosis.[39-41] In general, diurnal fluctuations greater than 8–10 mm Hg are considered a risk for glaucoma. As discussed in Chapter 3, there are many different influences on IOP that should be considered in the evaluation of an individual patient who is suspected of having glaucoma. Although elevated IOP is certainly an important risk factor in the development of glaucoma, it is not the only one; IOP measurements should only be used in conjunction with other patient data.[42]

Gonioscopy

Gonioscopic examination is mandatory before making a diagnosis of any form of glaucoma. Even if the anterior chamber angles appear wide open with the van Herrick estimation, gonioscopy must be performed to rule out iridocorneal angle abnormalities. The specific angle structures visualized should be recorded appropriately for each eye. Additional comments are used to describe the width of the angle approach, the amount of trabecular pigmentation, and the presence or absence of iris processes, peripheral anterior synechiae, and neovascularization. Secondary open-angle glaucomas are thus identified and managed appropriately.

Visual Fields

A reduction of the visual field is the functional manifestation of the progressive loss of optic nerve fibers. In conjunction with tonometry and optic nerve head assessment, modern perimetry plays a vital role in the diagnosis and management of glaucoma. Available testing methods have improved dramatically over the past several decades. Automated static threshold perimetry currently has become the preferred method for complete visual field analysis. This brief discussion of visual fields and glaucoma will highlight the glaucomatous changes seen with automated perimeters.

Changes that characterize the glaucomatous visual field can be classified into two categories: generalized depressions and localized depressions. In general, diffuse depression of the visual field threshold may be the earliest detectable change.[43,44] This type of alteration does not occur in every glaucoma patient, nor is it a very specific change. After establishing a baseline with one to three visual field tests and after eliminating other potential causes, a documented reduction in the mean deviation (average decibel value) can indicate early glaucomatous damage.[45,46] Asymmetry between the two fields and correlation of visual field defects with ipsilateral elevated IOP or nerve head changes can help confirm this subtle finding.[47]

Localized visual field defects are caused by loss or impairment of the retinal nerve fiber bundles at the optic nerve head. These defects have a characteristic shape and location that are determined by the anatomic organization of the retinal nerve fiber layer.[48] Localized defects are easier to recognize than generalized depressions and will appear when only a small percentage of nerve fibers are destroyed. Nerve fiber bundle defects may present in a variety of patterns depending on which axons are dam-

aged and the extent of the damage. Paracentral defects, arcuate defects, and nasal steps are among the earliest localized scotomas to develop in glaucoma.[49,50] Among others, optic nerve drusen, disc edema, and optic neuritis are distinct congenital and pathologic causes of nerve fiber bundle defects that must be ruled out in these cases. Progression of axonal damage at the optic nerve causes an increase in the size and depth of these defects, eventually forming a dense arcuate or even an altitudinal field defect. Differing rates of axonal death at the superior and inferior poles of the optic nerve cause asymmetry between the superior and inferior visual hemifields. The earliest of depressions may be recognized by comparing mirror-image points in the two hemifields across the horizontal midline.[51]

There has been research demonstrating that the visual field defects found in low-tension glaucoma are slightly different than those found in primary open-angle glaucoma. Low-tension glaucoma may be characterized by field defects that are denser, steeper, and closer to fixation[52–54] (Figure 25-1). The exact cause of this is uncertain. Some studies have found no such significant differences.[55]

A central island or temporal island of vision may be all that remains after extensive glaucomatous atrophy. The temporal island is often not detected with automated perimetry programs that concentrate only on the central 30 degrees.

After characteristic glaucomatous defects to the visual field are identified, it is perhaps of even greater importance to monitor the field for progression. Unfortunately, this can often be a difficult task. Various factors, both disease-related (glaucoma) and patient-related, cause a fluctuation or variability in the visual field on repeated testing. Improved statistical analysis of numeric decibel values on multiple field examinations has attempted to correct for these fluctuations, allowing isolation of changes in the visual fields that are solely caused by the disease itself.[56,57]

Since clinically detectable nerve head changes precede visual field defects, it is usually possible to demonstrate a correlation between these two findings.[58,59] Patients with notching of the inferior neuroretinal rim will most likely have a superior arcuate scotoma. If there is not a good correlation, other potential causes or artifacts should be investigated. Relying on automated visual fields alone to diagnose early glaucoma can result in a significant delay in diagnosis.[60] When a repeatable loss of only 5 dB in retinal sensitivity is detected on automated perimetry, up to 20% of the ganglion cells may be destroyed in that area.[61] It is clear that damage is taking place before the perimetry is able to demonstrate a change in visual function. Thus, the emphasis should be on optic nerve head assess-

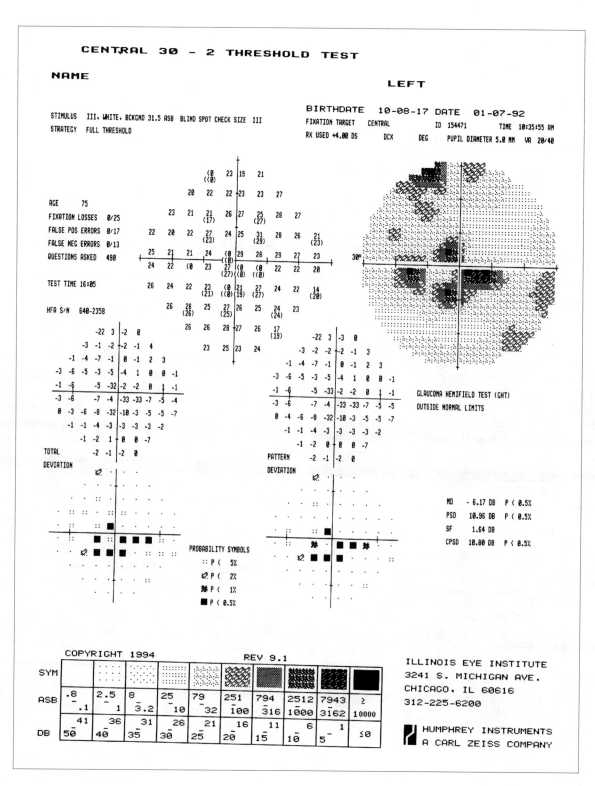

FIGURE 25-1

Automated visual field of a patient with low-tension glaucoma. The associated scotomatous defects are dense and close to fixation.

ment. Progressive field changes are more helpful in the advanced stages of glaucoma, whereas optic nerve head changes are more helpful in the early stages.

Short wavelength automated perimetry (SWAP) has been found to be more sensitive to early glaucomatous damage than traditional testing methods.[62] Here, a blue stimulus is projected onto a yellow background of a specially modified bowl perimeter. By targeting the short wavelength–sensitive (SWS) neural pathway, investigators have found defects appearing 3–5 years before they appear in white-on-white perimetry. The SWS pathway is therefore possibly more sensitive to increases in IOP. There are some difficulties with blue-yellow visual fields, including the current lack of normative data, influences from cataracts, and variable testing results. Its future role in clinical practice will be defined when these and other questions are answered.

The reversibility of glaucomatous visual field defects has been reported in several studies.[63] Although it does not occur in all patients, it can be seen in those with early glaucomatous field loss who have a dramatic reduction in IOP at the beginning of therapy.

Optic Nerve Examination

Ophthalmoscopic evaluation of the optic nerve provides the most reliable evidence of early glaucomatous change. It must be remembered that the use of IOP alone to differentiate between healthy and glaucomatous eyes is not always effective, and the search for early glaucomatous visual field defects is confounded by patient variability and subjectivity. Much attention has thus been directed at the identification of early changes in the retinal nerve fiber layer and optic nerve head in glaucoma. There is now sufficient clinical evidence demonstrating that damage to these structures occurs before the development of measurable and reproducible visual field defects.[64–66] Knowledge and recognition of these morphologic changes is thus an essential component of every glaucoma workup.

Proper evaluation techniques require that the optic nerve be examined with stereopsis and magnification.[67] Any of the currently available slit lamp indirect fundus lenses that achieve this are satisfactory. Diagrams that emphasize the contour, depth of cupping, and integrity of the neuroretinal rim (not just the cup-to-disc [C/D] ratio) should be regularly included in the record. Color photography of the optic nerve, preferably stereoscopic, is also essential in monitoring progressive atrophy.[59] Without detailing the normal anatomy of the optic nerve head and retinal nerve fiber layer, further discussion of the patterns of early and late glaucomatous optic atrophy will be given.

Glaucomatous Excavation   Cupping of the optic nerve is the most well known and distinguishing feature of glaucoma. The excavation of ganglion cell axons, glial tissue, and vascular tissue produces a backward bowing of the lamina cribrosa and an enlargement in the cup-to-disc ratio. This type of tissue loss and excavation is rarely seen in optic neuropathies other than glaucoma.[68] Early changes in glaucoma are the result of the loss of nerve fiber bundles at the optic nerve head. This loss is recognizable as thinning as well as other visible changes in the neuroretinal rim. The loss of rim tissue may be either localized or generalized, and the location of damaged rim tissue will correlate with its respective visual field projection (Figure 25-2). As the neuroretinal rim becomes thinner, the optic cup increases. Because all disc changes in glaucoma are typically asymmetric and progressive, these features can be helpful in the differentiation of normal versus abnormal optic nerves.[69–71]

Localized Thinning   Loss of neuroretinal rim tissue may occur over a focal area of the cup rim. This selective loss of tissue creates a "notching" of the rim (Figure 25-3). Focal notching of the neuroretinal rim most commonly occurs at the superior and inferior poles of the optic nerve head, although it can be detected at other locations along the temporal rim as well. This focal loss of tissue is highly specific for glaucoma, which must be strongly considered regardless of other findings (e.g., IOP and visual field results). With progression, focal notching may extend all the way outward until there is complete atrophy of the nerve fiber tissue, leaving a "sharpened disc margin." With prominent notching in the superior or inferior disc region, there is typically a corresponding visual field loss opposite to the focal excavation (i.e., a superior notch causes an inferior visual field defect). Selective loss at the superior and inferior poles of the neuroretinal rim is characteristic of glaucoma and frequently produces "vertical elongation" of the cup.

Generalized Enlargement   In contrast to focal notching, glaucomatous nerves may also show a concentric or generalized thinning of the neuroretinal rim 360 degrees around. This may present a difficult diagnostic dilemma, because large, normal physiologic cups may have a very similar appearance.[72,73] Fortunately this uniform loss of axonal tissue is a less common glaucomatous change than the easier to identify localized changes. In cases of generalized enlargement, it is important to compare the affected eye with the fellow eye for symmetry and to study serial photographs for evidence of progressive change. Asymmetry greater than 0.2 in the cup-to-disc ratio is found in only 1% of the normal population; thus, this finding is highly indicative of glaucoma.[74]

FIGURE 25-2
Diagram of a left optic nerve head illustrating the neural rim (top) and a corresponding schematic showing the anatomic origin of retinal nerve fiber axons (bottom). Localized damage to the nerve head will correspond to the respective visual field projection.

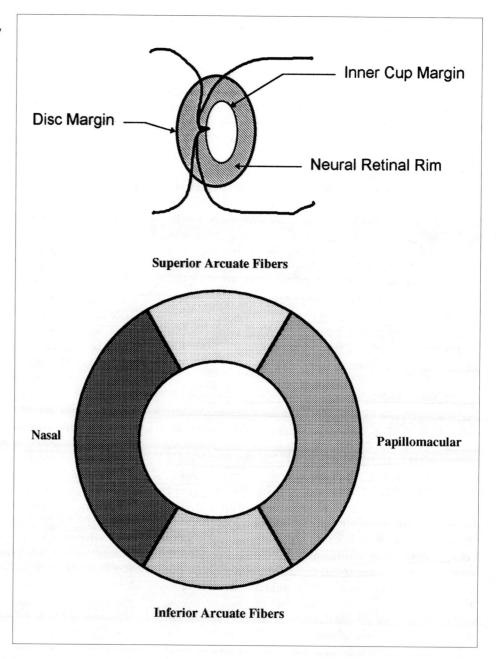

Deepening of the Cup Often in glaucoma, exposure of the lamina cribrosa to elevated IOP causes a backward bowing of the cup base. As the layers of the lamina collapse on one another and nerve fiber bundles atrophy, there is increased visualization of the gray laminar fenestrations. This is termed the *laminar dot sign.* Laminar dots that are striate in appearance are more specific for glaucoma, whereas round dots are more likely to be physiologic.[75,76] Stereoscopic viewing readily demonstrates this morphologic deepening of the optic cup.

A frequently confusing issue in glaucomatous optic neuropathy involves the development of pallor from the atrophy of axonal tissue. Central pallor of the physiologic cup is a normal finding resulting from light reflection off the lamina cribrosa. Pallor of the neuroretinal rim, when the rim tissue has not atrophied away, is 90% specific for nonglaucomatous optic atrophy.[68] In glaucoma, the neural rim will lose some of its healthy color but will not become completely pale and atrophic. A "pallor/cup" discrepancy develops when atrophy and

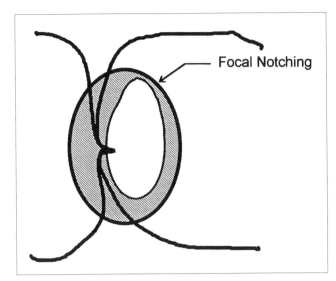

Focal Notching

A

FIGURE 25-3
A. Schematic illustrating focal notching of the superior neuroretinal rim tissue. B. Photograph showing superior notching in a left optic nerve head.

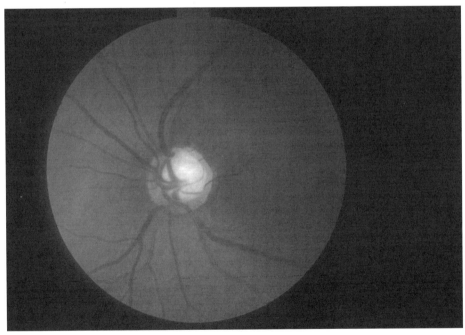

B

loss of the rim progresses ahead of the central area of pallor, which will also eventually progress outward to the disc margin (Figure 25-4).[13] Grading the size of the cup or the integrity of the neuroretinal rim based on color changes and monocular cues can often result in highly erroneous measurements.

Vascular Changes of the Glaucomatous Nerve Observation of the surrounding vessels may be helpful in the diagnosis of glaucoma. "Baring" of the circumlinear ves-

sels refers to the exposure of small branch vessels that run along the inside of the cup margin, which are normally in contact with the neural rim. Circumlinear vessels are present in about 50% of normal eyes. When glaucomatous atrophy causes outward expansion of the inner rim margin, the vessel remains behind and becomes "bared." Pallor, indicating loss of tissue, is then noted in the space between the vessel and the inner cup margin (Figure 25-5). This finding is relatively specific for glaucoma.[77]

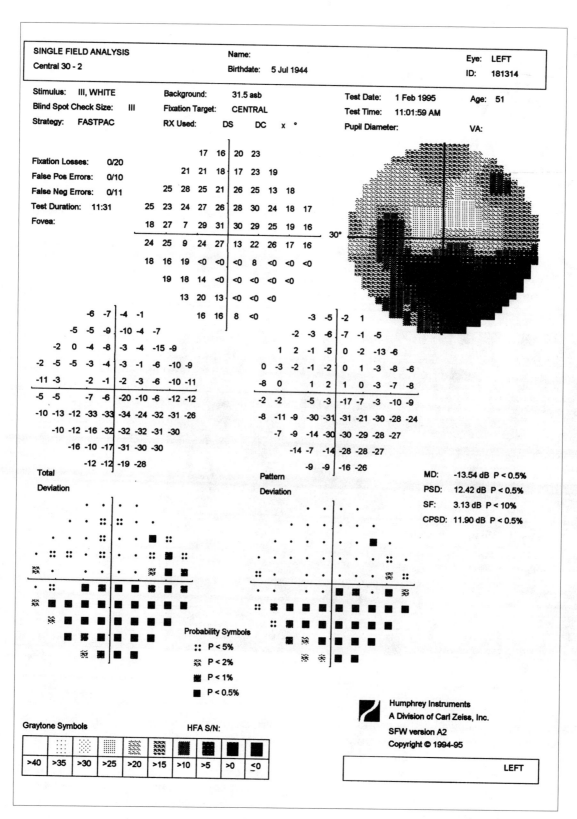

SINGLE FIELD ANALYSIS
Central 30 - 2

Name:
Birthdate: 5 Jul 1944

Eye: LEFT
ID: 181314

Stimulus: III, WHITE
Blind Spot Check Size: III
Strategy: FASTPAC

Background: 31.5 asb
Fixation Target: CENTRAL
RX Used: DS DC x °

Test Date: 1 Feb 1995
Test Time: 11:01:59 AM
Pupil Diameter:

Age: 51

VA:

Fixation Losses: 0/20
False Pos Errors: 0/10
False Neg Errors: 0/11
Test Duration: 11:31
Fovea:

```
                17  16  20  23
            21  21  18  17  23  19
        25  28  25  21  26  25  13  18
    25  23  24  27  26  28  30  24  18  17
    18  27   7  29  31  30  29  25  19  16
    24  25   9  24  27  13  22  26  17  16
    18  16  19  <0  <0  <0   8  <0  <0  <0
        19  18  14  <0  <0  <0  <0
            13  20  13  <0  <0  <0
                16  16   8  <0
```

30°

Total Deviation

```
            -6  -7  -4  -1
        -5  -5  -9 -10  -4  -7
    -2   0  -4  -8  -3  -4 -15  -9
-2  -5  -5  -3  -4  -3  -1  -6 -10  -9
-11 -3      -2  -1  -2  -3  -6 -10 -11
-5  -5      -7  -6 -20 -10  -6 -12 -12
-10 -13 -12 -33 -33 -34 -24 -32 -31 -26
    -10 -12 -16 -32 -32 -32 -31 -30
        -16 -10 -17 -31 -30 -30
            -12 -12 -19 -28
```

Pattern Deviation

```
            -3  -5  -2   1
        -2  -3  -6  -7  -1  -5
     1   2  -1  -5   0  -2 -13  -6
 0  -3  -2  -1  -2   0   1  -3  -8  -6
-8   0       1   2   1   0  -3  -7  -8
-2  -2      -5  -3 -17  -7  -3 -10  -9
-8 -11  -9 -30 -31 -31 -21 -30 -28 -24
    -7  -9 -14 -30 -30 -29 -28 -27
       -14  -7 -14 -28 -28 -27
            -9  -9 -16 -26
```

MD: -13.54 dB P < 0.5%
PSD: 12.42 dB P < 0.5%
SF: 3.13 dB P < 10%
CPSD: 11.90 dB P < 0.5%

Probability Symbols
:: P < 5%
※ P < 2%
▥ P < 1%
■ P < 0.5%

Humphrey Instruments
A Division of Carl Zeiss, Inc.
SFW version A2
Copyright © 1994-95

LEFT

Graytone Symbols | | | | | | | | | |
HFA S/N:

>40	>35	>30	>25	>20	>15	>10	>5	>0	≤0

FIGURE 25-3 (Continued)

C. Visual field of the left eye shown in B. There is a dense inferior defect corresponding to the superior notch.

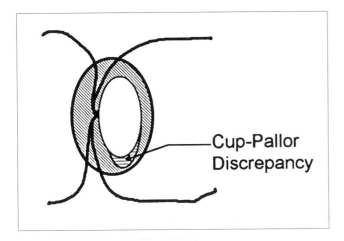

FIGURE 25-4

Atrophy of the neuroretinal rim, which progresses outward at a rate ahead of the progression of pallor is characteristic of glaucoma. In this example, shallow excavation extends nearly out to the disc margin inferiorly, whereas the region of overt cup pallor lags considerably behind.

Drance hemorrhages are small splinter hemorrhages that occasionally occur at the disc margin or on the neural rim in patients with glaucoma. They are transient in nature and are more commonly seen in low-tension glaucoma.[78] These hemorrhages are not specific for glaucoma, so other causes must be ruled out (e.g., hypertension, posterior vitreous detachment). There is some evidence that these hemorrhages signify impending nerve damage and visual field loss regardless of apparent past IOP control.[79] Patients should be monitored carefully after this observation.[80]

Nasalization of the vessels within the cup occurs in normal eyes and is not considered to be a specific change in glaucoma. It therefore has a minimal role in the diagnosis of glaucoma.[81] Bayonetting of vessels is another term used in glaucoma to describe the sharp kinking of vessels as they exit a deep cup onto the retinal surface. It appears with advanced cupping when the rim tissue is completely obliterated. This vascular change also is not helpful in the diagnosis of early glaucoma.

Retinal Nerve Fiber Layer Defects In addition to the optic nerve head, the retinal nerve fiber layer (RNFL) is readily observable in many patients and has been repeatedly found to demonstrate some of the earliest glaucomatous clinically detectable changes.[66,82,83] The striations of the RNFL are best viewed when a red-free filter and specialized black-and-white photography are used for enhancement. They are most prominent as they course in an arcuate fashion from the superior and inferior poles of the optic nerve across the temporal retina. The death of axonal fibers and bundles in the nerve cause large defects in the RNFL. These defects appear as dark/black stripes in the normally white reflective nerve fiber layer. Both localized and diffuse patterns may appear.[58,83] These defects have been regularly found to precede recognizable changes in the optic nerve head and visual fields.[64,66,82,83] Unfortunately, media opacities can significantly degrade the view of the RNFL, making its observation much less useful in elderly patients. Some investigators are now measuring the thickness of the RNFL at the disc margin and have noted that thinning of the RNFL is another early glaucomatous change.[84,85] The challenge is to find a method that is clinically feasible for obtaining these measurements.

All of the preceding glaucomatous changes emphasize one important concept: When evaluating a patient for glaucoma, greater emphasis must be placed on the health and integrity of the neuroretinal rim than on the cup-to-disc ratio. Evidence of focal neuroretinal rim tissue loss and progressive thinning of the rim is much easier to detect and much more reliable in glaucoma diagnosis than an increase in the C/D ratio.[67,86]

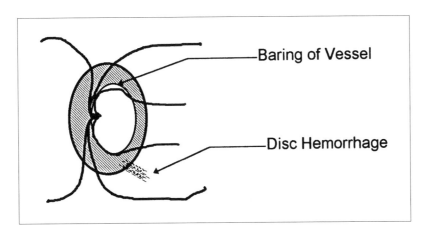

FIGURE 25-5

Schematic illustrating "baring" of a superior circumlinear vessel, as well as a typical position of small splinter hemorrhages that occasionally form at the disc margin in glaucomatous eyes.

To improve our capabilities for the earliest possible detection of these optic nerve changes, new instruments are being developed that provide a computerized scanning laser image analysis of the optic disc. These devices use a variety of techniques in providing quantitative information about the topography of the nerve head. Three-dimensional analysis can provide numerical data on the depth of cupping, the width and area of the neuroretinal rim, the thickness of the nerve fiber layer, and several other calculations that may prove to be specific for glaucoma. In the future an affordable, reliable, and easy to use instrument may be developed to dramatically change the way glaucoma is diagnosed.[87]

PRIMARY GLAUCOMAS

Primary Open-Angle Glaucoma

Primary open-angle glaucoma (POAG) is the most common form of glaucoma, accounting for approximately 70% of all cases.[88] Since there is no way to restore damaged nerve fibers, it is crucial that the disease be detected as early as possible. In many patients with equivocal findings, early and accurate detection requires a thorough and complete examination and evaluation of risk factors.

Three main areas must be evaluated in a glaucoma patient: the optic nerve head, visual fields, and tonometry findings. Glaucomatous changes occur to the optic nerve before the appearance of glaucomatous visual field defects, and the clinical detection of these nerve head changes dictates initiation of therapy regardless of IOP or visual field changes.[86,89]

Whereas older definitions of POAG often stipulated IOP readings consistently over 21 mm Hg, there is now substantial evidence to show that many patients can develop glaucoma with normal pressure. Thus, whereas multiple IOP readings or diurnal curves can facilitate a diagnosis or initiation of therapy, greater emphasis must be placed on the stereoscopic evaluation of the optic nerve and awareness of the possibility of low-tension glaucoma.

Ocular Hypertension

Ocular hypertension (OHTN) is defined as a repeatedly elevated IOP in patients who do not demonstrate any glaucomatous optic nerve or visual field changes. Commonly, IOP readings over 21 mm Hg are considered elevated based on the concept that this pressure level is greater than two standard deviations above the mean.[13,90] The suggestion is that these patients are at risk for developing glaucomatous damage at some point in the future. It is difficult to say exactly how much of a risk is present. Certainly not all of these patients will go on to develop glaucoma, and in fact most ocular hypertensives will never develop glaucoma. There are no absolute indicators or predictors of which patients will develop glaucoma. As in POAG, all risk factors must be evaluated together and the clinician and patient should discuss the costs and benefits of medical intervention.

Patients with few or no additional risk factors other than OHTN often can be followed on a regular basis with careful and repeated observation of the optic nerve head and visual field testing. Typically these patients are monitored every 3–6 months, and treatment is initiated when changes to the nerve or visual field are reliably demonstrated.[91]

Other patients, either because of additional risk factors and clinician or patient preference, may elect for early prophylactic therapy. For these cases the medication must be effective and well tolerated without significant side effects.

There may be an upper level of IOP above which all patients should receive treatment. A value of 30 mm Hg is often identified as the cutoff point where the risk for future optic neuropathy is considered too great to leave the elevated IOP untreated.[92]

Another group of patients are those who have IOPs between 21 mm Hg and 25 mm Hg and who have two or three additional risk factors for glaucoma. When these factors include a positive family history for glaucoma, diabetes, or hypertension, treatment is usually initiated. In these patients the accumulated risk factors dictate early therapy.

The fourth type of ocular hypertensive patient is one whose IOP is repeatedly between 25 and 30 mm Hg and who does not have any other risk factors. After discussing the pros and cons of treatment with the patient, a trial of prophylactic therapy can be initiated. Therapy can be continued in patients who respond well to a trial of topical medication without side effects. For those patients who do not respond, alternative medications should be used. If no medications are found to be effective without tolerable side effects, and no signs of glaucomatous damage develop, then the patient can be followed without treatment until definitive changes appear and more aggressive therapy is mandated.[92,93]

Low-Tension Glaucoma

Low-tension glaucoma (LTG), sometimes termed *normotensive glaucoma*, is characterized by glaucomatous optic atrophy, corresponding visual field defects, normal-appearing and open anterior chamber angles, and IOPs that never exceed the upper limit of statistically normal.

Commonly this value is considered to be 20 or 21 mm Hg. No other medical or neurologic disease that could cause the neuropathy should be identifiable.[52,53,94]

No single mechanism has been discovered to satisfactorily explain low-tension glaucoma. Numerous theories have attempted to mold the mechanical and vascular theories of POAG to fit the unique conditions of low IOP and optic neuropathy. Mechanically, patients with LTG could have a structurally weak lamina from a connective tissue abnormality, making it susceptible to backward bowing even in the normal pressure range.[95,96] Vasospasm and chronic vascular ischemia could also contribute significantly to the disease process in LTG; however, it must be a localized process at the optic nerve head because a definitive link between generalized vascular disease (atherosclerotic or hyperviscosity) has not been found.[97-100]

LTG is often misdiagnosed because a lower index of suspicion is applied to patients with normal intraocular tension. Greater emphasis must be placed on the optic nerve head examination for proper diagnosis. The prevalence of LTG ranges from 6% to 65% among all patients with glaucoma, depending on the definition used and patient population studied.[94] It is now generally accepted that LTG constitutes a significant proportion of all glaucoma cases and that it is not a rare condition.

There are several clinical findings that characterize some patients with LTG. Optic disc cupping tends to be shallow with gentle temporal sloping compared with the findings in patients with POAG.[101] Some studies, however, have not found these differences to be significant.[102,103] Visual field defects may demonstrate a higher frequency of dense, isolated scotomas close to fixation, more often in the superior hemifield.[53-55] Again some studies have not found these differences between LTG and POAG.[52]

LTG is often considered to be a diagnosis of exclusion. An ocular and medical workup must rule out any other potential causes of optic neuropathy and visual field loss. Diurnal measurement of IOP may detect spikes not previously recorded, thus eliciting a diagnosis of true POAG. Secondary glaucomas that have wide fluctuations in IOP such as pigmentary and exfoliative glaucoma should be excluded. Congenital disc anomalies such as optic pits, colobomas, optic nerve drusen, or oblique nerve insertion may also be mistaken for LTG. Other nonglaucomatous optic neuropathies such as anterior ischemic optic neuropathy, optic neuritis, compressive lesions, and disc edema generally do not produce excavation and cupping of the nerve head and can often be distinguished by clinical examination. A notable exception to this may be giant cell arteritis; patients with this entity have shown glaucomatous-like cupping.[104,105]

Medical workup of patients suspected of having LTG should include a complete physical examination to rule out vascular disease, endocrine and neurologic abnormalities, and blood dyscrasias. Further investigation with computed tomography or magnetic resonance imaging is somewhat controversial for patients suspected of having LTG. Careful stereoscopic examination, which detects characteristic glaucomatous cupping and corresponding visual field loss, may be all that is necessary to confirm the diagnosis. When clinical data are less conclusive, cranial imaging may be performed. Guidelines for imaging may include (1) patients under 65–70 years of age; (2) patients with rapidly progressing field loss; and (3) patients with unusual visual field loss or significant pallor to the neuroretinal rim tissue that is inconsistent with the amount of cupping.[91,94]

The treatment of LTG is also controversial. There has not been a study to demonstrate the benefit of treatment in LTG. Several investigators claim that since up to 60% of patients with LTG do not show progression, treatment should be withheld until progression is documented.[106,107] Hitchings studied patients with LTG who were surgically managed in one eye while the fellow eye remained untreated. He found no difference in the progression of visual field loss between the two eyes 15 months later.[108]

Most sources agree, however, that medical or surgical therapy is prudent, if not definitively beneficial.[109] The treatment goal is to obtain the lowest IOP possible and prevent further vision loss. Medical therapy usually begins with a beta-blocker because these provide the greatest reduction in IOP. However, some claim that topical beta-blockers will cause vasoconstriction and reduce blood flow to the optic nerve head, thereby worsening the hypoxic state and contributing to reduced axonal transport.[110] A prostaglandin agonist such as latanoprost, the topical carbonic anhydrase inhibitor dorzolamide, pilocarpine, or dipivefrin, if effective, might then have some theoretical role as first-line agents in LTG. Some researchers are investigating the use of systemic calcium channel blockers, which could dilate arterioles to the optic nerve head and improve blood flow and possibly reverse visual field defects.[111] Oral antiglaucoma agents can be used in LTG when they are tolerated by the patient. Argon laser trabeculoplasty is less effective in LTG and may not halt the progression of the disease.[112,113] Its ease of application and infrequent side effects often prompt its use despite the short-lasting reduction in IOP. Filtration surgery may be the best option for patients with LTG, because it can provide the greatest lowering of IOP and avoid chronic topical therapy.[114] In summary, the treatment of LTG is difficult and controversial, and a stepwise approach similar to that for POAG may be most judicious for those LTG patients with progressive disease.

Clinical Approach to the Medical Management of Primary Open-Angle Glaucoma

The selection of a regimen of medications used to manage a patient with glaucoma often follows a relatively well-established sequence (Figure 25-6). Decisions about the best pharmacologic agent are based on numerous systemic and ocular factors. Often a "therapeutic goal" is established. This is a target IOP that once attained would most likely prevent any further glaucomatous change. This theoretical pressure is based on the analysis of pretreatment IOP, the percentage of visual field loss, and optic nerve damage. Patients with greater amounts of glaucomatous damage require a more substantial lowering of pressure. Medications must be evaluated for their potential ocular and systemic side effects on the patient. The goal is always to use the lowest effective dose possible that also halts progressive glaucomatous damage.

Nonselective beta-blockers are the most frequently chosen agents for initiation of therapy. They provide significant reduction in IOP, are relatively convenient with once or twice per day administration, and potentially significant side effects are infrequently encountered with proper patient selection. If beta-blockers alone do not provide sufficient IOP control, then dorzolamide 2%, a topical carbonic anhydrase inhibitor generally is the next agent added because of its good additivity. Dipivefrin, an epinephrine derivative, has been shown to have only a minor (1–3 mm Hg) effect in lowering IOP when added to nonselective beta-blockers.[115] Although this pressure reduction is small, the decrease may be enough for some patients. It must be weighed against the cost and potential side effects of the agent. In many cases it is a better decision to add pilocarpine as a third glaucoma medication. Ocular side effects are common with pilocarpine, but its additive effects with topical beta-blockers is usually quite significant. If tolerated by the patient, increasing concentrations of pilocarpine can be substituted when the IOP rises above the target pressure.

Oral carbonic anhydrase inhibitors (e.g., acetazolamide) are the next class of medications typically added to the therapeutic regimen. These medications are quite valuable in lowering of IOP. Some practitioners choose to avoid the agents altogether because of the associated systemic side effects and offer laser trabeculoplasty to their patients as an alternative. Decisions such as this are made on an individual basis and should be made after a discussion of the future implications with the patient. A trial period of oral carbonic anhydrase inhibitors is a possibility before recommending laser therapy.[116]

A prostaglandin analog of PGF$_{2\alpha}$, latanoprost, has recently been developed. Latanoprost significantly lowers the IOP by increasing uveoscleral outflow. As such, it may have an additive effect with the beta-blockers. In comparison to timolol, latanoprost gives a statistically greater reduction in IOP.[117] A possible side effect of the drug is increased pigmentation of light-colored irides.

Once treatment has been instituted, the task of determining the efficacy of treatment begins. The frequency of follow-up visits should be influenced by the degree of optic nerve and visual field damage and by the level of compliance exhibited by the patient. Newly diagnosed cases are followed more frequently during the first few months to monitor the hypotensive effects of the drugs, as would be the case when medications are changed. Established cases of early to moderate glaucoma with controlled pressure are often monitored at 4- to 6-month intervals. Cases of advanced glaucoma, especially those with danger of central vision loss, should be monitored more frequently (e.g., every 2–3 months). Adequacy of treatment is gauged by evaluating the same data that were used in making the diagnosis. As previously stated, visible changes to the optic nerve supersede tonometry and visual field findings.

Monitoring of IOP levels during treatment should be conducted at various times of the day to reflect both diurnal IOP fluctuations and the ocular hypotensive effect of treatment. Stereoscopic disc evaluations should be performed at least yearly and more frequently in advanced cases. Fundus photographs of the optic nerve head (preferably also stereoscopic) should be taken before treatment to establish a baseline appearance and repeated annually or when any change in disc appearance is detected during follow-up care.

Threshold perimetry should be conducted at intervals commensurate with the degree of optic nerve damage. Established cases of long-term ocular hypertension without documented visual field loss may appropriately be tested every 8–12 months. Patients with moderate disease should have their visual fields tested every 6 months. Advanced cases often require that perimetry be performed every 3–6 months. Patients with very advanced disease will show greater changes to their visual field relative to visible optic nerve head changes because the significant axonal loss and large cupping precludes the detection of any further morphologic changes to the nerve.

Patient compliance with medical therapy is an important issue in a chronic disease such as glaucoma. A patient's failure to properly adhere to the treatment regimen can have a significant impact on the course of the disease. Patient education can help convey the significance of proper drug administration. Awareness of the possibility of noncompliance is very important, and taking steps to correct it is a considerable effort in the management of glaucoma.[118]

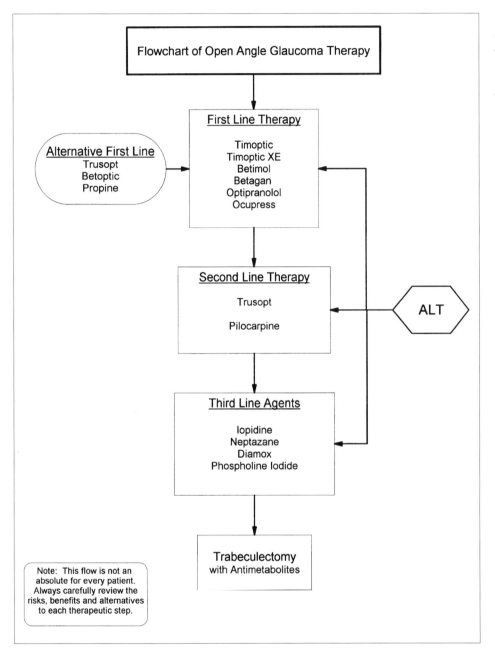

FIGURE 25-6
An overview of a typical sequence of glaucoma management. Each case must be approached individually, and significant alterations in the selection of medications and the organization of this chart are possible.

At any point during follow-up care, a decision may need to be made to modify the treatment when disease progression is recognized or the effectiveness of therapy in controlling the IOP is diminished. If it is determined that medications currently being used are still effective in lowering IOP, then additional medications are added to treat the advancing disease. If it is suspected that a certain medication has lost its effectiveness in lowing IOP, then the medication should be discontinued and a new one substituted. It is best to add a single agent at a time so that its solitary effectiveness can be evaluated.[13]

Primary Angle-Closure Glaucoma

Primary angle-closure glaucoma is defined as increased IOP and obstruction of aqueous outflow resulting from closure of the drainage angle by the peripheral iris. It primarily affects elderly persons and those with predisposing narrow angles. Primary angle-closure glaucoma can be classified as acute, subacute, and chronic. There is a continuum among these three forms in signs and symptoms.

Pupillary block is the underlying mechanism in the acute, subacute, and chronic forms of primary angle closure. This term refers to the functional block between the posterior iris and the anterior lens surface. Most commonly in the mid-dilated state, direct contact between these structures can prevent aqueous from flowing into the anterior chamber. As pressure increases in the posterior chamber, the peripheral iris is pushed farther up against the trabecular meshwork. Pupillary block is the underlying mechanism in all types of primary angle closure, except the plateau iris syndrome.[18,119]

Acute Angle Closure   In acute angle closure there is a sudden and significant rise in IOP resulting from complete or extensive closure of the anterior chamber angle. The patient notices blurred, foggy vision with halos, a red, painful eye, and there may be nausea and vomiting. If not treated properly, loss of vision may occur within hours.

Subacute Angle Closure   In subacute angle closure, there are brief, repeated attacks of increased IOP. A portion of the angle temporarily closes, elevating the pressure. The attack is self-resolving. The patient is often symptomatic. Subacute angle closure can cause glaucomatous changes to the optic nerve head and may lead to acute angle closure. Repeated attacks may cause the progressive development of peripheral anterior synechiae (PAS) from the iris coming in contact with the trabecular meshwork and anterior chamber angle. The development of PAS can lead to gradual closure of the entire filtration angle; in blacks this may progress to chronic angle closure.[18,119,120]

Chronic Angle Closure   In chronic angle closure, there is a slow, insidious rise in IOP as there is progressive closure of the angle. The patient is usually asymptomatic because of the eye's adaptation to high pressure. The eye is often white and quiet. Unless gonioscopy is performed, chronic angle closure may be mistaken for open-angle glaucoma.

Plateau Iris Configuration   Plateau iris configuration is a rare condition and refers to eyes with an unusual anatomic configuration to the angle. Just beyond its insertion into the ciliary body, the iris root angles forward, creating a narrow iridocorneal recess. After a forward angulation within the angle, the iris then courses centrally creating a plateau-like configuration. The anterior chamber remains relatively deep centrally but is narrow peripherally. Because of the anomalous configuration of the peripheral iris, obstruction of the trabecular meshwork occurs with pupillary dilation, despite the absence of pupillary block (see Figure 6-4). It is very difficult to diagnose this condition with gonioscopy. Rather, the diagnosis is usually made when angle closure occurs despite the presence of a patent iridotomy. Here pupillary block has been eliminated but the structural relationship between the peripheral iris and inner wall of the eye still leads to occlusion of the trabecular meshwork.[121]

In most populations, primary angle closure is much less common than open-angle glaucoma. Whereas 6% of the population may have narrow angles (gonioscopic grade II or less), only 2% are critically narrow, and less than 1% ever go on to develop angle closure. The typical angle-closure patient is over 60 years old, white, female, and hyperopic. Family history is generally not contributory.

Clinical Examination

Patient symptoms in acute angle closure are typically very characteristic, thus allowing for a rapid diagnosis. They include deep, aching pain around the eye; diffuse redness; blurred vision, possibly with halos around lights; and often nausea and vomiting. Symptoms for patients with subacute angle closure are similar, but to a milder degree; the symptoms are also always self-resolving after a couple of hours. Chronic angle closure is asymptomatic unless IOP becomes exceedingly high.

In an acute angle closure attack, there is pronounced conjunctival hyperemia and circumlimbal injection; a cloudy, edematous cornea; an oval mid-dilated pupil; and, if visible, cells and flare in a shallow anterior chamber. IOP is usually between 40 and 70 mm Hg or even higher.

It is essential to confirm the diagnosis of angle closure by viewing a closed anterior chamber angle with gonioscopy. Topical glycerin may be necessary to reduce corneal edema. Gonioscopy of the fellow eye should also show a narrowed angle when primary angle closure is present. While a three-mirror lens gives a reliable view, the Zeiss four-mirror lens can be used for indentation gonioscopy to distinguish between synechial and appositional closure (see Figure 6-24).[122,123]

Differential Diagnosis

The sudden onset of pain, redness, and blurred vision with high IOP is almost always secondary to acute angle closure; however, other forms of glaucoma must be ruled out. Open-angle glaucoma may occasionally present as an acute attack when associated with uveitis or hemorrhage. In patients with narrow but open angles, it may be difficult to distinguish the underlying cause. A laser iridotomy will obviously remove any pupillary block that may be causing angle closure. Secondary angle closure has several different mechanisms and may be associated with neovascularization, tumors, ciliary body swelling, central retinal vein occlusion, and other disorders.[18,119,124]

Management

There are three goals to managing a patient with acute angle closure: (1) rapidly reducing the IOP, (2) opening the filtration angle, and (3) preventing further attacks. Medical therapy is the first step, the goal of which is to lower the IOP and prepare the patient for laser treatment. Hyperosmotics (e.g., glycerin, isosorbide), oral carbonic anhydrase inhibitors (e.g., acetazolamide), and, to a lesser extent, miotics and beta-blockers, make up the arsenal of medical therapy for angle-closure glaucoma (Table 25-2).

Acetazolamide is administered orally in a single 500-mg dose (250 mg × 2). It lowers IOP by decreasing aqueous production. It is also available in intravenous form for patients who become nauseous or are already nauseous. Adverse reactions are rare for this one-time dose.

Beta-blockers also decrease aqueous production but not significantly enough to be used alone in an acute angle-closure attack. Typically, one or two drops of 0.5% timolol maleate or betaxolol can be given during the course of medical therapy. Caution must be used with all patients, taking care to avoid any medication when there is a contraindication to its use.

Apraclonidine has also been used in addition to other medications in treating acute angle closure. Despite the limited clinical experience with this agent, it appears to provide an additional effect in the acute lowering of IOP.[125]

Hyperosmotics act by raising serum osmotic pressure, thereby causing a rapid withdrawal of fluid from the vitreous. Because of the greater side effects with these medications, they should be reserved for patients with more intense attacks of angle closure. They might be necessary to break attacks where the pressure is significantly elevated or has gone untreated for several days. Patients are typically first treated with acetazolamide and a beta-blocker; then, if those agents are not successful in breaking the attack, hyperosmotics are administered. In addition to lowering the pressure, dehydration of the vitreous allows the iris-lens diaphragm to move posteriorly, thereby physically opening the angle.[126]

Miotics are usually ineffective at high IOP levels because of iris ischemia. In addition they may worsen an attack by causing further shallowing of the anterior chamber angle due to a forward rotation of the iris-lens diaphragm. The use of pilocarpine is generally withheld until IOP is reduced to below 40 mm Hg with other agents. After this reduction, 2% pilocarpine may be used to help pull the peripheral iris away from the trabecular meshwork.[127–129]

Topical steroids such as prednisolone acetate are given to reduce inflammation and vascular congestion from an angle-closure attack. They can be continued during the course of laser therapy (see Table 25-2).

TABLE 25-2
Suggested Approach to Acute Angle-Closure Glaucoma

1. The patient history should be consistent with variables including symptoms associated with acute angle closure, medications that may precipitate an attack, a possible history of subacute attacks, and the patient's activity before the attack.
2. Completely examine the involved eye and fellow eye. Evaluate central and peripheral anterior chamber depth, shape of peripheral iris. The fellow eye must also exhibit narrow anterior chamber angles.
3. Applanation tonometry results = 40–70 mm Hg.
4. Medical therapy (include some or all of the following):
   A. Acetazolamide (Diamox), 250 mg × 2 tablets PO
   B. Isosorbide/glycerol (3–6 oz), when intraocular pressure is more than 60 mm Hg
   C. Topical beta-blocker 1–2 gtt
   D. Prednisolone acetate 1%
   E. Apraclonidine 1%
5. Recline patient for 1 hour, repeat slit lamp and gonioscopic examination.
6. If intraocular pressure is reduced (< 40 mm Hg), may add 1–2 gtt 2% pilocarpine.
7. Reassess in 30 min:
   A. Angle open, intraocular pressure lowered: continue medical treatment (beta-blocker, 2% pilocarpine, topical steroid) until laser iridotomy can be scheduled (usually within 24 hours).
   B. Angle closed, intraocular pressure unchanged: continue medical therapy, refer for immediate laser or surgical iridectomy. Suspect lens-related angle closure.

Note: There is no exact or single treatment plan for acute angle-closure glaucoma; each case must be treated on an individual basis.
Source: Adapted from R Ritch, RF Lowe, A Reyes. Therapeutic Overview of Angle Closure Glaucoma. In R Ritch, MB Shields, T Krupin (eds), The Glaucomas (Vol. 2). St. Louis: Mosby, 1989;855–64.

Laser Therapy After IOP has been brought under control with medical therapy, or after maximum medical therapy has been delivered, then arrangements should be made for a laser iridotomy. This relatively safe, effective, and easy procedure is preferred over surgical iridectomy for all forms of primary angle closure. The laser is used to create an opening in the iris that allows aqueous to freely flow from the posterior chamber into the anterior chamber, thereby allowing the peripheral iris to fall away from the angle. Both argon and YAG lasers can be used. The YAG laser is favored because fewer light pulses need to be delivered and it is effective regardless of iris color. Complications are rare, but include corneal damage, hyphema, uveitis, cataract formation, and a transient increase in IOP.[130–132] After successful treatment of one eye with primary angle closure, the fellow eye should have a prophylactic laser iridotomy, because attacks become bilateral in up to 70% of patients.[132,134]

In eyes with extensive, permanent synechial angle closure, a laser iridotomy may not be completely successful in opening the angle and lowering the IOP. In these cases, the patient will need traditional glaucoma filtration surgery (trabeculectomy) to establish an outflow pathway for aqueous humor.[135] Overall, laser iridotomy is a simple and cost-effective, in-office procedure that provides prompt relief to patients with angle-closure glaucoma.

SECONDARY GLAUCOMAS

Pigmentary Glaucoma

Pigmentary glaucoma is a bilateral condition most commonly seen in younger, slightly myopic males. Pigment is liberated and dispersed throughout the anterior chamber as a result of a mechanical rubbing between the posterior iris epithelium and the lens zonules and ciliary processes. Pigment granules are deposited on the corneal endothelium, crystalline lens, and trabecular meshwork. A triad of clinical signs is typically seen in these patients including a central, vertical band of corneal endothelial pigmentation (Krukenberg's spindle, Figure 25-7), heavy trabecular meshwork pigmentation, and radial iris trans-illumination defects. The pigment dispersion syndrome (PDS) is used to refer to those individuals with these typical findings but without elevated IOP and changes to the optic nerve head or visual field. Pigmentary glaucoma may develop in up to 50% of patients with the pigment dispersion syndrome.[13,136]

Myopia is a risk factor for the development of pigmentary glaucoma possibly because of a posterior position of the peripheral iris that allows for touch between the lens zonules and posterior iris surface.[137-139] The pigment dispersion is more common in whites than in blacks or Asians; however, the disease may be underdiagnosed in blacks because of a densely pigmented iris stroma masking the iris defects.[140] Although there is good evidence to support the theory of iris pigment liberation via the rubbing of lens zonules against the iris pigment epithelium, the pathophysiologic development of increased pressure is not as well understood.[141,142] It is known that heavy iris pigment deposition in the trabecular meshwork can cause an elevation of IOP from obstruction of aqueous outflow. Endothelial cells in the meshwork must work harder to phagocytize excess pigment to allow for proper aqueous outflow. This extra phagocytosis of pigment may cause a premature death of these endothelial cells and ultimately a decreased facility of outflow and a rise in IOP. However, because there are individuals who never show pressure elevation with pigment release and because the disease is less common in darkly pigmented individuals, there are probably other factors involved as well.[13,136,140]

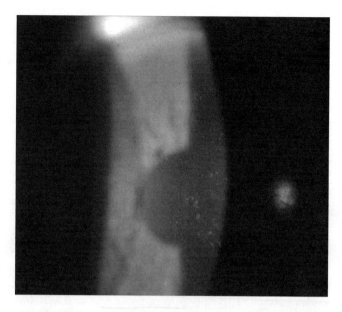

FIGURE 25-7
Krukenberg's spindle in a patient with pigment dispersion syndrome.

In addition to the clinical signs mentioned, patients with pigmentary glaucoma are known to have a wide diurnal fluctuation in IOP. Dramatic increases in pressure may also be noted after physical activity.[143] There appears to be an active stage of the disease between the third and fifth decades, with pigment dispersion then declining in later years. Age-related miosis and thickening of the crystalline lens are believed to move the peripheral iris away from the zonules, thus decreasing pigment liberation.[141,142,144] Depending on the ability of the trabecular meshwork to regain proper functioning, IOP may return to normal.

Treatment of patients with PDS and prolonged elevation of IOP is warranted in order to prevent glaucomatous optic nerve head damage. Given the relatively young age of patients with pigmentary glaucoma and an understanding of its pathophysiology, there are several factors to consider before initiating treatment.

With the understanding of the anatomic relationship responsible for pigment liberation, cholinergic agonists have two theoretical advantages. First, miosis from cholinergic stimulation will possibly help pull the peripheral iris off the lens zonules and decrease the rate of liberation. Second, by increasing aqueous outflow through the trabecular meshwork, removal of excess pigment may be enhanced.[139,140,145] Unfortunately, miotics are usually poorly tolerated in younger patients because of their visual side effects. Low concentration pilocarpine 0.5–1.0%, Pilopine 4% gel, and Ocuserts may be accepted as alternatives by the patient.

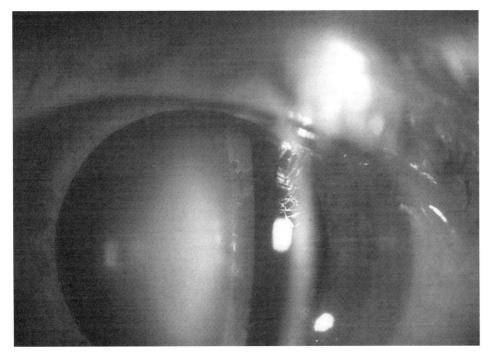

FIGURE 25-8
Exfoliative material on the anterior lens capsule. A bull's-eye pattern occurs due to rubbing away of exfoliation debris in a midperipheral zone by the posterior iris surface.

Topical beta-adrenergic blockers are often a successful medication choice for younger patients. They offer convenient dosing, minimal visual side effects, and can significantly reduce IOP. There are potential arguments against their selection. First, they decrease aqueous production, which may allow a greater accumulation of pigment in the trabecular meshwork. Second, reduced aqueous flow into the posterior chamber may increase peripheral iris bowing posteriorly and increase rubbing against the lens zonules. The benefits of IOP reduction should be weighed against these theoretical risks.

Dipivefrin has been recommended as a first choice medication in pigmentary glaucoma.[145] There are few systemic side effects and easy twice-a-day administration. Topical irritation and blurred vision secondary to pupillary dilation are possible ocular side effects. Although it may improve aqueous outflow, it does not pull the peripheral iris away from the zonules.

Laser iridotomy has been proposed as a method for flattening the peripheral iris and minimizing pigment liberation without the use of miotics.[146] The iridotomy allows for direct aqueous flow from the posterior to the anterior chamber, thus avoiding any build-up of pressure in the anterior chamber that might exacerbate peripheral iris bowing. Further study is needed to compare this treatment to others. Argon laser trabeculoplasty can be considered for those patients whose medical therapy does not adequately control glaucomatous progression.[147] Trabeculoplasty is more effective in younger patients (versus older

patients for POAG) and can provide continued IOP reduction for several years.[148,149] Surgical trabeculectomy may still be required for as many as one-third of patients 5 years after a diagnosis of pigmentary glaucoma.[150]

Exfoliative Glaucoma

The terms *exfoliation syndrome* and *pseudoexfoliation syndrome* identify a relatively common disorder of elderly persons that may lead to increased IOP and thus exfoliative/pseudoexfoliative glaucoma. Both terms refer to the same clinical condition. The use of the "pseudo" prefix helps to differentiate this idiopathic condition from a true lens capsular delamination, which is associated with the craft of glass blowing and exposure to infrared radiation.[13] Exfoliation syndrome has about a 3% prevalence in the United States but is more common (up to 75%) in Scandinavian countries and populations.[151,152] It is characterized by the accumulation of a flaky, grayish-white protein material on the crystalline lens and other intraocular structures. Persistent deposition of the material within the trabecular meshwork can result in decreased aqueous outflow and increased IOP.[153]

Many cases go undiagnosed because an undilated iris hides most of the anterior lens capsule, where much of the exfoliative material prominently collects (Figure 25-8). With mydriasis and slit lamp examination a typical bull's-eye pattern on the anterior surface of the lens can be detected. This bull's-eye pattern results from three distinct zones: (1) a central disc of exfoliative material, (2) a relatively clearer, midperipheral ring, and (3) a peripheral zone of exfoliative material. The clear annular zone most likely results from contact and rubbing between the posterior iris and anterior lens surfaces during normal pupillary movement. Also common to this condition is excessive pigment dispersion, leading to iris transillumination at the pupillary border and abnormal accumulation of pigmentation in the trabecular meshwork. Similar to the pigment dispersion syndrome, heavy trabecular pigmentation may be accompanied by the collection of pigment along Schwalbe's line (Sampaolesi's line).

Exfoliative glaucoma does not develop in all patients with exfoliation syndrome.[154,155] Ocular hypertension occurs in 22–81% of all individuals with the syndrome, and it has been noted that glaucoma may develop in 9–24% of patients over a 10-year period.[156] These percentages reflect the considerable variation in the literature. All patients with exfoliation syndrome should be monitored closely for increased IOP.

The source of exfoliative material is not certain. Most research indicates that the lens epithelium produces most of the material that accumulates on the lens surface and other structures. Because exfoliative material is also noted in aphakic eyes, the iris, trabecular meshwork, and blood vessel walls probably also produce the material.[153]

Exfoliative material is a fibrillar protein, similar to amyloid. Some studies suggest that it is a basement membrane proteoglycan, and the production and deposition of this material may represent an ocular manifestation of a systemic disease.[13,153,157]

Management of exfoliative glaucoma is essentially the same as for primary open-angle glaucoma. Medical therapy proceeds in the standard fashion, from beta-blockers to adrenergic agonists to cholinergics. Oral therapy and laser procedures may also be used but have risks and benefits, as in the treatment of POAG. Some investigators report that laser surgery is more effective for exfoliative glaucoma than for POAG; however, this effect is not long lasting. The success of trabeculectomy may be better compared with medical treatment.[158] Overall, treatment of exfoliative glaucoma is generally considered to be less efficacious than treatment of POAG. Patients therefore need to be followed more closely and perhaps treated more aggressively.

Angle-Recession Glaucoma

Glaucoma develops in a relatively small number of patients after a blunt ocular injury. Increased IOP results from tissue disruption or tearing in the trabecular meshwork and subsequent scarring, which decreases aqueous outflow.

An angle recession, which may accompany this injury, refers to a splitting of the ciliary body between the longitudinal and circular muscles. Blunt trauma may also create tears of the iris root (iridodialysis) or separation of the ciliary body from the scleral spur (cyclodialysis). Gonioscopically the anterior chamber angle appears deepened in each of these conditions, but the exact location of the splitting is often difficult to determine because scarring of the tissue masks identification of structures.[13,159]

Blunt trauma that causes a hyphema is more likely also to cause an angle recession. Between 2% and 20% of patients with angle recession will later develop glaucoma.[160] Patients with visible damage to greater than two-thirds of the angle are also more likely to develop glaucoma, and the glaucoma associated with angle recession may develop months to years after the injury.[160] It is interesting to note that many patients with angle-recession glaucoma also have primary open-angle glaucoma in the nontraumatized eye. This suggests that those patients who do develop angle-recession glaucoma have an underlying predisposition for elevated IOP.[161,162]

Management of angle-recession glaucoma is more difficult than that of POAG. After initiation of topical therapy with a beta-blocker, treatment options become much more limited. Since miotic and laser therapy rely on normal tissue and structure for good effectiveness, these therapies are usually much less effective because of the physical damage to the trabecular meshwork. Filtration surgery done in conjunction with an antimetabolite may be best at controlling more severe cases.[163]

Neovascular Glaucoma

Neovascular glaucoma (NVG) frequently occurs in association with several common retinal conditions. Central retinal vein occlusion and proliferative diabetic retinopathy are the leading causes; however, it is also found with central retinal artery occlusion, Coats' disease, sickle cell retinopathy, Eales disease, uveitis, ocular ischemic syndrome, retinal detachment, intraocular tumor, and after intraocular surgery. Retinal hypoxia is the major underlying risk factor. Chronic retinal hypoxia is theorized to initiate the production of an angiogenic substance that elicits the growth of new blood vessels. The iris is the primary site for this neovascularization, which is commonly known as "rubeosis iridis."[13,164,165]

Neovascular glaucoma usually progresses through several stages leading to its dramatic presentation. Initially, tiny tufts of new vessels appear at the pupillary margin. They are quite small and can be difficult to detect. IOP is normal at this point, and diagnosis and proper treatment can avoid further progression and glaucoma. Next, the vessels extend out onto the iris surface, eventually leading into the anterior chamber angle (Figure 25-9). These radial vessels may join with circumferential vessels in the angle and cross over the ciliary body and scleral spur to invade the trabecular meshwork. The progression of rubeosis does not always follow this exact sequence. There can be multifocal origins of the vessels, including an initial development in the angle. Gonioscopy is required to rule out the presence of angle rubeosis.

At this point the angle is still open, but the IOP may begin to rise quite dramatically. Inflammation, photophobia, pain, and hyphema can develop during this later phase. Contracture of the fibrovascular membrane overlying the trabecular meshwork forms synechial adhesions in the angle. Continued coalescence of the synechiae and traction of the membrane lead to intractable angle closure. The glaucoma is usually quite severe at this stage and requires prompt intervention. Ectropian uvea, a dilated pupil, decreased vision, corneal edema, conjunctival hyperemia, and pressures as high as 60–70 mm Hg frequently occur at this stage.[166–168]

The time frame for the progression is variable. Neovascular glaucoma is often referred to as "90-day glaucoma" because it commonly develops within 3 months after an ischemic CRVO. Not all cases follow this pattern, however, and rubeosis iridis may progress to NVG within days to years. The difficulty in treating the advanced angle-closure stage dictates that proper treatment be delivered as soon as rubeotic vessels are noted.

The primary treatment for NVG is to eliminate the underlying cause, retinal ischemia. This is accomplished with panretinal photocoagulation (PRP). At any stage of the disease, photocoagulation of the peripheral retina may help reduce or even eliminate anterior segment neovascularization. Regression of the rubeotic vessels often leads to a reduction of IOP as long as the anterior chamber angle has not developed synechial closure. Timely application of PRP at the earliest sign of rubeosis can prevent the development of complicated NVG.[169,170] Goniophotocoagulation involves argon laser therapy to new vessels in the angle. This procedure can be helpful in preventing synechial angle closure but does not remove the initiating factors.[171]

The initial medical management of neovascular glaucoma is directed at lowering the IOP and reducing the ocular inflammation. When pressures are extremely elevated, a combination of acetazolamide, hyperosmotics, and topical beta-blockers should be administered. Pilocarpine should not be used because of the ocular inflammation. Prednisolone acetate 1% and cycloplegia with atropine are also given to improve comfort and prepare the eye for PRP.[172] Filtering surgery has produced very

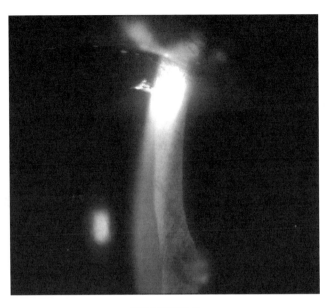

FIGURE 25-9

Pronounced rubeosis iridis in a patient with neovascular glaucoma that developed after a central retinal vein occlusion. (Courtesy of Mary McGehee, O.D., and Indre Rudaitis, O.D.)

limited success; however, the use of a seton (a surgically implanted device to facilitate greater aqueous drainage) may improve results.[173] In many advanced cases of NVG there is little or no chance of visual recovery and the patient can be managed conservatively. Blind, painful eyes with NVG may require cyclocryotherapy or cyclophotocoagulation to destroy the ciliary body and provide relief from the ocular pain.[174,175]

Uveitic Glaucoma

Glaucoma is a well-known complication of uveitis. Many of the numerous types of uveitis have some potential for the development of glaucoma. Although aqueous production typically decreases in anterior uveitis, the balance between inflow and outflow may be disturbed such that IOP becomes elevated. There are several mechanisms for the elevation of IOP. Reduction of normal aqueous outflow may be caused by inflammation and swelling of the trabecular meshwork and aqueous outflow channels. Inflammatory debris (fibrin, macrophages, etc.) can accumulate and become entrapped in the meshwork, overwhelming its capacity to act as a biological filter, thus causing a decrease in aqueous outflow.[176]

Glaucoma may also develop from two structural changes that arise from chronic inflammation. Posterior synechiae may prevent the flow of aqueous from the posterior chamber to the anterior chamber causing iris bombé and

FIGURE 25-10
Posterior synechiae formation at the pupillary margin due to anterior uveitis can lead to iris bombé and secondary angle-closure glaucoma. (Courtesy of Scott Robison, O.D.)

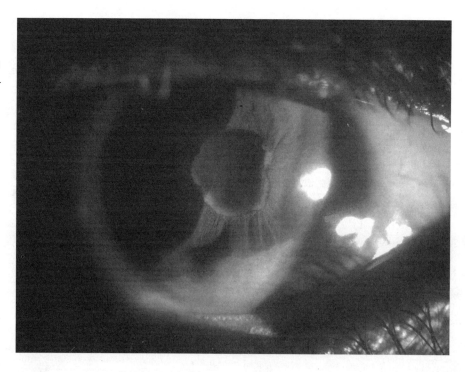

angle closure (Figure 25-10). This will usually not develop unless the synechial adhesions involve the pupillary margin 360 degrees. Finally, in chronic or repeated episodes of uveitis, peripheral anterior synechiae (PAS) can develop that may progress to overt angle closure. Even without angle closure the PAS may damage the trabecular meshwork and significantly decrease outflow facility.[177]

Acute, subacute, and chronic forms of nonspecific iridocyclitis may all lead to pressure elevation. Chronic uveitis and glaucoma are seen in systemic inflammatory diseases such as sarcoidosis, Behçet's disease, and juvenile rheumatoid arthritis, among many others.[176] Most cases of chronic anterior uveitis have periods of exacerbation and remission. Glaucoma may also be transient or chronic depending on the severity and duration of inflammation, as well as on the eye's ability to withstand damage from inflammation.

The treatment of uveitic glaucoma is first directed toward controlling the inflammation and reducing its effect on aqueous outflow. If the inflammation can be brought under control, the pressure often will return to normal as long as substantial damage to the trabecular meshwork has not taken place. Cycloplegia and topical, periocular, or oral steroids may be indicated to treat the inflammation depending on its severity and other factors. When the IOP is elevated to the point that optic nerve damage may occur, then antiglaucoma therapy should be initiated. Beta-blockers, dorzolamide, apraclonidine, and

acetazolamide in various combinations are all used in uveitic glaucoma. Miotics are contraindicated since they aggravate inflammation by causing increased vascular permeability and promote ciliary spasm that will worsen patient discomfort.

If maximal medical therapy fails to control IOP, then filtering surgery may be required. However, operating on an inflamed eye has many potential complications and a significantly lower success rate. In some cases the implantation of a seton may be required to allow continued aqueous outflow and a satisfactory IOP.[178] Laser trabeculoplasty is not effective in eyes with glaucoma secondary to uveitis and should not be used. Laser iridotomy is used when pupillary block and secondary angle closure develops.

Glaucomatocyclitic Crisis (Posner-Schlossman Syndrome)

Glaucomatocyclitic crisis is a unique disease characterized by recurrent attacks of marked elevation of pressure associated with signs of mild anterior uveitis. This condition is unilateral, affects adults 25–50 years of age, and is also characterized by mildly reduced vision, slight ocular discomfort, and the appearance of halos around lights from corneal edema. Slit lamp examination reveals open angles, mild ciliary flush, occasional keratic precipitates, and mild flare. IOP typically ranges between 40 and 60 mm Hg. Episodes usually last from hours to days

TABLE 25-3
Glaucoma Medication Chart

Medication	Concentration	Cap Color	Dose
Beta-blockers			
Nonselective			
Timoptic (timolol maleate)	0.25%	Light blue	qd/bid
	0.5%	Yellow	qd/bid
Timoptic XE (gel-forming solution)	0.25%	Light blue	qd
	0.5%	Yellow	qd
Betimol (timolol hemihydrate)	0.25%	White	qd/bid
	0.5%	White	qd/bid
Betagan (levobunolol)	0.25%	Light blue	qd/bid
	0.5%	Yellow	qd/bid
Optipranolol (metipranolol)	0.3%	Light blue	bid
Ocupress (carteolol)	1.0%	Clear	bid
Selective			
Betoptic S (betaxolol)	0.25%	Light blue	bid
Betoptic	0.5%	Dark blue	bid
Adrenergic stimulators			
Propine (dipivefrin)	0.1%	Purple	bid
Iopidine (apraclonidine)	0.5%	White	bid/tid
Miotics			
Pilocarpine	1.0–6.0%	Green	qid
Carbachol	1.5–3.0%	Green	tid
Phospholine iodide (echothiophate)	0.03–0.125%	Green	qd/bid
Carbonic anhydrase inhibitors			
Trusopt (dorzolamide)	2%	Orange	bid/tid
Diamox (acetazolamide)	125 mg	White tablets	qid
	250 mg		
Diamox sequels	500 mg	Orange capsules	bid
Neptazane (methazolamide)	25 mg	White tablets	bid/tid
	50 mg		

but may be longer. The glaucoma appears to be related to inflammatory changes within the trabecular meshwork. Treatment consists of beta-blockers or carbonic anhydrase inhibitors to decrease aqueous humor production and topical anti-inflammatory agents to quell the mild inflammation.[179,180] Patients wtih glaucomatocyclitic crisis have a propensity to eventually develop chronic elevation of IOP in the involved eye as well as the uninvolved eye. Therefore, there may be a greater likelihood of this syndrome to develop in patients who already have a tendency to develop primary open-angle glaucoma. All patients with glaucomatocyclitic crisis should therefore be monitored as glaucoma suspects.

OVERVIEW OF ANTIGLAUCOMA MEDICATIONS

Beta-Adrenergic Antagonists

Table 25-3 lists the drugs commonly used to treat glaucoma and their pertinent characteristics. The use of beta-blockers in glaucoma began in 1978 with the introduction of timolol maleate.[181] Today, topical beta-blockers are the most frequently prescribed agents for treating glaucoma in this country. They are considered the initial drugs of choice for the majority of patients with various forms of open-angle glaucoma. Although these agents have serious potential side effects in some patients, they lack many ocular side effects common to a number of other ocular hypotensive medications and are therefore well tolerated.

Beta-blockers have an ocular hypotensive effect by reducing aqueous humor formation. Various investigations in both animals and humans have supported this theory. Beta-blockers have minimal to no effect on aqueous outflow facility.[182] By blocking normal circulating catecholamines (i.e., norepinephrine, epinephrine, dopamine) at the level of the ciliary epithelium, beta-blockers reduce sympathetic activity, which causes their ocular hypotensive effects.[183] Beta-blockers, unlike most other topical glaucoma agents, have hypotensive effects on the contralateral eye, which is likely a result of systemic absorption and circulation. This contralateral hypotensive effect is significantly weaker than the response in the ipsilateral eye, thus supporting the direct effect on the ciliary epithelium as opposed to systemic vascular effects indirectly affecting aqueous production.[184]

The local ocular side effects associated with topical beta-blockers are relatively uncommon and in most cases not of major concern. The most common ocular complication is that of mild burning or stinging on instillation. Findings and symptoms consistent with dry eye and keratoconjunctivitis sicca have also been reported with the use of timolol. Other less common ocular side effects reported with topical beta-blockers include corneal anesthesia, corneal erosion in contact lens wearers, allergic conjunctivitis, and ptosis.[185–187] Ocular toxicity is rare.

Systemic side effects associated with topical beta-blocking drugs are by far more significant and potentially dangerous than their local ocular complications. The likelihood of systemic side effects is directly related to the ability of these agents to reach the systemic circulation. The relatively low serum concentrations that are found after the use of topical beta-blockers have been shown to be sufficient to produce a variety of undesirable systemic side effects in susceptible patients.[188] Caution should be used to reduce the likelihood of these complications. Suggestions include ensuring that only one drop is used per instillation, using punctal occlusion while keeping the lids closed after instillation, using the lowest effective concentration and number of administrations of the drug, and very careful screening of patients for systemic risk factors.

Some of the most common systemic findings with topical beta-blockers are central nervous system symptoms such as depression and concentration and memory problems. These symptoms often occur quite early after initiation of therapy, ranging from days to months. Although commonly transient, these symptoms may persist and require cessation of treatment. Cardiovascular side effects are also of concern with the use of topical beta-blockers, which include bradycardia, systemic hypotension, arrhythmia, syncope, and heart block.[185,186] Cardiovascular effects should be of concern especially in the care of patients with preexisting heart block, hypotension, or a history of heart failure. Beta-blockers can alter symptoms of hypoglycemia, and in some instances increase hypoglycemic episodes and alter the response to glucose administration. Therefore, they should be used with caution in patients with labile diabetes where blood glucose levels fluctuate greatly.[189] Respiratory side effects induced by topical beta-blockers are also of major significance. Secondary bronchial constriction can induce dyspnea, wheezing, pulmonary failure, asthma, and bronchitis, especially in susceptible patients with preexisting chronic obstructive pulmonary disease (COPD). Selective beta-blockers such as betaxolol

have been shown to induce fewer minimal respiratory side effects and therefore can be used, albeit cautiously, for some patients with mild airway disease.[190]

Topical beta-blockers are additive in their ocular hypotensive effects with most other glaucoma medications including miotics, carbonic anhydrase inhibitors, prostaglandin analogs, and, to a significantly smaller degree, adrenergic agonists such as epinephrine and dipivefrin.

Timolol Maleate (Timoptic)

Timolol is a nonselective beta-1 and beta-2 antagonist. Timolol was the first topical beta-blocker to be approved and has become the most frequently prescribed glaucoma medication. It is available in concentrations of 0.25% and 0.50%, both in solution form. The suggested dosage is twice per day at 12-hour intervals. Reports indicate greater effectiveness of the 0.5% concentration for dark irides.[191] Often, the 0.5% concentration is no more effective than the 0.25% concentration in light irides, but it may have a longer duration of effect.[192] Reduction in IOP begins within 1 hour of administration and maximum effect is achieved by 2 hours. Gradual return of baseline IOP is reached within 24–48 hours of instillation, but complete elimination of its ocular hypotensive effect may not occur for up to 2 weeks or more, especially after long-term use.[193] Timoptic XE is a "gel-forming solution" that is designed specifically for once-a-day administration. Initially a solution, the medication becomes a gel upon contact with the tear film, which lengthens contact time and thus penetration of the cornea.

The vast majority of patients will respond to topical timolol. The initial response over the first few weeks can be a reduction of up to 40% from the baseline IOP, but this degree of effect decreases during the first 6 months to a sustained ocular hypotensive effect that is approximately 23–33% below the pretreatment baseline level. This phenomenon is known as *short-term escape*. After timolol has been used for more than 1 year, some patients will demonstrate a further progressive loss of effect. This phenomenon is known as *long-term drift*.[194]

Some controversy exists over whether timolol is additive in its hypotensive effect with epinephrine or dipivefrin. If there is an additive hypotensive effect, the additional reduction in IOP is usually small, ranging from 1 to 3 mm Hg. The short-term additive effect is often greatest, but generally it will decline to a minimum within a few weeks.[195,196]

Timolol Hemihydrate (Betimol)

Timolol hemihydrate is a slightly different formulation of timolol maleate in which the maleate anions have been left off. Clinically, this agent performs very similarly to

Timoptic, and side effects and contraindications essentially remain the same. The medication's prime advantage lies in its lower cost.

Levobunolol (Betagan)

Levobunolol is a nonselective beta-1 and beta-2 antagonist. Levobunolol is available as 0.25% and 0.5% solutions. It is quite similar to timolol with respect to its efficacy in reducing IOP, drug to drug interactions, and systemic side effects. What distinguishes levobunolol from other approved topical beta-blockers is its duration of effect. A number of studies have suggested that levobunolol administered once daily is often effective in sustaining a desired ocular hypotensive result. Because of individual variations in response, levobunolol most often is used as a twice-a-day drug administered at 12-hour intervals.[197-200]

Metipranolol (Optipranolol)

Metipranolol is a nonselective beta-1 and beta-2 antagonist that was approved by the U.S. Food and Drug Administration in 1990. Metipranolol is available as a 0.3% solution. Suggested administration is twice daily at 12-hour intervals. Metipranolol is slightly less effective in lowering IOP compared with timolol while having similar side effects. Presently a distinguishing factor regarding metipranolol is its lower price in comparison with other topical beta-blockers.[201]

Carteolol (Ocupress)

Carteolol is another nonselective beta-blocker used for topical glaucoma therapy.[202] The indications and effectiveness for this agent are similar to the other nonselective beta-blockers. Carteolol's distinguishing factor is its pharmacologic property of "intrinsic sympathomimetic activity" (ISA). ISA allows for some small amount of beta receptor stimulation. This may reduce the systemic side effects commonly associated with this class of medications. However, this has not yet been clearly demonstrated. Carteolol does not lower high-density lipoprotein levels as much as timolol maleate. It is postulated this might lower the risk of myocardial infarction in some patients. Topically, carteolol is reported as being a more comfortable agent to instill.[202]

Betaxolol (Betoptic)

Betaxolol is a selective beta-1 antagonist. Betaxolol is available topically as a 0.5% solution and as a 0.25% suspension (Betoptic S). The 0.25% suspension offers equivalent IOP reduction along with greater patient comfort compared with the 0.5% solution.

Reported ocular hypotensive effects of topical betaxolol range from approximately 11-29% using the suggested administration schedule of twice a day at 12-hour intervals. Clinical experience as well as numerous investigations suggest that betaxolol is not as effective in its ocular hypotensive effects as timolol or levobunolol.[203-205] Because of its relative beta selectivity, betaxolol is less likely than nonselective beta-blockers to induce respiratory complications, and as such may be an acceptable drug for patients with mild COPD. The beta-1 selectivity of betaxolol is not absolute and therefore still has the potential to cause respiratory complications in at-risk individuals.[206] There are reports that betaxolol is less likely to induce CNS and cardiovascular complications compared with other beta-blockers. This is perhaps a result of poor systemic availability.[207]

Betaxolol has been shown to have better additive effects with topical adrenergic agonists such as epinephrine and dipivefrin compared with the other beta-blockers. Although not conclusively proven, the beta-1 selectivity of betaxolol is thought not to block the beta-2 effects of epinephrine, which may be responsible for increased aqueous outflow.[208]

Prostaglandin Agonist: Latanoprost (Xalatan)

Latanoprost is a prostaglandin $PGF_{2\alpha}$ analog that reduces IOP effectively with only minimal side effects. Latanoprost has the ability to lower IOP by an average of 31-35% when used in a concentration of 0.005%. Given once daily, it seems to be at least as effective and probably superior to a twice-daily dose regimen. Since latanoprost lowers IOP by increasing uveoscleral outflow, it has an additive effect with other glaucoma medications that have a different mechanism of action (e.g., timolol). It is additive with pilocarpine but to a lesser extent. Systemic side effects are essentially nonexistent with latanoprost. Ocular side effects include conjunctival hyperemia that resolves within several days of use in the majority of patients, as well as the development of increased iris pigmentation in some who have used the medication.[117]

Adrenergic Agonists

Epinephrine and its pro-drug, dipivefrin, are direct-acting sympathomimetics that stimulate both alpha and beta receptors. In addition to lowering IOP, these agents can also cause vasoconstriction and mydriasis.

Determination of the exact mechanism by which epinephrine reduces IOP remains controversial. Traditional theories hold that early decreases in IOP are a result of beta-adrenergic–mediated effects of reduced aqueous production, followed by alpha-adrenergic–mediated effects of increased aqueous outflow.[209] A number of more recent studies provide evidence in conflict with this traditional theory. The majority of evidence suggests that the primary ocular hypotensive effect for epinephrine is through increased uveoscleral and trabecular aqueous outflow.[210] Some recent studies using fluorophotometry suggest that epinephrine may induce a small short-term increase in aqueous production that is overwhelmed by the concomitant increase in outflow, thus producing a net ocular hypotensive effect.[211]

Most of the side effects reported with the topical use of adrenergic agents are ocular. Common findings include hyperemia, burning, irritation, tearing, and blepharoconjunctivitis.[212] Secondary mydriasis is a contraindication to the use of epinephrine or dipivefrin in patients with narrow angles. One of the most significant ocular side effects of adrenergic agents is the formation of cystoid macular edema in aphakic eyes, occurring in over 20% of those treated.[213] The onset of macular edema varies from months to years after institution of treatment. Vision loss is often gradually reversible with the discontinuation of the medication, although permanent visual alterations may occur in some cases.

Systemic side effects associated with the topical use of adrenergic agonists are less common. They include secondary systemic hypertension, premature ventricular contractions, tachycardia, palpitations, anxiety, headache, and browache. Epinephrine treatment for glaucoma is contraindicated for patients with severe hypertension, cardiovascular disease, and hyperthyroidism.[214] With the development of newer topical agents for glaucoma, the adrenergic agonists are no longer as popular due to their weaker effectiveness and ocular side effects.

Dipivefrin (Propine)

Dipivefrin (dipivalyl epinephrine) is a pro-drug of epinephrine. It is a synthetic compound that has much greater lipid solubility than epinephrine, and as such has 17 times greater corneal penetration. Therefore, low concentrations of dipivefrin can be used to achieve effective intraocular concentrations of epinephrine after biotransformation by naturally occurring ocular esterases. Because of lower topical concentrations, dipivefrin produces fewer systemic side effects than epinephrine. Dipivefrin is available only as a 0.1% solution. The suggested administration schedule is twice per day at 12-hour intervals. IOP reduction begins within 1 hour after administration and reaches its maximum effect by 4–8 hours. Baseline IOP is reached after 12–24 hours. The reported ocular hypotensive effect ranges from 15–26%.[215–218]

Apraclonidine (Iopidine)

Apraclonidine is an alpha-2 agonist and derivative of the alpha stimulator, clonidine. The ocular hypotensive effect

of apraclonidine can reduce aqueous humor production by 35%. The 1% concentration, available in single-dose form, is regularly used in anterior segment laser procedures including iridotomy, trabeculoplasty, and capsulotomy.[219,220] A 0.5% concentration is available to be used for adjunctive short-term therapy in open-angle glaucoma patients who require additional topical therapy. When added to timolol, apraclonidine produces an additional decrease in IOP of 17–22%. Contact dermatitis and tachyphylaxis appear to be the most significant ocular side effects limiting its long-term use.[221,222]

Cholinergic Agents

Cholinergic agents are used in the management of open-angle glaucoma for their ocular hypotensive effects, which are achieved by increasing aqueous outflow facility. This occurs via mechanical forces acting on the scleral spur and trabecular meshwork following ciliary muscle contracture. The ocular hypotensive effect of cholinergic agents is independent of pupillary miosis. Parasympathomimetics have been used in the treatment of glaucoma for several decades. Despite their visual side effects, they still play an important role in the medical management of glaucoma.[164,223,224]

Direct-acting cholinergics behave in the same manner as the endogenous neurotransmitter acetylcholine by stimulating parasympathetic receptors. Topical cholinergic agents cause a concomitant reduction of aqueous outflow via the uveoscleral route, but the effect on the trabecular route is much greater and therefore the net result is a reduction of IOP.

Ocular effects of cholinergic agents can be quite significant. The most commonly reported of these effects is reduced vision in dim illumination because of miosis, especially in patients with central lens opacities. Accommodative ciliary muscle spasm with resultant browaches and fluctuating vision tends to be more commonly reported in individuals under 40 years of age who have more active accommodative mechanisms.[225] Secondary angle closure with pupillary block can actually be induced by the topical use of cholinergics in patients with narrow angles and advancing lens intumescence. The combination of the forward displacement of the lens-iris diaphragm, common with advancing cataracts, and the miotic effects of cholinergics may precipitate pupillary block and cause an angle-closure episode.[226]

Although definitive evidence does not exist, there is a significant amount of circumstantial evidence that suggests an association between retinal detachment and the use of topical cholinergic agents. The theory is that ciliary muscle stimulation pulls on the retina and choroid peripherally. Patients with retinal detachment risk factors may be more prone to detachment if placed on cholinergic therapy, and therefore caution is advised with these patients. Pretreatment peripheral retinal examination and periodic follow-up evaluations should be performed.[227]

Pilocarpine

Pilocarpine is the cholinergic agent most commonly used for the treatment of glaucoma. Although pilocarpine is available in a wide variety of solution concentrations, ranging from 0.25% to 10%, the most commonly prescribed solution concentrations are 1%, 2%, and 4%. Various studies indicate that the maximum reduction of IOP achieved by various pilocarpine concentrations is dependent on the degree of ocular pigmentation.[164] This is thought to be due to the tendency of pilocarpine to bind to melanin. Individuals with light irides often have a maximum response with a 2% solution, those with brown irides with a 4% solution, and some very dark individuals may achieve a maximum response with a 6% or 8% solution. Increasing the solution concentrations above the maximum response level may extend the duration of action, but also increases the risks of ocular and systemic side effects.[228]

Topical application of pilocarpine solution results in a reduction in IOP within 1 hour. The duration of action ranges from 4 to 8 hours. The most commonly prescribed frequency of administration is four times daily at 6-hour intervals. Pilocarpine in all its forms is additive with other antiglaucoma agents such as beta-blockers, adrenergic agonists, and carbonic anhydrase inhibitors.

Pilocarpine is also available in a gel form, commercially known as Pilopine HS Gel. The gel provides extended contact between the drug and the eye and thus improves penetration.[229] Application of 4% pilocarpine gel once per day at bedtime provides a therapeutic effect that is approximately equal to 2% pilocarpine solution applied four times daily. There is some question whether pilocarpine gel provides adequate IOP reduction over a full 24-hour period. The gel form is often quite useful in controlling IOP spikes found in the early morning hours.[230] Many practitioners find that Pilopine Gel loses it effectiveness about 14–18 hours after administration. It is best to check the IOP at this time interval and, if necessary, have the patient add a single drop of 2% pilocarpine solution. This will improve around-the-clock IOP control. The advantages of once-a-day therapy and reduced ocular side effects may make Pilopine gel an attractive alternative for many glaucoma patients.

Carbachol

Carbachol is a direct-acting cholinergic agent that on a dose-for-dose basis is somewhat more potent than an equivalent concentration of pilocarpine. Carbachol has a longer duration of action than pilocarpine and therefore can be effective in doses given three times per day. Carbachol is available in 0.75%, 1.5%, 2.25%, and 3% concentration solutions. Carbachol is an effective cholinergic agent in its ability to lower IOP. It is usually considered as a replacement for pilocarpine should resistance or allergy develop.

Carbachol has systemic and ocular side effects that are similar to those of other direct-acting cholinergic agents. Accommodative spasm and associated headaches may be greater in intensity than with an equally effective concentration of pilocarpine.

Carbonic Anhydrase Inhibitors

Carbonic anhydrase inhibitors (CAIs) are most often used in the treatment of open-angle glaucoma. Their ocular hypotensive effect is additive with all topical glaucoma agents and in combination can reduce IOP by over 60%.[231] The greatest problem with the long-term use of carbonic anhydrase inhibitors is their side effects. Studies indicate that less than 50% of patients can be maintained on long-term CAI therapy.[232] The proper selection of a CAI can limit these side effects and improve compliance.

CAIs reduce IOP by reducing the formation of aqueous humor. They reversibly bind with carbonic anhydrase, an enzyme that catalyzes a key step in the formation of aqueous humor.

All significant side effects of CAIs are systemic. The most common of these are paresthesias of the extremities, altered kidney metabolism with secondary renal stones, and CNS effects such as depression, malaise, confusion, and decreased libido. Many of the side effects are related to the development of systemic acidosis. Patients taking potassium-depleting diuretics, patients treated with digitalis, those suffering from liver cirrhosis, chronic obstructive pulmonary disease, and sickle cell hemoglobinopathies are at greater risk for these side effects and must be monitored carefully.[232-234]

Dorzolamide (Trusopt)

After many years of research, the first topical carbonic anhydrase inhibitor, dorzolamide, was approved for use in 1995. To avoid the variety of systemic side effects of oral CAIs, a topical CAI was very desirable in the treatment of glaucoma. The mechanism of action is the same as oral CAIs (i.e., the reduction of aqueous humor formation). Dorzolamide is a potent antiglaucoma agent, with three times a day administration of the 2% concentration showing a peak (2 hours post-administration) IOP reduction of 18–26%. After 52 weeks of use in clinical trials, dorzolamide continued to show a 15–21% reduction in IOP.[235]

Topical side effects with dorzolamide are minimal but include mild stinging and burning. A bitter taste immediately following administration is noted in some patients. Systemic side effects are being evaluated. Dorzolamide is contraindicated in any patient with a history of sulfa allergy.[236]

Dorzolamide is labeled for three times a day dosing; however, clinical use with twice-a-day dosing may be similarly effective. When added to timolol, dorzolamide has shown an additional 13–21% reduction in IOP.[237] Although beta-blockers may remain the best first-line agents in open-angle glaucoma, dorzolamide appears to be an excellent alternative. If not used initially, it may be a good secondary agent.

Acetazolamide (Diamox)

Oral acetazolamide is available in tablet form in 125-mg and 250-mg preparations or in a timed-release 500-mg capsule form (Diamox Sequels). The standard administration schedule is four times daily for the 125-mg or 250-mg tablets and twice daily for the 500-mg Sequel. It is advisable to consider beginning with a reduced administration schedule such as twice daily for the tablets and once daily for the capsule in order to minimize potential side effects. If the desired hypotensive effect is not achieved, more frequent administration can then be instituted. Patients have fewer side effects with the 500-mg Sequels and are likely to be more compliant with the twice-per-day dosage.

IOP begins to fall within 60 minutes and reaches a maximum effect within 2–4 hours after oral administration. Duration of action of the tablets ranges from 4 to 6 hours. The timed-release capsule has an onset of action that is delayed by about 2 hours, reaches a maximum hypotensive effect within 8 hours, and maintains its duration of action for 12–24 hours.[238,239]

Methazolamide (Neptazane)

Methazolamide has gained popularity in recent years as a first choice CAI because of its relatively lower chance of causing renal disease or complications in patients with cardiopulmonary problems, compared with acetazolamide.

Methazolamide is available in 25-mg and 50-mg tablets. The administration schedule for oral methazolamide is two to three times daily. As is customary, the lowest dose and least frequent administration should be evaluated first for therapeutic effects. The ocular hypotensive effect begins within 1–2 hours after oral administration. Maximum hypotensive effect is reached within 6 hours, and the duration of action ranges from 12–14 hours. Oral use of met-

hazalomide, 50 mg bid, is slightly less effective than acetazolamide, 500-mg capsules bid or 250-mg tablets qid.[240,241]

LASER AND SURGICAL MANAGEMENT OF OPEN-ANGLE GLAUCOMA

Argon Laser Trabeculoplasty

Argon laser trabeculoplasty (ALT) has made a major contribution in the treatment of open-angle glaucoma. It is a technique that falls into place between insufficient-acting medical therapy and the use of filtration surgery. Laser trabeculoplasty consists of the application of laser burns to the inner surface of the trabecular meshwork. Successful ALT results in a lowering of the IOP via an increase in aqueous outflow. Aqueous production remains the same. Mechanical, cellular, and biochemical responses of the trabecular meshwork to the laser photocoagulation are possible explanations for why this treatment is effective.[242,243]

Argon laser trabeculoplasty is indicated when the patient's IOP is no longer adequately controlled with maximal medical therapy. Inadequate control implies increased IOP and progressive damage to the optic nerve and visual field. In some patients who for various reasons cannot be placed on medical therapy, ALT may be a first-line therapy.[244,245]

Treatment generally consists of approximately 50 laser spots being delivered to 180 degrees of the anterior trabecular meshwork. If this produces inadequate lowering of IOP, the second 180 degrees can also be treated.[246] In some cases 360 degrees of the meshwork may be treated in a single session, but this has a greater risk of significant inflammation and postoperative IOP spiking. Repeated laser therapy is usually not as effective as primary therapy, and there is some controversy over whether it should be administered.[247,248]

Postoperative complications are usually minor and easily controlled. They can include transient visual alterations, acute spiking of IOP, iritis, hemorrhage, and corneal burns. Topical steroids (prednisolone acetate 1%) are given for 7–10 days after the procedure to control inflammation. To reduce the amount of pressure elevation associated with laser treatment, apraclonidine 1% is administered preoperatively and postoperatively.[242,243] Argon laser trabeculoplasty is generally a very safe procedure, usually without any significant complications.

It is necessary to wait 4–6 weeks before a patient achieves the full response to ALT to determine if the procedure was successful. Approximately 80% of patients will have a significant (20–30%) lowering of IOP.[249] The patient's medical therapy may be reduced or eliminated if the magnitude of IOP reduction is great enough. Generally this is not the case, and ALT is used as an additional therapy to lower IOP in order to attain the target pressure. The success of ALT significantly decreases with time. With an average failure rate of 10% per year, after 5 years more than 50% of treated patients will no longer demonstrate a clinically significant IOP-lowering effect.[250]

Laser trabeculoplasty has been studied in patients with many types of glaucoma. Its success varies among different types of glaucoma. The best success rates occur for patients over 60 years of age with POAG, pigmentary glaucoma, and exfoliative glaucoma. Moderate success is found in pseudophakic, angle-recession, and the low-tension forms of glaucoma. Argon laser trabeculoplasty is contraindicated in the treatment of patients with juvenile glaucoma, active uveitis, and neovascular glaucoma.

The use of ALT as an initial or early therapeutic option has stimulated much discussion.[251,252] The Glaucoma Laser Trial (1989) demonstrated that early laser treatment of POAG was no better than medical (pharmacologic) therapy.[253] Although this is still a controversial point, with some practitioners preferring early laser intervention, ALT should generally only be recommended when medical therapy is no longer sufficient or cannot be tolerated by the patient. Exceptions are made for elderly patients, those with a history of poor compliance, or medical contraindications to topical or oral therapy.[254-256]

Filtration Surgery

The most common surgical procedure performed for open-angle glaucoma is a trabeculectomy.[257] It consists of creating a partial thickness scleral flap, a sclerostomy (opening) into the anterior chamber through the trabecular meshwork, and a conjunctival filtration bleb. Aqueous humor passes through the fistula, pushes open the scleral flap, and flows into the subconjunctival space, where it is ultimately drained away via surrounding lymphatic vessels and vasculature.[13]

Traditionally this procedure is used in the treatment of patients who are on maximal medical therapy and have had ALT yet continue to demonstrate glaucomatous progression.[258,259] In addition to open-angle glaucoma, the procedure is also successful for a wide variety of secondary glaucomas. In some instances it may be used early on in the course of therapy.[260,261] As a primary surgical treatment it is successful in about 75% of glaucoma patients.[262-264] It tends to be less successful in younger patients, blacks, some secondary glaucomas, and patients who have had prior intraocular surgery. Antimetabolite agents such as 5-fluorouracil and mitomycin C can significantly improve the success rate by working to decrease postoperative scarring, which will decrease aqueous outflow through the filtration bleb.[265-267]

Complications of trabeculectomy procedures include conjunctival bleb leak, hyphema, suprachoroidal hemorrhage, choroidal detachment, hypotony and flat anterior chamber, cataract development, endophthalmitis, IOP elevation, and malignant glaucoma. Diligent postoperative follow-up is critical for surgical success.[268,269]

REFERENCES

1. Wilson MR. Primary open-angle glaucoma: Magnitude of the problem in the United States. J Glaucoma 1992;1:64–7.
2. Leibowitz WM, Krueger DE, Maunder LR, et al. The Framingham Eye Study Monograph. Surv Ophthalmol 1980; 24(Suppl):335–610.
3. Tielsch JM, Sommer A, Katz J, et al. Racial variations in the prevalence of primary open angle glaucoma: The Baltimore Eye Survey. JAMA 1991;266:369–74.
4. Klein BE, Klein R, Sponsel WE, et al. Prevalence of glaucoma: The Beaver Dam Eye Study. Ophthalmology 1992; 99:1499–1504.
5. Bengtsson B. The prevalence of glaucoma. Br J Ophthalmol 1981;65:46–9.
6. Hollows FC, Graham PA. Intraocular pressure, glaucoma, and glaucoma suspects in a defined population. Br J Ophthalmol 1986;50:510–86.
7. Viggosson G, Bjornsson G, Ingvason JG. The prevalence of open-angle glaucoma in Ireland. Acta Ophthalmol 1986;64:138–41.
8. Armaly MF. On the distribution of applanation pressure. I. The statistical features and the effects of age, sex and the family history of glaucoma. Arch Ophthalmol 1965;73:11–8.
9. Linner E, Strombergo U. Ocular Hypertension. A Five Year Study of the Total Population in a Swedish Town, Skovde. In W Leytdhencker (ed), Glaucoma Symposium. Basel: Karger 1966;187–214.
10. Perkins ES. The Beford glaucoma survey. I. Long term follow-up of borderline cases. Br J Ophthalmol 1973;57: 179–85.
11. Graham PA. The definition of pre-glaucoma, a prospective study. Trans Ophthalmol Soc UK 1968;88:153–65.
12. Armaly MF. Ocular pressure and visual fields, a ten-year follow-up study. Arch Ophthalmol 1969;81:25–40.
13. Shields MB. Textbook of Glaucoma (3rd ed). Baltimore: Williams & Wilkins, 1992;84–125, 172–97, 264–76, 287–93, 307–17, 393–6, 431–45, 548–58.
14. Bankes JLK, Perkins ES, Tsolakis S, et al. Bedford glaucoma survey. Br Med J 1968;1:791–6.
15. Kahn HA, Milton RC. Alternative definitions of open-angle glaucoma: Effect on prevalence and associations in the Framingham Eye Study. Arch Ophthalmol 1980;98:2172–7.
16. Arkell SM, Lightman DA, Sommer A, et al. The prevalence of glaucoma among Eskimos of Northwest Alaska. Arch Ophthalmol 1987;105:482–5.

17. Loh RCK. The problems of glaucoma in Singapore. Singapore Med J 1968;9:76.

18. Lowe RF, Ritch R. Angle Closure Glaucoma. In R Ritch, MB Shields, T Krupin (eds), The Glaucomas. St. Louis: Mosby, 1989;825–53.

19. Jocson VL, Sears ML. Experimental aqueous perfusion in enucleated eyes. Arch Ophthalmol 1972;86:65–71.

20. Alvarado J, Murphy C, Juster R. Trabeular meshwork cellularity in primary open-angle glaucoma and nonglaucomatous normals. Ophthalmology 1984;91:564–79.

21. Fine BS, Yanoff M, Stone RA. A clinicopathologic study of four cases of primary open-angle glaucoma compared to normal eyes. Am J Ophthalmol 1981;91:88–105.

22. Rohen JW. Why is intraocular pressure elevated in chronic simple glaucoma. Anatomical considerations. Ophthalmology 1983;90:758–62.

23. Tripathi RC. Mechanism of the aqueous outflow across the trabecular wall of Schlemm's canal. Exp Eye Res 1971;11:116–21.

24. Johnson MC, Kamm RD. The role of Schlemm's canal in aqueous outflow from the human eye. Invest Ophthalmol Vis Sci 1983;24:320–5.

25. Anderson DR, Quigley HA. The Optic Nerve. In RA Moses, W Hart (eds), Adler's Physiology of the Eye (8th ed). St. Louis: Mosby, 1985;616–41.

26. Radius RL. Anatomy and Pathophysiology of the Retina and Optic Nerve. In R Ritch, MB Shields, T Krupin (eds), The Glaucomas. St. Louis: Mosby, 1989;89–132.

27. Minckler DS, Spaeth GL. Optic nerve damage in glaucoma. Surv Ophthalmol 1981;26:128–48.

28. Maumenee AE. Causes of optic nerve damage in glaucoma. Ophthalmology 1988;95;3–8.

29. Hayreh SS. Pathogenesis of optic nerve head changes in glaucoma. Semin Ophthalmol 1980;1:1–13.

30. Jonas JB, Naumann GOH. Parapapillary retinal vessel diameter in normal and glaucomatous eyes. II. Correlations. Invest Ophthalmol Vis Sci 1989;30:1604–11.

31. Lampert PW, Vogel MH, Zimmerman LE. Pathology of the optic nerve in experimental acute glaucoma. Electron microscopic studies. Invest Ophthalmol Vis Sci 1968;7:199–213.

32. Emery JM, Landis D, Paton D, et al. The lamina cribrosa in normal and glaucomatous human eyes. Trans Am Acad Ophthalmol Otolaryngol 1974;78:290–7.

33. Anderson DR, Hendrickson AE. Failure of increased intracranial pressure to affect rapid axonal transport at the optic nerve head. Invest Ophthalmol Vis Sci 1977;16:423–6.

34. Tielsch JM, Katz J, Sommer A, et al. Family history and risk of primary open angle glaucoma. Arch Ophthalmol 1994;112:69–73.

35. Shin DH, Becker B, Kolker AE. Family history in primary open-angle glaucoma. Arch Ophthalmol 1977,95:598–600.

36. Brown RH, Zillis JD, Lynch MG, Sanborn GE. The afferent pupillary defect in asymmetric glaucoma. Arch Ophthalmol 1987;105:1540–3.

37. McMenemy MG, Stamper RL. Psychophysical Testing in Glaucoma. In J Caprioli (ed), Contemporary Issues in Glaucoma. Philadelphia: Saunders, 1991;699–709.

38. Starreds ME. The measure of intraocular pressure. Int Ophthalmol Clin 1979;19:9–11.

39. Drance SM. The significance of the diurnal tension variations in normal and glaucomatous eyes. Arch Ophthalmol 1960;64:494–501.

40. Kitazawa Y, Horie T. Diurnal variation of intraocular pressure in primary open-angle glaucoma. Am J Ophthalmol 1975;79:557–65.

41. Shiose Y. Intraocular pressure—new perspectives. Surv Ophthalmol 1990;34:413–35.

42. Sommer A. Intraocular pressure and glaucoma. Am J Ophthalmol 1989;107:186–8.

43. Anctil J-L, Anderson DR. Early foveal involvement and generalized depression of the visual field in glaucoma. Arch Ophthalmol 1984;102:363–70.

44. Airaksinen J, Drance SM, Douglas G, et al. Diffuse and localized nerve fiber loss in glaucoma. Am J Ophthalmol 1984;98:566–71.

45. Anderson DR. Automated Static Perimetry. St. Louis: Mosby-Year Book, 1994;40–68.

46. Werner EB. Manual of Visual Fields. New York: Churchill Livingstone 1991;125–55.

47. Zeimer RC, Wilensky JT, Gieser DK, Viana MA. Association between intraocular pressure peaks and progression of visual field loss. Ophthalmology 1991;94:64–9.

48. Drance SM. Glaucomatous Visual Field Defects. In R Ritch, MB Shields, T Krupin (eds), The Glaucomas. St. Louis: Mosby, 1989;393–402.

49. Werner EB, Drance SM. Early visual field disturbances in glaucoma. Arch Ophthalmol 1977;95:1173–5.

50. Hart WM, Becker B. Onset and evolution of glaucomatous visual field defects. Ophthalmology 1982;89:268–79.

51. Werner EB, Piltz-Seymour J. What constitutes a glaucomatous visual field defect. Semin Ophthalmol 1992;7:110–29.

52. Levene RZ. Low tension glaucoma. A critical review and new material. Surv Ophthalmol 1980;24:621–64.

53. Caprioli J, Spaeth GL. Visual field defects in low-tension glaucoma: comparison of visual field defects in the low-tension glaucomas with those in high-tension glaucoma. Am J Ophthalmol 1984;97:730–7.

54. Chauhan BC, Drance SM, Douglas GR, Johnson CA. Visual field damage in normal-tension and high-tension glaucoma. Am J Ophthalmol 1989;108:636–42.

55. Motolko M, Drance SM, Douglas GR. Comparison of defects in low-tension and chronic open-angle glaucoma. Arch Ophthalmol 1982;100:1074–79.

56. Zulauf M, Caprioli J. What constitutes progression of glaucomatous visual field defects. Semin Ophthalmol 1992;7:130–46.

57. Boeglin RJ, Caprioli J, Zulauf M. Long-term fluctuation of the visual field in glaucoma. Am J Ophthalmol 1992; 113:396–400.

58. Quigley HA, MIller NR, George T. Clinical evaluation of nerve fiber layer atrophy as an indicator of glaucomatous optic nerve damage. Arch Ophthalmol 1980;98:1564–71.

59. Quigley HA, Addicks EM, Green WR. Optic nerve damage in human glaucoma: quantitative correlation of nerve fiber layer loss and visual field defects in glaucoma, ischemic

neuropathy, papilledema, and toxic neuropathy. Arch Ophthalmol 1982;100:135–46.

60. Sommer A, Pollack I, Maumenee AE. Optic disc parameters and onset of glaucomatous field loss. I. Methods and progressive changes in disc morphology. Arch Ophthalmol 1979;97:1444–8.

61. Quigley HA, Dunkelberger GR, Green WR. Retinal ganglion cell atrophy correlated with automated perimetry in human eyes with glaucoma. Am J Ophthalmol 1989;107: 453–64.

62. Johnson CA. Early losses of visual function in glaucoma. Optom Vis Sci 1995;72:359–70.

63. Flammers J, Drance SM. Reversibility of a glaucomatous visual field defect after acetazolamide therapy. Can J Ophthalmol 1983;18:139–41.

64. Airaksinen PJ, Drance SM, Douglas GR, et al. Visual field and retinal nerve fiber layer comparisons in glaucoma. Arch Ophthalmol 1985;103:205–7.

65. Caprioli J, Miller JM, Sears M. Quantitative evaluation of the optic nerve head in patients with unilateral visual field loss from primary open angle glaucoma. Ophthalmology 1987;94:1484–7.

66. Sommer A, Katz J, Quigley HA, et al. Clinically detectable nerve fiber atrophy precedes the onset of glaucomatous field loss. Arch Ophthalmol 1991,109:77–83.

67. Boeglin RJ, Caprioli J. Contemporary Clinical Evaluation of the Optic Nerve in Glaucoma. In J Caprioli (ed), Contemporary Issues in Glaucoma. Philadelphia: Saunders, 1991;711–31.

68. Trobe JD, Glasser JS, Cassady J, et al. Nonglaucomatous excavation of the optic disc. Arch Ophthalmol 1980,98: 1046–50.

69. Airaksinen PJ, Drance SM, Schulzer M. Neuroretinal rim area in early glaucoma. Am J Ophthalmol 1985;99:1–4.

70. Cheri T, Robinson LP. Thinning of the neural rim of the optic nerve head. Trans Ophthalmol Soc UK, 1973;93: 213–43.

71. Caprioli J, Spaeth GL. Looking for better ways to measure the optic disc. Ophthalmic Surg 1987;18:866.

72. Jonas JB, Zach FM, Gusek GC, Naumann GOM. Pseudoglaucomatous physiologic large cups. Am J Ophthalmol 1989;107:137–44.

73. Tomita G, Takamoto T, Schwartz B. Glaucoma like disks without increased intraocular pressure or visual field loss. Am J Ophthalmol 1989;108:496–504.

74. Armaly MF. Genetic determination of cup/disc ratio of the optic nerve. Arch Ophthalmol 1967;78:35–43.

75. Read RM, Spaeth GL. The practical clinical appraisal of the optic disc in glaucoma: The natural history of cup progression and some specific disc-field correlations. Trans Am Acad Ophthalmol Otolaryngol 1974;78:255–74.

76. Susanna R Jr. The lamina cribrosa and visual field defects in open angle glaucoma. Can J Ophthalmol 1983;18: 124–6.

77. Herschler JH, Osher RH. Baring of the circumlinear vessel. An early sign of optic nerve damage. Arch Ophthalmol 1980;98:865–9.

78. Kitazawa Y, Shiroaki S, Tetsuya Y. Optic disc hemorrhage in low-tension glaucoma. Ophthalmology 1986;93:853–7.

79. Drance SM, Fairclough M, Butler DM, Kottler MS. The importance of disc hemorrhage in the prognosis of chronic open angle glaucoma. Arch Ophthalmol 1977;95:226–8.

80. Drance SM. Disc hemorrhages in the glaucomas. Surv Ophthalmol 1989;33:331–7.

81. Armaly MF. The optic cup in the normal eye. I. Cup width, depth, vessel displacement, ocular tension and outflow facility. Am J Ophthalmol 1969;68:401–7.

82. Sommer A, Miller NR, Pollack T, et al. The nerve fiber layer in the diagnosis of glaucoma. Arch Ophthalmol 1977,95:2149–56.

83. Sommer A, Quigley HA, Robin AL, et al. Evaluation of nerve fiber layer assessment. Arch Ophthalmol 1984;102: 1766–71.

84. Caprioli J, Miller JM. Measurement of relative nerve fiber layer surface height in glaucoma. Ophthalmology 1989;96: 633–41.

85. Takamoto T, Schwartz B. Photogrammetric measurement of nerve fiber layer thickness. Ophthalmology 1989;96: 1315–9.

86. Zeyen TG, Caprioli J. Progression of disc and field damage in early glaucoma. Arch Ophthalmol 1993;111:62–5.

87. Fechtner RD, Weinreb RN. Examining and Recording the Appearance of the Optic Nerve Head. In RJ Starita (ed), Clinical Signs in Ophthalmology (Vol. XII). St. Louis: Mosby-Year Book, 1991;5:2–15.

88. Leske MC, Rosenthal J. The epidemiologic aspects of open-angle glaucoma. Am J Epidemiol 1979;109:250–72.

89. Pederson JE, Anderson DR. The mode of progressive disc cupping in ocular hypertension and glaucoma. Arch Ophthalmol 1980;98:490–5.

90. Hart WM Jr. The Epidemiology of Primary Open-Angle Glaucoma. In R Ritch, MB Shields, T Krupin (eds), The Glaucomas. St. Louis: Mosby, 1989;789–95.

91. Phelps CD. The "no treatment" approach to ocular hypertension. Surv Ophthalmol 1980;25:175–82.

92. Mills KB. Ocular hypertension. Semin Ophthalmol 1986;1: 41–5.

93. Taylor JDN, Weinreb RN. Management of ocular hypertension. Ophthal Pract 1992;10:119–22.

94. Werner EB. Low-tension Glaucoma. In R Ritch, MB Shields, T Krupin (eds), The Glaucomas. St. Louis: Mosby, 1989;797–812.

95. Cockburn DM, Gutteridge IF. Low-tension glaucoma: an optometric view point. Clin Exp Opt 1991;74:89–95.

96. Quigley HA, Addicks EM, Green WR, Maumenee AE. Optic nerve damage in human glaucoma—2. The site of injury and susceptibility to damage. Arch Ophthalmol 1987;99:635–49.

97. Drance SM, Sweeney VP, Morgan RW, Feldman F. Factors involved in the production of low tension glaucoma. Can J Ophthalmol 1974;9:399–403.

98. Gasser P. Ocular vasospasm: A risk factor in the pathogenesis of low-tension glaucoma. Int Ophthalmol 1989;13: 281–90.

99. Phelps CD, Corbett JJ. Migraine and low-tension glaucoma. A case-control study. Invest Ophthalmol Vis Sci 1985;26:1105–8.

100. Carter CJ, Brooks DE, Doyle DL, Drance SM. Investigations into a vascular etiology for low-tension glaucoma. Ophthalmology 1990;97:49–55.

101. Caprioli J, Spaeth GL. Comparison of the optic nerve head in high- and low-tension glaucoma. Arch Ophthalmol 1985;103:1145–9.

102. Fazio P, Krupin T, Feitl ME et al. Optic disc topography in patients with low-tension and primary open angle glaucoma. Arch Ophthmol 1990;108:705–8.

103. Miller KM, Quigley HA. Comparison of optic disc features in low-tension and typical open-angle glaucoma. Ophthalmol Surg 1987;18:882–9.

104. Radius RL, Maumenee AE. Optic atrophy and glaucomatous cupping. Am J Ophthalmol 1978;85:145–53.

105. Sebag J, Thomas JV, Epstein DL, Grand WM. Optic disc cupping in arteritic anterior ischemic optic neuropathy resembles glaucomatous cupping. Ophthalmol 1986;93:357–61.

106. Chumbley LC, Brubaker RF. Low-tension glacuoma. Am J Ophthalmol 1976;81:761–7.

107. Drance SM, Sweeny VP, Morgan RW, Feldman F. Studies of factors involved in the production of low-tension glaucoma. Arch Ophthalmol 1973;89:457–65.

108. Hitchings RA. Low tension glaucoma—is treatment worthwhile? Eye 1988;2:636–40.

109. Caprioli J. Low tension glaucoma. Curr Opin Ophthalmol 1990;1:122–6.

110. Grunwald JE. Effect of timolol maleate on the retinal circulation of human eyes with ocular hypertension. Invest Ophthalmol Vis Sci 1990;31:521–6.

111. Kitazawa Y, Shirai H, Go FJ. The effect of a Ca^{2+} antagonist on visual field in low-tension glaucoma. Graefes Arch Clin Exp Ophthalmol 1989;227:408–12.

112. Schwartz AL, Perman KI, Whitten M. Argon laser trabeculoploasty in progressive low-tension glaucoma. Ann Ophthalmol 1984;16:560–6.

113. Watson PG, Allen ED, Graham CM, et al. Argon laser trabeculoplasty or trabeculectomy—a prospective randomized block study. Trans Ophthalmol 1985;104:55–61.

114. De Jong N, Greve EL, Hoyng PFJ, Geijssen HC. Results of a filtering procedure in low-tension glaucoma. Int Ophthalmol 1989;13:131–8.

115. Parrow KA, Mong YJ, Shin DH, et al. Is it worthwhile to add dipivefrin HCl 0.1% to topical β_1 β_2 blocker therapy? Ophthalmology 1989;1338–42.

116. Schumer RA, Podos SM. Medical treatment as the initial therapy for open-angle glaucoma. Semin Ophthalmol 1992;7:81–91.

117. Alm A, Stjernschantz J, The Scandinavian Latanoprost Study Group. Effects on intraocular pressure and side effects of 0.005% latanoprost applied once daily, evening or morning: a comparison with timolol. Ophthalmology 1995;102:1743–52.

118. Weinreb RN. Compliance with medical treatment of glaucoma. J Glaucoma 1992;1:134–6.

119. Greenidge KC. Angle-closure glaucoma. Int Ophthalmol Clin 1990;30:177–86.

120. Alper MG, Laubach JL. Primary angle-closure in the American Negro. Arch Ophthalmol 1968;79:663–8.

121. Galin MA. Angle-closure glaucoma. Semin Ophthalmol 1986;1:50–2.

122. Spaeth GL. Gonioscopy uses old and new, the inheritance of occludable angles. Ophthalmology 1978;85:222–32.

123. Forbes M. Gonioscopy with corneal indentation. Arch Ophthalmol 1966;76:488–92.

124. Fourman S. Diagnosing acute angle-closure glaucoma: A flow chart. Surv Ophthalmol 1989;33:491–4.

125. Krawitz PL, Podos SM. Use of apraclonidine in the treatment of acute angle closure glaucoma. Arch Ophthalmol 1990;108:1208–9.

126. Ritch R, Lowe RF, Reyes A. Therapeutic Overview of Angle Closure Glaucoma. In R Ritch, MB Shields, T Krupin (eds), The Glaucomas. St. Louis: Mosby, 1989;855–64.

127. Ganias F, Mapstone R. Miotics in closed angle glaucoma. Br J Ophthalmol 1975;59:205–6.

128. Airaksinsen PJ, Saari KM, Tiainen TJ, Jaanio EAT. The management of acute closed-angle glaucoma with miotics and timolol. Br J Ophthalmol 1979;63:822–5.

129. Greenidge KC. Angle-closure Glaucoma: Definitions, Detection Distinctions, Decisions and Dissolution. In RJ Starita (ed), Clinical Signs in Ophthalmology. St. Louis: Mosby-Year Book, 1990;10:2–15.

130. David R. The management of primary acute glaucoma. Glaucoma 1985;8:64–8.

131. Hyams S. Laser iridotomy—think first. Glaucoma 1991;13:122–5.

132. Del Priore LV, Robin AL, Pollack JP. Neodymium:YAG and argon laser iridotomy: long-term follow-up in a prospective, randomized clinical trial. Ophthalmology 1988,95:1207–11.

133. Lowe RF. Acute angle-closure glaucoma. The second eye: An analysis of 200 cases. Br J Ophthalmol 1962;46:641–50.

134. Mapstone R. The fellow eye. Br J Ophthalmol 1981;65:410–2.

135. Salmon JF. The roles of trabeculectomy in the treatment of advanced chronic angle-closure glaucoma. J Glaucoma 1993;2:285–90.

136. Richardson TM. Pigmentary Glaucoma. In R Ritch, MB Shields, T Krupin (eds), The Glaucomas. St. Louis: Mosby, 1989;981–95.

137. Davidson JE, Brubaker RF, Ilstrup DM. Dimensions of the anterior chamber in pigment dispersion syndrome. Arch Ophthalmol 1983;101:81–3.

138. Strasser G, Hauff W. Pigmentary dispersion syndrome: A biometric study. Acta Ophthalmol 1985;63:721–3.

139. Potash SD, Tello C, Liebmann J, Ritch R. Ultrasound biomicroscopy in pigment dispersion syndrome. Ophthalmology 1994;101:332–9.

140. Farrar SM, Shields MB. Current concepts in pigmentary glaucoma. Surv Ophthalmol 1993;37:233–52.

141. Campbell DG. Pigmentary dispersion and glaucoma: A new theory. Arch Ophthalmol 1979;97:1667–72.

142. Kampik A, Green WR, Quigley HA, Pierce LH. Scanning and transmission electron microscopic studies of two cases of pigment dispersion syndrome. Am J Ophthalmol 1981;91:573–87.

143. Haynes WL, Johnson AT, Alward WL. Effects of jogging exercise on patients with pigmentary dispersion syndrome and pigmentary glaucoma. Ophthalmology 1992;999: 1096–103.

144. Ritch R. Pigmentary glaucoma: A self-limited entity? Ann Ophthalmol 1983; 15:115–6.

145. Ritch R, Campbell DG, Camras C. Initial treatment of pigmentary glaucoma. J Glaucoma 1993;2:44–9.

146. Karickhoff JR. Pigmentary dispersion syndrome and pigmentary glaucoma: A new mechanism concept, a new treatment and a new technique. Ophthalmic Surg 1992;23:269–77.

147. Lunde MW. Argon laser trabeculoplasty in pigmentary dispersion syndrome with glaucoma. Am J Ophthalmol 1983;96:721–5.

148. Traverso CE, Spaeth GL, Starita RJ, et al. Factors affecting the results of argon laser trabeculoplasty in open-angle glaucoma. Ophthalmic Surg 1986;17:554–9.

149. Ritch R, Liebmann J, Robin A, et al. Argon laser trabeculoplasty in pigmentary glaucoma. Ophthalmology 1993; 100:909–13.

150. Farrar SM, Shields MB, Miller KN, Stoup CM. Risk factors for the development and severity of glaucoma in the pigment dispersion syndrome. Am J Ophthalmol 1989; 108:223–9.

151. Layden WE, Shaffer RN. Exfoliation syndrome. Am J Ophthalmol 1974;78:835–41.

152. Lindblom B, Thorburn W. Observed incidence of glaucoma in Halsingland, Sweden. Acta Ophthalmol 1984; 62:217–22.

153. Layden WE, Exfoliation Syndrome. In R Ritch, MB Shields, T Krupin (eds), The Glaucomas. St. Louis: Mosby, 1989; 997–1015.

154. Kozart DM, Yanoff M. Intraocular pressure status in 100 consecutive patients with exfoliation syndrome. Ophthalmology 1982;89:214–8.

155. Sugar S. Pigmentary glaucoma and the glaucoma associated with the exfoliation pseudoexfoliation syndrome—update. Ophthalmology 1984;91:307–10.

156. Hansen E, Sellevold OJ. Pseudoexfoliation of the lens capsule. II. Development of the exfoliation syndrome. Acta Ophthalmol 1969;47:161–73.

157. Schlotzer-Schrehardt UM, Koca MR, Nauman GO, et al. Pseudoexfoliation syndrome: Ocular manifestation of a systemic disorder. Arch Ophthalmol 1992;110:1752–6.

158. Konstas AGP, Jay JL, Marshall GE, Lee WR. Prevalence, diagnostic features and response to trabeculectomy in exfoliation glaucoma. Ophthalmology 1993;100:619–27.

159. Herschler J, Cobo M. Trauma and Elevated Intraocular Pressure. In R Ritch, MB Shields, T Krupin (eds), The Glaucomas. St. Louis: Mosby, 1989;1225–37.

160. Kaufman JM, Tolpin DW. Glaucoma after traumatic angle recession: A ten-year prospective study. Am J Ophthalmol 1974;78:648–54.

161. Herschler J. Trabecular damage due to blunt anterior segment injury and its relationship to traumatic glaucoma. Trans Am Acad Ophthalmol Otolaryngol 1977;83:239–48.

162. Tesluk GC, Spaeth GL. The occurrence of primary open angle glaucoma in the fellow eye of patients with unilateral angle-cleavage glaucoma. Ophthalmology 1984;92: 904–11.

163. Mermoud A, Salmon JF, Burron A et al. Surgical management of post traumatic angle recession glaucoma. Ophthalmology 1993;100:634–42.

164. Ben Ezra D. Neovasculogenesis: Triggering factors and possible mechanisms. Surv Ophthalmol 1979;24:167–76.

165. Hoskins HD, Kass MA. Becker-Shaffer's Diagnosis and Therapy of the Glaucomas (6th ed). St. Louis: Mosby, 1989;242–8, 422–4.

166. Gartner S, Henkind P. Neovascularization of the iris. Surv Ophthalmol 1978;22:291–312.

167. Wand M. Neovascular glaucoma. In R Ritch, MB Shields, T Krupin (eds), The Glaucomas. St. Louis: Mosby, 1989;1063–110.

168. Smith RJH. Rubeotic glaucoma. Br J Ophthalmol 1981;65:606–9.

169. Jacobson DR, Murphy RP, Rosenthal AR. The treatment of angle neovascularization with panretinal photocoagulation. Ophthalmology 1979;86:1270–5.

170. Magargal LE, Brown GC, Ausburger JJ, et al. Efficacy of panretinal photocoagulation in preventing neovascular glaucoma following ischemic central retinal artery obstruction. Ophthalmology 1982;89:780–4.

171. Simmons RJ, Depperman SR, Dueker DK. The role of gonio-photocoagulation in neovascularization of the anterior chamber angle. Ophthalmology 1980;87:79–82.

172. Weber PA. Neovascular glaucoma: Current management. Surv Ophthalmol 1981;26:149–53.

173. Mermoud A. Salmon JF, Alexander P et al. Molteno tube implantation for neovascular glaucoma: long-term results and factors influencing the outcome. Ophthalmology 1993;100:897–902.

174. Caprioli J, Strang SL, Spaeth GL, Poryzees EH. Cyclocryotherapy in the treatment of advanced glaucoma. Ophthalmology 1985;92:947–54.

175. Schuman JS, Puliafito CA, Allingham RR, et al. Contact transscleral continuous wave neodymium:YAG laser cyclophotocoagulation. Ophthalmology 1990;97:571–80.

176. Krupin T, Dorfman NH, Spector SM, Wax MB. Secondary glaucoma associated with uveitis. Glaucoma 1988;10:85–90.

177. Krupin T, Feitl ME. Glaucoma Associated with Uveitis. In R Ritch, MB Shields, T Krupin (eds), The Glaucomas. St. Louis: Mosby, 1989;1205–23.

178. Hill RS, Nguyen QH, Baerveldt G, et al. Trabeculectomy and molteno implantation for glaucomas associated with uveitis. Ophthalmology 1993;100:903–8.

179. Kass MA, Becker B, Kolker AE. Glaucomatocyclitic crisis and primary open-angle glaucoma. Am J Ophthalmol 1973;75:668–73.

180. Raitta C, Vannas A. Glaucomatocyclitic crisis. Arch Ophthalmol 1977;95:608–12.

181. Radius RL, Diamond GR, Pollack IP, Langham ME. Timolol. A new drug for management of chronic simple glaucoma. Arch Ophthalmol 1978;96:1603-8.

182. Zimmerman TJ, Harbin R, Pett M, Kaufman HE. Timolol and facility of outflow. Invest Ophthalmol Vis Sci 1977;16:623-4.

183. Sonntag JR, Brindley GO, Shields MB. Effect of timolol therapy on outflow facility. Invest Ophthalmol Vis Sci 1978;17:293-6.

184. Martin XD, Rabineau PA. Intraocular pressure effects of timolol after unilateral instillation. Ophthalmology 1988; 95:1620-3.

185. Van Buskirk EM. Adverse reactions from timolol administration. Ophthalmology 1980;87:447-50.

186. McMahon CP, Schaffer RN, Hoskins HD Jr, Hetherington J Jr. Adverse effects experienced by patients taking timolol. Am J Ophthalmol 1979;88:736-8.

187. Zimmerman TJ, Bauman JD, Hetherington J Jr. Side effects of timolol. Surv Ophthalmol 1983;28:243-9.

188. Van Buskirk EM, Fraunfelder FT. Ocular beta-blockers and systemic side effects. Am J Ophthalmol 1984;98:623-4.

189. Velde TM, Kaiser FE. Ophthalmic timolol treatment causing altered hypoglycemic response in a diabetic patient. Arch Intern Med 1983;143:1627-30.

190. Schoene RB, Abuan T, Ward RL, Beasley CH. Effects of topical betaxolol, timolol and placebo on pulmonary function in asthmatic bronchitis. Am J Ophthalmol 1984;97:86-92.

191. Katz IM, Berger ET. Effects of iris pigmentation on response of ocular pressure to timolol. Surv Ophthalmol 1979;23:395-8.

192. Mills KB. Blind randomized non-crossover longterm trial comparing topical timolol 0.25% with timolol 0.5% in treatment of simple chronic glaucoma. Br J Ophthalmol 1983;67:216-9.

193. Zimmerman TJ, Kaufman HE. Timolol: Dose response and duration of action. Arch Ophthalmol 1977;95:605-7.

194. Steinhart RF, Thomas JV, Boger WP III. Long term drift and continued efficacy after multiyear timolol therapy. Arch Ophthalmol 1981;99:100-3.

195. Plane C, Steen C, Borrmann L, et al. Additive ocular hypotensive effect of dipivefrin and timolol. Glaucoma 1990;12:16-9.

196. Thomas JV, Epstein DL. Timolol and epinephrine in primary open angle glaucoma: Transient additive effect. Arch Ophthalmol 1981;99:91-5.

197. Cinotti A, Cinotti D, Grant W, et al. Levobunolol vs. timolol for open-angle glaucoma and ocular hypertension. Am J Ophthalmol 1985;99:11-7.

198. Wandel T, Charap AD, Lewis RA, et al. Glaucoma treatment with once daily levobunolol. Am J Ophthalmol 1986;101:298-304.

199. Rakofsky SI, Almog Y, Lazar M, et al. Efficacy and safety of once daily levobunolol for glaucoma therapy. Can J Ophthalmol 1989;24:2-6.

200. Rakofsky SI, Melamed S, Cohen JS, et al. A comparison of the ocular hypotensive efficacy of once-daily and twice-daily levobunolol treatment. Ophthalmology 1989;96:8-11.

201. Serle JB, Lustgarten JS, Podos SM. A clinical trial of metipranolol, a noncardioselective beta-adrenergic antagonist, in ocular hypertension. Am J Ophthalmol 1991;112:302-7.

202. Zimmerman TJ. Topical ophthalmic beta blockers: a comparative review. J Ocular Pharmacol 1993;9:373-84.

203. Stewart RH, Kimbrough RL, Ward RL. Betaxolol vs. timolol: a six month double blind comparison. Arch Ophthalmol 1986;104:46-8.

204. Radius RL. Use of betaxolol in the reduction of elevated intraocular pressure. Arch Ophthalmol 1983;101:898-900.

205. Berry DP, Van Buskirk EM, Shields MB. Betaxolol and timolol. A comparison of efficacy and side effects. Arch Ophthalmol 1984;102:42-5.

206. Dunn TL, Gerber MJ, et al. The effect of topical ophthalmic instillation of timolol and betaxolol on lung function in asthmatic subjects. Ann Rev Respir Dis 1986;133:264-8.

207. Lynch MG, Whitson JT, Brown RH, et al. Topical beta-blocker therapy and central nervous system side effects. A preliminary study comparing betaxolol and timolol. Arch Ophthalmol 1988;106:908-11.

208. Allen RC, Epstein DL. Additive effect of betaxolol and epinephrine in primary open angle glaucoma. Arch Ophthalmol 1986;104:1178-84.

209. Garner LL, Johnstone WW, Ballintine EJ, Carroll ME. Effect of 2% levo-rotary epinephrine on the intraocular pressure of the glaucomatous eye. Arch Ophthalmol 1959;62:230-8.

210. Richards JSF, Drance SM. The effect of 2% epinephrine on aqueous humor dynamics in the human eye. Can J Ophthalmol 1967;2:259-63.

211. Townsend DJ, Brubaker RF. Immediate effect of epinephrine on aqueous formation in the normal human eye as measured by fluorophotometry. Invest Ophthalmol Vis Sci 1980;19:256-66.

212. Drance SM, Ross RA. The ocular effects of epinephrine. Surv Ophthalmol 1970;14:330-5.

213. Thomas JV, Gragoudas ES, Blair NP, Lapus JV. Correlation of epinephrine use and macula edema in aphakic glaucomatous eyes. Arch Ophthalmol 1978;96:625-8.

214. Ballin N, Becker B, Goldman ML. Systemic effects of epinephrine applied topically to the eye. Invest Ophthalmol 1966;5:125-9.

215. Kass MA, Mandell A, Goldberg I, et al. Dipivefrin and epinephrine treatment of elevated intraocular pressure: A comparative study. Arch Ophthalmol 1979;97:1865-6.

216. Kriegelstein GK, Leydhecker W. The dose-response relationships of dipivalyl epinephrine in open angle glaucoma. Graefes Arch Klin Exp Ophthalmol 1978;205:141-6.

217. Mandell AI, Stenz F, Kitabicki AE. Dipivalyl epinephrine: A new pro drug in the treatment of glaucoma. Trans Am Acad Ophthalmol Otolaryngol 1978;85:268-74.

218. Kohn AN, Moss AP, Hargett NA, et al. Clinical comparison of dipivalyl epinephrine and epinephrine in the treatment of glaucoma. Am J Ophthalmol 1979;87:196-201.

219. Gharagozloo N, Relf S, Brubaker RF. Aqueous flow is reduced by the alpha-adrenergic agonist apraclonidine hydrochloride. Ophthalmology 1988;95:1217-20.

220. Silverstone DE, Brint SF, Olander KW, et al. Prophylactic use of apraclonidine for intraocular pressure increase after Nd:YAG capsulotomies. Am J Ophthalmol 1992;113:401–5.

221. Nagasubramanian S, Hitchings RA, Demailly P, et al. Comparison of apraclonidine and timolol in chronic open-angle glaucoma. A three-month study. Ophthalmology 1993;100: 1318–23.

222. Cardakli UF, Smythe BA, Eisele JR et al. Effect of chronic apraclonidine treatment on intraocular pressure in advanced glaucoma. J Glaucoma 1993;2:271–8.

223. Grierson I, Lee WR, Abraham S. Effects of pilocarpine on the morphology of the human outflow apparatus. Br J Ophthalmol 1978;62:302–13.

224. Bill A, Phillips CI. Uveoscleral drainage of aqueous humor in human eyes. Exp Eye Res 1971;12:275.

225. Abramson DH, Franzen LA, Coleman DJ. Pilocarpine in the presbyope. Arch Ophthalmol 1973;89:100–3.

226. Abramson DH, Coleman DJ, Forbes M, Franzen LA. Pilocarpine: Effect on the anterior chamber and lens thickness. Arch Ophthalmol 1972;87:615–20.

227. Alpar JJ. Miotics and retinal detachment: A survey and case report. Ann Ophthalmol 1979;11:395–401.

228. Drance SM, Nash PA. The dose response of human intraocular pressure to pilocarpine. Can J Ophthalmol 1971;6:9.

229. Johnson DH, Epstein DL, Allen RC, Boys-Smith J, et al. A one-year multicenter clinical trial of pilocarpine gel. Am J Ophthalmol 1984;97:723–9.

230. March WF, Stewart RM, Mandell AI, Bruce LA. Duration of effect of pilocarpine gel. Arch Ophthalmol 1973;100:1270–2.

231. Dailey RA, Brubaker RF, Bourne WM. The effects of timolol maleate and acetazolamide on the rate of aqueous formation in normal human subjects. Am J Ophthalmol 1982;93:232–7.

232. Lichter PR, Newman LP, Wheeler NC, Beall OV. Patient tolerance to carbonic anhydrase inhibitors. Am J Ophthalmol 1978;85:495–502.

233. Becker B. Carbonic anhydrase and the formation of aqueous humor. Am J Ophthalmol 1959;47:342–61.

234. Epstein DL, Grant WM. Carbonic anhydrase inhibitor side effects. Serum chemical analysis. Arch Ophthalmol 1977;95:1378–82.

235. Wallace TR, Fraunfelder FT, Petrusson GJ, Epstein DL. Decreased libido—a side effect of carbonic anhydrase inhibitor. Ann Ophthalmol 1979;11:1563–6.

236. Serle JB, Podos SM. Topical Carbonic Anhydrase Inhibitors in the Treatment of Glaucoma. In DA Less (ed), Ophthalmology Clinics of North America. Philadelphia: Saunders, 1995;315–25.

237. Nardin G, Lewis R, Lippa EA, et al. Activity of the topical CAI MK-507 bid when added to timolol bid. Invest Ophthalmol Vis Sci 1991;32(Suppl):989–91.

238. Yakatan GJ, Frome EL, Leonard RB, et al. Bioavailability of acetazolamide tablets. J Pharm Sci 1978;67:252–6.

239. Berson FG, Epstein DL, Grant WM, et al. Acetazolamide dosage forms in the treatment of glaucoma. Arch Ophthalmol 1980;98:1051–4.

240. Dahlen K, Epstein DL, Grant WM, et al. A repeated dose-response study of methazolamide in glaucoma. Arch Ophthalmol 1978;96:2214–8.

241. Stone RA, Zimmerman TJ, Shin DH, et al. Low-dose methazolamide and intraocular pressure. Am J Ophthalmol 1977;83:674–9.

242. Van Buskirk EM. Pathophysiology of laser trabeculoplasty. Surv Ophthalmol 1989;33:264–72.

243. Higginbotham EJ, Shahbazi MF. Laser therapy in glaucoma: An overview and update. Int Ophthalmol Clin 1990; 30:187–97.

244. Schwartz AL, Del Priore LV. The Evolving Role of Argon Laser Trabeculoplasty in Glaucoma. In J Caprioli (ed), Contemporary Issues in Glaucoma. Philadelphia: Saunders, 1991;827–38.

245. Savitt ML, Wilensky JT. Should laser trabeculoplasty be the initial mode of treatment in open-angle glaucoma. Semin Ophthalmol 1992;7:92–6.

246. Weinreb RN, Ruderman J, Juster R, Wilensky JT. Influence of the number of laser burns administered on the early results of argon laser trabeculoplasty. Am J Ophthalmol 1983;95:287–92.

247. Feldman RM, Katz LJ, Spaeth GL, et al. Long-term efficacy of repeat argon laser trabeculoplasty. Ophthalmology 1991;98:1061–5.

248. Weber PA, Burton GD, Epitropoulos AT. Laser trabeculoplasty retreatment. Ophthalmic Surg 1989;20:702–6.

249. Robin AL, Pollack IP, House B, Enger C. Effects of ALO 2145 on intraocular pressure following argon laser trabeculoplasty. Arch Ophthalmol 1987;105:646–50.

250. Reiss GR, Wilensky JT, Higginbotham EJ. Laser trabeculoplasty. Surv Ophthalmol 1991;35:407–28.

251. Shingleton BJ, Richter CU, Dharma SK, et al. Long-term efficacy of argon laser trabeculoplasty. Ophthalmology 1993;100:1324–9.

252. Thomas JV, El-Mofty A, Handy EE, et al. Argon laser trabeculoplasty as initial therapy for glaucoma. Arch Ophthalmol 1984;102:702–3.

253. Searle AET, Rosenthal AR, Chaudhuri PR. Argon laser trabeculoplasty as primary therapy in open-angle glaucoma: A long-term follow up. Glaucoma 1990;12: 70–5.

254. Beckman H, Meinert CL, Ritch R, et al. The Glaucoma laser trial. 2. Results of argon laser trabeculoplasty versus topical medicines. Ophthalomology 1990;97:1403–13.

255. Lichter PR. Practice implications of the glaucoma laser trial. Ophthalmology 1990;97:1401–2.

256. Van Buskirk EM. The laser step in early glaucoma therapy. Am J Ophthalmol 1991;112:87–90.

257. Schwartz AL. Argon laser trabeculoplasty in glaucoma: What's happening? J Glaucoma 1993;2:329–35.

258. Watson PG. The role of trabeculectomy in the management of glaucoma. Semin Ophthalmol 1986;1:46–9.

259. Miller E, Caprioli J. The Basis for Surgical Treatment of Open-Angle Glaucoma. In J Caprioli (ed), Contemporary Issues in Glaucoma. Philadelphia: Saunders, 1991; 839–51.

260. Sherwood MB, Migdal CS, Hitchings RA. Filtration surgery as the initial therapy for open angle glaucoma. J Glaucoma 1993;2:64–7.

261. Jay JL, Allan D. The benefit of early trabeculectomy versus conventional management in primary open-angle glaucoma relative to severity of disease. Eye 1989;3:528–35.

262. D'Ermo F, Bonomi L, Doro D. A critical analysis of the long-term results of trabeculectomy. Am J Ophthalmol 1979;88:829–35.

263. Freedman J, Shen E, Ahrens M. Trabeculectomy in a Black American glaucoma population. Br J Ophthalmol 1976;60:573–4.

264. Wilson P. Trabeculectomy: Long-term follow-up. Br J Ophthalmol 1977;61:535–8.

265. Rockwood EJ, Parrish RK, Heurer DK et al. Glaucoma filtering surgery with 5-fluorouracil. Ophthalmology 1987;94:1071–8.

266. Palmer SS. Mitomycin as adjunct chemotherapy with trabeculectomy. Ophthalmology 1991;98:317–21.

267. Liebmann JM, Ritch R, Marmor M, et al. Initial 5-fluorouracil trabeculectomy in uncomplicated glaucoma. Ophthalmology 1991;98:1036–41.

268. Katz LJ, Spaeth GL. Filtration Surgery. In R Ritch, MB Shields, T Krupin (eds), The Glaucomas. St. Louis: Mosby, 1989;653–96.

269. Greenidge KC, Allison K. Filtration blebs: Formation, development, maturation, and complications. Ophthalmic Pract 1990;8:188–92.

Appendix

Appendix

Common Ocular and Medical Abbreviations

ā	before	ASCVD	atherosclerotic cardiovascular disease
A	assessment or alternating (AET, alternating esotropia, etc.)	ASHD	atherosclerotic heart disease
		assn	association
AAU	acute anterior uveitis	astig	astigmatism
abd	abdominal	ATR	against-the-rule (astigmatism)
ABK	aphakic bullous keratopathy	AU	anterior uveitis
abn	abnormal	AVM	arteriovenous malformation
ac	before meals	A/V	arteriolar/venous (ratio, nicking)
AC	anterior chamber	BAK	benzalkonium chloride
ACC	accommodation	bas	basophils
ACE	angiotensin-converting enzyme	BC	base curve
ACG	angle-closure glaucoma	BCC	basal cell carcinoma
ACIOL	anterior chamber intraocular lens	BCP	birth control pill
add	adduction or bifocal power	BCR	base curve radius
ad lib	as desired	BD	base down
adv	advanced	BDR	background diabetic retinopathy
AIDS	acquired immunodeficiency syndrome	BI	base in
AKS	ankylosing spondylitis	bid	twice a day
AL	argon laser	bilat	bilateral
ALT	argon laser trabeculoplasty	BINO	bilateral internuclear ophthalmoplegia
AMA	against medical advice	BIO	binocular indirect ophthalmoscope (ophthalmoscopy)
ambl	amblyopia		
AMD	age-related macular degeneration	BK	bullous keratopathy
AMPPE	acute multifocal placoid pigment epitheliopathy	bleph	blepharitis
ANA	antinuclear antibody	BM	basement membrane
ant	anterior	BO	base out
AODM	adult-onset diabetes mellitus	BP	blood pressure
AP	anteroposterior	BRAO	branch retinal artery occlusion
APD	afferent pupillary defect	BRVO	branch retinal vein occlusion
approx	approximately	BU	base up
APTT	activated partial thromboplastin time	BUN	blood urea nitrogen
ARC	anomalous retinal correspondence	BUT	break-up time
ARMD	age-related macular degeneration	BVA	best visual acuity
ARN	acute retinal necrosis	bx	biopsy
art t	artificial tears	c̄	with
AS	anterior synechiae	C	cornea
ASA	aspirin (acetylsalicylic acid)	CA	carcinoma
ASAP	as soon as possible	CABG	coronary artery bypass graft
ASC	anterior subcapsular cataract	CAD	coronary artery disease

CAI	carbonic anhydrase inhibitor	DD	disc diameter
cap(s)	capsule(s)	DDx	differential diagnosis
cat	cataract	DFE	dilated fundus examination
CAT	computed axial tomography	D&I	dilation and irrigation
CB	ciliary body	dia	diameter
CBC	complete blood count	disp	dispense
$\overline{cc}$	with correction	DJD	degenerative joint disease
CC	chief complaint	Dk/L	oxygen transmissibility of a contact lens
CCA	common carotid artery	DM	diabetes mellitus
CCC	central corneal clouding	DME	diabetic macular edema
c/d or C/D	cup-to-disc ratio	DO	direct ophthalmoscopy
CF	count fingers	DPE	dipivalyl epinephrine
C&F	cells and flare	DR	diabetic retinopathy
CHF	congestive heart failure	DRS	Duane's retraction syndrome or Diabetic
CHRPE	congenital hypertrophy of the retinal pigment epithelium		Retinopathy Study
		DV	distance vision
Cil	Ciloxin (ciprofloxacin)	DW	daily wear
CL	contact lens *or* clear	Dx	diagnosis
cm	centimeter	E	esophoria at far
CME	cystoid macular edema	E'	esophoria at near
CMV	cytomegalovirus	EBMD	epithelial basement membrane dystrophy
CN	cranial nerve	ECA	external carotid artery
CNB	cranial nerve (CN) bevel	ECCE	extracapsular cataract extraction
CNS	central nervous system	ED	electrodiagnostic (testing)
CNVM	choroidal neovascular membrane	EDTA	ethylenediaminetetraacetic acid
c/o	complaining of	EEG	electroencephalogram
COAG	chronic open-angle glaucoma	EF	eccentric fixation
cong	congenital	EKC	epidemic keratoconjunctivitis
conj	conjunctiva	EKG or ECG	electrocardiogram
COP	cicatricial ocular pemphigoid	ELISA	enzyme-linked immunosorbent assay
COPD	chronic obstructive pulmonary disease	endo	endothelium
CP	cerebral palsy	ENT	ear, nose, throat
CPK	creatine phosphokinase	EOG	electro-oculography
CPR	cardiopulmonary resuscitation	EOM	extraocular muscles
CR	chorioretinal	eos	eosinophils
CRAO	central retinal artery occlusion	epith	epithelium
CRF	chronic renal failure	ER	emergency room
CRV	central retinal vein	ERG	electroretinography
C&S	culture and sensitivity	ERM	epiretinal membrane
CSF	cerebrospinal fluid	ESR	erythrocyte sedimentation rate (sed rate)
CSME	clinically significant macular edema	ET	constant esotropia at far
CSR	central serous chorioretinopathy	ET'	constant esotropia at near
CSW	corneoscleral wound	E(T) or IET	intermittent esotropia at far
CT	cover test	E(T)' or IET'	intermittent esotropia at near
CT scan	computed tomographic scan	ETOH	ethyl alcohol
CV	color vision	EUA	examination under anesthesia
CVA	cerebrovascular accident	EV	eccentric viewing
CVD	cardiovascular disease	EW	extended wear
CWS	cotton-wool spot	EXT	external ocular examination, including adnexa
Cx	culture		
CXR	chest x-ray film	exoph	exophthalmos
cyl	cylinder	FA or FANG	fluorescein angiography
d	days	FAZ	foveal avascular zone
D_{250}	Diamox 250-mg tablets	FB	foreign body
D	diopter or diameter	FBS	fasting blood sugar
D/C	discontinue	FC	finger count
D&C	deep and clear	FD	fixation disparity

FH or FHx	family history		ICE	iridocorneal endothelial syndrome
FHI	Fuchs' heterochromic iridocyclitis		ICP	intracranial pressure
fl	fluorescein		ICU	intensive care unit
FMHx	family medical history		I&D	incision and drainage
FML	fluorometholone		IDDM	insulin-dependent diabetes mellitus
FOHx	family ocular history		IDU	idoxuridine
FR	foveal reflex		IFIOL	iris-fixated intraocular lens
FROM	full range of motion		Ig	immunoglobulin
FTA-ABS	fluorescent treponemal antibody absorption test		IK	interstitial keratitis
FTFC	full-to-finger counting		IM	intramuscular
FTMH	full-thickness macular hole		Imp	impression
f/u	follow-up		inf	inferior
GC	gonorrhea or gonococcus		inj	injection
GCA	giant cell arteritis		INO	internuclear ophthalmoplegia
gent	gentamicin		INQ	inferonasal quadrant
GI	gastrointestinal		int	intermittent
GLC	glaucoma		IOH	intraocular hemorrhage
G0, GI, GII, GIII, GIV	grades of anterior chamber angle: G0 = closed; GIV = wide open		IOL	intraocular lens
			ION	ischemic optic neuropathy
gonio	gonioscopic examination		IOP	intraocular pressure
GPC	giant papillary conjunctivitis		IP	iris process
gr	grain		IR	infrared
gt	drop (plural, gtt)		IRMA	intraretinal microvascular abnormality
GTT	glucose tolerance test		ITQ	inferotemporal quadrant
GVF	Goldmann visual field		IU	international unit or intermediate uveitis
h	hour		IV	intravenous
HA	headache		JODM	juvenile-onset diabetes mellitus
hab	habitual		JRA	juvenile rheumatoid arthritis
Hb, Hgb	hemoglobin		K	potassium
HCL	hard contact lens		KCS	keratoconjunctivitis sicca
Hct	hematocrit		kg	kilogram
HCTZ	hydrocholorothiazide		KP	keratic precipitate
hem	hemorrhage		L	left or lens
HHP	Hollenhorst plaque		lab	laboratory
HIV	human immunodeficiency virus		lac	lacrimal
HLA	histocompatibility locus antigen or human leukocyte antigen		LASIK	laser in situ keratomileusis
			LD	learning disabled
h/o	history of		LI	laser interferometry
H_2O	water		LK, LKP	lamellar keratoplasty
HM	hand motion		LIO	left inferior oblique
H&P	history and physical		LIR	left inferior rectus
hs	at bedtime		LL	lids and lashes or lower lid
HSK	herpes simplex keratitis		LLR	left lateral rectus
HSV	herpes simplex virus		LMR	left medial rectus
HT	hypertropia at far		LN	lymph node
HT′	hypertropia at near		LND	light-near dissociation
HTN	hypertension		LP	light perception, light projection, or lumbar puncture
HVF	Humphrey visual field			
Hx	history		LS	lid scrubs
HZO	herpes zoster ophthalmicus		LSO	left superior oblique
I	iris or intermittent (IAET, intermittent alternating esotropia, etc.)		LSR	left superior rectus
			LTP	laser trabeculoplasty
I&A	irrigation and aspiration		LTQ	lower temporal quadrant
IBx	incisional biopsy		LVA	low vision aids
IC	iridocyclitis		lymph	lymphocytes or lymphatic
ICA	internal carotid artery		m	meter
ICCE	intracapsular cataract extraction		M	manifest refraction

mac	macular	NVE	neovascularization of the retina elsewhere
mand	mandibular	NVG	neovascular glaucoma
max	maximum or maxillary	NVI	neovascularization of the iris
μg	microgram	NS	nuclear sclerosis
MCH	mean corpuscular hemoglobin	O	objective
MCHC	mean corpuscular hemoglobin concentration	O_2	oxygen
MCV	mean corpuscular volume	OAD	overall diameter
meds	medications	OAG	open-angle glaucoma
MEM	monocular estimate method	OBS	organic brain syndrome
mEq/L	milliequivalent per liter	OD	right eye
MEWDS	multiple evanescent white dot syndrome	ODM	ophthalmodynamometry
MFS	monofixation syndrome	OFHx	ocular family history
M.G.	Marcus Gunn	OGTT	oral glucose tolerance test
mg	milligram	OHTN	ocular hypertension
MGD	meibomian gland dysfunction	OHx	ocular history
MHx	medical history	OKN	optokinetic nystagmus
MI	myocardial infarction	ON	optic nerve
min	minute or minimum	ONA or OA	optic nerve atrophy or optic atrophy
ml	milliliter	OP	outpatient
mm	millimeter	OR	operating room
MM	malignant melanoma	ortho-K	ortho-keratology
mm Hg	millimeters of mercury	OS	left eye
M&N	Mydriacyl (tropicamide) and Neo-synephrine (phenylephrine)	OTC	over the counter
		OU	both eyes
mon	monocytes	OZ	optical zone
mot	motility	P	pupil
MRI	magnetic resonance imaging	$\bar{p}$	post, after
MS	multiple sclerosis	PA	posteroanterior
MVA	motor vehicle accident	PAM	potential acuity meter
N	Neptazane	PAN	preauricular node
N/A	not applicable	PAS	peripheral anterior synechia
NaCl	sodium chloride	pat or pt	patient
NAG	narrow-angle glaucoma	path	pathology
NAP	no apparent pathology	P4, P2, etc.	pilocarpine 4%, 2%, etc., drops
NCT	noncontact tonometer (tonometry)	PBK	pseudophakic bullous keratopathy
neg	negative	pc	after meals
neo	neovascularization	PC	posterior capsule
NFL	nerve fiber layer	PCF	pharyngoconjunctival fever
NFLD	nerve fiber layer defect	PCIOL	posterior chamber intraocular lens
NG	nongranulomatous	PCN	penicillin
NI	no improvement	PCP	*Pneumocystis carinii* pneumonia
NIDDM	non–insulin-dependent diabetes mellitus	PD	pupillary distance
NKA	no known allergies	PDR	proliferative diabetic retinopathy
nl	normal	PDS	pigment dispersion syndrome
NLP	no light perception	PE	physical examination
non repet	not to be repeated (refilled)	PEE	punctate epithelial erosions
NPA	near point of accommodation	PEK	punctate epithelial keratitis
NPC	near point of convergence	PERRLA	pupils equal, round, reactive to light and accommodation
NPDR	nonproliferative diabetic retinopathy		
NQ	nasal quadrant	PF	Pred Forte
NR	no refill	Pg	pregnant
NRC	normal retinal correspondence	ph	pinhole
NSAID	nonsteroidal anti-inflammatory drug	phako	phakoemulsification
NTG	normotensive glaucoma	PHNI or NIph	pinhole no improvement
NV	near vision or neovascularization	PHPV	persistent hyperplastic primary vitreous
N/V	nausea and vomiting	PI	present illness, peripheral iridotomy, or peripheral iridectomy
NVD	neovascularization of the disc		

PI 1/8, 1/4	Phospholine iodide drops, 1/8%, 1/4%, etc.		RTO	return to office
PKP or PK	penetrating keratoplasty		Rx	prescription
PMMA	polymethylmethacrylate		s̄	without
PMN	polymorphonuclear neutrophil		S	subjective
po	per os, by mouth		s̄c̄	without correction
POAG	primary open-angle glaucoma		SC	secondary curve
POHS	presumed ocular histoplasmosis syndrome		SCC	squamous cell carcinoma
post	posterior		SCL	soft contact lens
PPD	purified protein derivative or posterior polymorphous dystrophy		SCr	secondary curve radius
			SCw	secondary curve width
PPDR	preproliferative diabetic retinopathy		Sed rate	erythrocyte sedimentation rate
PPLOV	painless progressive loss of vision		SEI	subepithelial infiltrate
PPVx	pars plana vitrectomy		SGOT	serum glutamic oxaloacetic transaminase
prep	preparation		SGPT	serum glutamic pyruvic transaminase
PRK	photorefractive keratectomy		SI	sector iridectomy
prn	take as needed		sibs	siblings
PRP	panretinal photocoagulation		sig	write on label
PS	posterior synechia		SJS	Stevens-Johnson syndrome
PSC	posterior subcapsular cataract		SL	Schwalbe's line or serum lysozyme
PT	prothrombin time		SLE	systemic lupus erythematosus or slit lamp examination
PTMH	partial thickness macular hole			
PVA	polyvinyl alcohol		SLEx	slit lamp examination
PVD	posterior vitreous detachment		SLK	superior limbic keratoconjunctivitis
Px	prognosis		Sn	sign
PXE	pseudoxanthoma elasticum		SNQ	superonasal quadrant
q	every		SOB	shortness of breath
qd	every day		sol	solution
q2h, etc.	every 2 hours, etc.		S/P	status post
qid	four times a day		SPK	superficial punctate keratitis
qod	every other day		SR	subjective refraction
R	right		SRF	subretinal fluid
RA	rheumatoid arthritis		SRNVM	subretinal neovascularization membrane
RB	rose bengal		SRx	spectacle prescription
RBC	red blood cell		SS	scleral spur or sickle cell disease
RBON	retrobulbar optic neuritis		stat	immediately
RCE	recurrent corneal erosion		STD	sexually transmitted disease
RD	retinal detachment		STQ	superotemporal quadrant
Ret	retinoscopy		strab	strabismus
RF	rheumatoid factor		subcu or sub Q	subcutaneous
R-G	red-green		sup	superior
RGP	rigid gas permeable		susp	suspension
RI	rubeosis iridis		SVP	spontaneous venous pulsations
RIO	right inferior oblique		Sx	symptom
RIR	right inferior rectus		synech	synechia
RK	radial keratotomy		T 1/4, T 1/2	Timoptic drops 1/4%, 1/2%
RLF	retrolental fibroplasia		TA	temporal arteritis
RLR	right lateral rectus		tab(s)	tablet(s)
RMR	right medial rectus		Tap	applanation tonometry
R/O	rule out		TB	tuberculosis
ROP	retinopathy of prematurity		tbs	tablespoon
RP	retinitis pigmentosa		TBUT	tear break-up time
RPE	retinal pigment epithelium		TDx	tentative diagnosis
RS	Reiter's syndrome		TED	thyroid eye disease
RSO	right superior oblique		TF	trial frame
RSR	right superior rectus		TIA	transient ischemic attack
RT	return		tid	three times a day
RTC	return to clinic		TM	trabecular meshwork

Tnct	noncontact (air puff) tonometry
TOV	transient obscuration of vision
TPR	temperature, pulse, respiration
trab	trabeculectomy
TSH	thyroid-stimulating hormone
tsp	teaspoon
Tx	treatment or traction
UA	urinalysis
UCT	unilateral cover test
UL	upper lid
ung	ointment
UNQ	upper nasal quadrant
URI	upper respiratory infection
ut dict	as directed
UTI	urinary tract infection
UTT	unable to test
UV	ultraviolet
V	vitreous
VA	visual acuities
V$\overline{cc}$	vision with correction
V$\overline{ccl}$	vision with contact lens
VD	venereal disease
VDRL	Venereal Disease Research Laboratory
VEP	visual evoked potential
VF	visual fields
VKC	vernal keratoconjunctivitis
VKH	Vogt-Koyanagi-Harada syndrome
V$\overline{sc}$	vision without correction
VZV	varicella-zoster virus
W-4-D	Worth-four-dot
WBC	white blood cell
WC	warm compresses
W/C	wheelchair
WC/LS	warm compresses and lid scrubs
WD	wound or working distance
Wk	week
WL	wound leak
WNL	within normal limits
WRA	with-the-rule
wt	weight

X	exophoria at far or axis
X'	exophoria at near
XT	constant exotropia at far
XT'	constant exotropia at near
X(T) or IXT	intermittent exotropia at far
X(T)' or IXT'	intermittent exotropia at near
YAG	yttrium aluminum garnet
YLI	YAG laser iridotomy
y/o	years old
YPC	YAG laser posterior capsulotomy

Symbols

φ	orthophoric (lateral) at far
φ'	orthophoric (lateral) at near
⊖	orthophoric (vertical) at far
⊖'	orthophoric (vertical) at near
⊕	orthophoric (lateral and vertical) at far
⊕'	orthophoric (lateral and vertical) at near
♀	female
♂	male
−	minus or negative
+	plus or positive
=	equal to
≠	not equal to
≈	approximately equal
1°	primary
2°	secondary
◯	combined with
∅	none or no
> (≥)	greater than (greater than or equal to)
< (≤)	less than (less than or equal to)
Δ	change or prism diopter
∴	therefore
$\dot{\text{i}}$	one (drops, tablets, etc.)
$\overline{\text{ii}}$	two (drops, tablets, etc.)
$\overline{\text{iii}}$	three (drops, tablets, etc.)
↑	increased
↓	decreased
#	number or pound

Index

The abbreviation t refers to a table and the abbreviation f refers to a figure.